W9-BLC-415

Health Assessment in Nursing

Lina K. Sims, RN, MSN, CS
Assistant Professor
St. Joseph's College of Nursing
Joliet, Illinois

Donita D'Amico, RN, EdM
Assistant Professor/RN Program Coordinator
Department of Nursing
William Paterson College
Wayne, New Jersey

Johanna K. Stiesmeyer, RN, MS, CCRN
Cardiovascular Education Specialist
El Camino Hospital
Mountain View, California

Judith A. Webster, RN, MSN
Manager, Corporate Health and Wellness Program
Applied Materials
Santa Clara, California

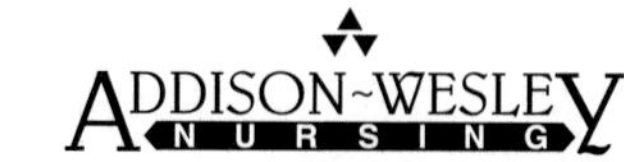

A DIVISION OF
THE BENJAMIN/CUMMINGS PUBLISHING COMPANY, INC.

Redwood City, California • Menlo Park, California
Reading, Massachusetts • New York • Don Mills, Ontario
Wokingham, UK • Amsterdam • Bonn • Sydney
Singapore • Tokyo • Madrid • San Juan

Executive Editor: Patricia L. Cleary
Acquisitions Editor: Erin Mulligan
Developmental Editor: Laura Bonazzoli
Production Supervisor: Wendy Earl
Production Coordinator: Bradley Burch
Editorial Assistant: Suzanne Rotondo
Text Designer: Mark Ong/Side by Side Studios
Cover Designer: Yvo Riezebos Design
Art Coordinators: Betty Gee and Suzanna Gee
Principal Artists: Biomed Arts Associates, Todd A. Buck, Barbara Cousins, Nea Hanscomb, Romaine LoPrete, Kristin N. Mount
Photo Coordinators: Bradley Burch and Elena Dorfman
Photo Researcher: Alisa Guttman
Principal Photographer: Richard Tauber
Copy Editor: Antonio Padial
Proofreader: John Hammett
Indexer: Elinor Lindheimer
Compositor: Side by Side Studios
Prepress Supplier: GTS Graphics
Manufacturing Coordinator: Merry Free Osborn
Text Printer and Binder: R. R. Donnelley and Sons/Willard
Cover Printer: Color Dot Litho

This book is printed on recycled paper. The cover is printed with soy-based inks.

Photographic and art credits may be found on page 741.

Care has been taken to confirm the accuracy of information presented in this book. The authors, editors and the publisher, however, cannot accept any responsibility for errors or omissions or for the consequences from application of the information in this book and make no warranty, express or implied, with respect to its contents.

The authors and publisher have exerted every effort to ensure that drug selections and dosages set forth in this text are in accord with current recommendation and practice at time of publication. However, in view of ongoing research, changes in government regulations, and the constant flow of information relating to drug therapy and drug reactions, the reader is urged to check the package inserts of all drugs for any change in indications of dosage and for added warnings and precautions. This is particularly important when the recommended agent is a new and/or infrequently employed drug.

The quilt pictured on the cover, "Spring: Garden Series #1," was designed by Glenne Stoll and photographed by Carina Woolrich.

Library of Congress Cataloging-in-Publication Data

Health assessment in nursing / Lina K. Sims . . . [et al.].
p. cm.
Includes bibliographical references and index.
ISBN 0–8053–7347–0
1. Nursing assessment. 2. Holistic nursing. 3. Physical diagnosis. I. Sims, Lina K.
[DNLM: 1. Nursing Assessment. 2. Medical History Taking—nurses' instruction. 3. Physical Examination—nurses' instruction. 4. Interview, Psychological—nurses' instruction. WY 18 H4344 1995]
RT48.H446 1995
610.73—dc20
DNLM/DLC
for Library of Congress 94-38953
CIP

ISBN 0-8053-7347
1 2 3 4 5 6 7 8 9 10–DOW–98 97 96 95 94

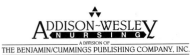

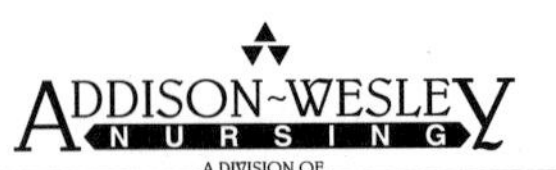

390 Bridge Parkway; Redwood City, California 94065

Contributors

Mary T. Boylston, RN, MSN, CCRN
School of Nursing
Eastern College
St. David's, PA

Darlene Nebel Cantu, RNC, MSN
School of Professional Nursing
Baptist Memorial Hospital System
San Antonio, TX

Kathleen A. De Lorenzo, RN, PhD, CS
Abilene Intercollegiate School of Nursing
Abilene, TX

Patsy Eileen Gehring, RNC, BSN, MS
Department of Nursing
Lakeland Community College
Mentor, OH

Janet S. Hickman, RN, EdD
Department of Nursing
West Chester University
West Chester, PA

Cynthia Holmgren, RN, MSN, OCN
Bellin College of Nursing
Green Bay, WI

Patricia A. O'Leary, RN, DSN
Department of Nursing
Middle Tennessee State University
Murfreesburo, TN

Mary M. Reeve, RN, EdD
School of Nursing
San Jose State University
San Jose, CA

Judith Schurr Salzer, RN, MS, CPNP
Children's Memorial Hospital
University of Illinois
Chicago, IL

Linda A. Spencer, RN, MPH, PhD
School of Nursing
Georgia Baptist College of Nursing
Atlanta, GA

Arlene M. Sperhac, RN, PNP, PhD
Children's Memorial Hospital
Clinical Faculty, Rush University School of Nursing
Loyola University
Chicago, IL

Jean Smith Temple, RN, MSN
College of Nursing
University of Southern Alabama
Mobile, AL

Eugenia H. Tickle, RN, EdD
Nursing Program
Midwestern State University
Wichita Falls, TX

Sharon C. Wahl, RN, EdD
School of Nursing/College of Applied Sciences and Arts
San Jose State University
San Jose, CA

Interview Strategies Contributors

Juanita K. Hunter, RN, EdD, FAAN (Homelessness)
State University of New York at Buffalo
Buffalo, NY

Maxine J. Kamlowski, RN, BSN (Substance Abuse)
Health Care for the Homeless
Mercy Hospital
Springfield, MA

Judith A. Mealey, RN, MSN, ANP (Substance Abuse)
Health Care for the Homeless
Mercy Hospital
Springfield, MA

Annie Lewis-O'Connor, RN, MS, NP, MPHc (Child Abuse)
Boston University
Neponset Health Center
Dorchester, MA

Anne Griswold Peirce, RN, PhD (Elder Abuse)
School of Nursing
Columbia University
New York, NY

Yvonne Campbell Ulrich, RN, PhD, ARNP
(Domestic Violence)
School of Nursing
Wichita State University
Wichita, KS

Reviewers

Michael H. Ackerman, RN, MS, DNS
School of Nursing
State University of New York
Buffalo, NY

Cynthia H. Allen, RN, MPH, MN
Charity School of Nursing
Delgado Community College
New Orleans, LA

Janet T. Barrett, RN, PhD
Deaconess College of Nursing
St. Louis, MO

Margaret Benz, RN
School of Nursing
Texas Christian University
Fort Worth, TX

Ellen Biebesheimer, RN, MSN, PNP
Beth-El College of Nursing
Colorado Springs, CO

Kathleen Koernig Blais, RN, EdD
School of Nursing
Florida International University
Miami, FL

Jeri L. Brandt, RN, PhD
School of Nursing
Nebraska Wesleyan University
Lincoln, NE

Kimberly Ferrin Carter, RN, MSN, CHES
School of Nursing
Radford University
Radford, VA

Katharine C. Cook, RN, MS, ANP
Department of Nursing
College of Notre Dame of Maryland
Baltimore, MD

Emily Cornett, RN, PhD
School of Nursing
University of Texas
Austin, TX

Patricia Dennis, RN, MSN
School of Nursing
Ohio Valley Hospital
Steubenville, OH

Patricia Ferris, RN, MS, PhD
Nursing Department
Seattle University
Seattle, WA

Christy Flory, RN, MS
Department of Dermatology
Beth Israel Hospital
Boston, MA

Merilyn Francis, RN, BSN
University of the District of Columbia
Washington, DC

M. K. Gaedeke, RN, MSN, CCRN, CS
Pediatric Critical Care
Children's Hospital of Buffalo
Buffalo, NY

Marian S. Gustafson, RN, MSN
Division of Nursing
Butler County Community College
Butler, PA

Bonnie L. Hammack, ARNP, MSN
Department of Nursing
Miami-Dade Community College
Miami, FL

Ann Harley, RN, EdD
Department of Nursing
Carson-Newman College
Jefferson City, TN

Marilyn Henning, RN, MSN
Nursing Department
Milwaukee Area Technical College
Milwaukee, WI

MaryAnne House-Fancher, ARNP, MSN, CCRN
Department of Cardiothoracic Surgery
University of Florida
Gainesville, FL

Elizabeth Miller Jenkins, RN, MS
College of Nursing
University of Delaware
Newark, DE

Patti Kay Kratzke, RN, MN, C
City University
Belleview, WA

Patsy S. McGeorge, RN, BSN, MS, FNP
College of Nursing
Arizona State University
Tempe, AZ

Mary Maggio, RN, MN, CNP
Department of Obstetrics and Gynecology
Palo Alto Medical Foundation
Palo Alto, CA

Martha A. Nelson, RN, MS
School of Nursing
Dominican College
San Rafael, CA

Kim Nichols-Rzeszewicz, RN, MSN
Department of Nursing
Tacoma Community College
Tacoma, WA

Julie C. Novak, RN, CPNP, DNSc
School of Nursing
University of Virginia
Charlottesville, VA

Constance O'Kane, RN, MS
College of Mainland
Texas City, TX

Nancy Otterness, RN, MS
College of Health Sciences
Boise State University
Boise, ID

Marilyn K. Overstreet, RN, MN
School of Nursing
Baker University
Topeka, KS

Cathy Patton, RN, MA
El Camino Health Care System
Mountain View, CA

Louise M. Rauckhurst, RN, CS, ANP, EdD
Phillip Y. Hahn School of Nursing
University of San Diego
San Diego, CA

Lois Rhodes
School of Nursing
Pacific Lutheran University
Tacoma, WA

Virginia Richardson, RN, DNS, CPNP
School of Nursing
Indiana University
Indianapolis, IN

Julia Marostica Robinson, RN, MS, ANP
Department of Nursing
California State University
Bakersfield, CA

Beth Rodgers, RN, MSN
School of Nursing
Baylor University
Dallas, TX

Karen Rotondo, RN, BSN
Director Department of Community Health
Mercy Hospital
Springfield, MA

Josephine Ryan, RN, DNSc
School of Nursing
University of Massachusetts
Amherst, MA

Gyneth Sanders, RN, MSN
Department of Nursing
Kansas City Comunity College
Kansas City, KS

Sarla Sethi, RN, PhD
Faculty of Nursing
University of Calgary
Calgary, Alberta, Canada

April Sieh, RN, MSN
School of Nursing
Delta College
Delta Center, MI

Susan J. Sorenson, RNC, MSN, FNP
Bellin College of Nursing
Green Bay, WI

Yvonne N. Stock, RN, BSN, MS
Nursing Education
Iowa Western Community College
Council Bluffs, IA

Lynn A. Templeton, RN, MSN, FNP
College of Nursing
Arizona State University
Tempe, AZ

Sandy L. Theis, RN, PhD
College of Nursing
University of Illinois
Chicago, IL

Carmel T. White, RN, BSN, MSN
Deaconess College of Nursing
St. Louis, MO

Judith M.Wilkinson, MA, MS, RNC
Nursing Program
Johnson County Community College
Overland Park, KS

Denise Yurick, RN, MS
School of Nursing
Cuesta College
San Luis Obispo, CA

Mary M. Ziemer, RN, DNSc
College of Nursing
Villanova University
Villanova, PA

Preface

The health care system in the United States is, as always, changing. Historically, health care has been illness-focused. As the pendulum swings toward the prevention of disease and the promotion of health, nurses are taking a more independent and far broader role in client care. Skill in health assessment is an integral part of that broader role. Nurses now perform assessments not only of acutely ill clients in hospitals, but also of clients with minor health problems and those who simply want to achieve wellness. The latter clients are seen in community clinics, schools, the wellness centers of businesses and industries, and in private homes.

The many changes on the horizon have created the need for a new text book. *Health Assessment in Nursing* was written to teach the basic skills of health assessment to nursing students. It will also be helpful to practicing nurses who wish to improve, review, or update their current skills.

Organization

Health Assessment in Nursing is organized in three units. Unit One presents fundamental concepts of holistic nursing care. Chapter 1 introduces health assessment as the first step in the nursing process and teaches the diagnostic reasoning process and the skill of documentation. Chapter 2 discusses the health history and presents interviewing strategies. Chapters 3 through 6 discuss the holistic dimensions of the client that the nurse considers when performing an assessment. These include: developmental stages, psychosocial factors, self-care factors, ability to perform activities of daily living, and the influence of the client's family, culture, and environment on overall health.

The chapters in Unit Two provide comprehensive background essential for conducting a holistic health assessment of a specific body region or system. Chapter 7 explains the basic assessment techniques and describes the general survey of the client. Chapters 8 through 18 describe the regional or systemic assessments. Each chapter begins with a full-color review of anatomy and physiology. A focused interview section presents specific questions with rationales appropriate to that region or system. Additional questions to be used with children, childbearing clients, and older adults are also provided. Assessment techniques are presented one step at a time, with bulleted substeps for additional information. Each step presents normal findings, and special considerations identifying common abnormalities are discussed in a separate column to the right of the technique. Thus, the student may focus on learning the proper technique and normal finding *first*, then return to the deviations from normal after the technique has been mastered.

Developmental variations are explored following the step-by-step techniques. Psychosocial considerations, self-care practices, and family, cultural, and environmental considerations are explored as they influence health and physical findings. A special nursing diagnosis section clusters data and identifies the most common nursing diagnoses for each region or system. Additionally, to help students apply the nursing process to real-world situations, *Diagnostic Reasonings in Action* boxes present case studies and demonstrate how to cluster data to generate nursing diagnoses.

Common alterations in health are described in text and illustrated tables. Sections on health promotion and client education close each chapter in Unit Two, emphasizing the importance of the nurse's teaching role.

Chapters 19 through 21 in Unit Three provide guidelines for assessing infants, children, adolescents, childbearing clients, and older adults. These chapters are organized much like the chapters in Unit Two and contain many of the same features. The final chapter in the book is a checklist for one possible adult exam sequence.

Our Philosophy

We wrote *Health Assessment in Nursing* with the following goals in mind:

- To provide a truly holistic approach. While other assessment books may claim to present a holistic approach, *Health Assessment in Nursing* is the only text that makes this approach meaningful for students by including extensive content and features that support holistic assessment. Separate chapters in Unit One focus on development, psychosocial health, self-care, and family, culture, and environment. In addition, Unit Two chapters each open with a figure summarizing the interrelationship of other body systems with a region or system being assessed, as well as the holistic factors (such as self-care practices) to consider when assessing that particular region or system. These holistic factors are grouped and color-coded to match comprehensive discussions that follow the assessment techniques sections in each chapter.

- To promote wellness and prevent illness. Our approach to wellness is demonstrated in all three units of this text. Wellness is defined and discussed in Chapter 1, and it is a fundamental consideration in the remaining chapters in Unit One. This emphasis continues in Units Two and Three, in which each chapter contains interview questions that support wellness. As mentioned earlier, the techniques sections focus on normal findings. Most chapters contain *Diagnostic Reasoning in Action* boxes that help students apply the concepts of wellness, health promotion and client teaching to clinical situations.
- To empower nurses to teach. We believe that client teaching is a vital part of nursing care. The emphasis of client teaching is always to support the client's existing strengths and to assist the client in reducing or eliminating behaviors or conditions that limit health. This goal is supported in Chapters 8 through 21 in the sections on health promotion and client teaching, and by *Diagnostic Reasoning in Action* boxes that conclude with the nurse providing appropriate client teaching.
- To help students master the diagnostic reasoning process. As educators, we are familiar with students' difficulties in making the leap from assessment data to nursing diagnoses. To help students master this skill, we provide in Chapter 1 an overview of the diagnostic reasoning process. Chapters 8 through 21 provide tables of appropriate NANDA nursing diagnoses with defining characteristics and related factors. Finally, the *Diagnostic Reasoning in Action* boxes in each of these chapters provide case studies in which nurses cluster the assessment data and identify appropriate diagnoses.
- To demystify the health assessment process. Health assessment can be overwhelming for the student or recent graduate. Chapters 8 through 21 of *Health Assessment in Nursing* contain specific questions—not just topics—for the nurse to use during a focused interview. Rationales for each question are also provided. The assessment techniques are designed as main steps numbered and in bold type, with bulleted substeps. At a glance, students can see exactly what they need to do when, and how to do it. In close proximity to these written steps, we provide students with full-color photos and illustrations, and special considerations are placed in a column alongside the corresponding techniques. Finally, *Alert!* boxes remind students to proceed with caution during assessment techniques that have the potential for harming the client, and *Referral* boxes identify situations in which the nurse should immediately refer the client to a physician or to social services.

Summary of Features

- Figures showing essential considerations for holistic assessment
- Illustrated tables presenting alterations in health
- Nursing diagnosis tables
- *Diagnostic Reasoning in Action* boxes
- *Alert!* boxes
- *Referral* boxes

In addition, *Health Assessment in Nursing* provides students with:

- A preparation page for each physical assessment section, listing the equipment needed and providing tips to follow just before and during the assessment.
- Pain assessment tables in selected chapters, which help the student compare the client's description of pain to pain parameters typical of common medical diagnoses.
- Chapter summaries
- Lists of key points
- An appendix of articles that present interview techniques for situations requiring particular skill. These include tips for uncovering cases of substance abuse and domestic violence (including elder and child abuse) and assessing homeless clients.

Acknowledgments

Our special thanks to Laura Bonazzoli, our developmental editor, for her unending creativity, patience, and assistance throughout this process. For helping us realize our potential and giving us savvy guidance and unflagging support, we thank Patti Cleary, executive editor.

Wendy Earl, managing editor, did an incredible job managing all aspects of the production of this book. Our special thanks for the beautiful photos shot by Richard Tauber! Bradley Burch masterfully managed all of the photo sessions as well as our tireless models, Eric DeMello and Armida Quiñonez. Other key production team members include Antonio Padial, copy editor, who made often wordy prose succinct yet friendly and Mark Ong who provided a clean page design.

Thanks also to our professional colleagues for their continued support and encouragement, and to our families and friends for their understanding and for giving us the time we needed to explore this new adventure. Our gratitude also goes to typist Minnie Lynch.

We are grateful to have the opportunity to finally and publicly thank our many contributors and reviewers for lending their expertise in numerous content areas and for their hard work in writing or critiquing for us with deadlines always approaching!

Finally, we would like to thank our students for giving us the inspiration to help them achieve their educational and professional goals. This book is dedicated to them.

Lina Sims
Donita D'Amico
Johanna Stiesmeyer
Judith Webster

Contents

Unit Three

Integrated Health Assessments

Chapter 19

Assessing Infants, Children, and Adolescents 583

Chapter 20

Assessing the Childbearing Client 634

Chapter 21

Assessing the Older Adult 666

To the Student

This book contains a number of learning devices to help you learn to perform holistic assessment with skill and confidence.

ALERT! boxes. Identifiable *ALERT!* boxes are integrated throughout the physical assessment sections, identifying key precautions.

184 UNIT TWO Physical Assessment

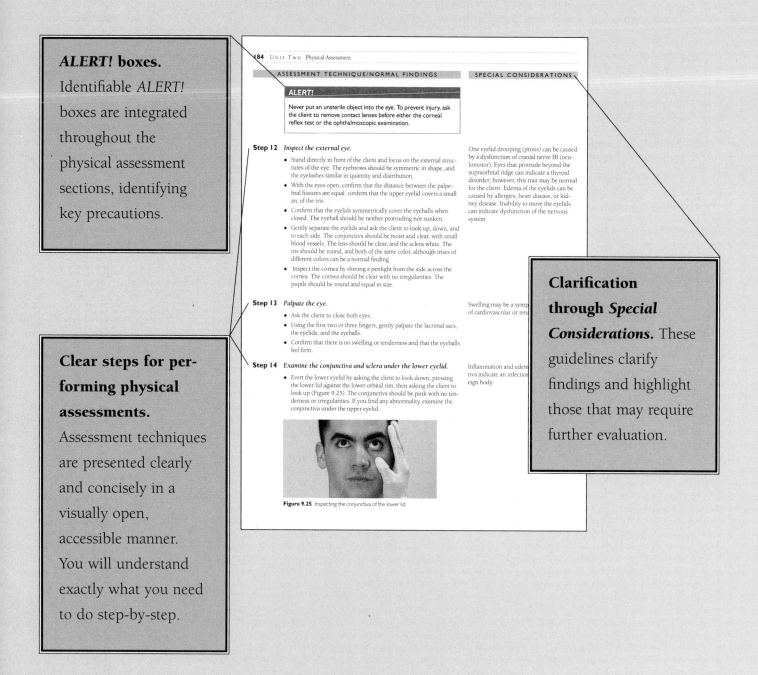

ASSESSMENT TECHNIQUE/NORMAL FINDINGS	SPECIAL CONSIDERATIONS

ALERT!

Never put an unsterile object into the eye. To prevent injury, ask the client to remove contact lenses before either the corneal reflex test or the ophthalmoscopic examination.

Step 12 *Inspect the external eye.*

- Stand directly in front of the client and focus on the external structures of the eye. The eyebrows should be symmetric in shape, and the eyelashes similar in quantity and distribution.
- With the eyes open, confirm that the distance between the palpebral fissures are equal. confirm that the upper eyelid covers a small arc of the iris.
- Confirm that the eyelids symmetrically cover the eyeballs when closed. The eyeball should be neither protruding nor sunken.
- Gently separate the eyelids and ask the client to look up, down, and to each side. The conjunctiva should be moist and clear, with small blood vessels. The lens should be clear, and the sclera white. The iris should be round, and both of the same color, although irises of different colors can be a normal finding.
- Inspect the cornea by shining a penlight from the side across the cornea. The cornea should be clear with no irregularities. The pupils should be round and equal in size.

One eyelid drooping (ptosis) can be caused by a dysfunction of cranial nerve III (oculomotor). Eyes that protrude beyond the supraorbital ridge can indicate a thyroid disorder; however, this trait may be normal for the client. Edema of the eyelids can be caused by allergies, heart disease, or kidney disease. Inability to move the eyelids can indicate dysfunction of the nervous system.

Step 13 *Palpate the eye.*

- Ask the client to close both eyes.
- Using the first two or three fingers, gently palpate the lacrimal sacs, the eyelids, and the eyeballs.
- Confirm that there is no swelling or tenderness and that the eyeballs feel firm.

Swelling may be a symp of cardiovascular or ren

Step 14 *Examine the conjunctiva and sclera under the lower eyelid.*

- Evert the lower eyelid by asking the client to look down, pressing the lower lid against the lower orbital rim, then asking the client to look up (Figure 9.25). The conjunctiva should be pink with no tenderness or irregularities. If you find any abnormality, examine the conjunctiva under the upper eyelid.

Inflammation and edem tiva indicate an infectio eign body.

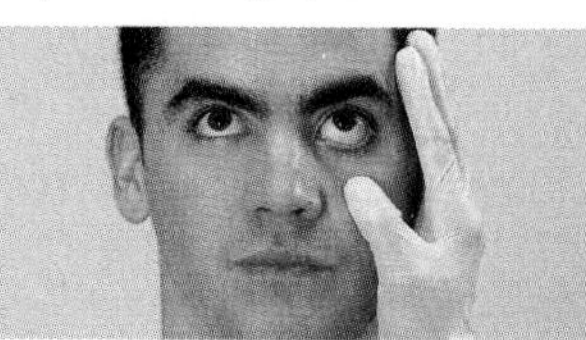

Figure 9.25 Inspecting the conjunctiva of the lower lid.

Clear steps for performing physical assessments. Assessment techniques are presented clearly and concisely in a visually open, accessible manner. You will understand exactly what you need to do step-by-step.

Clarification through *Special Considerations.* These guidelines clarify findings and highlight those that may require further evaluation.

Focused Interview. In the comprehensive *Focused Interview* section found in each assessment chapter, you are given a detailed list of what questions to ask, as well as rationales for *why* they need to be asked. The result: you gather more data and formulate more accurate nursing diagnoses.

Gathering the Data

As with all other systems, you review the database completed during the client's initial interview to identify what additional information you need before you assess the head and neck. Any diagnostic test results that are available should be reviewed. Tests may include imaging studies (X-ray films, CT scans, MRI studies), hearing and sight tests, and blood studies.

Focused Interview

The focused interview is as important as the physical assessment. It provides a wealth of information that leads to nursing diagnoses addressing health promotion, illness prevention, client teaching (eg, teaching correct administration of medication and teaching self-care for chronic, acute, and potential problems). If the client presents with a problem of the head or neck, or if there is a family history of a problem in this area, a more thorough history of each complaint must be obtained. In data collection, questions related to the respiratory, gastrointestinal, neurological, and musculoskeletal systems are important. For a description of the full health history, see Chapter 2.

Questions Related to the Head

1. Tell me why you are here today. Please describe how you are feeling generally, and tell me about any health problems you have and any treatments you are receiving.
2. Do you have headaches? If so, please tell me about
   a. Frequency: How often?
   b. Onset: How long have you been bothered with this type of headache? When does the headache begin?
   c. Duration: How long does a typical headache last? .
   d. Location: Where is the pain? On one side of the head, behind the eyes, in the sinus area?
   e. Character: Is the pain throbbing, steady, dull, sharp? On a scale of 1 to 10 with 10 being the strongest, how severe is the pain?
   f. Associated symptoms: Do you experience any nausea, vomiting, sensitivity to light or noise, muscle pain, or other symptoms along with the headache?
   g. Precipitating factors: Do you feel that the headaches usually are triggered by stress, alcohol intake, menstrual cycle, allergies, or any other factors describe.

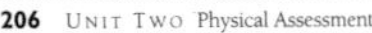

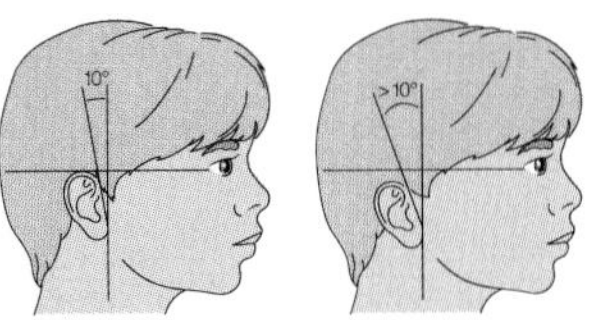

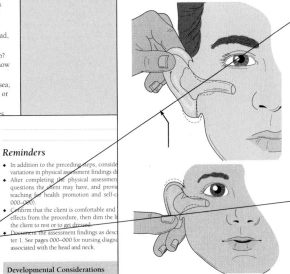

Figure 9.49 Normal alignment of a child's ears.

and continues throughout adolescence. Count the number of teeth the child has and ascertain whether they are appropriate for age. Infants frequently have small white pearly patches on the gums and hard palate. Called *Epstein's pearls*, they are small cysts that disappear a few weeks after birth.

Assess the range of motion of the neck by turning the infant's head from side to side. Then gently flex and extend the neck. When examining older children, ask them to look in different directions. An infant should be able to hold the head at a 90-degreee angle from a prone position by 2 months of age and be able to hold the head up in a seated position by 3 months. The thyroid is difficult to palpate on an infant, but it can be accomplished on a child using two or three fingers. Lymph nodes are usually not palpable in infants, but a child's nodes may be very prominent. Nodes up to 1 cm in size are considered normal, but they should be nontender, movable, and discrete.

Childbearing Clients

The childbearing client may develop blotchy pigmented spots on her face, facial edema, and enlargement of the thyroid. All of these symptoms are considered normal and subside after childbirth. She may also complain of headaches during the first trimester, which may be related to increased hormones, but severe persistent headaches should be evaluated.

The childbearing client may complain of dry eyes and may discontinue wearing contact lenses during her pregnancy. The client may also describe vision changes due to shifting fluid in the cornea. These symptoms are usually not significant and disappear after childbirth. Changes in eyesight, especially blurred or double vision, distorted color perception, or temporary blindness, should be reported to an ophthalmologist.

Nasal congestion and nosebleeds due to increased estrogen levels during pregnancy are common. The client may also become aware of a sense of fullness in the ears, resulting in some degree of hearing loss. This condition is also due to the elevated levels of estrogen, which cause increased vascularity of the upper respiratory tract. Bleeding gums with normal toothbrushing is also related to the increase in estrogen levels, which produces increased vascularity of the gums.

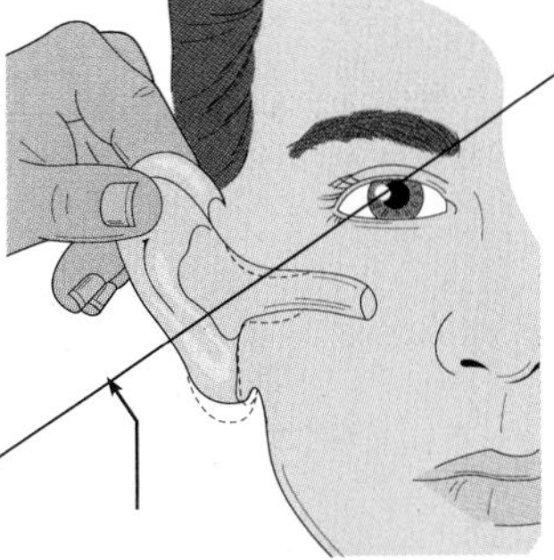

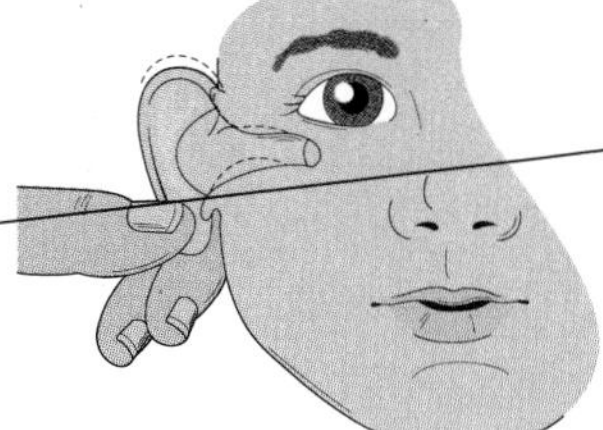

Figure 9.50 Procedure for pulling the pinna before inserting the otoscope in the adult and the child.

Older Clients

Mild rhythmic nodding of the head due to *senile tremors* is usually a normal finding. Senile tremors may also cause slight protrusion of the tongue.

By age 45, the lens of the eye loses elasticity, and the ciliary muscles become weaker, resulting in a decreased ability of the lens to change shape to accommodate for near vision. This condition is called *presbyopia*. The loss of fat from the orbit of the eye produces a drooping appearance. The lacrimal glands decrease tear production, and the client may complain of a burning sensation in the eyes. The cornea of the eye may appear cloudy, and you may detect a deposit of white-yellow

Reminders

- In addition to the preceding steps, conside[…] variations in physical assessment findings d[…]
- After completing the physical assessmen[…] questions the client may have, and provi[…] teaching for health promotion and self-c[…] 000–000).
- Confirm that the client is comfortable and […] effects from the procedure, then dim the li[…] the client to rest or to get dressed.
- Document the assessment findings as desc[…] ter 1. See pages 000–000 for nursing diagno[…] associated with the head and neck.

Strong lifespan coverage. Developmental Considerations summarize common health risks for each age group, reinforcing the text's coverage of lifespan issues and health promotion strategies.

Developmental Considerations

Infant, Children, and Adolescent[…]

An infant's head should be measured at each vi[…] of 2 years. It should be symmetric from all angl[…] larger than the chest until the age of 2. Any abn[…] in head size or failure to grow should be noted. […] skull is shown in Figure 9.48. Suture lines in the skull should be palpable until the age of 6 months. Palpable suture lines in a child older than 6 months of age can indicate hydrocephalus or Down syndrome. Fontanels should be firm and even with the surface of the skull. Slight pulsations of the fontanels are normal. An indented fontanel may indicate dehydration. Bulging fontanels may indicate increased intracranial pressure. It is common to discover bruits when auscultating the skull in children under the age of 4 or 5. After age 5, bruits are an indication of increased intracranial pressure.

(Figure 9.50).

A nasal speculum is usually not used to examine the nose of an infant or small child. The preferred method is to push the tip of the child's nose with your thumb, then shine a penlight into the nares. In children younger than 8 years, the sinus area is too small to evaluate by palpation, so it is not necessary to do so.

Both sets of teeth develop before birth. The deciduous teeth begin to erupt between 6 months of age and 2 years of age. Eruption of the permanent teeth begins at about age 6

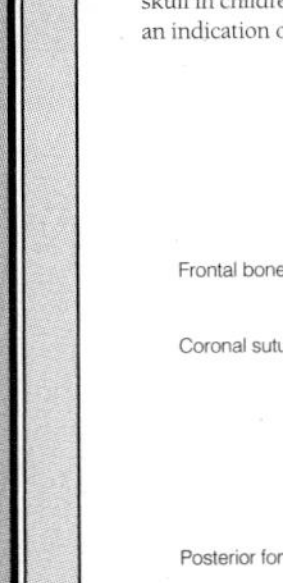

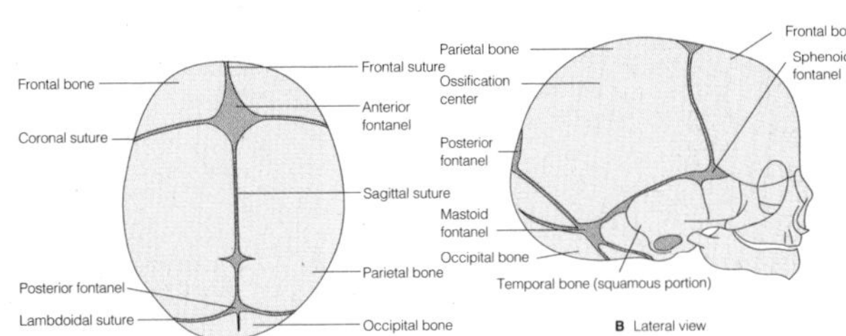

Figure 9.48 The newborn's skull.

Health Promotion and Client Education

At the conclusion of the assessment, answer any questions the client may have. All clients need information on promoting the health of the head and neck. Information about the care of chronic disease may also be appropriate, as well as information to prevent any current health problems from progressing. All clients also need information on self-monitoring and reporting of signs and symptoms of cancer of the head and neck.

Promoting the Health of the Head and Neck

The following are the cancer warning signs which apply to the head and neck, as identified by the American Cancer Society:

- Any unexplained lump or thickening
- Changes in the size or color of warts or moles
- Difficulty in swallowing
- Unusual bleeding or discharge
- Any sore that does not heal
- Persistent hoarseness or cough

Caution the client to wear protective head gear during participation in any potentially dangerous activity. Some examples are skateboarding, riding a motorcycle, bicycle riding, rollerskating, or rollerblading, skydiving, bungee jumping, playing football or hockey, and working in construction sites.

When riding in an automobile, make sure that everyone, driver and passengers, is wearing a seat belt. Protect the cervical spine by ensuring that head rests are at the proper height. Be certain that any child under the age of 4 years is secured properly in a carseat each time the child rides in an automobile. Do not use the infant seat in the front seat of a car equipped with a passenger-side air bag, because upon opening the bag can injure the child.

Stress the importance of compliance with any instructions for medications intended to increase cerebral perfusion, or to treat convulsive or thyroid disorders. Teach relaxation techniques as one method of dealing with chronic headaches, jaw pain, or neck pain.

Explain when to seek medical care for any problem of the head, neck, and inclusive structures.

Concrete health promotion strategies. In support of the nurse's expanding role in promoting health, every assessment chapter presents strategies for client teaching and care.

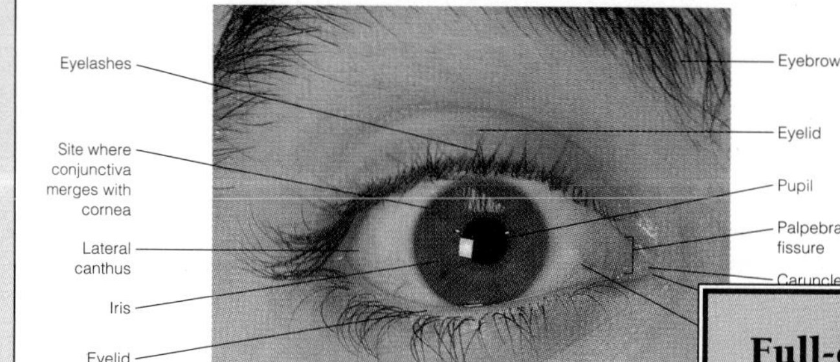

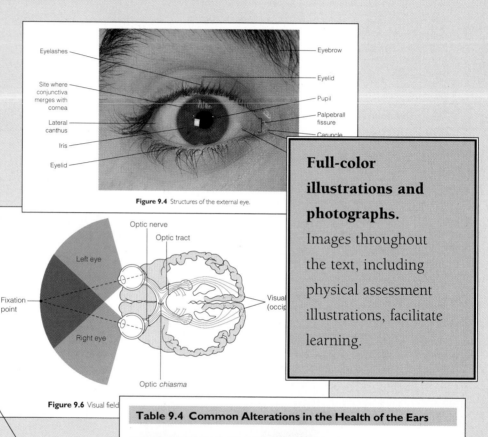

Figure 9.4 Structures of the external eye.

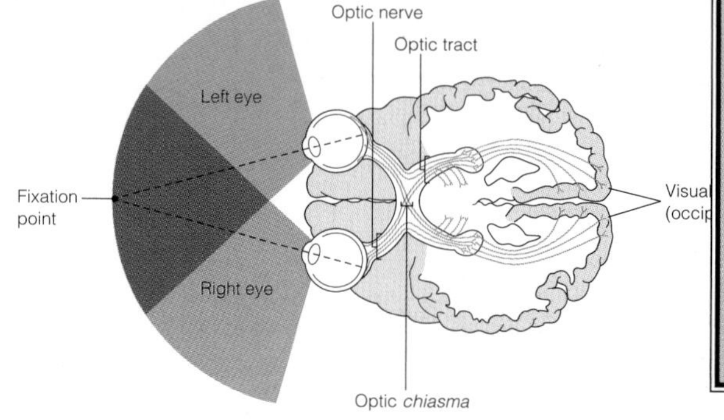

Figure 9.6 Visual field

Full-color illustrations and photographs. Images throughout the text, including physical assessment illustrations, facilitate learning.

DIAGNOSTIC REASONING IN ACTION

Ellen Dodson is a 28-year-old banking executive who comes to the wellness clinic for assistance in the management of "tension headaches." She describes her headaches as a dull, bandlike constricting pain in the occipital and temporal area of the head. Her appetite has decreased, and she experiences diarrhea about two times per month when she is especially nervous. Ms Dodson states that she has "been under a lot of pressure at work lately," and her physician has told her that her headaches are related to tension. The physician has suggested that she investigate some stress-management strategies.

The nursing assessment of Ms Dodson reveals a well-developed, well-nourished female in no acute distress at this time. The nursing diagnosis is health-seeking behaviors, stress reduction.

Ed Masters, RN, suggests the following methods for reducing stress:

- Time management: a m... more efficiently
- Regular exercise at least ... ness clinic's fitness cent...
- Guided imagery: a tec... trates on a relaxing ima... image
- Progressive relaxation: ... learns to constrict and ... tematic fashion
- Biofeedback: a method ... ence physiologic respo... tary control
- Yoga: a discipline in w... breathing techniques ar...

After considerable discu... would like to set up a regu... ness center and also try gu... Ms Dodson arrange a ti... guided-imagery sessions, ... to evaluate Ms Dodson's stress level and number of headaches one month from the first session.

Diagnostic Reasoning in Action. These boxes show you how to think critically and cluster assessment data in order to formulate nursing diagnoses.

Table 9.4 Common Alterations in the Health of the Ears

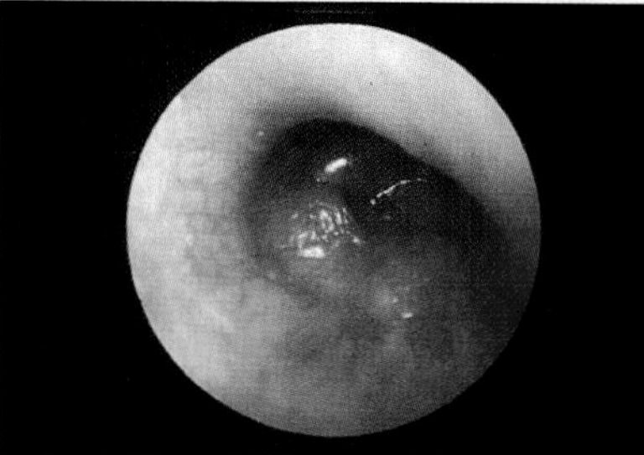
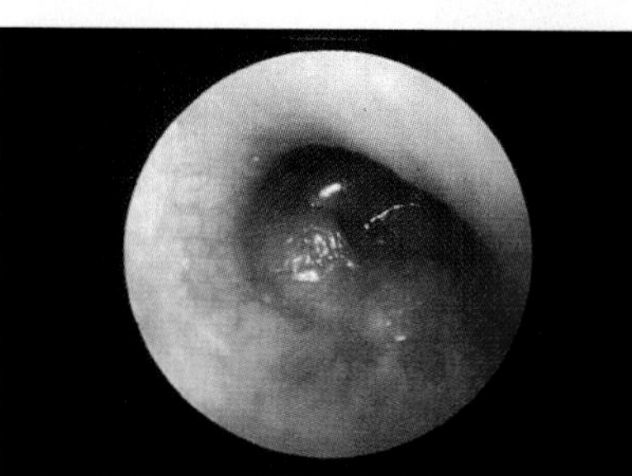

Otitis Media

Infection of the middle ear producing a red, bulging eardrum, fever, and hearing loss. The otoscopic examination reveals absent light reflex. More common in children, whose auditory tubes are wider, shorter, and more horizontal than those of adults and thus allow easier access for infections ascending from the pharynx.

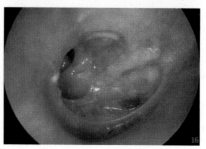

Perforation of Tympanic Membrane

A rupturing of the eardrum due to trauma or infection. During otoscopic inspection, the perforation may be seen as a dark spot on the eardrum.

CHAPTER 9 Assessing the Head and Neck 207

material around the cornea, called *arcus senilis*. This is a deposition of fat, but it is considered normal and has no effect on vision. The pupillary light reflex is slower with age, and the pupils may be smaller in size.

Within the eye, the blood vessels are paler in color, and you may detect small round yellow dots scattered on the retina. They do not interfere with vision. As the client ages, the lens continues to thicken and yellow, forming a dense area that reduces lens clarity. This condition is the beginning of a *cataract* formation. Macular degeneration can occur in the older client, resulting in a loss of central vision. The ophthalmoscopic examination may reveal narrowed blood vessels with a granular pigment in the macula.

The client may have coarse hairs at the opening of the auditory meatus. The ears may appear more prominent, because cartilage formation continues throughout life. The tympanic membrane may be paler in color and thicker in appearance. Assessment of hearing may reveal a loss of high-frequency tones, which is consistent with aging. With time, this loss often progresses to lower-frequency sounds as well. Gradual hearing loss with age is called *presbycusis*.

As the adult ages, many changes occur inside the mouth. The lips and buccal mucosa of the mouth become thinner and less vascular, with a shiny surface. Gums are paler in color. The tongue develops more fissures, and motor function may become impaired, resulting in problems with swallowing. A decreased sense of taste and smell may contribute to a diminished appetite and poor nutrition. There may also be a decrease in saliva production. This decrease may be due to atrophy of the salivary glands, but is often due to side effects from medication. Gums begin to recede, and some tooth loss may occur due to osteoporosis. If teeth are lost, the remaining teeth may drift, causing malocclusion of the maxilla and mandible. This condition can produce headaches and muscle spasms of the jaw. You may notice lesions in the mouth that may be due to ill-fitting dentures, or marked deterioration of old dental restorations. Refer the client to a dentist.

Psychosocial Considerations

A client who is under a great deal of stress may be prone to headaches, including tension headaches, neck pain, and mouth ulcers. Pain in the temporomandibular joint may be due to unconscious clenching of the jaw during stressful situations, such as driving in heavy traffic or taking an exam. Chronic TMJ syndrome may eventually result in a wearing down of the teeth, and the client may need to consult a dentist. Other indications of psychosocial disturbances include tics (involuntary muscle spasms), hair twisting or pulling, biting the lips, and excessive blinking. Relaxation techniques such as meditation and guided imagery may help relieve head and neck symptoms related to stress. If appropriate, refer the client to a mental health professional for assistance.

Self-Care Considerations

It is essential to consider the client's self-care when you assess the head and neck. Most clients spend more time caring for this unique and highly visible region than any other part of the body. The way the client cares for the hair, face, and teeth may afford clues to the client's overall health status or may indicate musculoskeletal problems, neurologic impairments, or psychosocial disturbances.

There may be a link between the client's food consumption and the onset of headaches. Some clients find that eating chocolate or cheese, for example, triggers their headaches. Alchohol ingestion may also lead to headaches.

Helmets are absolutely essential for people riding motorcycles or bicycles, and those participating in certain sports such as hockey or football. The use of seatbelts in automobiles decreases the client's risk of head injury.

Excessive sun exposure without the use of sunglasses may promote cataract formation. A deficiency of vitamin A may cause night blindness. Some medications have side effects that may cause excessive corneal dryness, vision changes, or increased intraocular pressure. When assessing a client who wears contact lenses, ask how long the client wears the lenses each day and evaluate the client's cleansing routine. Sharing eye makeup increases the risk for infection and should be avoided.

Cleaning the ears with invasive instruments can result in trauma. Even cleaning with cotton-tipped swabs may impact cerumen and result in hearing loss. Note that certain medications may cause hearing disturbances such as ringing in the ears.

Clients may have a knowledge deficit related to poor hygiene if teeth have tartar buildup. Some medications, especially if used in childhood, cause permanent discoloration of the teeth. Teeth may also yellow with use of tobacco. Smoking and chewing tobacco increases the risk of oral cancers. Some medications, such as anticholinergics, decrease saliva production and may cause the client's oral mucosa to feel particularly dry. Mouth odors may be due to poor dental hygiene, heavy smoking, or alcohol consumption. Mouth odors may also be affected by the client's diet, especially the use of certain spices.

Family, Cultural, and Environmental Considerations

Asian clients have epicanthic folds (a vertical fold of skin) covering the inner canthus of the eye. Dark-skinned people may have dark pigmented spots on the sclera, and their retinas may be darker. People with light-colored eyes typically have lighter retinas and better night vision but are more sensitive to bright sunlight and artificial light. Dark-skinned clients may also have darker cerumen in the ear, and their oral mucosa may be darker.

Guidelines for evaluating all dimensions of individual health. Sections throughout the text help you integrate basic assessment skills with other considerations that affect individual health. Every assessment chapter incorporates developmental, psychosocial, self-care, family, cultural, and environmental factors.

Ideal for the Clinical Setting

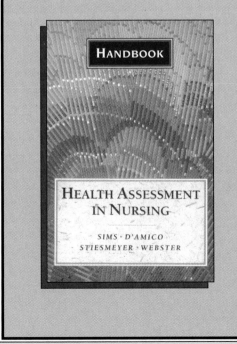

Health Assessment Handbook

A unique resource for students that distills the basics and provides a perfect reference for performing health assessment in the clinical setting. This concise, 256-page, pocket-sized guide can be used as a complement to the text or on its own. Chapters review health assessment from a wellness perspective and focus on the following areas:

- Focused interviews and history taking
- Step-by-step explanations of assessment techniques and special considerations for each body system and region
- Client education for health promotion

In addition, this sourcebook includes over 125 detailed drawings and photos and end-of-chapter Physical Assessment Summaries to aid learning and reinforce correct assessment techniques.

ISBN 0-8053-7349-7

Unit One

The Foundation of Health Assessment in Nursing

1. Introduction to Health Assessment 2. The Interview and Health History 3. Assessing Growth and Development 4. Assessing Psychosocial Health 5. Assessing Self-Care and Wellness Activities 6. Assessing the Family, Culture, and Environment

Chapter 1

Introduction to Health Assessment

Health assessment may be defined as a systematic method of collecting data about a client for the purpose of determining the client's health status. Its significance to nursing was first described by Florence Nightingale, an English nurse and educator: "The most important practical lesson that can be given to nurses is to teach them what to observe—how to observe—what symptoms indicate improvement—what the reverse—which are of importance—which are of none—which are the evidence of neglect—what kind of neglect" (Nightingale 1860).

The data gathered during the health assessment is like the pieces of a jigsaw puzzle, which fit together to form a complete picture (Barker 1987). When key assessment data—the pieces of the puzzle—is missing, the picture of the client's health status is incomplete. Similarly, when data is grouped incorrectly, the final picture of the client's health status is inaccurate. This chapter introduces you to the skills you need to make a complete and accurate health assessment.

In Chapter 2, you'll learn about the first step of assessment, the health history and interview. The remaining chapters in Unit One will help you to gather data related to the client's developmental stage, psychosocial health, self-care habits, and family, culture, and environment. Unit Two describes the process of gathering physical data. Finally, the chapters of Unit Three present holistic assessments of three client populations: infants through adolescents, the childbearing client, and the older adult. Unit Three concludes with a comprehensive health assessment checklist.

Health Assessment in Nursing Practice

You probably have performed rudimentary health assessments many times without even knowing it. Here is an example that might sound familiar: Megan Larson is a nursing student. She is at home studying one Saturday when Walter Kraus, her elderly neighbor, stops by. Megan knows that Walter's wife died of colon cancer 4 months ago.

Megan notices that Walter is pale and has circles under his eyes. His clothing is not as neatly pressed as usual, and he hasn't shaved that day. She offers him some lunch. He says, "I'm not hungry, but I'll have a cup of coffee." As he sips his coffee, she notices that his hands are trembling. She sits down with him and asks him if anything is wrong. He says no and tells Megan that he just stopped in to see how she was doing. She wonders if he has been socializing much since his wife's death and asks him about his golf game. He tells her that he hasn't played for the past few weeks because "I'm no good lately." Megan continues to talk with Walter, and after a while he reveals that he has been having trouble sleeping. "I don't seem to sleep more than 1 or 2 hours a night. My thoughts keep going around and around." She asks him what he thinks about, and he confesses that he blames himself for his wife's death because he didn't insist she go to the doctor "when there was still a chance."

Megan tells Walter that the hospital where she works has a support group for people who have lost a spouse to cancer, and she gives him the phone number. Because she also suspects that the caffeine he consumes might be keeping him up at night, she asks him how much coffee he drinks each day and whether he drinks it at night. He says he usually has a cup after dinner, and another cup while he's watching television, around ten o'clock. Megan reminds Walter that caffeine is a stimulant and tells him that its effects can last for up to 7 hours. She suggests that he not drink any coffee after mid-afternoon, and he promises, "This will be my last cup for today!"

Megan's interaction with Walter illustrates many of the components of health assessment that you will be learning about. For instance, Megan gathered data by asking Walter a number of questions. At first these questions were general, but once she had guessed that Walter's sleeplessness might be related to his wife's recent death and his consumption of coffee, her questions became more specific. She observed physical cues, such as his trembling hands, pallor, and the dark circles under his eyes, and clustered these cues into groups. And once she had guessed the nature of his problem, she offered him a referral to a counseling group and health teaching about the effects of caffeine.

The process of health assessment in nursing practice is certainly more complex and requires a much more highly developed set of skills than indicated in this example. But the same keen observation and critical thinking shown in the example form the basis for effective health assessments in nursing practice, and they are among the most important skills you will bring with you to your clinical practice.

Historical Perspective

Nurses have always conducted assessments (Figure 1.1). Harriet Newton Phillips, considered the first trained nurse in America, assessed individuals in the community setting in the 1860s (Lange 1976). Mary Breckenridge, who founded the Frontier Nursing Service in 1925, performed assessment while giving care to the poor of rural America (Pletsch 1981). Battlefield assessments of soldiers and civilians were done not only by Florence Nightingale during the Crimean War and Dorthea Lynde Dix during the U.S. Civil War but also by nurses in World Wars I and II, the Korean and Vietnam Wars, and the Persian Gulf War.

Even though nurses have always performed assessment on clients as part of giving nursing care, until recently assessment was considered the official domain of the physician via the physical examination. Today, this perspective has changed.

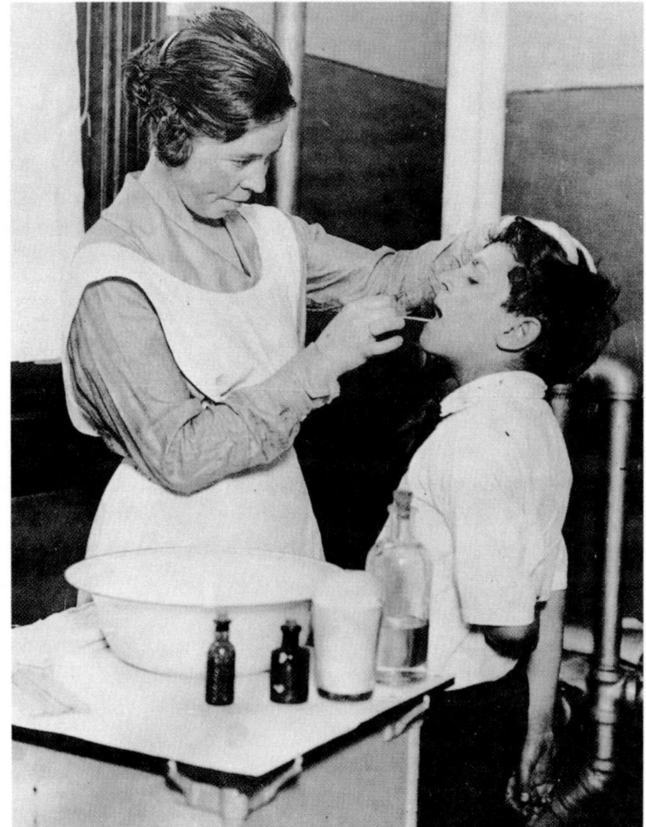

Figure 1.1 Assessment has always been part of the nurse's role.

Nurses perform health assessments, including the health history and physical assessment, that are comprehensive and holistic in nature. The nursing assessment of today is aimed as much at preventing illness and maintaining health as at curing disease.

Today's nurse may gather data not only through the traditional health history, the health interview, and the physical assessment traditionally performed in an examinatioon room but also through a brief focused interview, a questionnaire, a health risk assessment or lifestyle assessment tool, or a review of computerized data about the client. How the nurse performs the nursing assessment varies as the settings for data collection vary. For instance, a nurse teaching a class in smoking cessation, stress management, or nutrition may find opportunities to collect data about class participants during the class session.

Don't forget that, in spite of nursing's emphasis on maintaining health, the best opportunity for assessment in many instances is the client's seeking out of health care because of a current illness. As you address the current problem, keep in mind that this illness-precipitated episode is an opportunity to identify ways to support, promote, and enhance the client's state of health.

The Health Assessment Setting

Most students recognize the hospital as the usual setting of health assessment. However, because nurses are responsible for providing comprehensive health care services, including health promotion and illness prevention, they may carry out health assessment in a variety of settings. In recent years employment opportunities for nurses have shifted from hospitals, and many nurses today practice in outpatient clinics, surgical centers, schools, the workplace, and the client's home. In fact, home care is one of the fastest growing segments of the health care industry (Weinstein 1993).

Nurses working in ambulatory settings typically do not care for clients with acute diseases. Instead, their work tends to focus on *health promotion*, which may be defined as activities directed toward achieving a higher level of wellness. During health promotion, nurses use assessment data to encourage self-care practices and identify resources that support the client's wellness. Nurses in ambulatory settings may also focus on *health protection,* activities that make the client's environment healthier, and *disease prevention*, actions to prevent specific diseases or conditions.

Nurses who perform health assessment in such settings as community hospitals, nursing homes, rehabilitation centers, or mental health residential homes typically use health assessment as a foundation on which to base care plans for early discharge and stronger home management.

In brief, health assessment is practiced wherever the client happens to be at the moment of nurse-client interaction.

Health Assessment and the Nursing Process

When caring for the sick, infirm, and aged, nurses have always employed methods that reflected the values, mores, beliefs, and technical advances of the society in which they lived. Because there were no proven scientific theories or conceptual models for the practice of nursing, each nurse or group of nurses developed their own methods based on experience, intuition, or trial and error. It was not until the mid 1800s that a theoretic basis for the practice of nursing was proposed. At that time, Florence Nightingale wrote a treatise entitled *Notes on Nursing: What It Is, and What It Is Not*. In this work, which was to become the foundation for modern nursing practice, Nightingale espoused basic principles for the practice of nursing care. It took almost another 100 years, however, before a standard method for providing nursing care, the nursing process, was developed.

Evolution of the Nursing Process By the early 1950s, nurse scholars had begun to analyze how nurses function. In 1955, Lydia Hall introduced the concept and terminology of the nursing process (George 1985). Between 1955 and 1973, nurse practitioners, researchers, and educators began to delineate the steps of the process that would guide future nursing practice. In 1973, the American Nurses Association sanctioned the nursing process as the framework for the delivery of care by professional nurses (ANA 1973). The five steps of the process are **assessment, diagnosis, planning, implementation,** and **evaluation** (Figure 1.2). The nursing process is still used as the standard for providing nursing care today.

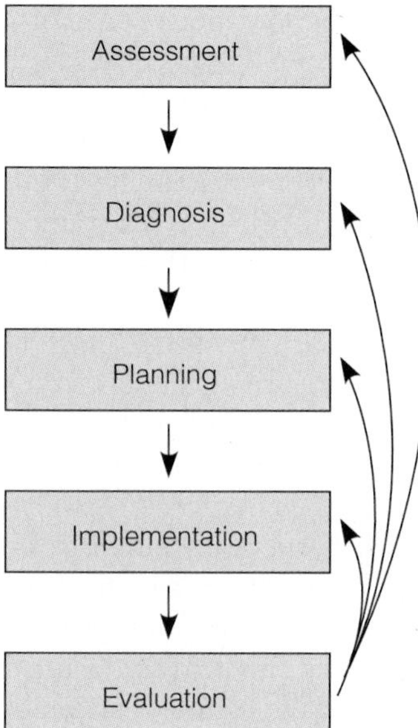

Figure 1.2 The nursing process.

Standards of Care for Assessment and Diagnosis

Standard I. Assessment

THE NURSE COLLECTS CLIENT HEALTH DATA.

Measurement Criteria

1. The priority of data collection is determined by the client's immediate condition or needs.
2. Pertinent data are collected using appropriate assessment techniques.
3. Data collection involves the client, significant others, and health care providers when appropriate.
4. The data collection process is systematic and ongoing.
5. Relevant data are documented in a retrievable form.

Standard II. Diagnosis

THE NURSE ANALYZES THE ASSESSMENT DATA IN DETERMINING DIAGNOSES.

Measurement Criteria

1. Diagnoses are derived from the assessment data.
2. Diagnoses are validated with the client, significant others, and health care providers, when possible.
3. Diagnoses are documented in a manner that facilitates the determination of expected outcomes and plan of care.

The Relationship of Health Assessment to the Nursing Process Health assessment is the vital first step of the nursing process. The remaining steps of the process—diagnosis, planning, implementation, and evaluation—cannot be effective if the quality of the assessment data is in question. Accurate nursing diagnoses require accurate and complete assessment data. When planning nursing interventions, you will use assessment data to determine whether you have prioritized client goals correctly and whether the nursing interventions you've identified are realistic in view of the client data.

Although the steps of the nursing process are identified and described as discrete actions, they are actually interrelated and overlap to some degree. This is particularly true for assessment, which is an ongoing activity. In caring for a client, whether over a period of hours in a critical care setting or over a period of months in a rehabilitation setting, the nurse continuously updates and reinterprets assessment data in response to the changing health status of the client. For example, the condition of a client with labile (constantly changing) blood pressure may change from hour to hour as the blood pressure fluctuates from very high to very low readings. In situations such as this, the client is constantly assessed, and nursing interventions are modified to accommodate changes in the client's condition. The American Nurses Association's Standard Assessment Factors for General Professional Nursing Practice are provided in the box above.

The Process of Assessing a Client's Health

Developing the Database

Figure 1.3 on page 6 illustrates the process of assessment. The critical first step in this process is developing the database. The health assessment begins at the moment you first gather information about the client, whether in person, over the

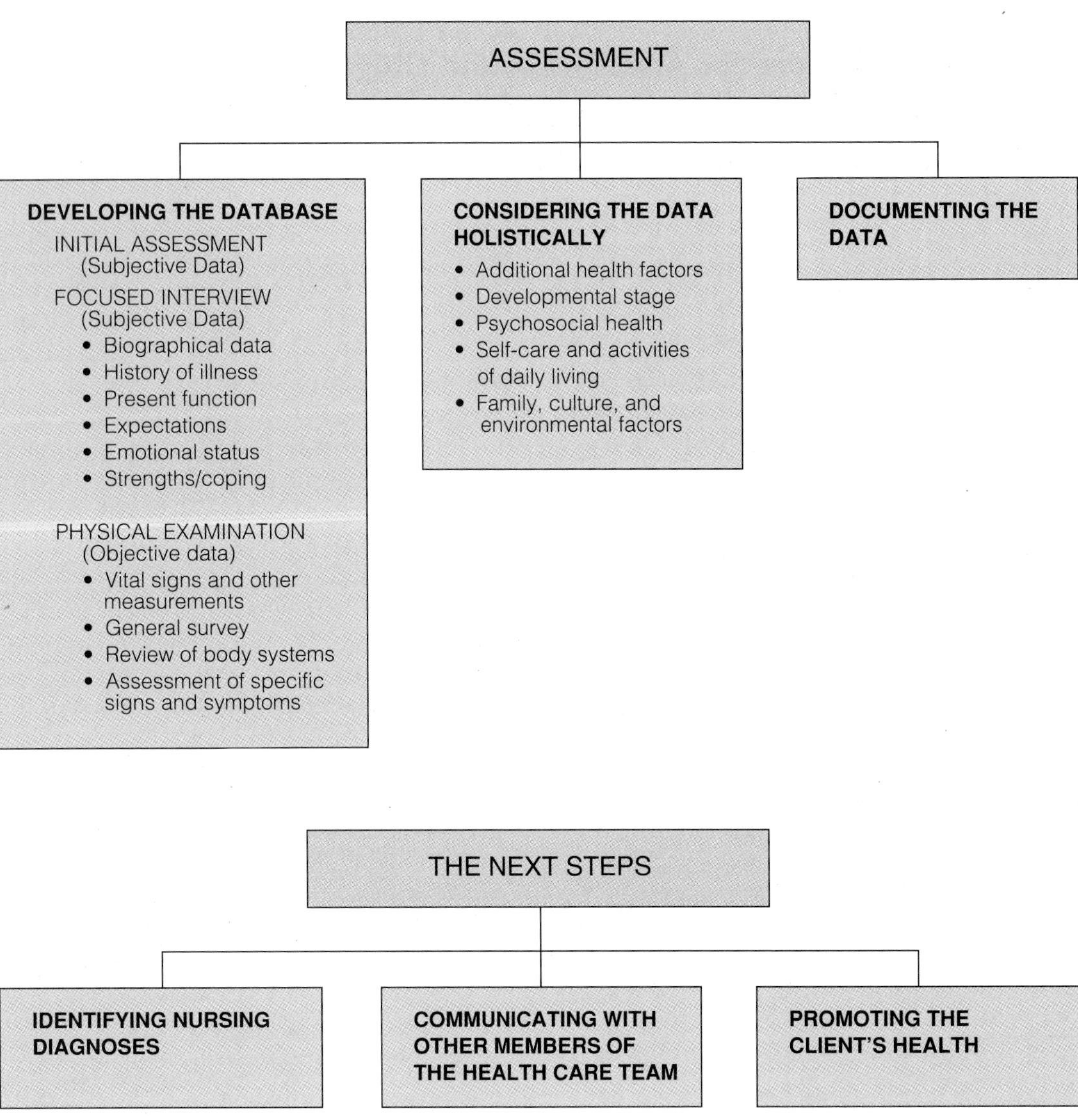

Figure 1.3 The process of assessing a client's health.

phone, or even during a review of the client's medical records. The **database** is the collected "bits" of information, or **data**, that are gathered and compiled during the assessment phase of the nursing process. Each "bit" of information collected about a client is referred to as a **cue**, because it hints at the possibility of a health problem.

The database is collected in two phases: General information is recorded during the initial contact with the client. This general information is called **baseline data** and is used as a yardstick during future assessments. Most institutions and agencies designate specific formats for recording baseline data. More information about the initial client interview is provided in Chapter 2. Any health problems revealed during the initial interview are then assessed in greater detail during a *focused interview* and *physical assessment*. The chapters in Unit Two provide focused interview questions and physical assessment techniques for specific body regions and systems.

Sources of Data The essential content of the database includes physiologic, developmental, psychosocial, self-care, family, cultural, and environmental information derived from a variety of sources. The **primary** (or *direct*) **source** from which data is collected is the client. The client's family or friends, other health personnel, medical records, and literature are **secondary** (or *indirect*) **sources** of data.

Types of Data You collect two major types of information during the assessment: *subjective data* and *objective data*. **Subjective data** is information that the client experiences and communicates to an observer. Perceptions of pain, nausea, dizziness, or nervousness are examples of subjective data that only the client can describe. Subjective data is usually referred to as **covert** (hidden) **data**, or as a **symptom**, when it is perceived by the client and cannot be observed by others.

You can also obtain subjective data from family members, friends, or other health care personnel. They may relate subjective data that the client has shared with them, or they may voice their own opinion on some aspect of the client's condition. Information obtained from family members or those who are close to the client is especially helpful when the client is an infant or child, is very ill, or is unable to communicate. However, to ensure accuracy, you should validate subjective data obtained from sources other than the client with at least one other source.

Objective data is observed or measured by a health care professional, usually during a physical examination. It may be referred to as **overt data** or a **sign** because the finding is obvious or apparent to others. You may gather objective data from the medical records or laboratory or diagnostic tests as well as from the physical assessment. It is determined by noting and comparing client responses to accepted standards. An elevated temperature, absent reflexes, a slow pulse, decreased range of motion, and low specific gravity in the urine are some examples of objective data.

Other Descriptors of Data Both subjective and objective data may further be categorized as *constant* or *variable*. **Constant data** is information that does not change over time, whereas **variable data** may change within minutes, hours, or days. The client's race, sex, or blood type are examples of constant data. Blood pressure, blood counts, and a client's age are all examples of variable data.

Historical data is information about what happened in the past. A previous surgical intervention, the birth of a child, or an injury from a car accident are examples of historical data. **Current data** is information about what is occurring now. Current data may reveal why the client is seeking assistance. Some examples of current data include fever, headache, and acute pain.

Increasing the Accuracy of Data The accuracy of your subjective data depends on your ability to clarify the information you gather with follow-up questions and to obtain supporting data from other pertinent sources. The accuracy of your objective data depends on your ability to avoid reaching conclusions without substantive evidence. For example, if you observe a client who appears to be overweight, you cannot automatically assume that the client has an alteration in nutrition and eats more than the body requires. Before you could accept or reject this assumption, you would need to ask a number of questions about the client's general health status and nutritional habits, to measure the client's height and weight, and to perform a physical assessment.

The accuracy of your objective data is also increased by attention to detail and verification. For example, one blood pressure measurement alone may not provide an accurate picture of a client's cardiovascular status. You can increase your accuracy by measuring the blood pressure with the client sitting, standing, and lying down, or by taking the blood pressure reading at different times of the day. Remain aware of the possibilities for error and misinterpretation of both subjective and objective data, and organize the assessment to build an accurate and complete representation of the client's health status.

The Focused Interview A **focused interview** is a brief exchange between you and your client during which you make a concentrated effort to uncover more information about a specific health problem. In general, the focused interview is less formal than the initial history-taking interview, concentrates on the client's subjective responses, and is performed any time additional information is needed. However, you should always conduct a focused interview before a physical assessment to gain a better understanding of the client's health problems and to help determine the focus of the physical assessment. For example, if a client tells you that the joint pain previously described seems to be worst in the left shoulder, you would give this area careful attention during the physical assessment.

You also conduct focused interviews throughout the physical assessment, gathering more information as needed about each part of the body and any new signs and symptoms. For example, suppose you are about to perform a physical assessment of a 45-year-old woman who has been complaining of chest pain on exertion. During the focused interview, you concentrate on questions related to her breathing and activity patterns and related signs and symptoms. However, while examining her chest wall, you notice a black, irregularly shaped, raised, molelike lesion over her left scapula. You recognize that the lesion is a potential health hazard, and you immediately begin to gather more specific data about it, asking the client questions about it, measuring it, and so on, even though the client's major complaint is chest pain. This situation is typical of how you implement focused interviews whenever you need new or more specific information.

The focused interview is one of your most effective assessment tools because it gives you additional insights into clients' feelings and expectations, pinpoints more specific information about signs and symptoms, and keeps information about the client's health status current. Conducting a focused interview is a difficult task, however, because you cannot prepare a formal set of questions in advance. During a focused interview, you need to "think on your feet" to determine what kinds of questions you should ask next and what avenues of information you should pursue.

The Physical Assessment The **physical assessment** is the hands-on assessment of the client during which you use special skills to confirm the absence of health problems or to uncover unexpected findings. You usually perform the physical assessment after compiling a complete database from interviews with the client, significant others, and health care providers who have cared for the client as well as reviews of the medical records and relevant literature. (Of course, in emergency or urgent situations compiling a database may not be possible.) The physical assessment is an essential component of the health assessment process because it helps you verify or discredit the hypothetical or probable nursing diagnoses. The chapters in Unit Two present the skills and techniques you'll use in performing thorough physical assessments.

Considering the Data Holistically

Nurses who assess only the client's physiologic alterations are seeing only the "tip of the iceberg," a small part of the whole. Physiologic health is the most easily assessed aspect of a client's overall health; it includes signs and symptoms, lab results, physical findings, and the client's stated reason for seeking health care. The remaining aspects of the client's health status, like the submerged portion of an iceberg, usually are not as easily observed. Nonetheless, they are just as critical to the integrity of the data gathered in the health assessment. If you do not view the client holistically, your assessment and the plan of care you derive from it will not help the client to move toward optimum health and well-being.

Holistic theory describes the human organism as a composite of interacting parts that together make up more than the sum of these parts (Krieger 1981). In health assessment, the nurse who uses a holistic approach incorporates all the components that make up the client. This means that, in addition to assessing a client's physiologic health status in relation to the client's current health problem, the nurse considers other health factors that may seem unrelated to the client's current health problem, as well as developmental, psychosocial, self-care, family, cultural, and environmental aspects (Smith 1984). For example, Mr. Chang, who works at a computer manufacturing company, requests a visit to the company's occupational health nurse. He states that he is concerned that the chemicals he works with are harming his health. The nurse begins by assessing Mr. Chang's physical status in relation to his health concern, looking for cues that may indicate a physiologic reaction to the chemicals, such as skin rash, irritation of mucous membranes, or breathing difficulties.

The nurse continues the assessment, additionally gathering data about Mr. Chang's psychosocial, family, and cultural status. Mr. Chang states that he is married and tells the nurse that his wife just gave birth a week ago to their fourth daughter. The nurse knows that some individuals, and some cultures in general, place a higher value on male children than female children. Upon further assessment, the nurse learns that Mr. Chang's concern regarding the chemicals is not that they are making him feel ill but that they may somehow be preventing him from having a male child.

This example illustrates the importance of a holistic approach to assessment. If the nurse had not collected holistic data about the client, the client's true health concern might not have been identified. The accompanying box lists the major factors to consider for a holistic health assessment.

Factors to Consider for a Holistic Health Assessment

- **Additional health factors**. These may seem unrelated to the client's present problem yet may yield information that could affect the progress or outcome of your assessment. *For example*, when you assess an elderly client with multiple bruises, poor vision is a significant factor, because it may contribute to frequent falls.
- **Developmental factors**. The client's developmental stage profoundly influences the collection and interpretation of assessment data. *For example*, the health assessment of a pregnant 13-year-old is markedly different from the health assessment of a woman of 37 who is pregnant for the third time. Chapter 3 discusses growth and development.
- **Psychosocial factors**. Clients' emotional health, level of stress and anxiety, and general satisfaction with life can have a significant influence on their physiologic health. In the same way, physiologic problems can affect the client's psychosocial health. *For example*, a client's severe job stress may contribute to her ulcers. On the other hand, an adolescent client's severe acne may contribute to his body image disturbance. Chapter 4 discusses psychosocial health assessment.
- **Self-care factors.** Self-care factors include nutrition; exercise; hygiene; grooming; use of tobacco, alcohol, and other legal and illegal drugs; safety practices; rest and recreation; and many other factors related to a client's health practices. Self-care factors can greatly influence a client's health status, both positively and negatively, and are essential to consider in a holistic assessment. *For example*, a client's recurring urinary tract infections may be related to her self-care practice of taking hot bubble baths. Chapter 5 discusses self-care factors.
- **Family, culture, and environmental factors**. A client's family structure, cultural group, religious practices, socioeconomic status, educational level, job, and living environment are also important to consider when performing the holistic health assessment. *For example*, a client's diabetes may be exacerbated by an inability to afford nourishing food and prescribed medications. Chapter 6 discusses family, culture, and environmental factors.

Documenting the Data

The primary purpose of documentation is to communicate accurately and thoroughly the data gathered in the health assessment to others involved in the care of the client. Complete and accurate documentation of the assessment data increases the effectiveness of the entire health care team. It also prevents the client from having to repeat identical information to more than one team member. The sharing of information helps to prevent gaps or overlaps in data and reduces the chance of errors occurring because of incorrect or incomplete information.

Clear, objective documentation also serves to protect the client, the nurse involved, and the health care agency. Written documentation serves as legal proof and a permanent record of the client's health status at the time of the documentation.

What to Document It is often difficult to decide what health assessment data to document. If you document everything you observe about the client, the result is likely to be an unwieldy and unusable collection of data. If you document too little information, the health assessment may not provide a good foundation for the remaining phases of the nursing process. You should strive to strike a balance: Review the objectives for client care and use them as guidelines for what you should document. If you need the information to formulate the nursing diagnosis, plan nursing interventions, or provide nursing care, then you should record it. As you study this text, you will learn in each chapter to identify the physical cues and related factors for each body system or region. This knowledge will help you decide what information you should document and what information you can safely disregard.

When and How to Document Data collected during the health assessment should be recorded as soon as possible. The accuracy of recall fades as time passes, and delaying the documentation of information may compromise its integrity. You may find that the best time to document is immediately after you complete the physical assessment, while the client is getting dressed or, in the case of hospitalized clients, while the client is resting after the procedure.

You should document not only the initial assessment data but also information from the focused interview, physical assessment, and any ongoing assessment you perform. All documentation should be clear, accurate, objective, specific, concise, and current. For example, "Client has diarrhea," is less accurate than "Client states he has had 10 liquid greenish yellow stools in the past 8 hours." By recording the data as a statement by the client, you identify it as subjective. In addition, recording the specific number, color, and firmness of the stools and the duration makes it possible to determine whether the client's condition is improving or deteriorating over time.

The Next Steps

Identifying Nursing Diagnoses

Nursing diagnoses are statements used by nurses to describe a client's response to health problems that nurses are educated about and licensed to treat. **Health problems** are situations in which a client needs help to promote, maintain, or regain health. Some examples of nursing diagnoses that describe a client's response to a health problem are *Pain, Fear,* and *Sleep pattern disturbance.*

Nurses who are being introduced to the nursing process for the first time frequently have difficulty understanding how nursing diagnoses are derived from the assessment of the client. Identifying nursing diagnoses requires an ability to perform an accurate and thorough health assessment, an understanding of nursing diagnosis, and the ability to engage in critical thinking.

Critical Thinking **Critical thinking** may be defined as the ability to think in a logical manner in order to analyze information, draw correct conclusions, make decisions, and evaluate difficult situations (Risner 1986). It is the use of careful judgment to examine ideas, inferences, assumptions, and even conclusions about data in order to increase understanding.

Two cognitive skills are essential to critical thinking: analysis and synthesis. **Analysis** is the ability to separate a situation into its component parts so that they can be carefully studied. **Synthesis** is the ability to reassemble the component parts of a situation into a logical whole. In simple terms, the function of analysis and synthesis is to take a situation apart, study it carefully, and then put it back together in a logical manner so that valid judgments and decisions can be made. Nurses experienced in health assessment use the skills of analysis and synthesis many times throughout the day as they carefully study the assessment data and then reassemble the findings into clusters that lead to nursing diagnoses.

In addition to analysis and synthesis, these characteristics are important for critical thinking in health assessment:

- Critical thinking is reasonable and rational. It is based on reason and logic rather than prejudice, preference, self-interest, or fear.
- Critical thinking is reflective. Rather than making a hurried decision, the nurse who thinks critically takes the time to collect thorough and accurate data, then thinks the matter through in a disciplined manner, weighing facts and evidence.
- Critical thinking inspires an attitude of inquiry. A critical thinker is constructively skeptical, asking questions in an effort to know more.

- Critical thinking is autonomous. A critical thinker does not passively accept the beliefs or conclusions of others, but analyzes the issues and reaches conclusions independently.
- Critical thinking is creative. A critical thinker is able to originate ideas by making connections between varied bits of data.
- Critical thinking is fair. Critical thinkers attempt to remove bias from their own thinking and to recognize bias in the thinking of others (Kozier et al 1995).

Although critical thinking plays an important role in most clinical judgments, it is the very foundation of the method you will use to identify nursing diagnoses from assessment data. This method is known as the *diagnostic reasoning process*.

Diagnostic Reasoning For most experienced nurses, the thinking process used to develop nursing diagnoses is unconscious and intuitive. It has become "second nature" with time, experience, and education. If you are identifying nursing diagnoses for the first time, however, you may find it helpful to use the step-by-step approach called the **diagnostic reasoning process**.

The diagnostic reasoning process includes the following steps:

1. Gather preliminary data.
2. Formulate diagnostic hypotheses.
3. Gather supporting data.
4. Organize and cluster the data.
5. Select and validate the nursing diagnoses.
6. Identify etiologic or related factors.

The accompanying box describes the critical thinking that takes place during each step of the diagnostic reasoning process. You may wish to follow this box as you read the following discussion of the six steps.

Gathering Preliminary Data During the first phase of the diagnostic reasoning process, you gather preliminary data derived from an initial interview of the client and significant others, the review of the medical records, and discussion with other health professionals caring for the client. During the initial interview, you take a *health history*, which is a detailed account of the client's past and present health status and problems. The health history is discussed more fully in Chapter 2.

If necessary, you review the literature. The goals of a review of the literature are:

- To research expected norms for comparison with client data
- To review relevant anatomy and physiology in order to understand client data
- To explore probable nursing diagnoses

All of the information that is collected about the client then becomes part of the preliminary database and is used as a baseline against which to compare future changes in the client's condition.

Formulating Diagnostic Hypotheses Although it is too early to identify nursing diagnoses, it is not too early to formulate **diagnostic hypotheses**, which are educated guesses made to explain the presence of the cues identified in step 1. The hypothesis is stated in the form of a probable or possible nursing diagnosis, and is developed from one of two actions: by comparing the client data to standards, or by making inferences.

- Comparison to standards. A diagnostic hypothesis may be developed when a cue does not compare to an accepted standard. A cue that deviates from the normal is a signal that the client is responding abnormally and that you should consider the possibility of a nursing diagnosis. When this happens, you begin to look for other cues that commonly occur along with the cue that you observed. Consider the following situation: John Valek, a 15-year-old high school student, visited the school nurse one morning stating that he felt "hot and sweaty." The school nurse checked his oral temperature and found it to be 101.6F, 3 degrees higher than normal. Once this cue was identified, the nurse began to look for additional cues associated with an elevated temperature. In John's case, these cues included flushed skin, elevated pulse and respirations, and nausea. From this information, a probable nursing diagnosis of *Hyperthermia* was identified.
- Making inferences. Hypotheses are also generated from inferences arrived at through the process of *inductive reasoning*. Nurses demonstrate inductive reasoning when they use known or observed facts to draw conclusions about a condition that is not directly observable. For example, a nurse caring for a client who has blood-saturated surgical dressings, a plummeting blood pressure, and elevated pulse would infer that the client is hemorrhaging with impending shock. "Impending shock" is not a condition that can be directly measured or seen. Experience and recall play an important role in this process because the nurse relates past clinical experiences to the present situation to derive appropriate nursing diagnoses. In fact, inductive reasoning is possible only when the nurse has developed a body of knowledge through study and clinical experience.

Gathering Supporting Data During the third phase of diagnostic reasoning, data is collected to support or reject the diagnostic hypotheses (the probable nursing diagnoses). This data is collected by conducting the focused interview and performing a physical assessment. The process of gathering supporting data during a focused interview and a physical assessment was described previously. They are also discussed in detail throughout the chapters of Unit Two.

Examples of Critical Thinking during the Diagnostic Reasoning Process

Step 1 Gather preliminary data.

- Have I seen, read, studied, or heard about these types of cues before? If so, what nursing diagnoses were they associated with?
- Are these cues associated with a psychologic or physiologic deviation? If so, is the deviation related to a nursing diagnosis?
- Does this client have a medical diagnosis? If so, are the signs and the symptoms of the medical diagnosis also related to a nursing diagnosis?
- Have diagnostic tests yielded findings? Do these abnormal findings point to a nursing diagnosis?
- Have I collected all of the information needed to look for tentative nursing diagnoses at this point?
- Do I need to review nursing literature to determine whether or not identified cues represent a probable diagnosis?

Step 2 Formulate diagnostic hypotheses.

- Are there cues present that do not fit acceptable standards?
- Is a pattern of cues developing that points to a probable diagnosis?
- Could I make assumptions concerning this client's health problem?
- Do I have preconceived ideas or biases that maybe interfering with clear thinking?
- Is there enough evidence to support a probable diagnosis?
- Are data present that would support an alteration in health requiring collaborative management?

Step 3 Gather supporting data.

- What information do I need to support the probable nursing diagnoses I have made?
- Have I overlooked other health problems during the initial contact with the client that I should address at this time?
- Have I overlooked any other factors that may be contributing to the client's health problems?
- Does the client exhibit responses during the physical assessment that I have not seen before? How do these responses relate to the total picture seen so far?
- Do the physical findings corroborate the information I obtained from the medical record, initial interview, and family and friends?
- Are there expected pieces of information that are not present? Is there an explanation for the missing information?

Step 4 Organize and cluster the data.

- What nursing model should I use to sort and group the data?
- Is one nursing model better than another to sort the data for this client?
- Is there any information that is insignificant and should not be used?
- Is there any information that is missing?
- Which cues seem related? Why?

Step 5 Select and validate a nursing diagnosis.

- Do any of the groups of diagnostic cues look familiar?
- Does the group of diagnostic cues fit the major defining characteristics of the nursing diagnosis that I've chosen?

Step 6 Identify etiologic or related factors.

- What factors have contributed to the development of this nursing diagnosis?
- Do the factors that are present correlate with the contributing factors suggested by NANDA?

Organizing and Clustering the Data After gathering the supporting data, the nurse sorts and groups all of the diagnostic cues collected according to the defining characteristics of specific nursing diagnoses. For example: Kathleen Magruder is a 21-year-old college student injured in a car accident 2 weeks before. She went to the college infirmary because of pain in her mouth. She had lost two teeth in the car accident, and her gums did not seem to be healing. She told Ms Collings, the infirmary nurse, "My mouth is so sore that I can't eat." When further questioned, she admitted that she had not carried out the oral hygiene the dentist had recommended after the injury because "it hurts too much." As Ms Collings sought more information from the student and completed the physical assessment, she saw a group of related diagnostic cues emerge. These included yellow, indurated patches throughout the mouth, cracked lips, a coated tongue, halitosis, and severe discomfort. The nurse recognized these findings as defining characteristics for the nursing diagnosis *Altered oral mucous membrane* related to the previous mouth injury and poor oral hygiene.

Selecting and Validating the Nursing Diagnoses In this next step of the diagnostic reasoning process, the nurse determines the final nursing diagnoses. It is at this point that any *probable* nursing diagnoses become *actual* nursing diagnoses. The nurse compares each diagnostic cluster with the defining characteristics of the tentative nursing diagnosis earlier hypothesized. In the previous example of Kathleen Magruder, Ms Collings compared her assessment findings with the defining characteristics of *Altered oral mucous membrane.* When the two sets of data matched, she could confirm or validate the diagnosis.

Identifying the Etiology or Related Factors With this step, you identify and include etiologic or related factors in the nursing diagnoses to confirm the validity of the chosen nursing diagnoses. In most cases the nurse has already collected and identified this information along with the diagnostic cues. In the example of Kathleen Magruder, the related factors were the injury to her mouth in the accident and poor oral hygiene.

Applying the Diagnostic Reasoning Process Developing nursing diagnoses from health assessment data is a complex task requiring you to gather significant diagnostic data and draw logical conclusions from it. While you are still learning assessment and diagnostic skills, you should follow this diagnostic reasoning model until you can carry out the process automatically. The accompanying box provides a case study illustrating how the diagnostic reasoning process is put into action in the clinical setting. In addition, Chapters 8 through 18 each contain two case studies, called "Diagnostic Reasoning in Action," that help you apply the diagnostic reasoning process to clients with alterations in health for specific body regions and systems.

Communicating with Other Members of the Health Care Team

When you have completed the health assessment and organized and documented the information that you obtained, your next step is to communicate the data to the rest of the team who provide care for the client. Team members may include other nurses, physicians, or any other individuals involved in the client's care.

Communication of the data may be written or verbal and may take one of several forms. A **discussion** is an informal communication that may lead to a decision regarding the client's care. An example of a discussion is a nurse practitioner sharing data gathered about the client with a physician. A **report** is an oral or written account reviewing the information gathered. Data communication by report is often done at the change of shift by nursing personnel in acute care settings. A **record** is a written, formal, and legal document. Client charts and nursing progress notes are examples of records.

Some assessment findings require prompt communication with other members of the health care team. Alterations in health that require such collaborative management are discussed in each chapter of Unit Two. In addition, when you are learning the specific assessment techniques for each body region or system, special referral boxes will alert you to findings that require emergency collaboration or findings that require you to collaborate with nonphysician caregivers, such as social workers, psychotherapists, and physical therapists.

Promoting the Client's Health

Health assessment is applicable to promotion of health and wellness as well as prevention and treatment of disease. Health traditionally has been defined as the absence of disease. More recently, however, the World Health Organization defined **health** as a state of complete physical, mental, and social well-being (WHO 1947). **Wellness** describes a state of life that is balanced, personally satisfying, and characterized by health-enhancing behaviors; in other words, a state of optimal health. In a wellness perspective, health is seen on a contiuuum, with illness and premature death at one end, and optimal wellness, what we think of as being "fully alive," at the other (Figure 1.4).

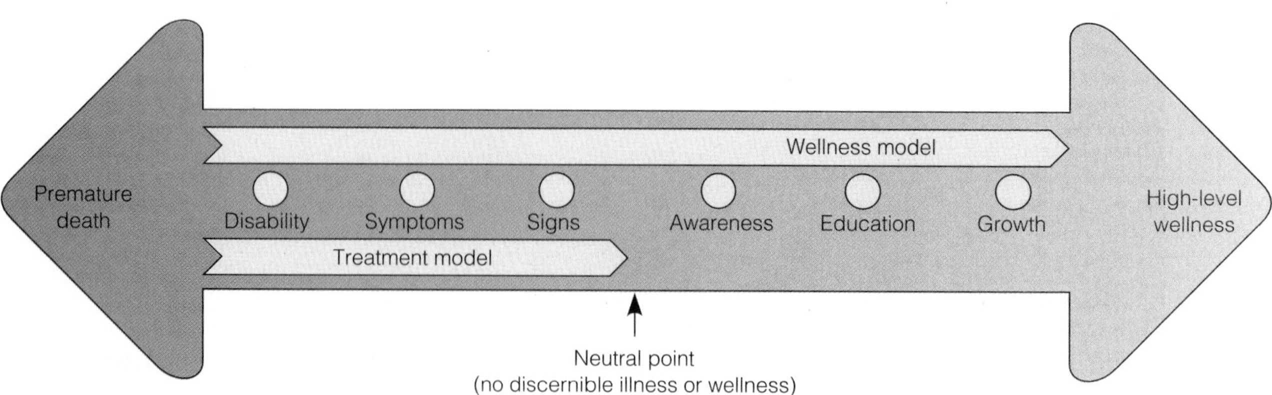

Figure 1.4 The wellness–illness continuum.

Applying the Diagnostic Reasoning Process

John McIntyre, a 42-year-old accountant, was admitted to Jamestown Medical Center with diarrhea, fever, and dehydration. He told the admitting nurse, Silvia Gonzales, that the diarrhea had started 5 days ago while the McIntyres were on vacation in South America. Although he tried to use over-the-counter medications to curtail the problem, the diarrhea became increasingly worse, requiring him to cut his vacation short and return home. His wife told Ms Gonzales that Mr. McIntyre had complained of weakness and dizziness during the plane trip home and had several bouts of vomiting. During the physical assessment, Ms Gonzales documented the following data:

Blood pressure: 98/42

Apical pulse: 104 and thready

Respirations: 24 per minute

Oral temperature: 102.2F

Color, flushed

Height and weight, 6'2", 180 pounds

Complains of cramplike pain in left lower abdominal quadrant during bowel movement

States he has had 10 liquid, greenish stools in the past 8 hours

Complains of nausea and vomiting

Has not tolerated liquids in the past 48 hours

Skin warm and dry

Abdomen slightly distended

Lips dry and parched

Oral mucosa pale and dry

Rectum red and irritated

Bowel sounds frequent and high-pitched

Tenderness in lower-left quadrant

Has had no recent history of diarrhea

States he has never been in a hospital

Appears anxious and confused

Diagnostic Reasoning Steps	Findings for Mr. McIntyre
1. Gather preliminary data	Elevated temperature. History of nausea and vomiting. Painful, frequent stools. Weakness and dizziness.
2. Formulate diagnostic hypotheses	1. *Hyperthermia* 2. *Pain* 3. *Diarrhea* 4. *High risk for injury*
3. Gather supporting data	*Hyperthermia:* Flushed, warm, dry skin. Increased pulse and respiratory rate. Confused and anxious.
4. Organize and cluster the data	*Pain:* Cramping pain during bowel movement. *Diarrhea:* Ten liquid, greenish, stool in last 8 hours. Frequent, high-pitched bowel sounds. Red, irritated rectum. *High risk for injury:* No supporting information noted.
5. Select and validate nursing diagnoses	*Hyperthermia:* The diagnostic cluster matched the defining characteristics for hyperthermia. *Pain:* Only one cue identified. Did not fit defining characteristics for nursing diagnosis of pain. *Diarrhea:* The diagnostic cluster matched the defining characteristics for diarrhea. *High risk for injury:* Did not match.
6. Identify etiologic or related factors	*Hyperthermia:* Dehydration, vomiting, inability to tolerate fluids for 48 hours. *Diarrhea:* Dietary changes, food intolerance, recent travel, increased intestinal motility secondary to possible infection by intestinal parasites.

In a wellness assessment, you and the client work together to examine the positive adaptations and previously successful behaviors that contribute to optimal health and well-being. Thus, the wellness assessment emphasizes the client's personal strengths and ability to enhance health. The goals for both you and your client may be to reinforce and continue health-promoting behaviors, prevent illness, identify acute or chronic needs and problems, and even to support the client in meeting death with dignity and spiritual wellness. Thus, even clients who are experiencing disease can be helped to achieve their optimal state of health, or wellness. For clients free from disease, a wellness assessment can reveal areas where health can be increased.

Using a wellness framework for health assessment implies that, unless there is a condition that prevents the client from making decisions, responsibility for the client's physiologic, psychologic, and spiritual well-being resides with the client. The emphasis is on the client's personal behavior, because behavior and health are strongly linked. For instance, elimination of behavioral risk factors such as use of tobacco, alcohol, and other drugs; lack of exercise; and poor nutrition could significantly improve the health of the client. It is critically important for nurses, as client advocates, to assess behavioral risks as part of the holistic health assessment.

Modeling wellness behaviors can enhance nurses' efforts to help their clients achieve wellness. For instance, a nurse assessing an anxious client might suggest that learning to relax will help reduce the client's blood pressure, but this message will have little impact if at the same time the nurse keeps looking at the clock, fidgeting, and speaking impatiently. In this case, the effectiveness of the health teaching is reduced because the nurse does not model behavior that reinforces the value of stress management.

In addition to being a role model for wellness, the nurse must demonstrate that health promotion is a priority when assessing the client and when providing care. For instance, consider a nurse who is performing a nursing assessment on a truck driver. Obviously the nurse addresses the physical complaint of back pain that initially led the individual to seek health care, but the nurse should pay equal attention to the use of seat belts. This focus on safety demonstrates to the client that the nurse values health-promoting behaviors and that these behaviors are as important to health as seeking care for a physical complaint.

The nurse must help individuals to take responsibility for their health. The nurse educates clients and encourages these self-responsible behaviors:

- Becoming informed about what options exist before making health-promoting lifestyle choices
- Seeking help from a nurse or other health resources when problems or situations become too complex for the individual to handle alone
- Knowing what community resources may help support lifestyle changes, such as community health education classes, self-care books and aides, support groups, counseling services, and not-for-profit organizations like the Red Cross, March of Dimes, and American Heart Association
- Setting reasonable goals for health-promoting behaviors
- Accepting responsibility for the decisions the individual makes about a healthy lifestyle
- Changing negative health practices in a slow and productive way, rather than all at once
- Knowing one's own health values and living by them, making sure that they fit into one's own life and environment
- Making decisions for themselves, not for others

For instance, deciding to exercise daily because family members insist on it will not result in a lasting behavior change for the individual. Lasting, positive change in health behaviors occurs only when individuals agree to take responsibility for their own health and well-being.

For your wellness assessment to be truly effective, you must fully attend to the wellness concerns of the client, even when they do not seem to you to be a high priority. For example, an obese client may communicate during the interview that stress management is a primary reason for seeking health care. Based on observations made during the physical assessment, you might feel that weight loss should be a priority. Nevertheless, you should recognize that the client's input has value. Then respond to the client's health concern by asking focused questions to gather more data about the client's feelings of excessive stress. After further data collection, you may find that the client sees a relationship between increased stress and overeating.

The following questions may be appropriate during a wellness assessment:

- What issues are you concerned with regarding your health?
- How does your health concern affect you and your lifestyle?
- What health goals do you want to begin moving toward?
- What do you see as your strengths?
- How do you think your care provider/nurse can help you?
- What do you think you need to do to help resolve this concern?

Summary

Throughout the history of nursing, assessment of the individual's health status has been the key to the remainder of the nursing process. By turning this key, the nurse sees what problems can be identified, which nursing diagnoses to formulate, and what interventions to implement.

Nursing assessment is the art of observing, of getting the facts first, before making any decisions. Nurses must use all their senses to observe all aspects—physical, psychologic, social, and environmental—of the client. The data gathered during the nursing assessment is the foundation on which nurses base all decisions regarding the client's care.

Key Points

- ✓ Health assessment is a systematic method of collecting data about a client for the purpose of determining the client's health status.
- ✓ Historically, nurses have performed assessment in a variety of settings, even though assessment was officially the domain of the physician.
- ✓ Health assessment may be carried out in a variety of settings, including hospitals, outpatient clinics, surgicenters, schools, the workplace, and the client's home.
- ✓ Health assessment is the first step of the nursing process and is continuous and ongoing through every phase of the nursing process.
- ✓ The database is the collected "bits" of information gathered during the assessment phase of the nursing process. It contains baseline data about a client's condition.
- ✓ The client is the primary source of assessment data. Secondary sources include the client's relatives, friends, other health care personnel, and the medical record.
- ✓ Subjective data is information that the client, a family member, or a friend experiences and communicates to an observer. Objective data is observed or measured by a health care professional, usually during a physical examination.
- ✓ Nurses taking a holistic approach to assessment recognize the client as a whole person; one whose health is affected by developmental, psychosocial, self-care, family, cultural, environmental, and physiologic factors.
- ✓ The purpose of documenting the assessment data is to communicate accurately and thoroughly the information gathered about the client to other members of the health care team.
- ✓ When deciding what assessment information to document, include anything you need to formulate nursing diagnoses and to develop a plan of care for the client.
- ✓ Complete your documentation as soon as possible after the health assessment. All documentation should be clear, accurate, objective, specific, concise, and current.
- ✓ The diagnostic reasoning process is a method for identifying nursing diagnoses from health assessment data. It consists of six steps: gathering the preliminary data, formulating diagnostic hypotheses, gathering supporting data, organizing and clustering the data, selecting and validating the nursing diagnoses, and identifying etiologic or related factors.
- ✓ After documenting the assessment data, the nurse communicates significant findings to the rest of the health care team. Three methods of communication are discussion, report, and record.
- ✓ Health assessment is applicable to promotion of health and wellness as well as prevention and treatment of disease. In a wellness assessment, the nurse and client work together to examine the positive adaptations and previously successful behaviors that contribute to optimal health and well-being.

Chapter 2

The Interview and Health History

The health assessment interview provides an opportunity to gather detailed information about events and experiences that have contributed to a client's current state of health. In addition, you explore clients' concerns, emotions, expectations, and knowledge about their health.

The nursing **health history** is a comprehensive record of the client's past and current health status. It is gathered during the initial health assessment interview, which usually occurs at the client's first visit to a health-care facility. The purpose of the health history is to document the response of the whole person to actual and potential health concerns. Thus, the health history includes a wellness assessment covering questions on how the client optimizes health and well-being in such areas as nutrition, stress management, and social interaction.

The health history performed by the nurse has a different focus from the medical history performed by the physician. Although both consist of subjective data, the focus of the medical history is to gather data about the cause and course of disease. Thus, the medical history focuses on the disease rather than on the client and the client's lifestyle practices. For example, the physician may ask a client to relate the details of the range of motion in the left hip to determine the cause of abnormal movement and to prescribe a specific treatment. The nurse obtains the same information but uses it to determine the extent to which the client will need support and teaching regarding ambulation and performance of activities of daily living (ADLs), such as getting dressed independently at home. The nurse and the physician gather the same information for different purposes. The nursing health history may produce information about a medical diagnosis, but its focus is on the client's response to the health concern as a whole person, not just on one or two body systems.

Communication Skills for Health Assessment

The nurse's knowledge of and skill with the communication process play an important role in developing a nurse-client relationship, conducting the health assessment interview, and collecting data for the health history. Communication is also important in educating, guiding, facilitating, directing, and counseling. You cannot develop trust, establish rapport, or carry out nursing interventions for clients without a knowledge of communication styles. For instance, you may need to modify your communication style when you deal with younger or older clients. The younger nurse teaching the elderly client ways to add fiber to the diet may need to use a serious and respectful communication style. Conversely, an older nurse counseling a teenage client regarding safe and responsible sexual practices may need to make special efforts to create an informal atmosphere that allows the teenager to open up and speak freely.

Communication is the exchange of information between individuals. During the communication process an individual, sometimes called the sender, develops an idea and transmits it in the form of a message to another person, or receiver. The receiver perceives the message (the sender's transmitted idea) and interprets it. Once the receiver interprets the meaning, the receiver formulates a response and transmits it back to the sender as feedback. *Encoding* is the process of formulating a message for transmission to another person. To encode an idea, the sender has to choose the words, body language, signs, or symbols that will be used to convey the message. *Decoding* is the process of searching through one's memory, experience, and knowledge base to determine the meaning of the intended message (Figure 2.1).

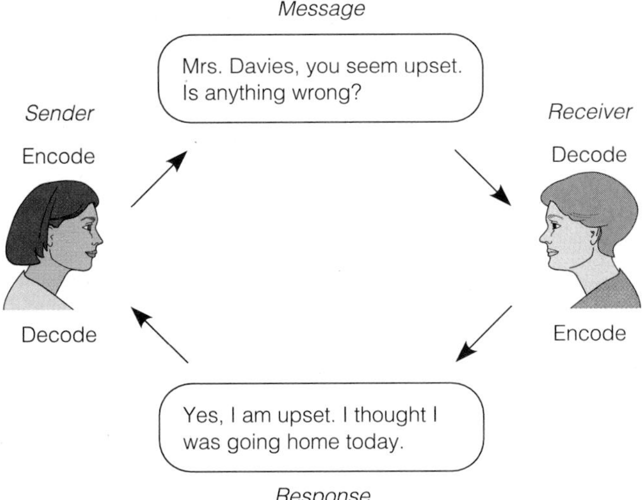
Message
Mrs. Davies, you seem upset. Is anything wrong?
Sender
Encode
Receiver
Decode
Decode
Encode
Yes, I am upset. I thought I was going home today.
Response

Figure 2.1 The communication process.

To communicate successfully, you must make sure the client can accurately decode the messages you send. For example, communication may break down if you use words the client doesn't understand or if you deliver a message in a manner that frightens the client. Communication may also break down if you fail to decode the client's messages accurately because, for example, you don't listen actively and attentively.

Interactional Skills

Interactional skills are actions that you use during the encoding/decoding process to obtain and disseminate information, develop relationships, and promote understanding of self and others. Nurses use a variety of interactional skills during the communication process to gather assessment data from the client, family, significant others, and health care personnel. Brammer (1988) has identified several categories of interactional skills that are helpful during an interview: listening, leading, reflecting, and summarizing (Table 2.1 on page 18).You use these interactional techniques to help the client communicate information thoroughly and also to confirm that you have understood the client's communication correctly.

Listening Listening is a basic part of the communication process and is the most important interactional skill. People who have not developed listening skills have problems relating to others and difficulty attaining their goals. Successful listening involves taking in the client's whole message; hearing words as well as interpreting body language. Successful listening is an active process requiring effort and attention on the part of the nurse (Figure 2.2 on page 19). You must push thoughts about the day's schedule or the next client from your mind while listening to a client. You must give your full attention, or you will miss some of the client's message. You should not only note the words the client speaks but also the tone of voice and even what the client does not say. The woman who states, "My mother died last week" and immediately moves on to another topic of discussion has told the nurse a lot about how she is dealing with a death in her family. Giving your full attention to verbal and nonverbal messages is called attending.

Mehrabian (1972) states that body language may be as much as 93% of the message a client sends. Body language, or nonverbal messages, also provides significant information that you might otherwise overlook and signals information that the client may have omitted intentionally or unintentionally. For example, a male client who feels expressing pain is a weakness might deny that he's in pain. However, his facial expression, guarded reaction to abdominal palpation, and drawn position in bed send a message of severe pain. Because body language can send messages such as hostility, defensiveness, or confusion, you should always tune in to the client's nonverbal as well as verbal messages. Nonverbal cues such as posture, eye contact, makeup, dress, accessories, and items in

Table 2.1 Interactional Skills

Skill/Definition	Technique	Examples
Listening **Attending** Giving the client undivided attention.	◆ Use direct eye contact if appropriate for culture. Look at the client during the conversation. ◆ Lean toward the client slightly. ◆ Select quiet area with no distractions for interview. ◆ Convey unhurried manner; avoid fidgeting and looking at watch.	Nurse arranges with peers for no interruptions during interview. Nurse sits facing client, remains alert, and focuses on what client is saying.
Paraphrasing Restating the client's basic message to test whether it was understood.	◆ Listen for the client's basic message. ◆ Restate the client's message in your own words. ◆ Ask the client if your words are an accurate restatement of the message.	*Client:* "I toss and turn all night. Sometimes I can't get to sleep at all. I don't know why this is happening. I've always been a deep sleeper." *Nurse:* "It sounds like you're not getting enough sleep. Is that right?"
Leading **Direct Leading** Directing the client to obtain specific information or to begin an interaction.	◆ Decide what area you want to explore. ◆ Tell the client what you want to discuss. ◆ Encourage the client to follow your lead.	"Let's discuss the pain in your back." "When did your symptoms begin?"
Focusing Helping the client zero in on a subject or get in touch with feelings.	◆ Use focusing when the client strays from the topic or uses tangential speech. ◆ Listen for themes, issues, or feelings in the client's rambling conversation. ◆ Ask the client to give more information about a specific theme, issue, or feeling. ◆ Encourage the client to emphasize feelings when giving this information.	"Describe how you feel when you can't sleep." "Did you say you were angry and frustrated before you went to bed? Go over that again."
Questioning Gathering specific information on a topic through the process of inquiry.	◆ Use open-ended questions whenever possible. Avoid using questions that can be answered with "yes," "no," "maybe," or "sometimes." ◆ Ask the client to express feelings about what is being discussed. ◆ Ask questions that help the client gain insight.	"What did you mean when you said your back was breaking?" "How did you feel after you talked to your boss?"
Reflecting Letting the client know that the nurse empathizes with the thoughts, feelings, or experiences expressed.	◆ Take in the client's feelings from verbal and nonverbal body language. ◆ Determine which combination of "cues" you should reflect back to the client. ◆ Reflect the "cues" back to the client. ◆ Observe the client's response to the reflected feelings, experience, or content.	*Feelings:* "It sounds like you're feeling lonely." "It must really be frustrating not to be able to get enough sleep." *Experience:* "You're yawning. You must be tired." "You act as if you're in pain." *Content:* "You think you're going to die." "You believe the medication is helping."
Summarizing Tying together the various messages that the client has communicated throughout the interview.	◆ Listen to verbal and nonverbal content during the interview. ◆ Summarize feelings, issues, and themes in broad statements. ◆ Repeat them to the client, or ask the client to repeat them to you.	"Let's review the health problems you've identified today."

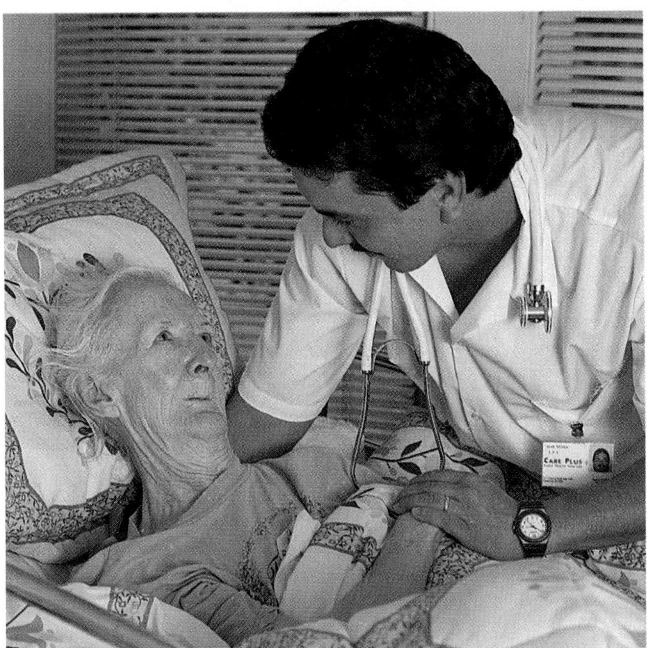

Figure 2.2 Successful listening includes hearing words as well as interpreting body language.

the client's environment (eg, books, a rosary, or photographs) also tell a significant story and add more depth to the intended message.

Attentive listening skills also include encouraging the client to speak by making comments such as "I see" and "Go on." They also include checking to make sure you have understood the client accurately by paraphrasing. See Table 2.1 for examples of these listening skills.

Leading Nurses use leading skills to encourage open communication. These skills are most effective when you start an interaction or are trying to get the client to discuss specific health concerns. They are especially helpful in getting clients to explore their feelings and to elaborate on areas already introduced in the discussion. The leading techniques nurses commonly use when interviewing a client include direct leading, focusing, and questioning (See Table 2.1).

An additional helpful technique is to use open-ended questions. These are purposefully general and encourage the client to provide additional information. Examples are "Tell me why you are here today." or "You said that your ankle hurts. Tell me more about that."

Reflecting Reflecting is a way of showing the client that you empathize or are in tune with the client's thoughts, feelings, and experiences. For example, Mr. Bates, a 60-year-old male with diabetes, is admitted to an outpatient clinic to be evaluated for a possible amputation of his right lower leg because of gangrene. During the clinic visit, Mr. Bates sits in a chair in the examination room with his head in his hands. When the nurse practitioner begins to question him, he looks up and says, "Leave me alone. Nothing you can do will help. I might as well be dead." The nurse's response might be: "Mr. Bates, may I sit here for awhile? I can see that you are upset" (reflecting feeling). "You must feel angry that this is happening to you" (reflecting content). As this example shows, thoughts, feelings, and experience are usually reflected at the same time. Table 2.1 gives examples of ways to use reflecting.

Summarizing Summarizing is the process of gathering the ideas, feelings, and themes that clients have discussed throughout the interview and restating them in several general statements. Summarizing is a useful tool because it shows clients that you have listened and understood their concerns, lets clients know that progress is being made in resolving their health concerns, and signals closure of the interview.

Barriers to Nurse-Client Communication

In some situations the nurse may unknowingly hinder the flow of information by using nontherapeutic interactions (interactions that are harmful rather than helpful). Nontherapeutic interactions interfere with the communication process by making the client uncomfortable, anxious, or insecure. Some interactions that can be most harmful if used during the health assessment interview include the following:

False Reassurance False reassurance occurs when the nurse assures the client of a positive outcome with no basis for believing in it. False reassurance robs clients of the right to communicate their feelings. Examples include "Everything will be all right." or "Don't worry about not being able to sleep at night. You'll be fine."

Interrupting or Changing the Subject Interrupting the client or changing the subject shows insensitivity to the client's thoughts and feelings. In most cases this happens when the nurse is ill at ease with the client's comments and is unable to deal with their content. Clients who show extreme emotion (eg, anger, weeping) during the interview, ask intimate questions about the nurse's personal life, or are sexually aggressive in the presence of the nurse may make the nurse uncomfortable during the interview. In these instances, you should recognize what about the client's behavior is making you uncomfortable and deal with the situation at hand in a professional manner rather than changing the subject. "Your questions about my personal life are making me feel uncomfortable. We need to talk about what is concerning you today instead."

Passing Judgment Judgmental statements convey a strong message that the client must live up to the nurse's value system to be accepted. These statements imply nonacceptance and discourage further interaction. Examples include "Abortion is the same as murder." or "You're not following your diet."

Cross-Examining Asking question after question during an assessment interview may cause the client to feel threatened, and the client may seek refuge by revealing less and less information. Because all interviews include lots of questions, you must be careful not to make clients feel that they are being "grilled" with an endless barrage of questions. You can pause between questions and ask how the client is tolerating the interview to this point. Encouraging clients to express their feelings about the pace and nature of the interview makes them feel more at ease.

Technical Terms Whenever possible, you should use lay rather than technical terms and avoid jargon, slang, or cliches. Terms such as *anterior* and *posterior* are useful for nursing and medical personnel but are more confusing to the client than the terms *front* and *back*. Also avoid the use of initials and acronyms unless they are commonly accepted as everyday language. For instance, most clients will understand the term *AIDS* but not *PRN*.

Sensitive Issues You will often need to ask clients questions that are sensitive and personal. The client may feel uncomfortable providing information about such concerns as abuse, homelessness, emotional and psychologic problems, self-image, sexuality, religion, or use of drugs and alcohol. See "Interviewing Strategies for Special Situations" beginning on page 715 for more information on conducting successful interviews with homeless and abused clients. Discomfort with these issues may cause the client to lapse into silence. You need to be sensitive to the client's need for silence. The client may need to reflect on what was said or to come to grips with emotions the question has evoked before proceeding. Also watch for nonverbal signs, such as tear-filled eyes or wringing of hands, which indicate the client's need to pause for a moment. After a period of silence, if the client does not resume the conversation, you may need to prompt the client by saying, "After that what happened?" or "You were saying . . ."

Certain questions may cause a client to cry. You should let the client cry and wait until the client is ready to proceed before asking additional questions. Offer tissues. Some clients may feel that they need your permission to cry. If you see that the client is choking back tears, you should give the client permission to cry: "I know that you are upset. It's OK to cry." If the client reacts to questions about sensitive issues with anger, you should acknowledge what the client is feeling: "I can see that you are angry. Please tell me why." When you make a client angry, you should acknowledge the anger and apologize. Don't resume the interview until the client's anger dissipates. Also recognize that asking the client sensitive questions may make you uncomfortable. If you anticipate being uncomfortable with certain questions, take time to reflect upon and come to terms with your feelings before you begin the interview. Role playing the situation with another nurse as the client or mentally visualizing how to react in the anticipated situation will help you avoid feeling uncomfortable during the interview. When asking sensitive questions, be direct and honest with the client: "I feel uncomfortable asking you such personal questions, but I need the information to complete your plan of care." Communication strategies like these will help you conduct a thorough and effective interview in these sensitive situations.

Cultural Considerations

Diversity

How a sender encodes a message and a receiver decodes it depends on a combination of factors. These include culture, ethnicity, religion, nationality, level of intelligence, education, and health status. When two people differ in any of these ways, each must be more open to the other person's way of thinking and foster mutual understanding.

Be careful not to bring cultural stereotypes to the communication process. Each individual, whether client or nurse, has some degree of ethnocentrism, that is, the individual sees a culturally specific way of life as being the "normal" way. You must not impose your own culturally specific values on your clients. Avoiding cultural bias requires effort because these values may be so ingrained that they may surface unconsciously during communication. All people have a right to have their cultural heritage recognized as valuable. No one culture is better than another. The nurse who works in a community with other cultures and nationalities should learn as much as possible about the culture, values, and belief systems of the clients who come for health care. The best way to learn is by asking and observing the "cultural experts": your clients and their families.

In the United States, many individuals are often uncomfortable with silence and speak constantly to avoid any lag in the conversation. In Vietnam, a talkative individual could be perceived as impatient, inconsiderate, and superficial. The nurse who makes a lot of small talk while interviewing a client of Vietnamese descent may find it difficult to obtain information from the client. A Cantonese client using English as a second language may misplace stress on syllables and use short vowels. A nurse from a different cultural background may think this client is angry, curt, impatient, or rude, resulting in miscommunication.

Consider the following situation: Myrtle Robinson, a 76-year-old African-American woman who has lived most of her life in the rural South, had her blood pressure checked at the local senior citizen center while visiting her daughter in Detroit. The nurse who checked Mrs. Robinson told her that her blood pressure was high and suggested that she see her family physician as soon as possible. Mrs. Robinson interpreted the nurse's statement to mean that she had "high blood," a simple condition the "old folks talked about." Mrs. Robinson believed she could treat "high blood" by drinking

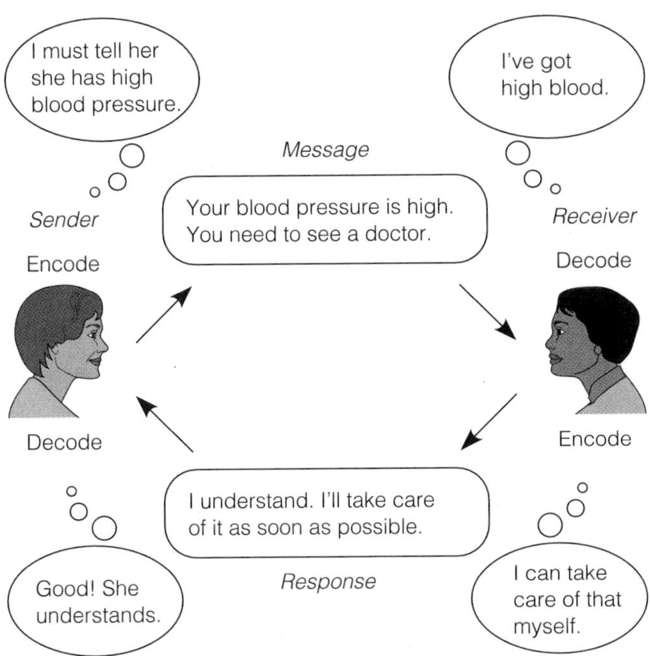

Figure 2.3 Differences in cultural or regional background may become barriers to effective nurse-client communication.

vinegar and water and eating salty foods. In this situation, the difference in cultural and regional background between Mrs. Robinson and the nurse contributed to the difference in the way each one encoded and decoded the term "high blood pressure" (Figure 2.3).

Your body language is extremely important when you are developing the nurse-client relationship. If you and the client are from different cultures, your body language is an even more critical part of the communication process. Simple body movements such as eye contact, handshakes, or posture may carry different messages in different cultures. For example, some Native American communities consider direct eye contact an invasion of privacy and a firm handshake aggressive. The nurse of Northern European descent might believe that a client who avoids direct eye contact is suspicious and cannot be trusted, and that a weak handshake translates into a weak personality. The nurse of Asian descent might believe that the outgoing and talkative client of Italian descent is being rude.

Although nurses should attempt to individualize communication styles to ethnic groups, they must not make assumptions about the ethnicity of clients. The differences among individuals in a group are often greater than the differences between the groups themselves. For example, a client or nurse of Japanese descent who is a fourth-generation American differs little in communication style from an American of European descent. As another example, consider the reverse of the earlier situation with Mrs. Robinson. The client, Mrs. Robinson, is a well-educated urban black woman, but the nurse assumes that, simply because Mrs. Robinson is of African-American descent, she must believe in the concept of "high blood." The potential for miscommunication in this situation is even greater than in the first example. Never stereotype clients because they are of a different culture, country, or religion. Rather, it is your responsibility to learn about a client's culture and use this knowledge as a basis for developing a meaningful nurse-client relationship.

Communicating with the Client Who Speaks Another Language

Communication is further challenged if the client does not speak the same language as the nurse or uses the language of the dominant culture, such as English, as a second language.

If you know that the client does not speak the same language, bring in a translator to assist with the interview. If possible, meet with the translator before approaching the client to discuss the purpose of the interview, the terms you need to use, and the kinds of information you need to collect. Learning a few key health related terms in the client's language contributes to developing trust and an effective nurse-client relationship.

During the interview, arrange the seating so that the client can see you and the translator at the same time without turning the head from side to side. As the interview progresses, look at the client, not the translator. Don't fall into the habit of discussing the client with the translator, leaving the client out of the conversation. Throughout the interview, ask questions one at a time using clear, concise terms. Even clients who are not bilingual may understand some of the words that are used. See the box on page 22 (Guidelines for Interviewing Clients Who Do Not Speak English).

Although some clients speak English extremely well as a second language, they may have some difficulty communicating their thoughts when overcome by extreme stress. It is not uncommon for clients who speak fluent English to revert back to their native tongue during times of stress. If this is the case, follow the recommendations for clients who do not speak English. A translator is usually not needed unless the client is extremely stressed or in severe pain. Some clients communicate better in writing or understand the written word better than the spoken word. If this is the case, have a pencil and paper readily available. See the box on page 22 (Guidelines for Interviewing the Client Who Speaks English as a Second Language).

Establishing the Nurse-Client Relationship

Clients are more willing to discuss their health issues if they perceive that they are in a trusting, helping relationship and have developed a sense of rapport or mutual trust and under-

Guidelines for Interviewing Clients Who Do Not Speak English

- Be open to ways you can communicate effectively. Imagine yourself entering a care setting where few people speak your language. Your sensitivity to this fear and unease will be your greatest strength in providing quality care for your client.
- Determine what language your client speaks. Your first assumption may not be correct. For example, South American immigrants may speak one of a variety of Native American dialects, Portuguese, or Spanish.
- Make sure the client can read and write, as well as speak, in the native language. Be alert for any confusion.
- Learn key foreign phrases that will help you communicate with the client.
- Find friends, relatives, neighbors, or other nurses who can help you translate. Try to obtain a phone number for this person. You may need immediate help with a question or emergency.
- Find out if your health care facility has access to translators. It is best to have an official translator when you give instructions or obtain consent.
- Look at your *client* while telling the translator what to say. This helps your client feel connected to you and conveys meaning through body language and facial expression.
- Use clear, simple language. For example, don't tell the translator to ask for a clean-catch specimen; instead, explain what you mean step by step.
- Pause frequently for the translator.
- Ask the translator to provide the proper context for any colloquial expressions your client may use.

If You Can't Find a Translator

- Develop cards with phrases or illustrations to aid communication. Have several translators review the cards before using them.
- Use written handouts for client teaching. These can be developed or purchased. Look for handouts with plenty of diagrams.

Guidelines for Interviewing the Client Who Speaks English as a Second Language

- Use clear, simple language. Omit technical terms, slang, and jargon.
- Speak in a slow, distinct, natural tone. Do not raise your voice.
- Use paper and pen if the client can write better than he or she speaks.
- Watch the client's facial expression for feedback related to your message.
- Give the client extra time to respond. The client may need time to translate your question before formulating an answer.
- Don't assume that the client who answers "yes" or nods agreement has understood your message. To validate understanding, have the client repeat the information.

standing with the interviewing nurse. Carl Rogers defines the helping relationship as one "in which at least one of the parties has the intent of promoting the growth, development, maturity, improved functioning and improved coping with life of the other" (1957, pp. 39–40). Most nurses who establish helping relationships with their clients, however, believe that the positive aspects of the helping relationship are mutual, shared by the nurse (perhaps to a lesser degree) as well as the client.

The nurse interviewer's attitude plays an important role in the success of the interview. The client is more likely to cooperate if you convey a willingness to help and assist the client. Rogers (1951), Brammer (1988), Carkhuff and Anthony (1979), and other social psychologists agree that a helping person possesses the following characteristics: positive regard, empathy, genuineness, and concreteness.

Positive Regard

Positive regard is the ability to appreciate and respect another person's worth and dignity with a nonjudgmental attitude. Nurses who respect their clients value their individuality and accept them regardless of race, religion, country of origin, or cultural or ethnic background. Clients sense positive regard in nurses by their demeanor, attitudes, and verbal and nonverbal communication.

Empathy

Empathy is "the capacity to respond to another's feelings and experiences as if they were your own" (Cormier et al 1984, p. 22). Nurses demonstrate empathy by showing their understanding and support of the client's experience or feelings through actions and words. Empathy allows the nurse to see the issues through their clients' eyes, fostering understanding of their clients' health concerns.

Genuineness

Genuineness is the ability to present oneself honestly and spontaneously. People who are genuine present themselves as "down-to-earth" and "real." To be genuine, nurses must convey interest in, and focus on, the situation at hand, giving the client their full attention. They use direct eye contact, facial expressions appropriate to the situation, and open body language. Facing the client, leaning forward during conversation, and sitting with arms and legs uncrossed are examples of open body language.

A genuine person communicates in a congruent manner, making sure that verbal and nonverbal messages are consistent. The nurse who tells a client to "take your time" during the interview but constantly looks at the clock gives a mixed or incongruent message. Genuineness and congruent communication promote rapport and trust with the client.

Concreteness

For the nurse, concreteness means speaking to the client in specific terms rather than in vague generalities. For instance, tell the client "I need this information to help you to plan a diet to lower your cholesterol level" rather than "I need this information to plan your nursing care." The more specific statement promotes understanding and a sense of security in the client. Speaking to the client in concrete terms implies that you respect the client's ability to understand and recognize the client's right to know the details of the plan of care.

The Health Assessment Interview

The health assessment interview is the exchange of information between the nurse and the client. You use this information along with the data you learn from the physical assessment to develop nursing diagnoses and design the nursing care plan. Unlike other types of interviews nurses conduct, the health assessment interview is a formal, planned interaction in which you inquire about the client's health patterns, activities of daily living, past health history, current health issues, self-care activities, wellness concerns, and other aspects of the client's health status. In most situations, nurses use a special health history tool to collect assessment data (see "The Health History" on page 27). The health history is a critical component of the comprehensive health interview.

Sources of Information

The Primary Source The client is the primary and best source of information for the health assessment interview because the client is the only one who can describe personal symptoms, experiences, and factors leading to the current health concern. In some situations the client might be unable or unwilling to provide information. For example, a client who has had a cerebral vascular accident (stroke) may not be able to understand what you say or verbalize a response. You should carefully evaluate the client who is unable to give accurate and reliable information and use another source of information if indicated. The following clients may be unable to provide accurate and reliable information:

Infants or children

Clients who are seriously ill, comatose, sedated, or in substantial pain

Mentally deficient clients

Clients disoriented to person, place, or time

Emotionally disturbed clients

Clients who cannot speak the common language

Aphasic clients

In some situations an adult client is able but unwilling to provide certain types of information because of fear, anxiety, embarrassment, or distrust. Some reasons why clients may be hesitant to share information include:

- Fear of a terminal diagnosis. A client may not be ready to cope with the stress of a terminal illness and deny its possibility.
- Fear of undergoing further physical examination. For instance, a claustrophobic client might deny problems because of fear of a magnetic resonance imaging (MRI) scan.
- Embarrassment. For instance, a male client may refuse to discuss urinary problems because he fears catheterization or rectal examination.
- Fear of legal implications. For instance, an alcoholic client involved in a car accident might fear revealing the addiction to alcohol.
- Fear of losing a job. For instance, an airline pilot might not admit visual problems or hearing loss.
- Lack of trust. For instance, a client with AIDS who wishes the diagnosis to remain private may fear a breach in confidentiality.

Secondary Sources A secondary source is a person or record that provides additional information about the client. The nurse uses secondary sources when the client is unable or unwilling to communicate or to augment and validate previously obtained data. The most commonly used secondary sources are significant others to whom the client has expressed thoughts and feelings about lifestyle or health status and medical and other records, containing descriptions of the client's subjective experience. The interviewing nurse should not overlook the attending physician and other health care personnel who have cared for the client as excellent secondary sources of information.

Significant Others Clients often share their personal experiences, feelings, and emotions with significant others. A significant other is a person who has won the client's respect and who holds a position of importance in the client's life. A significant other might be a family member, lover, cohabitant, legal guardian (if the client is a minor or legally incompetent), close friend, coworker, pastor, teacher, or health professional. These individuals often provide a different viewpoint or perspective about the client's stresses and thoughts, attitudes, and concerns about daily life and illness. The significant other who has the closest relationship with the client is usually the best and most accurate source of information when the client is unable or unwilling to speak.

Whenever possible, you should obtain the client's permission before requesting information from another person. This simple act of courtesy demonstrates respect for the client's privacy and goes a long way in establishing a mutual sense of trust. Obtaining the client's verbal and written permission also prevents potential accusations concerning invasion of privacy.

Be cautious when collecting client data from another person. This information may be prejudiced by that person's own bias, life experience, and values and may not be a true reflection of the client's own thinking. You should make every attempt to validate secondary information by verifying it with the client, by observation, or by confirming the information with at least one other source. Do not seek secondary information if the client is competent but unwilling to provide personal information and has not granted you permission to explore information with secondary sources.

Medical Record The medical record is an excellent source of accurate subjective and objective information about the client. The subjective statements made by the client and recorded in the nursing progress notes provide insight about the client's symptoms and feelings. Nursing progress notes, descriptions of client responses to treatment, physicians' progress notes, treatment plans, medical histories, laboratory results, and vital signs are examples of excellent secondary resources you can use to develop the nursing care plan. You should also investigate medical records from previous hospitalizations or clinic visits. If the medical record is available, you should review it before the health assessment interview because it "cues" you to actual and potential health problems to explore. During the interview, always validate any information from a secondary source, especially if it conflicts with the client's statements during the interview.

Phases of the Health Assessment Interview

The health assessment interview is divided into three phases: preinteraction, initial or formal interview, and the focused interview. The first two phases provide information you use along with information from the physical assessment to develop the total client database, formulate nursing diagnoses, and initiate the nursing care plan. The third phase, the focused interview, occurs throughout all stages of the nursing

Table 2.2 Phases of the Health Assessment Interview

Phase	Activities
Phase I: Preinteraction	Gather data from medical records, other health personnel. Review relevant literature. Plan the setting and time for the initial interview.
Phase II: Initial interview	Establish a nurse-client relationship. Describe the purposes of the interview. Interview client. Document health history data. Validate data with secondary sources if necessary. Use information to plan the physical exam.
Phase III: Focused interview	Collect data supporting hypothesized nursing, medical, or collaborative diagnoses. Clarify previously obtained data. Gather data that is new or missing. Update information about specific health problems.

process. Its purpose is to gather, clarify, and update additional client data as it becomes available (Table 2.2).

You also use the focused interview to validate probable or hypothetical nursing or collaborative diagnoses. After the initial interview, you develop several hypothetical nursing diagnoses. Before making a final diagnosis, you conduct a focused interview along with a physical assessment to gather additional data. Then you compare this additional data with defining characteristics of the probable diagnoses to determine the most appropriate nursing diagnosis for the client. The chapters in Unit 2 contain focused interview questions for each body region or system.

Phase I: Preinteraction

Purpose of the Preinteraction Phase The preinteraction phase is the period before your first meeting with the client. During this time, you collect data from the medical record; previous health risk appraisals; health screenings; therapists, dieticians, and other health personnel who have cared for, taught, or counseled the client; and family members or friends. Review the client's name, age, sex, nationality, medical and social history, and current health concern. If necessary, also review literature describing recent research, new treatments, medication, prevention strategies, and self-care interventions that might have a bearing on the client's care.

You use information obtained during the preinteraction phase to plan and guide the direction of the initial interview. You are more likely to conduct a successful interview if you know in advance, for example, that the client has an emotional problem, is deaf, speaks a foreign language, or is a triathlete.

Information about the client is not the nurse's only consideration during the preinteraction stage. Northouse and Northouse (1992) state that the interviewer should "assess one's own strengths and limitations" during this period. For example, a nurse opposed to abortion may have difficulty interviewing a client who is considering an abortion. In this situation, the nurse's anxiety could interfere with the collection of data and the provision of nursing care. Nurses should be aware of their own feelings and prejudices and plan how to interact with the client. For instance, you need to decide whether or not to reveal to the client that you have had an experience similar to the client's, if that were the case.

Planning for the Initial Interview You should choose the setting and time before the initial interview takes place. A quiet, private place where few distractions or interruptions will occur is most conducive to a successful interview. The client will feel more relaxed and comfortable if the area has subdued lighting, moderate temperature, and comfortable seating. Provide more chairs if family members or an interpreter will be present. A glass of water and tissues should be available for the client's use.

The most ideal setting is private, because the presence of another person might hinder the client's ability to be free and open. If the client is hospitalized, you can hold the interview in a private conference room if one is available. You can also hold the interview in the client's room, preferably with no roommates present. If this is not possible, select a quiet time of day for the interview, draw bedside curtains or place a screen for privacy, and use a subdued level of speech. In the home setting, a quiet room in the house or even the backyard may be used as long as the client is comfortable and no distractions are present.

You should sit facing the client at a comfortable distance. Don't use a table, desk, or any other barrier that might make communication difficult. When possible, you and the client should be on the same level. If you sit in a chair that is higher than the client's or stand at the bedside, you place the client in an inferior position that might make the client uncomfortable Keep a distance of approximately 1½ to 4 feet between you and the client. This is the distance that is most likely to make the client feel at ease communicating with another person. If you move closer than 1½ feet you may invade the client's intimate space, and clients from some cultures may consider this impingement on private space aggressive or seductive. Although 1½ to 4 feet is the average distance, each person's personal space differs slightly. If the client moves back in the chair, suddenly crosses arms and legs, or seems anxious, you may be invading the client's intimate space. If so, move back until the client seems more relaxed. A translator or family member who is present to assist with the interview should sit on one side of the client so that conversation flows easily (Figure 2.4).

Schedule the interview at a time that is convenient for you and the client. The interview should not interfere with cooking dinner, picking up the children after school, or work. If the client is hospitalized, take care not to schedule the interview at the same time diagnostic tests or treatments are scheduled, or during mealtimes or visiting hours. Postpone the

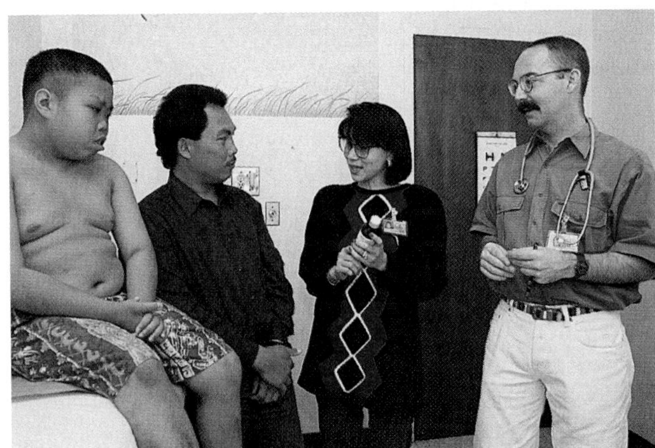

Figure 2.4 A translator may help facilitate interaction with a client who does not speak English.

interview if the client is in pain, has been sedated recently, is upset, or is confused.

Phase II: The Initial Interview The initial interview is a planned meeting in which the nurse interviewer gathers information from the client. In most cases, you use a health history form to collect the data to avoid overlooking any area of information. Gather information about every facet of the client's health status and state of wellness at this time. You will use this data to develop hypothetical nursing diagnoses. In addition to providing data, the initial interview also helps establish a nurse-client relationship based on mutual trust and communication, and gives you insight into the client's lifestyle, values, and feelings about wellness, health and illness. See the accompanying box.

Beginning the Interview The health assessment interview is an anxiety-producing situation for most clients. In few other situations is a person required to tell a stranger such intimate details about personal history, health habits, or physical and emotional problems. You have a great responsibility to allay these fears and anxieties so that the client can communicate as effectively as possible. One way to make clients feel at ease is to address them by their family names rather than given names. Always ask permission to use the client's given name, because otherwise some clients may feel you are being overly familiar or inappropriate. In this case, the client will be reluctant to divulge personal information.

Begin by describing the interviewing process to the client. Explain its importance, and tell the client what to expect. You might say something like this:

"Good morning, Mr. Bradley. I'm Janet Goebel, the nurse responsible for your care today. To plan the care, I need some additional information. For about the next 45 minutes I would like to find out as much as possible about you and why you are here. Since we will be talking about a variety of things, I'll be jotting down some notes as we speak. Please stop me at any time if you don't understand a question or need more information about something. Everything we discuss will be held in strict confidence, and you don't have to reveal any information you do not wish to."

Notice several things about these introductory remarks. First, the nurse introduced herself and described the purpose of the interview in a friendly caring tone intended to make the client feel at ease. Second, the nurse gave the client a time frame and said that she would be jotting down information. This advance notice is important, because some clients become threatened or anxious when the nurse writes down information. Third, the nurse encouraged the client to interrupt or ask questions at any point during the interview. Finally, the nurse reinforced the privacy and confidentiality of the interview.

After making the introductory comments, begin to seek information about the client's health status. The opening questions are purposely broad and vague, to let the client adjust to the questioning nature of the interview. You might say, for instance, "Why did you request a visit by a home health nurse?" or "What led up to your seeking assistance with your health?" If you begin the interview with a series of very specific personal questions, the client may begin to "shut down," giving less and less information, until no exchange takes place.

Continuously assess the client's anxiety level as the interview continues. Restlessness, distraction, and anger are signs that the client perceives the interview as threatening. You will elicit the best information from clients by asking carefully thought out and clearly stated, open-ended questions throughout the interview.

Closing the Interview When you have gathered sufficient information, proceed with closure of the interview. Indicate that the interview is almost at an end, and give the client an opportunity to express any final questions or concerns. For instance, you might ask, "Is there anything else you would like to discuss or ask about, since our time is just about at an end?"

Take a few minutes to summarize the information gathered in the interview and to identify key health strengths as well as concerns. Review what the client can expect next with regard

Guidelines for Conducting a Health Assessment Interview

- Provide a setting that is quiet, private, free from distractions, and comfortable for the client.
- Address the client by family name unless the client gives you permission to use a given name.
- Explain the purpose of the interview before beginning to ask questions. Use a calm, friendly, unhurried approach and allow clients enough time to answer at their own pace.
- Communicate at the client's level of understanding. Consider the client's age, sex, level of education, and culture when formulating assessment questions.
- Use open, attending body language that conveys your interest and concern.
- Make brief notations as you question the client. Use a predetermined format to record data if available.
- Interview a close family member, friend, or significant other if the client is unable to communicate.
- Use terminology that the client understands. Avoid jargon, slang, or cliches.

Stop, Look, and Listen

When conducting the health assessment interview, stop, look, and listen!

Stop: Take the time necessary to put the client at ease.

Look: Observe the client for additional nonverbal messages.

Listen: Hear the obvious as well as the hidden messages the client is sending.

to nursing care. Finally, thank the client: "I've appreciated your time and cooperation during the interview."

Phase III: The Focused Interview or Assessment The nurse uses the focused interview throughout the physical assessment, during treatment, and while caring for the client. The purpose of the focused interview is to clarify previously obtained assessment data, gather missing information about a specific health concern, update and identify new diagnostic cues as they occur, guide the direction of a physical assessment as it is being conducted, and identify or validate probable nursing diagnoses.

Consider the following situation: Mr. Bradley is a 36-year-old stockbroker who is a new client at the outpatient clinic. He tells the nurse practitioner during the initial interview that he experiences severe abdominal pain, nausea, and bloating after eating spicy foods and that this is why he has decided to seek help. Later that day when Mr. Bradley is admitted to the hospital, the same nurse practitioner uses a focused interview to elicit the following information from the client: He drinks at least 10 cups of coffee and smokes two packages of cigarettes a day, tends to forget to eat when feeling stressed, uses over-the-counter medication to treat his heartburn, and recently lost a large amount of money in the stock market. When questioned further, Mr. Bradley confirms that his pain sometimes occurs at times when he has not eaten spicy food. By using a focused interview, the nurse practitioner clarified information that had been previously obtained (the client's abdominal pain is not associated with spicy food), included additional needed information, and identified several new cues not observed before (caffeine and nicotine intake, stress, and anxiety). It is not unusual for clients like Mr. Bradley to fail to give adequate information during the initial interview because of anxiety, distrust, discomfort, or confusion.

You use the focused interview continuously to update diagnostic cues, because signs, symptoms, and client health concerns often change from moment to moment or day to day. Nurses perform most focused assessments during routine nursing care. For example, while bathing a man who recently had surgery, the nurse focuses on the client's discomfort by asking pertinent questions about his pain. Examples of focusing questions or statements a nurse might use in this situation to update information include: "Is the pain as severe as it was yesterday?" "Describe the pain you are experiencing now."

In some cases, the information you learn during the focused interview plays an important part in how you conduct the physical assessment. For example, if the client states that he is experiencing severe pain in the upper right quadrant of the abdomen, you would examine this area last.

In Mr. Bradley's situation, the nurse practitioner's initial hypothetical nursing diagnosis was *Pain* related to consumption of spicy foods, as evidenced by abdominal discomfort, nausea, and abdominal distention. However with the additional information obtained during the focused interview, the nurse practitioner changed the nursing diagnosis to *Pain* related to nicotine and caffeine intake, stress, and missed meals, as evidenced by abdominal discomfort, nausea, and abdominal distention. In view of the new information, the nurse practitioner added the following nursing diagnosis: *Anxiety* related to financial losses, as evidenced by chain smoking, forgetting meals, increased intake of coffee, and agitation.

The Health History

The goal of the interview process is to obtain a health history containing information about the client's health status. In many health care settings, both inpatient and outpatient, the nurse and physician complete separate health histories regarding the client.

The nursing health history focuses on the client's physical status, patterns of daily living, wellness practices, and self-care activities as well as psychosocial, cultural, environmental, and other factors that influence health status. As you gather information during the nursing history, you give your clients an opportunity to express their expectations of the health care staff as well as the agency or institution. You use the information in a nursing health history along with the subsequent data from the physical assessment to develop a set of nursing diagnoses that reflect the client's health concerns.

A medical history, by contrast, focuses on the client's past and present illnesses, medical problems, hospitalizations, and family history. The major aim of the medical history is to determine a medical diagnosis that accounts for the client's physiologic alteration.

Although nursing and medical histories tend to overlap in some areas, neither format alone presents a true picture of the client's total health status and health needs. Combining the nursing and medical history into one format, the complete health history, provides the most comprehensive source of information for assessing the client's total health needs (La Monica 1985).

The Health History

The health history, which is the format most commonly used in today's health care settings, is a comprehensive account of the client's past and present health. The completed health history is a combination of information collected by the nurse and the physician. It is combined with the nursing and medical physical assessments to form the total health database, which reflects a total picture of the client's past and present physical, social, and emotional status.

Integrating the salient features from the nursing and medical history has distinct advantages for both the client and the caregivers. The information in the health history directs coordinated or collaborative medical and nursing treatment plans that complement one another. The health history saves both the staff and the client time and energy, because the client has to provide significant information only once. Using a health history fosters communication among members of the health team, because they all share its contents. The health history, therefore, fosters effective communication and collaboration between the nurse, physician, and other health care providers.

Organization of the Health History

Most health care settings have developed nursing and medical health history forms for collecting the data, organizing it, and ensuring that the interviewer does not omit any information. The nursing health history form is organized differently in different institutions, and that organization often reflects a conceptual framework or nursing model used by that facility. However, regardless of which framework or nursing model is used, how the information is labeled, or how the data is categorized, the required information remains constant. For instance, Orem's model is organized according to self-care deficits (Orem 1980); Gordon's, according to 11 functional health patterns (Gordon 1987); and Doenges's, according to 13 diagnostic divisions (Doenges 1991). Nonetheless, all models focus on the current health concern along with an additional broad focus on all aspects of the client's lifestyle and response to the environment.

In general, health histories include the following groups of information (Table 2.3):

- Biographic data
- Reason for seeking care
- History of present concern
- Client health history
- Family history
- Review of the body systems
- Health patterns

Biographic Data The biographic data include the identifying information about the client as well as pertinent data concerning family members, occupation, and cultural and religious orientation. When possible, the client completes a form that elicits this data. Otherwise, the interviewing nurse records it.

Reason for Seeking Care and History of Present Concern The client usually gives the reason for seeking care when you ask "What brought you to seek help today?" or "What is bothering you?" The reason for seeking care is an important part of the health history picture, and you should explore it carefully because it provides the first indicators for possible nursing diagnoses and sets the direction of the rest of the health history interview. Be careful, however, not to attempt to develop nursing diagnoses at this point. The client has given minimal information, and no physical assessment or diagnostic testing has been performed. Instead, you should develop a list of statements that reflect the client's major reasons for seeking care. Each statement is a brief, concise, and time-oriented description of the client's concern. Here are some examples of statements describing reason for seeking care:

Substernal chest pain since 9:00 A.M.

Swelling in lower legs and feet for the past 2 weeks

Physical examination needed for football team by next Tuesday

10-pound weight gain since discontinuing daily walking regime

Use the client's own words to document the reason for contact whenever possible: "I've lost 15 pounds in the last 3 weeks." or "I've lost the feeling in my right arm and hand." Explore the onset and progression of each behavior, symptom, or concern the client relates. Also ask clients how their concern has affected their lives and what expectations they have for recovery and subsequent self-care. The answers to these questions provide valuable information about clients' ability to tolerate and cope with the stress brought on by their health concern and health care.

Client Health History The client health history includes information about childhood diseases, immunizations, allergies, blood transfusions, major illnesses, injuries, hospitalizations, labor and deliveries, and surgical procedures. Be sure to record dates and, when pertinent, locations. Many health history forms include a checklist of the most commonly occurring illnesses or surgical procedures to help the client recall information. A list of all medications, both prescription and over-

Table 2.3 Health History Data

Biographic Data

1. Full name (including maiden name if female, mother's maiden name if male)
2. Age and birth date
3. Place of birth
4. Sex
5. Race, nationality, culture, and ethnicity
6. Marital status
7. Family members and significant others living with client
8. Contact person's name and address
9. Occupation
10. Address
11. Telephone number
12. Social Security number
13. Religion
14. Educational level
15. Insurance coverage

Reason for Seeking Care and History of Present Health Concern

1. Why are you seeking care?
2. How do you feel about having to seek care?
3. Onset
4. Duration
5. Course of the health concern
6. Signs, symptoms, and related behaviors
7. What medications or treatments have you used? How effective were they?
8. What aggravates this health concern?
9. What alleviates symptoms?
10. What caused the health concern to occur?
11. Previous history and episodes of this condition
12. Related health concerns
13. How has concern affected life and daily activities?
14. Expectations for recovery
15. Expectations for self-care

Client Health History

1. Birth history
2. Growth and development history
3. Immunization history
4. Childhood diseases
5. Allergies
6. Previous health concerns
7. Previous hospitalizations
8. Surgical procedures
9. Pregnancies and deliveries
10. Accidents and injuries
11. Blood transfusions
12. Emotional or psychiatric problems
13. Ongoing medications: prescription medications, over-the-counter medications, recreational drugs, birth control use, caffeine use
14. Past alcohol use

Family History (Genogram)

1. Age and health status of living grandparents, parents, siblings, children, aunts, uncles, and cousins
2. Age and cause of death of deceased grandparents, parents, siblings, children, aunts, uncles, and cousins
3. Any family history of:
    - Heart disease
    - Lung disease
    - Cancer
    - Hypertension
    - Diabetes
    - Tuberculosis
    - Arthritis
    - Neurologic disease
    - Obesity
    - Mental illness
    - Genetic disorders

Review of the Body Systems

1. Integumentary system
2. Respiratory system
3. Cardiovascular system
4. Axillae and Breasts
5. Gastrointestinal system
6. Urinary system
7. Reproductive system
8. Peripheral vascular system
9. Musculoskeletal system
10. Neurologic system
11. Endocrine system

Health Patterns

1. Nutrition
2. Weight control
3. Activity/fitness/exercise
4. Sleep-rest
5. Self-perception/body image, self-concept/self-esteem
6. Role performance/relationship patterns
7. Sexuality-reproduction/sexual responsibility/breast and testicular self-examination
8. Coping, stress tolerance
9. Locus of control
10. Safety/accident prevention (home, work, driving)
11. Environmental hazards/exposure to air pollution, toxic chemicals, radiation
12. Psychosocial/communication style
13. Leisure and recreational activities
14. Substance use: drugs, alcohol, tobacco, caffeine
15. Medical self-care, selecting health care provider and facilities, dealing with minor illnesses

the-counter, should be included, as well as information on the client's use of any illicit drugs, vitamins, and birth-control pills.

The nurse asks the client to recall all childhood diseases. A history of German measles, polio, chickenpox, streptococcal throat infections, or rheumatic fever is especially significant, because these diseases have sequelae that may affect the client's health status and health concerns in adulthood. Also ascertain a history of the client's immunizations. If the client is a child, check whether the immunizations are up-to-date. If possible, verify the immunization data through immunization records. Question adult clients concerning the administration of recent tetanus immunizations or boosters, flu shots, or immunizations required for foreign travel.

Elicit information about any history of major illnesses, injuries, surgical procedures, hospitalizations, major outpatient care, or therapies. The client should describe each incident, including the date, treatment, health care provider, and any other pertinent information. If the client has had a surgical procedure, elicit specific information concerning the type of surgery and postoperative course. Complicated labor and deliveries are recorded here, as well as in the reproductive section of the review of the systems.

Obtain a thorough history of any chronic illness and major health concerns. Disease processes such as diabetes, heart disease, or asthma are examples of illnesses in this category. Record the onset, frequency, precipitating factors, signs and symptoms, method of treatment, and long-term effects so that you can use this information to meet the learning needs of the client and develop appropriate nursing interventions in the nursing care plan.

Family History The family history is a review of the client's family to determine if any genetic or familial patterns of health or illness might shed light on the client's current health status. For example, if the client has a family history of type I diabetes, question the client closely about signs of the disease. The family history begins with a review of the immediate family: parents, siblings, children, grandparents, aunts, uncles, and cousins. Encourage the client to recall as many generations as possible to develop a complete picture. If the client provides data about a genetic or familial disease, attempt to interview older members of the family for additional information. Although adopted children, spouses, and other individuals living with the client may not be related by blood, you may want to review their health history, because the client's concern may have an environmental basis. Document information collected from the client and the family in a family genogram. The family genogram is the most effective method of recording the large amount of data gathered from a family's health history (Figure 2.5).

Review of Body Systems The focus of this portion of the health history is to uncover current and past information about each body system and its organs. Ask the client about system

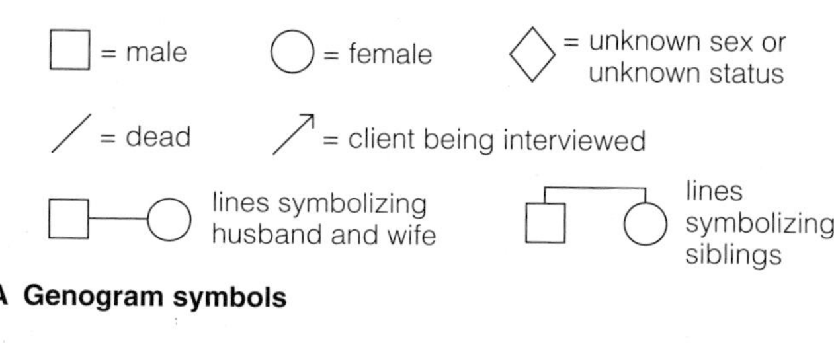

A Genogram symbols

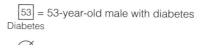

53 = 53-year-old male with diabetes
Diabetes

65 = 65-year-old female dead of colon cancer
Colon cancer

24 = 24-year-old female being interviewed

2 = two unknown individuals

B Combining symbols to provide additional information

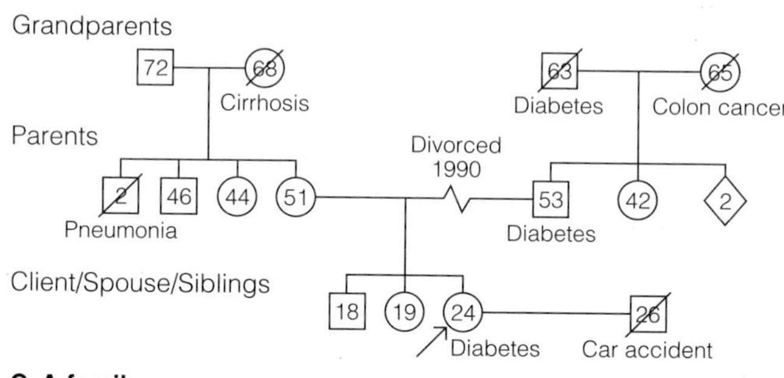

C A family genogram

Figure 2.5 A., Standard symbols used in constructing the family genogram. B, Combining symbols to provide additional information. C, A family genogram.

function and any abnormal signs or symptoms. Pay special attention to gathering information about the functional patterns of each system. For example, when assessing the gastrointestinal system, ask the client to describe digestive and elimination patterns ("How many bowel movements do you have each week?") as well as function ("Are your bowel movements usually hard or soft?"). Open-ended questions or statements are best for eliciting information about abnormal signs or symptoms: "Describe the abdominal pain you've been experiencing." "What other symptoms are associated with the pain?" Carefully explore characteristics and quality of each subjective symptom the client identifies to obtain a total picture of each system.

Some health history formats use a cephalocaudal or head-to-toe approach for collecting data. In this approach, you consider regions of the body rather than systems. Although there are several ways of dividing the body into regions, this is the most common: the head and neck, thorax, axillae and breasts, abdomen, pelvis, and the back and extremities. If you take this approach, you consider the body systems associated with the head and neck first. For example, you ask questions about the eyes, nose, ears, and mouth to evaluate neurologic and sensory function. Then you review the skin, hair, conjunctiva, and oral mucous membranes for integumentary function; the tongue, teeth, and salivary glands for digestive function, and so on. Review each area of the body until you cover all systems in each region. Many nurses who use a head-to-toe approach for the physical assessment prefer to collect health history data in the same way.

Health Patterns A health pattern is a set of related traits, habits, or acts that affects a client's health. The description of the client's health patterns plays a key role in the client's total health history because it is the "lifestyle thread" that, woven throughout the fabric of the health history, gives it depth, detail, and definition. For example, the number of hours a client sleeps, the time a client awakens and falls asleep, the number of times a client awakens during the night, and any dream activity are the set of behaviors that defines a client's sleep patterns. Inadequate sleep can contribute to client stress, which in turn can be related to gastrointestinal symptoms, such as upset stomach.

You can compare a client's health behavior to predetermined standard health patterns. For example, most people sleep 8–10 hours per night, seldom awaken once asleep, and can recall some dream activity. When assessing a client's rest and sleep patterns, you can compare the client's behavior to the health pattern standard. You usually collect information about a client's health patterns as you assess the system or section of the body with which the health pattern is associated. For example, you might collect information on patterns related to rest and sleep as you assess the neurologic system; on activity and exercise, as you assess the musculoskeletal system; on sexuality, as you assess the reproductive system; and so on. Some health patterns do not relate directly to a specific body system; assess these independently. Health patterns related to roles, relationships, health values and beliefs, self-care, and prevention fall into these categories.

Summary

You can use the health history and interview in various health care settings to create a comprehensive account of the client's past and present health. The completed health history is a compilation of all the client data you collect and it is combined with information obtained during the nursing physical assessment to form the total health database for the client. You can use this database, which provides a total picture of the client's past and present physical, psychologic, social, cultural and spiritual health, to formulate nursing diagnoses and plan the client's care.

Key Points

- ✓ The health assessment interview is a unique opportunity to obtain a comprehensive assessment of the client's health status.
- ✓ Interactional skills that facilitate the collection of assessment data include listening, leading, reflecting, and summarizing.
- ✓ Communication problems that hinder the exchange of information during a health assessment interview include false reassurance, interrupting or changing the subject, passing judgment, using technical terms, and cross-examining the client.
- ✓ Factors that affect the way the nurse and client send and receive messages include culture, ethnicity, religion, nationality, level of intelligence, education, health values, and health status.
- ✓ The nurse who works with clients from different cultures should learn about their language and cultural patterns but be sensitive to individual variations within the group.
- ✓ When interviewing a client who speaks little or no English, you should use a translator; speak slowly, clearly, and concisely; ask for feedback; and avoid the use of jargon, slang, or cliches.
- ✓ Qualities that help you establish a good relationship with the client are genuineness, positive regard, empathy, and concreteness.
- ✓ The setting for the interview should be private, quiet, comfortable, and free from distractions.
- ✓ The health history is a comprehensive account of the client's past and present health.
- ✓ Health history forms are organized according to various models of care.
- ✓ The health history documents biographical data, the client's reason for seeking care, the history of the present concern, the client health history, the family history, the findings after a review of the body systems, and the client's health patterns.

Chapter 3

Assessing Growth and Development

Knowledge of growth and development provides a framework for nursing assessment and planning effective nursing interventions. The focus of assessment is not a specific aspect of an individual's health. Rather, nursing assessment requires the ability to interpret how the complex interactions of physiologic, cognitive, and psychologic development, heredity, and environment affect an individual at a particular time. By developing an image of what is usual, or expected, of children and adults of various ages, the nurse has a basis for a comparison with the norm. This knowledge and an understanding of individual variations provide a foundation for assessment and appropriate nursing interventions that help individuals attain their maximum level of wellness.

Growth and development are dynamic processes that describe how people change over time. The two processes are interdependent and interrelated. **Growth** involves physical change that can be measured quantitatively. Indicators of growth include height, weight, bone size, and dentition. Growth is rapid during the prenatal, neonatal, infancy and adolescent stages of life; slows during childhood; and is minimal during adulthood. **Development** is an increase in functional complexity and skill acquisition. It involves the continuous, irreversible, complex evolution of intelligence, personality, creativity, sociability, and morality. Development is continuous throughout the life cycle as an individual progresses through stages in physiologic maturation, cognitive development, and personality development.

The pattern of growth and development is consistent in all individuals; however, the rate of growth and development varies as a result of heredity and environmental factors. Heredity is a determinant of physical characteristics such as stature, sex, and race. It may also play an important role in personality development as the determinant of temperament. Environmental factors affecting growth and development include nutrition, family, religion, climate, culture, school, community, and socioeconomic status.

Principles of Growth and Development

Four commonly accepted principles define the orderly, sequential progression of growth and development in all individuals:

1. Growth and development proceed in a *cephalocaudal*, or head-to-toe, direction. An infant's head grows and becomes functional before the trunk or limbs. A baby's hands are able to grasp before the legs and feet are able to be used purposefully.
2. Growth and development occur in a *proximal to distal* direction, or from the center of the body outward. A child gains the ability to use the hand as a whole prior to being able to control individual fingers.
3. Development proceeds from *simple to complex*, or from the general to specific. To accomplish an integrated act such as putting something in the mouth, the infant must first learn to reach out to the object, grasp it, move it to the open mouth, and insert it.
4. *Differentiated development* begins with a generalized response and progresses to a skilled specific response. An infant responds to stimuli with the entire body. An older child responds to specific stimuli with happiness, anger, or fear.

Theories of Development

Although the classic theories of human development provide the foundation for nursing assessment, researchers are continuously evolving developmental theories that further define and explain human behavior. Additionally, interpretation of the classic theories broadens as societal changes and advances in technology redefine individuals' relationships, expectations, and goals. Behavior that is widely accepted or even the norm today was often considered unusual or abnormal a generation ago. For instance, the family unit is no longer assumed to be two parents with children but may now consist of a single parent of either sex, stepsiblings, half-siblings, a surrogate mother, same-sex parents, or other configurations. What are the implications for development? Researchers also study innovations in technology. Children are bombarded with stimuli through television and videotapes, and they interact extensively with video games and computers. How do these affect the development of interpersonal skills? Advances in health care knowledge and technology have increased life expectancy, thus prolonging the span of productive years. This fact, too, profoundly affects development, which continues until the individual dies.

Three of the most influential classic theories of development are discussed here to provide a basic framework for nursing assessment. Although no one theory encompasses all aspects of human development, each is valuable as a framework for understanding, predicting, or guiding behavior.

Cognitive Theory

Cognitive theory explores how people learn to think, reason, and use language. Jean Piaget (1896–1980) theorized that cognitive development is an orderly, sequential process that occurs in four stages in the growing child. Each stage demonstrates a new way of thinking and behaving. Piaget believed that a child's thinking develops progressively from simple reflex behavior into complex, logical, and abstract thought. All children move through the same stages, in the same order, with each stage providing the foundation for the next. At each stage, the child views the world in increasingly complex terms. Piaget's stages of cognitive development are summarized below and discussed in more detail with each specific developmental stage later in the chapter.

Stage 1: Sensorimotor (Birth to 2 Years) The infant progresses from responding primarily through reflexes to purposeful movement and organized activity. *Object permanence* (the knowledge that objects continue to exist when not seen) and object recognition are attained.

Stage 2: Preoperational Skills (2 to 7 Years) Highly egocentric, the child is able to view the world only from an individual perspective. The new ability to use mental symbols develops. The child's thinking now incorporates past events and anticipations of the future.

Stage 3: Concrete Operations (7 to 11 Years) *Symbolic functioning*, the ability to make one thing represent a different thing that is not present, develops. The child is able to consider another point of view. Thinking is more logical and systematic.

Stage 4: Formal Operations (11 to Adulthood) The child uses rational thinking and deductive reasoning. Thinking in abstract terms is possible. The child is able to deal with hypothetical situations and make logical conclusions after reviewing evidence.

Psychoanalytic Theory

Sigmund Freud (1856–1939) was an early theorist whose concepts of personality development provided the foundation for the development of many other theories. Freud believed that people are constantly adjusting to environmental changes, and that this adjustment creates conflicts between outside forces (environment) and inner forces (instincts). The type of conflict varies with an individual's developmental stage, and personality develops through conflict resolution.

Psychoanalytic theory defines the structure of personality as consisting of three parts: the id, the ego, and the superego. The personality at birth consists primarily of the *id*, which is the source of instinctive and unconscious urges. The *ego*, a minor nucleus at birth, expands and gains mastery over the id. The ego is the seat of consciousness and mediates between the inner instinctual desires of the id and the outer world. In addition, it is the receiving center for the senses and forms the mechanisms of defense. The *superego* is the conscience of the personality, acting as a censor of thoughts, feelings, and behavior. The superego begins to form after age 3 or 4 years.

According to Freud's theory, children pass through five stages of psychosexual development, with each phase blending into the next without clear separation. Individuals may become fixated at a particular stage if their needs are not met or if they are overindulged. Fixation implies a neurotic attachment and interferes with normal development.

1. The *oral phase* occurs during the first year of life when the mouth is the center of pleasure. Sucking and swallowing give pleasure by relieving hunger and reducing tension.
2. The *anal phase* follows the oral phase and continues through about 3 years of age. The anus becomes the focus of gratification, and the functions of elimination take on new importance. Conflict occurs during the toilet-training process as the child is required to conform to societal expectations.
3. The *phallic phase* occurs during years 4 to 5 or 6, when the focus of pleasure shifts to the genital area. Conflict occurs as the child feels possessive toward the parent of the opposite sex and rivalry toward the parent of the same sex. These conflicts are referred to as the Oedipal and Electra complexes.
4. The *latency phase* occurring from 5 or 6 years of age to puberty. This is a time of relative quiet as previous conflicts are resolved and aggressiveness becomes latent. The child focuses energy on intellectual and physical pursuits and derives pleasure from peer and adult relationships and school.
5. The *genital stage* covers the period from puberty through adulthood. Sexual urges reawaken as hormonal influences stimulate sexual development. The individual focuses on finding mature love relationships outside the family.

Psychosocial Theory

Erik Erikson (b. 1902) includes cultural and societal influences in his developmental theory, which involves the entire life span. His **psychosocial theory** describes eight stages of ego development, but, unlike Freud, he believes the ego is the conscious core of the personality. Erikson views life as a sequence of tasks that must be achieved, with each stage presenting a crisis that must be resolved. Each crisis may have a positive or negative outcome depending on environmental influences and the choices that the individual makes. Crisis resolution may be positive, incomplete, or negative. Erikson believes that task achievement and positive conflict resolution are supportive to the person's ego. Negative resolution adversely influences the individual's ability to achieve the next task.

Stage 1 (birth to 1 year) presents the crisis of *trust versus mistrust*. The child who develops trust develops hope and drive. Mistrust results in fear, withdrawal, and estrangement.

Stage 2 (1 to 3 years), is the crisis of *autonomy versus shame and doubt*. The child who achieves autonomy develops self-control and will power. A negative resolution of the crisis results in self-doubt.

Stage 3 (4 to 5 years) challenges the child to develop *initiative versus guilt*. Initiative leads to purpose and direction, whereas guilt results in lack of self-confidence, pessimism, and feelings of unworthiness.

Stage 4 (6 to 11 years) is the crisis of *industry versus inferiority*. Industry results in the development of competency, creativity, and perseverance. Inferiority creates feelings of hopelessness and a sense of being mediocre or incompetent. Withdrawal from school and peers may result.

Stage 5 (12 to 20 years) presents the challenge of *identity versus inferiority*. Achieving ego identity results in the ability to make a career choice and plan for the future. Inferiority creates confusion, uncertainty, indecisiveness, and an inability to make a career choice.

Stage 6 (20 to 24 years) is the time of *intimacy versus isolation*. Successful resolution allows the individual to form an intimate relationship with another person. Isolation results in the development of impersonal relationships and the avoidance of career and life-style commitments.

Stage 7 (25 to 65 years) is the time of *generativity versus stagnation*. Positive crisis resolution results in creativity, productivity, and concern for others. Stagnation results in selfishness and lack of interests and commitments.

With stage 8 (65 years to death), *integrity versus despair*, individuals conclude life, either appreciating the uniqueness of their lives and accepting death or feeling a sense of loss, despair, and contempt for others.

Stages of Development

The most common and traditional approach used by developmental theorists to describe and classify human behavior is according to chronologic age. Theorists attempt to identify meaningful relationships in complex behaviors by reducing them to core problems, tasks, or accomplishments that occur during a defined age range, or stage of life. Because theorists vary in their definitions of life stages, the following stages have been delineated to best illustrate the concepts of sequential development. It is important to remember that the ages are somewhat arbitrary. It is the sequence of growth, development, and observed behaviors that is meaningful during nursing assessment. Table 3.2 on page 49 lists common developmental health risks that may be identified through nursing assessment of individuals during each life stage.

Infants (Birth to 1 Year)

During infancy, change is dramatic and occurs rapidly. The totally dependent newborn is transformed into an active child with a unique personality, all within the first year of life. The infant rapidly becomes mobile, often displaying a new skill each day. The developmental tasks of infancy are

- Forming close relationships with primary caregivers
- Interacting with and relating to the environment

Physiologic Growth and Development

Growth Height, weight, and head circumference are the measurements used to monitor infant growth. At birth, most term infants weigh 2.7 to 3.8 kg (6.0 to 8.5 lb). During the first few days of life, many infants lose up to 10% of their birth weight but usually regain it by 10 days of age. Infants gain weight at a rate of 5 to 7 ounces weekly during the first 6 months. Weight gain occurs in spurts rather than in a steady, predictable manner, with birth weight usually doubled in 4 to 6 months, and tripled by 1 year of age.

The average height of a normal term infant is 50 cm (20 in) at birth. Height increases at a rate of about 2.5 cm a month during the first 6 months. An infant's height increases 50% during the first year of life.

Head circumference reflects growth of the skull and brain. At birth, the average term infant's head measures 35 cm (13.75 in). Growth occurs at a monthly rate of 1.5 cm during the first 6 months, decreasing to 1 cm in the second 6 months. Ninety percent of head growth occurs during the first 2 years of life.

Physiologic Development Dramatic changes occur within the organ systems of infants during the first year. The brainstem, which controls functions such as respiration, digestion, and heartbeat, is relatively well developed but lacks maturity at birth. As a result, these vital functions tend to be irregular during the early months of infancy, becoming regular with brainstem maturation by 1 year. The infant's nervous system is extremely immature at birth. Tremors of the extremities or chin are normal, reflecting immature myelinization. Much of the young infant's physical behavior is reflexive (see Chapter 19). These reflexes, or infant automatisms, disappear as myelinization of the efferent pathways matures. Myelinization of the efferent nerve fibers follows the cephalocaudal and proximodistal principles discussed earlier.

At birth the infant's heart lies in an almost horizontal position and is large in relation to body size. With growth, the heart gradually shifts to a more vertical position. Although the ventricles are of equal size at birth, by 2 months of age the left ventricle develops better muscularity than the right. As the heart grows larger and the left ventricle becomes stronger, the low systolic blood pressure seen in the newborn rises, and the rapid heart rate of infants becomes slower.

At birth, the lungs are filled with fluid, which is quickly eliminated and absorbed as the lungs fill with air. The full complement of conducting airways is present, and the airway branching pattern is complete. The airways increase in size and length as the infant grows. Alveoli and respiratory bronchioles continue to grow after birth. The infant's thoracic cage is relatively soft, allowing it to pull in during labored breathing. Less tissue and cartilage in the trachea and bronchi also allow these structures to collapse more easily. Infants are obligatory nose breathers during the first few months of life. They gradually learn to breathe through their mouths by 3 or 4 months of age.

Development of the eyes and visual acuity occurs rapidly during infancy. The inability of the young infant to fixate consistently on an object, or not always being able to fixate the eyes together, is a result of immature eye muscles, which usually develop by 6 to 8 months of age. New babies see best at a distance of about 7½ inches and have a visual acuity of about 20/150. Visual acuity rapidly develops to 20/40 by age 2.

The ears and hearing are well developed at birth. The auditory (eustachian) tube, which connects the middle ear to the back of the throat in the nasopharynx, is shorter, wider, and more horizontal during infancy than during adult years. The size and position of the auditory tube gradually change with head growth.

Taste buds are present but immature at birth. Refined taste discrimination does not appear to develop until the infant is about 3 months old. Although the sense of smell is not refined in infancy, newborns are able to discriminate among distinctive odors and to recognize the smell of their mother's milk. The sense of touch is well developed at birth. Newborn infants show discriminating response to varied tactile stimuli.

Bone development, which begins before birth, continues during infancy. Ossification, the formation of bone, gradually occurs in the bony structures. While ossification is occurring, bones grow in length and width. Muscular growth occurs about twice as fast as that of bone from 5 months through 3 years. As muscle size increases, strength increases in response to appropriate stimulation.

Motor Development Gross and fine motor skills develop in a predictable sequence, following the direction of maturation in the nervous system. Motor skill attainment in infancy provides milestones that mark normal development. Delay of early milestones may be an early indication of a developmental or neurologic abnormality. Table 3.1 on page 36 shows how gross and fine motor skills develop during infancy. The age of skill attainment is an average, with some infants acquiring the skill somewhat earlier, some later. The Denver II is often used to assess the development of infants and children up to 6 years of age (see Chapter 19).

Language Development Undifferentiated crying in early infancy communicates infants' needs. By 1 month of age, crying becomes differentiated as the pitch and intensity of the cry communicates various needs such as hunger, discomfort, anger, or pain. Infants are cooing with pleasure by about 6 weeks and babbling by 4 months. They begin to imitate the sounds of others by 9 to 10 months, although infants do not necessarily understand the meaning of their sounds. By 1 year, most infants say several words with meaning.

Cognitive Development According to Piaget, infants are in the sensorimotor phase of cognitive development, during which the infant changes from a primarily reflexive response to being able to organize sensorimotor activities in relation to the environment. At birth, the infant responds to the environment with automatic reflexes. From 1 to 4 months, the infant perceives events as centered on the body and objects as an extension of self. By 4 to 8 months, infants gradually acknowledge the external environment (Figure 3.1). They begin to develop

Table 3.1 Motor Skill Development in Infancy

Age	Gross Motor Skills	Fine Motor Skills
1 month	Lifts head unsteadily when prone. Turns head from side to side. "Stepping" reflex when held upright. Symmetric Moro reflex.	Hands held in fists. Tight hand grasp. Head and eyes move together. Positive Babinski reflex.
2 months	Holds head erect in midposition. Turns from side to back. Can raise head and chest when prone.	Holds a toy placed in hand. Follows objects with eyes. Smiles.
3 months	Holds head erect and steady. Holds head at 45- to 90-degree angle when prone. Stepping reflex absent. Sits with rounded back with support. May turn from front to back.	Plays with fingers and hands. Able to place objects in mouth.
4 months	When prone, uses arms to support self at a 90-degree angle. Can turn from back to side and abdomen to back. Sits with support.	Spreads fingers to grasp. Hands held predominantly open. Brings hands to midline.
5 months	Head does not lag and back is straight when pulled to sitting position. Reaches for objects. Moro reflex disappearing. Rolls from back to abdomen.	Grasps objects with whole hand. Transfers object from hand to hand.
6 months	Sits briefly without support. May crawl on abdomen.	Bangs object held in hand. Can release an object from hand. Reaches, grasps, and carries object to mouth. Uses all fingers in apposition to thumb for grasping.
7 months	Sits briefly with arms forward for support. Bears weight when held in a standing position.	Uses tips of all fingers against the thumb. May grasp feet and suck on toes.
8 months	Sits well alone.	Uses index and middle fingers against the thumb to grasp.
9 months	Creeps and crawls. Pulls to standing position.	Uses pincer grasp (thumb and forefinger). Sucks, chews, and bites objects. Holds bottle and places it in mouth.
10 months	Stands, cruises (walks sideways holding onto something).	Can clap, wave, and bring hands together to play "peek-a-boo."
11 months	Tries to walk alone.	Puts objects into container. Very precise pincer grasp.
12 months	Walks alone.	Positive Babinski reflex beginning to fade. Can hold a cup.

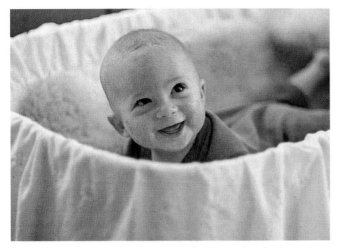

Figure 3.1 An infant begins to notice the external environment by the age of 4 to 8 months.

the notion of object permanence, the concept that objects and people continue to exist even though they are no longer in sight. The infant first learns to search for a partly hidden object but does not search for one completely out of sight. By 9 to 10 months, the infant learns to search behind a screen for an object if it was seen to be placed there.

Psychosocial Development According to Freud's psychoanalytic theory of personality, the id is present at birth. The unconscious source of motive and desires, the id operates on the "pleasure principle" and strives for immediate gratification. Infants are egocentric and do not differentiate themselves from the outside world; motivated by the id, they view the world as existing solely for their gratification. When gratification is delayed, the ego develops as infants begin to differentiate themselves from the environment.

Infants are in what Freud calls the oral stage of psychosexual development until 12 to 18 months of age. Most of their gratification is obtained from sucking nipples, hands, and objects, which satisfies the id's need for immediate gratification. Non-nutrient sucking on a pacifier, fingers, or thumb helps satisfy infants' need for oral gratification.

Erikson believed that the quality of care infants receive during the early months determines the degree to which they learn to trust themselves, other people, and the world in general. Erikson defines the primary task of infancy as developing a sense of trust or a sense of mistrust. Trust develops as the infant's basic needs are met through sucking, feeding, warmth, comfort, sensory stimulation, and other activities that convey the sense of love and security. The problem of basic trust versus mistrust is not resolved forever during infancy but is a component of each successive stage of development. A basically trusting child may later develop a sense of mistrust when lied to by someone the child respects. However, the foundation for all later psychosocial development is laid in infancy because, according to Erikson, the consistency and quality of the parent-infant interaction directly affect the infant's development of ego identity, or self-concept.

All theorists of infant psychosocial development acknowledge the significance of the manner in which infants' needs are met. Although the concept of infant needs and the best way to meet them varies from theorist to theorist, it is clear that infants' needs extend beyond the physiologic domain. Infants who lack sufficient social and cognitive stimulation exhibit signs of physical and affective imbalance. Children who receive adequate social and cognitive stimuli progress through sequentially more complex affective and social behaviors.

Attachment, a focused, enduring relationship between the infant and the primary caregivers, is imperative for the healthy attainment of infant goals and is a precursor for relating appropriately to others in the future. Occurring over a period of months, attachment requires consistent, intimate interaction between the infant and primary caregiver. Many factors affect attachment. The infant and the primary caregiver each bring a unique temperament, personality, and style to the relationship. In addition, the primary caregiver's previous life experiences and preconceived expectations of the infant and parenting experience influence the attachment process.

The quality of attachment depends on what is often referred to as goodness of fit of the infant and primary caregiver. Goodness of fit refers to the concept that both the infant and primary caregiver must receive positive feedback and evoke a positive response in the relationship in order for attachment to develop. The crying infant who quiets in response to being held by the primary caregiver makes the primary caregiver feel successful. The infant who is difficult to console gives negative feedback with continued crying, making the primary caregiver feel unsuccessful, and perhaps unloved. The primary caregiver transmits anxiety about parenting abilities to the infant, increasing the crying. By smiling and cooing in response to the primary caregiver's vocalizations, the infant encourages the caregiver to continue vocalizations, providing the infant with environmental stimulation.

By 3 months, the infant and primary caregiver achieve social synchrony, which is apparent in reciprocal vocal and affective exchanges. This mutually satisfying synchrony signals the end of the early adjustment period. The next step in attachment occurs at 3 to 5 months when the infant developments a clear preference for primary caregivers. As memory for absent objects emerges between 7 and 9 months, the infant's preference for primary caregivers creates the reaction of stranger anxiety.

Throughout the first year of life, the infant's crying serves as the signal of the need for comfort. Research has shown that infants whose mothers respond promptly to their cries in the first months of life cry less at 1 year. It is now well accepted that responding promptly to infants' cries helps establish a sense of internal security that fosters later independence. Concern over "spoiling" infants by promptly responding to their cries is no longer an accepted concept.

Chronically inconsistent nurturing of infants may result in infants and toddlers uninterested in exploring, even in the presence of the caregiver. Some such children appear unusually clingy, others appear actively angry and distrustful, ignoring or resisting caregivers' efforts to comfort them.

Assessment of Infants Frequent assessments during the first year provide opportunities to monitor the infant's rate of growth and development as well as to compare the infant with the norm for age. Height, weight, and head circumference measurements are plotted on an appropriate growth chart at each assessment. The three measurements often fall in approximately the same percentile. More importantly, each measurement should follow the expected rate of growth, following the same percentile throughout infancy.

Accurate assessment combining information obtained by history, physical assessment, and knowledgeable observation allows early identification of common problems that may easily be resolved with early intervention. Often basic parent education and support remedy problems that, left untreated, could result in significant health problems or disturbed parent-child interactions later.

Overnutrition and undernutrition are identified by weight that crosses percentiles; the rate of weight gain is accelerated or diminished. Overnutrition may occur when caregivers do not learn to read infants' cues but instead assume that every cry signals hunger. Cultural beliefs that a fat baby is a healthy baby may also lead caregivers to overfeed infants.

Undernutrition may be caused by inadequate caloric intake resulting from lack of knowledge of normal infant feeding, a lack of financial resources to obtain formula, or inappropriate mixing of formula. Some quiet or passive infants do not demand feedings, and caregivers may misinterpret this passivity as lack of hunger.

Head growth that crosses percentiles requires evaluation. Early diagnosis and intervention for rapid head growth prevents or diminishes serious neurologic sequelae.

Parents and caregivers generally enjoy relaying infants' new developmental milestones and can accurately describe infants' abilities. An infant who seems to be lagging behind on milestones may not be receiving appropriate stimulation. Assessing caregivers' expectations and knowledge of infant development may reveal a knowledge deficit. Suggesting specific activities for caregivers to do with their infants may be the only intervention required. Infants who continue to lag further behind and are not achieving normal milestones require evaluation.

Healthy attachment is observed as a caregiver holds the infant closely, in a manner that encourages eye contact. The caregiver looks at the infant, smiles, talks, and interacts with the infant. The infant responds by fixing on the caregiver's face, smiling, and cooing. The caregiver stays close to the infant, providing support and reassurance during examinations or procedures.

Failure to engage the infant through eye contact, to talk, or to smile, limits available opportunities for the caregiver to receive positive feedback from the infant. The infant, in turn, finds efforts to engage the parent futile, resulting in decreased attempts to interact. A negative pattern is quickly established, requiring more extensive intervention the longer it persists.

Table 3.2 on page 49 lists common developmental health problems encountered during infancy, along with nursing assessment and health promotion recommendations.

Toddlers (1 to 3 Years)

The toddler is a busy, active explorer who recognizes no boundaries. Maturing muscles and developing language increase the toddler's ability to interact with the environment, allowing the child to gather information and learn with every experience. The major developmental tasks of toddlerhood include

- Differentiating self from others
- Tolerating separation from primary caregivers
- Controlling bodily functions
- Acquiring verbal communication

Physiologic Growth and Development

Growth The rate of growth decreases during the second year. The expected weight gain is about 2.5 kg (5½ lb) between 1 and 2 years, and about 1 to 2 kg (2.2 to 4½ lb) between 2 and 3 years. The average 3-year-old child weighs about 13.6 kg (30 lb).

Height growth is about 10 to 12 cm (4 to 5 in) between 1 and 2 years, slowing to 6 to 8 cm (2½ to 3½ in) between 2 and 3 years.

The head circumference of the toddler increases about 3 cm (1.25 in) between the age of 1 and 3 years. By 2 years the head is four-fifths of the average adult size and the brain is 70% of the average adult size.

Physiologic Development Alterations in the toddler's body proportions create striking changes in appearance as the child develops. Young toddlers appear chubby with relatively short legs and large heads. After the second year, the toddler's head becomes better proportioned, and the extremities grow faster than the trunk. Young toddlers have pronounced lordosis and protruding abdomens. With growth, the abdominal muscles gradually develop, and the abdomen flattens.

Neurologic advances during the toddler years enable the toddler to progress developmentally. The increasing maturation of the brain contributes greatly to the child's emerging cognitive abilities. Myelinization in the spinal cord is almost complete by 2 years, corresponding to the increase in gross motor skills.

The toddler's cardiovascular system continues gradual growth. The gradual decrease in heart rate is related to the increasing size of the heart. The larger heart can pump blood more forcefully and efficiently. In addition, the toddler's capillaries constrict more efficiently to conserve body heat.

As the lungs grow in size, their volume and capacity for oxygenation increase. This increased productivity of the lungs results in a decreased respiratory rate.

Visual acuity is close to 20/40 at 2 years and close to 20/30 by 3 years. Accommodation to near and far objects becomes fairly well developed in toddlers and continues with age. Taste and smell are well developed; taste and odor preferences and aversions are clearly communicated.

The toddler's changing body proportions are the direct result of musculoskeletal growth. Muscle grows faster than bone during the toddler years as muscle fibers increase in size and strength in response to increased use. Ossification slows after infancy but continues until maturation is complete. Long-shafted bones contain red marrow, which produces blood cells. The legs and feet of toddlers grow more rapidly than their trunks. The bowlegged appearance of young toddlers diminishes between 18 months and 2 years as the small-shafted bones rotate and gradually straighten the legs.

Motor Development Gross and fine motor development continues at a rapid pace during the toddler years. The major accomplishments are listed below.

- 15 months: Creeps upstairs and is able to build a tower of two to three blocks.
- 18 months: Runs, climbs, pulls toys, and throws. Puts a block in large holes, scribbles, and builds a tower of four to five blocks.
- 2 years: Tries to jump, and can walk up and down stairs. Can turn doorknobs, imitates a vertical stroke with crayon, uses a spoon without spilling, turns pages of a book, unbuttons a large button, and builds a tower of six to seven blocks.
- 2½ years: Can stand on one foot for at least 1 second, can walk on tiptoe, jumps in place, and catches a ball with arms and body. Is able to make a tower of nine large blocks, likes to fill containers with objects, will take things apart, can take off some clothing, buttons a large button, twists caps off bottles, and places simple shapes in correct holes.
- 3 years: Pedals a tricycle, jumps from a low step, is toilet trained, can undress, goes up and down stairs using alternating feet, puts own coat on, and catches an object with both arms. Begins to use blunt scissors, strings large beads, can copy a circle, can help with simple household tasks, can wash and dry hands, and can pull pants up and down for toileting.

Language Development Language skills develop rapidly, progressing from a few single words at 1 year to hundreds of words used in sentences by 3 years. At 1 year children express entire thoughts by one word, saying, for instance, "out" to express "I want to go out." Simple phrases are characteristic of the speech of 2-year-olds, such as "go car." Although their speech is simple, these children understand most of what is said to them. By 3 years, sentences are more complex and include more parts of speech.

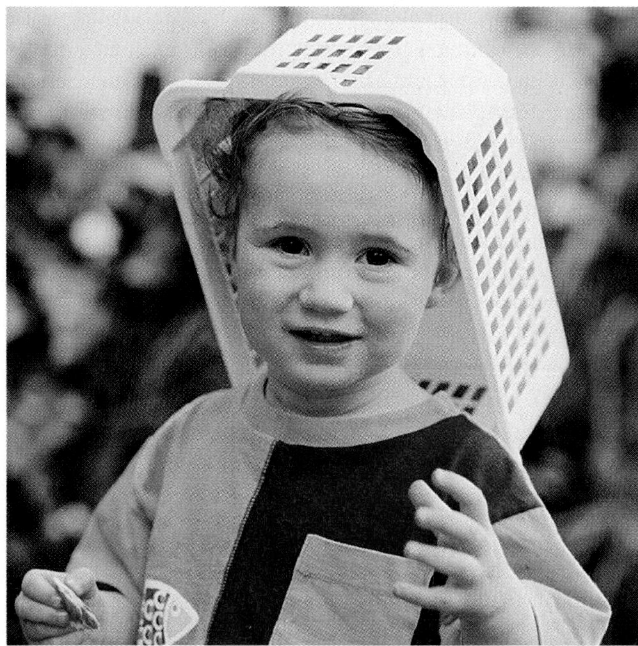

Figure 3.2 A toddler demonstrates symbolic play.

Cognitive Development The toddler continues in Piaget's sensorimotor stage until the age of 2 years, when the preoperational stage begins. Object permanence continues to develop, and by 18 to 24 months is fully developed. The toddler is then able to conduct a search in many places for objects hidden from sight. As object permanence develops, toddlers develop the understanding that they are separate from the environment.

By age 2 the toddler acquires the ability to think of an external event without actually experiencing it. This is called *mental representation*. As a result, the toddler is now able to think through plans to reach a goal, rather than proceeding by trial and error.

With the preoperational stage, the child enters into the use of *symbolic function*. Instead of tying thoughts to the actual, the present, or the concrete, the child is able to think back to past events, think forward to anticipate the future, and think about what might be happening elsewhere in the present. Symbolic function enables the child to demonstrate *delayed imitation*: the child witnesses an event, forms a mental image of it, and later imitates it. In *symbolic play*, the child makes one object stand for something else, such as pretending that a laundry basket is a hat (Figure 3.2).

Psychosocial Development According to Freud, the ego, which represents reason or common sense, continues to develop as the toddler experiences increased delays in gratification. The toddler years correspond to Freud's anal stage, during which the child takes great pleasure from expelling urine and, especially, feces. Toddlers may hold their stool, not wanting to give it up, or they may consider it a gift and object to its disposal. Toilet training takes on great significance as parents urge socially acceptable toileting while the child learns self-control and delayed gratification. Freud believed that the approach to toilet training and the child's reaction to it greatly influence the adult personality.

Toddlers' sense of trust developed during infancy leads them to a realization of their own sense of self. Realizing they have a will, they assert themselves in a quest for autonomy during Erikson's stage of autonomy versus shame and doubt. Parents are challenged to provide an environment in which toddlers may explore, while protecting them from danger and frustration above their level of tolerance. Parents provide a safe haven, with safe limits, from which the child can set out and discover the world, and keep coming back to them for support.

Erikson believed that toddlers who are not provided with safe limits by adults develop a sense of shame, or rage turned against themselves. Children who fail to develop a sense of autonomy, as a result of an overly controlling or permissive environment, may become compulsive about controlling themselves. Fear of losing self-control may inhibit their self-expression, make them doubt themselves, and make them feel ashamed.

Toddlers who have developed a firm attachment during infancy continue attachment behaviors during the toddler stage. Their repertoire of attachment behaviors becomes increasingly elaborate as they no longer seek prolonged body-to-body contact. Toddlers are sustained by only brief visual or physical contact with caregivers and can happily investigate new people and places. A secure attachment relationship in the first 2 years is characterized by the child's ability to seek and obtain comfort from familiar caregivers, and the child's willingness to explore and master the environment when supported by a caregiver's presence.

Assessment of Toddlers Although the rate of growth of toddlers decreases, it proceeds in an expected manner. Height and weight continue to follow a percentile, although slight variations are often seen. Assessing caloric intake by obtaining a 24-hour recall gives clues to inappropriate feeding patterns. Toddlers generally feed themselves and begin to interact with the family at meals. A favorite food one week may be refused the next, causing frustration and confusion in caregivers. Concern for the toddler's health may precipitate a power struggle as parents try to force the toddler to eat. Poor weight gain may result as the toddler exerts a new-found independence by refusing to eat. Excessive weight gain occurs when caregivers use food to quiet or bribe their toddlers. Discussing appropriate eating expectations and weight gain helps parents resolve eating problems.

Development of young toddlers is often assessed best by taking a health history since cooperation of the young toddler is unlikely. Older toddlers are more willing to play with developmental testing materials or explore the environment while in close proximity to a caregiver, enabling direct observations of development. Toddlers may not speak in a strange or threatening environment, making language assessment difficult. Listening to the child talk in a playroom or waiting room increases the probability of assessing the toddler's language.

The toddler wanders a short distance from a caregiver to explore, returning periodically to "touch base." After receiving reassurance and encouragement, the child is ready for further exploration. Exploration provides learning opportunities but also places the toddler at risk for accidental injury or poisoning.

Tantrums are a frequent occurrence, the result of unwanted limits or frustration. An attitude of calm understanding limits the duration of tantrums and keeps tantrums from becoming power struggles or attention-getting behavior.

Toddlers quickly turn to caregivers for comfort or when confronted with a stranger. Observing the adult-child interaction and listening to how the adult speaks to the child provides information on the quality of the relationship.

Continuous clinging of a toddler to a caregiver in a nonthreatening situation is unusual. Failure of the child to look to a caregiver for comfort and support may indicate that trust did not develop during infancy. Inappropriate caregiver expectations, such as expecting a toddler to sit quietly in a chair, show a lack of knowledge that may interfere with the normal progression of the child's development. Caregiver inattention to the activities of the child and failure to set limits, result in the child's inability to develop self-control.

Table 3.2 on page 49 lists common developmental health problems encountered during the toddler years, ways to assess them, and suggested interventions.

Preschool Children (3 to 6 Years)

The busy, curious preschooler has an appearance and proportions closer to those of adults. The preschooler's world expands as relationships include other children and adults in settings outside the home. Developmental tasks during the preschool period include

- Identifying sex role
- Developing a conscience
- Developing a sense of initiative
- Interacting with others in socially acceptable ways
- Learning to use language for social interaction

Physiologic Growth and Development

Growth Preschoolers tend to grow more in height than weight and appear taller and thinner than toddlers. Weight gain is generally slow at a rate of about 2 kg (4.5 lb) per year. The rate of height growth is about 7 cm (2.75 in) per year.

Physiologic Development The preschooler's brain reaches almost its adult size by 5 years. Myelinization of the central nervous system continues, resulting in refinement of movement. Most physiologic systems continue to grow and are nearing maturity. Visual acuity remains approximately 20/30 throughout the preschool years. The musculoskeletal system continues to develop. Muscles are growing, and cartilage is changing to bone at a faster rate than previously. From 4 to 7 years, the active red bone marrow of earlier ages is gradually replaced by fatty tissue.

Motor Development Gross and fine motor skills continue to be refined during the preschool years.

- 3½ years: Skips on one foot, hops forward on both feet, kicks a large ball, and catches an object with hands. Cuts straight lines with scissors, manipulates large puzzle pieces into position, places small pegs in a pegboard, and unbuttons small buttons.
- 4 years: Jumps well, hops forward on one foot, walks backward, and catches an object with one hand. Cuts around pictures with scissors, can copy a square, and can button small buttons.
- 5 years: Can jump rope, and alternates feet to skip. May be able to print own name, copies a triangle, dresses without assistance, threads small beads on a string, and eats with a fork.

Language Development Language becomes a tool for social interaction. As the preschooler's vocabulary increases, sentence structure becomes more complex, and the child becomes better able to understand another's point of view and share ideas. Sentences evolve from three or four words between 3 and 4 years to six to eight words in grammatically correct sentences by 5 to 6 years.

Cognitive Development Preschoolers are in the middle of Piaget's preoperational stage. Although symbolic thought is an immense milestone begun as a toddler, the preschooler's thinking continues to be rudimentary. Preschoolers continue to be egocentric and unable to see another's point of view. In addition, they feel no need to defend their point of view, because they assume that everyone else sees things as they do. Preschoolers demonstrate *centration*; they focus on one aspect of a situation and ignore others, leading to illogical reasoning. In addition, preschoolers believe that their wishes, thoughts, and gestures command the universe. The child believes that these "magical" powers of thought are the cause of all events.

Preschoolers enter Piaget's stage of intuitive thought at about 4 years. While egocentricity continues, older preschoolers are developing the ability to give reasons for their beliefs and actions and to form some concepts. They are limited by their inability to consider more than one idea at a time, making it impossible for them to make comparisons. Fantasy play begins to give way to play that imitates reality (Figure 3.3).

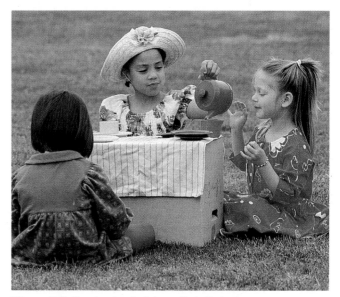

Figure 3.3 Preschoolers imitate reality in their play.

Psychosocial Development The superego, or conscience, develops as the preschooler becomes more aware of other people's interests, needs, and values. The child learns right from wrong, developing an understanding of the consequences of actions. At this stage, the child's conscience is rigid and often unrealistic. With maturity, the conscience becomes more realistic and flexible.

As preschoolers become further aware of their separateness, gender awareness develops. They learn what makes girls different from boys during what Freud called the phallic phase. At this time, Freud believed that children have a romantic attraction to the parent of the opposite sex, making them rivals with their same-sex parent. The resulting fear and guilt are resolved as children identify with the same-sex parent, realizing they are unable to compete with the bigger, powerful parent. According to Freud, sexual urges are repressed, and the sex-related behaviors, attitudes, and beliefs of the same-sex parent are imitated.

Erikson believes the child's primary conflict at this stage is between initiative, which enables them to plan and carry out activities, and guilt over what they want to do. Preschoolers are characterized by their high level of energy, eagerness to try new things, and ability to work cooperatively. Children who are encouraged, reassured, and cheered on in their pursuits learn self-assertion, self-sufficiency, direction, and purpose. They develop initiative. Children who are ridiculed, punished, or prevented from accomplishing develop guilt.

Preschoolers turn from a total attachment to their caregivers to an identification with them. A firm attachment during the early years allows preschoolers to detach from caregivers at this stage. This ability to detach enables children to explore new territory, learn new games, and form new relationships with peers.

Assessment of Preschoolers Preschoolers' slowed rate of growth is often of concern to caregivers. You can allay anxiety by showing the preschooler's growth chart and discussing eating expectations.

Preschoolers are generally pleasant, cooperative, and talkative. They continue to need the reassurance of a caregiver in view but do not need to return to the caregiver for comfort except in threatening situations. Talking with preschoolers about favorite activities allows you to assess language ability, cognitive ability, and development. Evaluate the child's use of language to express thoughts, sentence structure, and vocabulary. You may identify centration, magical thinking, and reality imitation as the child relays play activities. Lack of appropriate environmental stimulation may become evident, and you may need to educate caregivers about age-appropriate activities for their children.

A clinging, frightened preschooler in a nonthreatening situation may be a child who lacks trust. Lack of communication between caregiver and child limits the child's ability to learn appropriate social interaction. In addition, the child does not have the opportunity to practice language skills or to obtain information by having questions answered.

Table 3.2 on page 49 lists common developmental health problems encountered during the preschool years, ways to assess them, and health promotion recommendations.

School-Age Children (6 to 12 Years)

The school-age period begins about the age of 6 years, when deciduous teeth are shed, and ends with the onset of puberty at about 12 years. Tasks of the school-age child include:

- Mastering physical skills
- Building self-esteem and a positive self-concept
- Fitting in to a peer group
- Developing logical reasoning

Physiologic Growth and Development

Growth Most children during the years from 6 to 10 reach a relative plateau, with growth occurring in a slow but steady manner. The average child gains about 3 kg (6.5 lb) and grows about 5.5 cm (2 in) per year. Growth accelerates again at the onset of puberty, which occurs about age 10 for girls and age 12 for boys. During preadolescence (10 to 12 or 13 years), the growth of boys and girls differs. Growth in boys is generally slow and steady, and rapid in girls. Growth is variable, especially among girls at this age. Some girls of 11 years look like children, while others are starting to look like adolescents. By 12 years, some boys are beginning their growth spurt and demonstrating the onset of secondary sexual characteristics.

Physiologic Development The body proportions of the school-age child are different from those of the preschooler. Children often appear gangly and awkward because of their proportionately longer legs, diminishing body fat, and a lower center of gravity. As increases in organ maturity and size occur, the child responds physiologically to illness in a more adult manner. The continuing maturation of the CNS allows the child to perform increasingly complex gross and fine motor skills. Brain growth is slowed, with 95% of growth achieved by 9 years of age. Myelinization continues and is partly responsible for the transformation of the clumsy 6-year-old into the coordinated 12-year-old.

As cardiac growth continues, the diaphragm descends, allowing more room for cardiac action and respiratory expansion. The respiratory tissues achieve adult maturity, with lung capacity proportional to body size.

Most children achieve 20/20 vision by age 5 or 6 years. Visual maturity, including fully developed peripheral vision, is usually achieved by 6 or 7 years.

The most rapid growth during the school-age years occurs in the skeletal system. Ossification continues at a steady pace. Muscle mass gradually increases in size and strength, and the body appears leaner as "baby fat" decreases. As muscle tone increases, the loose movements, "knock-knees," and lordosis of early childhood disappear.

Motor Development The gross motor skills of the 6- to 7-year-old are far better developed than fine motor coordination. Children of this age greatly enjoy gross motor activity such as hopping, roller skating, bike riding, running, and climbing. The child seems to be in perpetual motion. Balance and eye-hand coordination gradually improve. The 6-year-old is able to hammer, paste, tie shoes, and fasten clothes. Right- or left-hand dominance is firmly established by age 6. By age 7, the child's hands become steadier. Printing becomes smaller, and reversal of letters during writing is less common. Many children have sufficient finger coordination to begin music lessons.

Less restlessness is seen in 7- and 8-year-old children, although they retain their high energy level. Increased attention span and cognitive skills enhance their enjoyment of board games. Improved reaction time increases sports ability.

Children between 8 and 10 years of age gradually develop greater rhythm, smoothness, and gracefulness of movements. They are able to participate in physical activities that require more concentrated attention and effort. They have sufficient coordination to write rather than print words, and they may begin sewing, building models, and playing musical instruments.

Energy levels remain high in children between 10 and 12 years of age, but activity is well directed and controlled. Physical skills are almost equal to those of the adult. Manipulative skills are also comparable to the precision exhibited by adults. Complex, intricate, and rapid movements are mastered with practice.

Language Development The school-age child uses appropriate sentence structure and continues to develop the ability to express thoughts in words. Comprehension of language continues to exceed the school-age child's ability of expression. Vocabulary increases as the child is exposed to a wider range of reading materials and ideas in school and through association with peers.

Cognitive Development Sometime around 6 or 7 years of age, children become what Piaget calls operational. They are now able to use symbols to carry out operations, or mental activities, enabling them to perform activities such as reading and using numbers. The child becomes able to serialize, that is, order objects according to size or weight. In addition, the child begins to understand how to classify objects by something they have in common. Children commonly practice this new skill by collecting and frequently sorting collections of rocks, sports cards, shells, or dolls (Figure 3.4).

The school-age child develops an understanding of the principle of *conservation*, the ability to tell the difference between how things seem and how they really are. The child is able to see that transformation of shape or position does not change the mass or quantity of a substance. For instance, the child understands that two equal balls of clay remain equal when one ball is rolled into a "hot dog." In contrast, a younger child who has not mastered the principle of conservation believes the cylindrical shape is bigger because it is longer.

School-age children develop logical reasoning and understand cause-and-effect relationships. They can consider various sides of a situation and form a conclusion. Egocentrism decreases as the child becomes able to consider another's point of view. Although able to reason, the child is still somewhat limited by the inability to deal with abstract ideas.

Psychosocial Development School-age children have resolved their sexual conflicts, accepted their sex roles, and are now able to turn their energies to acquiring new facts, mastering skills, and learning cultural attitudes. Freud termed this the latency stage, considering it a term of relative sexual quiet. Curiosity about sex, and sexual and bathroom jokes demonstrate the ongoing sexual awareness of school-age children; however, the sexual turbulence of earlier and later stages is absent.

Erikson describes the crises of this stage as industry versus inferiority. Motivated by activities that provide a sense of worth, children focus on mastering skills in school, sports, the arts, and social interaction. Approval and recognition for their achievements result in feelings of confidence, competence, and industry. When children feel that they cannot meet the expectations of family or of society, they lose confidence, lack the drive to achieve, and develop feelings of inferiority and incompetence. The challenge of caregivers and teachers is to praise accomplishments and encourage skill development while avoiding criticism in areas in which children fail to excel. Providing successful experiences and positive reinforcement for children increases their opportunities to achieve.

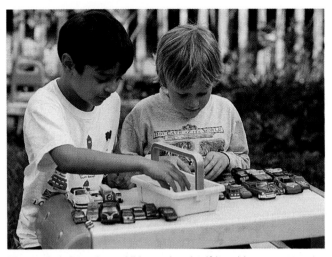

Figure 3.4 School-age children enjoy classifying objects.

Belonging to groups and being accepted by peers take on a new significance for school-age children. Children form clubs and gather in groups, often implementing strict rules or secret codes. They gradually become less self-centered and selfish as they learn to cooperate as part of a group. With this increased social exposure, children begin to question parental values and ideas. The family, however, remains the major influence on behavior and decisions.

As children enter the late school-age or preadolescent years (10 to 12 or 13 years), the caregiver-child relationship becomes strained as children begin to drift away from the family. Preadolescent children increasingly challenge parental authority and reject family standards as they discover that the family is not perfect and does not know everything. Identification with a peer group increases, and children form a close relationship with a best friend. Some children begin to show an interest in others of the opposite sex. Preadolescents continue to want and need some restrictions, because their immaturity makes determining their own rules too frightening.

Assessment of School-Age Children The slow, steady growth and changing body proportions of school-age children make them appear thin and gangly. Assessing children's intake of nutrients and calories and reviewing their growth charts reassures parents that their children are not too thin. You can relieve family stress resulting from parents pushing their children to eat by educating parents to evaluate objectively their children's diets during the early school-age years. Older school-agers have an increase in appetite as they enter the prepubertal growth spurt. During the growth spurt, height and weight increase and may normally cross percentiles.

School-age children are eager to talk about their hobbies, friends, school, and accomplishments. Increasing neurologic maturity allows them to master activities requiring gross and fine motor control, such as sports, dancing, playing a musical instrument, artistic pursuits, or building things. School-agers enjoy showing off newly acquired skills, and the family displays pride in their children's accomplishments.

School-agers frequently sort and classify collections of rocks, sports cards, dolls, coins, stamps, or almost anything. They are industrious in school, feeling pride in their accomplishments as they master difficult concepts and skills. The family provides positive feedback and encouragement to their children and speaks of their children's successes with pride.

Adult family members and school-agers communicate openly, with adults setting needed limits. Although peer relationships are becoming more important, the family remains the major influence during most of the school-age years. As children approach adolescence, the relationship with family may become strained as the children are drawn closer to peer groups and seek greater independence.

Children who lack hobbies or cannot think of any accomplishments may be environmentally deprived. Caregivers who are unable to think of anything positive to say about their children or who speak of them as a burden likely have a disturbed parent-child relationship. Children who lack encouragement and positive reinforcement at home for their achievements are at risk for gang recruitment. Gangs provide the "family" support children lack at home, increasing children's risk for violence, drug use, and illegal activity.

Problems in school may evolve at this time, with conflicts over grades and study time. Encourage the caregiver to help the child set a consistent place and time for homework, and to communicate actively with the child's teacher. Teachers, adults, family members, and health care providers may identify learning disabilities at this time by careful observation.

Table 3.2 on page 50 lists common developmental health problems encountered during the school-age years, ways to assess them, and health promotion recommendations.

Adolescents (12 to 19 Years)

Adolescence marks the transition from childhood to adulthood. Although all children undergo this transformation, passing through the stages of growth and development in a predictable sequence, the age and rate at which it occurs are highly variable. In a group of children of the same age, some look and act like children and some look and act like young adults. The search for one's unique self or identity is the foundation of the tasks of this stage.

- Searching for identity
- Increasing independence from parents
- Forming close relationships with peers
- Developing analytic thinking
- Forming a value system
- Developing a sexual identity
- Choosing a career

Physiologic Growth and Development

Growth An increase in physical size is a universal event during puberty, with maximum growth occurring prior to the onset of discernible sexual development. Pubertal weight gain accounts for about 50% of an individual's ideal adult body weight. The percentage of body fat increases in females during puberty and decreases in adolescent males. Pubertal height growth accounts for 20–25% of final adult height. The growth spurt generally begins between the ages of 12 and 14 in girls, and 12 to 16 in boys, and lasts 24 to 30 months. Girls experience their fastest rate of growth at about 12 years, gaining 4.6 kg (10 lb) to 10.6 kg (23.5 lb) and growing 5.4 cm (2 in) to 11.2 cm (4.5 in). Boys experience their fastest rate of growth at about 14 years, gaining 5.7 kg (12.5 lb) to 13.2 kg (29 lb) and growing 5.8 cm (2.25 in) to 13.1 cm (5.25 in).

Physiologic Development During puberty, the period of maturation of the reproductive system, primary and secondary sexual characteristics develop in response to endocrine changes. Primary sexual development includes the changes that occur in the organs directly related to reproduction, such as the ovaries, uterus, breasts, penis, and testes. Secondary sexual development includes the changes that occur in other parts of the body in response to hormonal changes, such as development of facial and pubic hair, voice changes, and fat deposits (see Chapters 15 and 19). Sebaceous and sweat glands in both boys and girls become active in response to androgen influence.

Brain tissue appears to reach maturity with puberty, and myelinization continues until the middle adult years. Because growth of the cerebrum, cerebellum, and brainstem is essentially complete by the end of the tenth year, the central nervous system does not experience substantial growth during the pubertal period.

A cardiac growth spurt occurs during the prepubertal growth period, increasing cardiac strength, elevating the blood pressure, and stabilizing the pulse at a lower rate.

During the growth spurt, rapid growth of the hands and feet occurs first, then growth of the long bones of the arms and legs, followed by trunk growth. Skull and facial bones

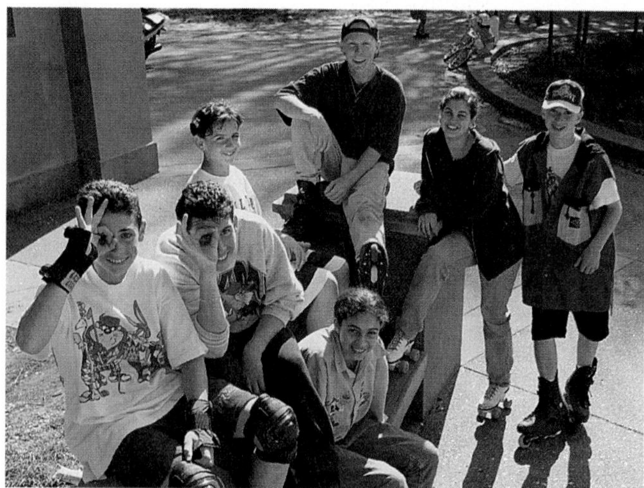

Figure 3.5 Adolescents develop comfort in social situations by participating in peer group activities.

change proportions as the forehead becomes more prominent and the jawbones develop. The growth rate slows after the onset of the external signs of puberty as ossification slows and the epiphyseal maturation of the long bones occurs in response to hormonal influences. Since androgen influences bone density, the bones of males become more dense than those of females. Androgen also appears to be directly related to the significant increase in male muscle mass.

Cognitive Development The period of adolescence corresponds to Piaget's stage of formal operations in which *abstract thinking* develops. Adolescents develop the ability to integrate past learning and present problems to plan for the future. They learn to use logic and solve problems by methodically analyzing each possibility. They use this new ability in scientific reasoning, and they create hypotheses and test them by setting up experiments. Analytic thinking extends to the adolescent's development of values. No longer content to accept what others say in an unquestioning manner, the adolescent can reason through inconsistencies and consider value options.

Psychosocial Development According to Freud, sexual urges repressed during latency reawaken as adolescents enter the genital stage. Sexual gratification comes with finding a partner outside of the family.

Erikson describes the conflict of adolescence as ego identity versus role diffusion. Homogeneous cliques support adolescents through the difficult search for their identity. They become very concerned with their bodies, their appearances, and their abilities, avoiding anything that would make them appear different. Erikson feels that the intolerance of others outside the clique displayed by adolescents is a temporary defense against identity confusion.

Adolescents' search for identity is stressful for adolescents and their families. The peer group becomes even more important than during the school-age years, providing a sense of belonging. Peer group participation allows adolescents to develop comfort in social participation (Figure 3.5). Peer group influence on clothing and hair styles, beliefs, values, and actions may create tension between adolescents and their families. As personal identity evolves, adolescents begin to plan for a future career and prepare to enter adulthood.

Assessment of Adolescents Unlike during earlier stages, caregivers rarely express concern that their adolescents are not eating. The pubertal growth spurt requires adolescents to increase their caloric intake dramatically, causing parents concern that they eat constantly but never seem full. Adolescents (particularly women) are at risk for developing eating disorders; feelings surrounding changes in the body should be explored.

Adolescents often communicate better with peers and adults outside of the family than with family members. Assessing adolescents with their parents, then alone, affords a more complete picture of their relationship and provides adolescents with an opportunity to freely express themselves and discuss concerns.

Adolescents are able to hold an adult conversation and are often happy to discuss school, friends, activities, and plans for the future. They tend to be anxious about their bodies and the rapid changes occurring. Often adolescents are unsure if what is happening to them is normal, and they frequently express somatic complaints.

As adolescents become more independent, adult family members become anxious over their evolving lack of control. Parents may be uncomfortable with adolescents' sexuality, rebellious dress and hair styles, and developing values which may differ from parents'. Communication between parents and adolescents is often challenging at this stage.

Severely restricting the activities and freedom of adolescents inhibits their ability to progress toward independence. Adolescents who lack social contacts and tend to spend much time alone may be depressed and at high risk for suicide. Acting out and risk-taking behaviors place adolescents at risk for serious injury from accidents or drug or alcohol use. Alliance with gangs places adolescents at risk for violence and participation in illegal activities.

Table 3.2 on page 50 lists common developmental health problems encountered during adolescence, ways to assess them, and health promotion recommendations.

Young Adults (20 to 40 Years)

The young adult establishes a new life on a chosen career path and in a lifestyle independent of parents. Tasks of this period include

- Leaving the family home
- Establishing a career or vocation
- Choosing a mate and forming an intimate relationship
- Managing one's own household
- Establishing a social group
- Beginning a parenting role
- Developing a meaningful philosophy of life

Physiologic Development During young adulthood, the body reaches its maximum potential for growth and development, and all systems function at peak efficiency. Skeletal system growth is completed around 25 years of age with the final fusion of the epiphyses of the long bones. The vertebral column continues to grow until about 30 years, adding perhaps 3 to 5 mm to an individual's height. Adult distribution of red bone marrow is achieved at about 25 years of age. Muscular efficiency reaches its peak performance between 20 and 30 years and declines at a variable rate thereafter.

Cognitive Development According to Piaget, by young adulthood, cognitive structures have been completed. During the formal operations stage in adolescence, abstract thinking

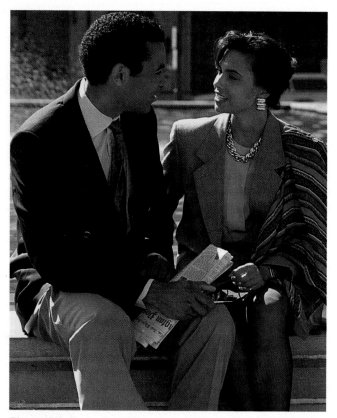

Figure 3.6 During their 30s, young adults typically strive to advance their careers.

has been achieved. Formal operations characterize thinking throughout adulthood. Young adults continue to develop, however, as egocentrism diminishes and thinking evolves in a more realistic and objective manner.

Psychosocial Development According to Erikson, the central task of young adults in their early 20s is intimacy versus isolation. During this stage, the young adult forms one or more intimate relationships. A secure self identity must be established before a mutually satisfying and mature relationship can be formed with another person. The mature relationship requires the ability to establish mutual trust, cooperate with another, share feelings and goals, and completely accept the other person.

Other theorists feel that young adulthood consists of several stages. The 20s are generally accepted as the time of establishing oneself in adult society by choosing a mate, friends, an occupation, values, and lifestyle. Around the age of 30, life is reassessed and the person either reaffirms past choices or deliberates changes. During the 30s, life again settles down, with the adult striving to build a better life in all aspects. It is a time of financial and emotional investment, and career advancement (Figure 3.6).

The decision whether to have children usually is made sometime during the young adult years. The addition of children requires major role adjustment and causes readjustment in a couple's relationship.

Assessment of Young Adults Young adults are busy, productive, and healthy. At their maximum physical potential, young adults actively pursue sports and physical fitness activities. They refine their creative talents and enjoy activities with peers.

Young adults form an intimate partnership with another in a mature, cooperative relationship. Traditionally this intimate relationship involved marriage. Increasingly, the relationship is formed and maintained without a formal marriage or between two people of the same sex. Developmentally, the important concept is the formation of the mature, intimate relationship.

The decision whether to have children is most often made during the young adult years. People deciding to have children have many more choices than previously: surrogate motherhood, artificial insemination, and test tube babies and other technologic innovations. Deciding not to have children or delaying having children is increasingly accepted, as is the decision of single women to have children.

Young adults have chosen an occupation, established their values, and adopted a lifestyle. Career advancement, financial stability, and emotional investment characterize the young adult years.

The young adult without a steady job may lack direction and self-confidence. Marital discord may trigger feelings of failure and insecurity. Failing to achieve intimacy may place the young adult at risk for depression, alcoholism, or drug abuse.

Table 3.2 on page 50 lists common developmental health problems encountered during the young adult years, ways to assess them, and health promotion recommendations.

Middle Adults (40 to 65 Years)

The middle years of life signal a halfway point, with as many years behind an individual as potentially ahead. This is a time of evaluation and adjustment, and its tasks include

- Accepting and adjusting to physical changes
- Reviewing and redirecting career goals
- Developing hobby and leisure activities
- Adjusting to aging parents
- Coping with children leaving home

Physiologic Development Functioning of the central nervous system during the early years of middle adulthood is normally maintained at the same high level achieved in young adulthood. Some individuals may experience a gradual decline in mental or reflex functioning as age advances past 50 because of changes in enzyme function, hormones, and motor and sensory functions. Decreased central nervous system integration may result in a slower, more prolonged, and more pronounced response to stressors.

Both men and women experience decreasing hormonal production during middle adulthood. During menopause, which usually occurs between ages 40 and 55, the ovaries decrease in size, and the uterus becomes smaller and firmer. Progesterone is not produced, and estrogen levels fall, resulting in the atrophy of the reproductive organs, vasomotor disturbances, and mood swings. Men experience a gradual decrease in testosterone, causing decreased sperm and semen production and less intense orgasms.

In individuals who become more sedentary over time, the heart begins to lose tone, and rate and rhythm changes become evident. Blood vessels lose elasticity and become thicker. Degeneration of cardiovascular tissues becomes a leading cause of death in individuals over age 45.

Lung tissues become thicker, stiffer, and less elastic with age, resulting in gradually decreased breathing capacity by age 55 or 60. Respiratory rates increase in response to decreasing pulmonary function.

Visual acuity declines, especially for near vision, and auditory acuity for high-frequency sounds decreases. Skin turgor, elasticity, and moisture decrease, resulting in wrinkles. Hair thins, and gray hair appears. Fatty tissue is redistributed in the abdominal area.

Bone mass decreases from age 40 until the end of middle adulthood. Calcium loss from bone tissues becomes pronounced in females. Muscle mass and strength are maintained in individuals who continue active muscle use. In those who lead a sedentary lifestyle, muscles decline in mass, structure, and strength. Muscle loss may also result from changes in collagen fiber, which becomes thicker and less elastic.

Cognitive Development The middle adult's cognitive and intellectual abilities remain constant, continuing the abilities characteristic in Piaget's stage of formal operations. Memory and problem solving are maintained, and learning continues, often enhanced by increased motivation at this time of life. Life experiences tend to enhance cognitive abilities as the middle adult builds on past experiences.

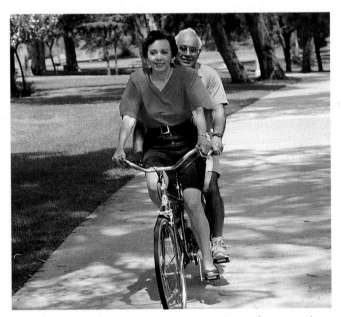

Figure 3.7 Middle adults usually have more time to focus attention on their relationship.

Psychosocial Development Erikson defined the developmental task of middle adulthood as generativity versus stagnation. He defined generativity as the concern for establishing and guiding the next generation. People turn from the self- and family-centered focus of young adulthood toward more altruistic activities such as community involvement, charitable work, and political, social, and cultural endeavors. Erikson believed that stagnation results if the need for sharing, giving, and contributing to the growth of others is not met. Stagnation refers to feelings of boredom and emptiness, which lead individuals to become inactive, self-absorbed, self-indulgent, and chronic complainers.

Some theorists believe the middle adult years begin with a transition during which a major reassessment of life accomplishments occurs. Typically the middle adult asks the question, "What have I done with my life?" People confront reality, accept that they cannot meet some goals, and emerge with redirected goals. Reassessment involves areas of career, personal identity, and family. The middle adult may reorder career goals or choose a new career path. Adjusting in a positive manner to children leaving home helps parents to focus attention on other relationships, find satisfying leisure activities, or pursue intellectual activities (Figure 3.7). Successful coping with the death of a parent helps people in middle adulthood come to terms with their own aging and death. Making financial plans and preparing for productive use of leisure time in retirement strengthen effective adaptation to retirement.

Assessment of Middle Adults The adult in the middle years of life is satisfied with past accomplishments and involved in activities outside the family. Adjusting to the physical changes of aging, individuals develop appropriate leisure activities in preparation for an active retirement. Good financial planning during the middle adult years ensures financial security during retirement.

The middle adult years signal the end of childbearing and, most often, the end of childrearing. Individuals adjust to never having had children or to children leaving home. Couples renew their relationships or sometimes find they have little in common and separate. Some women choose to delay childbearing until their late 30s or early 40s, after establishing their careers. They begin their childrearing years as many of their peers are completing this phase of life. Older mothers must make the transition from career women to mothers, even if they continue their careers.

The dissatisfied middle adult is unhappy with the past and expresses no hope for the future. Sedentary and isolated, the individual complains about life, avoids involvement, and fails to plan appropriately for retirement.

Table 3.2 on page 50 lists common developmental health problems encountered during the middle adult years, ways to assess them, and health promotion recommendations.

Older Adults (65+ Years)

Individuals in late adulthood vary greatly in their physical and psychosocial adaptation to aging. Developmental tasks of older adults include

- Adjusting to declining physical strength and health
- Forming relationships within one's peer group
- Adjusting to retirement
- Developing postretirement activities that maintain self-worth and usefulness
- Adjusting to the death of spouse, family members, and friends
- Conducting a life review
- Preparing for death

Physiologic Development During the later years, there is an inevitable decline in body functions. The body becomes less efficient in receiving, processing, and responding to stimuli. The central nervous system experiences a decrease in electrical activity, resulting in slowed or altered sensory reception and decreases in reactions and movement time.

The cardiovascular system demonstrates degenerative effects in old age. Fatty plaques are deposited in the lining of blood vessels, decreasing their ability to supply blood to tissues. Systolic blood pressure increases as a result of the inelasticity of the arteries and an increase in peripheral resistance. Endocardial thickening and hardening throughout the heart decrease the efficiency of its pumping action. The valves become more rigid and less pliable, leading to reduced filling and emptying abilities. Cardiac output and reserve diminish, resulting in an inability to react to sudden stress efficiently.

Efficiency of the lungs decreases with age, increasing the respiratory effort required to obtain adequate oxygen. Vital capacity decreases, and residual air increases with age. The bronchopulmonary tree becomes more rigid, reducing bronchopulmonary movements. Ciliary activity decreases, allowing mucous secretions to collect more readily in the respiratory tree. The ability to cough decreases as a result of diminished muscle tone and decreased sensitivity to stimuli.

Visual changes include loss of visual acuity, decreased adaptation to darkness and dim light, loss of peripheral vision, and difficulty in discriminating similar colors. Gradual loss of hearing is the result of changes in nerve tissues in the inner ear and a thickening of the eardrum. The sense of taste and smell decrease, and older adults are less stimulated by food than before. The gradual loss of skin receptors increases the threshold for sensations of pain and touch in the elderly.

Renal function is slowed by structural and functional changes associated with aging. Arteriosclerotic changes can reduce blood flow, impairing renal function. The kidney's filtering abilities become impaired as the number of functioning nephrons decreases with age. An enlarged prostrate gland causes urinary urgency and frequency in men, and in women the same complaints are often due to weakened muscles supporting the bladder or weakness of the urethral sphincter. The capacity of the bladder and its ability to empty completely diminish with age in both men and women.

All bones are affected by a decrease in skeletal mass. Decreased density causes bones to become brittle and fracture more easily. Range of motion decreases as the tissues of the joints and bones stiffen.

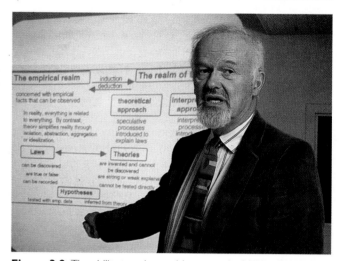

Figure 3.8 The ability to solve problems may be highly efficient in the older adult.

Cognitive Development Research continues into the effects of aging on cognitive abilities. Different kinds of cognitive functions seem to undergo different types, amounts, and rates of change in individual older adults. Functions dependent on perception rely on the acuity of the senses. When senses become impaired with aging, the ability to perceive the environment and react appropriately is diminished. Changes in the aging nervous system may also affect perceptual ability. Impaired perceptual ability diminishes the aging adult's cognitive capability.

Studies suggest that people who live in a varied environment that provides for continued use of intellectual function are often the ones who maintain or even strengthen these skills throughout life. Conversely, those who live in a static environment that lacks intellectual challenge may be the ones who most likely show some decline in intellectual ability with aging. Although learning and problem solving may not be as efficient in old age as in youth, both processes still occur to a greater extent than is often portrayed in stereotypes of older adults (Figure 3.8).

Psychosocial Development The developmental task of late adulthood, according to Erikson, is ego integrity versus self-despair. When a review of life events, experiences, and relationships makes the adult content with life, the person attains

Table 3.2 Common Health Risks by Age Group

Age Group	Problem	Assessment	Health Promotion Recommendations
Infancy 0–1 year	Overnutrition/ undernutrition	◆ Plot height and weight. ◆ If infant is breast-fed, ask about frequency and length of nursing; good letdown; mother's nutrition, fluid intake, and rest. ◆ If infant is bottle-fed, ask about formula (powder, concentrates, or ready-to-feed), how formula is mixed, how much is given, how often; how much is given in 24 hours; whether infant spits up solids (what, how much, how often). ◆ Ask about number, consistency of stools. ◆ Ask about urine: how many wet diapers? ◆ Ask: how do you know infant is hungry? ◆ Ask about infant's personality. ◆ Determine height and weight of family members.	◆ Breast-feed young infants every 2 hours; mother needs good nutrition with increased fluids, adequate rest, help from others, appropriate priority setting. ◆ Bottle-feed young infants every 3–4 hours, mix formula appropriately, provide resources for obtaining formula, change formula if necessary. ◆ Discuss: infant needs, reading infant cues, awakening quiet infant who may not cry for feeding.
	Developmental delay	◆ Perform Denver II. ◆ Ask where infant spends most of the day (crib, playpen, walker, infant seat). ◆ Ask about activities enjoyed, toys available, amount of interaction, and TV watching.	◆ Discuss infant's needs and abilities, stimulation, moving infant from room to room, placing infant in different positions, appropriate interactive play, appropriate toys, too young for TV.
	Disturbed attachment	◆ Determine if pregnancy was planned and access perceptions of infant, knowledge of infant abilities and needs, family stressors, support system, infant temperament and clarity of cues, parental fears.	◆ Discuss the infant's needs and abilities, cues, positive attributes, temperament; ask how the parent was raised. ◆ Establish support system, refer to early intervention programs or parent support groups, role model holding and talking to infant.
Toddler 1–3 years	Language delay	◆ Ask about language spoken at home, history of multiple ear infections, family history of hearing problems, how child communicates desires. ◆ Determine amount of interaction with others, TV time. ◆ Obtain hearing test.	◆ Discuss use of pictures, books, games in which the toddler names objects. ◆ Encourage teaching use of words to express wants, putting child in a play group, decreasing TV time.
	Developmental delay	◆ Perform Denver II ◆ Ask how child spends most of the day, activities enjoyed, toys available, amount of interaction and TV watching.	◆ Discuss toddler's needs and abilities, stimulation, appropriate interactive play, appropriate toys, limiting TV, parent/child play group. ◆ Refer for evaluation of significant delays.
	Behavior management	◆ Ask about problem behaviors, type of discipline used, child's response to discipline. ◆ Determine parent expectations, child's temperament.	◆ Discuss toddler expectations, use of time-outs and logical consequences, inappropriate corporal punishment.
Preschool 3–6 years	Language delay	◆ Ask about language spoken at home, history of multiple ear infections, family history of hearing problems, how child communicates desires. ◆ Determine amount of interaction with others, TV time. ◆ Obtain hearing test, speech evaluation.	◆ Dicuss reading books, having conversations with child, putting child in preschool, increasing interactive activities, decreasing TV time, speech therapy.
	Developmental delay	◆ Perform Denver II. ◆ Ask how child spends most of day, activities enjoyed, toys available, amount of interaction, TV time.	◆ Discuss preschool needs and abilities, use of play for learning, appropriate interactive play, appropriate toys, limiting TV, attendance in preschool. ◆ Refer for evaluation of significant delays.
	Social isolation	◆ Ask: How often does child get out of the house? Where does the child go? Who does the child see other than the family? Who babysits?	◆ Discuss need for contact outside of home and family, desirability of some separation from family, learning opportunities outside of home.

Table 3.2 Common Health Risks by Age Group (continued)

Age Group	Problem	Assessment	Health Promotion Recommendations
School Age 6–12 years	Lack of self-esteem	◆ Ask child about friends, activities, hobbies, interests. ◆ Ask parent about what child does well, school progress.	◆ Discuss need to pursue activities child is good at; need for positive feedback and encouragement, friends and group activities, increased independence, limit setting; danger of gang involvement.
	Learning problems	◆ Ask about school progress, repeated grades, last report card, the teacher's opinions, attendance in classes for special help, special testing.	◆ Discuss parent support for homework, consistent time and place for homework, communication between parent and teacher. ◆ Refer for learning disability testing if progress is not as expected or grades consistently poor.
Adolescence 12–19 years	Sexual conflict	◆ Ask about dating habits, sexual activity, STD history, birth control, feelings about sexuality, questions about sex.	◆ Discuss birth control, STD risk, HIV risk, pregnancy, feelings about sexuality.
	Parent-child conflict	◆ Ask parent and child separately about relationship, conflicts, how conflict is handled.	◆ Discuss normal parent-adolescent conflicts, conflict resolution, teen need for increasing independence, appropriate limits, need for professional intervention.
	Depression	◆ Ask child about school activities, friends, hobbies, plans for the future. ◆ Observe affect.	◆ Discuss risk behaviors, substance abuse, gangs. ◆ Refer for counseling.
Young Adulthood 20–40 years	Lack of direction	◆ Ask about employment, job changes, job satisfaction, goals, future plans, feelings about how life is going.	◆ Discuss how to define and achieve goals, need for satisfying work, hobbies that lead to employment, developing problem-solving skills.
	Continued dependence	◆ Ask about living situation, relationship with parents, social contacts, activities, hobbies.	◆ Discuss feelings about independence and parents, steps towards achieving independence, problem solving.
	Failure to establish intimacy	◆ Ask about relationships, friends, dating patterns, feelings about self and others of preferred sex.	◆ Discuss relationships, reasons for lack of intimate relationships, how to make social contacts, infuence of self-concept.
Middle Adulthood 40–65 years	Failure to prepare for future	◆ Ask about goals for the future, leisure activities, financial planning, retirement plans, feelings about retirement.	◆ Discuss need to prepare for retirement, developing enjoyable activities, planning activities to keep busy within financial means during retirement.
	Social isolation	◆ Ask about marriage, relationships, children and whether they have left home, social activities, hobbies, community involvement.	◆ Discuss options for developing new relationships, need for socializing, interests and possible hobbies, opportunites for community involvement. ◆ Refer to community resources.
Late Adulthood 65+ years	Failure to maintain self-worth	◆ Ask about recreational activities, social group, projects, hobbies, what is enjoyable, level of involvement with others.	◆ Discuss need for social interaction, developing or maintaining social group, developing hobbies or activities. ◆ Refer to community resources.
	Social isolation	◆ Ask about living situation; move from home; daily routine; deaths of friends, family, spouse; family contacts; support system. ◆ Determine physical limitations.	◆ Discuss need to get out and interact with others, interests, developing hobbies or activities; refer to community resources.

Adapted from: Fisher M, ed, 1989. *Guide to Clinical Preventive Services: An Assessment of the Effectiveness of 169 Interventions.* Report of the US Preventive Services Task Force. Baltimore: Williams and Wilkins, pp. xlii–lv.

ego integrity. Failure to resolve this last developmental crisis results in a sense of despair, resentment, futility, hopelessness, and a fear of death.

Late adulthood requires lifestyle changes as well as review of one's past life. The adult adjusting to retirement must develop new activities to replace work and the role of worker. New friendships are established with peers of similar interests, abilities, and means. The person may pursue projects or recreational activities deferred during the working years, but activities are limited to those compatible with the physical limitations of old age. Lack of adequate income limits the activities and lifestyle of many elderly; money enables them to be independent and look after themselves.

The lifestyle of later years is, to a large degree, formulated in youth. The person who was gregarious and spent time with people continues to do so, and the person who avoided involvement with others continues toward isolation. Those who learned early in life to live well-balanced and fulfilling lives are generally more successful in retirement. The later years can foster a sense of integrity and continuity, or they can be years of despair.

Through the late adult years, the deaths of friends, siblings, and partner occur with increasing frequency. Reminded of the limited time left, the older adult comes to terms with the past and views death as an acceptable completion of life.

Assessment of Older Adults Well-adjusted older adults maintain an active lifestyle and involvement with others and often do not appear their age. Lifestyle changes occur in response to declining physical abilities and retirement. Participation in activities that promote the elderly adult's sense of self-worth and usefulness also provides opportunities for developing new friendships with others of similar abilities and interests. Intellectual function is maintained through continued intellectual pursuits. Content with their life review, elderly adults enjoy their retirement years and accept death as the inevitable end of a productive life.

The older adult who has not successfully resolved developmental crises may feel that life has been unfair. Despair and hopelessness may be evident in the individual's lack of activity and bitter complaining.

Table 3.2 lists common developmental health problems encountered during late adulthood, ways to assess them, and health promotion recommendations.

Summary

A thorough nursing assessment includes an assessment of the client's growth and development. Early intervention in developmental crises prevents minor problems from developing into serious alterations in health, self-esteem, or interpersonal relationships. Accurate nursing assessment of growth and development and effective interventions assist individuals to function at their maximum level of wellness throughout life.

Key Points

- ✓ Nursing assessment requires the ability to interpret how complex interactions of physiologic, cognitive, and psychologic development, heredity, and environment affect an individual at a particular time.
- ✓ Knowledge of growth and development and an understanding of individual variations provide a foundation for assessment and nursing interventions that help individuals attain their maximum level of wellness.
- ✓ Growth and development proceed in an orderly, sequential progression.
- ✓ Researchers are continuously evolving developmental theories in an attempt to further define and explain human behavior.
- ✓ Cognitive theory explores the manner in which people learn to think, reason, and use language.
- ✓ Psychoanalytic theory describes how personality develops as individuals adjust to environmental changes and resolve conflicts occurring between environments and instincts.
- ✓ Psychosocial theory includes cultural and societal influences on ego development throughout the life span.
- ✓ The growth and development of infants and toddlers is rapid, transforming a totally dependent newborn into an active, verbal child with a unique personality.
- ✓ During the preschool and school-age years, children's knowledge and skills expand through learning experiences and relationships with other children and adults outside the home.
- ✓ Adolescence marks the transition from childhood to adulthood as children pass through the stages of growth and development in a predictable sequence, but at a highly variable age and rate.
- ✓ Growth and development continue throughout adulthood as individuals achieve independence and intimacy during young adulthood, attain career satisfaction and prepare for retirement during middle adulthood, and adjust to aging and participate in activities that promote their self-worth in late adulthood.

Chapter 4

Assessing Psychosocial Health

Psychosocial functioning includes the way a person thinks, feels, acts, and relates to self and others; the ability to cope and tolerate stress; and the capacity for developing a value and belief system. Holistic theorists describe this psychosocial component as part of an intricate set of subsystems making up the human organism. These subsystems are interrelated components that make up an individual who is greater than a sum of parts. Assessment of the human being must consider the interaction of body, mind, and spirit in their entirety rather than as separate body systems. When one part is missing or dysfunctional, all other parts of the organism are affected.

Illness, developmental changes, or life crises may bring about changes in psychosocial functioning. The client may become stressed, may lose self-esteem, or may experience positive changes such as greater closeness with family. Changes in psychosocial functioning may, in turn, affect the client's physical health or response to treatment. For example, a client who is extremely stressed may not be able to understand or remember instructions for self-care, and a client who is socially isolated may not be able to get needed help at home.

In addition, research has shown that psychosocial factors can play a direct role in the onset and course of many physiologic disorders (Fox 1989, Goodkin et al 1986, Pelletier 1992, Polonsky et al 1985, Smith et al 1985). Clinical evidence also demonstrates that psychosocial, emotional and behavioral interventions in some instances have at least as much proof of effectiveness as many purely medical interventions (Ornish et al 1990, Pelletier 1992, Spiegel et al 1989). Clients who are in a state of optimum psychologic, social, and spiritual well-being have faster recovery rates, better response rates to treatment modalities, and in some cases, lower mortality rates. There is an increasing body of scientific evidence supporting the theory that mind-body interactions play a key role in both health and illness. No matter what the source of the client's concern, a psychosocial assessment can provide significant insights that help you individualize client care.

Factors Affecting Psychosocial Wellness

To perform a comprehensive psychosocial assessment, you need to understand relevant aspects of the client's psychosocial health. Psychosocial health includes self-concept, roles and relationships, stress and coping, the senses and cognition, and spiritual and belief systems.

Self-Concept

Self-concept is the collection of feelings and beliefs a person holds about self at any given time. It develops throughout the lifetime as a person internalizes the reactions and feedback from significant others and accepts them. The self-concept includes four components: body image, self-ideal, self-esteem, and personal identity (Stuart and Sundeen 1991, p. 145). Body image includes both conscious and unconscious ideas, feelings, and attitudes about one's own body. The self-ideal is the expectations an individual has about how to behave and appear to others. Self-esteem may be described as an individual's feelings and beliefs about personal worth. Personal identity is the "conscious sense of individuality and uniqueness that is continually evolving throughout life" (Kozier et al 1995).

Roles and Relationships

A role is the set of behaviors that society or significant others expect of an individual in a certain position. Friend, parent, company manager, and student are all examples of roles an individual may assume. Each role carries with it a set of expected behaviors. Role performance describes how well an individual carries out that role in relation to societal expectations. Problems arise when individuals fail to master roles (role mastery failure), are unclear about how roles should be carried out (role ambiguity), or feel unsuited for a role (role strain).

Roles are closely tied to the client's relationships with other people. An important component of psychosocial health is having friends, neighbors, or family members that the client trusts, can call on for help, and feels close to (Figure 4.1).

Stress and Coping

Stress and coping patterns are the individual's physical and emotional response to psychosocial or physical threats to safety, called stressors. An automobile accident, a failing grade, an illness, or loss of a job are all examples of stressors. However, the stress is not the event itself, but the individual's response to it. Events that are highly stressful for one person may not be stressful for another. The stress response may include such familiar physical symptoms as sweaty palms and a pounding heart. The immediate physical reaction to stress is also referred to as the "fight-or-flight" response by stress researchers because its physiologic origins are thought to date back to an early human response to danger by fighting the perceived threat or taking flight to a safer environment. Physical reactions to long-term stress may include other symptoms, such as habitually cold hands or suppression of immune function. The emotional side of stress may include such reactions as difficulty sleeping, inability to concentrate, or anxiety.

Positive as well as negative events may be stressful. Winning ten million dollars in the lottery can be just as stressful and produce the same psychosocial and physiologic responses as being fired from one's job.

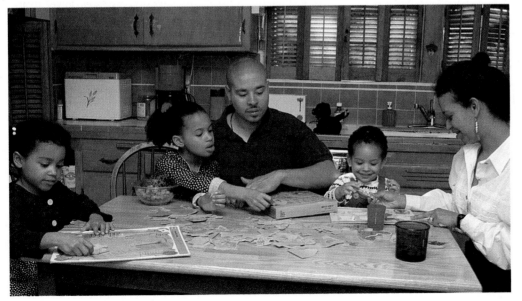

Figure 4.1 Clients with solid family support systems may have fewer problems with societal roles.

You can assess the physical signs of the client's stress response (see the accompanying box). Note that stress in itself is not necessarily bad. In fact, some stress can enhance and motivate performance. Consider the nursing student approaching a final exam. One week prior to the exam, the student may go out with friends for an evening of fun at the movies. However, the night prior to the test, the stress of knowing the exam is the next day will most likely motivate the student to give up an evening with friends in favor of studying for the test.

Coping behaviors are what an individual uses to deal with threats to physical and mental well-being and balance. Like other patterns of behavior, patterns of coping with stress stem from an individual's early development when significant people in the child's life role-modeled ways of coping and dealing with stress.

The Senses and Cognition

Sensory and cognition patterns are the logical sequencing of thoughts and feelings, and the ways an individual perceives and makes sense of the environment. Cognitive patterns include an individual's overall orientation to reality as well as general intelligence, insight, concrete and abstract thinking, and the ability to reason. Other cognitive patterns include an individual's attention, memory span, and concentration.

Spiritual and Belief Systems

Spiritual and belief patterns reflect an individual's relationship with a higher power, or with something, such as an ideal, a human group, or humanity itself, that the person sees as being larger than self and that gives meaning to life. Spiritual patterns also include the outward demonstration of that relationship. This outward demonstration may be reflected in a religion, lifestyle, or relationships with others. An individual's moral code may also be included in spiritual and belief patterns. A moral code is the internalized values, virtues, and rules learned from significant others and developed by oneself in order to distinguish between right and wrong. It includes the rules people use to determine what they should or should not do. An individual's spiritual and belief patterns are significantly affected by culture and ethnic background.

The Stress Response

The stress response, which occurs when an individual feels an internal (psychic) or external (environmental) danger, is initiated by the central and autonomic nervous systems. These systems initiate changes in the endocrine, respiratory, cardiovascular, gastrointestinal, and renal body systems. When the individual feels threatened, the stimulus triggers the limbic system of the cerebrum. The limbic system activates the hypothalamus, which in turn signals the parasympathetic and sympathetic portions of the autonomic nervous system and the pituitary gland to prepare for action. The following changes occur:

- Increased heart rate
- Decreased blood clotting time
- Increased rate and depth of respirations
- Dilated pupils
- Elevated glucose levels
- Dilated skeletal blood vessels
- Elevated blood pressure
- Dilated bronchi
- Increased blood volume
- Contraction of the spleen
- Increased blood supply to vital organs
- Release of T lymphocytes

Gathering the Data

When you conduct a psychosocial assessment, your goal is to take a holistic approach to both the well and distressed client as you gather data to assess the client's response to life experiences and the environment. You use this information to guide the formulation of nursing diagnoses. In each phase of the interview process, you determine which areas of psychosocial function you should explore further in the next phase. Psychosocial assessment begins before the initial interview when you gather information from the medical record relating to past emotional or psychiatric problems as well as physiologic illnesses that may have affected the client's psychologic or social functioning. For example, psychosocial problems may be related to brain tumors, multiple sclerosis, or Huntington's chorea.

During the initial interview, you gather more information about the client's social history (eg, marital status and occupation), history of growth and development, past emotional problems, response to crises and illnesses, and family history of emotional or psychiatric illness. If you discover an area of heightened concern, you may focus on that area during the initial interview. You may also conduct a focused interview at a later time during the course of the client's care. During the focused interview, you use information obtained from the medical history, the initial interview, and subsequent client

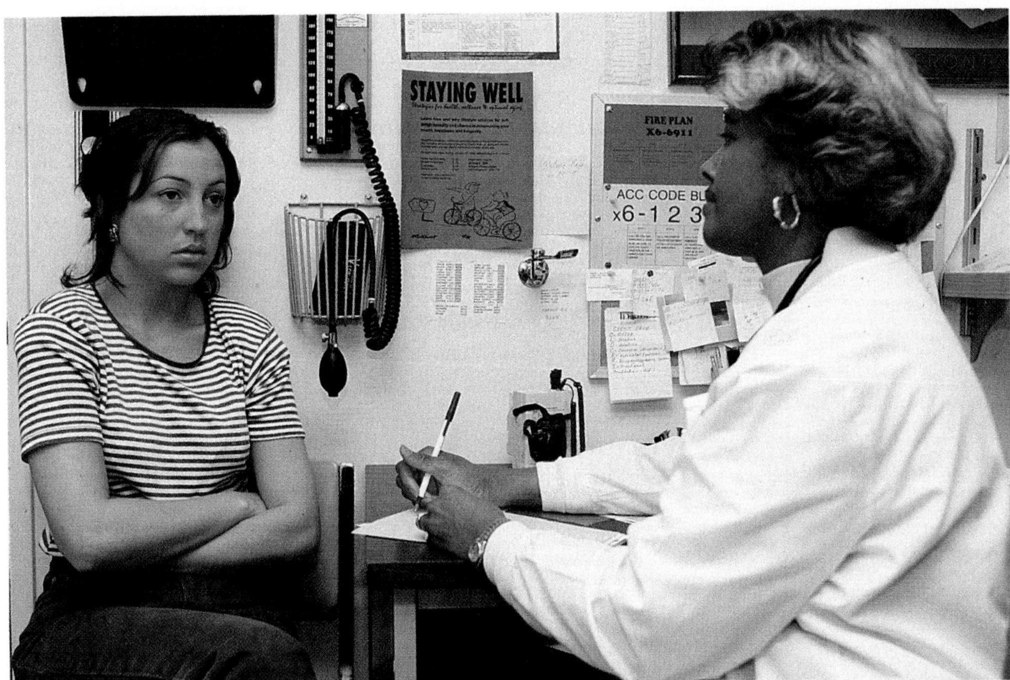

Figure 4.2 Clients may feel uncomfortable answering questions about themselves, especially if the data requested concerns psychosocial aspects of the client's life.

interactions to help the client do a careful inventory of past and current psychosocial health status.

Focusing the Interview on Psychosocial Well-Being

You conduct an interview focused on psychosocial well-being when

- the information you collect during the health history indicates psychosocial dysfunction
- the client's behavior during the initial interview is anxious, depressed, erratic, or bizarre
- you need more information to determine if any relationships exist between past disease processes and potential emotional or psychiatric concerns

In some situations a psychosocial concern is not apparent at the time of the initial interview but becomes apparent at a later time, such as when a client learns of a negative prognosis or undergoes disfiguring surgical procedures. In these cases, you should seek a focused psychosocial interview whenever the emotional problem becomes apparent. The case study on page 56 describes a situation where anxiety and fear impeded a client's recovery from a physical illness. Only after the nurse focused on the emotional impact of the illness was the client able to respond to therapy.

In some situations the client's primary health concern is psychosocial in nature. Clients with substance abuse, depression, neurosis, or psychosis fall into this category. In these situations, you should integrate the questions outlined here as part of the focused interview into the initial interview during the first contact with the client, family, or friends.

Structure the focused interview to obtain the most information with the fewest questions. Clients may feel uncomfortable answering questions about themselves, making it difficult for you to gather accurate and detailed data regarding the psychosocial aspects of the client's life (Figure 4.2). The following sections include a variety of questions that you can use as a guide for collecting information about the client's past history of psychosocial and physiological problems as well as the five areas of psychosocial functioning.

Past History of Psychosocial Concerns Some psychosocial concerns begin early in life and reappear whenever a client faces a major stressor or life crisis. The way the client coped with problems and treatment modalities in the past can be useful information for planning for the client's current problems. The following questions are helpful in eliciting this information:

1. Describe any emotions you find yourself frequently experiencing both currently and in the past. *When you assess clients, a complete psychosocial history is helpful in determining whether the current health problem is related to previous psychosocial dysfunction.*
2. If you have had an emotional problem in the past, were you treated for it? What kind of treatment did you have? Was the treatment successful? Who gave you the treatment? When? Do you still have the problem? *This information is helpful in developing the current nursing care plan if previous methods of treatment were successful.*
3. Do you use alcohol or drugs? If so, what do you use, how much, and how often? Have you had any treatment for substance abuse? What kind of treatment?

Case Study

Mrs. Ada Sweeney, a 54-year-old grandmother, was admitted to intensive care with gastrointestinal bleeding. Over the next few days Mrs. Sweeney was diagnosed with severe ulcerative colitis, anemia, and dehydration. Although the physician initiated an aggressive therapeutic medical regimen, Mrs. Sweeney failed to respond to therapy and continued to experience diarrhea accompanied by gastrointestinal bleeding, elevated temperatures, and severe abdominal pain. One evening the nurse on duty, Indira Singh, discovered Mrs. Sweeney crying in her room. Ms Singh then used a focused interview to gather information regarding the behavior Mrs. Sweeney was demonstrating. "I'm worried about my grandson," Mrs. Sweeney told the nurse. "I'm raising him and his sisters until their mother is able to come back for them." Mrs. Sweeney went on to tell Ms Singh that her daughter had been sent to prison on drug charges and there was no one else to care for her four children. "I do the best I can, but there's never enough money to go around, and I'm terrified the authorities will take the children away from me." Ms Singh questioned Mrs. Sweeney about her immediate and extended family, income, job, and available support systems. After Ms Singh reviewed the data she gathered during the focused interview, it became clear that Mrs. Sweeney's anxiety and fear over the future of her grandchildren was interfering with her recovery. Ms Singh developed the following nursing diagnoses:

1. *Anxiety* related to inadequate financial resources.
2. *Fear* related to inadequate supervision of client's grandchildren in client's absence.

Within the next few days the social service department at the hospital found a state program that provided a homemaker for the children until their grandmother recovered, assisted the family in obtaining food stamps, and began a search for better housing. Mrs. Sweeney immediately began to show a response to her nursing and medical treatment and was able to leave the hospital within 2 weeks.

Where? *Substance abuse may be the underlying cause of physiologic or psychosocial health problems or may be the result of some other underlying problem.*

4. Have you had any eating problems such as anorexia or bulimia? Were you treated? How? By whom? When? *A client who has an eating disorder may be in denial and unable to give accurate information on this question. If you suspect an eating disorder, look for the diagnostic cues during the physical assessment.*

Past and Current History of Physiologic Alterations or Diseases When being treated for medical-surgical conditions, clients and their families may be unaware that the physical problems may be related to or caused by an underlying psychosocial problem. An understanding of the interaction, both positive and negative, of the the body with the mind can help you and your clients realize when covert cognitive, perceptual, or affective problems are related to the overt signs and symptoms. Sometimes the underlying problem does not surface immediately but becomes apparent only after you have given several days of nursing care. The following questions are helpful for uncovering additional information:

1. Describe any chronic illnesses you have had. *Clients with recent onset of chronic illnesses often have problems complying with treatment or adjusting to living with the condition.*
2. How has your illness changed your mood or feelings? When you are nervous or anxious, how does your body feel? *A physiologic condition may be an underlying cause of anxiety, nervousness, or other abnormal behavior. Conversely, abnormal psychosocial behavior may aggravate or cause a physiologic condition.*
3. Have you had any of the following health problems? If so, describe how the condition has affected your life.

   Arthritis

   Asthma

   Bowel disorders

   Heart problems

   Glandular problems

   Headaches

   Stomach ulcer

   Skin disorders

   These conditions sometimes have both a psychologic and physiologic component. The presence of the condition may signal an underlying psychosocial disturbance.

Self-Concept It is difficult to gather significant data about self-concept, because most clients find it embarrassing to answer questions about themselves. Clients feel more comfortable divulging this information after you have established a positive nurse-client relationship and when you integrate questions into general conversation. The following questions are helpful in obtaining additional information about self-concept:

1. How would you describe yourself to others? *Asking clients to describe themselves is an excellent technique for determining how they perceive themselves.*

2. What are your best characteristics? What do you like about yourself?
3. What would you change about yourself if you could? *This is a positive way of asking a client to talk about negative self-perceptions.*
4. Would you describe yourself as shy or outgoing?
5. Do you consider yourself attractive? Sexually appealing? If no, why not? *The client's self-perception of attractiveness and sex appeal may reveal problems with self-image.*
6. Have your feelings about your appearance changed with this illness? If so, how? *Self-image may change if the illness or treatment has caused a change in appearance.*
7. Who comes first in your life: your spouse, children, friends, parents, or yourself?
8. Do you have difficulty saying no to others? *Clients who are depressed, feel hopeless, or feel powerless have difficulty with assertiveness.*
9. Do you like to be alone? *Clients with positive self-concept enjoy spending time by themselves, but those who indicate that they'd rather be alone most of the time may be experiencing emotional problems.*
10. Describe your social life. What do you do for fun? *Clients who are unable to answer this question may be depressed or out of touch with reality.*
11. What are your hobbies or interests? Do you spend much time pursuing them?
12. For heterosexuals only: Are you comfortable relating to the opposite sex? If no, why not? *Persons with self-concept or self-image problems may experience difficulty relating to the opposite sex.*
13. Are you comfortable with your sexual preference? If not, why not? *Clients who are homosexual and have not learned to accept their sexuality may experience a self-image problem.*
14. Do you have any concerns about your sexual function? If so, what?

Family History You should explore this area more fully if the health history indicates a family history of psychosocial dysfunction. Although no member of the family may have been diagnosed as being mentally ill, you should explore individual as well as family dysfunction. Ask the following questions in relation to the client's parents, siblings, and extended family when a child, and also in relation to the client's current family.

1. Describe any problems your family may have had with mental disorders. *Some mental disorders such as schizophrenia are familial, that is, the illness recurs in the same family over several generations.*
2. What were your major responsibilities in your family?
3. Describe your relationships with your parents. Extended family. *Look for family dysfunction problems such as schisms (families in chronic controversy), disengagement (detached relationships), or enmeshment (family interactions are intense and focus on power conflicts rather than affections) as the client describes his or her family life. (See Chapter 6 for more information on family dysfunction.)*
4. What is your birth order in your family? How many brothers and sisters? Are your sisters and brothers older or younger? *Age and gender birth order influence how an individual relates to other men and women throughout life.*
5. Describe your relationship with your siblings growing up at home. Did you and your siblings have problems getting along? If so, how did you solve them? *The way a client learned to handle stress and conflict with siblings as a child influences the way the client handles these issues throughout life.*
6. What members of your extended family (grandparents, aunts, uncles, cousins) were important to you as you grew up? How did they influence you? *Significant others shape an individual's self-concept and self-esteem. Descriptions of significant others help you understand why clients feel and act as they do.*
7. Did you have death or losses in your family as you grew up? How did your parents teach you to cope with the loss? How did they cope with the loss? *Clients who are depressed may not have learned how to deal with loss as a child and may have difficulty dealing with the loss of a loved one or with their own or a significant other's declining health status.*
8. Were your parents divorced and/or remarried during your childhood? If so, whom did you live with? Describe your life growing up with a single parent or step-parent. *Children who are products of a divorce may carry emotional scars into adulthood, affecting their psychosocial health and indirectly affecting their physical health status.*
9. Describe how your parents raised you. How did it affect you? *Clients who were raised by parents who had serious emotional problems, or who were abused by their parents, are more likely to have emotional problems as adults.*
10. How did your family deal with adversity and conflict? *Clients learn to deal with problems from their family. Knowing how the client learned to deal with problems as a child helps you understand how the client might deal with the present health problem.*
11. When disagreement arose in your family, how was it solved? Who sided with whom? *In dysfunctional families, schisms result causing family members to align themselves into coalitions against other family members, such as parents against children, father and sons against mothers and daughters, and sisters against brothers. (For more information see Chapter 6.)*

Other Roles and Relationships

1. Describe your relationships with your friends, neighbors, and coworkers.
2. Do you belong to any social groups? Community groups?
3. Who is your closest friend? How do you maintain your friendship? *An individual's ability to form close relationships indicates a healthy self-concept. Individuals who consistently fail to form close relationships may have a self-concept problem.*
4. Is your closest friend the most important person in your life? If not, who is the most important person in your life? Explain why.

Stress and Coping A person learns coping mechanisms from significant others during early childhood and throughout life. The ability to cope is also greatly affected by the number and severity of stressors that have occurred in a person's life. One method for assessing stress in a client's life is to administer the Holmes Social Adjustment Rating Scale (Table 4.1). The items on this scale represent stressors that may occur in a person's life. Since stress is a response to events, not the events themselves, not all people are equally stressed, or stressed in the same way, by these events. But, on average, the higher the individual's score, the more likely it is that the individual has responded with stress. As a result, the individual is more likely to experience stress-related disorders (eg, headaches, asthma, skin rashes, back pain, frequent colds, anxiety). The scale demonstrates that positive life events should also be part of a psychosocial assessment, because these positive events can be just as stressful as negative events in a person's life.

The following questions are helpful to gather additional information about the client's stress and coping mechanisms:

1. What do you do for relaxation? For recreation?
2. What is your greatest source of comfort when you are feeling upset? *This question identifies the client's coping mechanisms.*
3. Who do you call when you need help? *This question identifies important persons in the client's support system.*
4. What is the greatest source of stress in your life at the present time? How have you coped with similar situations in the past? *A person who has successfully coped with stress in the past may be able to call upon these coping skills to deal with current problems.*
5. Describe how you are dealing with your illness. Have you had difficulty adjusting to changes in your appearance, ability to carry out activities of daily living, or relationships? If so, describe how you feel. *Clients who have undergone severe, sudden changes that are apparent to others frequently have difficulty adjusting to these changes.*
6. Do you take any drugs, medications, or alcohol to cope with your stress? If so, describe what you are taking. *Clients who are experiencing stress are at risk for becoming addicted to these substances, especially if there is a family history of drug or alcohol abuse.*
7. Are you experiencing any of the following:

   Sadness

   Crying spells

   Insomnia

   Lack of appetite

   Weight loss

   Loss of sex drive

   Constipation

   Fatigue

   Hopelessness

   Irritability

   Indecisiveness

   Confusion

   Pounding heart or pulse

   Trouble concentrating

   These may indicate a high level of stress.
8. Have you ever considered taking your life? If so describe what you would do. *(See the box on page 60 for characteristics of the suicidal client.) Clients who are suicidal often admit their intentions if questioned directly. Clients are at high risk for suicide if they can describe a method for committing the suicide and have the necessary means at their disposal.*

The Senses and Cognition Clients who are out of contact with reality may display illusional, delusional, and hallucinatory speech and behavior, such as talking to themselves (auditory hallucinations); reacting to objects, noises, or other people in strange ways (illusions); or discussing false beliefs (delusions). Direct questioning may increase the client's anxiety and escalate the abnormal behavior or cause confusion. You should use direct questioning only when the client appears to be in control and in touch with reality. The following questions are helpful to gather additional information. You should preface these questions by first explaining to the client that some of the questions may seem silly or unimportant, but that they are helpful in assessing memory.

1. What is your name, age, and place of birth? *Questions 1–3 determine whether the client is oriented to person, place, and time.*
2. Where are you right now?
3. What day of the week is it? What is the date?

Table 4.1 Holmes Social Readjustment Rating Scale

Event	Event Value
1. Death of a spouse	100
2. Divorce	73
3. Marital separation	65
4. Jail term	63
5. Death of a close family member	63
6. Personal injury or illness	53
7. Marriage	50
8. Fired at work	47
9. Marital reconciliation	45
10. Retirement	45
11. Change in health of family member	44
12. Pregnancy	40
13. Sex difficulties	39
14. Gain of a new family member	39
15. Business readjustment	39
16. Change in financial state	38
17. Death of a close friend	37
18. Change to different line of work	36
19. Change in number of arguments	35
20. Mortgage or loan over $10,000	31
21. Foreclosure of mortgage or loan	30
22. Change in responsibilities at work	29
23. Son or daughter leaving home	29
24. Trouble with in-laws	29
25. Outstanding personal achievement	28
26. Spouse begins or stops work	26
27. Begin or end school	26
28. Change in living conditions	25
29. Revision of personal habits	24
30. Trouble with boss	23
31. Change in work hours or conditions	20
32. Change in residence	20
33. Change in schools	20
34. Change in recreation	19
35. Change in church activities	19
36. Change in social activities	19
37. Change in sleeping habits	16
38. Change in number of family get-togethers	15
39. Vacation	13
40. Christmas	12
41. Minor violations of the law	11
Total Points	______

Directions for completion: Add up the point values for each of the events that you have experienced during the past 12 months.

Scoring

Below 150 points:

The amount of stress you are experiencing as a result of changes in your life is normal and manageable. There is only a 1 in 3 chance that you might develop a serious illness over the next 2 years based on stress alone. Consider practicing a daily relaxation technique to reduce your chance of illness even more.

150 to 300 points:

The amount of stress you are experiencing as a result of changes in your life is moderate. Based on stress alone, you have a 50/50 chance of developing a serious illness over the next 2 years. You can reduce these odds by practicing stress management and relaxation techniques on a daily basis.

Over 300 points:

The amount of stress you are experiencing as a result of changes in your life is high. Based on stress alone, your chances of developing a serious illness during the next 2 years approaches 90%, unless you are already practicing good coping skills and regular relaxation techniques. You can reduce the chance of illness by practicing coping strategies and relaxation techniques daily.

From Holmes T, Rahe RJ. *J Psychosom Res* 11:213–218, 1967. Elsevier Science Ltd., Pergamon Imprint, Oxford, England.

Characteristics of the Client Who Is at the Highest Risk for Suicide

The following characteristics may indicate that a client is at increased risk for suicide. While one of the following items alone may not indicate a client is contemplating suicide, the more factors present, the more likely that the client is at increased risk.

- Single, divorced, or widowed
- Socially isolated, or little or no support system
- History of suicide attempts
- Family history of suicide
- Recent loss, ie, divorce; threat of or loss of a loved one; loss of a job, money, or social status
- History of drug abuse or alcoholism
- History of mental illness
- Depressed or recovering from depression
- Severe anxiety or fear
- Serious or physical illness, with impaired life-style or altered body image
- Sleep dysfunction
- Expressing feelings of hopelessness, powerlessness, rejection, or punishment
- Arranging personal affairs, ie, taking out an insurance policy, planning a funeral, canceling social engagements, preparing a will, or giving possessions away
- Verbalizing suicidal thoughts, ie, "Sometimes I think I'd be better off dead" or "I give up"
- Sudden or unexplained behavior change
- Feelings of ineffective communication, or family members rejecting attempts at communication
- Feelings of increased life responsibilities
- Crying for no obvious reason
- Certain demographic variables such as gender (suicide rates are higher for men), race (suicide rates are higher for Caucasians and Native Americans), age (suicide rates are higher between 15 and 24 years), both ends of the socioeconomic scale

4. What would you take with you if a fire broke out? *The client's ability to make a judgment is tested here.*
5. Count backwards from 10 to 1. *Tests cognitive function.*
6. What did you have for breakfast? *Tests recent memory.*
7. Who were the last two presidents? *Tests remote memory.*

Clinical Alert: Hallucinations and Delusional Systems

The content of a client's hallucinations and delusions is important to assess in order to provide for the client's safety and the safety of others. Command hallucinations tell clients to carry out acts against themselves or others that are usually harmful. The command hallucinations may be part of an elaborate delusional system clients hold in which they feel persecuted or in danger. In some cases clients are disturbed by these thoughts and share them with others. In other situations, however, clients keep their thoughts to themselves, and these thoughts do not become apparent until they commit some violent act. A client who demonstrates these symptoms should be referred to a psychiatric nurse clinical specialist who has the skill and expertise needed to uncover hallucinatory and delusional thinking without exacerbating the symptoms.

8. Describe what the following statement means "People who live in glass houses shouldn't throw stones." *Tests the client's ability to do abstract and/or symbolic thinking.*
9. Are you having any problems thinking? If so, describe what happens. *The client may not be able to answer this question if a thought disorder is present. Clients with manic disorders describe their thoughts as "racing."*
10. Do you have trouble making decisions? Describe what happens when you have to make a decision. *The inability to make decisions may indicate depression or low self-esteem.*
11. Do you ever hear voices, see objects, or experience other sensations that don't make sense? If so, describe your experiences. *The client who is out of contact with reality may experience auditory, visual, gustatory, somatic, and olfactory hallucinations (hearing, seeing, tasting, feeling, and smelling stimuli that are not real).*

    Discussing hallucinatory experiences in detail may reinforce them for the client; therefore do not dwell on these symptoms with the client.
12. If you hear voices, do they tell you what you must do? *Determine if the client is experiencing command hallucinations (see the Clinical Alert box above).*

    These are dangerous hallucinations that may lead the client to self-destructive behavior or to harm others.
13. Do you ever misinterpret objects, sounds, or smells? Describe. *Clients who are very anxious or out of contact with reality may experience illusions (misinterpretation of environmental stimuli).*

Spiritual and Belief Systems The questions in this section determine how clients' ethical, moral, and religious values affect their health status. Often the client's statements about values play an important role in how you should implement nursing care. Be sensitive to the client's reaction to these questions when assessing this area, because the client's spiritual life and belief systems may be very personal. Also be careful about querying a client who is hallucinating or is delusional, because your questions can exacerbate delusional or hallucinatory behavior.

The spiritual and belief systems of clients usually derive from their culture and ethnic background. A client who is not from the dominant culture may have beliefs about health and illness and their relationship to God or the supernatural; as the nurse, you may know nothing about these beliefs. You need to understand these issues to play an important role in helping the client to cope with a psychosocial health concern or illness.

Use the following questions when assessing the client's spiritual and belief systems and the culture and ethnic considerations surrounding them. As you collect this information, observe the client's verbal and nonverbal behavior, interpersonal relationships, and immediate environment.

1. Describe your ethnic and cultural background. *Clients from some ethnic and cultural groups are more likely to have health-related beliefs and practices that have an impact on nursing care. (See Chapter 6.)*
2. To whom do you go for help regarding your health (doctor, nurse practitioner, folk healer, medicine man, or other healer)? *You are more likely to gain the client's compliance if you include the client's folk healer in the planning stage.*
3. What are your beliefs about life, health, illness, and death? *You need this knowledge about the client's health-related beliefs to develop an individualized plan of care.*
4. Does religion or God play a part in your life? If so, what is it? *Incorporate the client's religion and faith in God in the plan of care if they are important to the client.*
5. What part do hope and faith play in your life? Is your faith helpful to you during times of stress?
6. Has your present health concern affected your spiritual life? If so, describe how.
7. Do your spiritual beliefs help you cope with illness or stress? If so, describe how.
8. Have you experienced any anger with God or a higher being or force because of things that have happened to you? If so, describe how you feel. *Clients who feel anger toward God or a higher force may project this anger toward family, friends, and health care providers.*
9. Do you believe your illness is a punishment for past sins or wrong doing? *Clients who feel they are being punished may feel guilty and lose the ability to cope with the illness.*
10. If you use prayer, describe how you use it to cope with life or stress. *Incorporate the client's use of prayer in the plan of care if it is meaningful to the client.*
11. Are you affiliated with any religion? If so, would you like to talk with your minister (priest, rabbi)? *Refusal to accept visits from clergy might indicate spiritual distress.*
12. Describe any religion-related nutrition or health practices that you must follow.
13. Are you concerned about the morality or ethical implications of any of the treatments planned for you?

Physical Observation

As you conduct the initial or focused interview, you should also observe the client's general appearance, posture, gait, body language, and speech patterns (Figure 4.3).

Observe the client's general appearance including the manner of dress, personal hygiene, and grooming.

- The client should be clean and well-groomed. The clothes should be clean, worn properly, and appropriate for the client's age and the time and place. Be careful not to impose your own standards, however, when judging the dress of another.

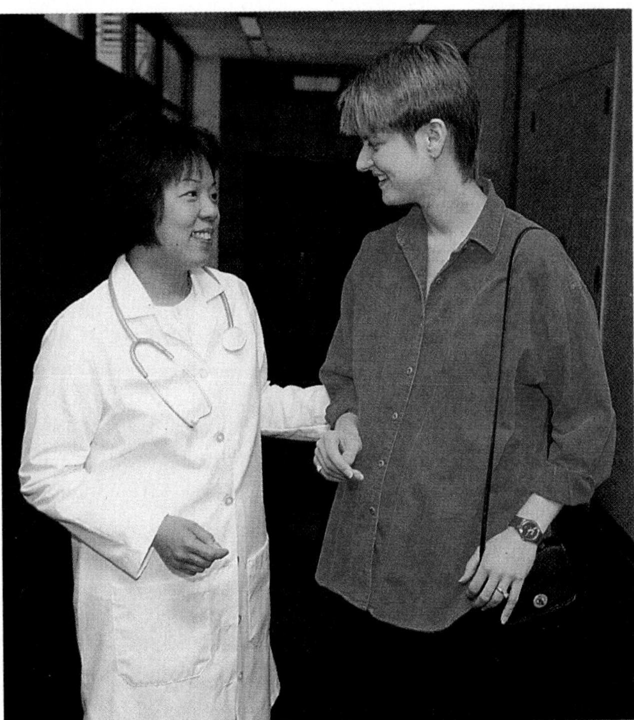

Figure 4.3 The client's general appearance, posture, gait, body language, and speech patterns may provide important clues to the client's psychosocial health status.

- The client who is dirty, disheveled, unshaven, or has a body odor may have a *Body image disturbance*, which may be caused by a *Self-care deficit*. Further assess the client for *Impaired skin integrity* due to unclean conditions. Look for signs of ringworm, pediculosis, or other skin problems. (See Chapter 8.)

Observe the client's posture, gait, and general body language.

- The client's posture should be erect and relaxed. The body language should be open with direct eye-contact unless inappropriate for the client's ethnic group. Movements should be fluid, relaxed, and spontaneous. A closed, guarded posture with poor eye-contact may indicate *Fear, Anxiety*, or *Defensive coping*. The client who paces, wrings hands, is restless, or exhibits tics (involuntary movements) may also be experiencing *Anxiety*. A slow, shuffling gait may indicate depression or poor contact with reality, signaling *Ineffective coping*.

Observe the facial expression and affect. The expression and affect should be appropriate for the conversation and circumstances.

- An unusually sad (depressed) or extremely happy (euphoric) demeanor that is inappropriate for the circumstances, labile (rapid) mood swings, or flat affect (absence of emotional expression) may indicate *Ineffective coping*.

Notice the content and manner of speech. The content, tone, pace, and volume of the speech should be appropriate for the situation.

Abnormal Speech Patterns Associated with Altered Thought Processes

- Loud, rapid, pressured, and high-pitched
- Circumlocution (inability to communicate an idea due to numerous digressions)
- Flight of ideas (jumping from one subject to another)
- Word salad (a conglomeration of multiple words without apparent meaning)
- Neologisms (coining new words that have symbolic meaning to the client)
- Clanging (rhyming conversation)
- Echolalia (constant repetition of words or phrases that the client hears others say)

- Abnormal speech patterns may indicate *Anxiety, Fear*, or *Altered thought processes* (see the box below). Observe the coherence and organization of the client's speech. The client's speech should be logical and sequential.
- Clients may demonstrate the following: talking to themselves (auditory hallucinations); reacting to objects, noises, or other people in strange ways (illusions); or manifesting erratic beliefs (delusions). The client may appear to be aphasic or incoherent. For such clients, consider the diagnoses *Altered communication, Altered thought processes,* and *Ineffective coping*.

Organizing the Data

Once you have collected the data from all of the various sources, you sort, group, and categorize the information. As you carry out this process, each diagnostic cue falls under one of the psychosocial functioning groups mentioned earlier in this chapter: self-concept, roles and relationships, stress and coping, the senses and cognition, and spiritual and belief systems. (See the accompanying box for a list of NANDA nursing diagnoses under each category.)

The Self-Concept Group

The self-concept group includes nursing diagnoses such as *Anxiety, Body image disturbance, Hopelessness, Powerlessness,* and *Low self-esteem*. Place a diagnostic cue in the self-concept group if it gives information on how the client:

- Feels about self
- Thinks other people feel about him or her
- Thinks other people see him or her
- Is able to be in control of his or her life

Table 4.2 on page 64 gives an example of a nursing diagnosis related to self-concept.

The Roles and Relationships Group

The roles and relationships group includes nursing diagnoses such as *Impaired verbal communication, Altered family processes, Dysfunctional grieving, Parental role conflict,* and *Social isolation*. Place a diagnostic cue in the roles and relationships group if it gives information about

- Family relationships and dynamics

Psychosocial Nursing Diagnoses Developed by NANDA

Self-Concept

- Anxiety
- Body image disturbance
- Altered growth and development
- Fatigue
- Fear
- Hopelessness
- Personal identity disturbance
- Powerlessness
- Self-esteem disturbance
- Chronic low self-esteem
- Situational low self-esteem

Roles and Relationships

- Impaired verbal communication
- Altered family processes
- Anticipatory grieving
- Dysfunctional grieving
- Parental role conflict
- Altered parenting
- High risk for altered parenting
- Impaired social interaction
- Social isolation
- Altered role performance

Stress and Coping

- Impaired adjustment
- Ineffective individual coping
- Ineffective family coping, compromised
- Ineffective family coping, disabling
- Family coping potential for growth
- Ineffective denial
- Defensive coping
- Post-trauma response
- Rape-trauma syndrome, compound reaction
- Rape-trauma syndrome, silent reaction
- High risk for violence, self-directed or directed at others

Sensory and Cognition

- Decisional conflict
- Sensory/perceptual alterations: visual, auditory, kinesthetic, gustatory, tactile, olfactory
- Altered thought processes

Spiritual and Belief Systems

- Spiritual distress

From: Proceedings of the Ninth National Conference of the North American Nursing Diagnosis Association, March 1994.

- The client's relationships with others
- The client's support systems

Table 4.3 on page 65 gives an example of a nursing diagnosis related to roles and relationships.

The Stress and Coping Group

Some of the nursing diagnoses that fall into the stress and coping group include *Impaired adjustment, Ineffective individual coping, Ineffective family coping, Rape-trauma syndrome,* and *High risk for violence*. A diagnostic cue belongs in the stress and coping group if it gives information about

- Sources of stress in the client's life
- Coping strategies and reactions to stressors (signs and symptoms)
- The client's use of chemical substances
- Losses of family or friends through death
- Other losses, such as loss of job or money
- Signs and symptoms of depression or suicidal ideation

Table 4.4 on page 65 gives an example of a nursing diagnosis related to the stress and coping group.

The Sensory and Cognition Group

Some of the nursing diagnoses included in the sensory and cognition group include *Decisional conflict, Sensory and perceptual alterations,* and *Altered thought processes*. A diagnostic cue belongs in the sensory and cognition group if it gives information about the client's

- Reality orientation
- Thinking processes
- Affective behavior

Table 4.2 Nursing Diagnosis Related to Self-Concept

ANXIETY	
Definition: A vague, uneasy feeling whose source is often nonspecific or unknown to the individual (NANDA).	
DEFINING CHARACTERISTICS	
Increased tension	Insomnia
Apprehension	Poor eye contact
Painful and persistent increased helplessness	Voice quivering
Uncertainty	Diaphoresis
Fearfulness	Concern about changes in life events
Anxiousness/worry	Restlessness
Overexcitement	Cardiovascular excitation
Nervousness	Pupil dilation
Feelings of inadequacy	Sympathetic stimulation
Trembling	Superficial vasoconstriction
Fear of unspecific consequences	
RELATED FACTORS	
Psychologic/Environmental	
Physiologic Alterations: Unconscious conflict about values and goals; threat or change in health status; threat to self-concept.	
Developmental: Threat of death; situational/maturational crises; threat to or change in interaction patterns; unmet needs; threat to or change in role functioning; threat to or change in environment.	

Table 4.5 on page 66 gives an example of a nursing diagnosis related to the sensory/cognition group.

The Spiritual Belief Group

At the present time NANDA has developed one nursing diagnosis in this group: *Spiritual distress*. A diagnostic cue belongs in this group if it gives information about the client's

- Relationship with a higher power
- Religious life
- Belief system

Table 4.6 describes *Spiritual distress*.

Identifying Nursing Diagnoses

After you have grouped and clustered the diagnostic cues under one of the five psychosocial groups, you determine final nursing diagnoses. Compare each cluster to the defining characteristics of each diagnosis in the group until you determine an appropriate fit. Consider the following examples:

Mr. Apostolu, a 35-year-old man, was admitted to the local hospital emergency room after being arrested for driving under the influence of alcohol, causing an accident, and disturbing the peace. On admission Nina Jones, the emergency room nurse, tentatively diagnosed Mr. Apostolu's problem as *Ineffective individual coping* based upon the behaviors (abusive language, agitated movements, and irritability) she observed while admitting the client. Upon interviewing the client, Ms Jones discovered that Mr. Apostolu had been drinking heavily and had been involved in three car accidents since losing his job several months ago. The client's wife, who was also present, volunteered that he had become irritable and abusive toward her and the children since he lost his job, blaming them for his bad luck. Ms Jones added the additional clues gathered during the focused interview of Mr. Apostolu and his wife (heavy drinking, car accidents, loss of job, irritability, and abusiveness) to the original information. Ms Jones then sorted and categorized this data under the stress and coping group.

Table 4.3 Nursing Diagnosis Related to Roles and Relationships

SOCIAL ISOLATION

Definition: A state in which an individual experiences aloneness, which is perceived as a negative or threatened state imposed by others (adapted from NANDA and Lederer).

DEFINING CHARACTERISTICS

Major	Minor
Expressed feelings of rejection	Preoccupation with own thoughts
Expressed feelings of aloneness	Withdrawal
Absence of supportive significant other, family, friends, group	Display of behavior unacceptable to dominant cultural group
	Sad, dull affect
	Evidence of physical/mental handicap

RELATED FACTORS

Physiologic Alterations

Treatment Related: Medical condition (specify); treatment imposed isolation; alteration in physical appearance.

Psychologic/Environmental: Chemical dependence; psychologic impairment (specify).

Table 4.4 Nursing Diagnosis Related to Stress and Coping

INEFFECTIVE INDIVIDUAL COPING

Definition: A state in which an individual is unable to problem-solve or use adaptive behaviors to meet life's demands and roles (NANDA).

DEFINING CHARACTERISTICS

Verbalization of inability to cope	Change in usual communication patterns
High illness rate	High rate of accidents
Inability to ask for help	Evidence of physical/psychologic abuse
Verbal manipulation	Expressing unrealistic expectations
Inability to problem-solve	Reported substance abuse
Inability to meet basic needs	Alteration in societal participation
Destructive behavior toward self	Inability to meet role expectations
Inappropriate use of defense and others mechanisms	

RELATED FACTORS

Psychologic/Environmental: Maturational crisis; situational crisis.

Table 4.5 Nursing Diagnosis Related to Sensory Cognition

ALTERED THOUGHT PROCESSES	
Definition: A state in which an individual experiences an impairment in cognitive operations, such as conscious thought, reality orientation, problem solving, and judgment. These impairments are a result of mental/personality or chronic organic disorders that may be exacerbated by situational crises (adapted from Carpenito and Lederer).	
DEFINING CHARACTERISTICS	
Fearful thoughts	Memory deficit/problems
Hallucinations	Inaccurate interpretation of environment
Irritability	Distractibility
RELATED FACTORS	
Psychologic/Environmental: Mental disorders; substance abuse; personality disorder; organic mental disorder.	

Table 4.6 Nursing Diagnosis Related to Spiritual Distress

SPIRITUAL DISTRESS	
Definition: A state in which an individual experiences a disruption in his/her belief and value system that is a usual source of security and strength for the person (NANDA).	
DEFINING CHARACTERISTICS	
Major	Requesting objects associated with worship
Expressing concern with meaning of life/death and/or belief system	Questioning existence or fairness of deity
Minor	Questioning moral/ethical implications of therapeutic regimen
Asking, "Why did this happen to me?"	Feelings of hopelessness/abandonment
Expressing concern about nonadherence to dietary laws	Disruption in sleep pattern
Inability to participate in usual spiritual rituals	Refusal to accept visits from priest, minister, rabbi, and so on
Seeking spiritual counseling	Anger toward God
RELATED FACTORS	
Psychologic/Environmental: Discrepancy between spiritual beliefs and prescribed treatment; separation from religious/cultural ties; challenge to belief and value system; test of spiritual beliefs.	

When compared to the defining characteristics of the nursing diagnoses in the stress coping group, Mr. Apostolu's cues pointed to the nursing diagnosis *Ineffective individual coping*, validating Ms Jones's original nursing diagnosis.

In this case the nurse relied on the client's significant other, his wife, for important information. The nurse may also want to teach the client or the significant other how to assess when they should seek professional help for the client (see the accompanying box).

Client Self-Assessment: Psychosocial Function

Teach the client and family to observe the client and seek professional assistance if the client

- Experiences severe mood swings
- Has a pronounced change in behavior
- Is out of contact with reality
- Has unusual lapses of memory
- Is anorexic or has unexplained weight loss
- Complains of insomnia or other sleep disorders
- Verbalizes suicidal thoughts or demonstrates other signs of impending suicide

The following case study also demonstrates how diagnostic cues obtained during the assessment lead to nursing diagnoses related to psychosocial well-being and function.

Mr. Johnson, a transient passing through town, was admitted to the local hospital emergency room after being arrested for disturbing the peace and possession of heroin. The guards at the jail had brought him to the hospital after they were unable to control his violent behavior. When approached by the admitting nurse, Ms Quan, Mr. Johnson shouted, "Don't come near me with that gas machine! The High Lord has told me that I control the secret of life and death, and if you touch me you must die." The nurse recognized that Mr. Johnson had seen the stethoscope she carried as a "gas machine." After observing Mr. Johnson's manner and tone for a few minutes, she also noted that he was hearing voices. Ms Quan knew that Mr. Johnson's behavior could become violent if he continued to experience command hallucinations. She removed the stethoscope from around her neck and showed it to Mr. Johnson. She said, speaking in a quiet calm voice, "This is the stethoscope that I use to listen to my patient's heart. Sometimes I use it to take blood pressures. Would you like to look at it?" As Mr. Johnson doubtfully held the stethoscope and rapidly and repeatedly turned it over, she said, "Most stethoscopes are black and silver but mine is white and gold. I think it's nice looking, don't you?" Mr. Johnson threw the stethoscope back at Ms Quan, mumbling "OK." After a few minutes she said, "You've been brought to the hospital, Mr. Johnson. I'm Ms Quan, your nurse, and I'm here to take care of you. Have you noticed that even though I've been helping you remove your clothes, nothing has happened to me?" In this situation, the nurse showed Mr. Johnson respect and concern for his feelings and well-being. She did not, however, validate his abnormal perceptions about the stethoscope or acknowledge the voices he heard. Instead, she reinforced reality for him by describing the white-and-gold stethoscope and pointing out that he had no special power to harm her.

Ms Quan reviews all the data and sees the following factors as contributing to Mr. Johnson's problems:

- Substance abuse
- Transient lifestyle

She then clusters the information gained from the assessment and identifies the significant diagnostic cues demonstrated by Mr. Johnson:

- Hallucinations
- Delusions
- Illusions
- Fearful thoughts
- Irritability
- Inaccurate interpretation of environment

Then, after reviewing the assessment data, identifying contributing factors, and clustering the information, Ms Quan identifies the nursing diagnosis: *Altered thought processes*.

Summary

The holistic approach to nursing holds as a basic premise that the individual must be viewed as a total being, which is body, mind, and spirit continuously interacting with self and with the environment. The psychosocial assessment is a key component that must be integrated into the nurse's holistic approach to data collection. This assessment guides the nurse toward a true and accurate picture of the client as a total human being.

Key Points

- ✓ Psychosocial functioning includes the way one thinks, feels, acts, and relates to oneself and others; the ability to cope and tolerate stress; and the capacity for developing a belief system.
- ✓ Psychosocial health patterns include self-concept, roles and relationships, stress and coping, sensory and cognition, and spiritual and belief systems.
- ✓ The self-concept is the collection of feelings and beliefs one holds about oneself at any given time. It includes four components: body image, self-ideal, self-esteem, and personal identity.

- ✓ Role performance is the set of behaviors society expects of an individual in a certain position.
- ✓ Stress and coping patterns are behaviors an individual uses to deal with psychosocial and physical threats to safety.
- ✓ Sensory cognition patterns include the way an individual perceives and makes sense of the environment and the logical sequencing of thought and feelings.
- ✓ Spiritual and belief patterns reflect an individual's relationship with a higher power and the outward demonstration of that relationship.
- ✓ The sources of information for a psychosocial assessment include the health history; medical record; family, friends, and health care providers; psychologic testing, information from the focused interview; and observations of the client's general appearance, posture, gait, body language, and speech patterns.
- ✓ The nurse sorts and clusters data collected during a psychosocial assessment in one of the psychosocial function groups.

Chapter 5

Assessing Self-Care and Wellness Activities

This chapter presents techniques for assessing the client's self-care and wellness activities. Although physical and psychosocial aspects of a client's lifestyle are interrelated and must be considered together when arriving at a nursing diagnosis, this chapter focuses mainly on the physical aspects. Psychosocial assessment is covered in Chapter 4. Self-care and wellness activities are important, because a client's behavior in this area can affect health and well-being. You collect data about personal habits and activities of the client and determine whether they support or are detrimental to health.

Health practices are areas over which clients have some control. Clients do not make a conscious choice to catch a cold, for instance, but they can choose to exercise or to make their home environment safer. For this reason, client self-responsibility is a key component to keep in mind when you assess ADLs, sleep and rest, nutrition, exercise, and safety. Responsibility can be thought of as the ability to accept personal accountability when making decisions and engaging in activities that affect one's own quality of life and health status.

This chapter focuses on five major areas of client lifestyle: activities of daily living (ADLs), nutrition, sleep and rest, exercise, and safety. The goals of assessing these areas are twofold: (1) to provide an opportunity for you and the client to determine the impact of the client's present activities on health, and (2) to educate the client about health behaviors and lifestyle changes that the client can use to maintain or increase the current level of wellness.

Environmental factors such as education, economic status, family influences, stress, religion, and culture also influence wellness. These aspects are covered in Chapter 6.

Factors Affecting Physical Wellness

Activities of Daily Living

In the adult client, activities of daily living (ADLs) are those skills or abilities that the client needs for independent performance of self-care, communication, and mobility. Examples include obtaining and preparing food, using the telephone, and moving about in and out of the home. The client's ability to perform these activities contributes either positively or negatively to total health. In assessing ADLs, you determine whether the individual is able to perform self-care activities independently or requires the assistance of another, and whether performance of these activities supports or hinders the client's overall health.

The performance of ADLs is influenced by the client's cultural, economic, and spiritual background. Communication is also an important part of performing ADLs. The client who is unable to communicate in the dominant language may be unable to indicate needs or desires. That person may not be able to understand safety information or directions for the use of household equipment such as stoves, microwave ovens, or heaters.

Economic factors also influence performance of ADLs. For example, a client may be physically able to go to the grocery store but may have insufficient money to buy needed food. See Chapter 6 for more information regarding the impact of cultural, economic, and spiritual factors on the client's total health status.

Sleep and Rest

Obtaining adequate sleep and rest significantly influences an individual's quality of life and well-being as well as the ability to cope with physiologic and psychologic stressors. People who get enough sleep and are well rested are more likely to function at an optimum level and to be free from anxiety. Inadequate sleep and rest can contribute to personality and pathophysiologic changes and cognitive deficits. Because sleep and rest have a major impact on the health status of an individual (Hales 1992), you always assess these health practices when planning care for the client.

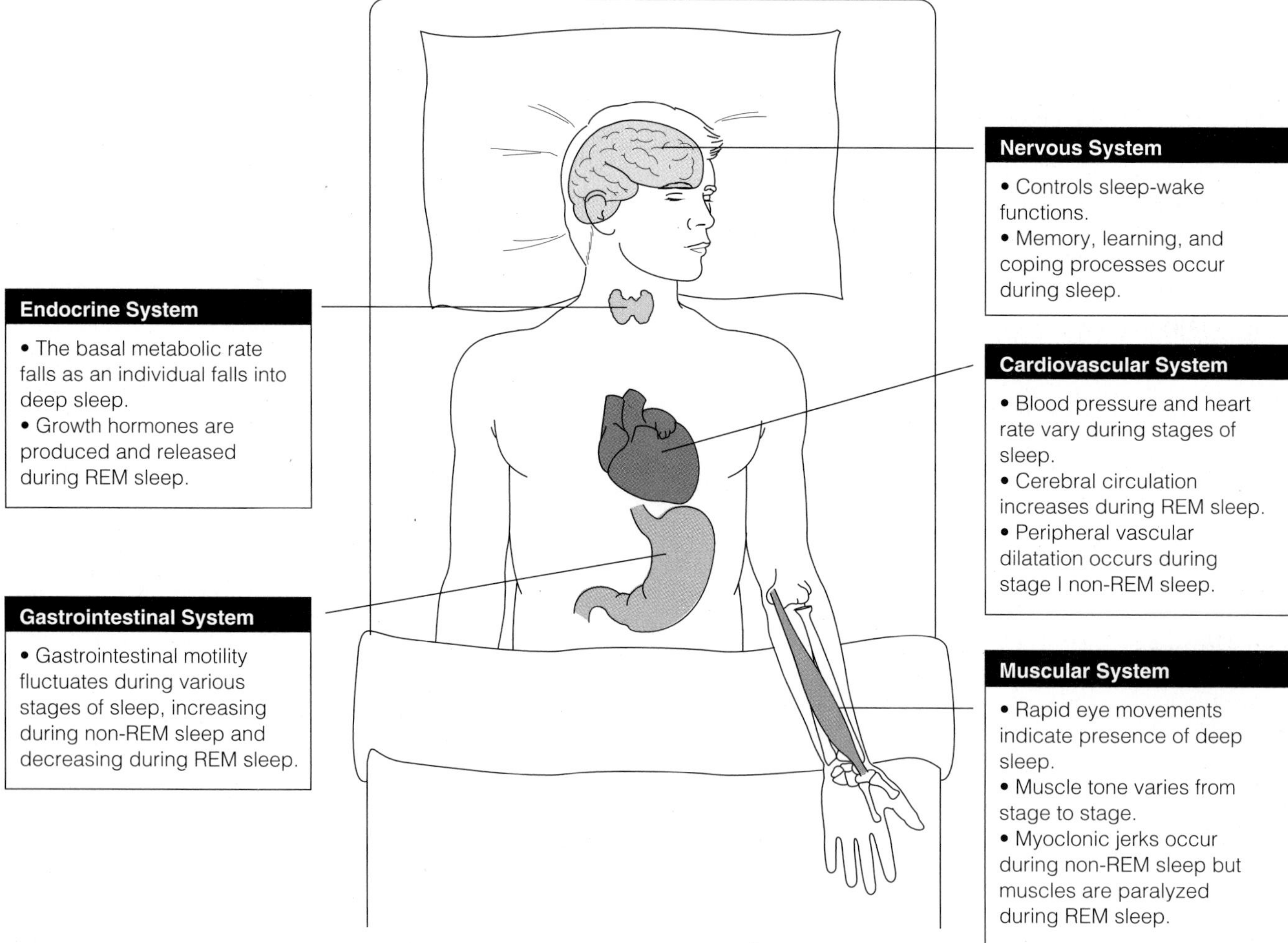

Nervous System
• Controls sleep-wake functions.
• Memory, learning, and coping processes occur during sleep.
Endocrine System
• The basal metabolic rate falls as an individual falls into deep sleep.
• Growth hormones are produced and released during REM sleep.
Cardiovascular System
• Blood pressure and heart rate vary during stages of sleep.
• Cerebral circulation increases during REM sleep.
• Peripheral vascular dilatation occurs during stage I non-REM sleep.
Gastrointestinal System
• Gastrointestinal motility fluctuates during various stages of sleep, increasing during non-REM sleep and decreasing during REM sleep.
Muscular System
• Rapid eye movements indicate presence of deep sleep.
• Muscle tone varies from stage to stage.
• Myoclonic jerks occur during non-REM sleep but muscles are paralyzed during REM sleep.

Figure 5.1 Relationship between body systems and sleep.

Sleep is a basic human need that involves both physiologic and psychologic restoration (Karvey and Anderson 1986). During sleep, a complex process occurs, mobilizing the neurologic, cardiovascular, endocrine, gastrointestinal, and musculoskeletal systems (Figure 5.1). Sleep and rest are associated with the build-up of body tissue (Adam and Oswald 1977), increased immune system function, increased production of growth hormones, and increased blood flow to the brain. Sleep also increases an individual's memory, learning powers, and stress-coping abilities.

You assess the client's sleep and rest patterns not only because sleep affects the client's overall health but also because health affects sleep. Sleep disturbances may signal other health problems.

Stages of Sleep Each sleep period is divided into two major categories differentiated by the presence of **rapid eye movements** (**REM sleep**) or their absence (**non-REM** or **NREM sleep**). During the first 60–90 minutes, the sleeper passes through gradually deepening non-REM sleep subdivided into stages I through IV. After the deep sleep of stage IV, the individual passes back through stage III and then stage II before entering REM sleep. The sleeping individual returns through stages II and III, and possibly IV, before ascending back up through the stages to repeat another REM phase. A complete cycle usually lasts approximately 60–90 minutes. Most adults repeat this cycle four or five times per night.

Although all stages of sleep are important for a person's well-being, stage IV and REM sleep are especially significant. In stage IV most of the body's restorative functions take place. Clients who are deprived of sleep do not benefit from these restorative effects. They may also exhibit erratic behavior, mood swings, and personality disorders.

Sleep Requirements The amount of sleep a person requires to function, carry out daily activities, and maintain health varies according to age and level of health as well as psychologic and environmental stressors. For instance, newborns and infants require the most sleep, spending from 12 to 16 hours in sleep per day (Olds et al 1992). As one grows older, sleep requirements gradually decrease; the older person may need as little as 5 or 6 hours a day to maintain health and function (Hoch and Reynolds 1986). The individual who is sick, overworked, or experiencing severe stress needs much more sleep than usual, probably because of the psychologic and physiologic restoration that takes place during sleep.

In assessing rest and sleep, determine whether the individual is able to obtain an adequate amount and quality of rest and sleep by collecting data on sleep and rest patterns as well as the client's subjective reports on how often she or he feels rested, tired, or exhausted.

Nutrition

Nutritional assessment is a very important component of the assessment of the whole person. Nutrition is evaluated in terms of the intake, storage, metabolism, and use of nutrients.

Function of Food Adequate intake of food contributes to the client's ability to maintain a high level of resistance to disease (Koop 1988). Clients require food that contains specific essential nutrients in order to repair body tissue and to promote growth (Barnett 1991). Food also supplies the energy needed for body processes and mobility.

Diet is influenced by many factors, including personal tastes, cultural practices, emotional factors, and level of knowledge regarding appropriate nourishment. Food also plays a role in family interactions and socialization, and some people view it as a reward or a source of emotional comfort. Dietary practices prevalent in North America include high intakes of "fast food," fat, and sugar. Thus, some degree of nutritional imbalance is common in North America, even though there is an abundance of nutritious food. Accurate assessment must include social and cultural influences on the client's current dietary practices. Cultural influences may be related to geographic region or to ethnic origin, or both. Chapter 6 includes additional information on assessment of cultural factors.

Dietary Guidelines In 1980 the United States Department of Agriculture (USDA) and the Department of Health and Human Services (DHHS) jointly recommended the following dietary guidelines for the general population:

- Eat a variety of foods.
- Maintain ideal body weight.
- Eat less fat, saturated fat, and cholesterol.
- Eat foods with adequate starch and fiber.
- Eat less sugar.
- Eat less sodium (including salt).
- If you drink alcohol, do so in moderation.

The USDA has also set forth a food-group plan, called the "food pyramid," to help individuals follow these guidelines (Figure 5.2 on page 72). The food pyramid is intended to emphasize the types and amounts of food that, in general, people should eat to remain healthy and reduce the risk of disease. This new food pyramid replaces the four basic food groups introduced by the USDA in 1956. The USDA recommends greater consumption of foods at the base of the pyramid and fewer servings of foods at the top of the pyramid.

When assessing the client's nutritional health practices, you should gather information regarding the client's understanding of and compliance with these guidelines. If the client does not follow the guidelines and is interested in improved nutrition, you should explore with the client what factors are interfering with good nutritional habits and how to overcome these barriers.

Exercise

Exercise is an important component of a healthy lifestyle. Regular physical exercise greatly benefits the individual: it

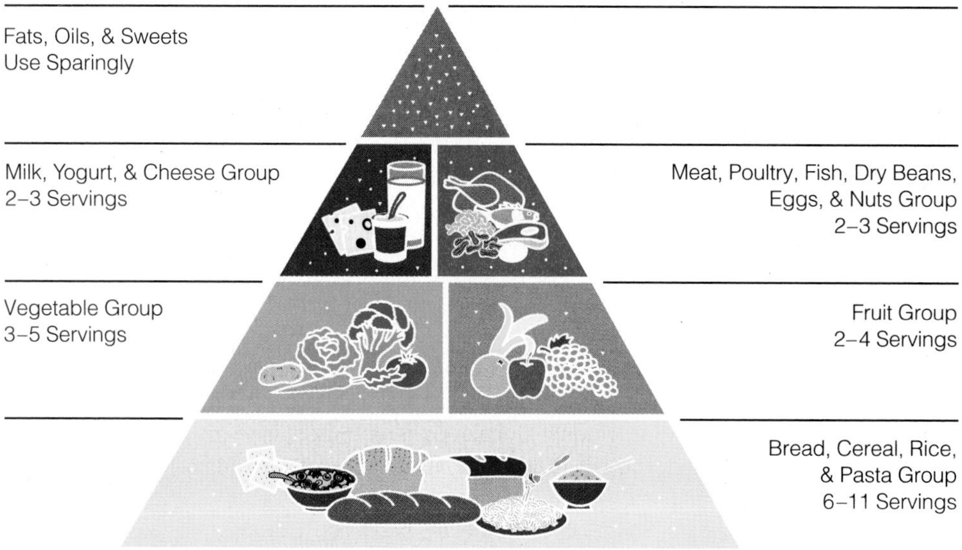

Fats, Oils, & Sweets
Use Sparingly

Milk, Yogurt, & Cheese Group
2–3 Servings

Meat, Poultry, Fish, Dry Beans, Eggs, & Nuts Group
2–3 Servings

Vegetable Group
3–5 Servings

Fruit Group
2–4 Servings

Bread, Cereal, Rice, & Pasta Group
6–11 Servings

Figure 5.2 The USDA food pyramid.

Table 5.1 Benefits of Physical Exercise

Musculoskeletal System

Increased muscle strength

Increased muscle tone

Muscle hypertrophy (increased muscle mass)

Increased muscular endurance

Increased muscular coordination and balance

Overall increase in lean muscle tissue

Increased joint mobility/flexibility

Bone density maintained or increased

Cardiovascular System

Decreased heart rate during rest and during exertion

Faster recovery of heart rate following exertion

Increased size of heart muscle, especially of left ventricle

Increased strength of heart muscle contraction

Increased stroke volume with each heartbeat

Increased collateral blood supply to heart muscle

Decreased systolic and diastolic blood pressure, especially if previously elevated

Increased efficiency of peripheral circulation, especially venous

Decreased potential for cardiac arrythmia

Respiratory System

Increased vital capacity and functional capacity at rest and with exertion

Increased diffusion of oxygen and carbon dioxide

Increased maximal oxygen consumption (increased effectiveness of muscle tissue in extracting oxygen from the blood)

Metabolism and Nutrition

Decreased serum triglyceride levels

Decreased serum cholesterol levels

Increased glucose tolerance

Improved perfusion of nutrients into body tissues and removal of metabolic wastes from body tissues

Overall decrease in body fat and improved long-term control of body fat

Bowel Elimination

Increased motility of gastrointestinal tract, decreasing the potential for constipation

Social, Emotional, and Intellectual

Decreased nervous tension related to psychologic stress

Increased ability to cope with stress

Improved self-concept and sense of well-being

Increased energy levels

Decreased tendency toward depression and anxiety reactions

Improved work performance

Improved quality of sleep

Source: Adapted from Cantu RC. *Toward Fitness: Guided Exercise for Those With Health Problems.* New York: Human Sciences Press, 1980.

prevents disease and improves physical and mental health and overall quality of life.

Benefits of Exercise A primary benefit of regular physical activity is protection against coronary artery disease (Marley 1982). In addition, exercise appears to provide some protection against such chronic diseases as hypertension, adult-onset diabetes, certain cancers, osteoporosis, and depression. It has positive effects on the functioning of the client's cardiovascular, respiratory, and musculoskeletal systems and enhances metabolism, nutrition, and bowel elimination. Exercise has also been found to enhance social, intellectual, and emotional status in individuals. See Table 5.1 for a description of the benefits of exercise.

Exercise Adherence Although the positive effects of exercise have been recognized in relation to enhancing individual health and supporting a healthy lifestyle, very few individuals include enough physical activity in their daily lives. Only 22% of adults in the United States engage in leisure-time physical activity at the recommended level. At least 24% of Americans are totally sedentary and never engage in beneficial physical exercise (U.S. Centers for Disease Control and Prevention and the American College of Sports Medicine 1993). You must not omit assessing this area of a client's lifestyle simply because the client looks healthy and physically fit, because lack of exercise is a risk factor for problems that may not appear for many years. You must assess the client's level of physical fitness to determine areas needing improvement to support a healthy lifestyle.

Exercise Recommendations You can use the following five criteria to assess physical fitness in the client: cardiorespiratory endurance, muscle strength and endurance, joint flexibility, body weight and composition, and motor skill performance. Table 5.2 describes criteria to observe in the client for each of these five areas.

In addition, you should also assess the client's exercise behavior in terms of frequency (how often), intensity (how hard), and duration (how long). The United States Centers for Disease Control and Prevention (CDC) and the American College of Sports Medicine (ACSM) have formulated the following recommendations for exercise:

1. Individuals should engage in a total of 30 minutes of moderate-intensity exercise over the course of most days of the week. The individual is not required to do all 30 minutes during one session, but can accumulate this total throughout the day. Walking, gardening, dancing, and walking up stairs (rather than taking the elevator) are all ways to incorporate more physical activity into daily life. People can also fulfill this recommendation through planned exercise or recreation such as tennis, swimming, or cycling.
2. Most individuals do not follow the recommendation of 30 minutes of moderate-intensity exercise daily, and almost all people should exercise more. People who do no exercise should begin by incorporating even a few

Table 5.2 Criteria for Distinguishing the Physically Fit and the Physically Unfit Person

Criterion	Physically Fit Person	Physically Unfit Person
1. Cardiorespiratory endurance	Decreased resting heart rate	Increased resting heart rate
	Increased resting stroke volume	Decreased resting stroke volume
	Can safely exceed baseline resting heart rate two or three times during strenuous exercise	No cardiorespiratory reserve with exercise; may overtax heart; danger of irregular heart rate with exercise
		Shortness of breath, chest pain, and skeletal muscle pain indicate inadequate perfusion of heart muscle and working skeletal muscle
2. Muscle strength and endurance	Firm muscle with increased tone	Flabby muscle with decreased tone
	Increased muscle size	Tone or muscle too tightly contracted, tight ligaments; decreased muscle size
	Increased muscle strength	Decreased muscle strength
	Increased muscle endurance	Decreased muscle endurance
3. Joint flexibility	Increased range of motion of joints (as measured in degrees of movement)	Decreased range of motion of joints (as measured in degrees of movement)
4. Body weight and composition	Ratio of weight to height is within normal limits	Ratio of weight to height is above normal limits (overweight)
	Percent of body fat is less than 15% in men, 25% in women	Percent of body fat is more than 16% in men, 26% in women
5. Motor skill performance	Performance demonstrates increased balance, power, agility, speed, reaction time, and coordination	Performance demonstrates decreased balance, power, agility, speed, reaction time, and coordination

Source: Kozier B, Erb G, Olivieri R. *Fundamentals of Nursing*, 4th ed. Redwood City, Calif.: Addison-Wesley Nursing, 1991.

minutes of exercise into their daily routine with the goal of eventually reaching 30 minutes per day (Figure 5.3). Activities to increase joint flexibility and muscle strength should also be included.

These guidelines are intended to encourage an increase in physical activity in all individuals. Assess the client's current level of activity to help the client identify and remove environmental and social barriers to exercise. You should also help the client identify how family and significant others as well as community agencies and resources can help support an active and thus more healthy lifestyle.

Safety

Clients' ability to protect themselves and prevent injury significantly contributes to a healthy lifestyle. Clients face actual and potential risks to personal safety every day, at home, work, and play. Each year, serious injuries have a greater impact on the overall health of individuals than the health effects of heart disease, cancer, and stroke combined (MacKenzie et al 1988).

Accidents and threats to personal safety may seem to happen by chance, but in fact the individual can control many of the risks to safety (Figure 5.4). Self-care, or the ability to take care of one's own personal health needs, includes the ability to identify and protect against actions and circumstances that can harm the individual.

When assessing safety, help the client to identify potential safety threats in several areas. Assess home safety, both inside the home (see the accompanying box) and in the yard and neighborhood, including use of yard equipment, air quality, neighborhood crime, and traffic. If the client is employed, also assess client safety in the workplace and collect data on actual and potential hazards, such as dangerous machinery, chemicals, loud noises, respiratory hazards, back and lifting injuries, radiation, cumulative trauma from improper workstation design, and extremes in temperature in the work environment.

As individuals work, so must they play. Remember to assess safety in regard to the client's leisure activities. Individuals who do not properly train for strenuous activities, or who

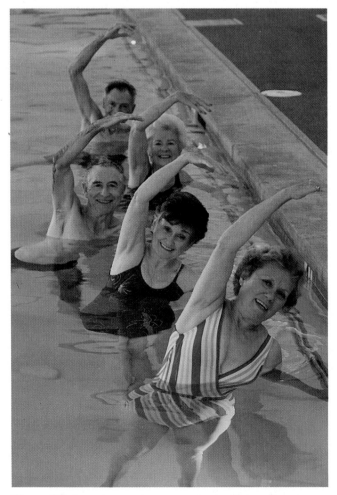

Figure 5.3 A regular exercise program has health benefits.

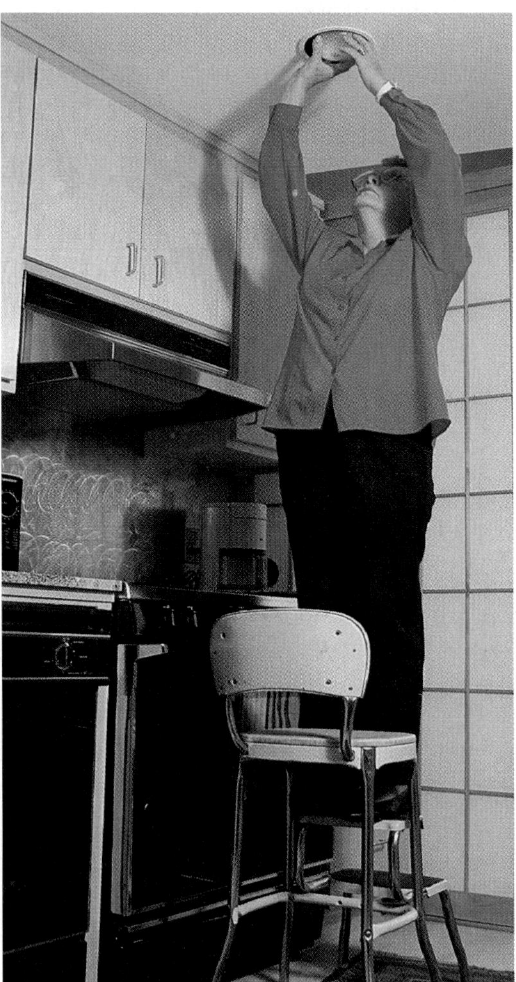

Figure 5.4 Clients often put their personal safety at risk when performing tasks around the home.

Adult Home Hazard Appraisal

Assess:

- *Walkways and stairways (inside and outside).* Note uneven sidewalks or paths, broken or loose steps, absence of handrails or placement on only one side of stairways, insecure handrails, congested hallways or other traffic areas, and inadequate lighting at night.
- *Floors.* Note uneven and highly polished or slippery floors and any unanchored rugs or mats.
- *Furniture.* Note hazardous placement of furniture with sharp corners. Note chairs or stools that are too low to get into and out of or that provide inadequate support.
- *Bathroom(s).* Note presence of grab bars around tubs and toilets, nonslip surfaces in tubs and shower stalls, adequacy of night lighting, adequacy of lighting for medicine cabinet, and need for raised toilet seat or bath chair in tub or shower.
- *Kitchen.* Note pilot lights (gas stove) in need of repair, inaccessible storage areas, and hazardous furniture.
- *Bedrooms.* Note adequacy of lighting, in particular the availability of night lights and accessibility of light switches. Assess floors and furniture as above.
- *Electrical.* Note unanchored and/or frayed electrical cords and overloaded outlets or those near water.
- *Fire protection.* Note presence or absence of fire extinguisher and fire escape plan, improper storage of combustibles, eg, gasoline, or corrosives, eg, rust remover (phosphoric acid), and accessibility of emergency telephone numbers (fire, police).
- *Toxic substances.* Note medications kept beyond date of expiration and improperly labeled cleaning solutions.

Source: Kozier B, Erb G, Olivieri R. *Fundamentals of Nursing*, 4th ed. Redwood City, Calif.: Addison-Wesley Nursing, 1991. Copyright ©1991 Addison-Wesley Publishing.

do not use appropriate safety equipment in high-risk activities such as hunting, horseback riding, skydiving, and rock climbing are at risk.

Finally, assess the client's attitude toward and knowledge of general safety practices. If the individual has self-care deficits in safety knowledge, gather data to help the client adopt healthy lifestyle behaviors.

Gathering the Data

Gather data regarding the client's lifestyle and health practices in each of the five areas described earlier: ADLs, sleep and rest, nutrition, exercise, and safety.

Gathering Data about ADLs

The purpose of gathering data about ADLs is to determine whether the client is able to use daily living skills independently. If the client needs assistance for some or all activities, determine whether assistance is available from family members, friends, neighbors, or professional caregivers. If the client is unable to function independently and assistance is not available, you must determine if alternative living arrangements are needed.

You assess ADLs most successfully by observing the client in the home. If you must conduct the assessment in a setting other than the client's home, you should ask the client or caregiver to provide historical information to supplement your observations. If you conduct the assessment in an institutional setting, include the use of any assistive devices (eg, eating utensils, grooming aides) in the assessment. The following questions will help you to gather data about the client's ability to perform basic ADLs:

Bathing/Hygiene Skills

1. Describe how you bathe or wash yourself.
2. Tell me about any problems you may have getting in and out of the shower or bath. *Clients with problems in balance or depth perception may be unable to lift the leg over the side of the bath.*
3. What safety equipment do you have available when taking a bath (eg, bath stool, nonslip mat)? *Safety equipment can prevent injury and increase the client's independence in bathing.*
4. Describe any assistance you need in bathing or washing. *Assistance may include the use of devices such as hand-held showers and/or human support for partial or complete bathing.*
5. Are you able to wash your hair? *Clients with arthritis, limited upper arm mobility, or poor vision may be unable to shampoo.*
6. After you have bathed, are you able to dry yourself completely? *Inability to dry all areas of the body and skin completely may result in skin breakdown from fungal or bacterial infections.*

Mobility and Transfer Skills

1. How do you get out of bed? Do you need assistance? *Clients with cardiovascular problems may experience dizziness if they get up from a lying position too quickly.*
2. Are you able to move around in bed without assistance? *Bedridden clients may have difficulty turning or changing positions in bed. This may lead to skin breakdown and the development of decubitus ulcers.*
3. Are you able to sit down in a chair without assistance? *Clients may have more difficulty sitting down in a deep, stuffed chair than a hard, straight-backed chair. If the client reports difficulty in sitting or getting up from a sitting position, identify if the difficulty is related to the type of chair.*
4. Are you able to get up from a sitting or lying position without assistance? *Clients with muscular weakness, hemiparesis, arthritis, or cardiorespiratory problems may have difficulty in moving to a standing position from a chair or bed.*
5. Are you able to walk without assistance? Do you have any discomfort when you walk? Short distances? Long distances? *Clients may report that they are able to walk unassisted but not be able to go very far. This might interfere with their ability to travel outside the home or to get adequate exercise.*
6. Do you use a cane, walker, or other assistive device to walk? How far are you able to walk with assistance? If you need assistance to walk, please describe the amount and type of assistance.
7. Are you able to climb stairs or steps without assistance? Do you use the handrail when climbing stairs? Are you able to manage the steps in your own home? If you have difficulty climbing stairs, describe the difficulty. *Sedentary clients and clients with cardiorespiratory problems may become short of breath when climbing stairs. Those with musculoskeletal or neuromuscular problems may have difficulty related to pain or muscle weakness when going up or down stairs. Use of the stair handrail prevents injury and increases the client's independence in stair climbing. Clients who are unable to manage the steps in their own home may have difficulty getting to an upstairs bathroom or may become socially isolated if they can't get out of their house.*
8. Do you require assistance for moving about? If so, describe the type and amount of assistance you require. *Clients may need assistive devices, such as a cane, walker, wheelchair, or human assistance for mobility.*
9. Do you use a prosthesis? How long have you used it?
10. Do you use a wheelchair?

Dressing Skills

1. Are you able to select your clothing and get it out of the closet or drawer without assistance? *Clients with visual problems may have difficulty selecting clothing. Those with muscle weakness may have problems taking the clothing out of the closet or drawers.*
2. Are you able to put on your clothing: underwear, socks or stockings, shoes, and outer clothes such as your dress, shirt, or trousers? *Female clients with limited range of motion in the upper extremities may have difficulty fastening a bra that hooks in the back. Clients with musculoskeletal limitations may not be able to reach their feet to put on socks or shoes.*
3. Describe any difficulty you have with buttons, zippers, or other fasteners on clothing. Do you have difficulty tying your shoelaces or buckling your shoes? *Clients with impaired manual dexterity related to arthritis or other musculoskeletal or neurologic problems may have difficulty fastening clothes or tying shoelaces. Clients with limited range of motion may not be able to fasten clothes with buttons or zippers in the back.*
4. If you require assistance in dressing or undressing, describe the amount and type of assistance needed.

Grooming Skills

1. Do you have difficulty brushing, combing, or styling your hair? Do you need assistive devices (eg, built-up brush handles)? *Clients with limited range of motion may have difficulty brushing, combing, or styling their hair. Older women may often adopt short hairstyles that are easier to maintain.*
2. If you wear makeup, do you have any difficulty applying it? *Clients with visual problems may have difficulty applying makeup.*
3. Are you able to shave? If not, who shaves you? *Clients with neurologic problems may not be able to manipulate a razor.*
4. Do you have difficulty caring for your fingernails or toenails? If so, does anyone help you? *Clients with limited range of motion or poor vision may have difficulty caring for their nails.*
5. Are you able to wash, iron, fold, and maintain your clothes? *Clients with decreased muscular strength, increased fatigue, cardiorespiratory illness, or musculoskeletal problems may have difficulty maintaining their clothing. Clients may adapt by purchasing clothing that doesn't require ironing and can be machine-washed.*

Eating Skills

1. Are you able to prepare your own meals? If not, where do you eat or how do you get your food? *Preparing meals requires the ability to hold pots and pans, manipulate the switches on the oven or stove, and turn faucets on the sink. Clients with muscular weakness or decreased dexterity may have difficulty performing these tasks.*

2. Describe any problems you may have feeding yourself. *Clients with physical limitations may have difficulty feeding themselves.*
3. Do you need assistance in cutting food?
4. Describe any difficulty in chewing or swallowing your food, including solid foods and liquids. Does food or drink get caught in your throat? *Clients who have suffered a stroke (cerebrovascular accident), have a disorder such as cerebral palsy, or experience dental problems may have difficulty swallowing solid foods or liquids. Solid foods may need to be cut in small pieces or pureed.*
5. Do you require any assistance for eating? Do you use any assistive devices such as built-up handles on your eating utensils? If you require assistance for eating or use assistive devices, describe the type and amount of assistance needed. *Clients who have limitations that affect eating may use adaptive devices to increase their independence. Clients who have paralysis or severe muscular weakness may need to be fed by another person.*

Shopping Skills

1. Are you able to get to the store to shop for food, clothing, and other basic needs? *Clients who have difficulty with ambulation or cannot drive or use public transportation will have difficulty shopping independently for basic needs.*
2. Are you able to walk through the grocery store, department store, mall, or other shops where you obtain your personal needs? *Clients who have difficultly in ambulation because of musculoskeletal, cardiorespiratory, neurologic, or psychosocial problems may be unable to ambulate for the time it takes to shop for personal needs.*
3. Are you able to select the items that you need? *Clients with visual problems may be unable to read labels.*
4. Are you able to carry your purchases home? *Clients with musculoskeletal, cardiorespiratory, or neurologic problems may be unable to carry purchases.*
5. Do you require any assistance for shopping? If so, describe the amount and type of assistance you need. *Clients who are unable to shop for personal needs may have family members, friends, or neighbors who assist them.*
6. Are you able to pay you bills independently by check? Are you able to balance your own checkbook? *Clients lacking manual dexterity or those with neurologic or psychologic problems may have difficulty performing these functions.*

Gathering Data About Sleep and Rest

In most cases, you gather little data about sleep and rest patterns during the initial interview unless the client indicates a problem in this area. If you identify a problem, gather additional information from the client, medical records, other health personnel (if the client is in a hospital or nursing home), family members, and from observations of the client. Sleep studies are another excellent source of information for assessing a client with sleeping problems. Electroencephalograms (EEGs), electromyograms (EMGs), and electrooculograms (EOGs) provide additional information about how the client progresses through the various stages of sleep, as well as the brain, muscle, and eye variations that occur during each stage.

The focused interview, however, is the most efficient way to obtain subjective information about the causes and effects of any sleep disturbances. During the interview, assess the client's sleep and rest history and patterns. If the client has kept a sleep diary, review it with the client at this time. The sleep diary should include complete information about the client's sleeping habits over the previous few weeks (see the accompanying box). The following are questions you can ask to collect data about the client's sleep and rest patterns.

Sleep Diary Contents

- Number of sleep periods during the previous 24-hour period
- Total number of hours of sleep (including naps)
- Length of time to fall asleep
- Time of onset of sleep at night
- Number of times awakened during the night
- Causes of awakening during the night
- Length of time required to go back to sleep
- Wake up time for the day
- Time, number, and length of daytime naps
- Location where sleep takes place
- Bedtime rituals (eg, warm bath, drinks, food, music)
- Usual sleeping position
- Unusual symptoms during sleep

Sleep History

1. Describe any past problems you have had sleeping.
2. Do you ever fall asleep in the middle of a conversation or some activity? *These behaviors may indicate an underlying neurologic disorder or a sleep and rest deficit.*
3. Does your spouse, family, or significant other complain that you have loud irregular snoring? *This behavior may be a sign of sleep apnea (the periodic cessation of breathing during sleep), especially when it is accompanied by frequent awakenings, irritability, and daytime drowsiness. Sleep apnea is most likely to occur during REM sleep.*

4. Have you ever walked in your sleep? If so, describe any incidence of this behavior that you remember or what others have told you about it. *Clients with a history of sleepwalking are at risk for injury during sleep.*

Sleep Patterns

1. Describe what you do to prepare for bed. What do you do to make yourself sleepy? *Knowledge of the client's bedtime rituals helps you plan activities to support and promote the client's sleep and rest.*
2. Describe the place where you sleep. *The client's sleeping environment may not be conducive to sleep.*
3. Have you recently changed the place where you sleep? *A change in the location, bed, or normal sounds a person hears at night may interfere with sleep and rest.*
4. What time do you go to bed? Get up?
5. How many hours of sleep do you average during the night?
6. In what position do you sleep during the night? *Clients who sleep propped up with pillows or in an upright position may have a respiratory condition that interferes with sleep. The client who sleeps in a supine position may experience respiratory obstruction due to the collapse of oropharyngeal soft tissues.*
7. How would you describe the quality of your sleep? Restful? Restless? *On the average, a person changes positions once every 20 minutes during stage IV sleep but seldom during REM sleep. Constant changing of position without periods of inactivity indicates that the person is getting little or no REM sleep.*
8. Do you feel rested after a full night's sleep? If not, describe how you feel.
9. Do you have trouble falling asleep? *Difficulty falling asleep can be a sign of anxiety or some other underlying disorder.*
10. Do you frequently awaken during the night or in the early morning and have difficulty returning to sleep? If so, describe the circumstances. *Frequent awakenings can be a sign of physical discomfort, mental stimulation, or anxiety.*
11. Do you take naps during the day? If so, how long do you sleep? *Frequent or long naps during the day tend to decrease the need for sleep at night.*
12. If you are having trouble sleeping, describe the circumstances surrounding the problem. When did the problem begin? How often does it occur? Have you tried to solve the problem?

Medications, Alcohol, and Substance Abuse

1. Are you taking any of the following drugs: hypnotics, barbiturates, sedatives, diuretics, amphetamines, or antidepressants? *These medications may contribute to disturbances in sleep and rest patterns.*
2. Do you eat or drink substances with caffeine or alcohol? *Heavy consumption of alcohol suppresses REM sleep, contributes to insomnia, and has been related to other sleep disturbances. Caffeine is thought to alter an individual's normal sleep-wakefulness patterns, resulting in insomnia and other sleep disorders.*
3. Do you wake up in the morning feeling "hung over" after taking sleeping pills? *Hypnotic drugs tend to cause excessive drowsiness and confusion during the day.*
4. Do you smoke? If so, describe your smoking habits. *Nicotine is a stimulant and disrupts sleep and rest patterns.*

Illnesses

1. Have you recently gained or lost weight? *Changes in weight appear to have an influence on the sleeping patterns of individuals.*
2. Do you have any illnesses that you know interfere with your sleep? If so, describe them. *The symptoms associated with some disease conditions may interfere with the client's normal sleep patterns.*
3. Do you have any of the following disease conditions:
   - Respiratory diseases, sinus problems, nasal congestion, asthma, or emphysema? *Respiratory problems that cause shortness of breath or impaired breathing interfere with a person's ability to sleep.*
   - Cardiac problems? *Chest pain and arrhythmias interrupt regular sleeping patterns. Clients with a history of heart disease may be afraid to sleep because they fear having a heart attack during the night. Periods of arrhythmias and hypertension are most likely to occur during REM sleep.*
   - Anxiety or depression? *Emotional disturbances interfere with a person's ability to fall asleep. Depression may cause early-morning awakening.*
   - Urinary problems? *Frequent urination during the night interrupts the sleep cycle.*
   - Arthritis or other rheumatoid disorders? *Painful joints may interfere with sleep.*
   - Hyper- or hypothyroidism? *Hypothyroidism reduces the time a client is in stage IV sleep. Hyperthyroidism may cause insomnia.*
   - Gastric ulcers? *Increased gastric motility and secretions occur during stage IV or non-REM sleep, resulting in gastric pain during each sleep cycle.*
   - Fever, liver or metabolic diseases, or migraine headaches? *These and a variety of other diseases cause anxiety, pain, or discomfort and may interfere with a client's ability to sleep.*

Lifestyle

1. Describe in detail any stress or major changes in your life that have happened recently. *Change or stress can interfere with the ability to sleep. Stressed individuals may not be able to relax enough to fall asleep. Stress can reduce the amount of stage IV and non-REM sleep.*
2. Would you describe your lifestyle as sedentary, moderately active, or very active? *Clients who lead an active lifestyle and include mild to moderate exercise in their routine tend to rest and sleep better.*
3. Has lack of sleep affected your ability to function during the day? If so, describe how. *Fatigue reduces REM sleep. REM periods become longer as the client rests.*
4. If you work, does your work schedule rotate between day and night shifts? If so, describe your work schedule over the past few months. *Changes in a person's sleeping routine may contribute to insomnia, emotional problems, and disturbances in coordination.*
5. Have you made any long-distance trips recently? Do you travel long distances routinely? *Long-distance trips may disrupt a client's normal sleep-wake patterns, reducing mental alertness and energy, and causing insomnia and gastrointestinal disturbances.*

Gathering Data about Nutrition

In addition to using a focused interview to collect information about the client's nutritional practices, you can use tools such as the 24-hour dietary recall and the dietary inventory. In the 24-hour dietary recall, the client records all food and fluid ingested during the previous 24 hours. The dietary inventory asks the client to record in a notebook or journal all food eaten over 1 week or 3 days. Use this information to supplement the information you collect during the focused interview. You can ask the following questions to obtain information regarding the client's nutritional practices.

Dietary Recommendations

1. How many servings of the following foods do you eat each day: bread, bagels, muffins, cereal, rice, bulgur, barley, kasha, pasta, pretzels, rice cakes, crackers, corn tortillas? *Individuals who do not eat at least a total of 6 to 11 servings of these foods from the "bread, cereal, rice, and pasta" group of the food pyramid may not be receiving adequate nutrients in their diet.*
2. What type of vegetables do you eat? How often? *In its food pyramid, the USDA recommends a total of 3 to 5 servings each day of vegetables, including the following: fresh vegetables such as broccoli, carrots, and peas served without cheese or butter; leafy vegetables such as romaine lettuce, spinach, and collard greens; and starchy vegetables such as corn, white potatoes, and sweet potatoes.*
3. What type of fresh fruit do you eat? How much? How often? *Individuals who do not eat of total of 2 to 4 servings daily of fresh fruit and fruit juice may not be receiving adequate nutrients in their diet.*
4. Do you eat dairy products like milk, yogurt or cheese? If so, how much and how often? *In its food pyramid, the USDA recommends a total of 2 to 3 servings daily of foods from the "milk, yogurt, and cheese" group, including nonfat or 1% milk, nonfat or low-fat yogurt and cheese, frozen yogurt, ice milk, and sherbet.*
5. Describe the amount of meat, fish, poultry, dried beans, eggs, and nuts you usually eat in one day. *In its food pyramid, the USDA recommends a total of 2 to 3 servings daily of foods from the "meat, poultry, fish, dried beans, eggs, and nuts" group, including lean cuts of meat, poultry with skin removed, fresh fish and shellfish, water-packed tuna, dried beans, dried peas, dried lentils, eggs, and unsalted nuts.*
6. Describe ways you limit the amount of fats, oils, and sweets in your diet. *In its food pyramid, the USDA recommends that these foods be consumed sparingly. Excess consumption of fats, oils, and sweets may increase the individual's risk of obesity.*

General Nutrition

1. Describe any recent problems you have had with eating. *Difficulty in eating may have a negative impact on nutrient intake and nutritional status.*
2. Have you had a change in appetite recently? *Changes in appetite can result in either under- or overconsumption of nutrients.*
3. Have you had a change in weight? If so, how many pounds? Over what period of time?
4. Have you had any recent surgery, trauma, burns, or infection? *These conditions may alter normal nutrient requirements.*
5. How is your diet influenced by cultural or religious factors? *Cultural and religious factors may influence the amount and type of food, and the nutrient intake of the individual.*
6. Describe your typical eating patterns. Describe what you usually eat at each meal/snack you have each day.
7. Are you on a special diet? Do you have any specific food likes or dislikes? Do you have any food allergies? *Any of these conditions may alter the nutritional intake of the individual.*
8. Where do you eat?
9. Do you drink alcohol? If so, how much per day or week? What kind? *Excessive alcohol consumption may reduce food intake.*

10. How much coffee, tea, cola, and cocoa do you drink each day? *Excess caffeine consumption can affect the individual's appetite.*

Food Preparation

1. What facilities are available for meal preparation? *Limited meal-preparation facilities may hinder the individual's ability to prepare food to meet nutritional requirements.*
2. Who prepares your meals?
3. Is your income adequate to buy the food you need? Do you use food stamps? *Clients with limited income may have difficulty purchasing the type and amount of food they need.*
4. Do you have adequate refrigeration and storage facilities? *Clients with inadequate storage and refrigeration facilities may be at risk for food-borne diseases.*

Associated Behaviors

1. Do you have sores in your mouth? Do you have problems with your teeth or dentures? *Individuals with oral problems may have difficulty ingesting food.*
2. Do you have difficulty chewing or swallowing? If so, is this associated with certain foods? With certain situations? *Difficulty in ingesting food may result in nutrition being less than required for optimal health.*
3. Have you had any nausea or vomiting? If so, is this associated with certain foods or situations?
4. Have you had any diarrhea or constipation? If so, for how long? *These conditions can prejudice nutritional status. They can also sometimes be reduced or eliminated by dietary changes.*
5. Do you take any prescription medications? Do you take any vitamin, mineral, or nutritional supplements? *Medications can interfere with absorption of nutrients. The individual may or may not need these vitamin and nutritional supplements.*
6. Have you had any surgery that may affect your nutritional status such as intestinal bypass?

Gathering Data about Exercise Patterns

You can use information from a focused interview along with clinical measures of physical fitness from the physical assessment to determine the client's exercise habits. You can ask the following questions to gather more information about the client's daily exercise patterns.

Activity Level

1. Describe your usual activity level: inactive, moderately active, or very active. *Most individuals do not get enough daily physical activity.*
2. Describe the amount of physical work you usually are required to do in the course of a day. Week. *People who engage in vigorous physical labor routinely exhibit higher fitness levels than those in sedentary jobs.*
3. List the types of physical activity you typically engage in during the day. Week. *Individuals who exercise infrequently do not derive enough benefits from that exercise to remain physically fit.*
4. Describe how you increase the amount of physical activity in your daily life (eg, taking stairs rather than an elevator). *Even daily activities may promote fitness in individuals.*

Duration of Activity

1. Do you engage in some sort of vigorous physical activity for a total of 30 minutes most days of the week? *A total of at least 30 minutes of moderate activity most days of the week has been shown to have health benefits.*
2. Do you regularly engage in some sort of recreational activity? If so, what and how often? *People are more likely to participate in enjoyable physical activity than routine formal exercise.*

Strength

- Describe what you do to improve and maintain your muscle strength. Back strength. *Exercise should include a strength component to prevent back problems and bone density loss, increase muscle strength and tone, and increase coordination and balance.*

Intensity of Exercise

- When you do engage in vigorous physical activity, does your pulse increase? Do you feel slightly out of breath? *To produce health benefits, physical activity must be vigorous enough to increase pulse rate to safe levels.*

Stretching

- Do you perform stretching exercises daily? *Stretching increases flexibility and reduces potential for injury.*

Gathering Data about Safety Practices

Because the ability of individuals to protect themselves against injury is critical to a healthy lifestyle, you must assess client practices in this area. You can ask the following questions during the focused interview to gather information on personal safety practices.

Safety in the Home

1. Describe how you maintain your home to reduce the risk of accidents to yourself and others (eg, adequate

lighting, uncluttered hallways, handrails on stairs, repairs to broken windows and flooring). *Proper repair and maintenance reduce the risk of accidents in the home.*

2. Have you placed fire extinguishers throughout the home? Do you have a plan to exit from your home in case of fire? *These measures reduce the risk of injury from household fires.*
3. Do you keep medications and household cleaning solutions in separate areas to reduce risk of poisoning? *Keeping medications and cleaning supplies separate reduces the chance of accidental poisoning. Individuals with vision problems may have difficulty distinguishing between labels.*
4. Describe what actions you would take if you or someone else was accidently poisoned or became ill in your home. *Knowing what to do in cases of accidental poisoning, such as calling 911, can save lives.*
5. Do you have a telephone? Are emergency phone numbers posted near your telephone?
6. If you have difficulty seeing, are you able to use the numbers on the telephone? *People with vision difficulties may have trouble using the telephone.*
7. If you live alone, does someone keep in touch with you daily?
8. Do you smoke in bed? *Smoking in bed significantly increases the risk of accidental fire in the home.*
9. If you spill or drop something, do you clean it up right away? *Slips and falls in the home are a serious safety risk, particularly among the elderly.*
10. Are carpets and rugs firmly attached to the floor or of the nonslip variety? *Loose floor coverings increase the risk of slips and falls.*
11. Describe what measures you take to avoid cooking accidents such as spills, burns, or fires.
12. If a family member or other member of your household harmed or injured you, what would you do?

Safety Outside the Home

1. Do you feel safe when walking alone in your neighborhood? If not, describe what you do, if anything, to protect yourself. *Individuals need to be aware of their surroundings. Failing to take precautions when needed, such as not walking alone or not learning how to reach emergency help, may increase their risk of injury.*
2. Do you live in a high-crime neighborhood or area of high gang activity? If so, what do you do to keep from becoming a victim? *Individuals living in high-crime or gang-dominated neighborhoods need to be aware of these threats to personal safety. You should help them explore ways of not becoming involved in crime or gang violence or the victim of it.*
3. Are you able to cross streets safely when traveling on foot? *In areas of high traffic, individuals with visual, musculoskeletal, or neurologic difficulties may be at increased risk when crossing busy streets.*
4. If you ride a bicycle, describe what you do to avoid accidents. Do you wear a bicycle helmet?
5. Do you feel safe when you take public transportation? If not, describe what steps you take to avoid being robbed, mugged, or assaulted? *If the client needs to use public transportation yet feels it is not safe, help the client explore ways to find alternative transportation or to reduce the risk of injury from violence when using public transportation, such as traveling with a companion or sitting close to the bus driver.*
6. If you drive a car, do you wear seat belts? Do you drive after you have been drinking? Do you obey the speed limit? *Speeding, driving after drinking, and not wearing seat belts increase the risk of accidents.*

Safety at Work

1. Do you work in what you would consider a dangerous job? If so, describe why you feel this way.
2. Do you work around machinery with moving parts? *Clothing or limbs may become caught in machinery, causing personal injury.*
3. Describe the noise level in your work environment. *Continued exposure to high levels of noise may eventually impair hearing. Clients need to use hearing-conservation equipment (eg, ear plugs) in these areas.*
4. Are you exposed to any chemicals or environmental hazards on the job (eg, smoke, radiation, acids, corrosive chemicals)? *These hazards may increase the individual's chance of becoming injured or ill on the job. Teach clients to use proper protective clothing and equipment and to follow safety procedures.*
5. Describe any lifting you do on the job. *Back injuries are a significant hazard when the job requires lifting.*
6. Does your job require a great deal of repetitive motions involving your hands or wrists? If so, describe them. *Individuals whose jobs require repetitive wrist or hand motion may be at increased risk for cumulative trauma injuries.*
7. Do you work in an extremely hot or cold environment? *Extremes in temperature may put the individual at risk for disorders such as frostbite or heat stroke.*
8. Describe what you would do if you or someone else were injured on the job. *If the individual does not know what to do in an emergency or how to obtain emergency help, you should help the client identify what to do in emergency situations at work.*

DIAGNOSTIC REASONING IN ACTION

Dorothy Stein, a 25-year-old mother of 6-week-old twin daughters, was returning to the Metropolitan Free Clinic for a routine 6-week postpartum checkup. On arrival she was greeted by Jesse Myers, the registered nurse practitioner who would be performing Mrs. Stein's examination that morning. During the initial interview, Mrs. Stein appeared anxious and tired. She stated that she had not had one full night's sleep since returning home from the hospital with the twins. "I can't get their schedules together," she said. "As soon as I get one baby to sleep, the other one wakes up. They never seem to sleep at the same time, day or night. Sometimes I can catch a nap but that's seldom."

Mrs. Stein also expressed concern that she had gained weight since the delivery of the twins. "I get so frustrated about being tired that I seem to just automatically go to the refrigerator and grab something to eat to make me feel better. I know that exercising, even going for a walk, would help me lose weight, but I don't seem to have time to do anything but take care of the twins."

Ms Myers observed Mrs. Stein wiping tears from her eyes as she related these incidents. Mrs. Stein appeared tired. Her clothes were wrinkled, and her hair was uncombed.

Ms Myers noted some significant diagnostic clues demonstrated by Mrs. Stein which led her to identify the nursing diagnosis of *Sleep pattern disturbance:* interrupted sleep, daytime napping, feeling tired, and irritability. Her disheveled appearance indicated a *Self-care deficit: dressing/grooming.* The weight gain and frequent snacking led Ms Myers to identify a nursing diagnosis of *Altered nutrition: more than body requirements.* Ms Myers also noted that Mrs. Stein's concern over not being able to find time to exercise combined with her weight gain could lead to a nursing diagnosis of *Body image disturbance,* if a focused interview reveals that she is distressed about her appearance.

Factors contributing to Mrs. Stein's problems included: newborn twins, new environment in the home, concern about weight and ability to exercise, and concern about fatigue.

Ms Myers discussed with Mrs. Stein the option of hiring a babysitter to care for the twins for a few hours during the week so that she could nap. She also suggested that Mrs. Stein discuss her fatigue with her husband and request his help in caring for the twins evenings and weekends. She also gave Mrs. Stein a copy of the food pyramid and recommended some healthy snacks such as fruit and carrot sticks that Mrs. Stein could eat for quick energy. As she left the clinic, Mrs. Stein remarked, "Maybe I can get my niece to babysit after school. Who knows? Maybe I could even find time to take a bubble bath!"

Identifying Nursing Diagnoses

After collecting information from the focused interview in each of the five areas, sort the data into groups of related data or clusters of data that point to nursing diagnoses and/or collaborative problems.

The case study above demonstrates how the nurse gathers information about the client's lifestyle and health practices, analyzes and groups the data into clusters, and formulates nursing diagnoses.

Summary

You assess lifestyle and health practices during the focused interview to gather information not only about the client's deficits and health problems but also about the client's strengths. You can use this information to support and optimize the individual's health status and to prevent potential problems. You can organize the data and use it to develop nursing diagnoses and subsequent nursing interventions that can take the client beyond the mere absence of disease to a higher state of optimal health and wellness.

Key Points

- ✓ All aspects of a client's lifestyle are interrelated, and you must consider them together when arriving at a nursing diagnosis.
- ✓ Clients' lifestyles and health practices can affect their health and well-being.
- ✓ You use data collected about the client's personal health habits to determine whether the client's lifestyle supports health.

- ✓ The five major areas of client lifestyle to assess are activities of daily living, sleep and rest, nutrition, exercise, and safety.
- ✓ Information gathered during the assessment can provide a basis for making decisions related to promoting the client's health.
- ✓ Lifestyle and health practices are an area over which clients can make conscious choices and over which they have some control.
- ✓ It is the responsibility of the client, supported by the nurse, to take positive steps to prevent health problems. The client and the nurse work collaboratively to develop a plan to support or modify existing self-care practices to promote individual health.
- ✓ Activities of daily living (ADLs) are those skills that the client needs for the independent performance of self-care.
- ✓ The client's performance of ADLs is influenced by cultural, economic, and spiritual factors.
- ✓ Clients' ability to secure adequate sleep and rest can influence their physical, psychologic, and social well being.
- ✓ Sleep fulfills a basic human need by providing both physical and psychologic restoration.
- ✓ Nutritional practices can affect the body's ability to maintain a high level of energy, resist disease, repair body tissue, and promote growth.
- ✓ Dietary practices are influenced by personal preferences, culture, emotional factors, and knowlege regarding appropriate diet.
- ✓ Client food choices should be guided by the USDA food pyramid.
- ✓ Regular exercise promotes improved physical and mental health as well as improved overall quality of life and disease prevention.
- ✓ Few individuals include enough vigorous physical activity in their daily lives.
- ✓ You should assess physical fitness in the client in terms of cardiorespiratory endurance, muscle strength, flexibility, body weight, and motor skill performance.
- ✓ Evaluate exercise in each of these areas for intensity, duration and frequency.
- ✓ Clients' ability to protect themselves from injury and promote a safe environment can significantly improve their health.
- ✓ Individuals can control many of the risks that lead to accidents and injury.
- ✓ Assess the client's potential threats to personal safety in the home, neighborhood, and workplace.
- ✓ Use the focused interview to gather data in each of the areas of the client's lifestyle.
- ✓ Information gathered during the assessment must be organized into groups of related data or clusters of data.
- ✓ From these clusters of data, you identify nursing diagnoses that help you promote a healthy lifestyle for the client.

Chapter 6

Assessing the Family, Culture, and Environment

The client's environment includes all of the external factors that affect life and health. It encompasses the limited physical geographic region where the client dwells, as well as the social environment, including the client's culture, community, work group, and family. People interact with and are influenced by their environment every moment of their lives.

Because environmental factors can significantly affect the client's lifestyle as well as the client's physiologic and psychosocial health, they are a critical part of the total health assessment.

Environmental influences on individual health and lifestyle are quite varied. They include physical environmental factors such as safety at home and in the community (see Chapter 5 for detailed information on assessing client safety). In addition, the individual's work environment can have a significant influence on health and wellness. For example, individuals who work in noisy, confined, hot, cold, or dusty environments can suffer significant alterations in health. Other environmental factors that can have either positive or negative effects on individual health include social, family, economic, religious, education, and cultural influences. This chapter examines in detail how you assess these areas to determine whether any actual or potential hazards to lifestyle and well-being exist. You can then use this information to identify aspects of the client's environment that may need to be enhanced or supported to promote or maintain health.

Relationship of Environmental Influences to Health and Well-Being

Environmental influences on individual behavior and lifestyle are particularly important in the areas of self-care, disease prevention, and health promotion. For example, individuals with low economic status may not be able to purchase adequate food to maintain nutritional status at an optimum level, increasing their risk for disease. Or, in a family environment where the father is the decision maker, other family members may not be encouraged to make decisions that promote health.

The relationship of environmental influences to health has been acknowledged since the earliest days of nursing practice. Florence Nightingale focused on assessing the impact of the physical environment on health by providing clean air, fresh water, light, and good hygiene for those under her care. Today, environmental influences are looked at more holistically and include the social and cultural environment. In addition, nurses do not wait until a client is ill as Florence Nightingale did to gather data to determine if environmental factors enhance or inhibit health. Instead, the nurse is concerned with whether the environment supports wellness and disease prevention, even for the currently healthy client. The nurse then develops nursing diagnoses and interventions to move the client toward optimal health and wellness.

The relationship of health and wellness to environmental influences is illustrated in Figure 6.1. This model proposes two axes: the health axis and the environmental axis. The health axis extends from death to peak wellness. Between these two points lie serious illness, minor illness, absence of illness, and good health. The environmental axis extends from a very unfavorable environment to an extremely favorable one and reflects physical, biologic, and psychosocial factors affecting the individual's health (Dunn 1959). The two axes form four quadrants:

1. Poor health in an unfavorable environment (eg, a sick baby whose mother is afraid to take the child to see a community clinic because of neighborhood violence).
2. Poor health in a favorable environment (eg, a brittle diabetic who has access to medications, proper diet, and health care teaching).
3. High-level wellness in an unfavorable environment (eg, a mother who despite family responsibilities and demands on her time still takes the time to eat sensibly and to make healthy food choices for herself and her family).
4. High-level wellness in a favorable environment (eg, a physically fit individual who has the time, family support, and financial resources to eat wholesome food and exercise daily).

In this model of environmental influences on health, the goal of high-level wellness for an individual is a lifestyle and method of functioning that maximizes health potential within the individual's environment (Dunn 1959). People can also take steps to improve an environment that does not promote their personal health and wellness. For instance, a busy mother with numerous family demands and limited time for personal exercise could improve her environment by obtaining child care so that she has time to exercise.

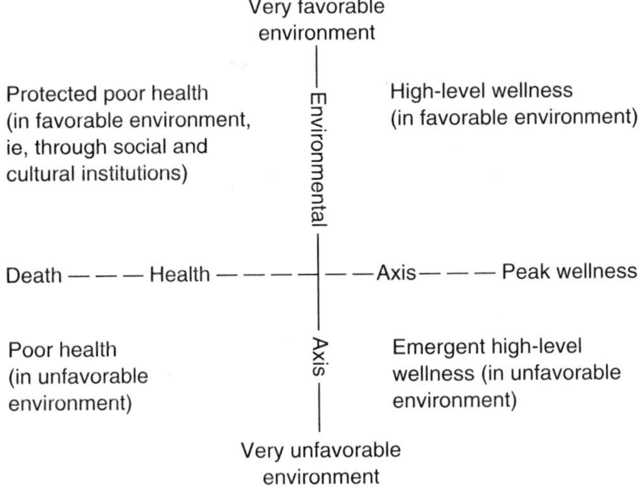

Figure 6.1 Dunn's Model of Wellness.

Assessing Major Environmental Influences

Socioeconomic

Social Influences The individual's social environment consists of people and organizations with which the individual interacts. It includes family (which is reviewed in detail in the next section), friends, peers, and coworkers. It also includes the community, because the individual's interaction with the community and neighborhood can influence health status. For example, people living in a neighborhood dominated by gangs may be unwilling to go to the store to secure needed food because they fear for their personal safety. This fear could prejudice their nutritional status and overall health. The community can also support and enhance individual health. Strong neighborhood social groups and community clinics can provide services that enhance physical and mental health.

Human beings are social creatures. Individuals need interaction with other individuals to achieve an optimum state of wellness. An individual's social network and support systems have a positive impact on physical and psychologic health (Muhlenkamp and Sayles 1986).

Remember that social factors not only influence other areas of the client's lifestyle (eg, the late-night social habits of an individual's peers may affect that person's sleep and rest patterns) but also interact with other environment influences. For example, in some cultures adolescent girls may not go out unchaperoned, and this practice may define the type of social relationships an adolescent female is allowed to have with her peers.

Family Influences The family environment, because it is one of the primary contexts in which health-promoting activities can occur, is therefore potentially the most immediate source of health-related support and education for the individual. Assess whether family attitudes and behavior regarding nutrition, sleep and rest, exercise, hygiene, and safety practices are affecting the individual's health and wellness. For instance, children from families who expect people to eat everything on their plates may consume more food than needed for good nutrition. These children are at risk for obesity.

When you perform the health assessment, remember that family health attitudes and behaviors are embedded in the family's cultural background. Some Native Americans with traditional cultural orientations do not believe in the germ theory of disease. In this instance, you would need to assess whether this cultural viewpoint might affect attitudes toward childhood immunization.

Family health attitudes and behaviors may also be positively or negatively affected by socioeconomic influences. For example, even in a family that values health highly, prenatal or well-child care may still be deferred if obtaining food or shelter becomes a higher priority. By contrast, in a family that values health and has ample financial resources, a health club membership for all family members may be a priority.

Assessment of the family means looking at how family members interact, depend on each other, and function as a social unit. It includes assessment of whether the family's internal and external relationships support health and wellness or are dysfunctional, perhaps requiring intervention. Also assess coping styles of the family group as well as of individual members to determine family stress levels, which could inhibit both individual and family health and wellness.

The U.S. Bureau of the Census (1985) defines family as, "two or more people related by birth, marriage, or adoption who reside in the same household." Friedman (1992) expands the definition of family to "two or more persons who are joined together by bonds of sharing and emotional closeness and who identify themselves as being part of a family." This definition allows for a wider range of family composition and more closely describes today's varied family lifestyles (Figure 6.2). Family structures in contemporary society are diverse and include but are not limited to the following structures.

The Traditional Nuclear Family The decline of the traditional nuclear family (mother-nurturer, father-provider, and children) is one of the most dramatic social transformations in recent history. According to the 1990 U.S. Census, the nuclear family represents only 26% of all households (U.S. Bureau of the Census 1991). Nontraditional nuclear families (which include a married couple but differ from the traditional model) include the dual-worker family, the childless family, the adoptive family, and the stepfamily.

The Extended Family In an extended family, the nuclear family shares the home with parents, siblings, or other close relatives. The children are then reared by a large network of adults. Extended families are common in some Native American, Chinese, and Middle Eastern cultures.

The Single-Parent Family It is estimated that over 50% of children in the United States live in a single-parent family: a home headed by one adult. The adult may be single by choice or because of divorce, death of a spouse, or separation. Single-parent families are most likely to be headed by a female who balances parenting and provider roles.

Nontraditional Family Forms Nontraditional family structures include but are not limited to communal families (two or more families living together in one dwelling), gay and lesbian families, and families in which the children are raised by grandparents or by older siblings.

Family Roles Family roles describe the divisions of labor in the family and its communication patterns. Each individual in the family occupies a role (eg, husband-father, wife-mother, daughter-sister, or son-brother). Each of these roles is associated with behavioral expectations. These expectations are affected by both family structure and culture. Roles also change over time as the family grows and develops. The advent of multiple family structures has meant a blurring of roles. In today's society, many roles are less closely identified with gender than previously. For example, the father who stays at home to care for children assumes the traditionally female nurturer role, whereas the mother who works outside the home assumes the traditionally male provider role.

Assess the individual's family environment to determine whether it supports or detracts from the individual's physiologic and psychologic health and wellness. For instance, a single working mother raising three children may not have the time to prepare a nutritionally balanced evening meal for the family as she struggles to balance parenting and provider roles, thus potentially endangering the nutritional status of the entire family.

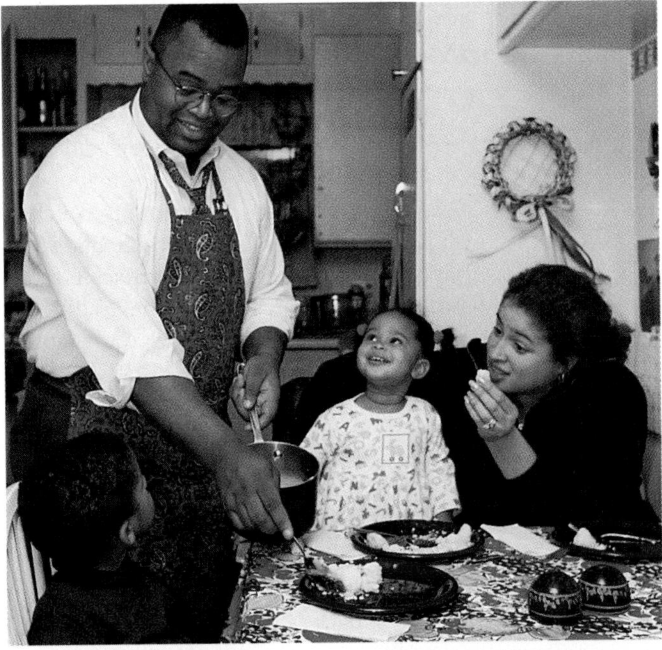

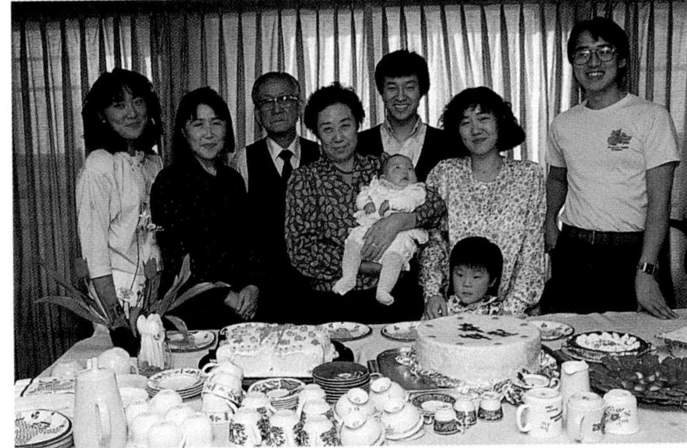

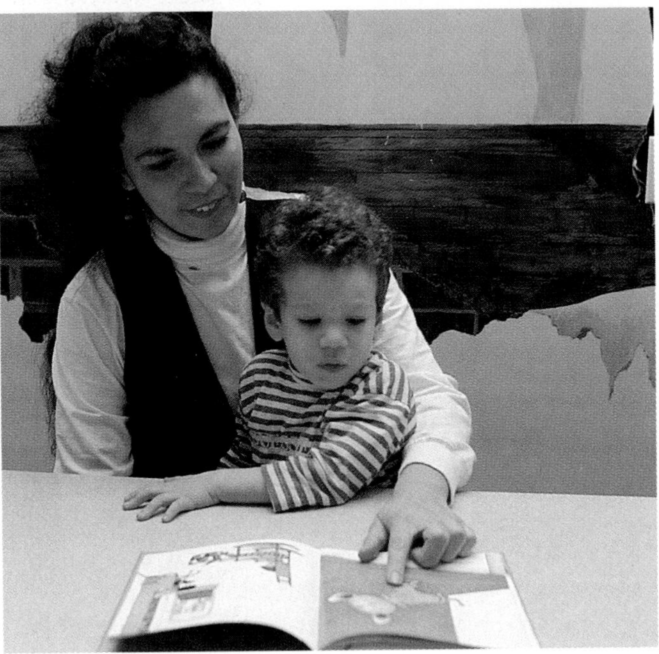

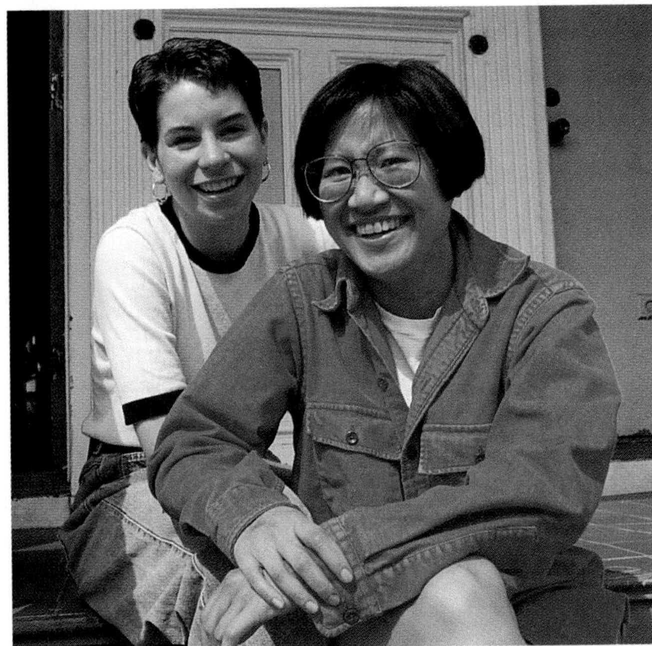

Figure 6.2 Modern family lifestyles include diverse structures and a wider range of family composition.

Economic Influences Individuals need the financial resources to meet basic needs of food, clothing, and shelter along with basic living expenses.

Lower-income individuals and families are generally at greater risk for developing health problems. Health disparities between low-income individuals and those with higher incomes are almost universal for all dimensions of health. The incidence of cancer increases as family income decreases. The risk of death from heart disease is 25% higher for low-income individuals than for the overall population. Low-income individuals have higher incidence of cancers of the lung, esophagus, mouth, prostate, and stomach (USHHS-PHS 1992). Individuals in low-income populations are also more likely to have some of the risk factors for poor health. Higher-than-average rates of obesity and high blood pressure, which are major risks for heart disease and stroke, have been linked directly to low economic status. Smoking is 20% more prevalent among low-income individuals than in the general population (USHHS-PHS 1992).

Economic influences on lifestyle are not limited to those with low incomes. The mental health and well-being of families in middle- and upper-income brackets may be affected by unemployment, layoffs, or unrelenting pressure to get ahead on the job. Elderly clients may have to get by on fixed incomes, which are eroded by inflation.

Religion

Religion can affect the individual's health and lifestyle in all phases of the person's life. It may play a significant role during health and illness, influencing the course of action an individual chooses and the person's feelings about life and death.

Religion is the organized set of beliefs pertaining to the cause and purpose of life and the universe held by a group of individuals. Group members practice common rituals and ceremonies. Religion may or may not include a belief in a higher being.

Spirituality is often closely related to religion. Spirituality is an individual's concept of the purpose and meaning of life and includes one's individual beliefs about right and wrong. It influences the decisions made by the individual and is closely integrated with and often manifested in the individual's religious practices.

Religious rituals often mark milestones in life, such as birth, attainment of adulthood, marriage, and death. They also can govern daily activities such as eating and maintenance of nutritional status. Some religions prohibit certain foods. Hinduism prohibits all meats. Islam prohibits pork and alcohol. Mormons (Church of Jesus Christ of Latter Day Saints) and Seventh-Day Adventists prohibit alcohol, tobacco, and caffeine. Catholics and Mormons practice fasting. Orthodox Jews follow dietary laws based on the Talmud. Foods selected and prepared correctly are called kosher—from the Hebrew word *kashar,* meaning right or fit.

You need to assess the influence of the individual's religion on health and lifestyle because the client often uses religious beliefs to explain the cause of illness and to determine the course of action to ensure both mental and physical health. Religious beliefs can also affect individuals' choice of healers, their perception of the severity of their health concern or illness, and the role, if any, that they can play in preventing illness and promoting a healthy lifestyle. For example, an individual who believes that a higher being controls all that happens may see prayer as the most important health-promoting activity.

Sometimes, religious influences and beliefs can be in conflict with accepted medical practices. For example, Jehovah's Witnesses generally won't accept blood transfusions even when the condition is life-threatening.

Education

You must assess the client's educational status when performing a comprehensive health assessment.

Characteristics of Culture

- *Culture is learned.* It is not instinctive or innate. It is learned through life experiences after birth.
- *Culture is taught.* It is transmitted from parents to children over successive generations. All animals can learn, but only humans can pass on culture. Language is the chief vehicle of culture.
- *Culture is social.* It originates and develops through the interactions of people.
- *Culture is adaptive.* Customs, beliefs, and practices change slowly, but they do adapt to the social environment and the biologic and psychologic needs of the people.
- *Culture is integrative.* The elements in a culture tend to form a consistent and integrated system. For example, religious beliefs are influenced by family organization, economic values, and health practices.
- *Culture is ideational.* Ideational means forming images or objects in the mind. The group habits that are part of culture are to a considerable extent ideal norms or patterns of behavior. People do not always follow those norms. The norms of their culture may be different from the norms of society as a whole.
- *Culture is satisfying.* Cultural habits persist only as long as they satisy people's needs. Once they no longer bring gratification and satisfaction, they disappear.

From: Kozier B, Erb G, Olivieri R. *Fundamentals of Nursing,* 4th ed. Redwood City, CA: Addison-Wesley Nursing, 1991, p. 745. Copyright © 1991 Addison-Wesley Publishing.

Low levels of literacy may prevent individuals from accessing the health care system because they may have difficulty communicating in writing, reading instructions, or filling out forms needed to enter the hospital or to receive services at a medical clinic.

Information about the educational level of the individual also helps you to know how to conduct the health history and interview. Low literacy in clients may limit the tools you use when assessing. For instance, if the client has poor reading and writing skills, you should not ask the client to fill in questionnaires to supplement the data you gathered during the verbal interview.

You also use the information you collected about the client's educational level when you plan nursing interventions to support the client's health and wellness. For example, suppose that while performing the health assessment, the nurse notes that the client has a knowledge deficit regarding ways to manage personal stress. In this case, the nurse needs to take the client's educational level into account when planning interventions to educate the client about stress-management techniques. If the client's reading and writing skills are limited, the nurse may choose a video on stress management or personally demonstrate some stress-management techniques. However, if the client's educational level indicates that the client can comprehend written materials, the nurse may instead select stress-management pamphlets and books, or written self-assessment tools.

Cultural Influences

Lifestyle and health practices are influenced by the individual's cultural environment. **Culture** is the set of beliefs and life practices followed by a group of individuals and passed down from generation to generation. It originates and changes through the interactions of individuals in the cultural group. Culture should not be confused with **race,** which denotes a system for classifying humans by physical characteristics. Culture is a learned rather than an innate set of behaviors. Culture includes beliefs, practices, rituals, objects, dress, art, language, and social institutions peculiar to the group. The box on page 88 lists characteristics of culture.

North American society has often been described as a cultural melting pot (in which people from diverse cultures come together to form one common culture), but most contemporary sociologists consider American society to be multicultural, with many cultures existing side by side. The cultural diversity of the American people continues to increase. *Healthy People 2000* (USHHS-PHS 1992) reports that by the year 2000 non-Hispanic whites will decrease from 76% of the population to 72%. The Hispanic population is expected to increase from 8 to 11.3%. The African-American population is expected to increase from 12.4 to 13.1%, and the Native American and Asian-American population will increase from 3.5 to 4.3% (USHHS-PHS 1992).

The individual's cultural environment can affect how the client defines health and illness as well as the practices that will be effective in promoting health and treating illness. Individuals learn from their own cultural environments how to be healthy, how to recognize illness, and how treat illness. Understanding how the cultural environment influences health helps you to gain an accurate and holistic view of the client's health status. Table 6.1 gives examples of some health-related beliefs and practices that may be practiced by some individuals in different cultural groups.

Table 6.1 Examples of Some Beliefs and Practices of Different Cultural Groups*

	Native American	Latino/Chicano	Asian-American	African-American	European-American
Views of health	Holistic view: spiritual forces give life and health	Holistic view: as a state of equilibrium; children may wear amulets for protection	Seen as a balance of energy, called yin and yang	Health means being able to work productively, being in a state of harmony with others in the universe	Health means being physically fit and free from illness
Views of illness	Tied into religion	Has spiritual, social ramifications; good or "natural" diseases due to imbalance; "supernatural" diseases due to satanic forces	Seen as an imbalance of energy	Seen as a state of incapacitation, sense of disharmony, lack of communication	Seen as a disturbance in body functioning, usually marked by physical symptoms and caused by external agents, eg, virus, toxins, and so on
Resource person for treatment	Healing specialists, herbalists, diagnosticians	*Curanderos,* other types of healers	Healers, herbalists	Older woman with experience; the caregiver must develop a healing relationship with the ill person	Physician, nurse, or other licensed health care provider
Treatments	Herbs; sweat baths; a family conference if necessary to decide if a family member enters a hospital (Navajo)	Folk medicine; prayers; herbs; hot-cold foods and fluids to offset specific illnesses classified as derived from "hot" or "cold" causes	Herbs; nutrition; meditation; spiritual healing; massage; acupressure; acupuncture; hot-cold foods and fluids to counteract illnesses; moxibustion	Religious healing; folk remedies; herb teas; poultices	Medication, surgery, physical therapy, or other prescribed treatments

*These are examples only. It is important not to make assumptions about a client's beliefs and practices because cultural norms vary greatly within a culture and from one individual to another. Observe the client carefully and take the time to ask questions. Your client will benefit greatly from your awareness of differences.

From Servonsky/Opas: *Nursing Management of Children.* Boston: Jones and Bartlett Publishers, 1987 p. 293.

Gathering the Data

Settings

Environmental assessment should be done as part of a comprehensive nursing assessment. If, during the health history and interview, you find that you need more information on the client's environment, then you should conduct a focused environmental assessment. For instance, if the preliminary data you have gathered leads you to believe that the client's family environment may be affecting the client's health and contributing to the client's current health concern, you may need to do a focused environmental assessment in the client's home with the family present to collect additional data.

Environmental assessment can occur in any setting. Common settings for assessing environmental influences on health and lifestyle include clinics, schools, hospitals, medical offices, and homes. In fact, the individual's family and community environment is best assessed in the client's home, where you can evaluate the environment firsthand. Family members should also be present.

The time for an environmental assessment should be planned, and sufficient time should be allotted. For an initial contact, you may need 1 to 2 hours.

Tools for Collecting Data

Data may be collected in a variety of ways. The best way is to collect it directly from the individual, family members, or significant others. You can use structured assessment guides in an interview approach, leaving self-assessment guides with the individual or family, or use a questionnaire. During the initial contact, you should provide an overview of those environmental areas to be assessed. You should also assure the individual of the confidentiality of the data. The following are some questions you can ask when assessing environmental influences on the client's health and lifestyle.

Social Influences

1. List the members of your social network (family members, friends, peers).
2. What is the role of these individuals when you are ill?
3. What community activities are you involved in?
4. What community services are available to you? How close are you to community resources (transportation, stores, schools)?
5. Describe the neighborhood you live in.
6. Is crime a problem in your neighborhood?

Family Influences

1. Describe your family members in detail (age, sex, occupation, education).
2. How do members of the family communicate with each other?
3. Do they show interest in each others' activities? Do they listen to each other?
4. Describe how you feel your family could improve communication.
5. Have there been any major changes in the family (eg, birth of child, loss of job)? If so, how have family members handled these changes?
6. Who makes the decisions in the family?
7. How are important decisions made? By one person, or by the group?
8. If one or more family members disagree, how are disputes resolved?

There are also a variety of family assessments available to the nurse. Smilkstein (1978) developed an assessment tool of family function called the Family APGAR (Figure 6.3 on page 92). This is a screening tool that can be completed by one or all family members.

Economic Influences

1. Who is the main wage earner in the family?
2. Is there more than one wage earner in the family?
3. Are there other sources of income (investments, relatives)?
4. What is the total approximate income of the individual or family group? Do you feel that this amount is sufficient to meet your current needs? Future needs?
5. Can you describe the impact your financial status has had on your standard of living? Place you live? Ability to stay healthy?
6. Do you feel any financial stress in your life at present (loss of job, large debt)? If so, describe it.
7. What plans have you made, if any, in case you lose part or all of your current income?

Religion

1. Describe your religious beliefs and those of your family.
2. Do all members of the family group have the same religious background?
3. What role do your religious beliefs and practices play when you are healthy? When you are ill?
4. Do you use any religious healers or support networks when you are ill?
5. Describe any religious practices you use to help you stay well. To help you get better when ill.

Education

1. What is the primary language that you speak? Write?
2. What is the primary language used in your home?
3. Describe any formal schooling/education you have had.
4. Is it easier for you to learn something if you read about it? Have someone show it to you? Explain it to you?

Cultural Influences

1. Do you identify with any specific ethnic group? If so, which one? Do all members of your family belong to this group?
2. Describe the cultural groups in your neighborhood.
3. Where were you born? What countries have you lived in?
4. Describe any customs or beliefs that affect important events in your life (births, deaths, marriage, illness).
5. Do you have any cultural food preferences? Are any foods forbidden to you because of your cultural beliefs?
6. Describe why you think you get sick. Is there anything you can do to keep from getting sick? Is there anything you can do to stay healthy?
7. What things are most important to you in life?

A more comprehensive guide to help you gather data regarding cultural influences is the Heritage Assessment Tool (Figure 6.4 on page 94).

Documentation

When documenting environmental assessment findings, you need to describe all data carefully, accurately, and objectively. You will use this information with the rest of the data you gather during the nursing health history and assessment to evaluate the client's health status and potential for supporting and promoting health. This information helps you determine the need for nursing interventions and referrals to other professionals or agencies and serves as a baseline for future assessments. Include in the assessment documentation aspects of the environment that support the client's health as well as those that do not.

Organizing the Data

After collecting information by assessing environmental influences on the client's health and well-being, you sort it into groups of related data. Then you evaluate cues for their significance, discarding irrelevant cues. You may need to reassess other cues to gather further information about that environmental area. The resulting data groupings, along with information from others areas of assessment, point to nursing diagnoses. Analyze this information to identify actual or potential nursing diagnoses related to environmental influences, which may include such areas as social networks, family function, economic status, or religious or cultural practices. For instance, data gathered about nutritional status and exercise patterns and information about cultural eating patterns may be grouped to support the nursing diagnosis *Altered nutrition: more than body requirements* related to cultural eating patterns and sedentary lifestyle.

Identifying Nursing Diagnoses

One way to identify nursing diagnoses related to environmental strengths and weaknesses is to cluster the assessment data under commonly used nursing diagnoses for that area. For example, some commonly used nursing diagnoses for families are listed in the box below.

Another method for categorizing diagnostic cues is to divide them into clusters representing either strengths or weaknesses in promoting and supporting client health. For example, a nurse assesses a client, 10-year-old Kate, who lives with her father, 33-year-old Mark, her mother, 31-year-old

Nursing Diagnoses for Family Care

Altered family processes
Health-seeking behaviors (specify)
High risk for injury
Altered parenting
Parental role conflict
Ineffective family coping: disabled
Compromised family coping
Family coping: potential for growth
Altered growth and development
Altered health maintenance
Knowledge deficit

Family APGAR Questionnaire

PART I

The following questions have been designed to help us better understand you and your family. You should feel free to ask questions about any item in the questionnaire.

The space for comments should be used when you wish to give additional information or if you wish to discuss the way the question is applied to your family. Please try to answer all questions.

Family is defined as the individual(s) with whom you usually live. If you live alone, your "family" consists of persons with whom you now have the strongest emotional ties.*

For each question, check only one box.

	Almost always	Some of the time	Hardly ever
I am satisfied that I can turn to my family for help when something is troubling me. *Comments:* ______	☐	☐	☐
I am satisfied that my family talks over things with me and shares problems with me. *Comments:* ______	☐	☐	☐
I am satisfied that my family accepts and supports my wishes to take on new activities or directions. *Comments:* ______	☐	☐	☐
I am satisfied that my family expresses affection and responds to my emotions, such as anger, sorrow, and love. *Comments:* ______	☐	☐	☐
I am satisfied with the way my family and I share time together. *Comments:* ______	☐	☐	☐

Scoring. The patient checks one of three choices which are scored as follows: "Almost always" (2 points), "Some of the time" (1 point), or "Hardly ever" (0). The scores for each of the five questions are then totaled. A score of 7 to 10 suggests a highly functional family. A score of 4 to 6 suggests a moderately dysfunctional family. A score of 0 to 3 suggests a severely dysfunctional family.

*According to which member of the family is being interviewed the nurse may substitute for the word "family" either spouse, significant other, parents, or children.

Carol, and her brother, 8-year-old Jeremy. The nurse finds the following diagnostic cues:

Mark: High school math teacher

Carol: Part-time secretary

Kate: 5th-grade student

Has fever of 101F.

Complains of ear pain in both ears.

Ear drums red and bulging.

Swims 5 times/week at the YWCA, on the swim team.

A average in school.

Family APGAR Questionnaire

PART II

Who lives in your home?* List the persons according to their relationship to you (for example, spouse, significant other,[†] child, or friend).

Well	Fairly	Poorly

Check the column that best describes how you now get along with each member of the family listed.

Well	Fairly	Poorly

If you don't live with your own family, list the persons to whom you turn for help most frequently. List according to relationship (for example, family member, friend, associate at work, or neighbor).

Well	Fairly	Poorly

Check the column that best describes how you now get along with each person listed.

Well	Fairly	Poorly

*If you have established your own family, consider your "home" as the place where you live with your spouse, children, or "significant other" (see next footnote for definition). Otherwise, consider home as your place of origin, for example, the place where your parents or those who raised you live.

†Significant other is the partner you live with in a physically and emotionally nurturing relationship but to whom you are not married.

Figure 6.3 The Family APGAR Questionnaire. Modified from Smilkstein G: The family APGAR: A proposal for family function test and its use by physicians, *J Fam Prac* 6(6), 1978. Copyright ©1978 Appleton & Lange, Inc. Reprinted by permission of the publisher.

Jeremy: 3rd-grade student

Enjoys playing soccer with friends.

B+ average in school.

Is a cub scout.

From this set of data about the health requirements of the family, both as a group and individually, the nurse develops the following clusters based on knowledge of the nursing diagnoses related to families:

Cluster 1 (strengths)	*Cluster 2 (weaknesses)*
Parents employed	Kate: Temperature 101
Children successful in school	Earache
Children involved in sports and organizations outside of the home	Ear drum red and bulging

The nurse compares these clusters to the defining characteristics of each of the possible nursing diagnoses. In this situation cluster 1 consists of diagnostic cues relating to *Growth and Development* of the entire family group. Cluster 2 consists of diagnostic cues related to *Altered health maintenance* of an individual family member, Kate. In this situation cluster 1 (which relates to family growth and development) indicates that family members are successfully meeting both their individual and family developmental tasks; therefore, no nursing diagnosis is indicated. In cluster 2, the diagnostic cues indicate a nursing diagnosis for Kate of *Altered health maintanence* related to otitis media.

Heritage Assessment Tool

This set of questions is related to a given client's—or your—ethnic, cultural, and religious background. It can help you perform a heritage assessment to determine how deeply a person identifies with her or his traditional heritage.

1. Where was your mother born? ____________
2. Where was your father born? ____________
3. Where were your grandparents born? ____________
   a. Your mother's mother? ____________
   b. Your mother's father? ____________
   c. Your father's father? ____________
   d. Your father's mother? ____________
4. How many brothers _____ and sisters _____ do you have?
5. What setting did you grow up in?
   Urban _____ Rural _____
6. What country did your parents grow up in?
   Mother ____________ Father ____________
7. How old were you when you came to the U.S.? _____
8. How old were your parents when they came to the U.S.?
   Mother ____________ Father ____________
9. When you were growing up, who lived with you?
   ____
10. Have you maintained contact with
   a. Aunts, uncles, cousins? ____________
   b. Brothers and sisters? ____________
   c. Parents? ____________
   d. Your own children? ____________
11. Did most of your aunts, uncles, and cousins live near to your home? ____________
12. Approximately how often did you visit your family members who lived outside of your home?
   Daily _____ Weekly _____ Monthly _____
   Once a year or less _____ Never _____
13. Was your original family name changed? _____
14. What is your religious preference?
   Catholic _____ Jewish _____ Protestant _____
   Other _____ None _____
15. Is your partner the same religion as you? _____
16. Is your partner the same ethnic background as you? _____
17. What kind of school did you go to?
   Public _____ Private _____ Parochial _____
18. As an adult, do you live in a neighborhood where the neighbors are the same religion and ethnic background as yourself? _____
19. Do you belong to a religious institution? _____
20. Would you describe yourself as an active member? _____
21. How often do you attend your religious institution? _____
22. Do you practice your religion at your home? If so, please specify
   Praying _____ Bible reading _____ Diet _____
23. Do you prepare foods that reflect your ethnic heritage? _____
24. Do you participate in ethnic activities? If so, please specify
   Singing _____ Festivals _____ Costumes _____
   Other _____
25. Are your friends from the same religious background as you? _____
26. Are your friends from the same ethnic background as you? _____
27. What is your native language? ____________
28. Do you speak this language?
   Prefer _____ Occasionally _____ Rarely _____
29. Do you read your native language? _____

Figure 6.4 Heritage Assessment Tool. Adapted from Rachel E. Spector, *Cultural Diversity in Health and Illness*, 3rd ed. Norwalk, CT: Appleton & Lange, 1991, pp. 331–333. Copyright © 1991 Appleton & Lange, Inc. Reprinted by permission of the publisher.

After assessing a client's religious and spiritual beliefs and practices the nurse may formulate a nursing diagnosis of *Spiritual distress* related to such factors as the crisis of illness, inability to practice religious beliefs, or conflict between religious belief and prescribed course of health care.

Clustering data obtained from assessing educational influences on the client's lifestyle may result in a nursing diagnosis of *Knowledge deficit* (specify) or *Impaired verbal communication*.

Cultural factors may lead to such nursing diagnoses as *Impaired verbal communication* related to language barrier, *Social isolation* related to cultural rituals, or *Ineffective individual coping* related to change in environment. Economic influences can lead to such nursing diagnoses as *Impaired Home maintenance management* related to low income level.

Environmental factors may be incorporated into the nursing diagnosis or be an etiologic factor in the nursing diagnosis.

Summary

You should use information from the environmental assessment, especially information pertaining to socioeconomic, religious, and cultural influences, if any actual or potential problems are present that may affect the client's health or increase risk of disease. Health problems are frequently related to environmental factors in the client's lifestyle. For example, a dysfunctional family environment may contribute to sleep pattern disturbances. Limited economic status may contribute to inability to purchase prescribed medications or nourishing food. Environmental data can inform the choice of nursing diagnosis or can be used to formulate the second part of the nursing diagnosis statement (eg, *Ineffective individual coping* related to unstable family environment).

Never underestimate the importance of assessing the influence of environmental factors on the client's health. You also need to consider how these factors interact and influence other areas of client functioning. The individual's environment interacts constantly and in totality with the individual. If you don't assess environmental influences on the client's health, you will have only a partial picture of the total lifestyle and health status of the individual.

Key Points

- ✓ Environment comprises all the factors that affect individual life and health.
- ✓ Individuals are influenced by their environment every moment of their lives.
- ✓ Environmental influences on individual health and lifestyle are a critical part of the comprehensive health assessment.
- ✓ Environmental influences on health and wellness include social, family, economic, educational, religious, and cultural factors.
- ✓ Dunn's model of wellness describes environmental influences on health in order to maximize health potential within the environment in which the individual lives.
- ✓ The individual's social environment consists of people and organizations with which the individual interacts.
- ✓ Assessment of the family includes the family as a group and encompasses how the family members interact with and relate to each other.
- ✓ Economic status may be correlated to health.
- ✓ The nurse needs to assess religious influences in the client's life. Clients may have religious explanations of the causes of illness, and religion may guide clients' practices to ensure health and prevent illness.
- ✓ Information about the client's educational level can help the nurse conduct the health history and interview.
- ✓ Culture is the set of life practices followed by a group of individuals. The cultural environment of an individual can strongly influence health practices.
- ✓ Environmental assessment can occur in any setting.
- ✓ After collecting information about environmental influences on individual health and lifestyle, the nurse clusters this information into groups of related data in order to identify nursing diagnoses.

Unit Two

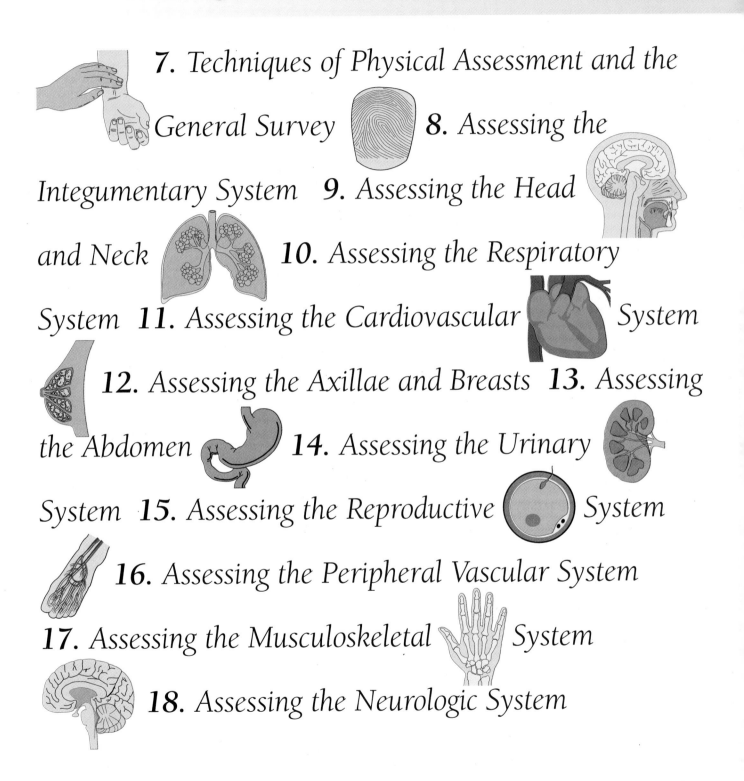

Physical Assessment

Chapter 7

Techniques of Physical Assessment and the General Survey

In Unit One, we discussed a variety of important areas to consider when assessing a client's overall health status, including developmental stage, psychosocial health, self-care, and family, culture, and environment. Much of this data is subjective and is gathered through client interviews, as, for example, when a client reports feeling grief over an impending divorce, or tells you of an inability to maintain a prescribed diet. In this unit, in addition to gathering subjective data through client interviews, you will learn how to gather objective data through an examination of the client's body. For example, you will learn to take the client's vital signs, determine the size and location of internal organs, and classify the various sounds of the client's heart, lungs, and bowels. You'll gather this critical objective data by directly observing the client, by touching the client, and by listening to the client's body sounds. Thus, your senses are important tools for performing the physical assessment.

In this chapter, you will learn about the basic skills and equipment used in physical assessment. You'll also learn how to prepare a comfortable setting for your client. We will share some tips for interacting with clients, and you will learn how to conduct the general survey of the client, including a vital signs assessment.

Basic Assessment Skills

You'll use four basic assessment skills throughout the physical assessment. These are inspection, palpation, percussion, and auscultation. Cue recognition and interpretation are additional skills that help the nurse gather and classify assessment findings.

Inspection

Inspection is the skill of observing the client in a deliberate, systematic manner. It begins the moment you meet the client and continues until the end of the client-nurse interaction. During the general survey, you will carefully inspect the client's whole body (Figure 7.1); during the focused assessments that follow, you'll inspect individual organs such as the eyes, regions such as the head, or systems such as the integumentary system (Figure 7.2).

Inspection always precedes the other assessment skills and is never rushed. Most beginning nurses feel uncomfortable simply staring at the client; nevertheless, such careful scrutiny provides critical assessment data. Avoid the temptation to touch the client right away or listen immediately to the client's heart or lung sounds. These observations will be much more focused and effective if they are preceded by a thorough inspection.

The inspection begins with a survey of the client's appearance and a comparison of the right and left sides of the client's body, which should be nearly symmetric. As you assess each body system or region, inspect for color, texture, size, shape, contour, symmetry, movement, and any eruptions, ulcerations, or drainage. When inspecting a large body region, proceed from a survey to a closer examination. For example, when inspecting the leg, survey the entire leg first, then examine each part, including the thigh, knee, calf, and ankle, in succession.

Throughout the inspection, use your critical-thinking skills to analyze the observations and to determine whether the findings are significant to the client's overall health. The box on page 100 provides examples of the critical thinking that takes place during an inspection.

Although you will perform most of the inspection of the client without the help of instruments, some special tools for visualizing certain body organs or regions are important. These include the ophthalmoscope, the otoscope, and a variety of lights such as a transilluminator and a Wood's lamp. These instruments are described later in this chapter.

Adequate lighting, either daylight or strong, direct artificial light, is essential for a successful inspection. See "Preparing the Setting" on page 108.

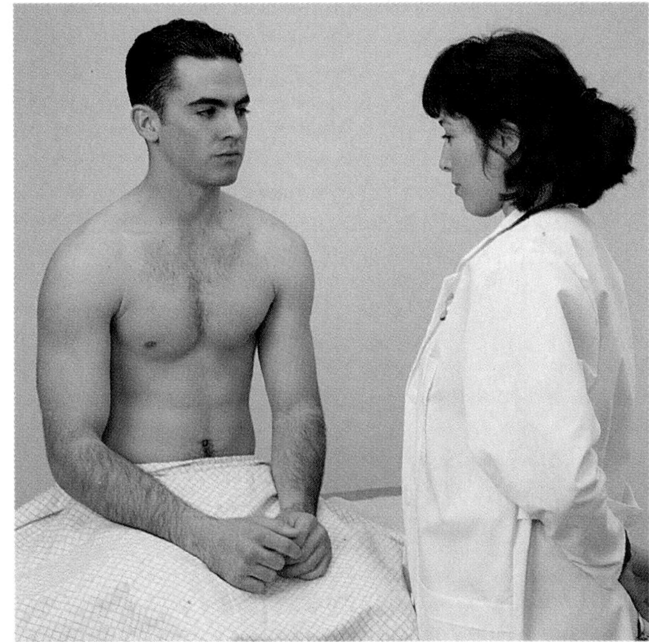

Figure 7.1 During the general survey, inspect the client as a whole person.

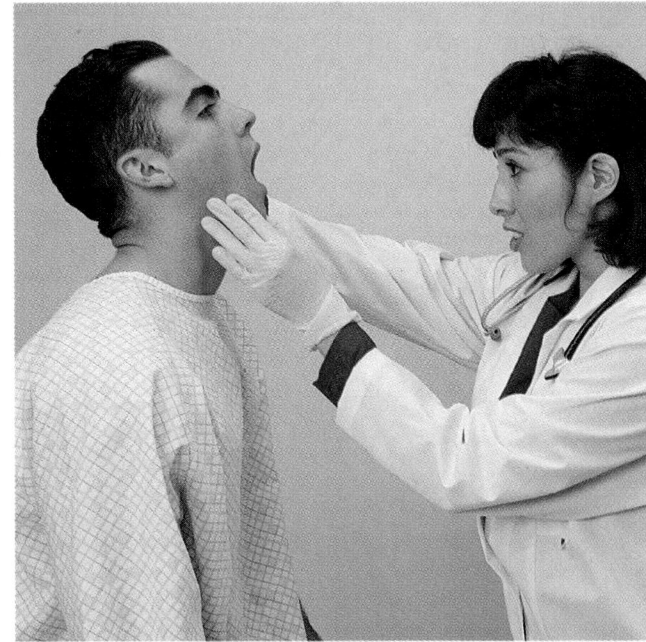

Figure 7.2 During a focused assessment, inspect individual regions, such as the oral cavity.

Critical Thinking during Inspection

- What do I expect to *see* as I perform this inspection?
- Do I *see* any alterations in color, size, texture, symmetry, contour, drainage, lesions, or movement?
- Are my findings normal data, variations from the norm, or unexpected findings?
- How do these findings match up with other diagnostic cues I have gathered so far?
- Am I asking the client focused questions to elicit more information about these findings?
- Based on the data gathered from this inspection, is there anything I should pay special attention to in my focused assessments of other body regions or systems?

Palpation

Palpation is the skill of assessing the client through the sense of touch. By palpating, you can determine skin temperature, texture, and moisture; sense pulses, vibrations, pain, tenderness, the presence of fluid or edema, or organ distention; and determine the position, size, shape, and mobility of organs, masses, and cysts.

Use different parts of your hands to assess for different qualities: The finger pads and palmar surface are more sensitive than the fingertips and are used for palpating skin texture, moisture, and pulses, as well as superficial lymph nodes and masses. The palmar aspects of the fingers are used to determine areas of pain and tenderness, the configuration of organs and abnormal growths, the presence of fluid accumulations, and body vibrations in the chest and abdomen. The metacarpophalangeal joint of the hand is used to assess the chest wall for vibrations. Although not as accurate as a thermometer, the dorsum (back) of the hand, which is very sensitive to heat and cold, can be used to determine body temperature. The thumb and index finger are used to assess the elasticity of the skin and the thickness of skin folds.

During palpation, use light, moderate, or deep pressure depending on the depth of the structure being assessed and the thickness of the layers of tissue overlying the structure.. Begin with *light palpation* because it is the safest, least uncomfortable method and allows the client to become accustomed to your touch. You also use light palpation to assess surface characteristics, such as skin texture, a pulse, or a tender, inflamed area near the surface of the skin. For light palpation, place the dominant hand perpendicular to the skin surface with the fingertips lightly touching the area being assessed and move the fingers gently in a circular motion (Figure 7.3*A*).

Use *moderate palpation* to assess most of the other structures of the body. For moderate palpation, place the palmar surface of the fingers of the dominant hand over the structure to be assessed and press downward approximately 1 to 2 cm, rotating the fingers in a circular motion (Figure 7.3*B*). With moderate palpation, you can determine the depth, size, shape, consistency, and mobility of most organs and masses, as well as any pain, tenderness, or pulsations that might be present.

Use *deep palpation* to palpate an organ or mass that lies deep within a body cavity or when overlying musculature is thick, tense, or rigid. For deep palpation, place the extended

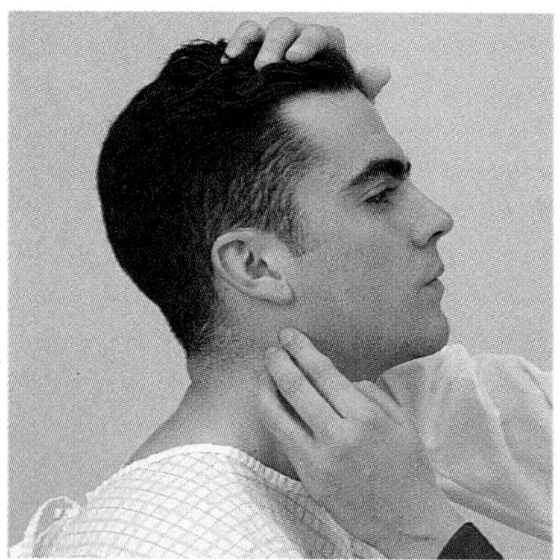
A

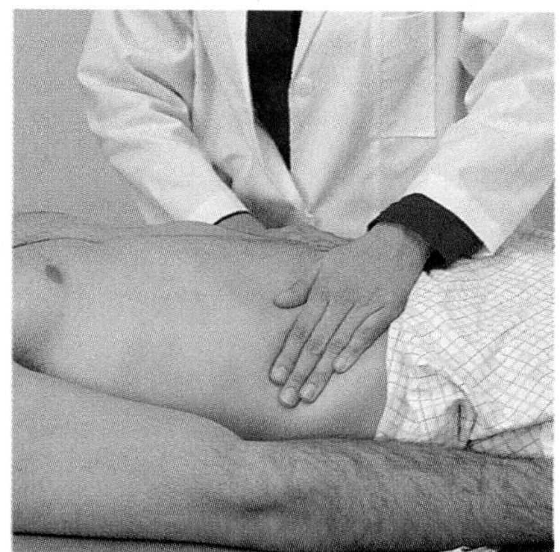
B

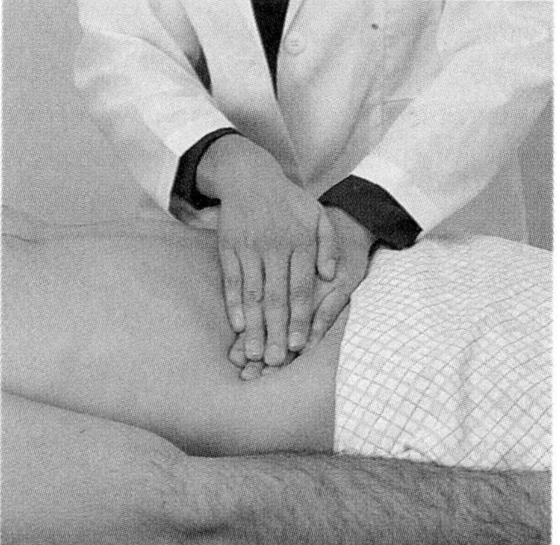
C

Figure 7.3 *A*, Light palpation. Press the fingertips lightly in a circular motion. *B*, Moderate palpation. Press the palmar surface of the fingers downward approximately 1 to 2 cm, rotating the fingers in a circular motion. *C*, Deep palpation. Use the top hand to press the bottom hand downward approximately 2 to 4 cm, in the same circular pattern used for moderate palpation.

Palpating Masses

To assess a mass, place the hands at opposite edges of the mass. Using both hands, gently palpate the circumference of the mass, while visualizing its size, shape, and depth. It may be helpful to mark the edges of the mass with a skin-marking pen. Next, determine if the mass is fixed or mobile by gently attempting to move the mass slightly from side to side. Then palpate the surface of the mass to determine if it is smooth or irregular, noting any lumps or thickened areas. Finally, palpate for the consistency of the mass: a mass may be solid, in which case it will feel firm to the touch, or it may be filled with fluid, in which case it will feel resilient, like a balloon.

Some critical-thinking questions to ask while palpating masses include:

- Should I use light, moderate, or deep palpation? Why?
- Have I fully determined the size, shape, depth, mobility, texture, and consistency of this mass?
- Do I detect any movement or pulsation within the mass?
- Are there any contraindications to further palpation of this mass?
- Am I asking the client focused questions to elicit more information about this mass?
- What other assessment data might be related to this mass?

fingers of the dominant hand on the skin surface of the abdomen. These fingers will be more sensitive to perception of touch than those on the nondominant hand. Place the extended fingers of the nondominant hand over the fingers of the dominant hand, pressing and guiding the fingers downward. This technique provides extra support and pressure and allows you to palpate at a deeper level, from 2 to 4 cm (Figure 7.3C). Use deep palpation with caution, because it can disseminate infections or cancerous cells or rupture underlying masses, such as cysts. The box above describes the technique and critical thinking you should use when palpating masses.

Before palpating the client, explain what you are about to do. Because it is difficult to feel underlying structures if the client is tense or frightened, try to make the client relaxed and comfortable before proceeding with the examination. To prevent discomfort, warm your hands, keep your fingernails smooth and trim, and do not wear jewelry. Put on gloves if you notice open skin areas, sinus formations, or drainage.

Critical Thinking during Palpation

- What do I expect to feel as I perform this palpation?
- Should I use light, moderate, or deep palpation? Why?
- Do I feel any alterations in consistency, texture, temperature, moisture, elasticity, or movement?
- Does the client report any discomfort during the palpation? If so, how could this be described?
- Are my findings normal data, variations from the norm, or unexpected findings?
- How do these findings match up with other diagnostic cues I have gathered so far?
- Am I asking the client focused questions to elicit more information about these findings?
- Based on the data gathered from this palpation, is there anything I should pay special attention to in my focused assessments of other body regions or systems?

Proceed slowly, using smooth, deliberate movements, and avoid abrupt changes. Most clients will be more relaxed if you talk to them during the examination, explaining each movement in advance. For example, during an abdominal assessment, you might say, "I'm going to place my hand on your abdomen next. Tell me if you feel any discomfort and I'll stop right away. How does it feel when I press down on this area?" It is a good idea to touch each area before palpating it. This touch informs the client that examination of the area is about to begin and may prevent a startled reaction.

Critical thinking plays an important role as you palpate the client. The box above lists examples of critical thinking you should use during palpation.

Percussion

Percussion involves striking or tapping the body to produce sound waves. As these waves travel toward underlying structures, they can be heard as characteristic tones. The procedure is similar to a musician striking a drum, creating a vibration heard as a musical tone. Use percussion to determine the size and shape of organs and masses and to determine whether underlying tissue is solid or filled with fluid or air. Percussion is used most commonly to assess thoracic and abdominal structures.

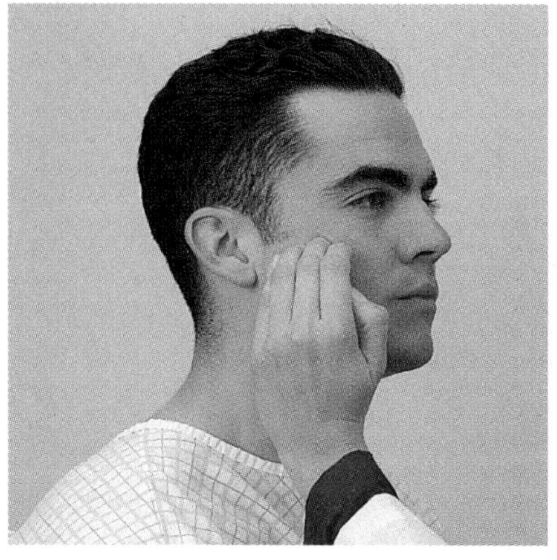

A

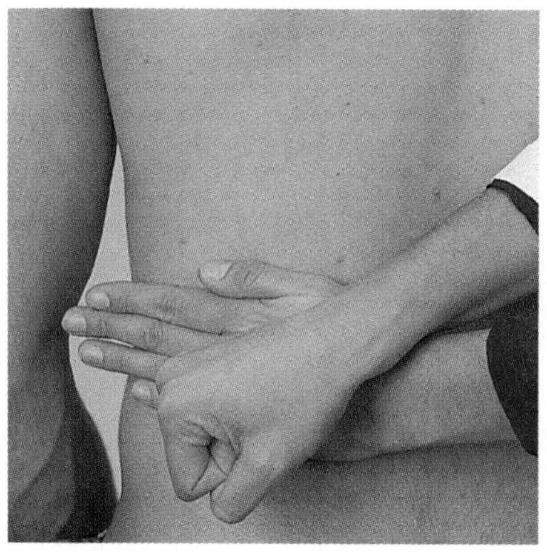

B

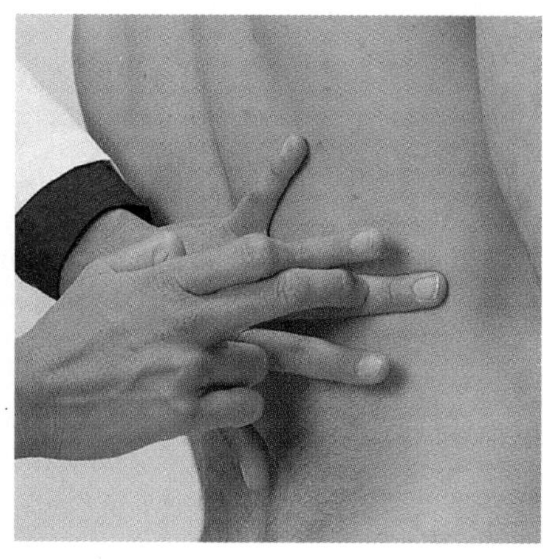

C

Figure 7.4 *A*, Direct percussion. Tap the body with the fingertips of one hand. *B*, Blunt percussion. Place the palm of one hand flat against the body and strike against it with the other hand, closed in a fist. *C*, Indirect percussion. Strike the distal end of the middle finger of the nondominant hand with the middle fingertip of the dominant hand.

Three methods of percussion can be used: direct percussion, blunt percussion, and indirect percussion. The area to be percussed governs the choice of percussion method.

Direct percussion is the technique of tapping the body with the fingers of one hand (Figure 7.4*A*). It is used mostly to assess the sinuses or examine an infant's thorax.

Blunt percussion involves placing the palm of one hand flat against the body surface and striking against it with the other hand, closed in a fist (Figure 7.4*B*). It is used for assessing pain and tenderness in the gallbladder, liver, or kidney.

Indirect percussion is the technique most commonly used because it produces tones that are clearer and more easily interpreted. To perform indirect percussion, place the middle finger of the nondominant hand *firmly* over the area being examined. This finger becomes the "drum." It is important to keep the other fingers and the palm of the hand raised to avoid contact with the body surface, because pressure from the other fingers and palm on the adjacent surface muffles the tones. Next, position the forearm of the dominant hand close to the body surface, keeping the upper arm and shoulder steady and the muscles relaxed. Using only the wrist of the dominant hand to generate the motion, bring the middle fingertip of the dominant hand swiftly down against the "drum" finger at the interphalangeal joint, and immediately back up again (Figure 7.4*C*). If the striking finger remains against the "drum" finger, the sound waves are muffled. Note that you should bring the striking finger down with enough force to set up vibrations in the body tissues below but not so forcefully as to injure yourself or the client. The accompanying box lists some common errors in percussion technique.

Repeat the percussing motion several times as needed to assess the entire area. In most cases, you should percuss in a systematic manner, from side to side or from top to bottom, listening to changes in tone from one area to another.

Interpreting a percussion tone is an art that takes time and experience to develop. The rule to remember is that the denser the tissue, the softer and shorter the tone; the less dense the tissue, the louder and longer the tone. Percussion sounds are usually classified as follows:

- *Tympany* is a loud, high-pitched, drumlike tone of medium duration characteristic of an organ that is filled with air. It is heard commonly over the gastric bubble in the stomach or over air-filled intestines.
- *Resonance* is a loud, low-pitched, hollow tone of long duration that is a normal finding over the lungs.

Common Errors in Percussion Technique

- Generating the percussion stroke from the forearm, rather than from the wrist.
- Generating the percussion stroke from the finger, rather than from the wrist.
- Holding the striking finger against the positioned finger, rather than releasing it immediately after the impact.
- Failing to keep the other fingers from touching the "drum" finger.
- Striking with the pad rather than the tip of the striking finger.
- Using excessive force, particularly with children and elderly clients.
- Creation of the "woodpecker syndrome." This is the delivery of more than two rapid consecutive strikes to the "drum" finger.

- *Hyperresonance* is an abnormally loud, low tone of longer duration than resonance. It is heard when air is trapped in the lungs.
- *Dullness* is a high-pitched tone that is soft and of short duration. It is usually heard over solid body organs such as the liver.
- *Flatness* is also a high-pitched tone, but it is even softer than dullness and is of shorter duration. It occurs over solid tissue such as muscle or bone.

Like other assessment skills, percussion requires critical thinking. The accompanying box gives examples of critical thinking used while percussing a client.

Critical Thinking during Percussion

- What sounds do I expect to hear as I percuss this area?
- Do I hear any unusual sounds as I percuss here?
- Does the client complain of any pain or tenderness as I percuss this area?
- Are my findings normal data, variations from the norm, or unexpected findings?
- How do these findings match up with other diagnostic cues I have gathered so far?
- Am I asking the client focused questions to elicit more information about these findings?
- Based on the data gathered from percussing this area, is there anything I should pay special attention to in my focused assessments of other body regions or systems?

Auscultation

Auscultation is the skill of listening to the sounds produced by the body. Like inspection, it is used throughout the physical assessment. When auscultating, you use both the unassisted sense of hearing and special instruments such as a stethoscope (Figure 7.5). Body sounds that can be heard with the ears alone include speech, coughing, respirations, and percussion tones. Many body sounds are extremely soft, however, and you need to use a stethoscope to hear them. Stethoscopes work not by amplifying sounds but by blocking out other noises in the environment. Use of the stethoscope is described shortly.

Auscultating body sounds requires a quiet environment in which you can listen not just for the presence or absence of sounds but also for the characteristics of each sound. Turn off televisions, radios, and noisy equipment whenever possible and avoid rubbing against the client's clothes, drapes, or bedding or touching the stethoscope tubing, because these sounds obscure the body sounds. Additionally, keep your client warm, because shivering is not only uncomfortable but also obscures body sounds.

Sounds are described in terms of four characteristics: intensity, pitch, duration, and quality. For example, you might note that a client's respirations are loud, high-pitched, long, and raspy. Listen intently, concentrating on one sound at a time. Closing your eyes might help you to focus on the sound.

Specific guidelines for auscultating body sounds are discussed throughout the text. For example, auscultation of lung sounds is described in Chapter 10, and auscultation of heart sounds is discussed in Chapter 11. The box on page 104 gives examples of critical thinking used during auscultation.

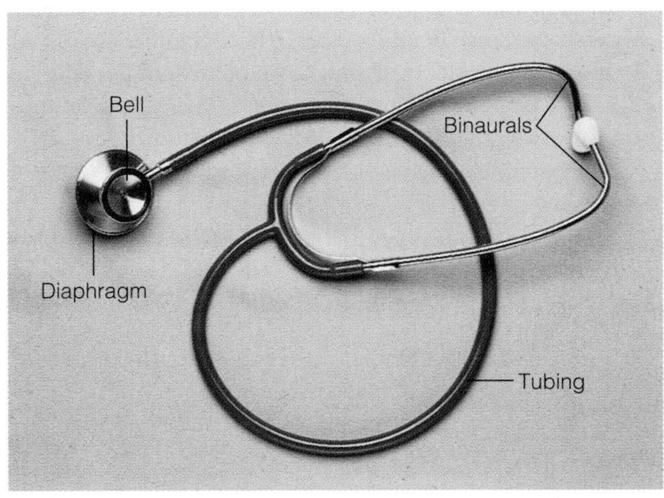

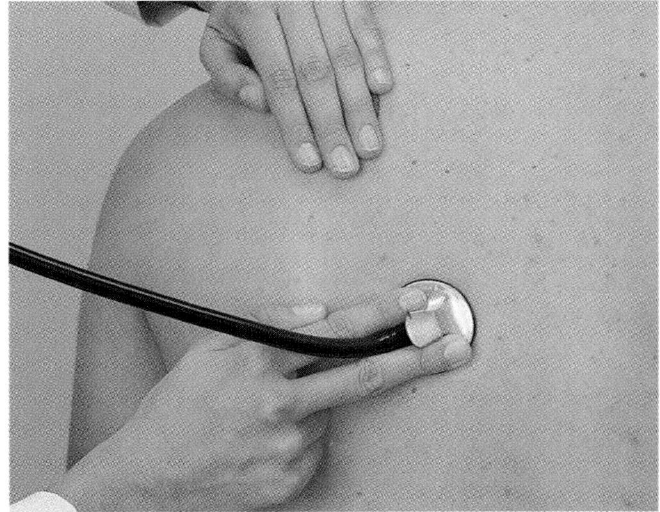

Figure 7.5 *A*, Stethoscope. *B*, Auscultation using a stethoscope.

Critical Thinking during Auscultation

- What sounds do I expect to hear as I auscultate this area?
- Do I hear any unusual sounds as I auscultate here?
- Are my findings normal data, variations from the norm, or unexpected findings?
- How do these findings match up with other diagnostic cues I have gathered so far?
- Am I asking the client focused questions to elicit more information about these findings?
- Based on the data gathered from auscultating this area, is there anything I should pay special attention to in my focused assessments of other body regions or systems?

Cue Recognition

In addition to developing the skills of inspection, palpation, percussion, and auscultation, you must be able to recognize the relative significance of the many visual, palpable, or auditory "cues" that may be present during an assessment. In other words, you need to know what to look for. To become skilled at **cue recognition**, cultivate your senses until they readily perceive even slight cues. Cue recognition develops with practice, but beginners can acquire the skill by observing an experienced nurse, by practicing on partners, by studying the visual aids in this text, and by using the many videotapes, films, and audiotapes available.

Interpretation

Once cues are recognized and data is collected, you must be able to **interpret** the findings. Is a particular finding normal, or does it indicate an alteration in the client's health? *Normal data* are assessment findings that fall within an accepted standard range for a specific type of data. For example, the normal range for the adult pulse rate is 60–90 beats per minute. A pulse of 76 is therefore considered normal. Some healthy individuals exhibit characteristics that are outside the standard range for a specific type of data. Such findings are considered *variations from the norm*. For example, a long-distance runner with a pulse of 48 resulting from regular cardiovascular conditioning exhibits a variation from the norm for pulse rate. Findings that are outside the range for a specific type of data and that may indicate a threat to the client's health are considered *unexpected findings* or *deviations from the norm*. For example, an irregular, thready pulse rate of 120 is an unexpected finding that could indicate the presence of a harmful condition. It is important to note that not all unexpected findings indicate the presence of a disease or disorder. For example, fatigue in a 20-year-old student may indicate anemia or infection, or it may be caused simply by a lack of sleep.

Gathering the Equipment

You'll use several different instruments during the physical assessment to help in visualizing, hearing, and measuring data. Before the exam, gather all the equipment together, organize it, and place it within easy reach. Table 7.1 gives a complete list of the equipment needed for a typical screening exam. Some of the more complex items on the list are discussed in greater detail below or in later chapters.

Stethoscope

Use the **stethoscope** to auscultate body sounds such as blood pressure, heartbeat, respirations, and bowel sounds. The stethoscope has three parts: the binaurals (earpieces), the flexible tubing, and the diaphragm and bell (Figure 7.5*A* on page 103).

To be effective in blocking out environmental noise, the stethoscope must fit the wearer. The binaurals should fit snugly but comfortably, sloping forward, toward the nose, to match the natural slope of the ear canals. Most manufacturers supply several different binaurals to choose from.

The tubing that joins the binaurals to the diaphragm and bell is thick, flexible, and as short as possible (approximately 30–36 cm, or 12–18 inches). Longer tubing may distort the sound.

The flat endpiece, called the *diaphragm*, screens out low-pitched sounds and therefore is best for transmitting high-pitched sounds such as lung sounds and normal heart sounds. Place the diaphragm evenly and firmly over the client's exposed skin. The deep, hollow endpiece, called the *bell*, detects low-frequency sounds such as heart murmurs. It is placed lightly against the client's skin so that it forms a seal but does not flatten to a diaphragm. Either endpiece may be held against the client's skin between the index and middle fingers (see Figure 7.5*B* on page 103). Friction on the diaphragm or bell from

Table 7.1 Equipment Used during the Physical Assessment

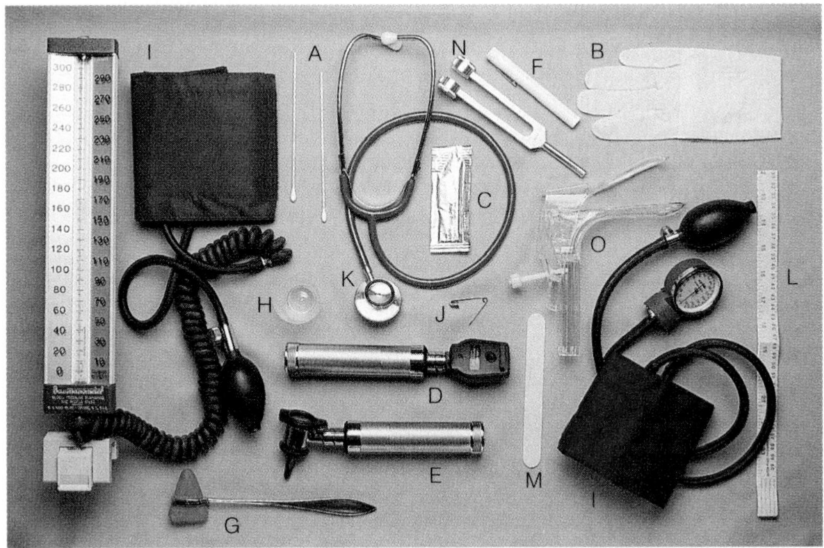

Equipment	Use
Cotton balls or wisps	Test the sense of touch
Cotton-tipped applicators (*A*)	Obtain specimens
Culture media	Obtain cultures of body fluids and drainage
Dental mirror	Visualize mouth and throat structures
Doppler ultrasonic stethoscope	Obtain readings of blood pressure, pulse, and fetal heart rate
Flashlight	Provide a direct source of light to view parts of the body
Gauze squares	Obtain specimens; collect drainage
Gloves (*B*)	Protect the nurse and client from contamination
Goggles	Protect the nurse's eyes from contamination by body fluids
Lubricant (*C*)	Provide lubrication for vaginal or rectal examinations
Nasal speculum	Dilate nares for inspection of the nose
Ophthalmoscope (*D*)	Inspect the interior structures of the eye
Otoscope (*E*)	Inspect the tympanic membrane and external ear canal
Penlight (*F*)	Provide a direct light source and test pupillary reaction
Reflex hammer (*G*)	Test deep tendon reflexes
Ruler, marked in centimeters	Measure organs, masses, growths, and lesions
Skin-marking pen	Outline masses or enlarged organs
Slides	Make smears of body fluids or drainage
Specimen containers (*H*)	Collect specimens of body fluids, drainage, or tissue
Sphygmomanometer (*I*)	Measure systolic and diastolic blood pressure
Sterile safety pin (*J*)	Test for sensory stimulation
Stethoscope (*K*)	Auscultate body sounds
Tape measure, flexible, marked in centimeters (*L*)	Measure the circumference of the head, abdomen, and extremities
Test tubes	Collect specimens
Thermometer	Measure body temperature
Tongue blade (*M*)	Depress tongue during assessment of the mouth and throat
Tuning fork (*N*)	Test auditory function and vibratory sensation
Vaginal speculum (*O*)	Dilate the vaginal canal for inspection of the cervix
Vision chart	Test near and far vision
Watch with second hand	To time heart rates, fetal pulse, or bowel sounds when counting

Table 7.1 Equipment Used during the Physical Assessment (continued)

Special Equipment	Use/Description
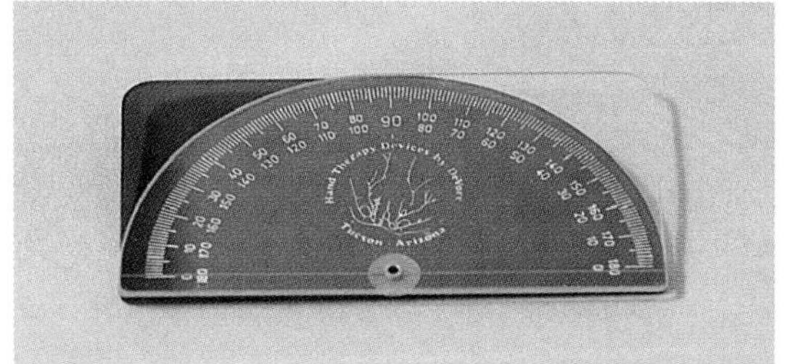 Goniometer	Measures the degree of joint flexion and extension. Consists of two straight arms of clear plastic usually marked in both inches and centimeters. The arms intersect and can be angled and rotated around a protractor marked with degrees. The nurse places the center of the protractor over a joint and aligns the straight arms with the extremity. The degree of flexion or extension is indicated on the protractor.
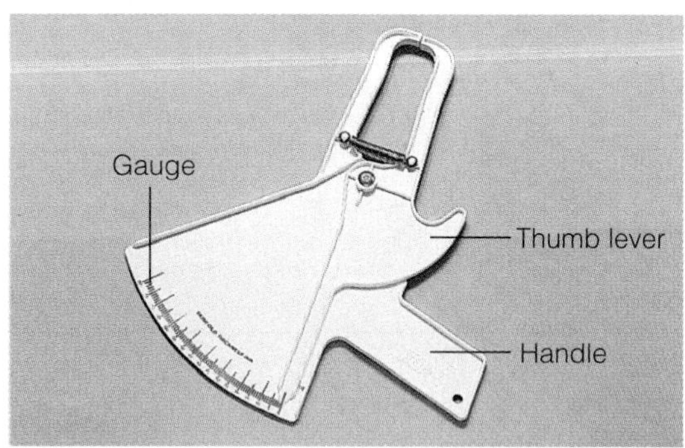 Skinfold calipers	Measures the thickness of subcutaneous tissue. The nurse grasps a fold of skin, usually on the upper arm, waist, or thigh, keeping the sides of the skin parallel. The edges of the caliper are placed at the base of the fold and the calipers tightened until they grasp the fold without compressing it.
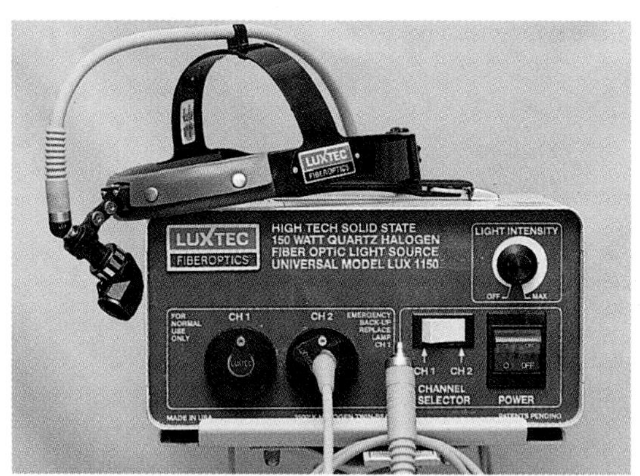 Transilluminator	Detects blood, fluid, or masses in body cavities. Instruments manufactured for transillumination are available, or a flashlight with a rubber adaptor may be used. In either case, the light beam produced is strong but narrow. When directed through a body cavity, the beam produces a red glow that reveals the presence of air or fluid.
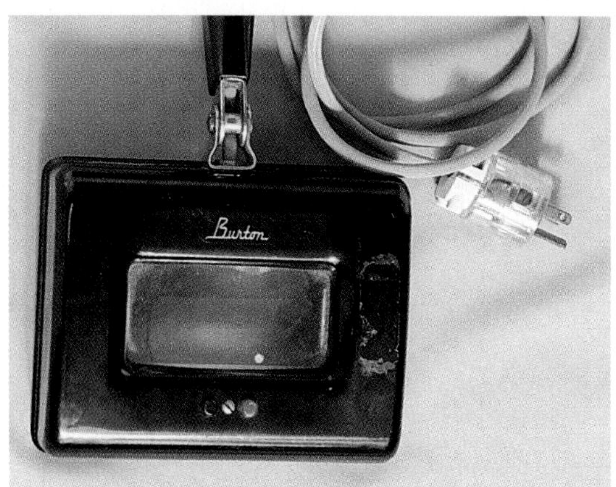 Wood's lamp	Detects fungal infections of the skin. The Wood's lamp produces a black light, which the nurse shines on the skin in a darkened room. If a fungal infection is present, a characteristic yellow-green fluorescence appears on the skin surface.

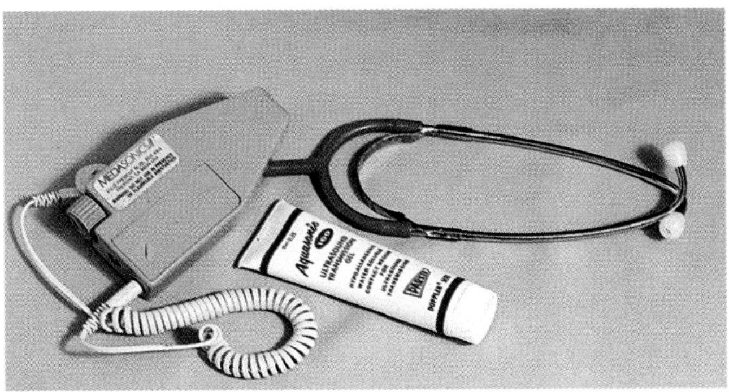

Figure 7.6 Doppler ultrasonic stethoscope.

coarse body hair may cause a crackling sound easily confused with abnormal breath sounds. To avoid this problem, wet the hair before auscultating the area. Stethoscopes usually include an assortment of interchangeable diaphragms and bells in different sizes for different purposes; for example, smaller diaphragm pieces are used for examining children.

Doppler Ultrasonic Stethoscope

A **Doppler ultrasonic stethoscope** uses ultrasonic waves to detect sounds that are difficult to hear with a regular stethoscope, such as fetal heart sounds and peripheral pulses (Figure 7.6). It operates on a principle discovered in the nineteenth century by the Austrian physicist, Johannes Doppler, who found that the pitch of a sound varies in relation to the distance between the source and the listener. To the listener, the pitch sounds higher when the distance from the source is small, and lower when the distance from the source is great.

To eliminate interference, apply a small amount of gel to the end of the Doppler probe (the transducer), which may resemble a wand or a disk. Turn the Doppler stethoscope on, and place the probe gently against the client's skin over the artery to be auscultated. Avoid heavy pressure, because it may impede blood flow. The probe sends a low-energy, high-pitched sound wave toward the underlying blood vessel. As the blood ebbs and flows, the probe picks up and amplifies the subtle changes in pitch, and you will hear a pulsing beat.

Ophthalmoscope

Use an **ophthalmoscope** to inspect internal eye structures. Its main components are the handle, which holds the battery; and the head, which houses the the aperture selector, viewing aperture, lens selector disk, lens indicator, lenses of varying powers of magnification, and mirrors (Figure 7.7A).

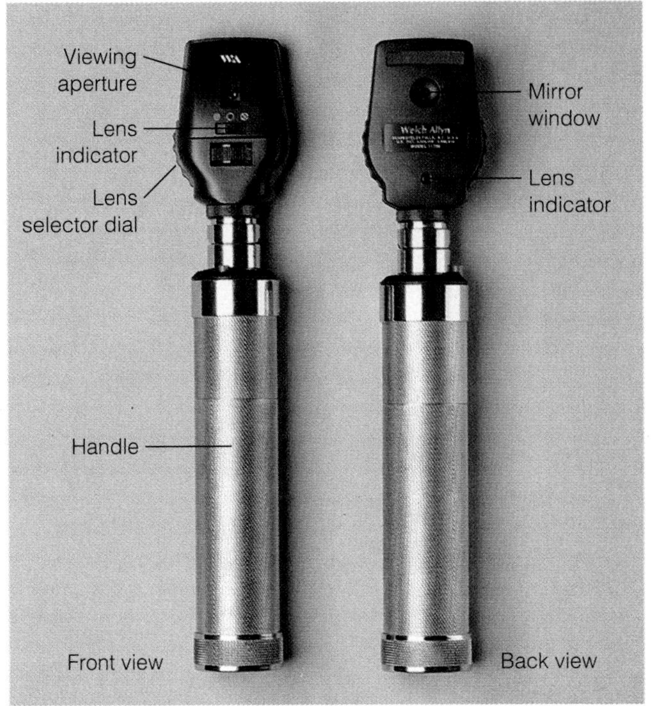

A

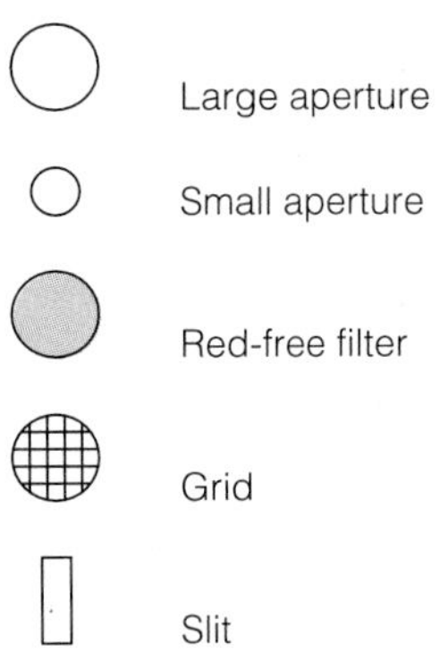

B

Figure 7.7 A, Ophthalmoscope. B, The five apertures contained within the viewing aperture.

The light source shines light through the viewing aperture, which is adjusted to select one of five apertures (Figure 7.7b):

- The large aperture is used most often. It emits a large, full spot for viewing dilated pupils.
- The small aperture is used for undilated pupils.
- The red-free filter shines a green beam used to examine the optic disc for pallor or hemorrhaging, which appears black with this filter.
- The grid allows the examiner to assess the size, location, and pattern of any lesions.
- The slit allows for examination of the anterior eye and aids in assessing the elevation or depression of lesions.

Rotate the lens selector dial to bring the inner eye structures into focus. While looking through the viewing aperture,

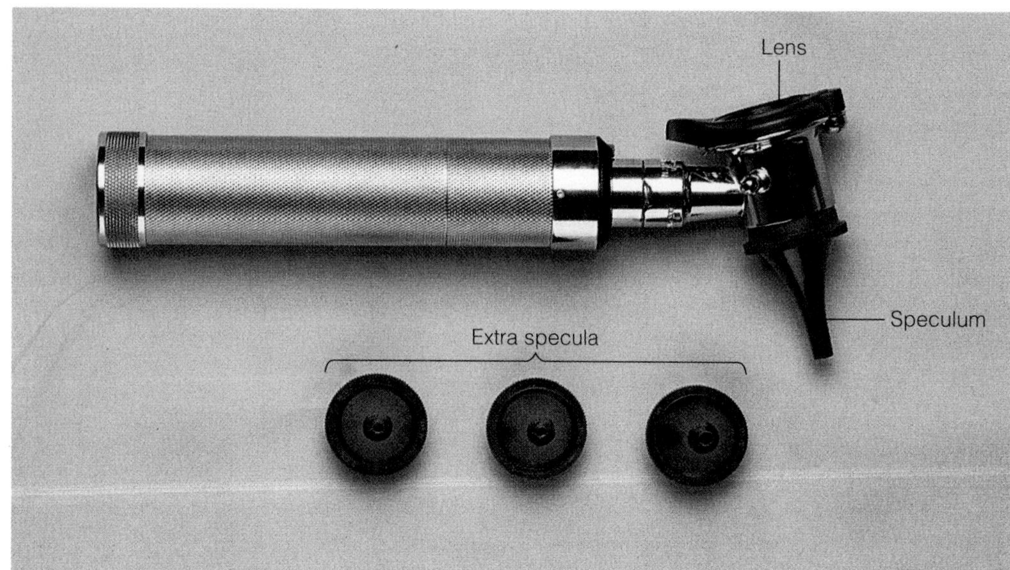

Figure 7.8 Otoscope.

rotate the lens selection dial to adjust the convergence or divergence of the light. At the zero setting, the lens neither converges nor diverges the light. Move the lens dial clockwise to access the numbers in black, which range from +1 to +40. These lenses improve visualization in a client who is farsighted. Move the lens dial counterclockwise to access the red numbers, which range from –1 to –20. These lenses improve visualization if the client is nearsighted. See Chapter 9 for a more detailed discussion of assessment of the eye.

Otoscope

Use the **otoscope** to inspect internal ear structures. The main components of the otoscope are the handle, which is similar to that of the ophthalmoscope, the light, the lens, and specula of various sizes (Figure 7.8). The specula are used to narrow the beam of light. Select the largest one that will fit into the client's ear canal. If a nasal speculum is not available, the otoscope can be used to inspect the nose. In this case, use the shortest, broadest speculum and insert it gently into the client's naris. See Chapter 9 for a more detailed discussion of assessment of the ears and nose.

Preparing the Setting

The physical assessment may be performed in a variety of settings, including a clinic, a hospital room, a school nurse's office, a corporate health services office, or a client's home. No matter where the location, you are responsible for preparing a setting that is conducive to the client's comfort and privacy. The examination room should be warm, private, and free from distractions and interruptions. Adequate overhead lighting that ensures good visibility and is free of distortion is essential, as is a portable lamp to highlight body surfaces and contours.

Position the client on a sturdy examination table with a firm surface. Though not as efficient, a firm bed will suffice if an examination table is not available. Place the table so that you have easy access to both sides of the client's body. Raise it to a height that allows you to perform the exam without stooping.

You should also have a stool to sit on during certain parts of the exam and a small table or stand to hold the examination equipment.

Interacting with the Client

When conducting the physical portion of the health assessment, it is important to avoid focusing solely on the client's body. Throughout the exam, continue to consider the client's needs holistically.

Respecting the Client's Individuality

Individualize the examination according to the client's personal values and beliefs. Some clients, for example, may request that a family member be present during the examination. Some may ask for a nurse of the same sex. Some female clients may object to breast and vaginal examinations, regardless of the gender of the examiner, and some male clients may refuse penile, scrotal, and rectal examinations. A thorough assessment of the client's culture, religious beliefs, and environment, as described in the previous chapter, may help you to anticipate these needs. Although explaining the reason for a certain procedure may help the client understand its benefit, never attempt to influence or coerce the client to agree to any procedure. In all cases, document which procedures took place and any that were refused.

Providing for the Client's Comfort and Safety

Many clients experience anxiety before and during a physical examination. Their feelings may stem from fear of pain, embarrassment at being looked at and touched by a stranger, or worry about the outcome of the exam. Alleviate the client's anxiety by approaching the examination gradually, first by chatting with the client, then by performing simple measurements such as height, weight, temperature, and pulse, which most clients find familiar and nonthreatening. As these measurements are taken, the client will have the opportunity to ask additional questions and to become accustomed to your presence.

In most cases, clients should urinate before the examination. Voiding helps clients feel more comfortable and relaxed and facilitates palpation of the abdomen and pubic area. If a urinalysis is to be done, instruct the client in obtaining a clean-catch specimen and give the client a container for the urine sample.

After ensuring that the examination room is warm, show the client how to put on the examination gown, and leave the client to undress in privacy. You may want to assure the client that it is all right to leave the underpants on until just before the genital examination. Before you reenter the examination room, knock to alert the client.

Use drapes to preserve the client's privacy and to provide warmth. When invasive procedures such as vaginal or rectal examinations are performed, drapes provide an aseptic field. When used properly, a drape exposes only the part of the body being examined and covers the surrounding area. Drapes are available in a variety of shapes and materials from simple rectangular sheets made of linen, to disposable drapes made of paper lined with waterproof plastic.

The physical examination may be an exhausting experience for a client who is elderly, debilitated, frail, or suffering from a chronic illness, since you must examine every part of the body and the client must make frequent changes in position. Consequently, consider the client's age, health status, level of functioning, and severity of illness at all times, and adapt the examination accordingly. In addition, conserve the client's energy by moving around the client during the exam, rather than asking the client to move, and by carrying out the exam as quickly and efficiently as possible.

Before beginning the physical examination, wash your hands in the presence of the client. Hand-washing not only protects you and the client but also signals that you are providing for the client's safety.

Some situations that arise during a physical examination pose a potential hazard for the client. For example, a client might become lightheaded and dizzy from taking deep breaths during a respiratory assessment, or fall when asked to touch the toes during a musculoskeletal assessment. A client who is frail, weak, debilitated, or suffering from a chronic illness is at greatest risk. Throughout the procedure, anticipate potential hazards and modify the examination as needed to prevent them. In addition, some examination techniques may injure the client if used indiscriminately. For example, vigorous, deep palpation of a throbbing mass might lead to a ruptured abdominal aneurysm. In this text, a special "alert" box appears alongside any technique that you should perform with caution.

Providing for the Client's Knowledge and Consent

Before beginning the examination, thoroughly explain to the client what is to follow and encourage the client to ask questions. If the client does not speak your language, secure the assistance of a translator. If the client's hearing is impaired, find someone who knows sign language.

During the examination, explain each step in advance so that the client can anticipate your movements. Clients are more relaxed and cooperative during the procedure when they understand what is about to happen. This is also an opportunity to provide client teaching. For example, as you are inspecting the client's skin, you may want to discuss the long-term effects of sun exposure. Sharing information with clients during the examination may alleviate their anxiety, enhance their understanding, and give them a sense of partnership in their health care.

At times, you may note an unexpected finding and want to call in another examiner to check the finding. In such instances, it is best simply to inform the client that you would like to ask another examiner to check your assessment. Because the finding may be normal for the client, it is best to avoid alarming the client.

In many health care institutions, the client is asked to sign a consent form for the physical examination, especially if invasive procedures such as a vaginal or rectal examination or blood studies are to be performed. Ensure that the client understands the procedures to be performed and that all necessary consent forms are signed.

Conducting the General Survey

The general survey is the initial phase of a complete physical assessment. During the general survey, you will gather preliminary data about a client's health status; assess the client's appearance, mental status, and behavior; and measure the client's height, weight, and vital signs. The general survey actually begins during the initial interview: while collecting subjective data, you observe the client, developing initial impressions about the client's health and formulating strategies for the ensuing examination. Clues that you uncover during the general survey may guide you during later assessments of discrete body regions and systems.

Guidelines for Conducting the General Survey

Positioning the Client

During the complete physical assessment, you will ask the client to assume special positions for assessment of certain body regions. These positions are described and illustrated in Table 7.2.

Following Universal Precautions

In 1987, the Centers for Disease Control and Prevention (CDCP) published a set of recommendations for universal precautions with all clients to reduce the risk of transmitting unidentified pathogens, especially blood-borne pathogens (US Department of Health and Human Services, 1987). These guidelines, which are essential for nurses performing physical assessments, are as follows:

Hand-Washing Wash your hands before and between clients. Wash your hands immediately and thoroughly with warm water and soap if you come in contact with blood or other body fluids or potentially contaminated articles. Wash your hands immediately after you remove your gloves, even if the gloves appear to be intact. When hand-washing facilities are not available, use a waterless antiseptic hand cleaner in accordance with the manufacturer's directions.

Gloves Wear gloves when touching blood and body fluids containing blood, as well as when handling items or surfaces soiled with blood or body fluids containing blood. Change gloves between clients. Wear gloves if you have cuts, scratches, or other breaks in the skin. Wear gloves in all situations in which contamination with blood may occur.

Other Protective Barriers Wear masks and protective eyewear (glasses, goggles) or face shields to protect the mucous membranes of your mouth, nose, and eyes during procedures that are likely to generate droplets of blood or other body fluids. Wear a disposable plastic apron or gown during procedures that are likely to generate splatters of blood or other body fluids and soil your clothing.

Sharps Disposal To prevent injuries, place used disposable needle-syringe units, scalpel blades, and other sharp items in puncture-resistant containers for disposal. Discard used needle-syringe units uncapped and unbroken. Place puncture-resistant containers as close as practicable to use areas.

Laundry Handle soiled linen as little as possible and with minimum agitation to prevent gross microbial contamination of the air and of persons handling the linen. Place linen soiled with blood or body fluids in leakage-resistant bags at the location where the linen is used.

Specimens Put all specimens of blood and body fluids in well-constructed containers with secure lids to prevent leakage during transport. When collecting specimens, take care to avoid contaminating the outside of the container.

Blood Spills Use a chemical germicide that is approved for use as a hospital disinfectant to decontaminate work surfaces after a spill of blood or other applicable body fluids. In the absence of a commercial germicide, a solution of sodium hypochlorite (household bleach) in a 1:100 dilution is effective.

Infective Wastes Follow agency policies for disposal of infective waste, both when disposing of, and when decontaminating, contaminated materials. Carefully pour bulk blood, suctioned fluids, and excretions containing blood and secretions down drains that are connected to a sanitary sewer.

The universal precautions are reviewed periodically by the CDCP and are subject to change. Be sure to check with your agency for CDCP updates.

Table 7.2 Client Positions and Body Areas Examined

	Position	Areas Examined
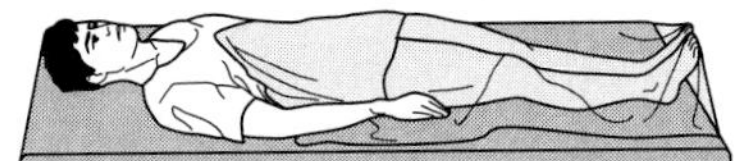 Dorsal Recumbent	Back-lying position with knees flexed and hips externally rotated; small pillow under the head. May be difficult for clients who have cardiopulmonary problems.	Head and neck, axillae, anterior thorax, lungs, breasts, heart, abdomen, extremities, peripheral pulses, vital signs, and vagina.
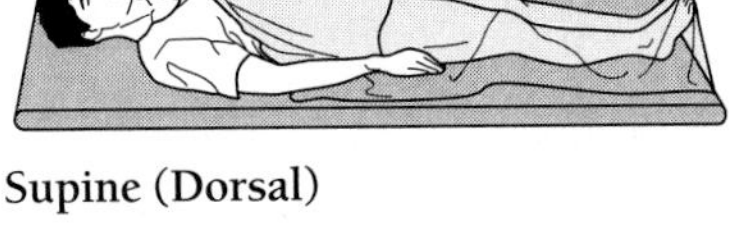 Supine (Dorsal)	Back-lying position without a pillow or with a small pillow. Tolerated poorly by clients with cardiovascular and respiratory problems.	Head, neck, axillae, anterior thorax, lungs, breasts, heart, extremities, abdomen, peripheral pulses.
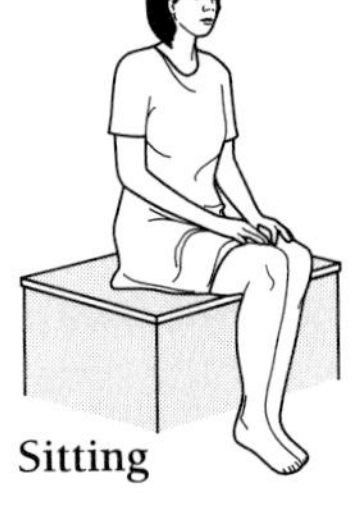 Sitting	A seated position, back unsupported and legs hanging freely. Weak clients may require support.	Head, neck, posterior and anterior thorax, lungs, breasts, axillae, heart, vital signs, upper and lower extremities, reflexes.
Lithotomy	Back-lying position with feet supported in stirrups; the hips should be in line with the edge of the table. May be difficult and tiring for older adults.	Female genitals, rectum, and female genital reproductive tract.
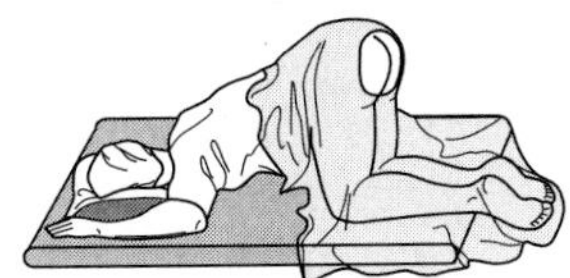 Genupectoral	Kneeling position with torso at a 90-degree angle to hips. Uncomfortable position tolerated poorly by clients who have respiratory problems.	Rectum.
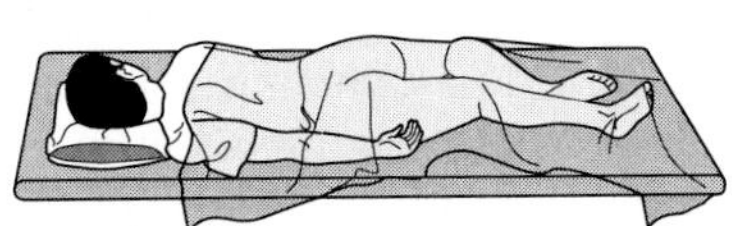 Sims'	Side-lying position with lowermost arm behind the body and uppermost leg flexed. Difficult for older adults and people with limited joint movement.	Rectum, vagina.
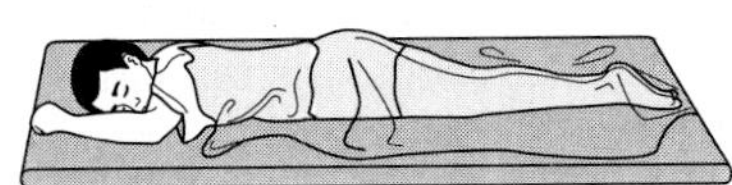 Prone	Face-lying position, with or without a small pillow. Often not tolerated by older adults and people with cardiovascular and respiratory problems.	Posterior thorax, hip movement.

Organizing the Steps of the Exam

Throughout the physical assessment, use a consistent pattern and routine. Two methods of examination commonly used are the head-to-toe (cephalocaudal) approach and the body systems approach. Many examiners find that a combination of these two methods allows for the most thorough assessment of the client, and a combined approach is adopted in this text. For example, the head and neck are most effectively assessed as a region, whereas the integumentary system is most effectively assessed over the entire body, as a system.

A *focused assessment* is an examination of a specific organ, system, or region. Usually, it is performed because of a client's complaint of a change in health status; for example, complaint of sunburn or wrist pain. Focused assessments also provide baseline data before a nursing intervention or medical procedure. For example, the nurse assesses a surgical site frequently during the immediate postoperative period.

Use a consistent method for performing the four assessment techniques: In all regions of the body except the abdomen, follow the sequence of inspection, palpation, percussion, then auscultation. When examining the abdomen, auscultate before percussing or palpating to prevent distortion of bowel sounds.

Documenting the Findings

Throughout the exam, make notations of findings. Many institutions use a checklist or form that the nurse completes during or soon after the examination. As described in Chapter 1, documentation of unexpected findings should be as complete and specific as possible. For example, rather than describing drainage as large or copious, give an approximate amount, eg, 500 cc. Rather than writing that a lesion is the size of a pea, state its approximate diameter. Also note any other signs associated with the unexpected findings. For example: *10:00 A.M. Perineal pad saturated with approximately 300 cc bright red vaginal drainage. Skin cool and clammy. Color pale. Client complains of dull pressure in lower abdominal area.* (See Chapter 1 for information on documenting findings.)

Assessing the Client's Appearance and Mental Status

The client's appearance and mental status provide you with immediate and important clues to the client's level of wellness. Thus, beginning with the initial meeting, note any factors about the client's appearance and mental status that are in any way unexpected. For example, you might note that a client appears undernourished, seems older than his or her stated age, walks slowly, has difficulty maintaining eye contact, talks incessantly, and so on.

When assessing the client's appearance, remember to consider the client's developmental stage, cultural background, socioeconomic status, job, level of intelligence, and other factors as described in previous chapters. Consider the following example: A 22-year-old male artist falls from a scaffold while painting scenery at the local theater. About an hour later, he begins feeling faint and nauseated and goes to a walk-in urgent care center. The admitting nurse, observing the client's age, dirty and disheveled clothing, dirty face and hands, confusion, slurred speech, and difficulty walking, may conclude that he is inebriated unless other factors, such as his job, are considered in the assessment.

An assessment of the client's appearance and mental status includes information about the following factors:

Dress and Grooming

The way clients dress may provide clues to their sense of self-esteem and body image. However, as discussed above, you must consider many factors before drawing conclusions based on a client's appearance. For example, a client who wears clothing that is uncoordinated or inappropriate for the situation or weather may be mentally ill or experiencing situational grief or anxiety, or such a client may be mentally fit but unable to afford to buy other clothes.

Personal Hygiene

Observe the client for cleanliness and personal hygiene. The client who is dirty or has a strong body odor or poor dental hygiene may be depressed, have poor self-concept, or lack knowledge about personal hygiene. However, as always, consider the client's environment before drawing conclusions. For example, a client who is dirty may have just come from working on a construction site.

Gait and Posture

Observe the client's gait and posture. Normally, the client walks in a rhythmic, straight, upright position with arms swinging at the sides. The shoulders are level and straight. Difficulty with gait and posture, such as stumbling, shuffling, limping, or inability to stand erect, calls for further evaluation. See Chapter 17 for information on assessing the musculoskeletal system.

Body Build

Body shape and build may indicate the client's general level of wellness. The body should be symmetric and the proportions regular: the client's arm span should approximate the height, and the distance from the pubis to the crown should roughly equal the distance from the pubis to the sole of the foot. The client's height and weight should be within normal ranges for age and body build (see pages 113–114 for information on measuring height and weight). Emaciation or obesity may indicate an eating disorder. Again, consider the client's lifestyle, socioeconomic level, and environment.

Behavior

Generally, you assess the client's behavior while the client is responding to questions and giving information about the health history. Note the client's affect and mood, level of anxiety, orientation, and speech. Findings in these areas may be evaluated further during the assessment of the client's psychosocial status (see Chapter 4) and neurologic system (see Chapter 18).

Affect and Mood Assess the client's emotional state by noting what the client says, the client's body language, facial expression, and the appropriateness of the client's behavior in relation to the situation and circumstances. The client should exhibit comfort in talking with the examiner. Giggling when answering questions about bowel movements may simply indicate embarrassment, whereas giggling when describing the death of a loved one may be an example of inappropriate affect.

Level of Anxiety Assess the client for apprehension, fear, and nervousness. Like affect and mood, the client's level of anxiety is revealed through speech, body language, and facial expression. During the health assessment, the client may exhibit anxiety due to embarrassment, fear of pain, or worry about the outcome of the exam. If the client's anxiety seems to have no cause, evaluate the client further. To obtain a relative impression of the level of anxiety, ask clients to rate their feelings of anxiety on a scale of 0 to 10. Use the client's response as an indicator of the need for further assessment and as a baseline for future assessment of anxiety levels.

Orientation Assess clients for orientation to person, place, and time; that is, clients should normally be able to state their name, location, and the date and time of day. In most cases, you will be able to sense a client's orientation during the initial interview; if the client seems confused, ask the client directly: "Tell me your name, where you are now, today's date, and the time." If the client cannot respond or responds incorrectly, perform a more detailed assessment of mental status. See Chapter 19 for details on how to perform this assessment.

Speech Assess the client's speech for quantity, volume, content, articulation, and rhythm. The client should speak easily and fluently to you or to an interpreter. Disorganized speech patterns, silence, or constant talking may indicate normal nervousness or shyness, or they may signal a speech defect, neurologic deficit, depression, or another disorder.

Special Considerations for Children and Adolescents

Consider the developmental stage of the child or adolescent when assessing for each of the above factors. Note that the appearance of the younger child reveals a great deal of information about the child's parents or caretakers, and the appearance of an older child gives clues about self-care. For instance, a child of 3 whose skin and clothes are dirty may be a victim of neglect, while a 13-year-old in the same condition may lack knowledge about proper hygiene.

Note the child's interaction with the parents or caretakers. Their relationship should exhibit mutual warmth and caring. Signs of child abuse include absence of separation anxiety in a child who, because of developmental stage, would ordinarily demonstrate it; avoidance of eye contact between caretaker and child; and a caretaker's demonstration of disgust with a child's behavior, illness, odor, or stool.

Special Considerations for Older Adults

The dress, grooming, and personal hygiene of an older adult may be affected by limitations in mobility from arthritis, cardiovascular disease, and other disorders, or by a lack of funds.

The gait of an older adult is often slower and the steps shorter. To maintain balance, the older adult may hold the arms away from the body or use a cane. The posture of an older adult may look slightly stooped because of a generalized flexion, which also causes the older adult to appear shorter. A loss in height may also be due to thinning of the intervertebral discs.

The behavior of the older adult may be affected by various disorders common to this age group, such as vascular insufficiency and diabetes. In addition, medications may affect the client's behavior: Some medications may cause the client to feel anxious, and others may affect the client's alertness, orientation, or speech. You should also consider overmedication when assessing the behavior of the older adult; thus, be sure to record every medication the client is taking.

Measuring the Client's Height and Weight

Measure the client's height and weight to establish baseline data and to help determine health status. Ask the client about height and weight before taking the measurements. Any large discrepancies between the stated height and weight and the actual measurements may provide clues to the client's self-image. Alternatively, discrepancies in weight may indicate the client's lack of awareness of a sudden loss or gain in weight that may be due to illness.

Height

To measure height, use a measuring stick attached to a platform scale or to a wall. Instruct the client to look straight ahead while standing as straight as possible with the heels together and the shoulders back. When using a platform scale, raise the L-shaped height attachment rod above the client's head, then extend and lower the right-angled arm until it rests on the crown of the head. Read the measurement from the height attachment rod (Figure 7.9). When using a measuring stick, place an L-shaped level on the crown of the client's head at a right angle to the measuring stick (Figure 7.10).

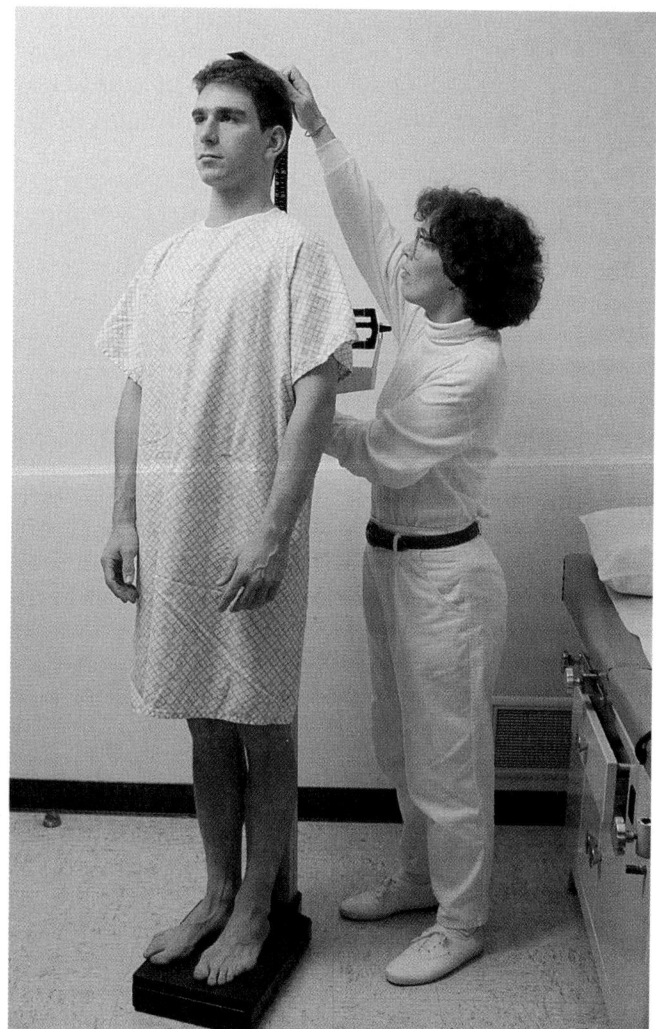

Figure 7.9 Measuring the client's height with a platform scale.

Weight

Use a standard platform scale to measure the weight of older children and adults. Whenever possible, use the same scale at each visit and weigh the client at the same time of day in the same kind of clothing (eg, the examination gown) and without shoes. If using a digital scale, simply read the weight from the lighted display panel. Otherwise, calibrate the scale by moving both weights to 0 and turning the knob until the balance beam is level. Move the large and small weights to the right and take the reading when the balance beam returns to level (Figure 7.11). Special bed and chair scales are available for clients who cannot stand.

Table 7.3 on page 116 lists average heights and weights for adult men and women. See Chapter 19 for height and weight tables and growth charts for infants and children. Although these standardized charts are useful as guidelines for assessing growth, development, and nutritional status, not all healthy clients fall within these ranges.

Special Considerations for Infants, Children, and Adolescents

Measure an infant's length by placing the child in a supine position on an examining table that is equipped with a ruler, headboard, and adjustable footboard. Position the head against the headboard. Extend the infant's leg nearest the ruler, and adjust the footboard until it touches the infant's foot. The space between the headboard and footboard represents the length of the infant. Alternatively, place the infant on a standard examination table, extend the infant's leg, mark the paper covering at the infant's head and foot, and measure the distance between the markings (Figure 7.12 on page 116).

Infants are weighed on a modified platform scale with curved sides to prevent injury. The scale measures weight in grams and in ounces. Place the unclothed baby on the scale on a paper drape and watch the baby to prevent a fall (Figure 7.13 on page 116). Measurements are taken to the nearest 10 g (½ oz).

Children over the age of 2 or 3 may be weighed on the upright scale or seated on the infant scale. Leave the child's underpants on. To measure height, use the platform scale or a measuring stick attached to the wall, as for an adult. By the age of 4, most children enjoy being weighed and measured and finding out how much they have grown. Chapter 3 discusses growth and development. Chapter 19 includes growth charts for boys and girls.

Special Considerations for Older Adults

The height of older adults may decline somewhat as a result of thinning of the intervertebral discs and a general flexion of the hips and knees. Body weight may decrease because of muscle shrinkage. In addition, the older client may appear thinner, even when well-nourished, because of loss of subcutaneous fat deposits from the face, forearms, and lower legs. At the same time, fat deposits on the abdomen and hips may increase.

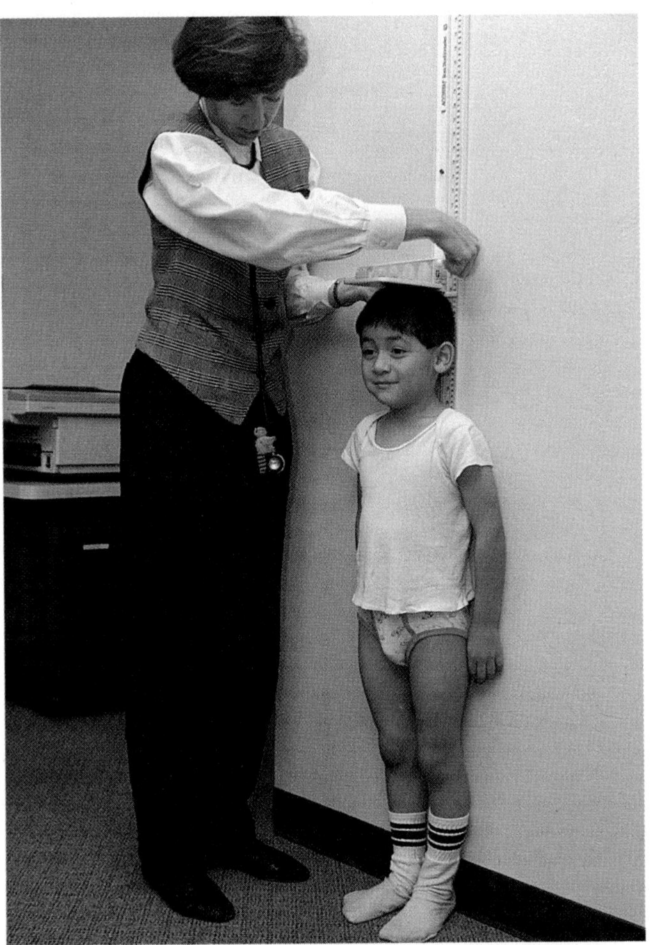

Figure 7.10 Measuring the client's height with a measuring stick.

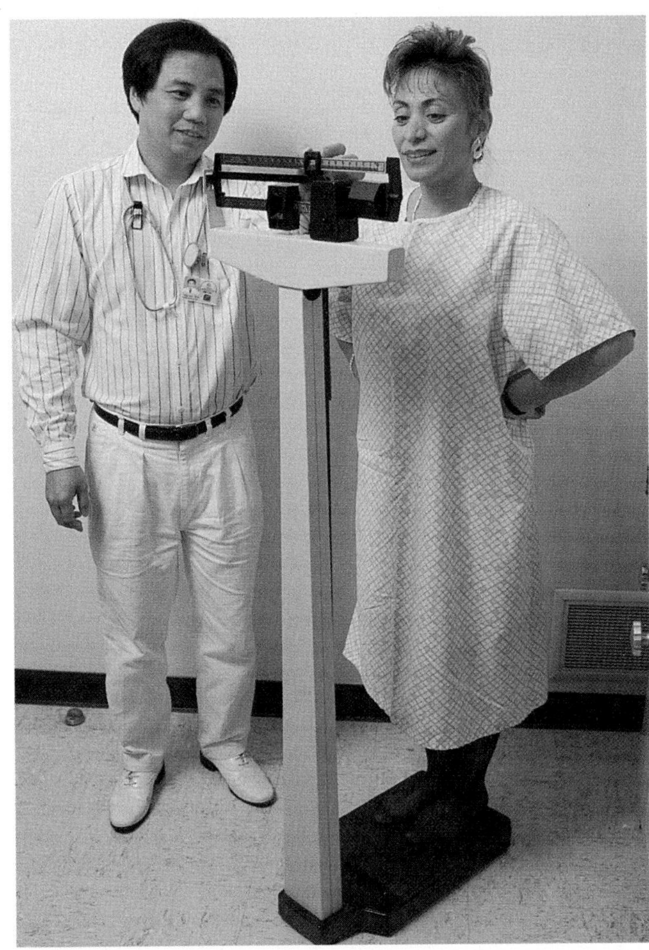

Figure 7.11 Measuring the client's weight with a standard platform scale.

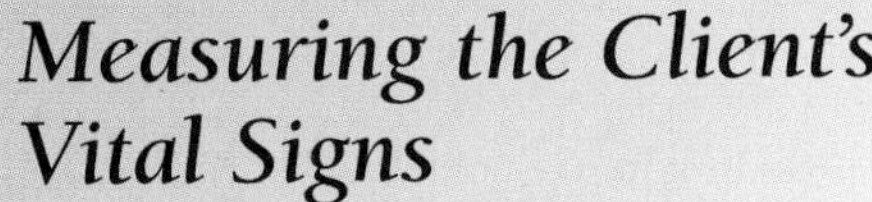

Measuring the Client's Vital Signs

Vital signs include body temperature, pulse, respirations, and blood pressure. Measure vital signs to obtain baseline data, to detect or monitor a change in the client's health status, and to monitor clients at risk for alterations in health.

Body Temperature

The body's *surface temperature*—the temperature of the skin, subcutaneous tissues, and fat—fluctuates in response to environmental factors and is therefore unreliable for monitoring a client's health status. Instead, measure the client's **core temperature**, or the temperature of the deep tissues of the body, eg, the thorax and abdominal cavity. This temperature remains relatively constant at about 37C, or 98.6F.

The body's core temperature is regulated by sensors in the hypothalamus. When these hypothalamic sensors detect heat, they signal the body to decrease heat production and increase heat loss, eg, by vasodilation and sweating. When sensors in the hypothalamus detect cold, they signal the body to increase heat production and decrease heat loss, eg, by shivering, vasoconstriction, and inhibition of sweating.

A variety of factors may influence normal core body temperature. These include:

- Age. The core temperature of infants is highly responsive to changes in the environment; therefore, infants need extra protection from even mild variations in temperature. The core body temperature of children is more stable than that of infants but less so than that of adolescents or adults. On the other hand, older adults are more sensitive than middle adults to variations in environmental temperature. This increased sensitivity may be due to the decreased thermoregulatory control and loss of subcutaneous fat common in older adults, or it may be due to environmental factors such as lack of activity, inadequate diet, or lack of central heating.

Table 7.3 1983 Metropolitan Height and Weight Tables, Men and Women, Ages 25 to 59

Men				Women			
	Weight (lb)*				Weight (lb)*		
Height	Small Frame	Medium Frame	Large Frame	Height	Small Frame	Medium Frame	Large Frame
5′ 2″	128–134	131–141	138–150	4′10″	102–111	109–121	118–131
5′ 3″	130–136	133–143	140–153	4′11″	103–113	111–123	120–134
5′ 4″	132–138	135–145	142–156	5′ 0″	104–115	113–126	122–137
5′ 5″	134–140	137–148	144–160	5′ 1″	106–118	115–129	125–140
5′ 6″	136–142	139–151	146–164	5′ 2″	108–121	118–132	128–143
5′ 7″	138–145	142–154	149–168	5′ 3″	111–124	121–135	131–147
5′ 8″	140–148	145–157	152–172	5′ 4″	114–127	124–138	134–151
5′ 9″	142–151	148–160	155–176	5′ 5″	117–130	127–141	137–155
5′10″	144–154	151–163	158–180	5′ 6″	120–133	130–144	140–159
5′11″	146–157	154–166	161–184	5′ 7″	123–136	133–147	143–163
6′ 0″	149–160	157–170	164–188	5′ 8″	126–130	136–150	146–167
6′ 1″	152–164	160–174	168–192	5′ 9″	129–142	139–153	149–170
6′ 2″	155–168	164–178	172–197	5′10″	132–145	142–156	152–173
6′ 3″	158–172	167–182	176–202	5′11″	135–148	145–159	155–176
6′ 4″	162–176	171–187	181–207	6′ 0″	138–151	148–162	158–179

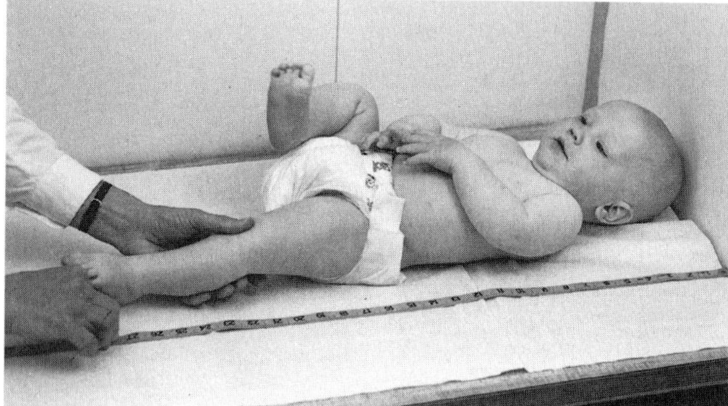

Figure 7.12 Measuring an infant's length.

- Diurnal variations. Core body temperature is usually highest between 8:00 P.M. and midnight, and lowest between 4:00 and 6:00 A.M. Normal body temperature may vary by as much as 1.0C or 1.8F between these times. Some individuals have more than one complete cycle in a day.
- Exercise. Strenuous exercise can increase core body temperature by as much as 2C or 5F.
- Hormones. A variety of hormones affect core body temperature. For example, in women, progesterone secretion at the time of ovulation raises core body temperature by about 0.35C or 0.5F.
- Stress. The temperature of a highly stressed client may be elevated as a result of increased production of epinephrine and norepinephrine, which increase metabolic activity and heat production.

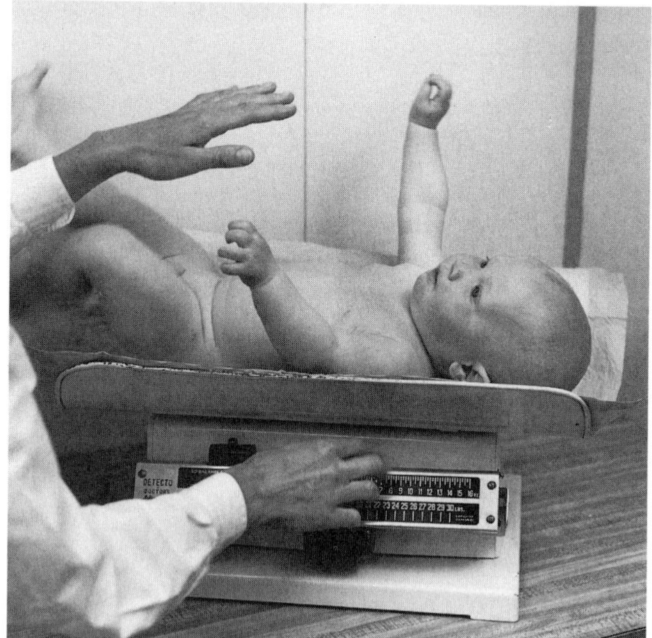

Figure 7.13 Weighing an infant.

- Illness. Illness or central nervous system disorder may impair the thermostatic function of the hypothalamus. *Hyperthermia*, also called fever, may occur in response to viral or bacterial infections, or from tissue breakdown following myocardial infarction, malignancy, surgery, or trauma. *Hypothermia* is usually a response to prolonged exposure to cold.

Until recently, core body temperature was measured usually with a mercury-in-glass thermometer. Today, nurses are more likely to use an electronic thermometer (Figure 7.14), which gives a highly accurate reading in only 2 to 60 seconds. These portable, battery-operated devices consist of an electronic display unit, a probe, and disposable probe sheaths. Attach the appropriate probe to the unit, cover it with a sterile sheath, and insert it into the body orifice. The probe is left in place until the temperature appears on the liquid crystal display (LCD) screen.

You may choose one of four routes for measuring core body temperature: oral, rectal, axillary, or tympanic:

- The *oral temperature* is the most accessible and convenient. If using a mercury-in-glass thermometer, shake the thermometer down to 35.5C or 96F. Place the thermometer at the base of the tongue in either of the sublingual pockets to the right or left of the frenulum (Figure 7.15) and instruct the client to keep the lips tightly closed around the thermometer. Leave the thermometer in place for 3 to 5 minutes, then remove the thermometer and either discard its plastic sheath or wipe it with a tissue toward the bulb. Hold the thermometer at eye level and rotate it until the mercury column is visible. The upper end of the column of mercury reflects the client's core body temperature.
- Take a *rectal temperature* if taking an oral temperature is not practical, eg, if the client is comatose, confused, or unable to close the mouth. For a rectal temperature, lubricate the thermometer, put on disposable gloves, ask the client to take a deep breath, then insert the thermometer from 1.5 cm to 4 cm into the anus. Do not force insertion of the thermometer. If using a mercury-in-glass thermometer, leave it in place for 3 minutes, holding onto the exposed end for safety.

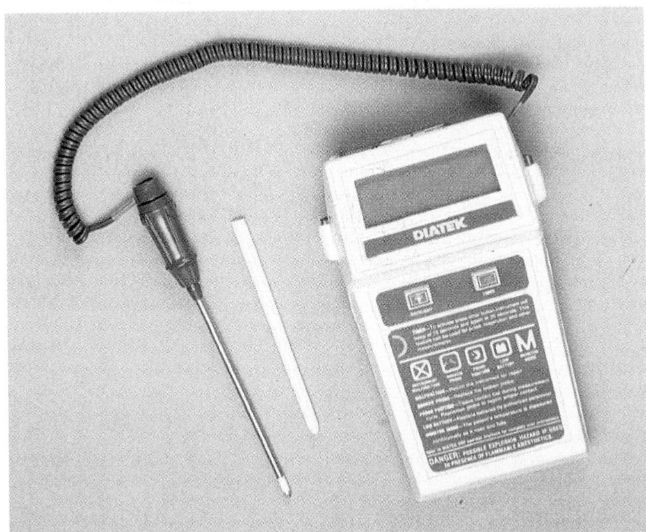

Figure 7.14 Electronic thermometer.

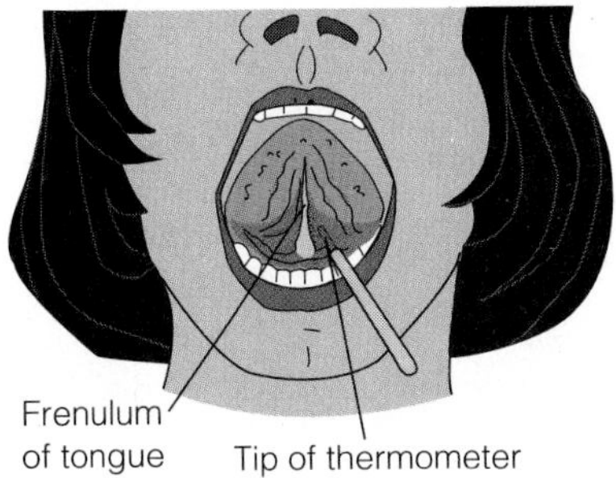

Figure 7.15 Placement of the thermometer for an oral temperature.

- Occasionally, you will need to take an *axillary temperature*. This is the safest method and is less invasive, but it is also the least accurate and, if using a mercury-in-glass thermometer, takes the longest time (9 minutes) to obtain a reading. For an axillary temperature, place the thermometer in the client's axilla, and assist the client in placing the arm tightly across the chest to keep the thermometer in place.
- The *tympanic temperature* can be taken only with an electronic thermometer. Using infrared technology, it measures a client's core body temperature quickly and accurately. This method is the most comfortable and less invasive for the client. The measuring probe resembles an otoscope. Place the covered tip of the probe at the opening of the ear canal. Be gentle: Don't force the probe into the ear canal or occlude the canal opening. After about 2 seconds, the client's temperature reading will appear on the LCD screen.

Pulse

The heart is a muscular pump. With every beat, the left ventricle of the heart contracts, forcing blood from the heart into the systemic arteries. The amount of blood pumped from the heart with each heartbeat is called the *stroke volume*. The force of the blood against the walls of the arteries generates a wave of pressure that is felt at various points in the body as a **pulse**. The ability of the arteries to contract and expand with the ebb and flow of blood is called *compliance*. When compliance is reduced, the heart must exert more pressure to pump blood throughout the body.

The *apical pulse* is the pulse as felt at the apex of the heart. Figure 7.16 on page 118 shows the location of the apical pulse for a child under 4 years, a child 4 to 6 years, and an adult. The *peripheral pulse* is the pulse as felt in the body's periphery, for example, in the neck, wrist, or foot. Figure 7.17 on page 119 shows eight sites where the peripheral pulse is most easily palpated. In a healthy client, the peripheral pulse rate is equivalent to the heartbeat. Alterations in the client's

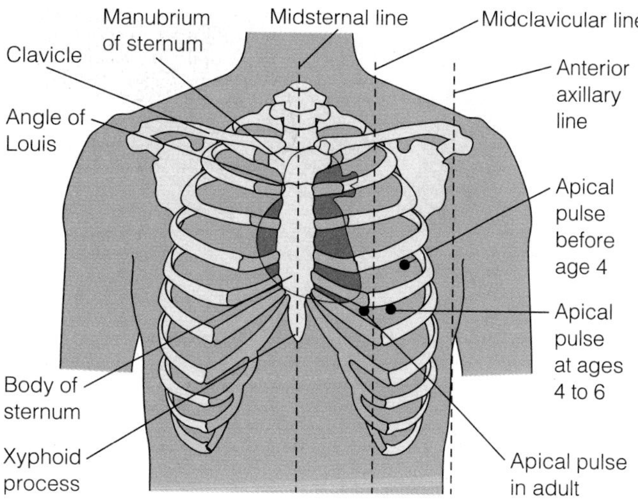

Figure 7.16 Location of the apical pulse in a child under age 4, a child age 4–6, and an adult.

health can weaken the peripheral pulse, making it difficult to detect. Thus, assessment of the peripheral pulse is an important component of a thorough health assessment.

A variety of factors may influence the normal pulse rate. These include:

- Age. The average pulse rate of infants and children is higher than that of teens and adults. After age 16, the pulse stabilizes to an average of about 70 beats per minute (BPM) in males and 75 BPM in females.
- Sex. As noted above, the average pulse rate of the adult male is slightly lower than that of the adult female.
- Exercise. The pulse rate normally increases with exercise.
- Stress. In response to stress, fear, and anxiety, the heart rate and the force of the heartbeat increase.
- Fever. The peripheral vasodilation that accompanies an elevated body temperature lowers systemic blood pressure, in turn causing an increase in pulse rate.
- Hemorrhage. Pulse rate increases in response to significant loss of blood from the vascular system.
- Medications. A variety of medications may either increase or decrease the heart rate.
- Position changes. When clients sit or stand for long periods, blood may pool in the veins, resulting in a temporary decrease in venous blood return to the heart and, consequently, reduced blood pressure and lowered pulse rate.

The peripheral pulse site most commonly used is the radial pulse. Palpate the radial pulse by placing the pads of the first three fingers on the anterior wrist along the radius bone (Figure 7.18). If the pulse is regular, count the beats for 30 seconds and multiply by two to obtain the total beats per minute (BPM). If the pulse is irregular, count the beats for a full minute.

When assessing the pulse, consider four factors: rate, rhythm, force, and elasticity. A pulse rate of less than 60 BPM, called *bradycardia*, may be found in a healthy, well-trained athlete. A pulse rate over 100 BPM, called *tachycardia*, may also be found in the healthy client who is anxious or has just finished exercising.

The pulse of a healthy adult has a relatively constant rhythm; that is, the intervals between beats are regular. Irregularities in heart rhythm are discussed fully in Chapter 11.

Assess the force of a pulse, or its stroke volume, by noting the pressure that must be exerted before the pulse is felt. A "full, bounding" pulse is difficult to obliterate. It may be caused by fear, anxiety, exercise, or a variety of alterations in health. A "weak, thready pulse" is easy to obliterate. It also may indicate alterations in health such as hemorrhage. For more information, see Chapter 11.

Palpate along the radial artery in a proximal-to-distal direction to assess the elasticity of the artery. A normal artery feels smooth, straight, and resilient.

Respirations

The human body continually takes in oxygen and gives up carbon dioxide through the act of **respiration**. Assess the client's respiratory rate by counting the number of breaths for 30 seconds, and then multiplying by two. If you detect irregularities or difficulty breathing, count the breaths for one full minute. Note that the respiratory rate in some clients may increase if they become aware that their breaths are being counted. For this reason, maintain the posture of counting the radial pulse while counting breaths per minute. Other factors that may increase respiratory rate include exercise, stress, increased temperature, and increased altitude. Some medications may either increase or decrease respiratory rate. Table 7.4 lists normal respiratory rates for newborns through older adults. See Chapter 10 for a more detailed discussion of respiration.

Blood Pressure

Blood ebbs and flows within the systemic arteries in waves, causing two types of pressure: The **systolic pressure** is the pressure of the blood at the height of the wave, when the left ventricle contracts. This is the first number recorded in a blood pressure measurement. The **diastolic pressure** is the pressure between the ventricular contractions, when the heart is "at rest." This is the second number recorded in a blood pressure measurement.

Measurements of arterial blood pressure reflect several factors:

- **Cardiac output** is the amount of blood ejected from the heart in one contraction. Cardiac output is equal to the *stroke volume*, or amount of blood ejected in one heartbeat

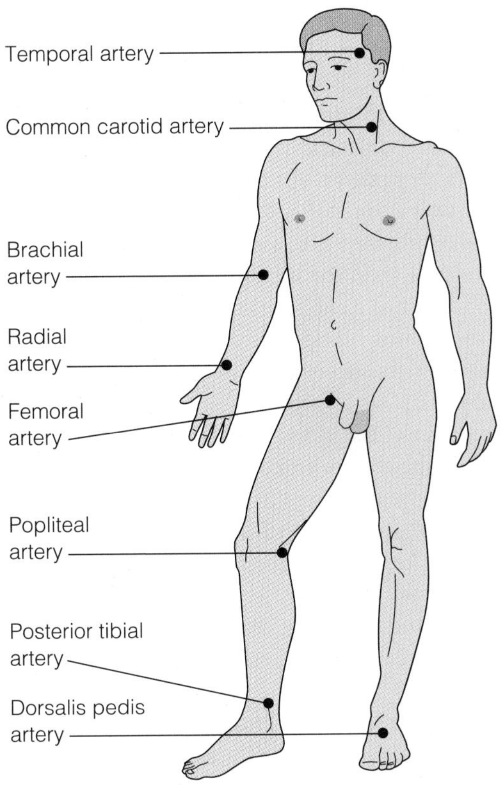

Figure 7.17 Body sites where the peripheral pulse is most easily palpated.

(measured in ml/beat), multiplied by the *heart rate* (measured in beats/min). Cardiac output averages about 5.5 L/min.

- **Blood volume** is the total amount of blood circulating within the entire vascular system. Blood volume averages about 5 L in adults. A sudden drop in blood pressure may signal sudden blood loss, as with internal bleeding.
- **Peripheral vascular resistance** is the resistance the blood encounters as it flows within the vessels. Peripheral resistance is in turn influenced by various factors, such as vessel length and diameter. Two of the most important factors influencing peripheral resistance are blood viscosity and vessel compliance:
  - *Blood viscosity* is the ratio between the blood cells (the formed elements) and the blood plasma. When the total amount of formed elements is high, the blood is thicker, or more viscous: the molecules pass one another with greater difficulty, and more pressure is required to move the blood.
  - *Vessel compliance* describes the elasticity of the smooth muscle in the arterial walls. Highly elastic arteries respond readily and fully to each heartbeat. Rigid, hardened arteries, as are found with arteriosclerosis, are less responsive, and greater force is required to move the blood along.

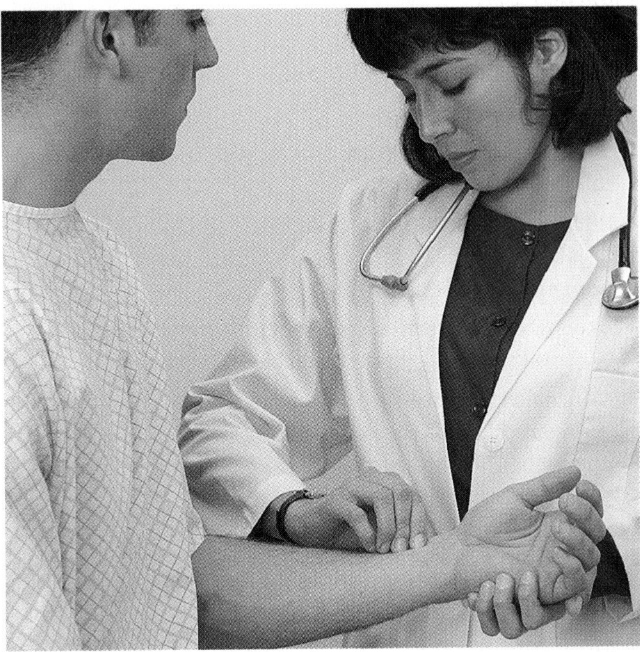

Figure 7.18 Palpating the radial pulse.

Table 7.4 Normal Respiratory Rates for Newborns through Older Adults

Age	Respirations per Minute
Newborn	30–80
3–9 years	20–30
10–15 years	16–22
16–adult	15–20
Adult	12–20
Older adult	15–25

Note that blood in the systemic circulation flows along a pressure gradient from central to peripheral; in other words, pressure is higher in the arterioles than in the capillaries, and higher still in the aorta.

The average blood pressure of a healthy adult is 120/80 mm Hg. Factors affecting blood pressure include:

- Age. Systolic blood pressure in newborns averages about 78 mm Hg. Blood pressure rates tend to rise with increasing age through age 18 and then tend to stabilize. In older adults, blood pressure rates tend to rise again as elasticity of the arteries decreases.
- Sex. After puberty, females tend to have lower blood pressures than males of the same age. This difference may be influenced by reproductive hormones, because blood pressure in women usually increases after menopause.

- Race. American males of African ancestry over the age of 35 tend to have higher blood pressures than American males of European descent.
- Obesity. Blood pressure tends to be higher in people who are overweight and obese than in people of normal weight of the same age.
- Physical activity. Physical activity (including crying in infants and children) increases cardiac output and therefore increases blood pressure.
- Stress. Stress increases cardiac output and arterial vasoconstriction, resulting in increased blood pressure.
- Diurnal variations. Blood pressure is usually lowest in the early morning and rises steadily throughout the day, peaking in the late afternoon or early evening.
- Medications. A variety of medications may increase or decrease blood pressure.

Blood pressure is also affected by alterations in health. Any condition that affects the cardiac output, peripheral vascular resistance, blood volume, blood viscosity, or vessel compliance can affect blood pressure.

An accurate measurement of blood pressure is an essential part of any complete health assessment. Note that client anxiety may cause a temporary elevation of blood pressure. Reassure the client that the procedure is quick and painless, and provide teaching as appropriate. The client should be at rest at least 5 minutes before you take the blood pressure, and up to 20 minutes if the client has been engaging in heavy physical activity.

Measure blood pressure with a blood pressure cuff, a sphygmomanometer, and a stethoscope. The *cuff* consists of an inflatable bladder, which is covered by cloth and has two tubes attached to it. One of these tubes ends in a rubber bulb with which to inflate the bladder. Air in the bladder is regulated by a small valve on the side of the bulb: when the valve is loosened, air in the bladder is released; when the valve is tightened, pumped air remains in the bladder.

The second tube attached to the bladder ends in a *sphygmomanometer*, a device that measures the air pressure in the bladder. There are two types of sphygmomanometers: aneroid and mercury (Figure 7.19). The aneroid sphygmomanometer has a small calibrated dial with a needle. It is more portable but less reliable than the mercury type. The mercury sphygmomanometer has a calibrated cylinder filled with mercury. To determine the blood pressure, read the measurement corresponding to the crescent-shaped top of the column of mercury.

The bladder of the blood pressure cuff must fit the length and width of the client's limb. If the bladder is too narrow, the blood pressure reading will be falsely high. The width of the bladder should equal 40% of the circumference of the limb. The length of the bladder should equal 80% of the circumference of the limb. Note that the circumference of the client's limb, and not the age of the client, determines the cuff used. Table 7.5 lists recommended cuff bladder dimensions by limb circumference.

Blood pressure measurements are usually taken by placing the cuff on the client's arm and auscultating the pulse in the brachial artery. Use common sense when choosing which arm to use for the measurement: for example, do not measure blood pressure in an arm on the same side as a mastectomy or an arm with a shunt. If blood pressure cannot be measured in either arm because of disease or trauma, a thigh blood pressure may be taken, using the popliteal artery, or a leg blood pressure may be taken, using the posterior tibial or dorsalis pedis arteries.

To measure the blood pressure in the client's arm:

- Place the client in a comfortable position in a quiet room.

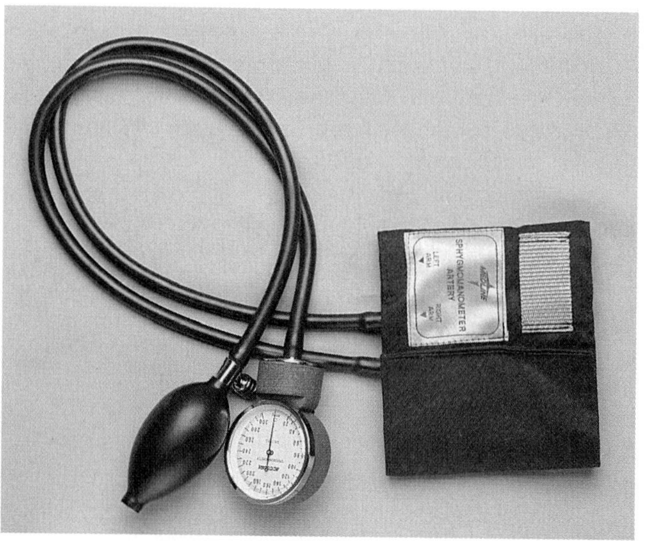

A

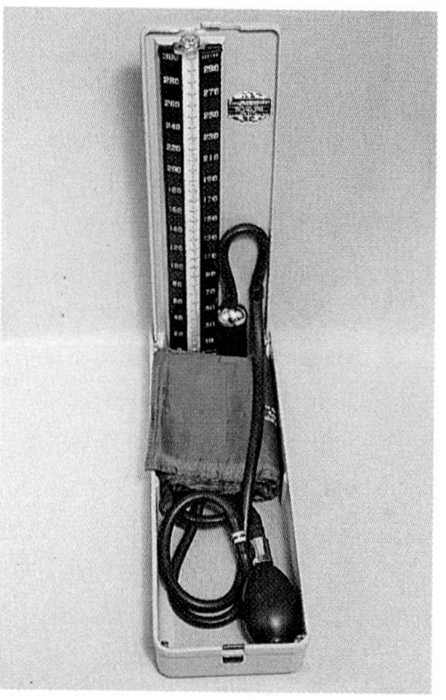

B

Figure 7.19 Sphygmomanometers. *A,* Aneroid. *B,* Mercury.

- Confirm that the blood pressure cuff is the appropriate size for the client's arm.
- Remove any clothing from the client's arm.
- Place the cuff on the arm with the lower border 1 inch above the antecubital area, making sure that the cuff is smooth and snug. One finger should fit between the cuff and the client's arm.
- Slightly flex the arm and hold it at the level of the heart with the palm upward.
- Palpate the brachial pulse.
- Place the diaphragm of the stethoscope over the brachial pulse (Figure 7.20).
- Pump up the cuff, listening for the disappearance of the brachial pulse, until the sphygmomanometer registers 30 mm Hg above the point at which the brachial pulse disappears.
- Release the valve on the cuff carefully so that the pressure decreases at the rate of 2 to 3 mm Hg per second.
- Note the manometer reading at each of the five phases described in the box on page 122.
- Deflate the cuff rapidly and completely.
- Remove the cuff from the client's arm.

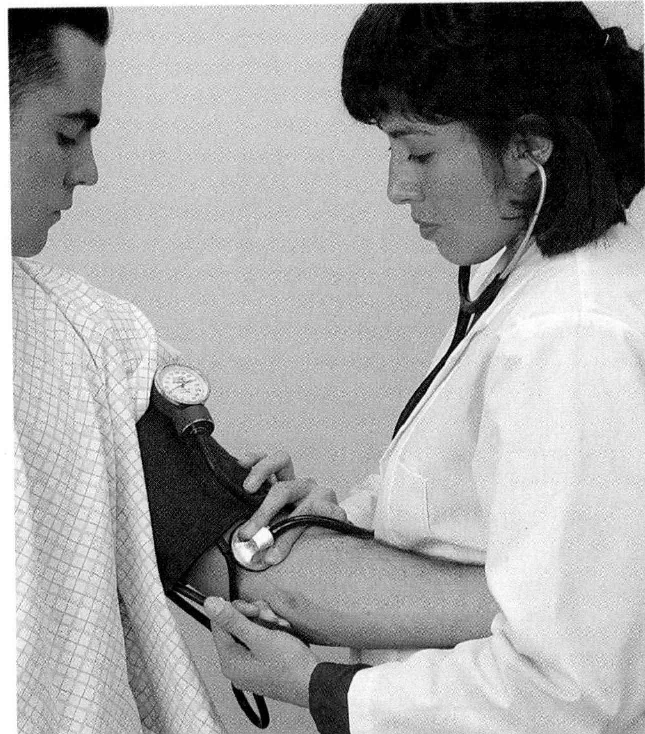

Figure 7.20 Measuring the client's blood pressure.

Special Considerations for Infants, Children, and Adolescents

Temperature Because taking a rectal temperature may cause an infant to cry, assess respirations and pulse rate before measuring rectal temperature in infants. Hold the infant in a lateral position with the knees flexed onto the abdomen, or prone on your lap. Separate the infant's buttocks with the nondominant hand and insert the thermometer with the dominant gloved hand. Use a blunt-tipped thermometer. Insert it no more than 2.5 cm or 1 inch, and hold onto the exposed end.

Table 7.5 Recommended Cuff Bladder Dimensions by Limb Circumference

Limb Circumference (in centimeters)	Cuff Size (in centimeters)
Less than 22	9 × 18
22–33	12 × 23
33–41	15 × 33
Greater than 41	18 × 36

Source: American Heart Asssociation. "Recommendations for Human Blood Pressure Determination by Sphygmomanometers," Publication number 701005 (1987), p. 10.

To avoid the risk of rectal perforation, take an axillary temperature rather than a rectal one in newborns. Take the axillary temperature also in toddlers and older children whenever possible, to eliminate their anxiety over the invasive rectal procedure. An oral route may be used as early as age 5, if the child is able to keep the mouth closed and does not bite on the glass thermometer. Electronic thermometers, which are unbreakable and register quickly, are particularly useful with children.

Pulse Use the apical site for children younger than age 2. In older children, use the radial site, and count the pulse for a full minute. Pay particular attention to any irregularities in rhythm, such as sinus arrhythmia, which is not uncommon in children. (See Chapter 11.)

Respirations Count respirations for one full minute in infants, because the breathing pattern may show considerable variation from a series of rapid breaths to brief episodes of apnea.

Blood Pressure Use a Doppler stethoscope when measuring blood pressure in infants and in children under the age of 2. In children over the age of 2, it is imperative that you use the correct size of cuff and a small diaphragm for the stethoscope. Note that the American Heart Association recommends that, in

Korotkoff's Sounds

When measuring blood pressure, auscultate to identify five phases in a series of sounds called Korotkoff's sounds, named after the Russian surgeon who first described them. These five phases are:

Phase 1: The period initiated by the first faint, clear, tapping sounds. These sounds gradually become more intense. To ensure that they are not extraneous sounds, identify at least two consecutive tapping sounds. *Rationale*: The tapping sounds occur when the cuff pressure has decreased enough to allow the first spurts of blood into the artery.

Phase 2: The period during which the sounds have a swishing quality. *Rationale*: The swooshing sounds occur as the blood flows turbulently through the partially occluded artery and the vessel walls vibrate from the impact.

Phase 3: The period during which the sounds are tapping sounds similar to Phase 1 sounds, but they are crisper, higher-pitched, and more intense. *Rationale*: During Phase 3, blood flows through the artery during systole, but the pressure in the cuff is still high enough to cause the artery to collapse during diastole.

Phase 4: The period during which the sounds become muffled and have a soft, blowing quality. *Rationale*: The pressure in the cuff is now low enough so that the artery no longer collapses completely during any part of the cardiac cycle.

Phase 5: The point at which the sounds disappear. *Rationale*: The absence of sound reflects the absence of pressure in the cuff: normal blood flow is inaudible.

Document the blood pressure measurements as follows:

- The systolic pressure is the point at which the first tapping sound is heard (Phase 1).
- In adults, the diastolic pressure is the point at which the sounds become inaudible (Phase 5).
- In children, the diastolic pressure is the point at which the sounds become muffled (Phase 4).
- Some institutions may require you to record readings at both Phase 4 and Phase 5 for all clients, regardless of age. In such cases, document the three readings as systolic pressure, first diastolic pressure, and second diastolic pressure. Note that the second diastolic pressure may be zero; that is, muffled sounds may be audible even when the cuff is completely deflated. Finally, in cases when muffled sounds (Phase 4) are never heard, record a dash for the Phase 4 reading.

Source: American Heart Association. "Recommendations for Human Blood Pressure Determination by Sphygmomanometers," Publication number 7001005 (1987) pp. 3–5.

children, diastolic pressure be read at the beginning of Korotkoff phase 4, when the sounds become muffled.

Special Considerations for Older Adults

Body temperature in the older adult may be reduced because of decreased thermoregulatory control and loss of subcutaneous fat. Older adults are more sensitive to environmental changes in temperature, possibly because of lack of physical activity, inadequate diet, or inability to afford adequate heating.

The pulse rate of the healthy older adult ranges from 60 to 100 BPM. The radial artery may feel rigid if there is loss of elasticity in the arterial walls.

The respiratory rate in older adults may be increased to accommodate a decrease in vital capacity and inspiratory reserve volume.

As the systemic arteries lose elasticity with increasing age, the heart pumps against increased resistance, and systolic blood pressure increases.

Special Considerations for Childbearing Clients

See Chapter 20.

Summary

The assessment techniques of inspection, palpation, percussion, and auscultation, combined with cue recognition and interpretation, form the foundation of the physical assessment of the client. This physical assessment begins with the general survey, during which you assess the client's appearance and mental status and measure the client's height, weight, and vital signs. But the general survey is more than just an introduction to the physical exam: Experienced nurses often uncover data during the general survey that help them recognize related data during the focused assessments that follow.

Key Points

- ✓ Inspection is the skill of observing the client in a deliberate, systematic manner.
- ✓ Palpation is the skill of assessing the client through the sense of touch.
- ✓ Percussion is the skill of striking or tapping the body to produce sound waves that are heard as characteristic tones.
- ✓ Auscultation is the skill of listening to the sounds produced by the body.
- ✓ To conduct a successful physical assessment, you must be able to recognize cues and interpret findings.
- ✓ Before the physical assessment, gather and organize all needed assessment equipment.
- ✓ Prepare an assessment setting that promotes the client's comfort, safety, and privacy and that facilitates the examination procedures.
- ✓ Interact with the client in a manner that respects the client's individuality and provides for the client's comfort, safety, knowledge, and consent.
- ✓ Alter the position of the client as needed for assessment of certain body regions.
- ✓ Follow universal precautions throughout the physical assessment.
- ✓ Use a consistent method of organizing the steps of the physical assessment, and document significant findings.
- ✓ During the general survey, assess the client's behavior and mental status and measure the client's height, weight, and vital signs.
- ✓ Assessment of the client's behavior and mental status includes assessment of dress and grooming, personal hygiene, gait and posture, body build, and behavior.
- ✓ Assessment of the client's vital signs includes measurement of temperature, pulse, respirations, and blood pressure.

Chapter 8

Assessing the Integumentary System

The integumentary system consists of the skin, the sweat and oil glands, the hair, and the nails. The largest organ of the body, the skin weighs approximately nine pounds and has a surface area of about 15–20 feet. Every square inch of the skin contains 10–15 feet of blood vessels and nerves, hundreds of sweat and oil glands, and over three million cells that are constantly dying and being replaced. This complex shield protects the body against heat, ultraviolet rays, trauma, and invasion by bacteria. In addition, it works with other body systems to regulate body temperature, synthesize vitamin D, store blood and fats, excrete body wastes, and help us sense the world around us.

A thorough assessment of the integumentary system provides valuable clues to a client's general health. The skin, hair, and nails can suggest the status of a client's nutrition, airway clearance, thermoregulation, and tissue perfusion and can reveal alterations in activity, sleep and rest, level of stress, and self-care ability. A client's ancestry, cultural practices, and physical environment both at home and at work can greatly influence integumentary health and are an integral part of the assessment data. Additionally, a client's developmental stage has a tremendous influence on the appearance and functioning of the integument. Figure 8.1 gives an overview of some important factors to consider when you assess the integumentary system.

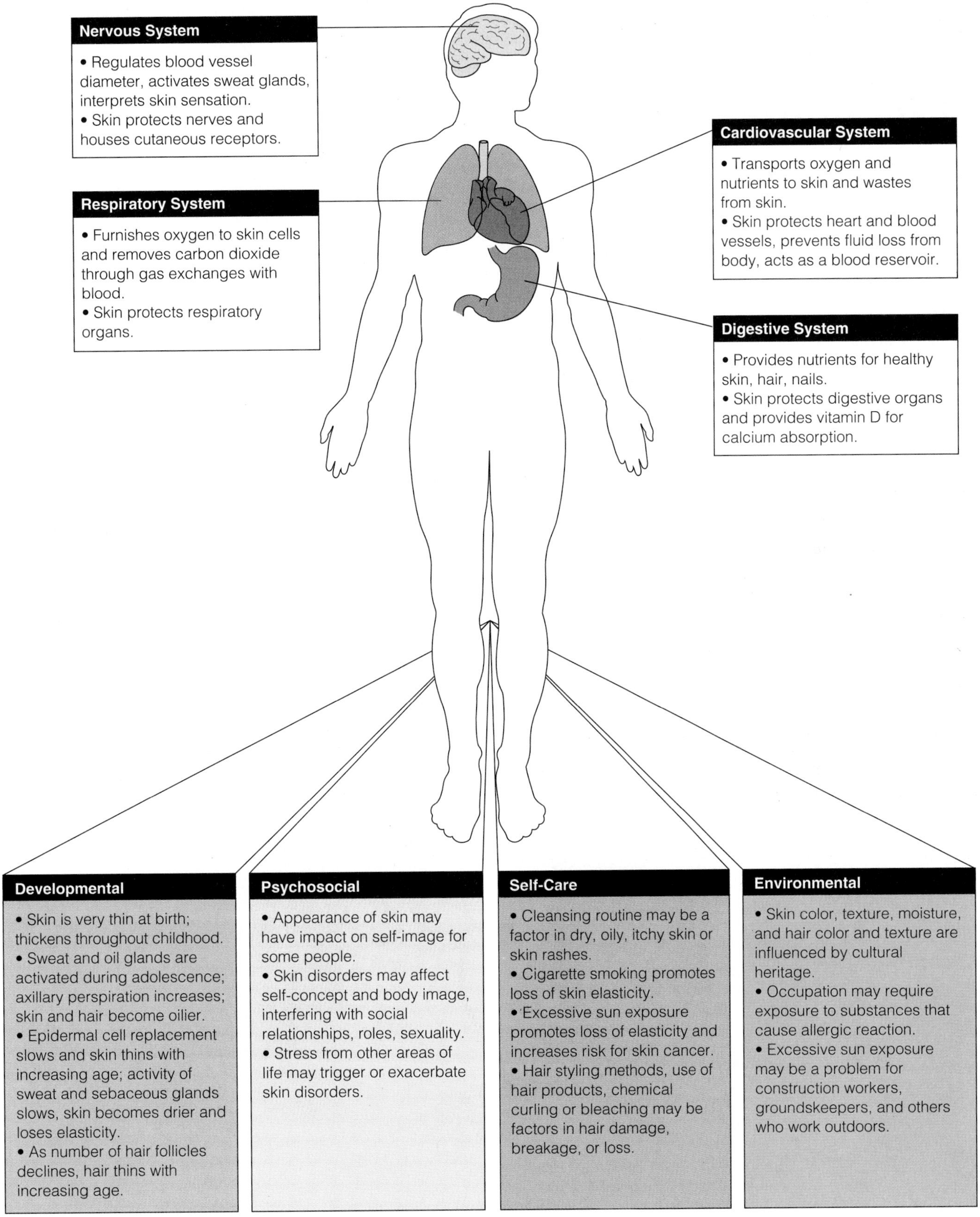

Nervous System
• Regulates blood vessel diameter, activates sweat glands, interprets skin sensation.
• Skin protects nerves and houses cutaneous receptors.
Respiratory System
• Furnishes oxygen to skin cells and removes carbon dioxide through gas exchanges with blood.
• Skin protects respiratory organs.
Cardiovascular System
• Transports oxygen and nutrients to skin and wastes from skin.
• Skin protects heart and blood vessels, prevents fluid loss from body, acts as a blood reservoir.
Digestive System
• Provides nutrients for healthy skin, hair, nails.
• Skin protects digestive organs and provides vitamin D for calcium absorption.
Developmental
• Skin is very thin at birth; thickens throughout childhood.
• Sweat and oil glands are activated during adolescence; axillary perspiration increases; skin and hair become oilier.
• Epidermal cell replacement slows and skin thins with increasing age; activity of sweat and sebaceous glands slows, skin becomes drier and loses elasticity.
• As number of hair follicles declines, hair thins with increasing age.
Psychosocial
• Appearance of skin may have impact on self-image for some people.
• Skin disorders may affect self-concept and body image, interfering with social relationships, roles, sexuality.
• Stress from other areas of life may trigger or exacerbate skin disorders.
Self-Care
• Cleansing routine may be a factor in dry, oily, itchy skin or skin rashes.
• Cigarette smoking promotes loss of skin elasticity.
• Excessive sun exposure promotes loss of elasticity and increases risk for skin cancer.
• Hair styling methods, use of hair products, chemical curling or bleaching may be factors in hair damage, breakage, or loss.
Environmental
• Skin color, texture, moisture, and hair color and texture are influenced by cultural heritage.
• Occupation may require exposure to substances that cause allergic reaction.
• Excessive sun exposure may be a problem for construction workers, groundskeepers, and others who work outdoors.

Figure 8.1 An overview of some important factors to consider when assessing the integumentary system.

Anatomy and Physiology Review

Skin and Glands

The skin is composed of two distinct layers: the outer layer, called the *epidermis*, is firmly attached to an underlying layer called the *dermis*. Deep to the dermis is a layer of *subcutaneous tissue* that anchors the skin to the underlying body structures.

Epidermis

The **epidermis** is a layer of epithelial tissue that comprises the outermost portion of the skin. Where exposure to friction is greatest, such as on the fingertips, palms, and soles of the feet, the epidermis consists of five layers (or strata), as shown in Figure 8.2. These include, from deep to superficial, the stratum basale, stratum spinosum, stratum granulosum, stratum lucidum, and stratum corneum. In other body regions, the stratum lucidum is absent.

New skin cells are formed in the *stratum basale*, or basal layer, which is also known as the stratum germinativum (germinating layer). These new skin cells consist mostly of a fibrous protein called *keratin*, which gives the epidermis its tough, protective qualities. About 25% of the cells in the stratum basale are melanocytes, which produce the skin pigment called *melanin*. All humans have the same relative number of melanocytes, but the amount of melanin they produce varies according to genetic, hormonal, and environmental factors.

Cells produced in the stratum basale gradually move through the layers of the epidermis toward the *stratum corneum*, where they are sloughed off. The abundance of keratin in this tough, "horny layer" protects against abrasion and trauma, repels water, resists water loss, and renders the body insensitive to a variety of environmental toxins.

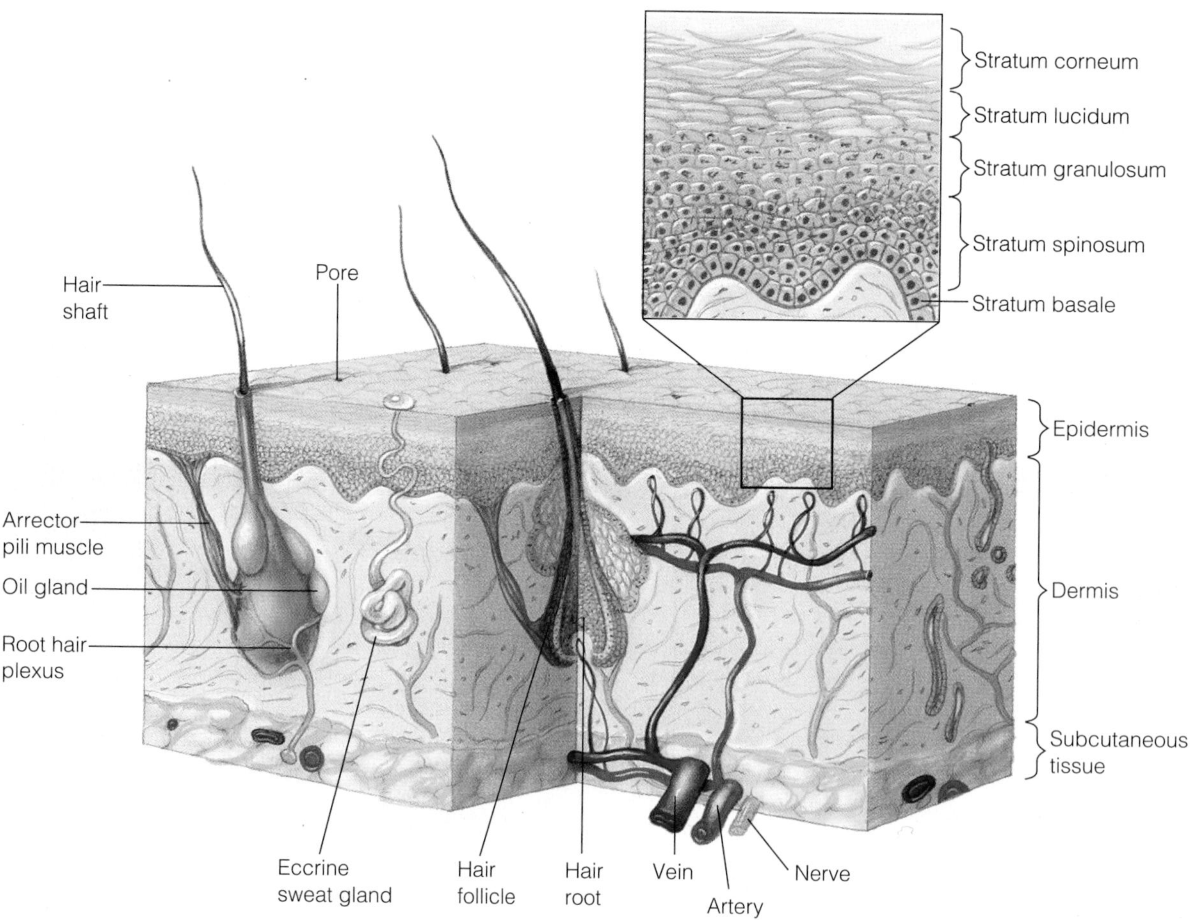

Figure 8.2 Skin structure. Three-dimensional view of the skin, subcutaneous tissue, glands, and hairs.

Dermis

The **dermis** is a layer of connective tissue that lies just deep to the epidermis. It consists mainly of two types of fibers: collagen, which gives the skin its toughness and enables it to resist tearing, and elastic fibers, which give the skin its elasticity. The dermis is richly supplied with nerves, blood vessels, and lymphatic vessels, and it is embedded with hair follicles, sweat glands, oil glands, and sensory receptors.

Subcutaneous Tissue

The **subcutaneous tissue** (or hypodermis) is a loose connective tissue that stores approximately half of the body's fat cells. Thus, it cushions the body against trauma and insulates the body from heat loss. Although not strictly considered part of the skin, it shares many of the same functions, described later.

Cutaneous Glands

The cutaneous glands are formed in the stratum basale and push deep into the dermis. They release their secretions through ducts onto the skin surface.

Sweat Glands There are two types of **sweat** (or **sudoriferous**) **glands**, eccrine and apocrine. *Eccrine glands* are more numerous and more widely distributed. They produce a clear perspiration mostly made up of water and salts, which they release into funnel-shaped *pores* at the skin surface. *Apocrine glands* are found primarily in the axillary and anogenital regions. They are dormant until the onset of puberty. Apocrine glands produce a secretion made up of water, salts, fatty acids, and proteins, which is released into hair follicles. When apocrine sweat mixes with bacteria on the skin surface, it assumes a musky odor.

Oil Glands **Oil** (or **sebaceous**) **glands** are distributed over most of the body except the palms of the hands and soles of the feet. They produce sebum, an oily secretion composed of fat and keratin that is usually released into hair follicles.

Functions of the Skin and Glands

The major functions of the skin are

- Perceiving touch, pressure, temperature, and pain
- Protecting against mechanical, chemical, thermal, and solar damage
- Protecting against loss of water and electrolytes
- Regulating body temperature
- Repairing surface wounds through cellular replacement
- Synthesizing vitamin D
- Allowing identification through uniqueness of facial contours, skin and hair color, and fingerprints

The major functions of the cutaneous glands are

- Excreting uric acid, urea, ammonia, sodium, potassium, and other metabolic wastes
- Regulating temperature through evaporation of perspiration on the skin surface
- Protecting against bacterial growth on the skin surface
- Softening, lubricating, and waterproofing skin and hair
- Resisting water loss from the skin surface in low-humidity environments
- Protecting deeper skin regions from bacteria on the skin surface

Hair

A **hair** is a thin, flexible, elongated fiber composed of dead, keratinized cells that grow out in a columnar fashion (Figures 8.2 and 8.3). Each hair shaft arises from a *follicle*. Nerve endings in the follicle are sensitive to the slightest movement of the hair. Each hair follicle also has an arrector pili muscle that causes the hair to contract and stand upright when a person is under stress or exposed to cold.

The deep end of each follicle expands to form a *hair bulb*. New cells are produced at the hair bulb. Hair growth is cycli-

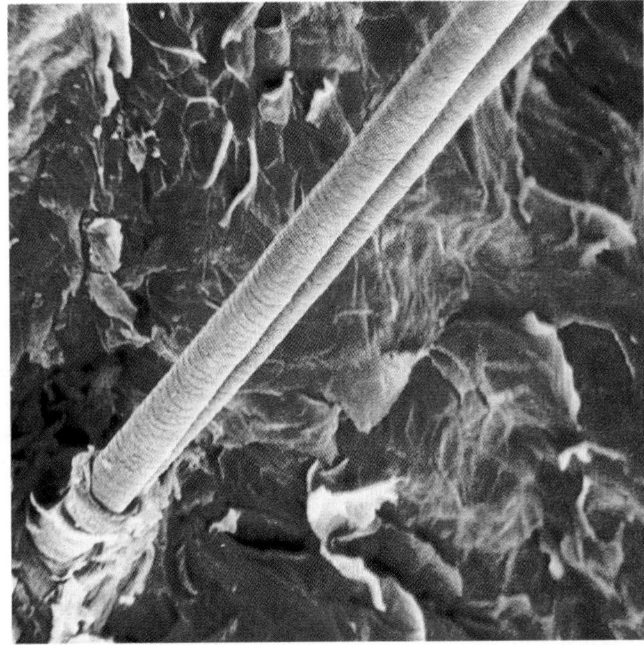

Figure 8.3 Scanning electron micrograph of a hair shaft emerging from a follicle at the epidermal surface.

cal: scalp hair typically has an active phase of about 4 years and a resting phase of a few months. Because these phases are not synchronous, only a small percentage of a person's hair follicles shed their hair at any given time.

Hair color is determined by the amount of melanin produced in the hair follicle. Black or brown hair contains the greatest amount of melanin.

The type and distribution of hair vary in different parts of the body. *Vellus hair*, a pale, fine, short strand, grows over the entire body except for the margins of the lips, the nipples, the palms of the hands and soles of the feet, and parts of the external genitals. The *terminal hair* of the eyebrows and scalp is usually darker, coarser, and longer. At puberty, hormones signal the growth of terminal hair in the axillae, pubic region, and legs of both sexes, and on the face and chest of most males.

The major functions of the hair are

- Insulating against heat and cold
- Protecting against ultraviolet and infrared rays
- Perceiving movement or touch
- Protecting the eyes from sweat
- Protecting the nasal passages from foreign particles

Nails

Nails are thin plates of keratinized epidermal cells that shield the distal ends of the fingers and toes (Figure 8.4). Nail growth occurs at the *nail matrix*, as new cells arise from the basal layer of the epidermis. As the nail cells grow out from the matrix, they form a transparent layer, called the *body* of the nail, which extends over the nail bed. The nail body appears pink because of the blood supply in the underlying dermis. A moon-shaped crescent called a *lunula* appears on the nail body over the thickened nail matrix. A fold of epidermal skin called a *cuticle* protects the root and sides of each nail.

The major functions of the nails are

- Protecting the tips of the fingers and toes
- Aiding in picking up small objects, grasping, and scratching

Gathering the Data

Focused Interview

Many people perceive themselves in relation to how they believe they appear to others; thus, the appearance of the skin may have a considerable impact on self-image. A person may feel a heightened sense of self-esteem from clear, healthy-looking skin; by contrast, some people experience anxiety over simple changes in the skin such as dryness or wrinkles, or marked changes such as rashes or other skin disorders. In fact, some people with visible chronic skin disorders isolate themselves, allowing the disorder to interfere with the development of meaningful relationships. In some people, the

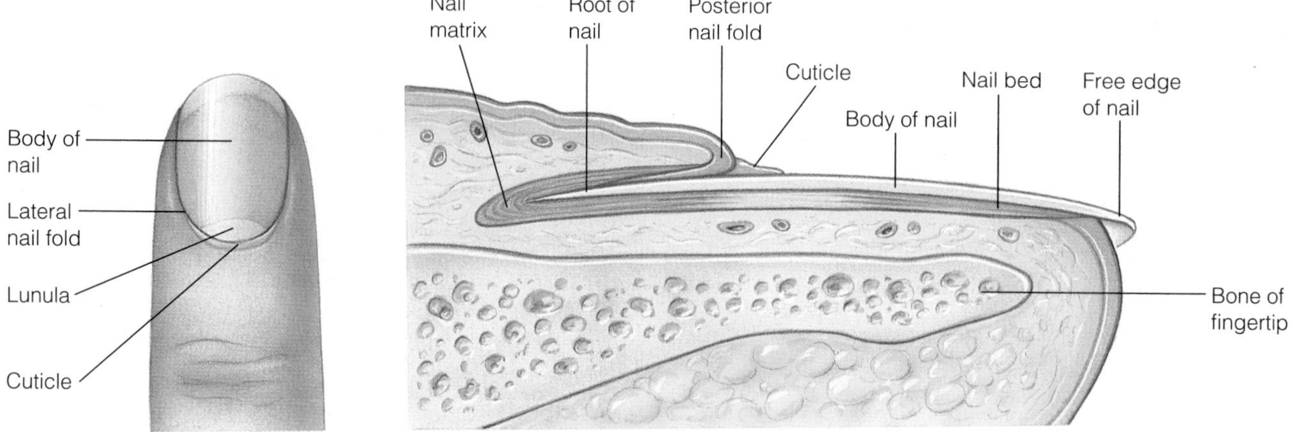

Figure 8.4 Structure of a nail. Longitudinal section shows nail matrix, cuticle, and body of nail.

stress of living with a skin disorder may even exacerbate the condition. Because the client with a skin disorder may be very sensitive about it, you should be especially considerate and careful when investigating the client's lifestyle, self-care, relationships with others, and methods of coping with the problem.

See Chapter 2 for a discussion of the general health history. The questions below are suggested as part of the focused assessment of the skin, hair, and nails.

Questions Related to the Skin and Glands

1. Describe your skin today; 2 months ago; 2 years ago. Have you ever had a skin problem? If so, please describe it, including any treatment and resolution.
2. Is there a history of allergies, rashes, or other skin problems in your family? *Some allergies and skin disorders are familial, and thus the client might be predisposed.*
3. How do you care for your skin? What kind of soap, cleansers, toners, or other treatments do you use? How do you clean your clothes? What kind of detergent do you use? How often do you bathe or shower? *Some skin products and laundry detergents may affect the skin of some clients. Infrequent cleansing of the skin increases the likelihood of skin infections, whereas excessive bathing decreases protective skin oils.*
4. Have you had an illness recently? If so, please describe it. *Some skin disorders are manifestations of systemic illness.*
5. Are you taking any prescription or over-the-counter medications? *Clients may experience rashes or other skin eruptions in response to various drugs. Some drugs, such as antibiotics, antihistamines, antipsychotics, oral hypoglycemic agents, and oral contraceptives, can cause an adverse effect if the client is exposed to the sun.*
6. Have you been exposed recently to extremes in temperature? If so, when? How long was the exposure? Where did this occur? Describe the temperature of your home environment. Of your work environment. *Extremes in environmental temperature may exacerbate skin disorders.*
7. [Female clients] Are you pregnant? If not, are you menstruating regularly? Describe your menstrual periods. *The skin may be affected by changes in hormonal balance.*
8. How would you describe your level of stress? Has it changed in the past few weeks? Few months? Describe. *Emotional stress may aggravate skin disorders.*
9. Please describe any skin pain or discomfort. Have you experienced any pain or discomfort in any body folds, for example, between the toes, under the breasts, between the buttocks, or in the perianal area? *Note that the warm, dark, moist environment in body folds may breed bacterial and fungal infections.*
10. Do you ever have trouble controlling body odor? If so, at what times? *Body odor becomes stronger during heavy activity because of increased excretion of uric acid. Body odor may also be related to diet. A change in body odor may indicate the presence of a systemic disorder.*
11. How much and how easily do you sweat? *Profuse sweating is a significant avenue for sodium chloride loss and may indicate the presence of a systemic disorder. Increased sweating is a side effect of some medications.*
12. Have you noticed any changes in the color of your skin? If so, did the change occur over your entire body or only in one area? *Widespread or localized color changes may indicate the presence of a disorder.*
13. Has your skin become either more oily or more dry recently, or have you noticed other changes in the way your skin feels? *Metabolic disorders or simple age-related changes in the production of sebum may produce changes in the texture of the skin.*
14. Does your skin itch? If so, where? How severe is it? When does it occur? *These questions may help in determining if the itching is due to an allergic reaction.*
15. Have you noticed any rashes on your body? If so, please describe. Where on your body did the rash start? Where did it spread? When did you first notice it? Does the rash happen at the same time as any other symptoms, such as fever or chills? *These factors may help in determining the cause.*
16. If you have a rash, do you notice it more after wearing certain clothes? Jewelry? Using certain skin products? Did it occur soon after starting a new medication? Does the rash happen during or after any other activities such as gardening or washing dishes? *Rashes related to clothing, jewelry, or cosmetics may be due to contact dermatitis, a type of allergy. Many medications cause allergic skin reactions. A drug reaction can occur even after the client has taken the drug a long time. Aspirin, antibiotics, and barbiturates are a few of the drugs that fall into this category.*
17. Have you changed your diet recently? Have you recently tried any unfamiliar types of food? Please describe. *Changes in diet or eating new foods may cause rashes and other skin reactions.*
18. How often do you travel? Have you traveled recently? If so, where? Have you come into contact with anyone who has a similar rash? *Suspect unfamiliar foods, water, plants, or insects as potential causes of rashes and other skin problems if the client has traveled recently. In addition, some rashes, such as measles and impetigo, are contagious.*
19. Do you have any sores or ulcers on your body that are slow in healing? Where are these? Do you have frequent boils or skin infections? *Delayed healing or frequent skin infections may be a sign of diabetes mellitus or inadequate nutrition.*

20. How does your skin react to sun exposure? Have you ever had a bad sunburn? If so, when? On what area of your body? *The ultraviolet radiation that accompanies a sunburn is capable of disabling cells that initiate the normal immune response. Individuals who burn easily or have a history of serious sunburns may have a greater risk for developing skin cancer.*
21. Do you sunbathe? Do you spend time in the sun exercising or playing sports? Do you work out of doors? If so, how often? For how long? Do you work in an environment where radioisotopes or X-rays are used? If so, are you vigilant about following precautions and using protective gear? *Excessive exposure to the ultraviolet radiation of the sun thickens and damages the skin, depresses the immune system, and alters the DNA in skin cells, predisposing an individual to cancer. Excessive exposure to X-rays or radioisotopes may predispose a client to skin cancer.*
22. Have you noticed a change in the size, color, shape, or appearance of any moles or birthmarks? When did you first notice this? Describe the change. Are they painful? Do they itch? Bleed? *Any changes in a mole or birthmark may signal a skin cancer.*
23. Have you noticed any other lesions, lumps, bumps, tender spots, or painful areas on your body? If so, when did you first notice them? Where? Describe how they have spread and where they are located now. *The time of onset and pattern of development may help determine the source of the problem. For instance, certain patterns of bruises may signal frequent falls or physical abuse.*
24. Does your job or hobby require you to perform repetitive tasks? To work with any chemicals? Does your job or hobby require you to wear a specific type of helmet, hat, goggles, gloves, or shoes? *Regular work with certain tools or regular wear of ill-fitting helmets, hats, goggles, or shoes may cause skin abrasions. Additionally, the skin absorbs some organic solvents used in industry, such as acetone, dry-cleaning fluid, dyes, formaldehyde, and paint thinner. Excessive exposure to these and other types of irritants may contribute to rashes, skin cancers, or other skin reactions.*
25. Have you noticed any drainage from any skin region? If so, where does the drainage come from? What does it look like? Does it have an odor? Is the drainage accompanied by any other symptoms? If so, please describe. *Diagnostic cues such as pain, chills, or fever may aid in identifying the source of the problem.*
26. Please describe anything you have done to treat your skin condition. When did you begin this treatment? How has your skin responded to the treatment?
27. Has the condition of your skin affected your relationships in any way? Has it limited you in any way? If so, how? *Skin problems may affect a person's self-concept and body image, interfering with social relationships, roles, and sexuality. This is especially true for adolescents and young adults. Serious skin problems may also affect a person's ability to function and maintain a job.*

Questions Related to the Hair

1. Describe your hair now; 2 months ago; 2 years ago. Have you ever had problems with your hair? If so, please describe the problem, including any treatment and resolution.
2. How often do you wash your hair? What kinds of shampoos do you use? Do you have excessive dandruff? Do you do anything to control it? *Excessive washing or washing with harsh shampoos can remove protective oils and dry the hair. Removal of natural scalp oils through shampooing also encourages dandruff. Excessive dandruff may also occur with protein and vitamin B deficiencies as well as a decrease in some essential fatty acids.*
3. Have you noticed an increased hair loss recently? If so, describe how the hair fell out. Have you been ill in the last few months? *The scalp typically sheds about 90 hairs each day, and so some hair loss is normal. Progressive diffuse hair loss is natural in some men. Hair loss in women that follows a male pattern may be due to an imbalance of adrenal hormones. When patches of hair fall out, suspect trauma to the scalp due to chemicals, infections, or blows to the head. Chemotherapeutic agents cause hair loss. Also, some people with nervous disorders pull or twist their hair, causing it to fall out. If hair loss is distributed over the entire head, suspect a systemic disease or fungal infection. Abnormal hair loss sometimes follows a feverish illness.*
4. Are you taking any prescription or over-the-counter medications? *Certain medications can change the texture of the hair or lead to hair loss. For instance, oral contraceptives may change the hair texture or rate of hair growth in some women, and drugs used in the treatment of circulatory disorders and cancer may result in a temporary generalized hair loss over the entire body.*
5. How do you style your hair? *Use of styling products can dry or damage hair, as can use of hair dryers, curling irons, and heated rollers. Some methods of setting hair, and sleeping in hair rollers, may cause breakage and lead to patchy hair loss. Repeated tight braiding may damage hair and lead to patchy hair loss.*
6. Do you bleach, color, perm, or chemically straighten your hair? If so, how often? When did you last have this done? *These chemical processes may damage the scalp and hair and may cause hair loss.*
7. Do you pluck your eyebrows or facial hair? Do you shave the hair on your face, legs, or under your arms? Do you use chemical hair removers or electrolysis? *Each*

of these hair removal methods can cause trauma to the skin. Use of unclean equipment can contaminate the skin. Plucking leaves an open portal for bacteria and may lead to infection if aseptic technique is not used.

8. Do you swim regularly? How often? For how long? Where? *Swimming regularly in salt water or chlorinated pools can dry the scalp and hair and may cause increased dandruff.*

Questions Related to the Nails

1. Describe your nails now; 2 months ago; 2 years ago. Have you ever had problems with your nails? If so, please describe the problem, including any treatment and resolution. *Ridged, brittle, split, or peeling fingernails may be caused by protein or vitamin B deficiencies. Changes in circulation may affect the nails. Newly acquired dark longitudinal lines may signal a nevus or melanoma in the nail root, although dark lines may be normal, especially in dark-skinned clients.*
2. Have you noticed any pain, swelling, or drainage around your cuticles? If so, when did you first notice this? What do you think might have caused it? *Infection of the cuticles could be due to an ingrown toenail, or to use of dirty instruments during a manicure or pedicure.*
3. Have you been ill recently? *Cancer, heart disease, liver disease, anemia, and other illnesses can cause various changes in the nails such as grooves, ridges, or discoloration.*
4. Have you been taking any prescription or over-the-counter medications? *Some medications may cause nail changes in some clients. For example, clients who have been treated with the antiviral drug zidovudine (Retrovir, AZT) can develop dark, longitudinal lines on all of their fingernails.*
5. Do you wear nail enamel? Do you wear artificial fingernails, tips, or wraps? *Prolonged use of nail polish may dry or discolor the nails. Additionally, some clients may have an allergic reaction to nail polish. Use of artificial nails may encourage the growth of fungi or damage the nail plate.*
6. Do you spend a great deal of time at work or at home with your hands in water? *Bacterial and fungal infections of the cuticles may occur in people who submerge their hands in water for long periods.*

Additional Questions with Infant, Children, and Adolescent Clients

1. Does the child have any birthmarks? If so, where are they?
2. Was there any change in the infant's skin color, such as jaundice, pallor, or redness, after birth?
3. Does your child have a rash? If so, what seems to cause it? Have you introduced any new foods into your child's diet? How do you clean your child's diaper area? How do you wash your child's diapers? *Many children may have allergic reactions to certain foods, especially milk, chocolate, and eggs. Infrequent changing of diapers may lead to diaper rash. Harsh detergents may cause skin reactions in some children.*
4. Has the child shared hair combs, brushes, or pillows with other children? *Sharing hair-care implements or pillows may expose the child to head lice.*
5. Does the child have any habits such as pulling or twisting the hair, rubbing the head, or biting the nails? *These habits may signal anxiety or emotional distress. Nail biting may also lead to impaired skin integrity.*

Additional Questions with Childbearing Clients

- What changes have you noticed in your skin since you became pregnant? *The hormonal changes of pregnancy may cause various benign changes in skin pigmentation, moisture, texture, and vascularity that are entirely normal.*

Additional Questions with Older Clients

1. What changes have you noticed in your skin in the past few years? *The normal changes of aging, such as increased dryness and wrinkling of the skin, may cause distress for some clients.*
2. Does your skin itch? *Pruritus (itching) increases in incidence with age. It is usually due to dry skin, which may in turn be caused by excessive bathing or use of harsh skin cleansers.*
3. Do you experience frequent falls? *Older adults bruise easily. Multiple bruises may result from frequent falls.*
4. Do you find it difficult to care for your skin, hair, and nails? If so, describe any difficulties you're experiencing. *Older adults with impaired mobility may have difficulty cleansing or grooming their skin, hair, and nails. Some older adults may have trouble reaching down to their feet to groom their toenails.*

Physical Assessment

Preparation

☑ **Gather the equipment:**

examination gown
examination light
examination gloves
centimeter ruler
magnifying glass
penlight
Wood's lamp (filtered ultraviolet light for special procedures)

☑ **Wash your hands.**

☑ **Ask the client to remove any items that would interfere with the physical assessment, including all clothing, jewelry, cosmetics, wigs, or hairpieces. If the client's visit is related to a problem with the nails, suggest that the client remove any artificial nails or nail enamel, if possible. Ask the client to put on the examination gown.**

☑ **Adjust the room lighting, if necessary. Direct sunlight is best for visualizing the skin, but if it is not available, ensure that artificial lighting is strong and direct.**

Remember

- Provide a warm, comfortable environment.
- Explain the procedure to the client to allay any fear or apprehension.
- Ensure the client's privacy.
- If at any time you notice open skin areas, sinus formations, or drainage on the skin surface, put on gloves before proceeding further with the assessment.

ASSESSMENT TECHNIQUE/NORMAL FINDINGS | SPECIAL CONSIDERATIONS

Skin

Step 1 *Position the client.*

- Place the client in a sitting position with all clothes removed except for the examination gown (Figure 8.5).

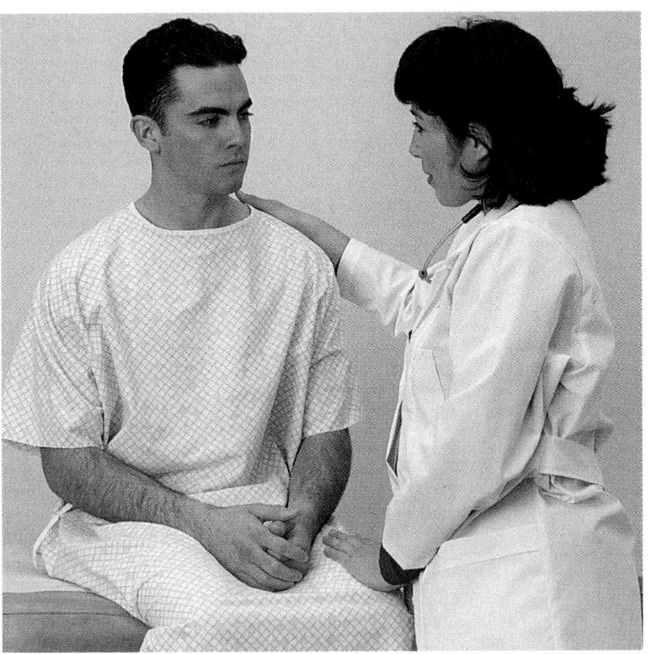

Figure 8.5 Positioning of client.

Step 2 *Confirm that the skin is clean and free from body odor.*

Body odor is produced when bacterial waste products mix with perspiration on the skin surface. During heavy activity, body odor increases because increased amounts of urea and ammonia are excreted in perspiration.

If the client has just come from work or has another reason not to be clean, body odor may be present.

Increased urea and ammonia may occur in clients with kidney disorders.

Step 3 *Observe the client's skin tone.*

- Evaluate any widespread color changes such as cyanosis, pallor, erythema, or jaundice. For example, always assess cyanotic clients for vital signs and level of consciousness.
- Use Table 8.1 on page 142 to evaluate color variations in light and dark skin.

Skin color is influenced by the amount of melanin and carotene pigments, the oxygen content of the blood, and the level of exposure to the sun. Dark skin contains large amounts of melanin, and fair skin has little. The skin of most Asians contains a large amount of carotene, which causes a yellow cast.

Cyanosis or pallor indicates abnormally low plasma oxygen, placing the client at risk for altered tissue perfusion.

Referral

Be alert for the possibility of impending shock if the client has pallor accompanied with a drop in blood pressure, increased pulse and respirations, and marked anxiety. If these cues are present, consult with a physician immediately.

ASSESSMENT TECHNIQUE/NORMAL FINDINGS	SPECIAL CONSIDERATIONS

Step 4 ***Inspect the skin for even pigmentation over the body.***

In most cases, increased or decreased pigmentation is caused by differences in the distribution of melanin throughout the body, and are normal variations. For example, the margins of the lips, areolae, nipples, and external genitalis are more darkly pigmented. Freckles (Figure 8.6) and certain *nevi* (congenital marks; Figure 8.7) occur in people of all skin colors in varying degrees.

For unknown reasons, some people develop patchy depigmented areas over the face, neck, hands, feet, and body folds. This condition is called *vitiligo* (Figure 8.8). Skin is otherwise normal. Vitiligo occurs in all races in all parts of the world but seems to affect dark-skinned people more severely. Clients with vitiligo may suffer a severe disturbance in body image

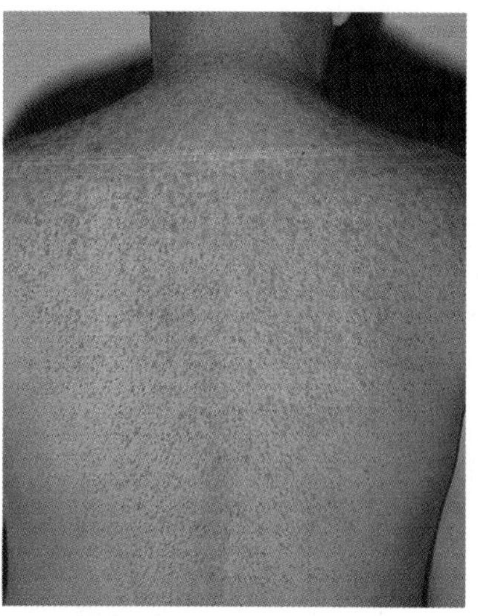

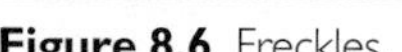

Figure 8.6 Freckles.

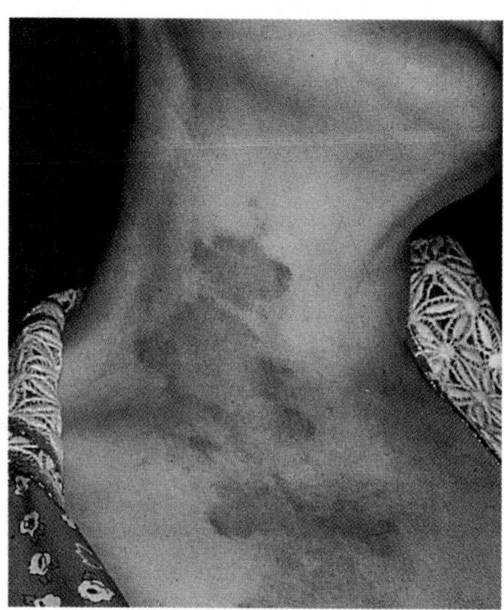

Figure 8.7 Nevus.

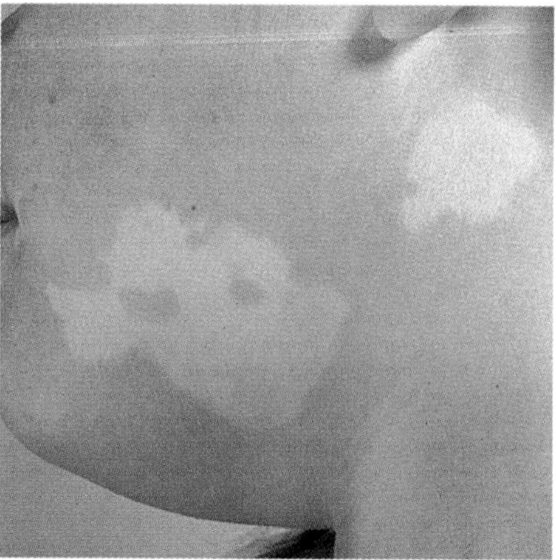

Figure 8.8 Vitiligo.

Step 5 ***Determine the client's skin temperature.***

- Use the dorsal surface of your hand, which is most sensitive to temperature.
- Palpate the forehead or face first, then continue to palpate inferiorly, including the hands and feet, comparing the temperature on the right and left side of the body (Figure 8.9).

The temperature of the skin is *higher* than normal in the presence of a systemic infection or metabolic disorder such as hyperthyroidism, after vigorous activity, and when the external environment is warm. Take the client's temperature if the skin feels very warm.

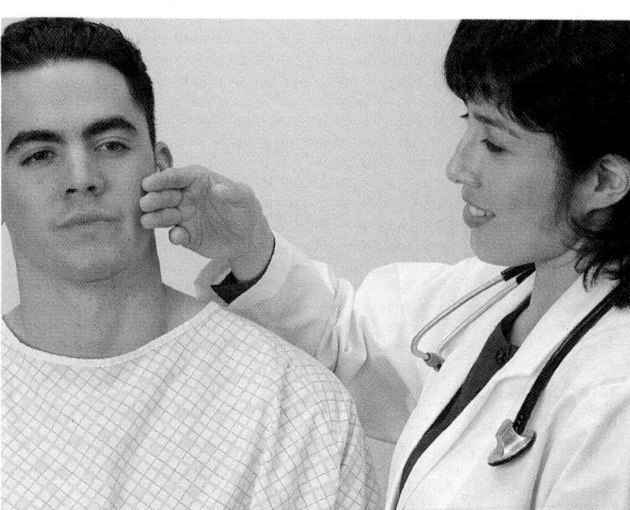

Figure 8.9 Palpating skin temperature.

ASSESSMENT TECHNIQUE/NORMAL FINDINGS | SPECIAL CONSIDERATIONS

Local skin temperature is controlled by the amount and rate of blood circulating through a body region. Normal temperatures range from mildly cool to slightly warm.

The skin on both sides of the body is warm when circulation is adequate. Sometimes the hands and feet are cooler than the rest of the body, but the temperature is normally similar on both sides.

The temperature of the skin is lower than normal in the presence of metabolic disorders such as hypothyroidism or when the external environment is cool. Localized coolness results from decreased circulation due to vasoconstriction or occlusion, which may occur from peripheral arterial insufficiency.

A difference in temperature *bilaterally* may indicate an interruption in or lack of circulation on the cool side due to compression, immobilization, or elevation. If one side is warmer than normal, inflammation may be present on that side.

Step 6 *Assess the amount of moisture on the skin surface.*

- Inspect and palpate the face, skin folds, axillae, palms, and soles of the feet, where perspiration is most easily detected.

A fine sheen of perspiration and/or oil is not an abnormal finding, nor is moderately dry skin, especially in cold or dry climates.

Diaphoresis (profuse sweating) occurs during exertion, fever, pain, emotional stress, and in the presence of some metabolic disorders such as hyperthyroidism. It may also indicate an impending medical crisis such as a myocardial infarction.

Severely dry skin typically is dark, weathered, and fissured. *Pruritus* (itching) frequently accompanies dry skin, and may lead to abrasion and thickening if prolonged. Generalized dryness may occur in an individual who is dehydrated or has a systemic disorder such as hypothyroidism.

Dry, parched lips and mucous membranes of the mouth are clear indicators of systemic dehydration. Check these areas if you suspect that the client is dehydrated. Dry skin over the lower legs may be due to vascular insufficiency. Localized itching may indicate a skin allergy.

Step 7 *Palpate the skin for texture.*

Use the palmar surface of fingers and finger pads when palpating for texture. Normal skin feels smooth, firm, and even.

The skin may become excessively smooth and velvety in clients with hyperthyroidism, whereas clients with hypothyroidism may have rough, scaly skin.

Step 8 *Palpate the skin to determine its thickness.*

The outer layer of the skin is thin and firm over most parts of the body except the palms, soles of the feet, elbows, and knees, where it is thicker. Normally, the skin over the eyelids and lips is thinner.

Very thin, shiny skin may signal impaired circulation.

Step 9 *Palpate the skin for elasticity.*

Elasticity is a combination of turgor (resiliency, or the skin's ability to return to its normal position and shape) and mobility (the skin's ability to be lifted).

When skin turgor is decreased, the skinfold "tents" (holds its pinched formation) and returns to the former position only slowly (Figure 8.11, *A* and *B* on page 136). Decreased turgor occurs when the client is

ASSESSMENT TECHNIQUE/NORMAL FINDINGS

- Using the forefinger and thumb, grasp a fold of skin beneath the clavicle or on the radial aspect of the wrist (Figure 8.10).

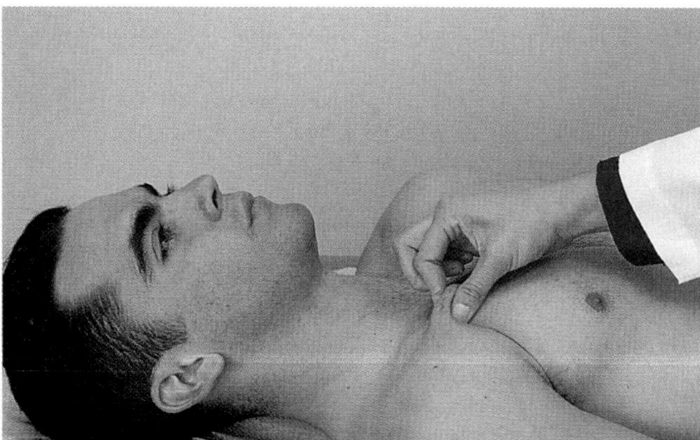

Figure 8.10 Palpating skin elasticity.

- Notice the reaction of the skin both as you grasp and as you release. Healthy skin is mobile, and returns rapidly to its previous shape and position.
- Firmly palpate the feet, ankles, and sacrum. Edema is present if your palpation leaves a dent in the skin.
- Grade any edema on a four-point scale: 1 indicates mild edema, and 4 indicates deep edema (Figure 8.13). Note that, because the fluid of edema lies above the pigmented and vascular layers of the skin, skin tone in the client with edema is obscured.

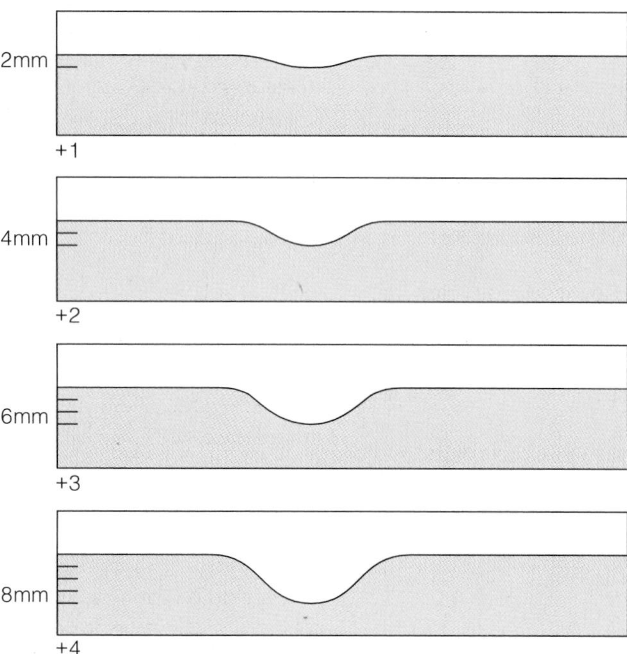

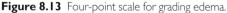

Figure 8.13 Four-point scale for grading edema.

SPECIAL CONSIDERATIONS

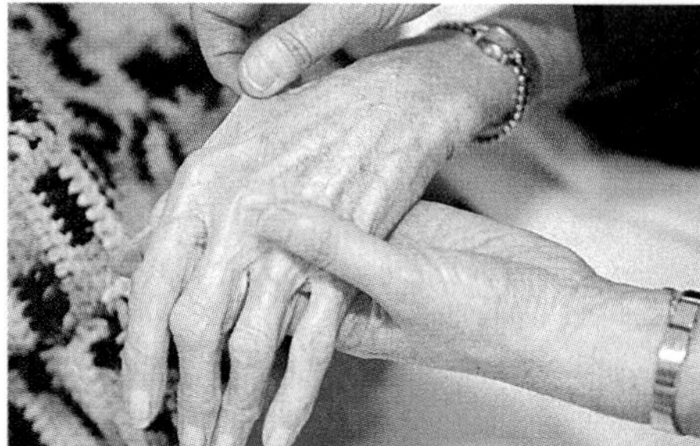

A

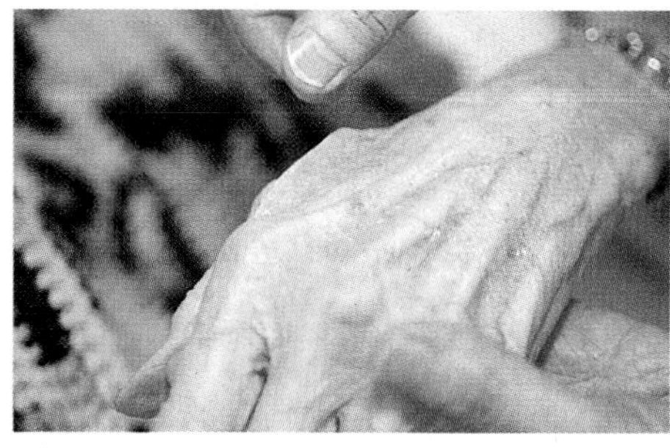

B

Figure 8.11 *A*, Testing for skin tenting. *B*, Example of tenting.

dehydrated or has lost large amounts of weight.

Increased skin turgor may be caused by scleroderma, literally "hard skin," a condition in which the underlying connective tissue becomes scarred and immobile

Edema is a decrease in skin mobility caused by an accumulation of fluid in the intercellular spaces. It is not a normal finding. Edema makes the skin look puffy, pitted, and tight. It may be most noticeable in the skin of the hands, feet, ankles, and sacral area (Figure 8.12).

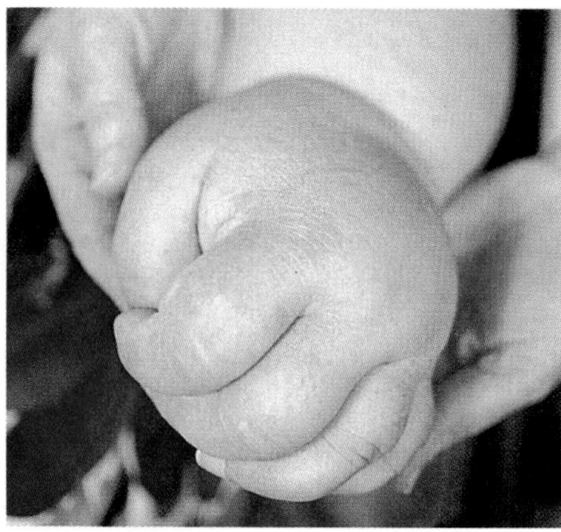

Figure 8.12 Edema of the hand.

ASSESSMENT TECHNIQUE/NORMAL FINDINGS

Step 10 *Inspect the skin for superficial arteries and veins.*

A fine network of veins or a few dilated blood vessels visible just beneath the surface of the skin are normal findings in areas of the body where skin is thin, eg, the abdomen and eyelids.

Step 11 *Inspect and palpate the skin for lesions.*

Lesions of the skin are changes in normal skin structure. *Primary lesions* develop on previously unaltered skin, and lesions that change over time or because of scratching, abrasion, or infection are called *secondary lesions*.

- Carefully inspect the client's body, including skin folds and crevices, under a good source of light.

ALERT!

If you notice drainage from any lesion, put on gloves before proceeding with the assessment.

- Palpate lesions between the thumb and index finger. Measure all lesion dimensions (including height, if possible) with a small, clear, flexible ruler.
- Document lesion size in centimeters. If necessary, use a magnifying glass and/or a penlight for closer inspection.
- Shine a Wood's lamp on the skin to distinguish fluorescing lesions.
- Assess any drainage for color, odor, consistency, amount, and location. If indicated, obtain a specimen of the drainage for culture and sensitivity.

Healthy skin is typically smooth and free of lesions; however, some lesions, such as freckles, insect bites, healed scars, and certain "birthmarks" are expected findings.

SPECIAL CONSIDERATIONS

Observe the periumbilical and flank areas of the body for the presence of *ecchymosis* (bruising). Ecchymoses in the periumbilical area may signal bleeding somewhere in the abdomen (Cullen's sign). Ecchymoses in the flank area are associated with pancreatitis or bleeding in the peritoneum (Grey Turner sign). Other vascular lesions of the skin are discussed in Table 8.2 on page 144.

Referral

Suspect physical abuse if the client has bruises or welts that appear in a pattern suggesting the use of a belt or stick; has burns with sharply demarcated edges suggesting injury from cigarettes, irons, or immersion of a hand in boiling water; has additional injuries such as fractures or dislocations; or has multiple injuries in various stages of healing. Be especially sensitive if the client is fearful of family members, is reluctant to return home, and has a history of previous injuries. When any of these diagnostic cues are evident, obtain medical assistance and follow your state's legal requirements to notify the police or local protective agency.

Certain systemic disorders may produce characteristic patterns of lesions on particular body regions. Widespread lesions may indicate systemic or genetic disorders, or allergic reactions, and localized lesions may indicate physical trauma, chemical irritants, or allergic dermatitis. You may wish to photograph the client's skin to document the presence, pattern, or spread of certain lesions. See Tables 8.3 and 8.4 on pages 146 and 147 for a description and classification of primary and secondary lesions.

ASSESSMENT TECHNIQUE/NORMAL FINDINGS | SPECIAL CONSIDERATIONS

Referral

The injection of drugs into the veins of the arms or other parts of the body results in a series of small scars called *track marks* along the course of the blood vessel. If you see track marks and suspect substance abuse, refer the client to a mental health or substance abuse professional.

Step 12 *Palpate the skin for sensitivity.*

ALERT!

Localized hot, red, swollen painful areas indicate the presence of inflammation and possible infection. Do not palpate these areas, because the slightest disturbance may spread the infection deeper into the skin layers.

- Palpate the skin in various regions of the body and ask the client to describe the sensations.
- Give special attention to any pain or discomfort that the client reports, especially when you are palpating skin lesions.
- Ask the client to describe the sensation as closely as possible, and document your findings.

The client should not report any discomfort from your touch.

Scalp and Hair

Step 1 *Confirm that the scalp and hair are clean.*

- Ask the client to remove any hairpins, hair ties, barrettes, wigs, or hairpieces and to undo braids. If the client is unwilling to do this, examine any strands of hair that are loose or undone.
- Part and divide the hair at 1-inch intervals and observe (Figure 8.14).

Excessive dandruff occurs on the scalp of clients with certain skin disorders, such as psoriasis or seborrheic dermatitis, in which large amounts of the epidermis slough away. Distinguish dandruff from head lice (see lesions of the scalp, step 5).

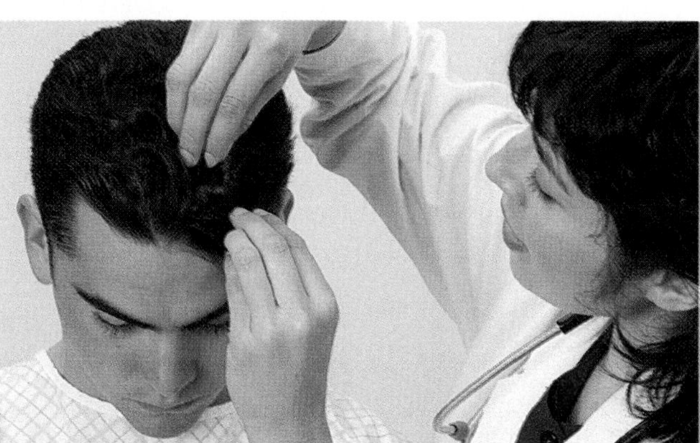

Figure 8.14 Inspecting the hair.

ASSESSMENT TECHNIQUE/NORMAL FINDINGS	SPECIAL CONSIDERATIONS

A small amount of dandruff (dead, scaly flakes of epidermal cells) may be present.

Step 2 ***Observe the client's hair color.***

Like skin color, hair color varies according to the level of melanin production. Graying is influenced by genetics and may begin as early as the late teens in some clients.

Graying of the hair in patches may indicate a nutritional deficiency, commonly of protein or copper.

Step 3 ***Assess the texture of the hair.***

- Roll a few strands of hair between your thumb and forefinger.
- Hold a few strands of hair taut with one hand while you slide the thumb and forefinger of your other hand along the length of the strand.

Hair may be thick or fine and may appear straight, wavy, or curly.

Hypothyroidism and other metabolic disorders, as well as nutritional deficiencies, may cause the hair to be dull, dry, brittle, and coarse.

Step 4 ***Observe the amount and distribution of the hair throughout the scalp.***

The amount of hair varies with age, sex, and overall health. Healthy hair is evenly distributed throughout the scalp.

In most men and women, atrophy of the hair follicles causes hair growth to decline by the age of 50. Male pattern baldness (Figure 8.15), a genetically determined progressive loss of hair beginning at the anterior hairline, has no clinical significance. It is the most frequent reason for hair loss in men.

Remember to assess the amount, texture, and distribution of body hair. Some practitioners prefer to perform this assessment with the regions of the body

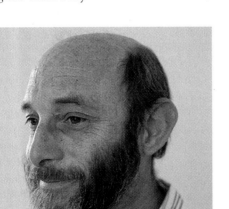

Figure 8.15 Male pattern baldness.

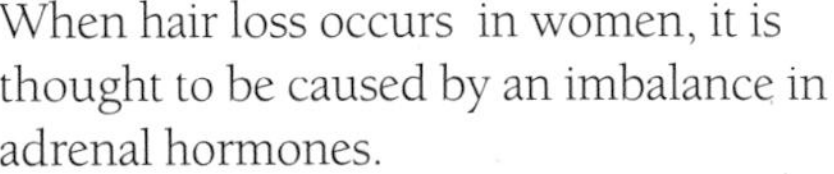

When hair loss occurs in women, it is thought to be caused by an imbalance in adrenal hormones.

Widespread hair loss may also be caused by illness, infections, metabolic disorders, nutritional deficiencies, and chemotherapy. Patchy hair loss (*alopecia areata*) may be due to infection (Figure 8.16).

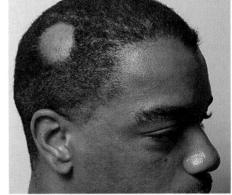

Figure 8.16 Alopecia areata.

Step 5 ***Inspect the scalp for lesions.***

- Dim the room light and shine a Wood's lamp on the client's scalp as you part the hair.

The healthy scalp is free from lesions and areas of fluorescent glow.

Gray, scaly patches with broken hair may indicate the presence of a fungal infection such as ringworm. Regions of infection will fluoresce when exposed to the ultraviolet light of a Wood's lamp.

ASSESSMENT TECHNIQUE/NORMAL FINDINGS | SPECIAL CONSIDERATIONS

Infestation by *head lice* (pediculosis capitis) is signaled by tiny, white, oval eggs (nits) that adhere to the hair shaft. Head lice usually cause intense itching; check the scalp for excoriation from scratching.

Nails

Step 1 *Confirm that the nails are clean and well-groomed.*

Dirty fingernails may indicate a self-care deficit but could also be related to a person's occupation.

Step 2 *Inspect the nails for an even, pink undertone.*

Small, white markings in the nail are normal findings and indicate minor trauma.

The nails appear pale and colorless in clients with peripheral arteriosclerosis or anemia. They appear yellow in clients with jaundice and dark red in clients with polycythemia, a pathological increase in production of red blood cells. Fungal infections may cause the nails to discolor. Horizontal white bands may occur in chronic hepatic or renal disease.

Referral

A darkly pigmented band in a single nail in any client may be a sign of a melanoma in the nail matrix and should be referred to a physician for further evaluation.

Step 3 *Assess capillary refill.*

- Depress the nail edge briefly to blanch, and then release. Color returns to healthy nails instantly upon release.

The nail beds appear blue, and color return is sluggish in clients with cardiovascular or respiratory disorders.

Step 4 *Inspect and palpate the nails for shape and contour.*

- Perform the Schamroth technique to assess clubbing.
- Ask the client to bring the dorsal aspect of corresponding fingers together, creating a mirror image.
- Look at the distal phalanx and observe the diamond-shaped opening created by the nails. When clubbing is present, the diamond is not formed and the distance increases at the fingertip (Figure 8.17).

The nails normally form a slight convex curve or lie flat on the nail bed. When viewed laterally, the angle between the skin and the nail base should be approximately 160 degrees (Figure 8.18).

Clubbing of the fingernails occurs when there is hypoxia or impaired peripheral tissue perfusion over a long period of time. It may also occur with cirrhosis, colitis, or thyroid disease. The ends of the fingers become enlarged, soft, and spongy, and the angle between the skin and the nail base is greater than 160 degrees (Figure 8.19).

Spoon nails form a concave curve and are thought to be associated with iron deficiency (Figure 8.20).

ASSESSMENT TECHNIQUE/NORMAL FINDINGS

SPECIAL CONSIDERATIONS

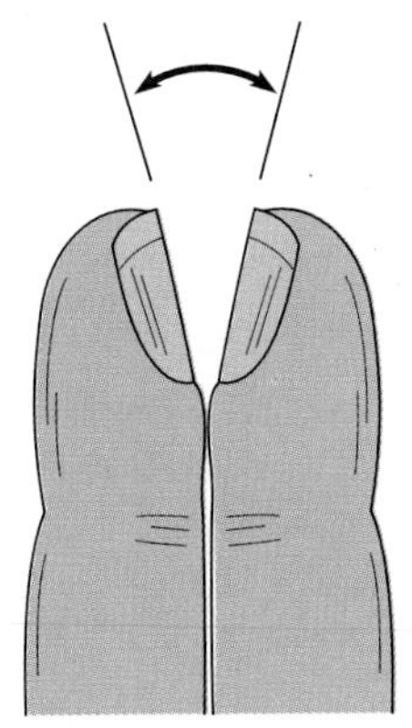

Figure 8.17 Schamroth technique to determine clubbing of fingers.

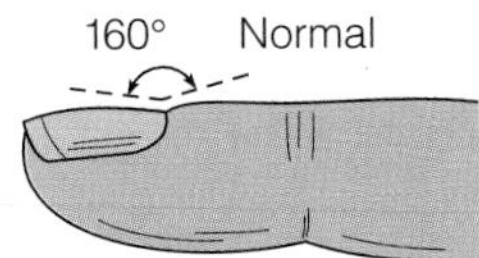

Figure 8.18 Curvature of the normal nail.

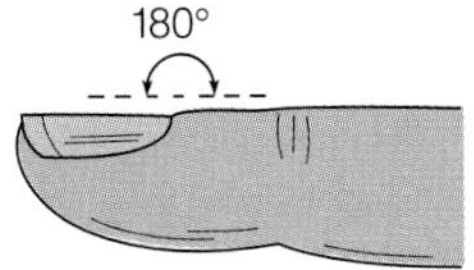

Figure 8.19 Clubbing of the nail.

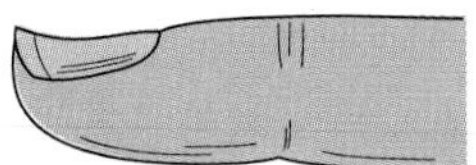

Figure 8.20 Spoon nail.

Step 5 ***Palpate the nails to determine their thickness, regularity, and attachment to the nail bed.***

Healthy nails are smooth, strong, and regular and are firmly attached to the nail bed, with only a slight degree of mobility.

Nails may be thickened in clients with circulatory disorders. *Onycholysis*, separation of the nail plate from the nail bed, occurs with trauma, infection, or skin lesions.

Step 6 ***Inspect and palpate the cuticles.***

The cuticles are smooth and flat in healthy nails.

Hangnails are jagged tears in the lateral skin folds around the nail. An untreated hangnail may become inflamed and lead to a *paronychia*, an infection of the cuticle.

Reminders

- In addition to the preceding steps, consider the common variations in physical assessment findings discussed in the following sections.
- After completing the physical assessment, answer any questions the client may have, and provide appropriate teaching for health promotion and self-care (see pages 152–158).
- Confirm that the client is comfortable and has no adverse effects from the procedure, then dim the lights and leave the client to rest or to get dressed.
- Document the assessment findings as described in Chapter 1. See pages 152 for nursing diagnoses commonly associated with the integumentary system.

Table 8.1 Color Variations in Light and Dark Skin

Color Variation/Localization	Possible Causes	Appearance in Light Skin	Appearance in Dark Skin
Pallor			
Loss of color in skin due to the absence of oxygenated hemoglobin. Widespread, but most apparent in face, mouth, conjunctivae, and nails.	May be caused by sympathetic nervous stimulation resulting in peripheral vasoconstriction due to smoking, a cold environment, or stress. May also be caused by decreased tissue perfusion due to cardiopulmonary disease, shock and hypotension, lack of oxygen, or prolonged elevation of a body part. May also be caused by anemia.	White skin loses its rosy tones. Skin with natural yellow tones appears more yellow; may be mistaken for mild jaundice.	Black skin loses its red undertones and appears ash-gray. Brown skin becomes yellow-tinged. Skin looks dull.
Absence of color			
Congenital or acquired loss of melanin pigment. Congenital loss is typically generalized, and acquired loss is typically patchy.	Generalized depigmentation may be caused by albinism. Localized depigmentation may be due to vitiligo or tinea versicolor, a common fungal infection.	Albinism appears as white skin, white or pale blond hair, and pink irises. Vitiligo appears as patchy milk-white areas, especially around the mouth. Tinea versicolor appears as patchy areas paler than the surrounding skin.	Albinism appears as white skin, white or pale blond hair, and pink irises. Vitiligo is very noticeable as patchy milk-white areas. Tinea versicolor appears as patchy areas paler than the surrounding skin.
Cyanosis			
Mottled blue color in skin due to inadequate tissue perfusion with oxygenated blood. Most apparent in the nails, lips, oral mucosa, and tongue.	Systemic or central cyanosis is due to cardiac disease, pulmonary disease, heart malformations, and low hemoglobin levels. Localized or peripheral cyanosis is due to vasoconstriction, exposure to cold, and emotional stress.	The skin, lips, and mucous membranes look blue-tinged. The conjunctivae and nail beds are blue.	The skin may appear a shade darker. Cyanosis may be undetectable except for the lips, tongue, and oral mucous membranes, nail beds, and conjunctivae, which appear pale or blue-tinged.
Reddish blue tone			
Ruddy tone due to an increased hemoglobin and stasis of blood in capillaries. Most apparent in the face, mouth, hands, feet, and conjunctivae.	Polycythemia vera, an overproduction of red blood cells, granulocytes, and platelets.	Reddish purple hue.	Difficult to detect. The normal skin color may appear darker in some clients. Check lips for redness.

Table 8.1 Color Variations in Light and Dark Skin (continued)

Color Variation/Localization	Possible Causes	Appearance in Light Skin	Appearance in Dark Skin
Erythema *Redness of the skin due to increased visibility of normal oxyhemoglobin.* Generalized, or on face and upper chest, or localized to area of inflammation or exposure.	Hyperemia, a dilatation and congestion of blood in superficial arteries. Due to fever, warm environment, local inflammation, allergy, emotions (blushing or embarrassment), exposure to extreme cold, consumption of alcohol, dependent position of body extremity.	Readily identifiable over entire body or in localized areas. Local inflammation and redness are accompanied by higher temperature at the site.	Generalized redness may be difficult to detect. Localized areas of inflammation appear purple or darker than surrounding skin. May be accompanied by higher temperature, hardness, swelling.
Jaundice *Yellow undertone due to increased bilirubin in the blood.* Generalized, but most apparent in the conjunctivae and mucous membranes.	Increased bilirubin may be due to liver disease, biliary obstruction, or hemolytic disease following infections, severe burns, or resulting from sickle-cell anemia or pernicious anemia.	Generalized. Also visible in sclera, oral mucosa, hard palate, fingernails, palms of hands, and soles of the feet.	Visible in the sclerae, oral mucosa, junction of hard and soft palate, palms of the hands, and soles of the feet.
Carotenemia *Yellow-orange tinge caused by increased levels of carotene in the blood and skin.* Most apparent in face, palms of the hands, and soles of the feet.	Excess carotene due to ingestion of foods high in carotene such as carrots, egg yolks, sweet potatoes, milk, and fats. Also may be seen in clients with anorexia nervosa or endocrine disorders such as diabetes mellitus, myxedema, and hypopituitarism.	Yellow-orange seen in forehead, palms, soles. No yellowing of sclerae or mucous membranes.	Yellow-orange tinge most visible in palms of the hands and soles of the feet. No yellowing of sclerae or mucous membranes.
Uremia *Pale yellow tone due to retention of urinary chromogens in the blood.* Generalized, if perceptible.	Chronic renal disease, in which blood levels of nitrogenous wastes increase. Increased melanin may also contribute, and anemia is usually present as well.	Generalized pallor and yellow tinge, but does not affect conjunctivae or mucous membranes. Skin may show bruising.	Very difficult to discern because the yellow tinge is very pale and does not affect conjunctivae or mucous membranes. Rely on laboratory and other data.
Brown *An increase in the production and deposition of melanin.* Generalized or localized.	May be due to Addison's disease or a pituitary tumor. Localized increase in facial pigmentation may be caused by hormonal changes during pregnancy or the use of birth control pills. More commonly due to exposure to ultraviolet radiation from the sun or from tanning booths.	With endocrine disorders, general bronzed skin. Hyperpigmentation in nipples, palmar creases, genitals, and pressure points. Sun exposure causes red tinge in pale skin, and olive-toned skin tans with little or no reddening.	With endocrine disorders, general deepening of skin tone. Hyperpigmentation in nipples, genitals, and pressure points. Sun exposure leads to tanning in various degrees from brown to black.

Table 8.2 Vascular Skin Lesions

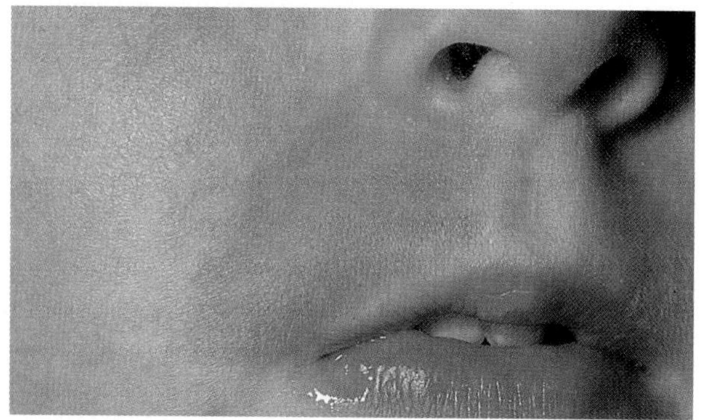

Port-Wine Stain

Flat, irregularly shaped lesion ranging in color from pale red to deep purple-red. Color deepens with exertion, emotional response, or exposure to extremes of temperature. It is present at birth and typically does not fade.

Cause A large, flat mass of blood vessels on the skin surface.

Localization/Distribution Most commonly appears on the face and head but may occur in other sites.

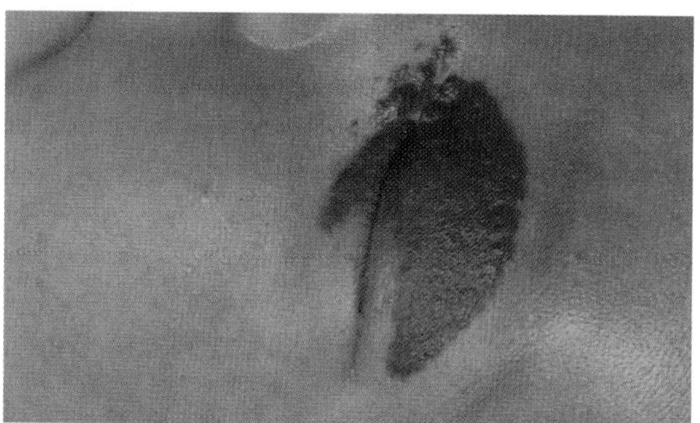

Strawberry Mark

A bright red, raised lesion about 2 to 10 cm in diameter. It does not blanch with pressure. It is usually present at birth or within a few months of birth. Typically, it disappears by age 3.The lesion pictured here is located on the upper and lower lid of the left eye.

Cause A cluster of immature capillaries.

Localization/Distribution Can appear on any part of the body.

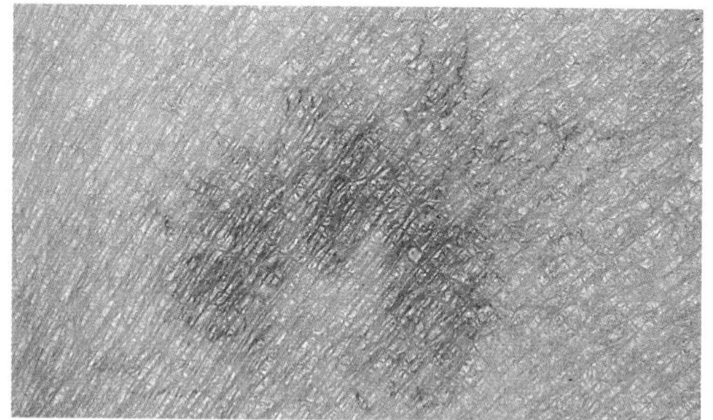

Spider Angioma

A flat, bright red dot with tiny radiating blood vessels ranging in size from a pinpoint to 2 cm. It blanches with pressure.

Cause A type of telangiectasis (vascular dilatation) caused by elevated estrogen levels, pregnancy, estrogen therapy, vitamin B deficiency, or liver disease, or may not be pathological.

Localization/Distribution Most commonly appear on the upper half of the body.

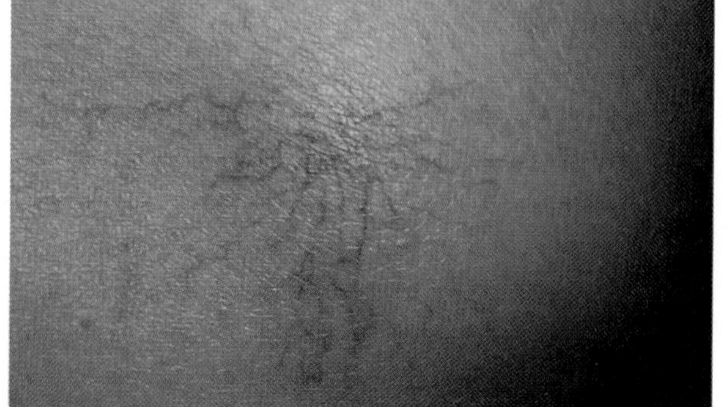

Venous Star

A flat blue lesion with radiating, cascading, or linear veins extending from the center. It ranges in size from 3 to 25 cm.

Cause A type of telangiectasis (vascular dilatation) caused by increased intravenous pressure in superficial veins.

Localization/Distribution Most commonly appear on the anterior chest and the lower legs near varicose veins.

Table 8.2 Vascular Skin Lesions (continued)

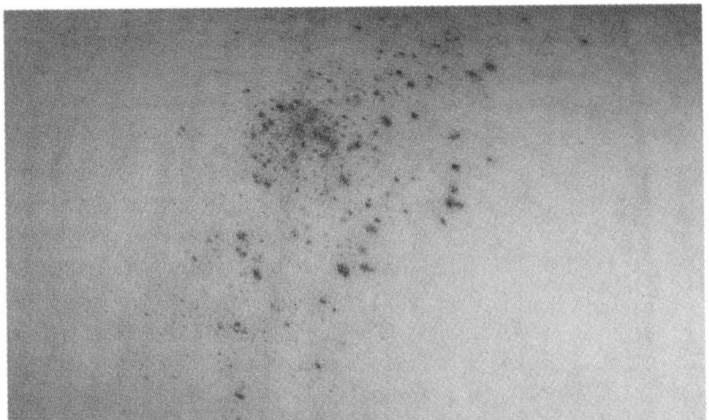

Petechiae

Flat red or purple rounded "freckles" approximately 1 to 3 mm in diameter. Difficult to detect in dark skin. Do not blanch.

Cause Minute hemorrhages resulting from fragile capillaries, petechiae are caused by septicemias, liver disease, or vitamin C or K deficiency. They may also be caused by anticoagulant therapy.

Localization/Distribution Most commonly appear on the dependent surfaces of the body, eg, back, buttocks. In the client with dark skin, look for them in the oral mucosa and conjunctivae.

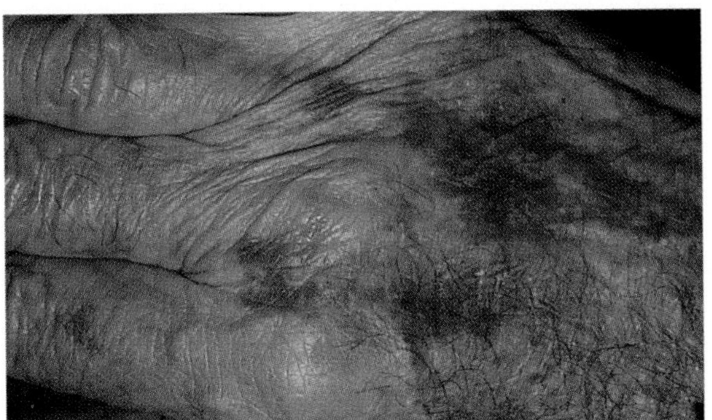

Purpura

Flat, reddish blue, irregularly shaped extensive patches of varying size.

Cause Bleeding disorders, scurvy, and capillary fragility in the older adult (senile purpura).

Localization/Distribution May appear anywhere on the body, but are most noticeable on the legs, arms, and backs of hands.

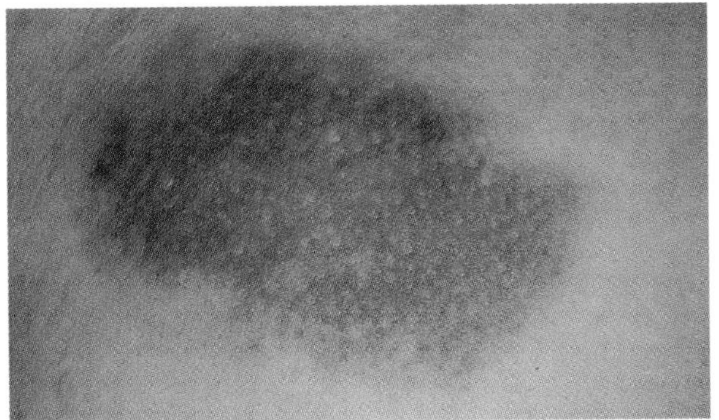

Ecchymosis

A flat, irregularly shaped lesion of varying size with no pulsation. Does not blanch with pressure. In light skin, it begins as bluish purple mark that changes to greenish yellow. In brown skin, it varies from blue to deep purple. In black skin, it appears as a darkened area.

Cause Release of blood from superficial vessels into surrounding tissue due to trauma, hemophilia, liver disease, or deficiency of vitamin C or K.

Localization/Distribution Occurs anywhere on the body at the site of trauma or pressure.

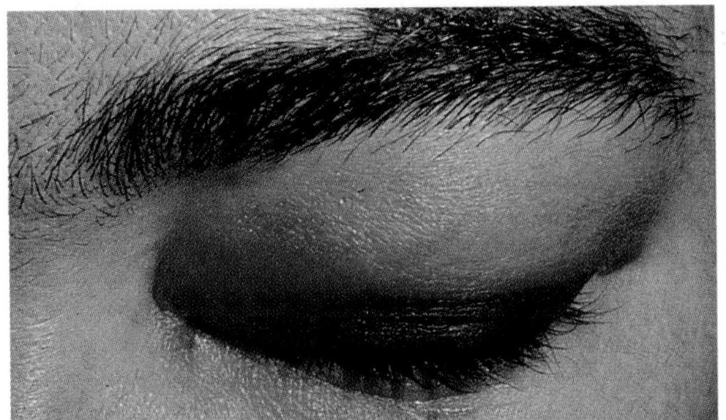

Hematoma

A raised, irregularly shaped lesion similar to an ecchymosis except that it elevates the skin and looks like a swelling.

Cause A leakage of blood into the skin and subcutaneous tissue as a result of trauma or surgical incision.

Localization/Distribution May occur anywhere on the body at the site of trauma, pressure, or surgical incision.

Table 8.3 Primary Skin Lesions

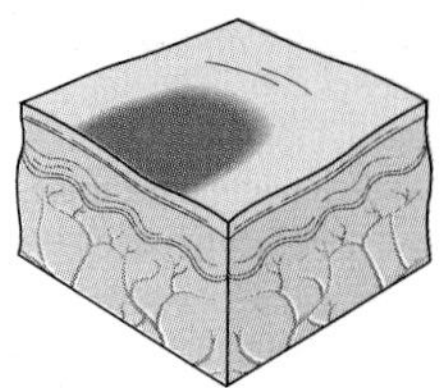

Macule, Patch

Flat, nonpalpable change in skin color. Macules are smaller than 1 cm, with a circumscribed border, and patches are larger than 1 cm and may have an irregular border.

Examples Macules: freckles, measles, and petechiae. Patches: mongolian spots, port-wine stains, vitiligo, and chloasma.

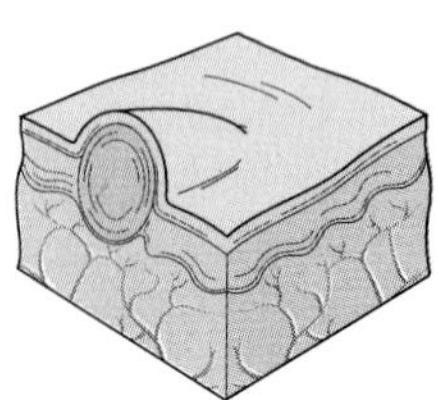

Papule, Plaque

Elevated, solid, palpable mass with circumscribed border. Papules are smaller than 0.5 cm; plaques are groups of papules that form lesions larger than 0.5 cm.

Examples Papules: elevated moles, warts, and lichen planus. Plaques: psoriasis, actinic keratosis, and also lichen planus.

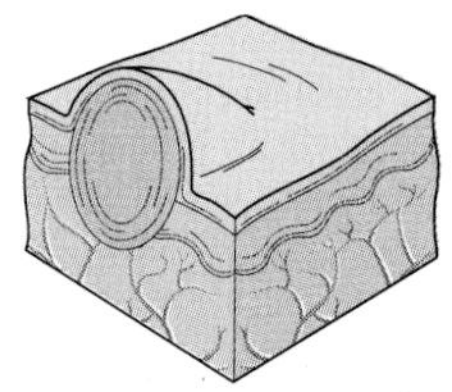

Nodule, Tumor

Elevated, solid, hard or soft palpable mass extending deeper into the dermis than a papule. Nodules have circumscribed borders and are 0.5 to 2 cm; tumors may have irregular borders and are larger than 2 cm.

Examples Nodules: small lipoma, squamous cell carcinoma, fibroma, and intradermal nevi. Tumors: large lipoma, carcinoma, and hemangioma.

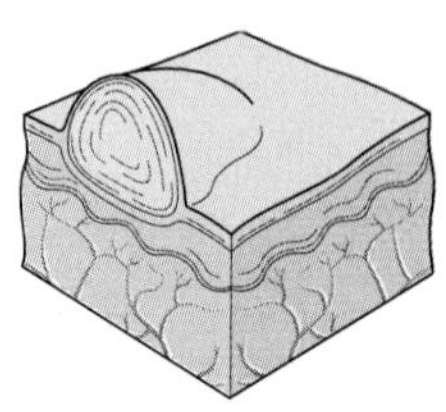

Vesicle, Bulla

Elevated, fluid-filled, round or oval shaped, palpable mass with thin, translucent walls and circumscribed borders. Vesicles are smaller than 0.5 cm; bullae are larger than 0.5 cm.

Examples Vesicles: herpes simplex/zoster, early chickenpox, poison ivy, and small burn blisters. Bullae: contact dermatitis, friction blisters, and large burn blisters.

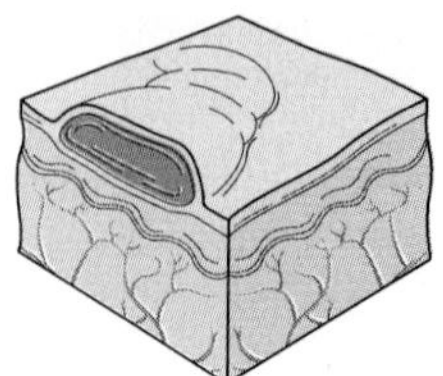

Wheal

Elevated, often reddish area with irregular border caused by diffuse fluid in tissues rather than free fluid in a cavity, as in vesicles. Size varies.

Examples Insect bites and hives (extensive wheals).

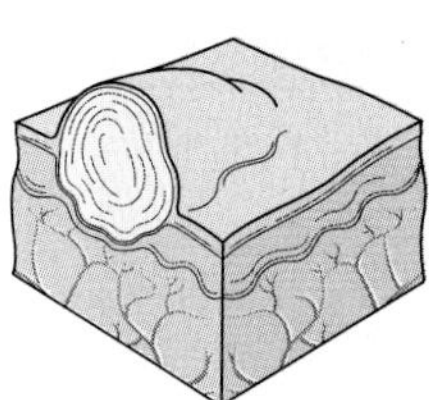

Pustule

Elevated, pus-filled vesicle or bulla with circumscribed border. Size varies.

Examples Acne, impetigo, and carbuncles (large boils).

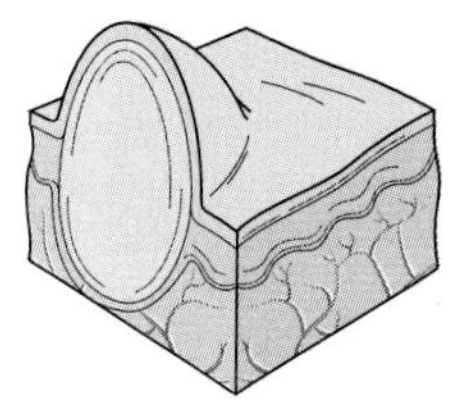

Cyst

Elevated, encapsulated, fluid-filled or semisolid mass originating in the subcutaneous tissue or dermis, usually 1 cm or larger.

Examples Varieties include sebaceous cysts and epidermoid cysts.

Table 8.4 Secondary Skin Lesions

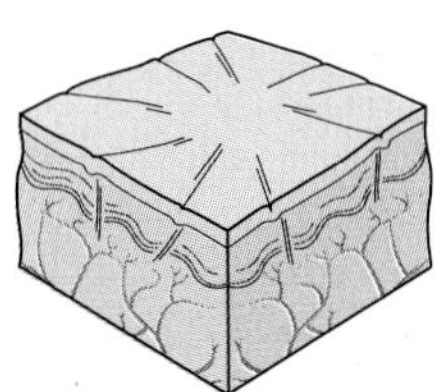

Atrophy

A translucent, dry, paperlike, sometimes wrinkled skin surface resulting from thinning or wasting of the skin due to loss of collagen and elastin.

Examples Striae, aged skin.

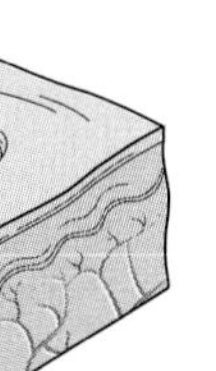

Erosion

Wearing away of the superficial epidermis causing a moist, shallow depression. Because erosions do not extend into the dermis, they heal without scarring.

Examples Scratch marks, ruptured vesicles.

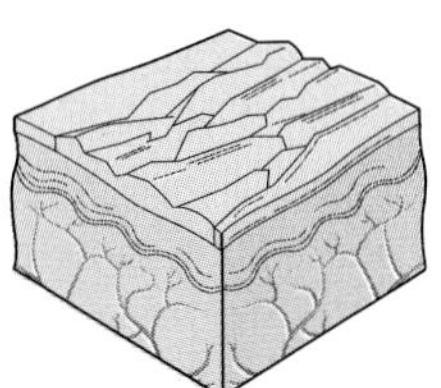

Lichenification

Rough, thickened, hardened area of epidermis resulting from chronic irritation such as scratching or rubbing.

Examples Chronic dermatitis.

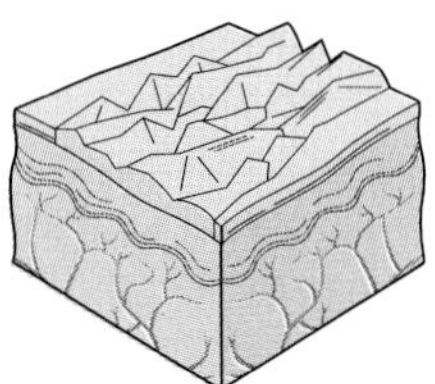

Scales

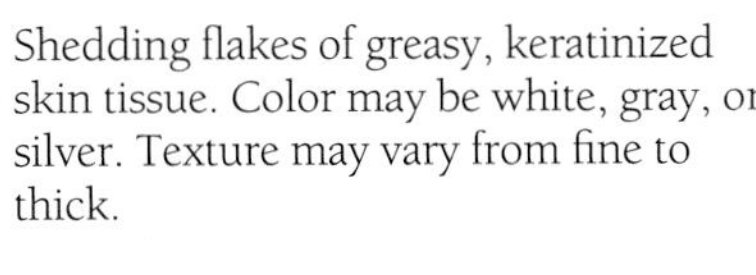

Shedding flakes of greasy, keratinized skin tissue. Color may be white, gray, or silver. Texture may vary from fine to thick.

Examples Dry skin, dandruff, psoriasis, and eczema.

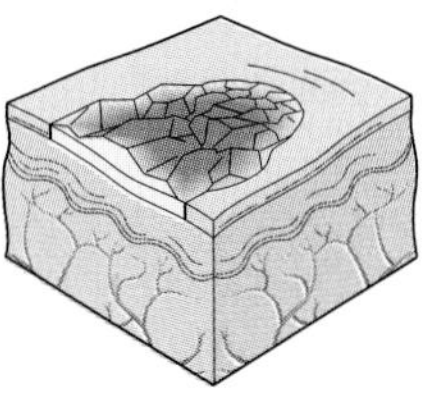

Crust

Dry blood, serum, or pus left on the skin surface when vesicles or pustules burst. Can be red-brown, orange, or yellow. Large crusts that adhere to the skin surface are called scabs.

Examples Eczema, impetigo, herpes, or scabs following abrasion.

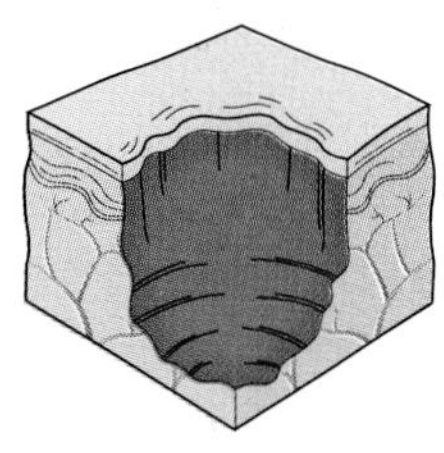

Ulcer

Deep, irregularly shaped area of skin loss extending into the dermis or subcutaneous tissue. May bleed. May leave scar.

Examples Decubitus ulcers (pressure sores), stasis ulcers, chancres.

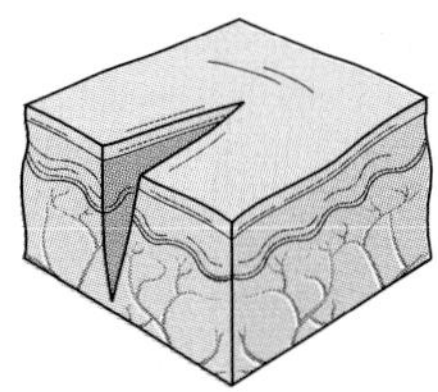

Fissure

Linear crack with sharp edges, extending into the dermis.

Examples Cracks at the corners of the mouth or in the hands, athlete's foot.

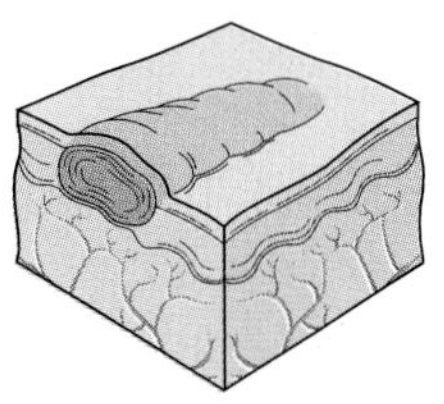

Scar

Flat, irregular area of connective tissue left after a lesion or wound has healed. New scars may be red or purple; older scars may be silvery or white.

Examples Healed surgical wound or injury, healed acne.

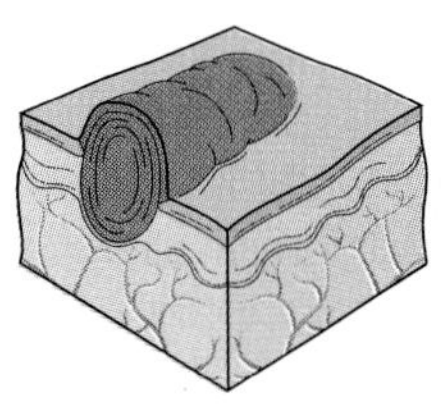

Keloid

Elevated, irregular, darkened area of excess scar tissue caused by excessive collagen formation during healing. Extends beyond the site of the original injury. Higher incidence in people of African descent.

Examples Keloid from ear-piercing or surgery.

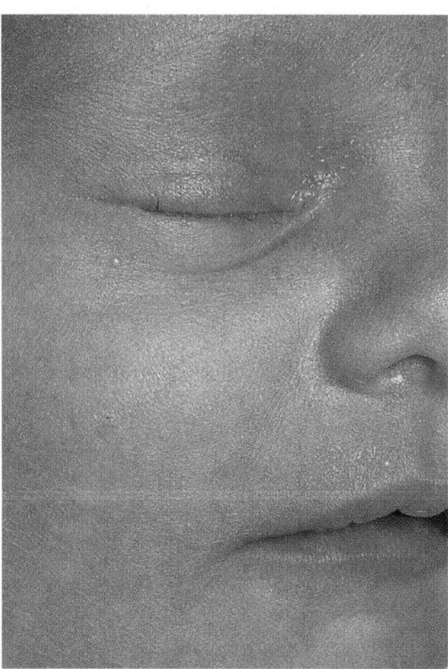

Figure 8.21 Milia.

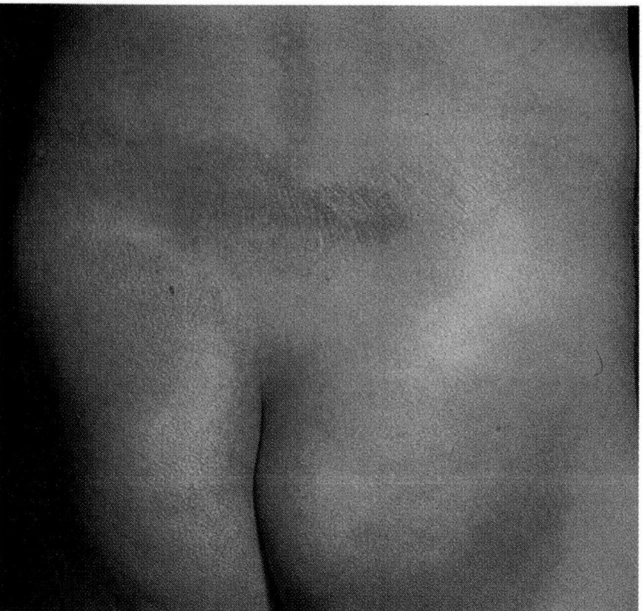

Figure 8.22 Mongolian spot(s).

Developmental Considerations

Infants, Children, and Adolescent Clients

At birth, the newborn's skin typically is covered with *vernix caseosa*, a white, cheeselike mixture of sebum and epidermal cells. The skin color of newborns is typically bright red for the first 24 hours of life, then fades. About half of all newborns develop *physiologic jaundice* 3 to 4 days after birth, resulting in a yellowing of the skin, sclera, and mucous membranes. The skin of dark-skinned newborns normally is not fully pigmented until 2 to 3 months after birth. An infant's skin is very thin, soft, and free of terminal hair.

Many harmless skin markings are common in newborns. For example, they may have areas of tiny white facial papules. These are called *milia* and are due to sebum that collects in the openings of hair follicles (Figure 8.21). Milia usually disappear spontaneously within a few weeks of birth. Vascular markings are also common. These may include *stork bites*, which are irregular red or pink patches found most commonly on the back of the neck. They disappear spontaneously within a year of birth. The newborn may also have transient mottling or other transient color changes such as *harlequin color change*, in which a side-lying infant becomes markedly pink on the lower side, and pale on the higher side. *Mongolian spots* are gray, blue, or purple spots in the sacral and buttocks areas of newborns (Figure 8.22). They occur in about 90% of newborns of African ancestry and in about 80% of newborns of Asian or Native American ancestry. They fade during the first year of life.

Diaper rash is common in infants and usually does not indicate neglect or other parenting problems. See the client teaching tips for diaper rash on page 158.

Because the subcutaneous fat layer is poorly developed in infants, and the eccrine sweat glands do not secrete until the first few months of life, their temperature regulation is inefficient.

The fine, downy hair of the newborn, called *lanugo*, is replaced within a few months by vellus hair. Hair growth accelerates throughout childhood. Head lice are relatively common in school-age children, as are skin rashes. Children may develop rashes after playing in areas overgrown with poison ivy or poison oak.

Throughout childhood, the epidermis thickens, pigmentation increases, and more subcutaneous fat is deposited, especially in females during puberty. During adolescence, both the sweat glands and the oil glands increase their production. Increased production of sebum by the oil glands predisposes adolescents to develop acne (Figure 8.23). Increased axillary perspiration occurs as the apocrine glands mature, and body odor may develop for the first time. Pubic and axillary hair appears during adolescence, and males may develop facial and chest hair. For a comprehensive health assessment of infants, children, and adolescents, see Chapter 19.

Childbearing Clients

Pigmentation of the skin commonly increases during pregnancy, especially in the areolae, nipples, vulva, and perianal area. Approximately 70% of pregnant women develop hyperpigmented patches on the face referred to as *chloasma* or "the mask of pregnancy" (Figure 8.24). This normal condition disappears after pregnancy in some women but may be permanent in others. Some pregnant clients may also have a dark line called a *linea nigra* running from the umbilicus to the pubic area (Figure 8.25), increased pigmentation of the areolae and nipples, and darkened moles and scars. These are all normal findings.

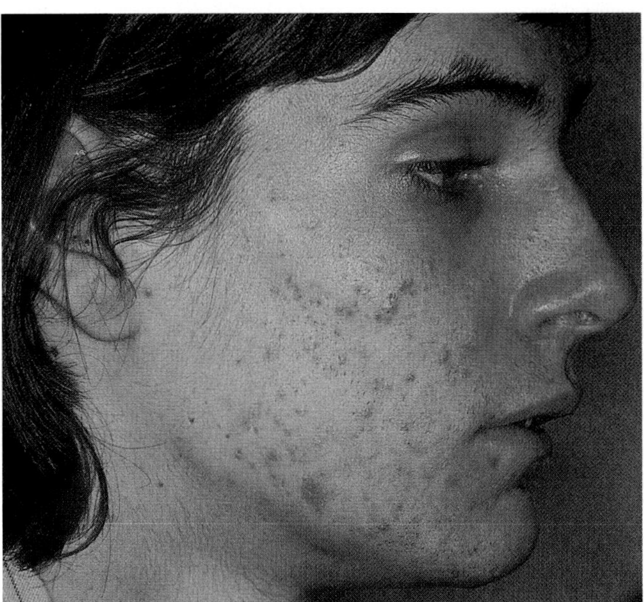

Figure 8.23 Acne.

Many pregnant women develop *striae* ("stretch marks") across the abdomen. These usually fade after pregnancy but do not disappear entirely. Cutaneous tags are not uncommon, especially on the neck and upper chest.

Hormonal changes may cause the oil and sweat glands to become hyperactive during pregnancy. This increased secretion may in turn lead to a worsening of acne in the first trimester of pregnancy, and an improvement in the third trimester. Hormonal changes also affect hair growth, and significant shedding is not uncommon 3 to 4 months after the birth of the child. For a comprehensive health assessment of childbearing clients, see Chapter 20.

Older Clients

As the skin ages, the epidermis thins and stretches out, and collagen and elastin fibers decrease, causing decreased skin elasticity and increased skin wrinkling. The skin becomes slack and may hang loosely on the frame. It may sag, especially beneath the chin and eyes, in the breasts of females, and in the scrotum of males.

The older client's skin is also more delicate and more susceptible to injury. Decreased production of sebum leads to dryness of both the skin and the hair. The skin may appear especially thin on the dorsal surfaces of the hands and feet and over the bony prominences. Tenting of the skin is common (see Figure 8.11, *B* on page 136). The sweat glands also decrease their activity, and the older adult perspires less. Decreased melanin production leads to a heightened sensitivity to sunlight, and skin cancer rates increase with age.

Some light-skinned older clients may appear pale because of decreased vascularity in the dermis, even though they may be healthy and well-oxygenated. The color of a dark-skinned elderly person may appear dull, gray, or darker for the same reasons.

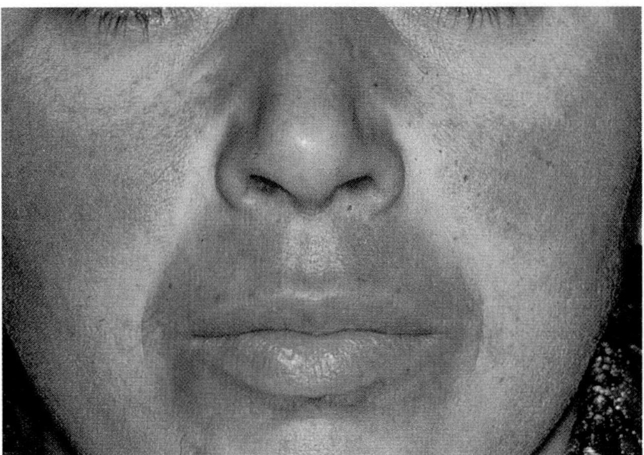

Figure 8.24 Chloasma.

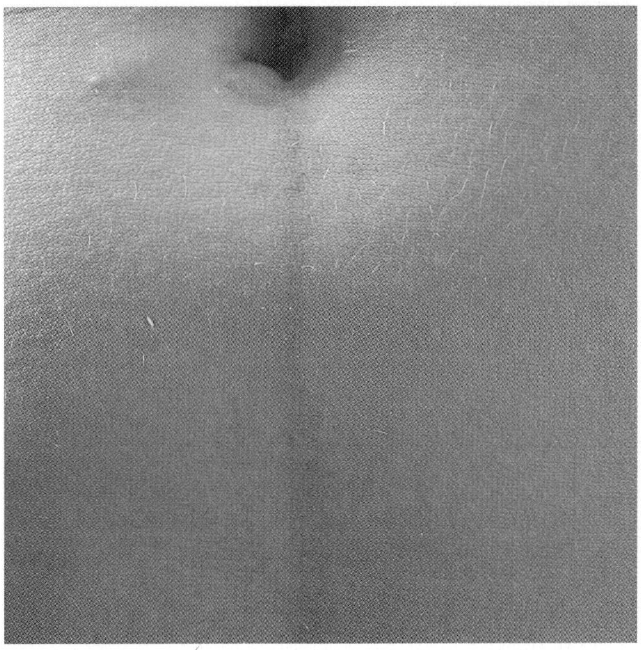

Figure 8.25 Linea nigra.

A variety of lesions are common in older adults. For example, the skin of many older clients may develop *senile lentigines* ("liver spots"), which look like hyperpigmented freckles, most commonly on the backs of the hands and the arms (Figure 8.26 on page 150). *Cherry angiomas* are small, bright red spots common in all older adults (Figure 8.27). They increase in number with age. *Cutaneous tags* may appear on the neck and upper chest (Figure 8.28), and *cutaneous horns* may occur on the face (Figure 8.29).

The hair becomes increasingly gray as melanin production decreases. Hair thins as the number of active hair follicles decreases. Facial hair may become more coarse.

The nails may show little change, or they may show the effects of decreased circulation in the body extremities, appearing thicker, harder, yellowed, oddly shaped, or opaque. They may be brittle and peeling, and may be prone to splitting and breaking. For a comprehensive health assessment of older clients, see Chapter 21.

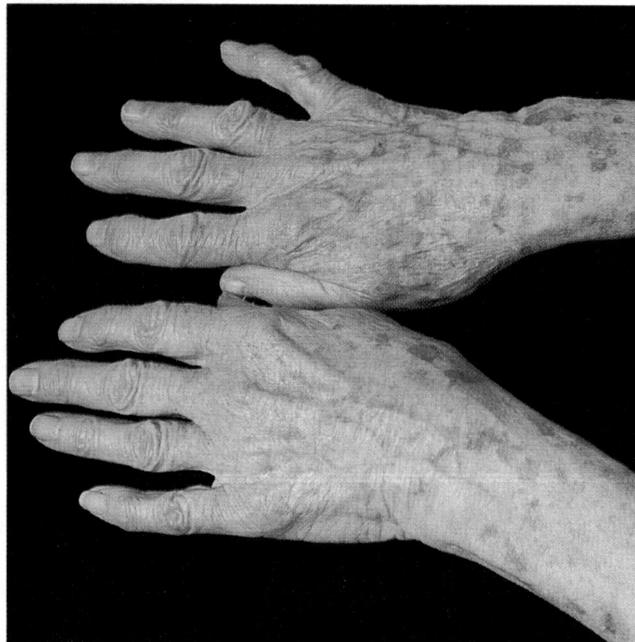

Figure 8.26 Senile lentigines.

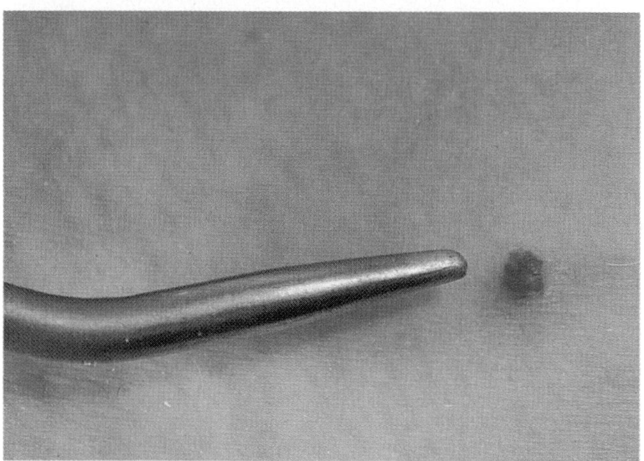

Figure 8.27 Cherry angioma.

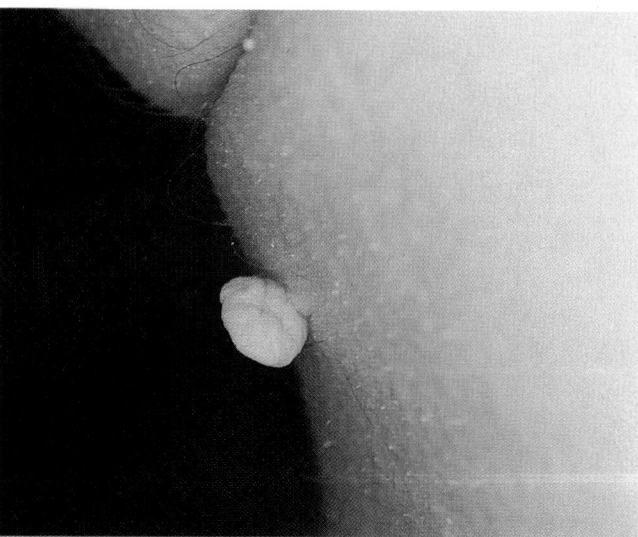

Figure 8.28 Cutaneous tag.

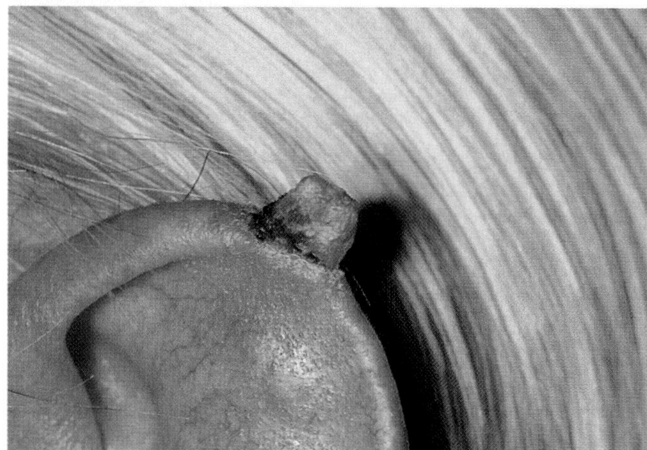

Figure 8.29 Cutaneous horn.

Psychosocial Considerations

Stress may exacerbate certain skin conditions such as rashes or acne. Stress may also be a factor in compulsive behaviors such as hair twisting and nail biting, signaled by nails that have no visible free edge, or have short, jagged edges. A lack of cleanliness of the skin, hair, or nails also may result from emotional distress, or it may indicate poor self-esteem or a disturbed body image. If appropriate, refer the client to social services or a mental health professional for assistance.

On the other hand, a visible skin disorder may trigger psychosocial health problems leading to social isolation, a body-image disturbance, or a self-esteem disturbance. If appropriate, assess the client further for the presence of emotional distress or anxiety related to the skin disorder.

Self-Care Considerations

Exercise, proper nutrition, and thorough, gentle cleansing all promote the health of the integumentary system. Consider the client's cleansing routine, as well as the use of makeup, perfumes, and other toiletries, when assessing for dry or oily skin, rashes, or lesions. Smoking may cause the skin to lose elasticity. Additionally, excessive sun exposure may result in loss of skin elasticity and may lead to skin cancer. Body odor may be affected by the client's diet, especially the use of certain spices that can be excreted via the skin. A prolonged use of topical steroids on any part of the body may cause the skin to become thin and fragile.

Some clients may be unwilling to undo special types of braids or other hair styles, especially if the style takes the client a long time to arrange or has religious or cultural significance. In these cases, examine any strands of hair that are loose or undone. Clients who regularly style their hair with hot rollers, curling irons, and blow dryers, use hair picks, or braid their hair tightly may experience hair breakage and patchy hair loss. Frequent use of permanent-wave solutions, chemical straighteners, bleaches, and dyes can also weaken hair and lead to hair loss. Many clients use a petroleum, lanolin, or glycerine hair dressing to add shine or control to their hair. Do not mistake the sheen from a hair product for overproduction of the oil glands in the scalp.

Regular use of tobacco may stain the nails. Staining may also occur with constant use of dark nail polish. Nail-polish removers containing acetone may cause excessive drying of the nails. Tight-fitting shoes may result in thickening of the toenails.

Family, Cultural, and Environmental Considerations

A client's culture, socioeconomic status, home environment, and means of employment may affect the health of the integument. If the client's skin, hair, and nails appear unclean, consider the client's job, socioeconomic status, and living situation. A client who seems unkempt may have just come from a physically demanding job or be ill, disabled, poor, or homeless and unable to maintain effective hygiene.

Changes in skin color may be difficult to evaluate in people with dark skin. Inspect areas of the body with less pigmentation, such as the lips, oral mucosa, sclerae, palms of the hands, and conjunctivae of the inner eyelids. Do not mistake the normal deposition of melanin in the lips of some olive-to-dark-skinned people for cyanosis. Some individuals with dark skin have increased pigmentation in the creases of the palms and soles, and yellow or brown-tinged sclerae. These are normal findings. (See Table 8.1 on page 142 for evaluating color variations in light and dark skin.)

Dry skin does not necessarily indicate dehydration and in fact may be normal for the dark-skinned client. By the same token, because many clients use petroleum-based products to lubricate their skin, ask about self-care before concluding that the client has oily skin.

The skin's response to stressors such as ultraviolet radiation is similar in all races. Dark-skinned clients tan, and their skin suffers the same damaging effects from the sun, although skin damage may take longer to occur. Assessment of color, texture, and moles and other lesions should therefore be as thorough as for light-skinned clients.

Calluses—circumscribed, painless thickenings of the epidermis—tend to form on parts of the body that are regularly exposed to pressure, weight-bearing, or friction. Common sites of calluses include the fingers, palms, toes, and soles of the feet.

Keep in mind that the client's occupation (eg, gardener, mechanic) may make it difficult to keep the fingers and nails unstained. Chemicals used in certain occupations also may stain the nails. The client's occupation may require frequent or prolonged immersion of the hands in water, which may lead to paronychia. The nail plates of dark-skinned clients may show darkly pigmented streaks, which are normal findings.

Organizing the Data

After carrying out the focused interview and conducting the physical assessment of the integumentary system, group the related data into clusters leading to either nursing diagnoses, which require nursing interventions such as client teaching (discussed on pages 152–158), or alterations in health, which require consultation with other members of the health care team.

Identifying Nursing Diagnoses

Nursing assessment of the integumentary system may lead to the diagnoses of *impaired tissue integrity* or *impaired skin integrity* (see Table 8.5 on page 152). The diagnoses are similar; however, impaired tissue integrity is a broader term involving the cornea, mucous membranes, and subcutaneous tissue as well as the skin, whereas impaired skin integrity involves simply the dermis and epidermis. For example, impaired tissue integrity effectively describes deep burns and surgical incisions, whereas impaired skin integrity is appropriate for rashes, hives, and abrasions.

The related factors and defining characteristics of the two diagnoses also differ. The defining characteristic for impaired tissue integrity is damaged or destroyed tissue, whereas the defining characteristics for impaired skin integrity are disruption of skin surface, destruction of skin layers, and invasion of body structures.

Other nursing diagnoses associated with the integumentary system include *pain; sleep pattern disturbance* related to pruritus; *potential for infection* related to bacteria, viruses, or fungi; *knowledge deficit* related to inadequate information about skin care; and *self-care deficit: bathing/hygiene.* Other nursing diagnoses may apply if the client with a skin problem is embarrassed, isolated, or contagious. These include *ineffective individual coping, body image disturbance, social isolation,* and *sexual dysfunction.*

Common Alterations in Health Associated with the Integumentary System

Common alterations in health associated with the integumentary system include allergic reactions, infectious rashes, skin cancer, and many others. (See Table 8.6 on page 153.)

Table 8.5 Nursing Diagnoses Commonly Associated with the Integumentary System

IMPAIRED TISSUE INTEGRITY	
Definition: A state in which an individual experiences damage to mucous membranes or to corneal, integumentary, or subcutaneous tissue (NANDA).	
DEFINING CHARACTERISTICS	
Damaged or destroyed tissue	
RELATED FACTORS	
Altered circulation, Nutritional deficit/excess, Fluid deficit/excess, Knowledge deficit, Impaired physical mobility, Chemical irritants (body excretions and secretions, medications), Thermal factors (temperature extremes), Mechanical factors (pressure, shear, friction), Radiation (including therapeutic radiation).	
IMPAIRED SKIN INTEGRITY	
Definition: A state in which the individual's skin is adversely altered (NANDA).	
DEFINING CHARACTERISTICS	
Disruption of skin surface Destruction of skin layer	Invasion of body structures
RELATED FACTORS	
External (environmental) Hyperthermia, Hypothermia, Chemical substance, Mechanical factors (shearing forces, pressure, restraint), Radiation, Physical immobilization.	*Internal (somatic)* Medication, Altered nutritional state (obesity, emaciation), Altered metabolic state, Altered circulation, Altered sensation, Altered pigmentation, Skeletal prominence, Developmental factors, Immunologic deficit, Alterations in skin turgor (change in elasticity).

Health Promotion and Client Education

At the conclusion of the assessment, answer any questions the client may have about skin care and skin health. Stress the following guidelines for maintaining healthy skin and preventing future skin problems as appropriate.

Promoting the General Health of the Skin

To maintain the general health of the skin

- Wash dry skin morning and night with a gentle soap. Apply a lotion with sunscreen daily.
- If your skin feels excessively dry, try applying lotion just after bathing.
- Wash oily skin two to three times daily with a warm washcloth and clear (glycerine) soap to remove skin oils and keratin plugs. Fatted soaps, greases, lotions, and creams should be avoided.

Table 8.6 Common Alterations in the Health of the Integumentary System

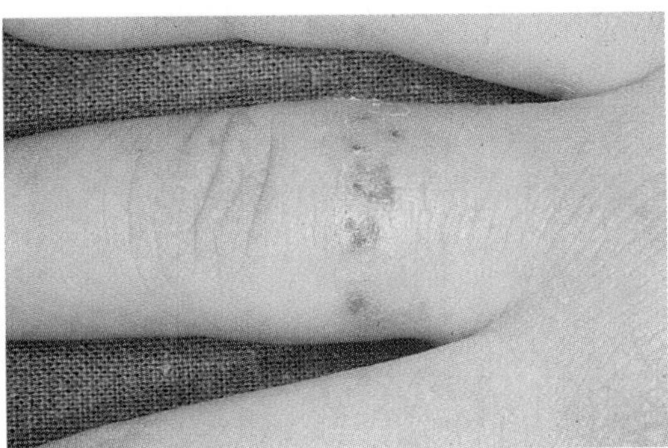

Contact Dermatitis

Inflammation of the skin due to an allergy to a substance that comes into contact with the skin, such as clothing, jewelry, plants, chemicals, or cosmetics. The location of the lesions may help identify the allergen. May progress from redness to hives, vesicles, or scales. Usually accompanied by intense itching.

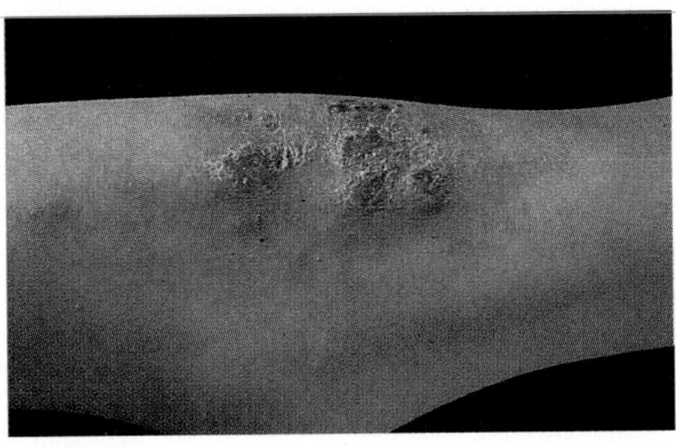

Eczema

Internally provoked inflammation of the skin causing reddened papules and vesicles that ooze, weep, and progress to form crusts. The lesions are usually located on the scalp, face, elbows and knees, and forearms and wrists. Eczema usually causes intense itching.

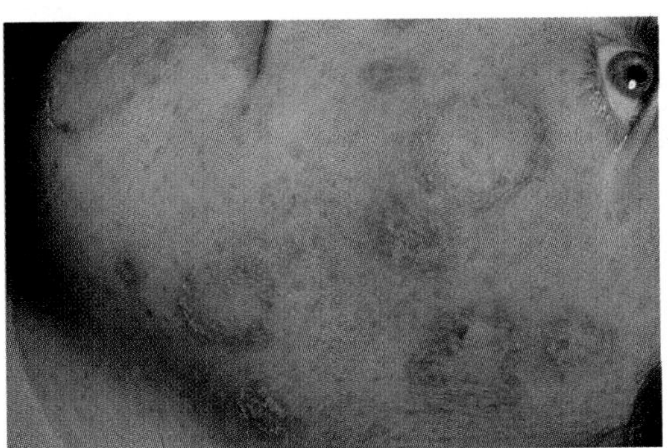

Impetigo

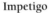

A bacterial skin infection that usually appears on the skin around the nose and mouth. It is contagious and common in children. May begin as a barely perceptible patch of blisters that breaks, exposing red, weeping area beneath. A tan crust soon forms over this area, and the infection may spread out from the edges.

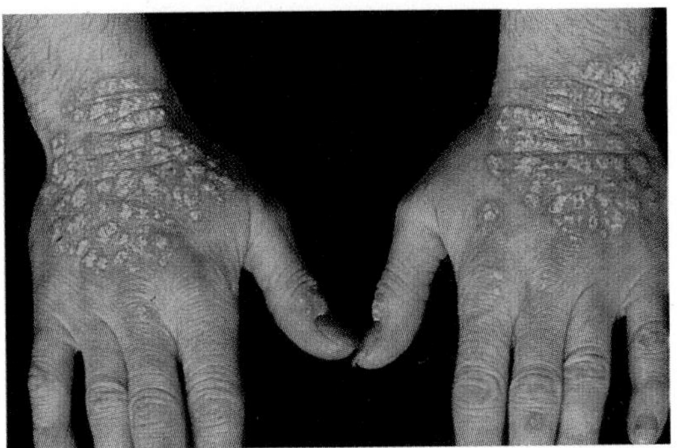

Psoriasis

Thickening of the skin in dry, silvery, scaly patches. Occurs with overproduction of skin cells resulting in build-up of cells faster than they can be shed. May be triggered by emotional stress or generally poor health. May be located on scalp, elbows and knees, lower back, and perianal area.

Table 8.6 Common Alterations in the Health of the Integumentary System (continued)

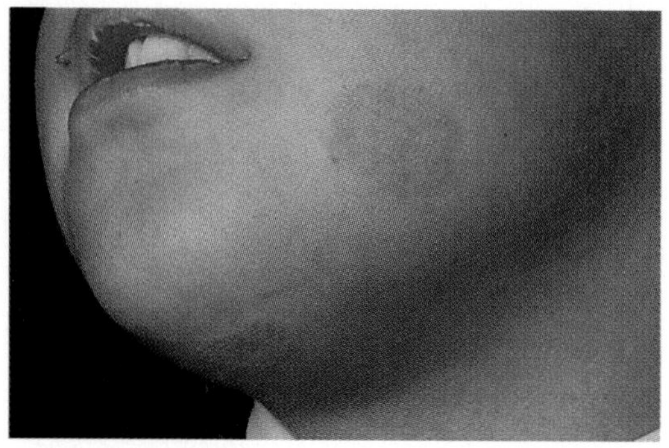

Tinea (Ringworm)

Fungal infection affecting the body (tinea corporis), the scalp (tinea capitis), or the feet (tinea pedis, also known as athlete's foot). Secondary bacterial infection may also be present. The appearance of the lesions varies, and they may present as papules, pustules, vesicles, or scales.

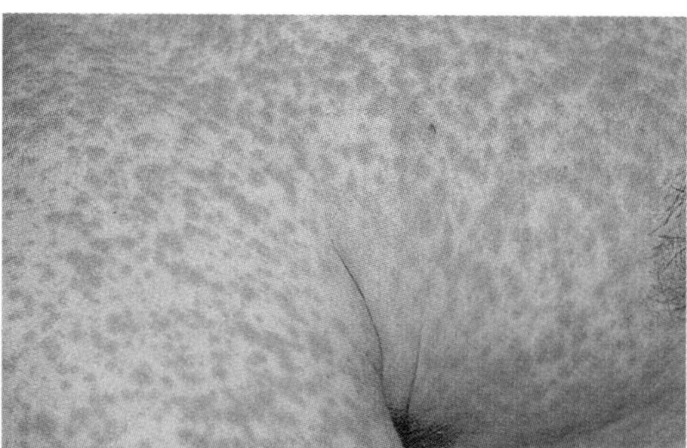

Measles (Rubeola)

Highly contagious viral disease that causes a rash of red to purple macules or papules. The rash begins on the face, then progresses over the neck, trunk, arms, and legs. It does not blanch. It may be accompanied by tiny white spots that look like grains of salt (called Koplik's spots) on the oral mucosa. Occurs mostly in children.

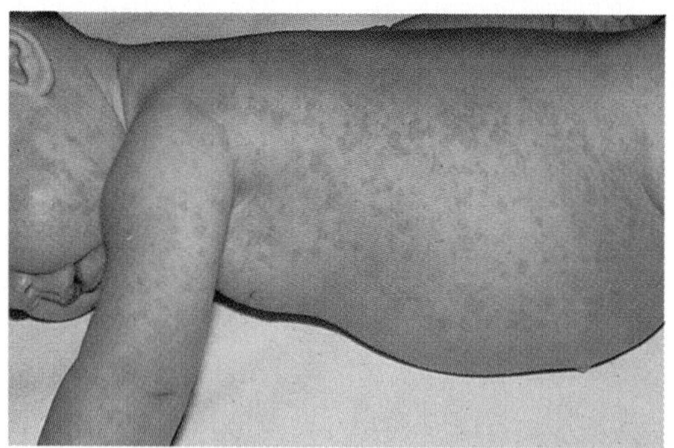

German Measles (Rubella)

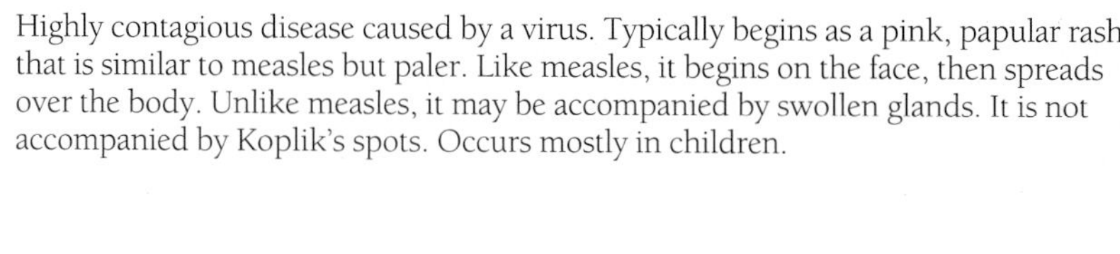

Highly contagious disease caused by a virus. Typically begins as a pink, papular rash that is similar to measles but paler. Like measles, it begins on the face, then spreads over the body. Unlike measles, it may be accompanied by swollen glands. It is not accompanied by Koplik's spots. Occurs mostly in children.

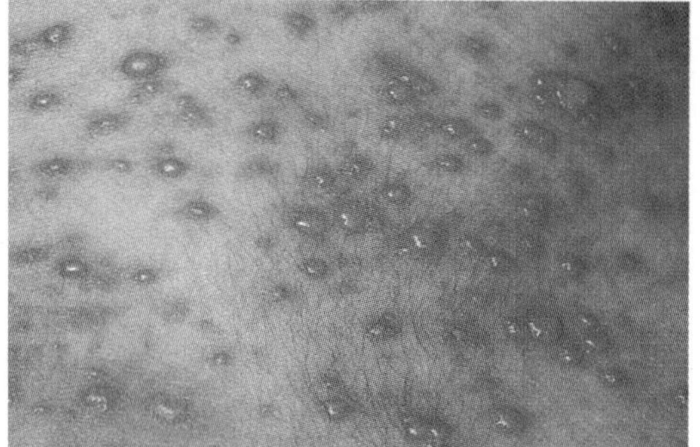

Chicken Pox (Varicella)

A mild infectious disease caused by the herpes zoster virus. Begins as groups of small, red, fluid-filled vesicles usually on the trunk. Progresses to face, arms, and legs. Vesicles erupt over several days, forming pustules, then crusts. The condition may cause intense itching. Occurs mostly in children.

Table 8.6 Common Alterations in the Health of the Integumentary System (continued)

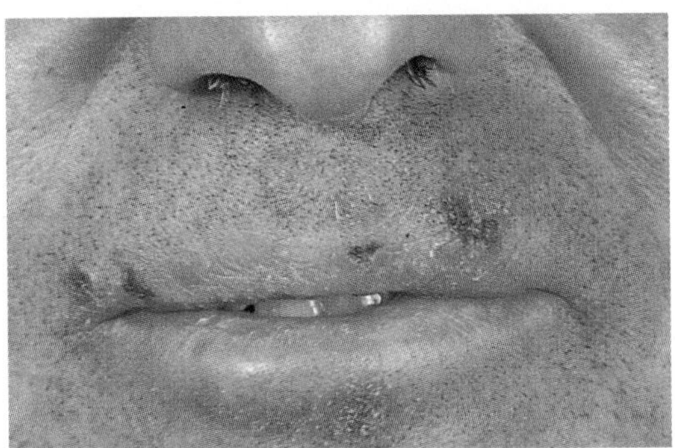

Herpes Simplex (Cold Sores)

Viral infection that causes characteristic lesions on the lips and oral mucosa. Lesions progress from vesicles to pustules, and then crusts. Herpes simplex also occurs in the genitals.

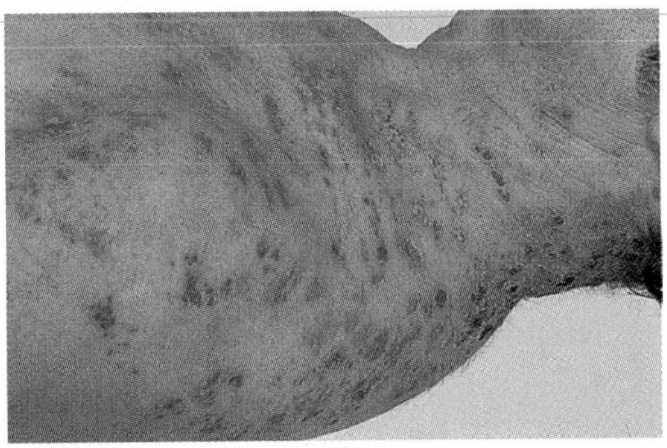

Herpes Zoster (Shingles)

Eruption of dormant herpes zoster virus, which typically has invaded the body during an attack of chicken pox. Clusters of small vesicles form on the skin along the route of sensory nerves. Vesicles progress to pustules and then crusts. Causes intense pain and itching. Condition is more common and more severe in older adults.

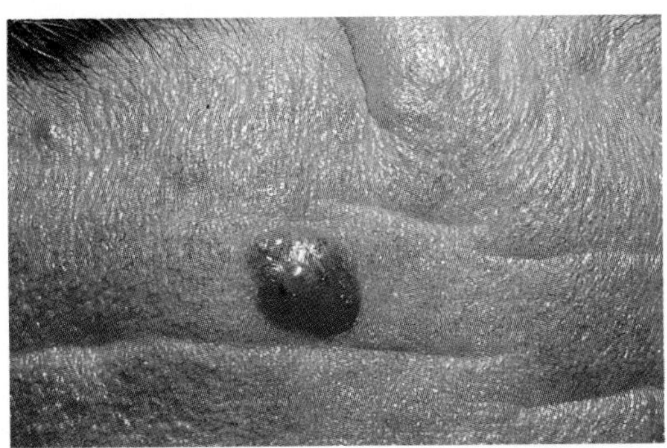

Basal Cell Carcinoma

The most common but least malignant type of skin cancer, basal cell carcinoma is a proliferation of the cells of the stratum basale into the dermis and subcutaneous tissue. The lesions begin as shiny papules that develop central ulcers with rounded, pearly edges. Lesions occur most often on skin regions regularly exposed to the sun.

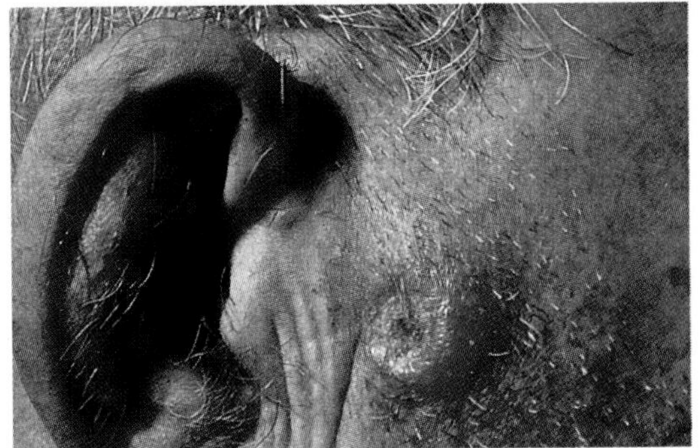

Squamous Cell Carcinoma

Squamous cell carcinoma arises from the cells of the stratum spinosum. It begins as a reddened, scaly papule, then forms a shallow ulcer with a clearly delineated, elevated border. It commonly appears on the scalp, ears, backs of the hands, and lower lip, and is thought to be caused by exposure to the sun. It grows rapidly.

Table 8.6 Common Alterations in the Health of the Integumentary System (continued)

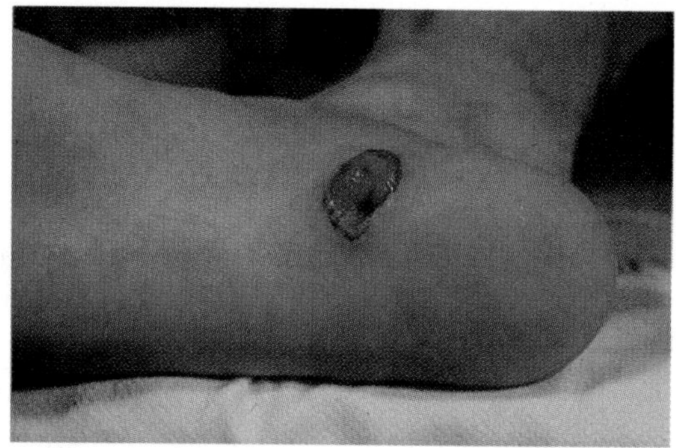

Malignant Melanoma

Malignant melanoma is the least common but most serious type of skin cancer, because it spreads rapidly to lymph and blood vessels. The lesion contains areas of varied pigmentation from black to brown to blue or red, the edges are often irregular, with notched borders, and the diameter is greater than 6 mm.

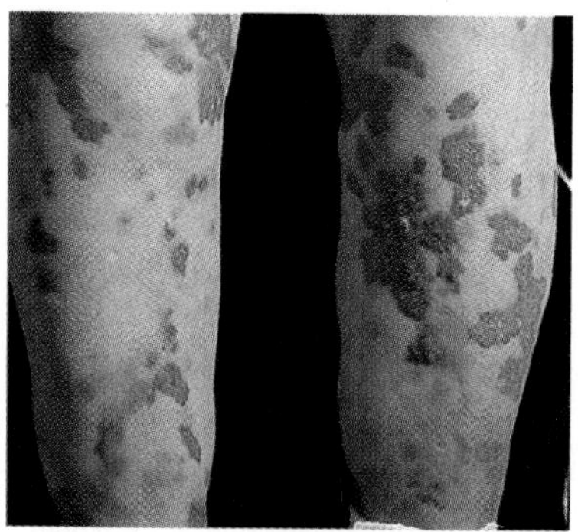

Kaposi's Sarcoma

A malignant tumor of the epidermis and internal epithelial tissues. Lesions are typically soft, blue to purple, and painless. Other characteristics are variable: they may be macular or papular and may resemble keloids or bruises. Kaposi's sarcoma is common in HIV-positive people.

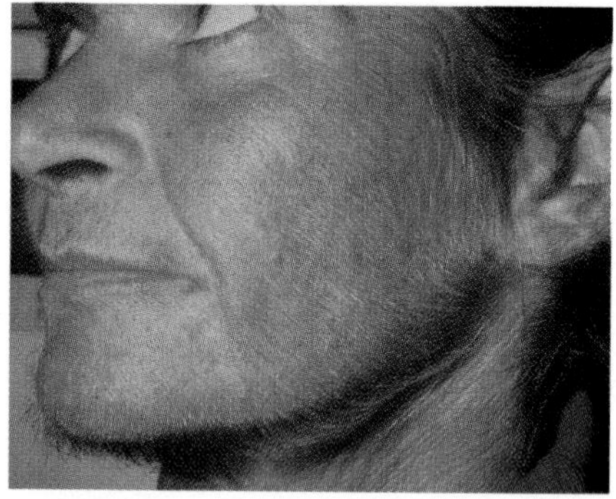

Hirsutism

Excess body hair in females on the face, chest, abdomen, arms, and legs, following the male pattern. Typically due to endocrine or metabolic dysfunction, though may be idiopathic.

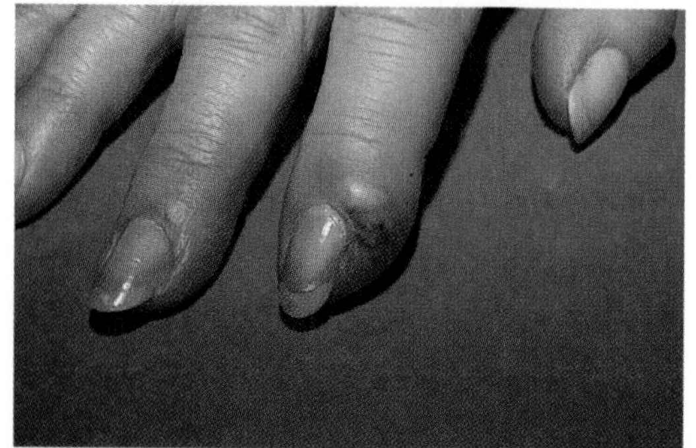

Paronychia

An infection of the skin adjacent to the nail, usually caused by bacteria or fungi. The affected area becomes red, swollen, and painful, and pus may ooze from it.

DIAGNOSTIC REASONING IN ACTION

Janine Gautier is a 28-year-old graphic artist who comes to a university health services office for evaluation of pain, burning, and itching in her axillary region. She has moved recently to the United States from France to study at the university. She tells Susan Liebowitz, RN, that the problem seemed to start about 3 weeks ago and has been getting progressively worse. She states that she can hardly keep from scratching the area, but when she does, it hurts even more.

Ms Liebowitz asks Ms Gautier to describe her bathing and skin-care habits, including any changes she has made in the last few weeks. Ms Gautier reports that since moving to the United States, she has begun to shave the hair under her arms, "like American women." She states that, immediately after shaving, she applies an antiperspirant. Ms Liebowitz asks Ms Gautier if she is using the same brand of antiperspirant she used in France, and she replies that after arriving in the United States, she switched to a new brand. She also reports taking birth control pills, and she uses aspirin about twice a month for headaches.

The nursing assessment of Ms Gautier's skin reveals patches of small red vesicles throughout the axillary region on both sides of her body. Ms Liebowitz also notes that, in general, Ms Gautier's skin, hair, and nails are clean and well hydrated, that the texture, thickness, and elasticity of her skin are normal, and that except in the axillary region, her skin is free from lesions.

The nursing assessment of Ms Gautier provides the following subjective and objective data:

- Pain, itching, and burning
- Change in self-care routine
- Use of chemical antiperspirant at site of rash
- Lack of exposure to information on proper techniques for shaving the axillary region
- Use of birth control pills and aspirin
- The client's skin is clean
- The client's skin is free of lesions except in the axillary region
- Disruption of skin surface in axillary region

To cluster the information, Ms Liebowitz:

- Considers the data regarding Ms Gautier's use of birth control pills and aspirin but disregards it because it is not likely to be related to the localized rash.
- Considers the data regarding Ms Gautier's change in antiperspirant and application immediately after shaving, and incorporates this information in her plan of care.
- Notes that a disruption of skin surface is a defining characteristic of the nursing diagnosis *Impaired skin integrity.*
- Notes that pain, chemical irritants, and knowledge deficit are related factors for the diagnosis *Impaired skin integrity.*

Ms Liebowitz arrives at the following nursing diagnoses:

1. *Impaired skin integrity* related to contact with a chemical substance
2. *Knowledge deficit* related to limited exposure to information about shaving and caring for the skin of the axillary region

Ms Liebowitz teaches Ms Gautier how to care for the skin in her axillary region. She advises her to refrain from applying any antiperspirant immediately after shaving and advises her to discontinue use of her antiperspirant until the rash resolves.

- Keep any hair conditioners, hair sprays, or other hair products from touching the face. Hair products that linger on the skin can cause acne and other skin reactions, especially on the forehead and around the hairline.
- Regular exercise increases circulation and oxygenation, and improves the health and appearance of the skin.
- Because smoking causes a loss in skin elasticity that leads to premature wrinkling, you should stop smoking.

Preventing Rashes and Allergic Reactions

To prevent rashes and allergic skin reactions

- If you must come in contact with strong chemicals or contaminants in your work, wear protective clothes, shoes, goggles, and a mask.
- Notify your doctor about any prescription medication that causes skin irritation.
- Avoid cosmetics, soaps, detergents, perfumes, after-shave lotions, antiperspirants, clothing, jewelry, foods, or other products that cause skin irritation.
- Some health care workers have allergic reactions to the powder in latex gloves. Gloves without powder can be ordered.

Preventing Sun Damage

To reduce the harmful effects of ultraviolet radiation on the skin

- Limit exposure to the sun to no more than 15 minutes at any time. Between 10:00 A.M. and 3:00 P.M., when the sun's rays are strongest, avoid sun exposure entirely.
- Always use a sunscreen with a sun protection factor (SPF) of 15 or more, even on overcast days. Sunscreen is especially important for infants, children, and older adults. Dark-skinned clients do need to wear sunscreen, because their skin suffers the same damage from the sun as light skin.
- Wear protective clothes such as wide-brimmed hats, long-sleeved shirts, and long pants.
- Take special precautions to prevent sun exposure if you are taking a medication that causes photosensitivity.
- Do not try to acquire or maintain a tan, either through sunbathing or use of tanning parlors. Accumulated ultraviolet exposure, whether from the sun or from a tanning booth, reduces skin elasticity and may cause skin cancer.

Make sure that clients understand the risk factors associated with skin cancer. These include:

- Age 50 or older
- Fair coloring
- Tendency to burn easily
- Personal history of sunburn
- Personal or familial history of skin cancer
- Geographic location near the equator or at high altitudes

Encourage clients who have had frequent sun exposure or have a personal or familial history of skin cancer to examine their skin once a month for moles or other lesions. Clients should report to their physician the appearance of a new mole or any change in a pre-existing mole. The following procedure for skin self-assessment is modified from the American Cancer Society:

- Use a room that is well-lighted and has a full-length mirror. Have a hand-held mirror and chair available. Remove all of your clothes.
- Examine all of your skin surface, front and back. Begin with your hands, including the spaces between your fingers. Continue with your arms, chest, abdomen, pubic area, thighs, lower legs, and toes. Next examine your face and neck. Make sure you inspect your underarms, the sides of your trunk, the back of your neck, the buttocks, and the soles of your feet.
- Next, sit down with one leg elevated. Use the hand-held mirror to examine the inside of the elevated leg, from the groin area to the foot. Repeat on the other leg.
- Use the hand-held mirror to inspect your scalp.
- Consult your physician promptly if you see any new pigmented area, or if any existing mole has changed in color, size, shape, or elevation. Also report sores that do not heal; redness or swelling around a growth or lesion; a change in sensation such as itching, pain, tenderness, or numbness in a lesion or the skin around it; and a change in the texture or consistency of the skin.

Preventing Diaper Rash

To prevent diaper rash, parents or caretakers should

- Change the baby's diapers frequently. Leave the diapers off altogether for as long as possible. Do not use plastic pants or disposable diapers with a thick plastic layer.
- Wash diapers in mild soap and rinse thoroughly. Adding vinegar to the last rinse cycle may help reduce the irritating ammonia.
- Try a protective ointment or petroleum jelly. Note: Do not apply ointments or jelly if a rash is already present, because it may delay healing.

Promoting Healthy Hair and Nails

To promote healthy hair and nails

- Avoid frequent chemical hair-styling procedures such as permanent waves, chemical straightening, bleaching, and coloring.
- Avoid vigorous brushing, combing, teasing, and picking of the hair, as well as tight braiding or "corn-rowing" of the hair.
- Do not share brushes, combs, or other hair implements.
- Keep toenails trimmed and wear shoes that allow room for toes to move.
- Avoid clipping the cuticles of the nails, to reduce the risk of infection.

Summary

The assessment of the integumentary system provides significant information about the client's total health status. Knowledge of the anatomy and physiology of the system helps you perform the assessment and understand the normal variations that occur in certain client groups. An interview focused on the skin allows you to consider the client's history of skin health and skin care, as well as developmental, psychosocial, and cultural and environmental factors that may influence skin health. Physical assessment of the skin, hair, and nails reveals a host of clues to the status of the body's oxygenation, circulation, fluid balance, hormone balance, and other factors. Nursing diagnoses commonly identified after assessment of the integumentary system include impaired tissue integrity and impaired skin integrity. After performing the health

DIAGNOSTIC REASONING IN ACTION

Mr. Shelley is a 54-year-old groundskeeper for a large corporation in the Southwest. He visits the company's health and wellness office saying, "My wife told me to have someone check my leathery skin."

Julieta Cadenas, RN, asks Mr. Shelley how much time he spends out of doors. He reveals that he is outside from about eight o'clock each morning until four o'clock each afternoon, except for his lunch break, which he usually takes in the cafeteria. He reports that he does not use sunscreen, and that in the summertime, he works in a short-sleeved shirt, shorts, and a baseball cap. He doesn't recall ever having had a bad sunburn. He states that he has a mole on his left thigh that has been present since birth, but that to his knowledge it has not changed. He is not aware of any other birthmarks or skin lesions. He has never performed a skin self-assessment. He reports no family history of skin cancer. He states that he never sunbathes or swims, and that he plays outdoor sports only at the annual family picnic. He showers each morning before work and again at the end of the work day before going home. He uses deodorant soap. He admits that his skin is often quite dry but says he feels that sunscreens and lotions "are for women."

The nursing assessment of Mr. Shelley's skin reveals the following data: his skin is clean. It is a ruddy brown color where frequently exposed to the sun and a pinkish tan elsewhere. His temperature is warm bilaterally, and he has a mild sheen of perspiration on his face, neck, and upper trunk. Where exposed to the sun, his skin is thick with decreased elasticity. There are no unexpected visible blood vessels or vascular lesions. There is a mole approximately 2 cm by 2 cm on the anterior surface of his left thigh. No drainage is noted. Mr. Shelley's scalp and hair appear dry but clean and free of lesions. Soil is embedded beneath the free edge of his nails. He states that he has been transplanting cuttings this morning.

Ms Cadenas clusters this information and arrives at the following nursing diagnoses:

1. *High risk for impaired skin integrity* related to regular exposure to the sun
2. *Knowledge deficit* related to lack of information about the prevention of skin cancer;
3. *Self-care deficit: bathing/hygiene* related to frequent showers with harsh soap.

Ms Cadenas advises Mr. Shelley to limit his exposure to the sun and teaches him how to perform a skin self-assessment, encouraging him to do so monthly. She also advises Mr. Shelley to avoid harsh soaps and to apply frequently a moisturizing lotion with an SPF of at least 15. Finally, she reviews with Mr. Shelley the risk factors for skin cancer and teaches him tips for limiting sun exposure and caring for his dry skin.

assessment and identifying any appropriate nursing diagnoses, provide the client with the information needed to promote skin health.

Key Points

- ✓ The skin is composed of two layers: the epidermis is the tough outer shell containing keratin and melanin; the dermis is a layer of underlying connective tissue containing collagen and elastin fibers. Subcutaneous tissue lies beneath the dermis. Its fat cells cushion the body against trauma and provide insulation. Sweat glands and oil glands are distributed in the dermis. The skin and its glands protect the underlying body structures against trauma, bacteria, chemicals, and water loss and help regulate the body's temperature.
- ✓ Hairs are fibers of keratinized cells that arise from follicles in the dermis. Nails are plates of keratinized cells that arise from the basal layer of the epidermis. The major functions of the hair and nails are protection and insulation.
- ✓ Conduct a focused interview to gather specific information about the client's skin, including history of the health of the skin, hair, and nails; any allergies, rashes, or lesions; and self-care practices, including sun exposure. Remember to consider the client's developmental stage, psychosocial factors, and factors related to the client's family, culture, and environment.
- ✓ Inspect and palpate the client's skin for hygiene, color, temperature, moisture, texture, thickness, elasticity, vascularity, and lesions.
- ✓ Inspect and palpate the client's scalp and hair for hygiene, color, texture, distribution, and lesions.
- ✓ Inspect and palpate the client's nails for hygiene, color, shape and contour, and thickness and integrity.
- ✓ Nursing diagnoses commonly associated with the integumentary system include impaired tissue integrity and impaired skin integrity.
- ✓ Provide the client with information needed to promote health of the skin, hair, and nails.

Chapter 9

Assessing the Head and Neck

Although all body regions and systems are linked and operate together as a whole, the head and neck region make up what is in many ways the most important region in the body. It houses our special senses of vision, hearing, smell, and taste, and it provides a means of identifying us from one another, through the uniqueness of our hair, eyes, and facial characteristics.

Because several body systems overlap in the head and neck region, you will be assessing several systems at the same time. For instance, the integumentary system provides covering and protection. The musculoskeletal system provides a bony shell for the brain and spinal cord and is responsible for movement of the head and neck and for facial expression. Food is taken in through the mouth, which is the beginning of the gastrointestinal system. Air enters the lungs through the nose, mouth, and trachea, which compose the upper respiratory system. The cardiovascular system carries oxygen and other nutrients to the region and transports wastes from the region. Consider this close interrelationship of systems as you assess the client's head and neck, and you may find clues to the client's nutritional status, airway clearance, tissue perfusion, metabolism, level of activity, sleep and rest, level of stress, and self-care ability.

When performing an assessment of the head and neck, you should also be aware of psychosocial factors, such as stress and anxiety, that can influence the health of this region. Consider as well the client's self-care practices: many clients spend a great deal of time caring for this region, and alterations in health may affect their ability to provide this care. A client's ancestry, cultural practices, socioeconomic status, and physical environment both at home and at work can greatly influence the health of the head and neck, and are an integral part of the assessment data. Additionally, a client's developmental stage has a tremendous influence on the appearance and functioning of the region. Figure 9.1 gives an overview of some important factors to consider when you assess the head and neck.

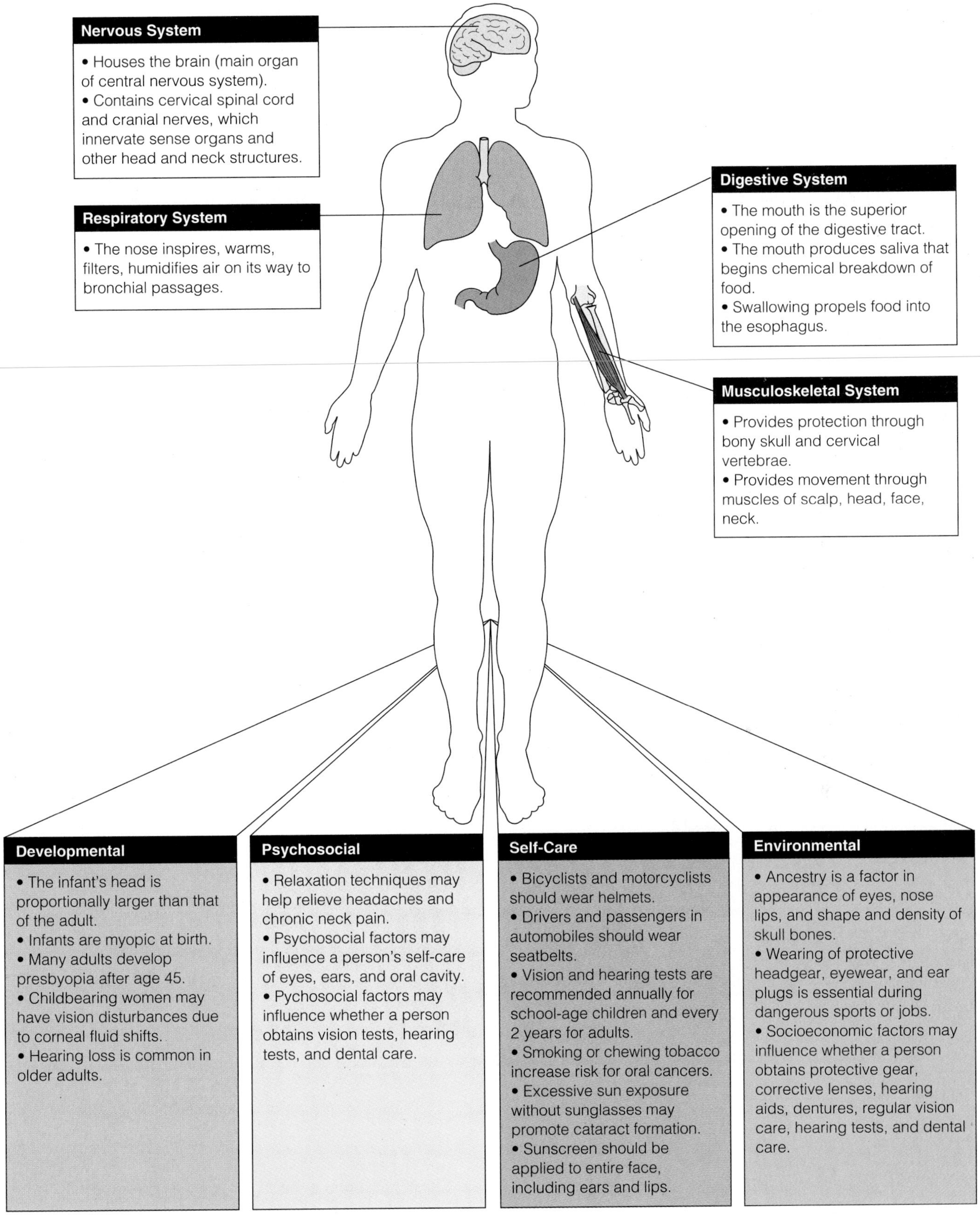

Nervous System
• Houses the brain (main organ of central nervous system).
• Contains cervical spinal cord and cranial nerves, which innervate sense organs and other head and neck structures.
Respiratory System
• The nose inspires, warms, filters, humidifies air on its way to bronchial passages.
Digestive System
• The mouth is the superior opening of the digestive tract.
• The mouth produces saliva that begins chemical breakdown of food.
• Swallowing propels food into the esophagus.
Musculoskeletal System
• Provides protection through bony skull and cervical vertebrae.
• Provides movement through muscles of scalp, head, face, neck.
Developmental
• The infant's head is proportionally larger than that of the adult.
• Infants are myopic at birth.
• Many adults develop presbyopia after age 45.
• Childbearing women may have vision disturbances due to corneal fluid shifts.
• Hearing loss is common in older adults.
Psychosocial
• Relaxation techniques may help relieve headaches and chronic neck pain.
• Psychosocial factors may influence a person's self-care of eyes, ears, and oral cavity.
• Pychosocial factors may influence whether a person obtains vision tests, hearing tests, and dental care.
Self-Care
• Bicyclists and motorcyclists should wear helmets.
• Drivers and passengers in automobiles should wear seatbelts.
• Vision and hearing tests are recommended annually for school-age children and every 2 years for adults.
• Smoking or chewing tobacco increase risk for oral cancers.
• Excessive sun exposure without sunglasses may promote cataract formation.
• Sunscreen should be applied to entire face, including ears and lips.
Environmental
• Ancestry is a factor in appearance of eyes, nose lips, and shape and density of skull bones.
• Wearing of protective headgear, eyewear, and ear plugs is essential during dangerous sports or jobs.
• Socioeconomic factors may influence whether a person obtains protective gear, corrective lenses, hearing aids, dentures, regular vision care, hearing tests, and dental care.

Figure 9.1 An overview of important factors to consider when assessing the head and neck.

Anatomy and Physiology Review

As mentioned above, the head and neck include many organs discussed in other chapters. For example, the skin is discussed in Chapter 8, and the brain and cranial nerves are discussed in Chapter 18. This chapter addresses the head, eyes, ears, nose and sinuses, mouth and throat, and neck. Each structure is discussed separately.

Head

The **skull** is a protective shell made up of the bones of the cranium and the face (Figure 9.2). The major bones of the cranium are 2 frontal bones, 2 parietal bones, 2 temporal bones, and 1 occipital bone. The face consists of 14 bones: the nasal, lacrimal, palatine, inferior conchae, zygomatic, and maxillary bones are paired. The mandible and vomer are unpaired.

Figure 9.3 shows the main muscles of the scalp, face, and neck. These muscles play a major role in expressing our emotions through our facial expressions. They also contribute to movement of the head and neck.

Movement of the facial muscles is controlled by the *facial nerve*, cranial nerve VII. Cranial nerve V, the *trigeminal nerve*, controls facial sensations and movement of the muscles for chewing. Cranial nerve I, the *olfactory nerve*, carries impulses for the sense of smell, whereas cranial nerve II, the *optic nerve*, carries impulses for vision. Cranial nerve VIII, the *vestibulocochlear nerve*, transmits impulses related to both equilibrium and hearing. The twelve cranial nerves are discussed fully in Chapter 18.

The *internal carotid artery* supplies blood to the orbits and most of the cerebrum. Branches of the *external carotid artery* supply most of the remaining tissues of the head. One of these branches, the superficial temporal artery, supplies most of the face. It describes a path anterior to the ear over the temporal bone and onto the forehead. Most blood from the head and neck drains through the *external* and *internal jugular veins* and the *vertebral veins*.

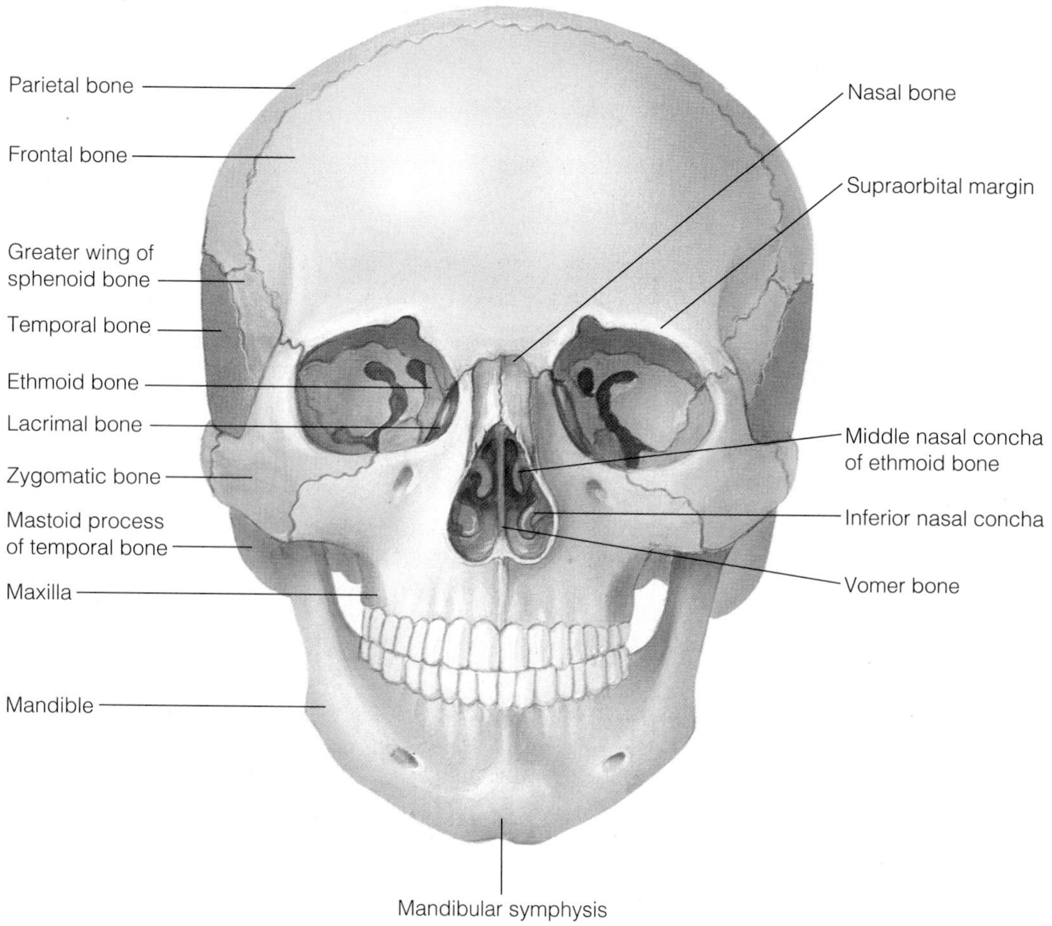

Figure 9.2 Bones of the skull.

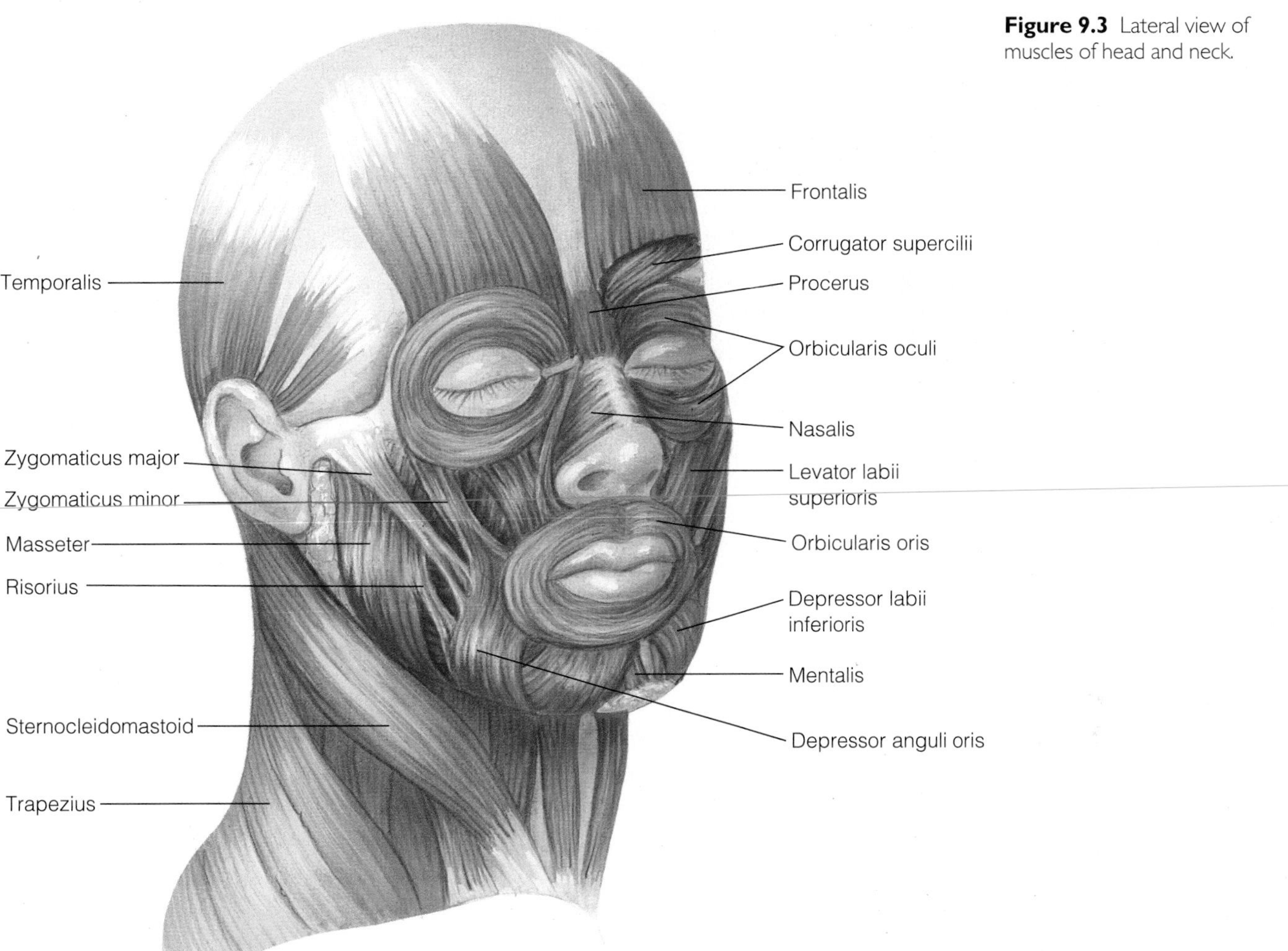

Figure 9.3 Lateral view of muscles of head and neck.

Eyes

The **eye** is a fluid-filled sphere that receives light waves and transmits them to the brain for interpretation as visual images. Figure 9.4 on page 164 shows the external structures of the eye. The **conjunctiva** is a thin mucous membrane that lines the interior of the eyelids and continues over the anterior portion of the eye. The outermost layer of the eye is composed of a tough white protective covering, called the **sclera**, and a transparent window over the center of the eye, called the **cornea** (Figure 9.5 on page 164). Light is transmitted through the cornea to the lens and then onto the retina.

The **iris** is a circular muscular membrane that controls the amount of light reaching the retina by dilating and constricting its opening, called the **pupil**. Light travels through the pupil to the **lens**, a transparent structure located behind the pupil that keeps images from varied distances in continual focus on the retina.

The lens divides the eye into the anterior and posterior segments. The anterior segment consists of the anterior chamber, the posterior chamber, and the aqueous humor. The aqueous humor is similar to the plasma of the blood. It is continuously formed, circulated in the segment, and drains through the canal of Schlemm. This helps maintain a constant normal pressure within the eye.

The posterior segment contains the vitreous humor, a gel-like clear substance that helps with the transmission of light rays and maintains the sphere shape of the eye with its constant intraocular pressure.

The **retina** is the innermost layer of the eye, on which light waves are transformed into nerve impulses that are transmitted through the optic nerve to the brain. Vision occurs by the refraction of light through the cornea and lens onto the retina. As light waves hit the retina, they generate neural impulses that are transmitted along the optic nerve and the *optic tract* to the *visual cortex* in the occipital lobe of the brain, where they are interpreted as images (Figure 9.6 on page 165). Notice that the medial, or nasal, fibers of each retina cross each other at the *optic chiasma*; thus, each optic tract contains fibers from both eyes: the left optic tract contains fibers from the left side of each retina, and the right optic tract contains fibers from the right side of each retina. The binocular vision

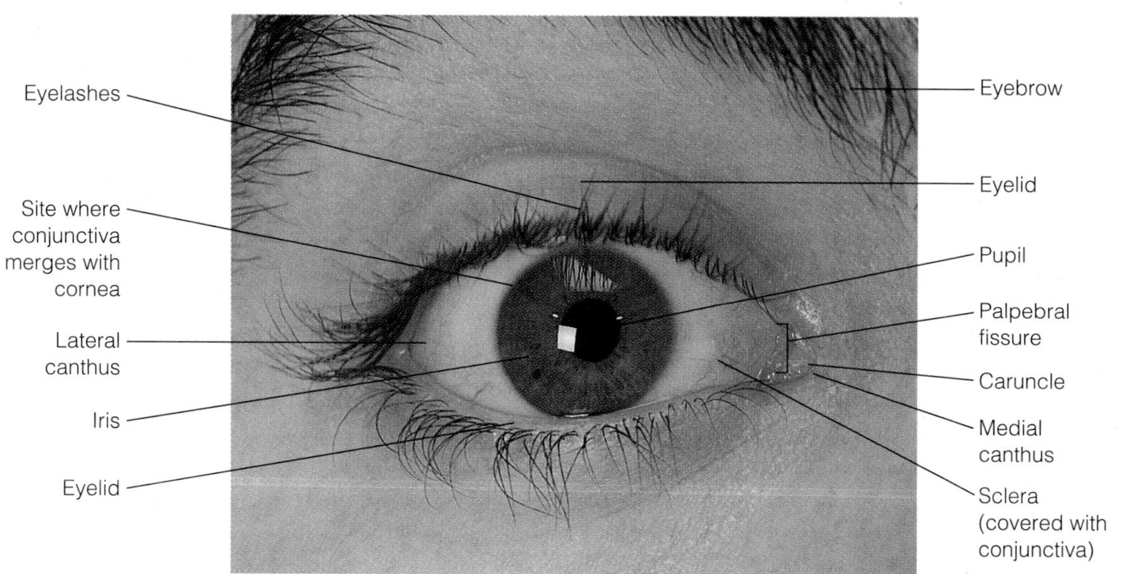

Figure 9.4 Structures of the external eye.

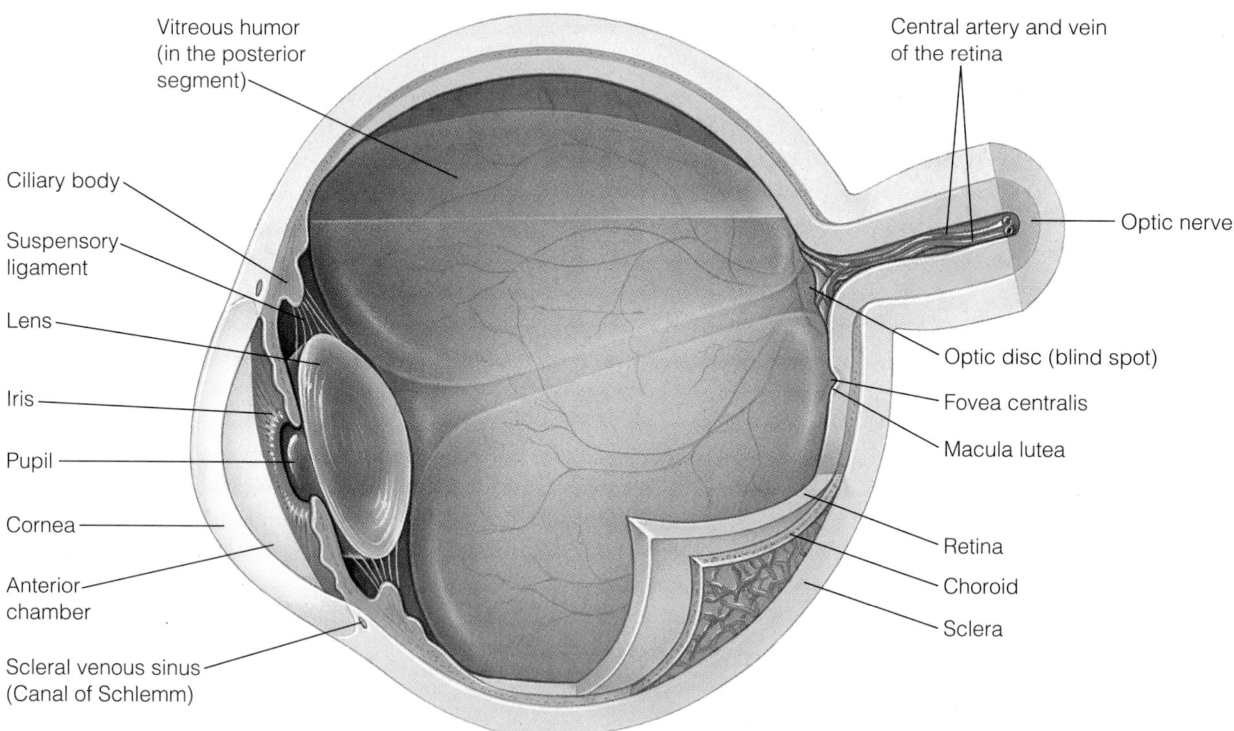

Figure 9.5 Interior of the eye.

of the human eyes is due also to the coordinated movements of six muscles: superior rectus, inferior rectus, medial rectus, lateral rectus, and the superior and inferior oblique muscles (Figure 9.7).

The **lacrimal glands**, located above and laterally to both eyes, secrete tears that keep the conjunctiva and cornea moist (Figure 9.8 on page 166). The tears also clean the eye with secretions that contain lysozyme, an antibacterial enzyme. The lacrimal ducts located in the inner canthus drain the tears into the nose.

The eyebrows, eyelids (or palpebrae), and eyelashes all serve as protectors for the eye. The opening between the upper and lower eyelid is called the palpebral fissure. The lids

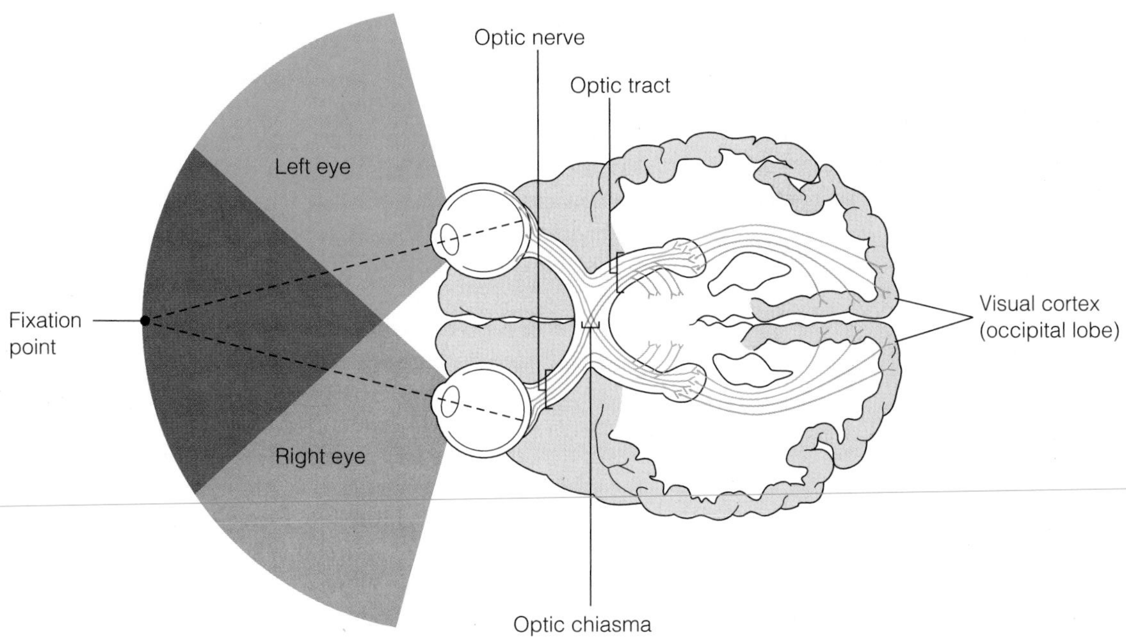

Figure 9.6 Visual fields of the eye and the visual pathway to the brain.

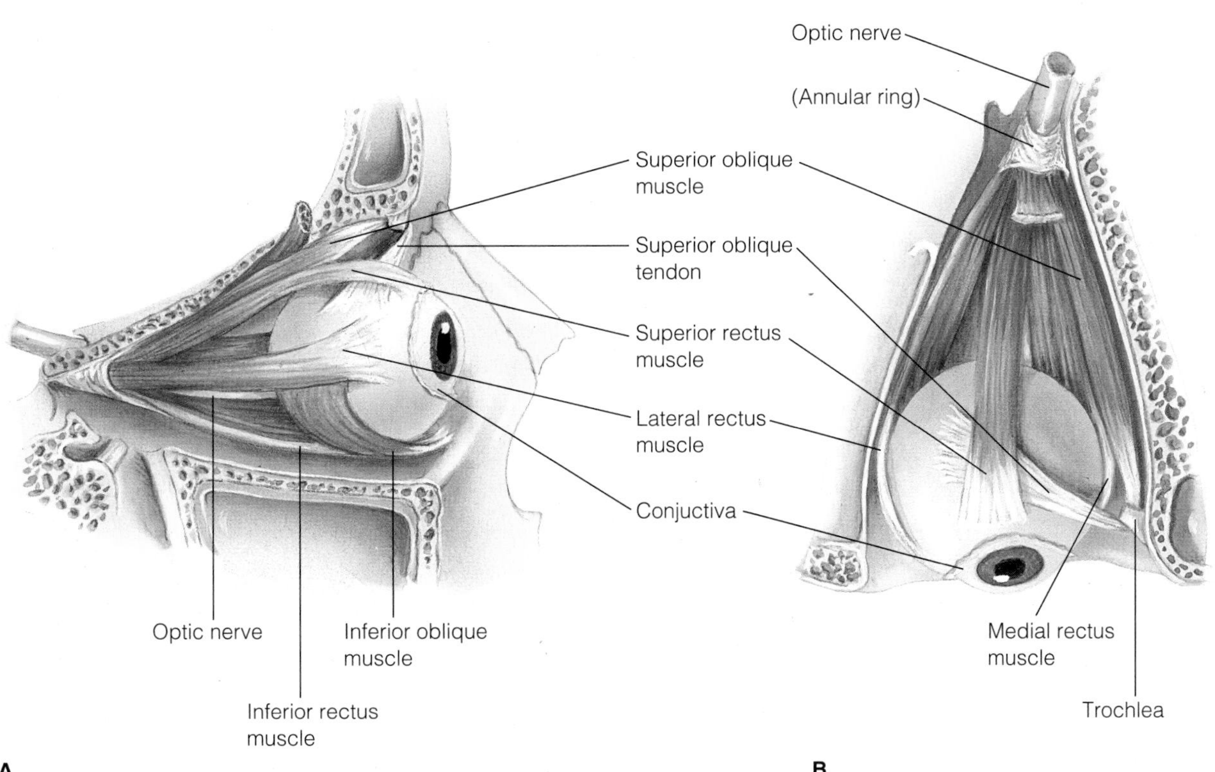

Figure 9.7 Extraocular muscles. *A*, Lateral view of the right eye. *B*, Superior view of right eye.

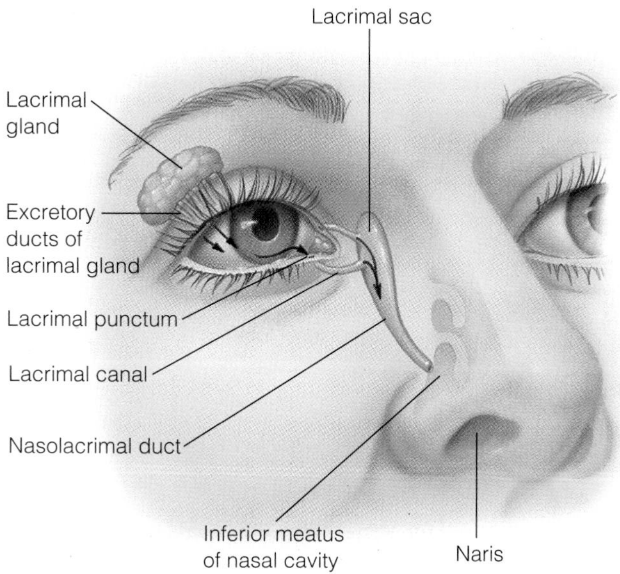

Figure 9.8 Lacrimal glands of the eye.

meet laterally and medially to form the lateral canthus and medial canthus.

The meibomian glands embedded in the lids are modified sebaceous glands that produce an oily substance to help lubricate the eyes and the eyelids.

The major functions of the eyes are

- Collecting and transmitting light waves to the brain
- Producing tears

Ears

The **ear** is the sensory organ that functions in hearing and equilibrium. It is divided into the external, middle, and inner ear. The external portion, or what most people think of as the ear, is called the **auricle**, or *pinna*. It is a shell of cartilage that funnels sound into the opening of the external auditory canal.

Figure 9.9 shows the surface anatomy of the external ear. An imaginary line from the top of the ear (the *helix*) extends horizontally across the lateral canthus of each eye to the helix of the other ear. The **external auditory canal** is about 1 inch long and lined with glands that secrete a yellow-brown wax called *cerumen*. These secretions lubricate and protect the ear. The *tragus* is a stiff projection that protects the anterior opening of the canal. The *lobule* of the ear is a small flap of flesh at the inferior end of the auricle.

The external ear and middle ear are separated by the **tympanic membrane** or *eardrum* (Figure 9.10). This thin, translucent membrane is pearly gray in color and lies obliquely in the canal. Sound waves entering the auditory canal strike the membrane, causing it to vibrate. The membrane transfers the vibrations to the tiny bones, or **ossicles**, of the middle ear: the *malleus*, the *incus*, and the *stapes*. The ossicles in turn transfer the sound vibrations to the *oval window*, through which they enter the inner ear. Note that the malleus projects inferiorly and laterally and can be seen through the translucent tympanic membrane when viewed with an otoscope. The **auditory** (*eustachian*) **tube** connects the middle ear with the nasopharynx and helps to equalize air pressure on both sides of the tympanic membrane.

The middle ear functions to conduct sound vibration from the external ear to the inner ear. It also protects the inner ear by reducing loud sound vibrations.

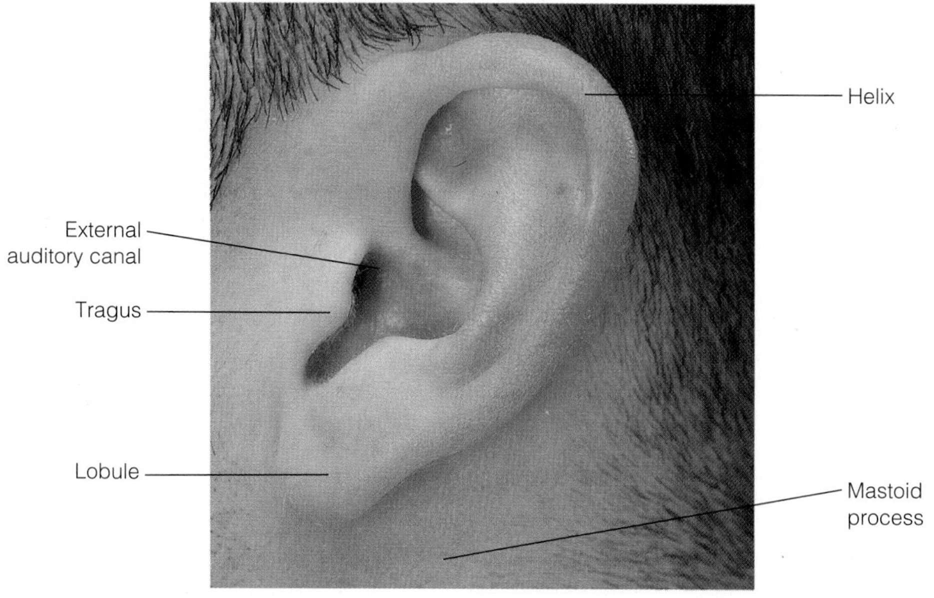

Figure 9.9 Structures of the external ear.

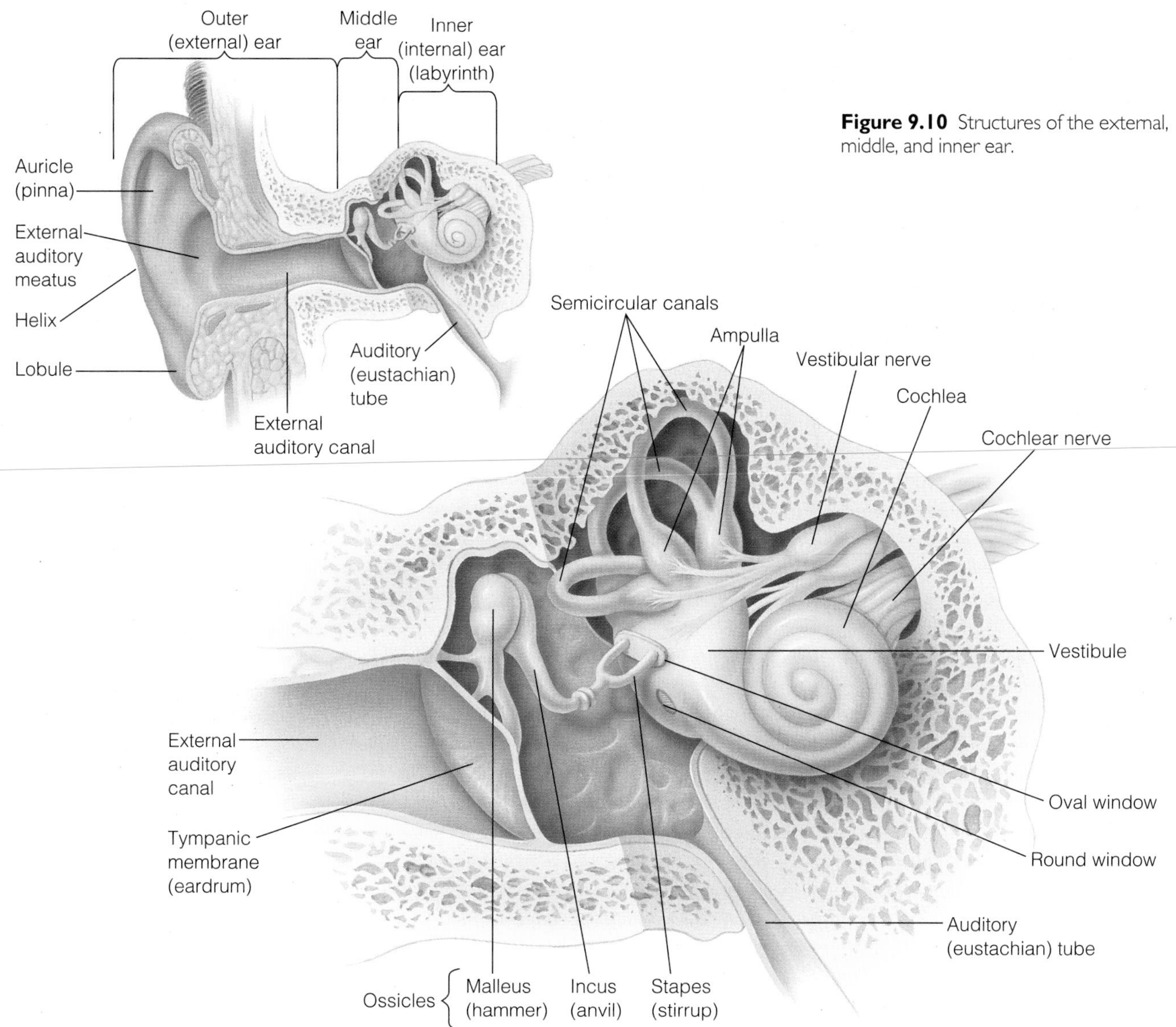

Figure 9.10 Structures of the external, middle, and inner ear.

The inner ear contains the **bony labyrinth,** which consists of a central cavity called the *vestibule*, three *semicircular canals* responsible for our sense of equilibrium, and the *cochlea*, a spiraling chamber that contains the receptors for hearing. The cochlea transmits sound vibrations to the auditory nerve, which in turn carries the impulses to the auditory cortex in the temporal lobe of the brain.

The major functions of the ears are

- Collecting and transporting sound vibrations to the brain
- Maintaining the sense of equilibrium

Nose and Sinuses

The **nose** is a projection of bone and cartilage situated in the midline of the face. It is the only externally visible organ of the respiratory system. During inspiration, air enters the nasal cavity through the *external nares*, or nostrils. The external and internal nares are divided into right and left sides by a *nasal septum*. Three *conchae* (or *turbinates*) project from the medial wall into each side of the nasal cavity, adding surface area for cleaning, moistening, and warming air entering the respiratory tract (Figure 9.11 on page 168). Each side of the posterior nasal cavity opens into the nasopharynx.

The **paranasal sinuses** are mucus-lined, air-filled cavities that surround the nasal cavity and perform the same air-processing functions (Figure 9.12 on page 168). They are named for the bones of the skull in which they are contained: sphenoid, frontal, ethmoid, and maxillary. The **mastoid sinus** lies in the temporal bone just behind the ear. It is easily located by the bony mastoid process.

The major functions of the nose and sinuses are

- Providing an airway for respiration
- Filtering, warming, and humidifying air flowing into the lungs
- Providing resonance for the voice
- Housing the receptors for olfaction

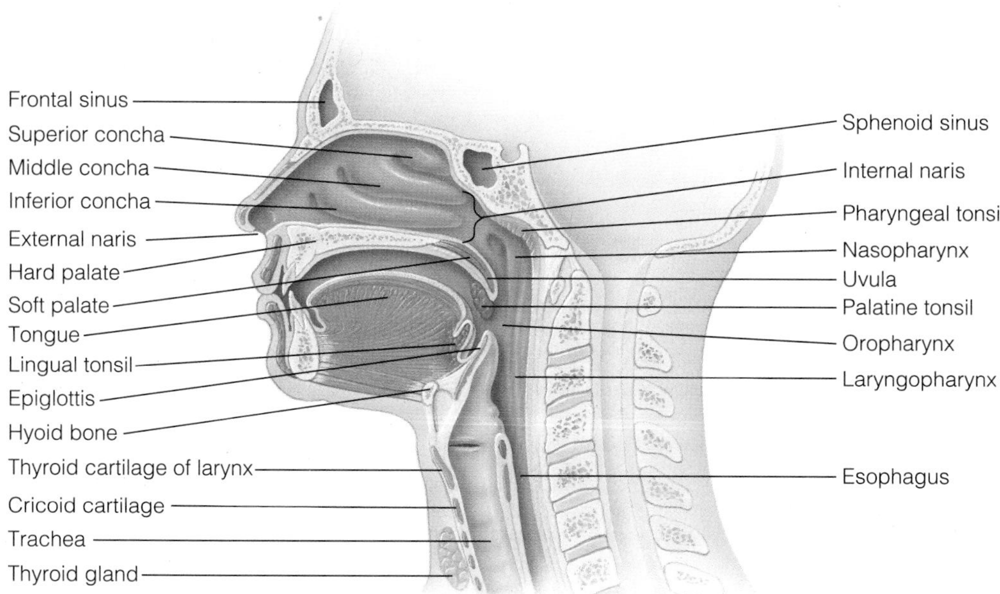

Figure 9.11 Structures of the upper respiratory system.

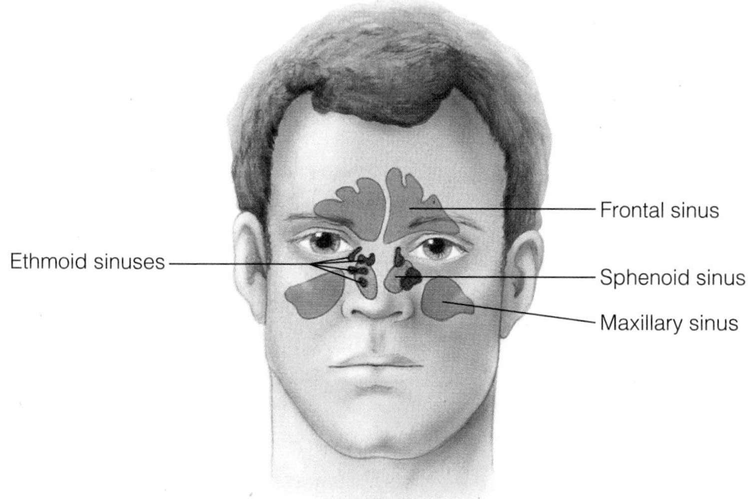

Figure 9.12 The paranasal sinuses, anterior view.

Mouth and Throat

The **oral cavity** is formed by the lips, the inside of both cheeks, the *palate*, or roof of the mouth, the mandible, and the maxilla (Figure 9.13). The **mouth** contains the teeth (32 in the adult), the tongue, the gums, openings for the salivary glands (parotid, submandibular, and sublingual) and the *uvula*, a projection of tissue suspended from the posterior margins of the soft palate.

The parotid gland is located anterior to the ear. Stensen's duct carries the saliva from the gland to the buccal mucosa. The ducts of the submandibular glands, called Wharton's ducts, open into the floor of the mouth near the midline close to the lingual frenulum. The sublingual glands have very short ducts that open directly into the floor of the mouth under the tongue. The tongue, a muscular organ, helps with speech, tastes, chewing and swallowing. The tongue is secured to the floor of the mouth by the frenulum.

The **tonsils** are large collections of lymphatic tissue named for their locations. The palatine tonsils are located in the bilateral posterior end of the oral cavity. The lingual tonsils lie at

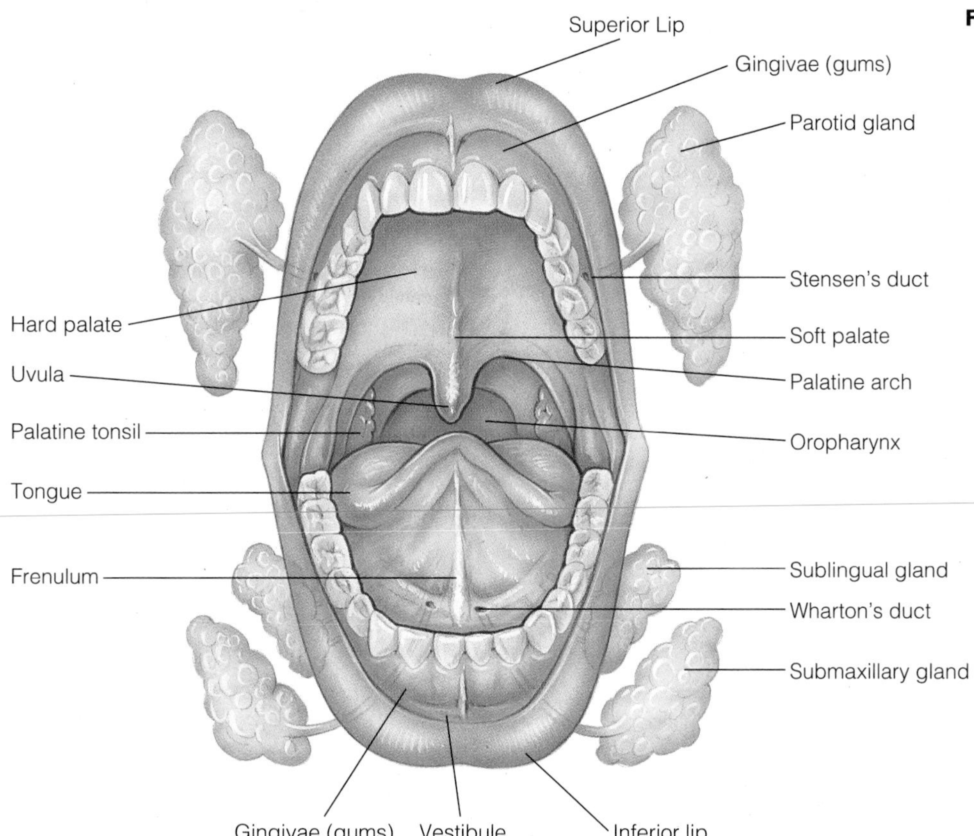

Figure 9.13 The oral cavity.

the bilateral base of the tongue. The pharyngeal tonsils (adenoids) lie in the posterior nasopharynx.

The anterior oral cavity is the entrance to the digestive tract, and the posterior oral cavity contains both the oral and nasal pharynx leading to the openings of the esophagus and trachea. Note that the soft palate rises to close off the nasopharynx when we swallow.

The muscles of mastication (chewing) are controlled by the trigeminal nerve (V). The tongue is innervated by the hypoglossal nerve (XII). The sensory receptors for taste are the glossopharyngeal nerve (IX) and the facial nerve (VII). Cranial nerves are discussed further in Chapter 18.

The major functions of the mouth and throat are

- Tasting, chewing, and beginning to digest food
- Providing the sense of taste
- Aiding in speech production

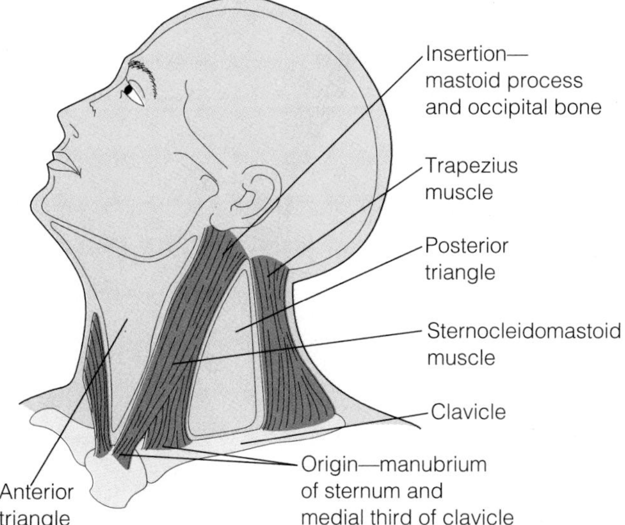

Figure 9.14 Triangles of the neck.

Neck

The two major muscles that provide support of the **neck** and make it mobile are the *sternocleidomastoid* and the *trapezius* muscles. These muscles divide the neck into two triangles: the anterior triangle and the posterior triangle (Figure 9.14). The anterior triangle is bordered by the mandible, the sternocleidomastoid muscle, and the trachea. The posterior triangle is

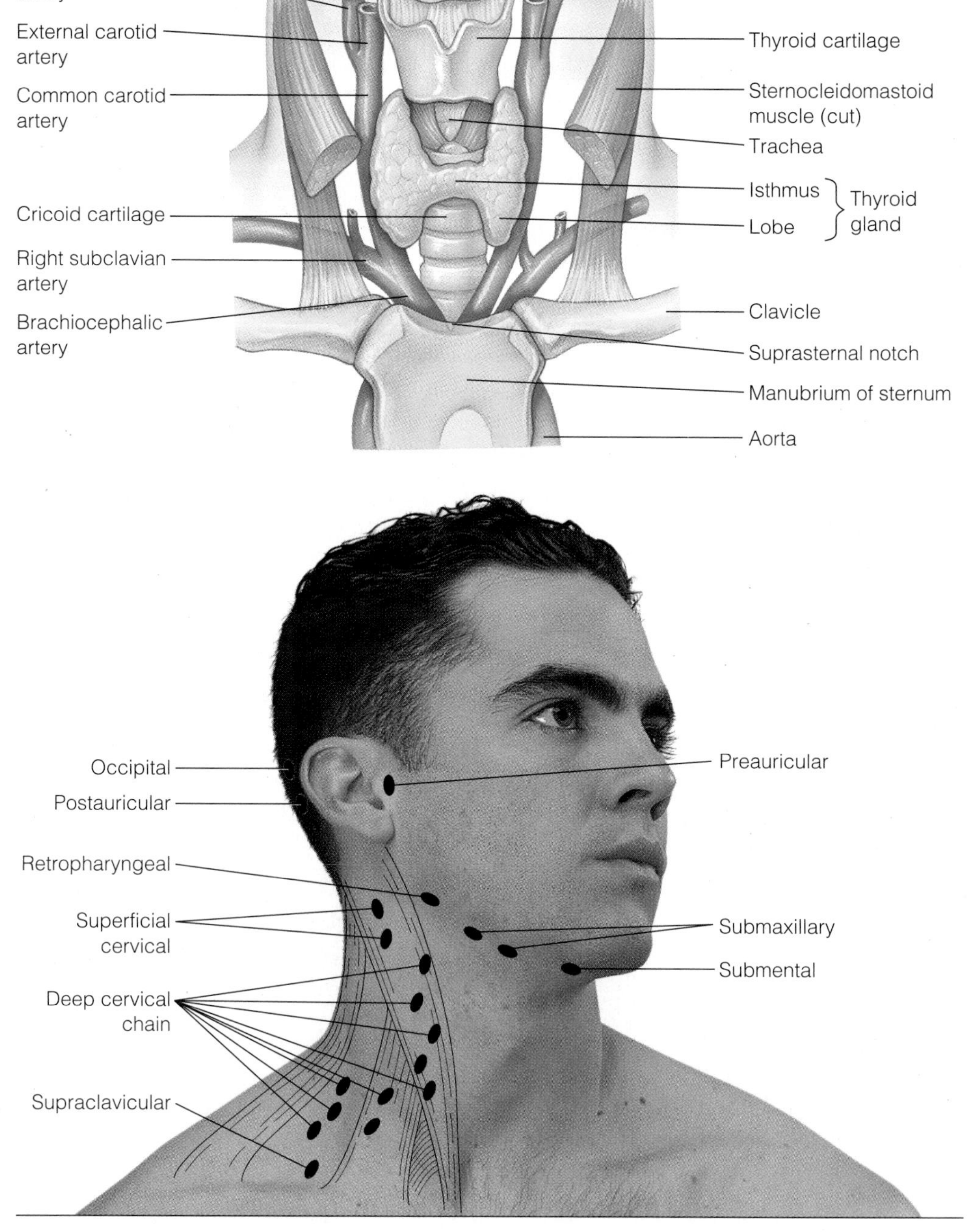

Figure 9.15 Location of the thyroid gland.

Figure 9.16 Cervical lymph nodes.

bordered by the sternocleidomastoid muscle, the trapezius muscle, and the clavicle.

The hyoid bone, located in the neck, is the only bone in the body that does not articulate directly with another bone. It is suspended in the neck, superior to the larynx. It serves as a movable base for the tongue and as an attachment for the muscles of the neck. It serves as a landmark when assessing the trachea.

The **thyroid gland** is found in the middle of the neck anterior to the trachea (Figure 9.15). It is shaped like a butterfly with two lobes lying on either side of the trachea and a body, called the *isthmus*, lying directly over the trachea. The thyroid produces thyroxine (T_4) and triiodothyronine (T_3), hormones, which influence cellular metabolism.

The greatest number of **lymph nodes** are in the head and neck. As described in Chapter 16, lymph nodes provide defense against invasion of foreign substances by producing antibodies and lymphocytes. The nodes are clustered along lymphatic vessels that infiltrate tissue capillaries and pick up excess fluid called *lymph.* The nurse palpates the neck looking for lymph nodes. Normally, the nodes are nonpalpable. Occasionally, you find one node. Nodes are palpable when infected or enlarged. This assessment may be significant in recognizing signs of early infection. Cervical lymph nodes are located in the following areas (Figure 9.16):

- Preauricular: in front of the ear
- Occipital: at the base of the skull
- Postauricular: behind the ear, over the outer surface of the mastoid bone
- Submental: behind the tip of the mandible at the midline
- Submaxillary: on the medial border of the mandible
- Retropharyngeal: at the junction of the posterior and lateral walls of the pharynx at the angle of the jaw
- Superficial cervical: anterior to and over the sternocleidomastoid muscle
- Deep cervical: posterior to and under the sternocleidomastoid muscle
- Supraclavicular: above the clavicle

Gathering the Data

As with all other systems, you review the database completed during the client's initial interview to identify what additional information you need before you assess the head and neck. Any diagnostic test results that are available should be reviewed. Tests may include imaging studies (X-ray films, CT scans, MRI studies), hearing and sight tests, and blood studies.

Focused Interview

The focused interview is as important as the physical assessment. It provides a wealth of information that leads to nursing diagnoses addressing health promotion, illness prevention, client teaching (eg, teaching correct administration of medication and teaching self-care for chronic, acute, and potential problems). If the client presents with a problem of the head or neck, or if there is a family history of a problem in this area, a more thorough history of each complaint must be obtained. In data collection, questions related to the respiratory, gastrointestinal, neurological, and musculoskeletal systems are important. For a description of the full health history, see Chapter 2.

Questions Related to the Head

1. Tell me why you are here today. Please describe how you are feeling generally, and tell me about any health problems you have and any treatments you are receiving.
2. Do you have headaches? If so, please tell me about
   a. Frequency: How often?
   b. Onset: How long have you been bothered with this type of headache? When does the headache begin?
   c. Duration: How long does a typical headache last?
   d. Location: Where is the pain? On one side of the head, behind the eyes, in the sinus area?
   e. Character: Is the pain throbbing, steady, dull, sharp? On a scale of 1 to 10 with 10 being the strongest, how severe is the pain?
   f. Associated symptoms: Do you experience any nausea, vomiting, sensitivity to light or noise, muscle pain, or other symptoms along with the headache?
   g. Precipitating factors: Do you feel that the headaches usually are triggered by stress, alcohol intake, anxiety, menstrual cycle, allergies, or any other factors? Please describe.
   h. Treatment: What seems to relieve the symptoms? Resting? Medication? Exercise?

   A detailed description of the headache is necessary to help determine the cause, type, and possible treatments.
3. Have you recently had an infection or cold? *These conditions may be accompanied by headaches.*
4. Have you had any dizziness, loss of consciousness, seizures, or blurred vision? When did each symptom occur? How long did the symptom last? What did you do to relieve the symptom? *These symptoms may indicate problems with carotid arteries, cerebral clots or bleeding, recent head injury, or neurologic disease.*
5. Have you noticed any swelling, lumps, bumps, or skin sores on your head that did not heal? *Swellings, masses, and lesions that don't heal may indicate cancer.*
6. Describe any recent injury you have had to your head.
   a. How did it occur?
   b. Did you lose consciousness? How long were you unconscious?

c. Did you have any symptoms afterwards? Describe them.

d. How and where were you treated for this injury?

Questions Related to the Eyes

1. Describe your vision. Please describe any changes in your vision in the past few months. Have you experienced any loss of vision? What measures have you taken to compensate for the loss, for instance, corrective lenses, large-print books, uncluttered living environment. Have the changes in your vision affected your ability to drive or perform other activities of daily living?
2. What was the date of your last eye examination? What were the results of that examination?
3. Do you wear glasses or contact lenses? How would you describe your vision with them? Without them? How do you clean your contact lenses? How long do you wear them?
4. Have you ever experienced any blurred vision, double vision, sensitivity to light, burning, or itching? *Blurred vision can be an indication of a neurologic problem or a need for corrective lenses. Double vision can be caused by muscle or nerve complications. Burning and itching can be caused by a decrease in the production of tears or allergies.*
5. Do you ever see small black spots that seem to move when you are looking at something? *These spots, called floaters, are common after middle age and are considered normal unless they obstruct vision.*
6. Do you ever see halos around lights? *Seeing halos around lights usually indicates glaucoma, a disorder marked by increased intraocular pressure.*
7. Have you had any eye pain? Please describe. *Eye pain can be superficial, affecting the outer eye only, or deep and throbbing, possibly associated with glaucoma. Any sudden onset of eye pain should be referred immediately to a physician.*
8. Have you ever had any eye injury or eye surgery? If so, describe it. *An eye injury or surgery can cause a distortion when the eye is examined by ophthalmoscope.*
9. Have you or any family member had diabetes, hypertension, or glaucoma? *All of these diseases can be hereditary and can cause visual difficulties. Hypertension can cause arteriosclerosis of the retina, a condition resulting in thickening of the walls and loss of elasticity of the arteries of the retina. Diabetes can cause bleeding in the capillaries of the retina, eventually affecting vision.*
10. Do you have trouble seeing or driving at night? *Night blindness can be caused by glaucoma, vitamin A deficiency, or miotic drugs, which keep the pupil constricted.*
11. What medications are you taking? Are they specific for the eye? *Some medications have side effects on the eye. Cortisone can increase intraocular pressure. Sulfa compounds, digitalis, barbiturates, and other drugs can cause color distortion.*
12. What kind of activities do you perform at work? What are your hobbies? *Prolonged work under bright lights or at a computer terminal may cause eye strain. Use of equipment such as weed eaters or welding tools without safety glasses can cause eye injury. Persons who spend a great deal of time in the sun without sunglasses are at risk for cataracts, opacities of the lens of the eyes.*
13. Have you been exposed to inhalants such as dust or pollen, chemical fumes, or flying debris that caused eye irritation? Describe.
14. How do you clean and care for your eye area? If you wear eye makeup, how do you remove it? *Certain eye makeup, skin care products, or cleansers may irritate the eye.*

Questions Related to the Ears

1. Describe your hearing. Have you noticed any change in your hearing? If so, tell me about:
   a. Onset: Gradual or sudden?
   b. Character: Just certain sounds or tones, or all hearing?
   c. Situations: When using a telephone? Watching television? During conversations?

   The client's failure to respond to questions, or asking you to repeat questions, may indicate a hearing loss. Hearing acuity decreases gradually with age. Any sudden loss of hearing should be investigated.
2. When was your last hearing test? What were the results? Does your hearing seem better in one ear than the other? Which ear? *Hearing tests should be conducted annually for children, older adults, and middle adults who live or work in noisy environments. Hearing loss in one ear could indicate an obstruction with earwax or a ruptured tympanic membrane.*
3. Has any member of your family had ear problems or hearing loss? *Hearing loss can be hereditary.*
4. Do you either own or use a hearing aid? *Some clients have hearing aids but will not use them because of increased background noise or embarrassment, or because they can't pay for the batteries for the hearing aid.*
5. Are you frequently exposed to loud noise? When? How often? For how long? Are protective devices available, and do you use them? *Long-term exposure to loud noise can result in hearing loss. At risk are clients with jobs in noisy factories; jobs at airports; jobs requiring the use of explosives, firearms, jackhammers, or other loud equipment; and jobs in nightclubs. Frequent exposure to loud music, either live or on stereos or headsets, can also contribute to hearing loss.*
6. Do you have any pain in your ears? Describe it. If so, have you recently had a cold or sore throat? Have you had any

problems lately with your sinuses or your teeth? Have you had any ear trauma or surgery? *Pain in one or both ears may be caused by a cold, ear or sinus infection, trauma, dental problems, or wax blockage.*

7. Have you had any ear drainage? Describe it. *Ear drainage may indicate an infection. Bloody or purulent drainage could indicate otitis media, infection of the middle ear. Serous drainage could indicate allergic reaction. Clear drainage could be cerebral spinal fluid following trauma.*
8. Have you had dizziness, nausea, vomiting, or ringing in your ears? *These symptoms could indicate a problem with the inner ear or a neurologic problem.*
9. Do you experience ear infections or irritations after swimming or being exposed to dust or smoke? If so, describe them. *Contaminated water left in the ear may cause otitis externa, or "swimmer's ear." Irritation of the ear after exposure to certain substances may indicate an allergy to such substances.*
10. Are you taking any medications? What are they? How often? *Certain medicines affect the ears. Aspirin can cause ringing in the ears (tinnitus). Some antibiotics can cause hearing loss and dizziness.*
11. How do you clean your ears? *Many people use cotton-tipped applicators to remove earwax. This practice can cause trauma to the eardrum and cause wax to become impacted.*

Questions Related to the Nose and Sinuses

1. Are you having any problems with your nose or sinuses? If so, describe them. Are you able to breathe through your nose? Can you breathe through both nostrils? Is one side obstructed? Describe any problems you have had breathing in the last few days. In the last few weeks. *A history of frequent respiratory problems may indicate an underlying respiratory problem such as allergies or recurring infections.*
2. Do you have nasal discharge? If so, is it continuous or occasional? Describe it. *A thin, watery discharge is the result of acute rhinitis from either a viral infection, such as the common cold, or an allergic reaction. Allergies that cause nasal discharge can also produce postnasal drip, sore throats, ear infections, or headaches. Some allergies are seasonal, others are constant.*
3. Do you have nosebleeds? How often? What is your usual blood pressure? Do you use nasal sprays? How do you treat your nosebleeds? *Nosebleeds can occur as a result of high blood pressure, overuse of nasal sprays, and certain blood disorders.*
4. Have you ever had any nose injury or nose surgery? Describe. How was the injury treated? Do you have any residual problems from the injury or surgery?
5. Describe your sense of smell. Are there any circumstances, objects, places, or activities that affect your sense of smell? If so, describe them. *Anosmia, the inability to smell, may be neurological, hereditary, or it may be due to a deficiency of zinc in the diet.*
6. What prescribed or over-the-counter drugs do you take to relieve your nasal symptoms? Do you use a nasal inhalant, oxygen, or humidifier to help you breathe? What other medications do you take regularly? *Certain medications can produce unpleasant side effects in the nose such as nasal stuffiness or nosebleeds. Many drugs administered by nasal inhalers may irritate the nasal mucosa and cause nosebleeds. Steroid inhalers can cause growth of* Candida *in the nose, mouth, or throat.*
7. Do you use recreational drugs? If so, what drugs? How often? *Some inhaled drugs, such as cocaine, gradually break down the nasal lining by vasoconstriction. A very pale color of the nasal septum, or holes in the septum, may indicate drug sniffing.*

Questions Related to the Mouth and Throat

1. How would you describe the condition of your mouth and teeth? Have you noticed any changes in the last few months?
2. Do you have any problems swallowing? *Dysphagia, or difficult swallowing, may be due to a neurologic or gastrointestinal problem, or it might be related to ill-fitting dentures or malocclusion. Achalasia, a chronic difficulty in swallowing caused by constriction of the esophagus, may be related to anxiety or stress. Finally, painful or difficult swallowing could be related to cancer of the throat or esophagus.*
3. Do you have any sores or lesions in your mouth or on your tongue? If so, describe them. Are they present constantly or do they come and go periodically? *Lesions of the mouth or tongue may be cold sores or mouth ulcers. They may also accompany viral infections and gum infections. Some lesions may be caused by ill-fitting dentures. Finally, any lesion of the mouth that does not heal should be evaluated for oral cancer.*
4. Do your gums bleed frequently? *Gum diseases such as gingivitis and periodontitis may cause gums to bleed easily. Gums may also bleed easily with ill-fitting braces or dentures.*
5. Have you noticed a change in your sense of taste recently? *Loss of the sense of taste commonly accompanies colds. A foul taste in the mouth may signal a gum infection or inadequate care of teeth or dentures.*
6. What dental problems, surgeries, or procedures have you had in the past? Describe them.

7. Do you wear dentures, partial plates, retainers, or any other removable or permanent appliance? Does it fit well? Is it comfortable? Why are you wearing the appliance? Does it help resolve the problem? Are any of your teeth capped? Which ones?
8. How often do you brush your teeth or dentures? Do you use floss regularly? *Regular mouth care is important in maintaining healthy teeth and gums and preventing gum diseases such as gingivitis and periodontitis.*
9. When was your last dental examination? Are you unable to eat some foods because of problems with your teeth? Do you have any pain in one or more teeth?
10. Do you have frequent sore throats? *A sore throat may be the result of irritation from sinus drainage, viral or bacterial infection, or the first sign of throat cancer.*
11. Have you noticed any hoarseness or loss of your voice? *Hoarseness is a common finding in disorders of the throat. Recurrent or persistent hoarseness may indicate cancer of the larynx. Hoarseness may also be due to anxiety, overuse of the voice, or a cold. Smoking and drinking alcohol can lead to inflammation of the vocal cords and result in hoarseness.*
12. Do you or did you ever smoke a pipe, cigarettes, or cigars? Chew tobacco or dip snuff? How much? How often? *Smoking, dipping snuff, or chewing tobacco may result in cancer of the lips, mouth, and throat.*

Questions Related to the Neck

1. Have you noticed any lumps or swellings on your neck? *Lateral neck masses are usually due to enlargement of the cervical lymph nodes, indicative of infection.*
2. Has your neck been weak, sore, or stiff? *Neck symptoms may indicate problems with the muscles of the neck or the cervical spinal cord, or an infectious problem such as meningitis.*
3. Have you ever had any problem with your thyroid gland? Have you had thyroid surgery? Are you taking thyroid medication? *Over- or undersecretion by the thyroid gland may cause rapid weight gain or loss, erratic temperature regulation, fatigue, dyspnea (painful breathing), mood swings, and other alterations in health.*

Additional Questions with Infants, Children, and Adolescents

1. Did you use alcohol or recreational drugs during your pregnancy? *Fetal alcohol syndrome causes some deformities of the face. Use of cocaine during pregnancy can result in neurologic problems in the infant.*
2. Did you have any vaginal infections at the time of delivery? *Vaginal infections in the mother can cause eye infections in the newborn.*
3. Was the infant full-term or preterm? *If the infant was born preterm, resuscitation and oxygen may have been required, which can cause damage to the eyes.*
4. Have you noticed any depression or bulging over the infant's "soft spots" (fontanels)? *A depressed fontanel can indicate dehydration, and a bulging fontanel can indicate an infection.*
5. Does your infant look directly at you? Have you noticed anything unusual about the infant's eyes? *The infant may have crossed eyes or eyes that move in different directions, possibly because of weakness of the muscles of the eye.*
6. Does your school-age child like to sit at the front of the classroom? *Poor eyesight may necessitate sitting at the front of the classroom.*
7. Is your child's vision tested routinely in school? How often? What were the results of the last vision exam?
8. Does your child rub the eyes frequently? *Rubbing eyes could be a symptom of visual disturbances, infection, or allergies.*
9. Does your child have recurrent ear infections? How many in the last 6 months? How were they treated? Has the child had any ear surgery such as insertion of ear tubes? When?
10. Does the child tug at the ears? *Tugging at the ears can be an early sign of infection.*
11. Does the child respond to loud noises? *A lack of response could indicate hearing loss.*
12. If the child is over 6 months of age, does the child babble? *A child who does not babble may have a hearing impairment.*
13. Have you ever had the child's hearing tested? What were the results?
14. Has your child had measles, mumps, or any disease with a high fever? Has your child been treated recently with any antibiotics such as streptomycin or neomycin? *High fevers and certain drugs can cause temporary hearing loss.*
15. How do you clean the child's ears? *Ascertain whether the procedure is harmful, such as cleaning ears with cotton swabs, which may cause impacted cerumen.*
16. Does your child put objects into the nose? *Foreign objects can cause trauma to nasal tissues.*
17. Does the child frequently have drainage from the nose? *Frequent drainage can indicate an infection or allergies.*
18. Does your child suck the thumb or a pacifier? *These behaviors can interfere with alignment of secondary teeth.*
19. When did the child's teeth begin to erupt? *Late eruption of teeth could indicate delayed development.*

20. Does your child go to bed with a bottle at night? What is in the bottle? *Frequent use of a bottle with milk or juice at night can cause decay of teeth.*
21. Does the child know how to brush the teeth? Does the child brush daily?
22. How often does the child go to the dentist? *Children should begin annual visits to the dentist between the ages of 3 and 4 years.*
23. Is the child's drinking water fluoridated? *Fluoride in the water supply helps prevent tooth decay.*
24. Have you noticed any swelling on the child's neck or below the angle of the jaw? *Swelling may be due to enlarged lymph nodes, indicating an infection.*
25. Was there any difficulty with the birth of the child? Were forceps used? *Trauma to the sternocleidomastoid muscle during birth may cause torticollis, or wryneck.*

Additional Questions with Childbearing Clients

1. Do you have frequent headaches? *Headaches are common during the first trimester, but it is important to rule out other possible complications of pregnancy.*
2. Have you had any changes in your eyesight during your pregnancy? *Any changes such as blurred vision, color distortion, or spots in front of the eyes should be referred to a physician or ophthalmologist.*
3. Have you had nosebleeds during your pregnancy? How often? *Nosebleeds and nasal congestion are common during pregnancy because of increased vascularity in the nasal passages.*

Additional Questions with Older Adults

1. Do you ever experience dryness or a burning sensation in your eyes? *Dryness is usually due to decreased tear production, which occurs with aging.*
2. Do you have any problems seeing at night? *Night blindness may be an indication of cataracts.*
3. Do bright glaring lights bother you? *With age, the lens of the eye begins to thicken, and accommodation to light is not as rapid.*
4. Are you tested routinely for glaucoma? What was the date of your last examination?
5. Do you wear a hearing aid? If so, is it effective? How often do you wear your hearing aid? *Many elderly persons have a hearing loss but cannot adjust to using a hearing aid, or cannot afford batteries for the hearing aid.*
6. Do you have any difficulty operating the hearing aid? How do you clean the hearing aid? *Some clients forget to clean the tubes of the hearing aid periodically.*
7. Are you able to chew all types of food? *If teeth are missing or dentures fit improperly, the client may not be able to chew meat or certain vegetables, resulting in undernutrition.*
8. Do you experience dryness in your mouth? *Certain medications may cause dryness, which may interfere with the client's appetite or digestion.*
9. Do you wear dentures? Do they fit properly? *Ill-fitting dentures can interfere with proper nutrition and can cause various problems in the mouth, such as lesions and bleeding gums.*

Physical Assessment

Preparation

☑ **Gather the equipment:**

examination gown	cotton-tipped applicator
examination gloves	opthalmoscope
Snellen eye chart or Tumble E Chart	otoscope
Jaeger card	tuning fork
cover card	nasal speculum
penlight	gauze square
sterile cotton balls	tongue depressor

☑ **Wash your hands.**

☑ **Ask the client to remove any items that would interfere with the physical assessment, including hats, veils, scarves, jewelry, wigs, and hairpieces. Ask the client to put on the examination gown. Clothing from the waist down and the female client's bra may be left on.**

☑ **Adjust the room lighting, if necessary.**

Remember

- Provide a warm comfortable environment.
- Explain the procedure to the client to allay any fear or apprehension.
- Ensure the client's privacy.
- Put on gloves before examining the eyes, nose, and mouth. If you notice open skin areas or drainage on the scalp or skin surface, put on gloves before proceeding with the assessment of these areas.

ASSESSMENT TECHNIQUE/NORMAL FINDINGS	SPECIAL CONSIDERATIONS

The Head

Step 1 *Position the client.*

- Ask the client to sit comfortably on the examination table (Figure 9.17).

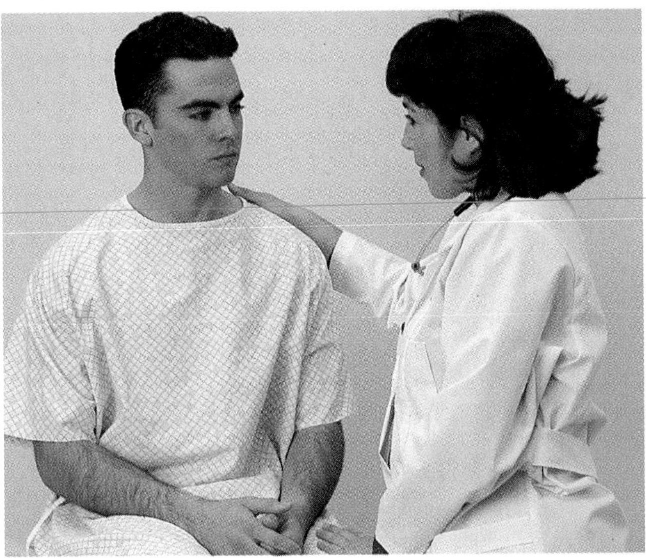

Figure 9.17 Positioning of client.

Step 2 *Inspect the head and scalp.*

- Note size, shape, symmetry, and integrity.

  Identify the prominences—frontal, parietal, and occipital—that determine the shape and symmetry of the head.
- Part the hair and look for scaliness of the scalp, lesions, or foreign bodies.
- Check hair distribution and hygiene.
- Inspect the face for symmetry and expression. The eyes, ears, nose, and mouth should be symmetrically placed.

See Table 9.2 on page 210 for some common alterations in the health of the head.

Step 3 *Observe movements of the head, face, and eyes.*

Jerky movements or tics may be the result of neurologic or psychologic disorders.

Step 4 *Palpate the head and scalp.*

- Note contour, size, and texture. Ask the client to report any tenderness as you palpate. Normally there is no tenderness with palpation.

Note any tenderness, swelling, edema or masses, which require further evaluation.

Step 5 *Confirm skin and tissue integrity.*

Note any alteration in skin or tissue integrity related to ulcerations, rashes, discolorations, or swellings.

ASSESSMENT TECHNIQUE/NORMAL FINDINGS	SPECIAL CONSIDERATIONS

ALERT!

If there is any open area or drainage, put on gloves before proceeding. Examine drainage for color, consistency, amount, and location. If indicated, obtain a specimen for laboratory analysis.

Step 6 *Palpate the temporal artery.*

- Palpate between the eye and the top of the ear (Figure 9.18).

The artery should feel smooth.

Any thickening or tenderness could indicate inflammation of the artery.

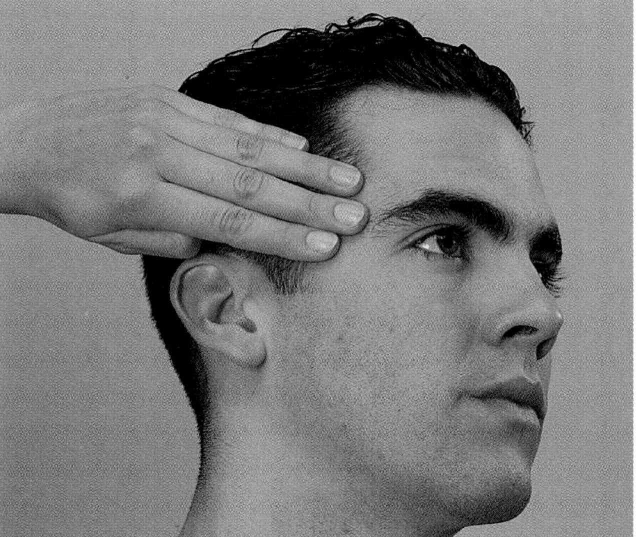

Figure 9.18 Palpating the temporal artery.

Step 7 *Auscultate the temporal artery.*

A swishing sound (bruit) may indicate a cardiac or vascular problem.

Step 8 *Test the range of motion of the temporomandibular joint.*

- Place your fingers in front of each ear and ask client to open and close the mouth slowly. There should be no limitation of movement or tenderness. You should feel a slight indentation of the joint. (For more detail on assessment of the temporomandibular joint, see Chapter 17.)

Any limitation of movement or tenderness upon movement requires further evaluation.

The Eyes

Step 1 *Test distant vision.*

Clients who wear corrective lenses for distance should be tested first with glasses/contacts, and then without glasses/contacts.

Inability to see objects at a distance is called **myopia**. The smaller the fraction, the worse the myopia. Vision of 20/200 is considered legal blindness.

ASSESSMENT TECHNIQUE/NORMAL FINDINGS

SPECIAL CONSIDERATIONS

- Ensure placement of the eye chart is at an appropriate height for the client and in a well-lit room.
- Position the client exactly 20 feet from the chart.
- Ask the client to cover one eye with a card and to read the smallest line of letters the client can see (Figure 9.19). Do not allow the client to use a hand to cover the eye, as this may put pressure on the eye.

Referral

If vision is poorer than 20/30, the client should be referred to an ophthalmologist, unless vision is corrected with glasses.

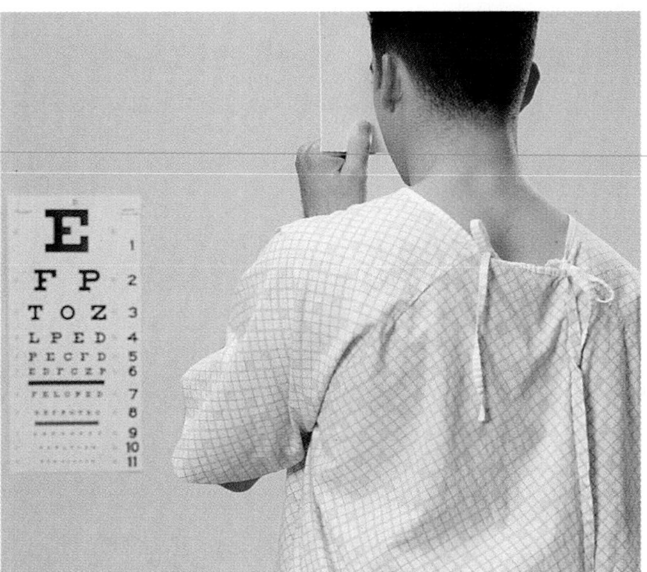

Figure 9.19 Testing distant vision.

- Repeat the process with the other eye, then with both eyes uncovered.
- Record the results as a fraction, using the numbers at the end of the last line read. The numerator indicates the distance of the client from the chart (20 feet). The denominator indicates the distance at which a person with **emmetropic** (normal) vision can read the last line the client read. Emmetropic vision is 20/20: at 20 feet the client can read the line numbered 20. If the client's vision is 20/30, the client reads at 20 feet what an emmetropic client can read at 30 feet. If the client is unable to read more than half of the letters on a line, record the number of the line above.
- Observe the client's behavior while reading the chart. You should determine whether the client is literate in English.

Frowning, leaning forward, and squinting indicate reading difficulty.

Step 2 *Test near vision.*

- Have the client hold a Jaeger card 14 inches from the client's eyes (Figure 9.20 on page 180).
- Have the client cover first one eye, then the other with a cover card, testing each eye separately.

Inability to see objects at close range is called **hyperopia**. In persons over the age of 45, inability to accommodate for near vision is called **presbyopia**. It is a common sign of aging.

ASSESSMENT TECHNIQUE/NORMAL FINDINGS

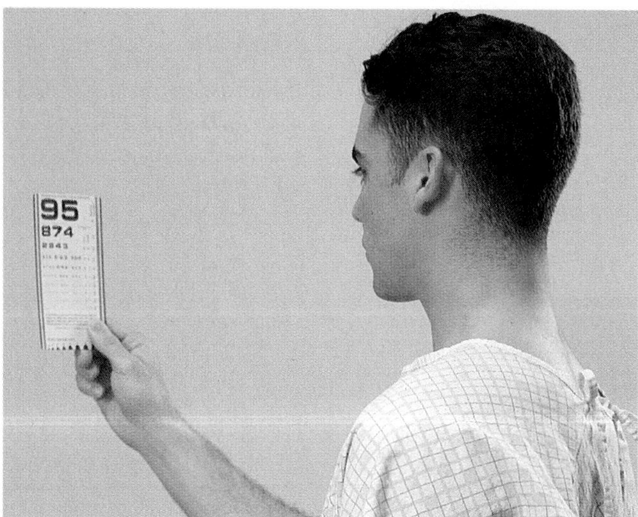

Figure 9.20 Testing near vision.

- Then test vision with both eyes uncovered.
- Ask the client to read with and without corrective lens if lenses are needed for near vision.

A normal result is 14/14 in each eye.

Step 3 *Test visual fields by confrontation.*

- Position yourself directly in front of the client, at eye level, at a distance of 2 to 3 feet.
- Ask the client to cover one eye with a card while you cover your opposite eye with a card.
- Holding a penlight in one hand, extend your arm upward, and advance it in from the periphery to the midline point (Figure 9.21).

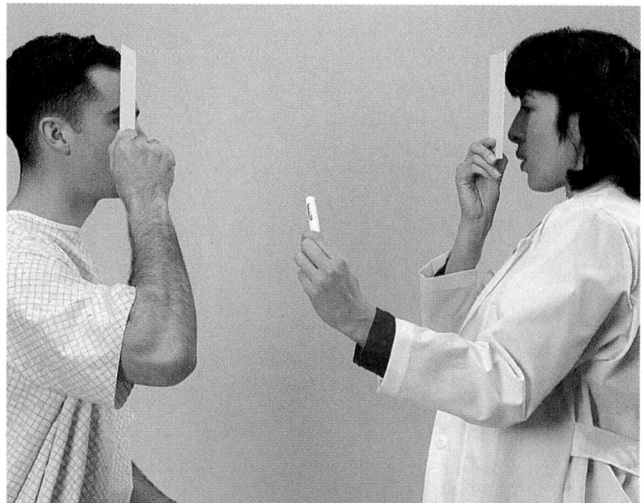
Figure 9.21 Testing visual fields by confrontation.

SPECIAL CONSIDERATIONS

Referral

If client is unable to read the letters at 14 inches, the client should be referred to an ophthalmologist.

If the client is not able to see the object at the same time that the examiner does, there may be some peripheral vision loss. The client should be evaluated further.

ASSESSMENT TECHNIQUE/NORMAL FINDINGS | SPECIAL CONSIDERATIONS

- Be sure to keep the penlight equidistant between the client and yourself.
- Ask the client to report when the object is first seen. Repeat the procedure upward, toward the nose, and downward. Then repeat the entire procedure with the other eye covered.

This test assumes the examiner has normal peripheral vision.

Step 4 ***Test the six cardinal fields of gaze.***

Examine eye movement controlled by the six extraocular muscles and by cranial nerves III (oculomotor), IV (trochlear), and VI (abducens), by testing the six cardinal fields of gaze.

- Standing about 2 feet in front of the client, ask the client to hold the head steady and to follow the movement of your penlight only with the eyes as the penlight moves through the *six cardinal fields of gaze*.
- Starting in the midline, move the penlight to the extreme left, then straight up, then straight down.
- Drop your hand. Position the penlight again in the midline.
- Now move the penlight to the extreme right, then straight up, then straight down.
- Assess the client's ability to follow your movements with the eyes (Figure 9.22). If the client moves the head to follow the penlight, hold the client's chin steady with your free hand.

If the eye movements are not parallel, or the eyes fail to follow in a certain direction, the client may have a weakness of an extraocular muscle or a dysfunction of a cranial nerve. *Nystagmus*, an involuntary, rapid, rhythmic movement of the eye, may indicate dysfunction of a cranial nerve.

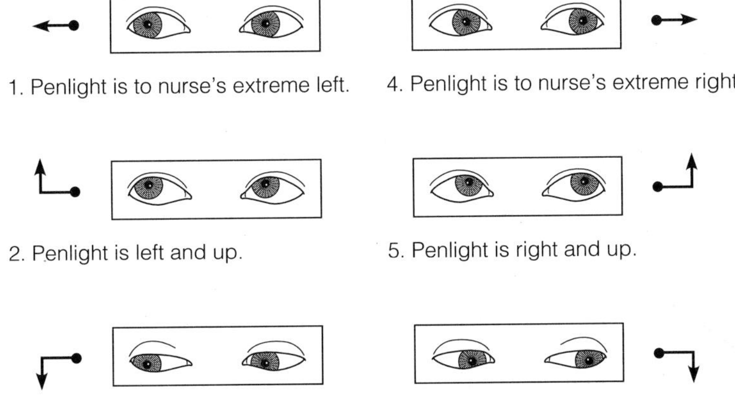
1. Penlight is to nurse's extreme left.
4. Penlight is to nurse's extreme right
2. Penlight is left and up.
5. Penlight is right and up.
3. Penlight is left and down.
6. Penlight is right and down.

Figure 9.22 Testing the six cardinal fields of gaze.

Step 5 ***Assess the corneal light reflex.***

- Ask the client to stare straight ahead as you shine a penlight about 12 inches from both eyes (Figure 9.23 on page 182).

The reflection of light should appear in the same spot on both pupils.

If the reflection of light is not symmetric, there could be a weakness in the extraocular muscles.

ASSESSMENT TECHNIQUE/NORMAL FINDINGS | SPECIAL CONSIDERATIONS

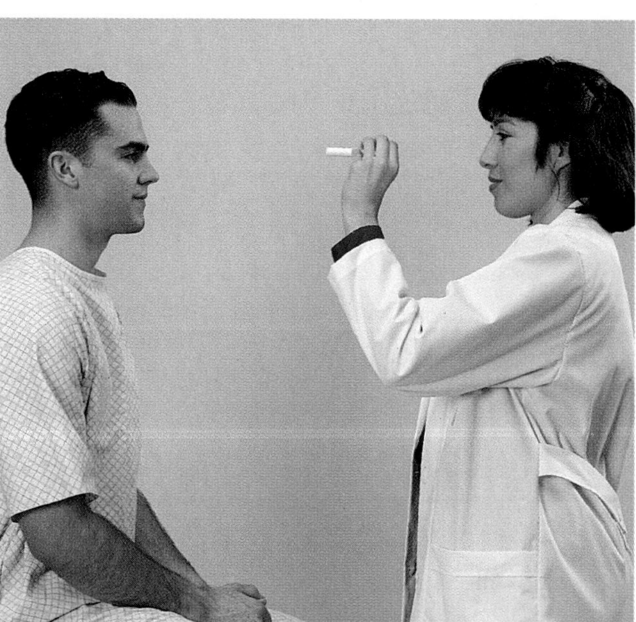

Figure 9.23 Testing the corneal light reflex.

Step 6 *Perform the cover test.*

- Ask the client to stare straight ahead at a fixed point.
- Cover one eye with a card and observe the uncovered eye, which should remain focused on the designated point.
- Remove the card from the covered eye and observe the newly uncovered eye for movement. It should focus straight ahead.
- Repeat the procedure with the other eye.

Movement of the covered or uncovered eye may indicate a weakness in the eye muscles.

This test detects an imbalance of the mechanism that keeps the eyes parallel (the fusion reflex). If there is a weakness in one of the eye muscles, the fusion reflex is blocked when one eye is covered and the weakness of the eye can be observed.

Step 7 *Inspect the pupils.*

The pupils should be round, equal in size and shape, and in the center of the eye.

Pupils that are not round and symmetric may indicate previous ocular surgery, increased intracranial pressure, or cranial nerve pathology.

Step 8 *Evaluate the pupillary response.*

Pupillary response is the direct and consensual reaction of the pupils to light.

- Dim the lights in the room so that the pupils dilate.
- Ask the client to stare straight ahead.
- Moving your penlight in from the client's side, shine light directly into one eye.

If the illuminated pupil fails to constrict, there is a defect in the direct pupillary response. If the unilluminated pupil fails to constrict, there is a defect in the consensual response, controlled by cranial nerve III (oculomotor). If the pupils fail to constrict, there is a problem in the pupillary response controlled by cranial nerve III (oculomotor).

ASSESSMENT TECHNIQUE/NORMAL FINDINGS	SPECIAL CONSIDERATIONS

- Observe the constriction in the illuminated pupil. Also observe the simultaneous reaction (consensual) of the other pupil. The direct reaction should be faster and greater than the consensual reaction.

Step 9 ***Test for accommodation of pupil response.***

- Ask the client to stare straight ahead at a distant point.
- Hold a penlight about 4 to 5 inches from the client's nose, then ask the client to shift the gaze from the distant point to the penlight.

The eyes should converge (turn inward) and the pupils should constrict as the eyes focus on the penlight.

Failure of the eyes to converge and the pupils to constrict indicates dysfunction of cranial nerves III, IV, and VI.

Step 10 ***Record the client's response to these tests.***

A normal response is recorded as: PERRLA (pupils equal, round, react to light and accomodation).

Step 11 ***Test the corneal reflex.***

The corneal reflex is controlled by cranial nerve V (trigeminal) and nerve VII (facial).

- Take a sterile cotton ball and twist it into a very thin strand.
- Using a lateral approach, gently touch the cornea on the outer aspect of each eye (Figure 9.24).

If one or both eyes fail to respond, there could be a problem with cranial nerve V, VII, or both, since cranial nerve V is sensory for this reflex, and cranial nerve VII is motor. Note that long-term use of contact lenses can diminish the corneal reflex.

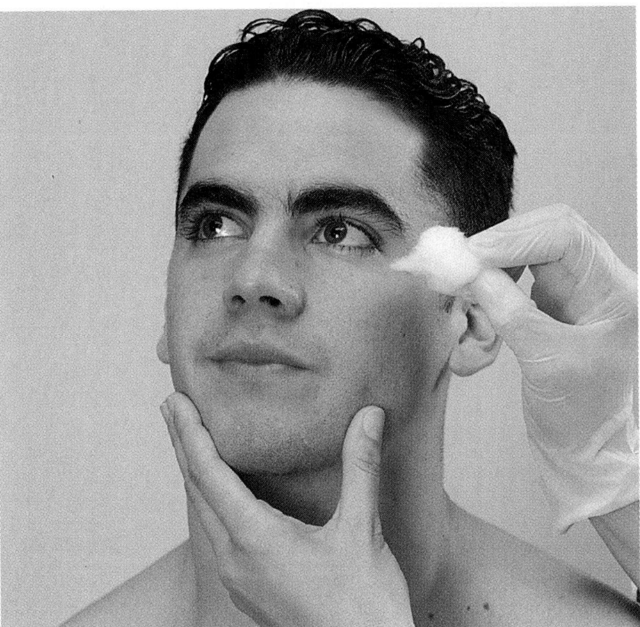

Figure 9.24 Testing the corneal reflex.

- Confirm that both eyes blink when either cornea is touched.
- Be sure not to touch the eyelashes or conjunctiva.

ASSESSMENT TECHNIQUE/NORMAL FINDINGS	SPECIAL CONSIDERATIONS

ALERT!

Never put an unsterile object into the eye. To prevent injury, ask the client to remove contact lenses before either the corneal reflex test or the ophthalmoscopic examination.

Step 12 *Inspect the external eye.*

- Stand directly in front of the client and focus on the external structures of the eye. The eyebrows should be symmetric in shape, and the eyelashes similar in quantity and distribution. The eyebrows and eyelashes should be free of flakes and drainage.
- With the eyes open, confirm that the distance between the palpebral fissures are equal. Confirm that the upper eyelid covers a small arc of the iris.
- Confirm that the eyelids symmetrically cover the eyeballs when closed. The eyeball should be neither protruding nor sunken.
- Gently separate the eyelids and ask the client to look up, down, and to each side. The conjunctiva should be moist and clear, with small blood vessels. The lens should be clear, and the sclera white. The iris should be round, and both of the same color, although irises of different colors can be a normal finding.
- Inspect the cornea by shining a penlight from the side across the cornea. The cornea should be clear with no irregularities. The pupils should be round and equal in size.

One eyelid drooping (ptosis) can be caused by a dysfunction of cranial nerve III (oculomotor). Eyes that protrude beyond the supraorbital ridge can indicate a thyroid disorder; however, this trait may be normal for the client. Edema of the eyelids can be caused by allergies, heart disease, or kidney disease. Inability to move the eyelids can indicate dysfunction of the nervous system.

Step 13 *Palpate the eye.*

- Ask the client to close both eyes.
- Using the first two or three fingers, gently palpate the lacrimal sacs, the eyelids, and the eyeballs.
- Confirm that there is no swelling or tenderness and that the eyeballs feel firm.

Swelling may be a symptom of infection or of cardiovascular or renal problems.

Step 14 *Examine the conjunctiva and sclera under the lower eyelid.*

- Evert the lower eyelid by asking the client to look down, pressing the lower lid against the lower orbital rim, then asking the client to look up (Figure 9.25). The conjunctiva should be pink with no tenderness or irregularities. If you find any abnormality, examine the conjunctiva under the upper eyelid.

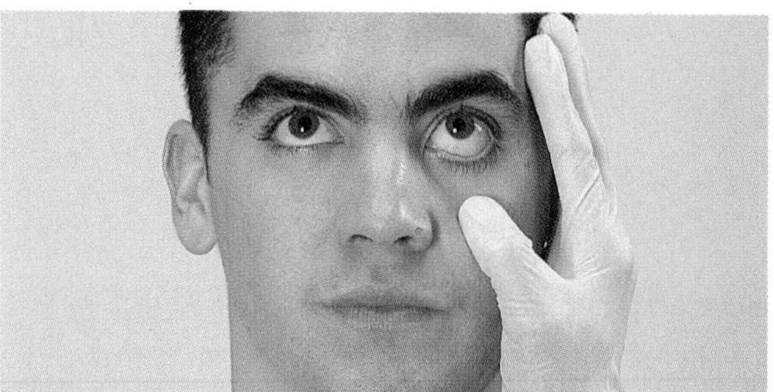

Figure 9.25 Inspecting the conjunctiva of the lower lid.

Inflammation and edema of the conjunctiva indicate an infection or possible foreign body.

ASSESSMENT TECHNIQUE/NORMAL FINDINGS

SPECIAL CONSIDERATIONS

- Ask the client to close the eye.
- Evert the upper eyelid by placing a cotton-tipped applicator against the upper lid (Figure 9.26, *A*).
- Grasp the eyelashes and pull the eyelid downward, forward, and up over the applicator (Figure 9.26, *B*).
- Gently release and return the eyelid to the normal position when finished.

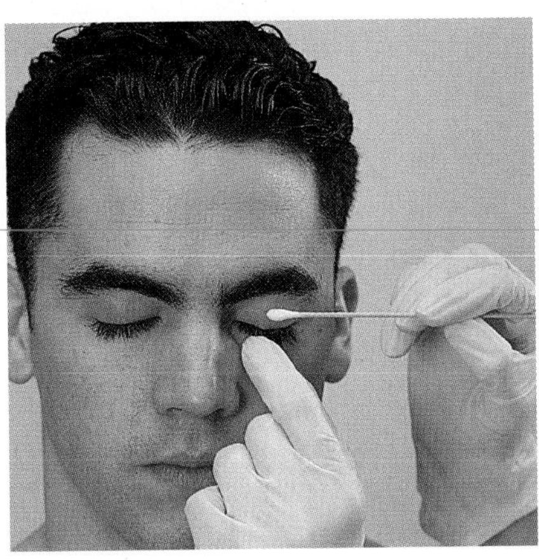

A

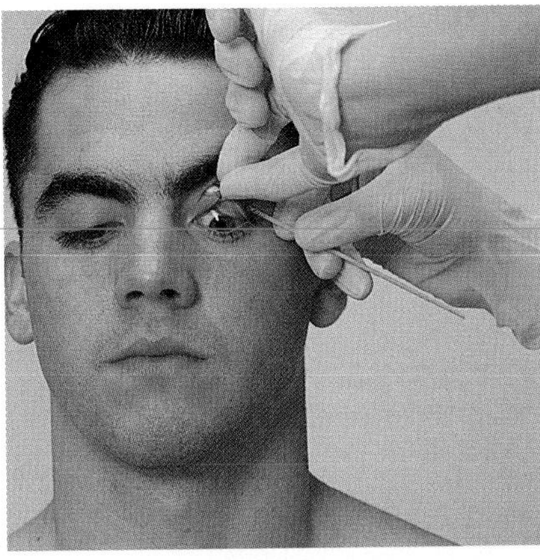

B

Figure 9.26 Eversion of the upper lid.

Step 15 ***Inspect the inner eye with the ophthalmoscope.***

The ophthalmoscopic examination allows for the retina, optic disc, and blood vessels of the eye to be viewed directly. It is used to diagnose neurologic, systemic, and ophthalmic disorders. See Chapter 7 for a description of the ophthalmoscope.

- Dim the lights in the room.
- Ask the client to look at a fixed point straight ahead and not to move.
- To examine the right eye, hold the ophthalmoscope in your right hand with the index finger on the lens wheel.
- Begin with the lens on the 0 diopter. With the light on place the ophthalmoscope over your right eye (Figure 9.27).

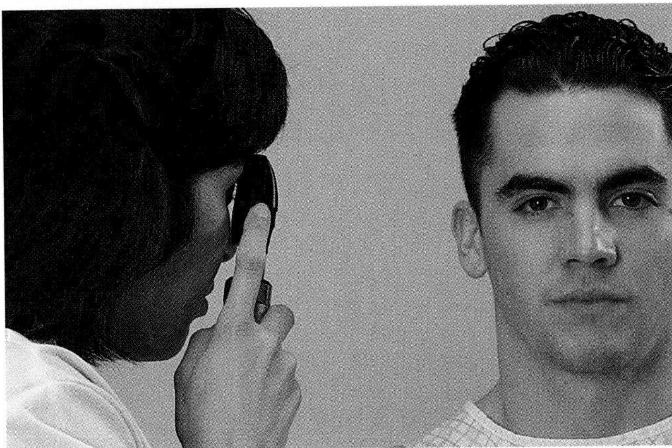

Figure 9.27 Approaching the client for the ophthalmoscopic exam.

ASSESSMENT TECHNIQUE/NORMAL FINDINGS	SPECIAL CONSIDERATIONS

- Stand at a slight angle lateral to the client's line of vision.
- Approach the client at about a 15-degree angle toward the nose.
- Place your left hand on the client's shoulder or forehead.
- Hold the ophthalmoscope against your head, directing the light into the client's pupil. Keep your other eye open.
- Advance toward the client.
- As you look into the client's pupil, you will see the *red reflex*,which is the reflection of the light off of the retina. Remember to examine your client's right eye with your right eye, and your client's left eye with your left eye. At this point you may need to adjust the lens wheel to bring the ocular structures into focus. Normally you will see no shadows or dots interrupting the red reflex. If the light strays from the pupil, you will lose the red reflex. Adjust your angle until you see the red reflex again.

Persistent absence of the red reflex may indicate a cataract, an opacity of the lens.

- Keep advancing toward the client until the ophthalmoscope is almost touching the client's eyelashes (Figure 9.28).

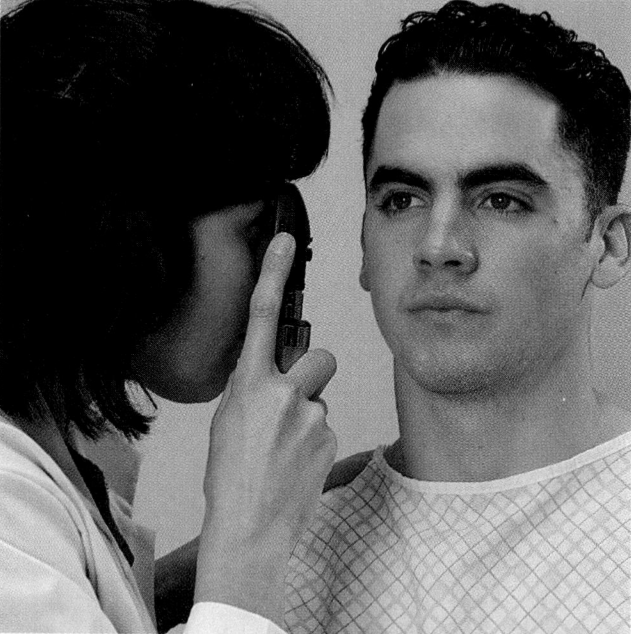

Figure 9.28 Examining the eye using the ophthalmoscope.

- Rotate the diopter wheel if necessary to bring the ocular fundus into focus.
- If the client's vision is myopic, you will need to rotate the wheel into the minus numbers (Figure 9.29).
- If the client's vision is hyperopic, rotate the wheel into the plus numbers.

ASSESSMENT TECHNIQUE/NORMAL FINDINGS

SPECIAL CONSIDERATIONS

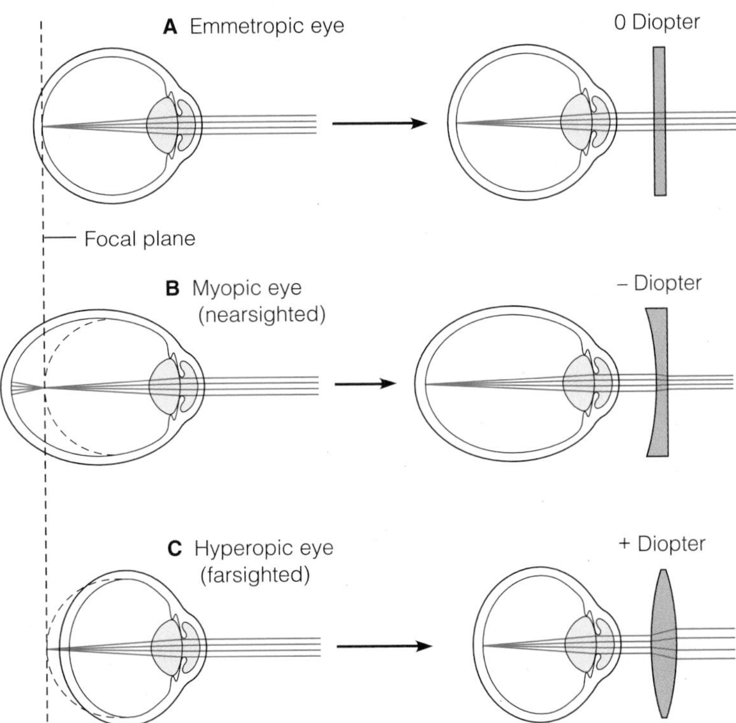

Figure 9.29 Use of diopter to adjust for problems of refraction. *A*, In the emmetropic (normal) eye, light is focused properly on the retina, and the 0 diopter is used. *B*, In the myopic eye, light from a distant source converges to a focal point before reaching the retina. Negative diopter numbers are used. *C*, In the hyperopic eye, light from a near source converges to a focal point past the retina. Positive diopter numbers are used.

- Begin to look for the *optic disc* by following the path of the blood vessels. As they grow larger, they lead to the optic disc on the nasal side of the retina (Figure 9.30). The optic disc normally looks like a round or oval yellow-orange depression with a distinct margin. It is the site where the optic nerve and blood vessels exit the eye.

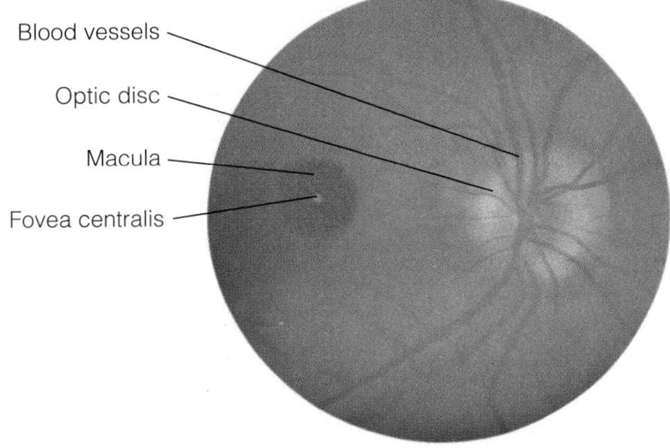

Figure 9.30 The optic disc.

ASSESSMENT TECHNIQUE/NORMAL FINDINGS	SPECIAL CONSIDERATIONS

- Follow the vessels laterally to a darker circle with only a few blood vessels. This is the *macula,* or area of central vision. The *fovea centralis*, a small white spot located in the center of the macula, is the area of sharpest vision.

Degeneration of the macula is common in older adults and results in impaired central vision. It may be due to hemorrhages, cysts, or other alterations.

- Systematically inspect these structures. A crescent shape around the margin of the optic disc is a normal finding. A *scleral crescent* is an absence of pigment in the choroid and is a dull white color, and a *pigment crescent*, which is black, is an accumulation of pigment in the choroid.

Abnormalities of the retinal structures present as dark or opaque spots on the retina, an irregularly shaped optic disc, and lesions or hemorrhages on the fundus.

- Use the optic disc as a clock face for documenting the position of a finding, and the diameter of the disc (DD) for noting its distance from the optic disc. For instance, "at 2:00, 2 DD from the disc" describes the finding in Figure 9.31.

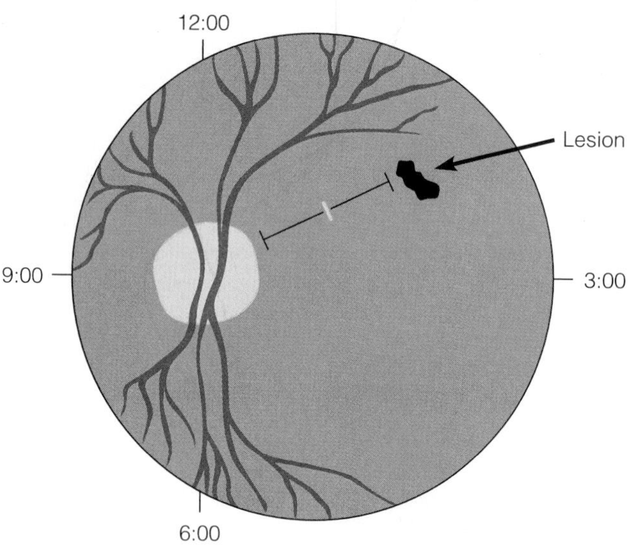

Figure 9.31 Documenting a finding from the ophthalmoscopic exam.

- Trace the path of a paired artery and vein from the optic disc to the periphery in the four quadrants of the eyeball.
- Note the number of major vessels, color, width, and any crossing of the vessels.
- Repeat the preceding procedure to examine the client's left eye, using your left hand and left eye.

An absence of major vessels in any of the four quadrants is an abnormal finding. Constricted arteries look smaller than two-thirds the diameter of accompanying veins. Crossing of the vessels more than 2 DD away from the optic disc requires further evaluation. Extremely tortuous vessels also require further evaluation.

The Ear

Note that you will have begun to evaluate the client's hearing while taking the health history. Did the client hear the questions you ask? Did the client answer appropriately? Generally, the formal evaluation of hearing is performed after otoscopic examination so that physical barriers to hearing, such as large amounts of cerumen, can be identified.

ASSESSMENT TECHNIQUE/NORMAL FINDINGS	SPECIAL CONSIDERATIONS

Step 1 ***Inspect the external ear for symmetry, proportion, color, and integrity.***

- Confirm that the external auditory meatus is patent with no drainage. The color of the ear should match that of the surrounding area and the face, with no redness, nodules, swelling, or lesions.

Any discharge, redness, or swelling may indicate an infection or allergy.

Step 2 ***Palpate the auricle and push on the tragus*** *(Figure 9.32).*

- Confirm that there are no hard nodules, lesions, or swelling. The tragus should be moveable.

This technique should not cause pain.

Pain could be the result of an infection of the external ear (otitis externa). Pain could also indicate temporomandibular joint dysfunction with pressure on the tragus. Hard nodules (tophi) are uric acid crystal deposits, which are a sign of gout. Lesions accompanied by a history of long-term exposure to the sun may be cancerous.

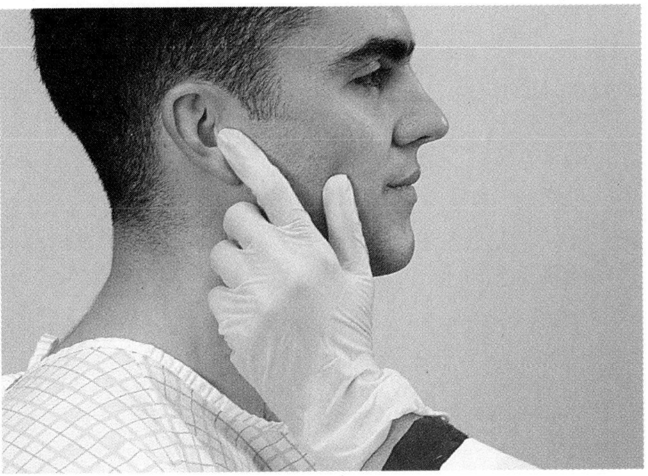

Figure 9.32 Palpating the tragus.

Step 3 ***Palpate the mastoid process lying directly behind the ear*** *(Figure 9.33).*

- Confirm that there are no lesions, pain, or swelling.

Mastoiditis is a complication of either a middle ear or throat infection. Mastoiditis is very difficult to treat. It spreads easily to the brain since the mastoid area is separated from the brain by only a thin, bony plate.

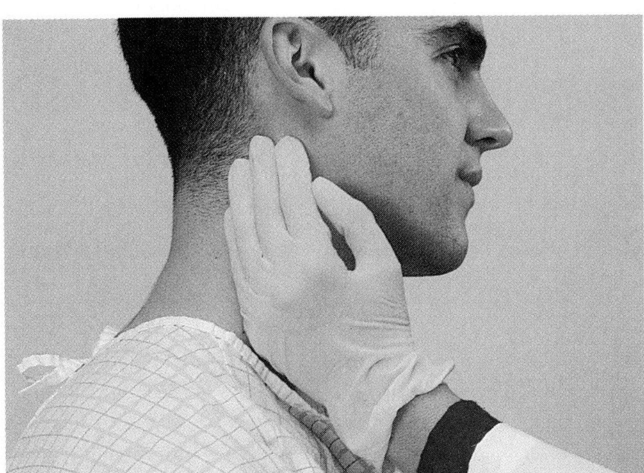

Figure 9.33 Palpating the mastoid process.

ASSESSMENT TECHNIQUE/NORMAL FINDINGS	SPECIAL CONSIDERATIONS

Step 4 ***Inspect the auditory canal using the otoscope.***

For the best visualization, use the largest speculum that will fit into the auditory canal.

- Ask the client to tilt the head away from you toward the opposite shoulder.
- Hold the otoscope between the palm and first two fingers of one hand. The handle may be positioned upward or downward.
- Use your other hand to stabilize the head and straighten the canal.
- In the adult client, pull the pinna up, back, and out to straighten out the canal (Figure 9.34). (See the next section for straightening the ear canal of a child.) Be sure to maintain this position until the speculum is removed.

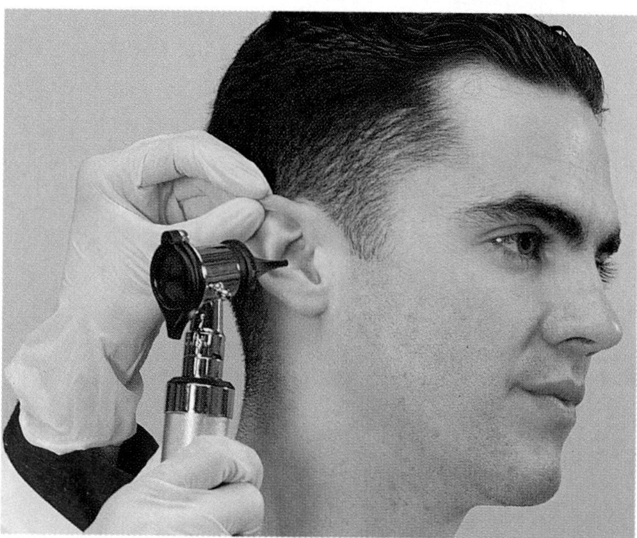

Figure 9.34 Inserting the otoscope for the adult client.

- With the light on, insert the speculum into the ear. The external canal should be open and without tenderness, inflammation, lesions, growths, discharge, or foreign substances.

ALERT!

Use care when inserting the speculum of the otoscope into the ear. The inner two-thirds of the ear are very sensitive, and pressing the speculum against either side of the auditory canal will cause pain.

- Note the amount of cerumen that is present, the texture, and the color.

If the ear canal is occluded with cerumen, it must be removed. Moist cerumen can be removed with a cerumen spoon; if the cerumen is dry, the external canal should be irrigated using a bulb syringe and a warmed solution of mineral oil and hydrogen peroxide, followed by warm water.

ASSESSMENT TECHNIQUE/NORMAL FINDINGS

Step 5 ***Examine the tympanic membrane using the otoscope.***

The membrane should be flat, gray, and translucent with no scars (Figure 9.35). A cone-shaped reflection of the otoscope light should be visible at the five o'clock position in the right ear and the seven o'clock position in the left ear. The short process of the malleus should be seen as a shadow behind the tympanic membrane. The membrane should be intact.

If you cannot visualize the tympanic membrane, remove the otoscope, reposition the auricle, and reinsert the otoscope. Do not reposition the auricle with the otoscope in place.

SPECIAL CONSIDERATIONS

White patches on the tympanic membrane indicate prior infections. If the membrane is yellow or reddish, it could indicate an infection of the middle ear. A bulging eardrum may indicate increased pressure in the middle ear, whereas a retracted eardrum may indicate a vacuum in the middle ear. (See Table 9.4 on page 215 for common alterations in the health of the ears.)

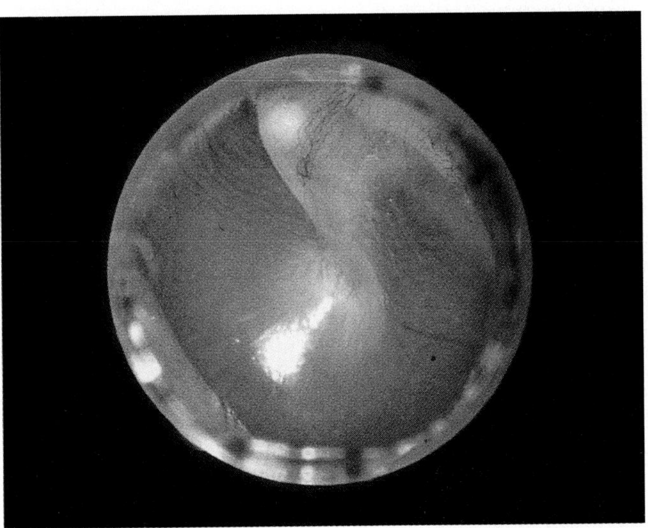

Figure 9.35 Normal tympanic membrane.

Step 6 ***While looking through the otoscope, instruct the client to perform the Valsalva maneuver.***

- Have the tympanic membrane in clear view.
- Ask the client to close the lips, pinch the nose, and gently blow the nose.

This maneuver lets you assess the mobility of the tympanic membrance and the patency of the eustachian tubes. The tympanic membrance should flutter toward the otoscope slightly as the client performs this manuever.

ALERT!

Do not ask an elderly client to perform the Valsalva manuever because it may result in dizziness. This manuever is also dangerous if the person has an upper respiratory infection, because it could force pathogenic organisms into the middle ear.

Rigidity of the tympanic membrane may be due to a variety of alterations and requires further evaluation.

ASSESSMENT TECHNIQUE/NORMAL FINDINGS

SPECIAL CONSIDERATIONS

Step 7 *Perform the whisper test.*

This test evaluates hearing acuity of high-frequency sounds.

- Ask the client to hold the heel of the hand over the left ear.
- Cover your mouth so that the client cannot see your lips.
- Standing at a distance of 1 to 2 feet, whisper a simple phrase such as, "The weather is hot today," and ask the client to repeat the phrase. Then do the same procedure to test the right ear using a different phrase.The client should be able to repeat the phrases correctly.

Inability to repeat the phrases may indicate a loss of the ability to hear high-frequency sounds.

Tuning forks are used to evaluate auditory acuity. The tines of the fork, when activated, produce sound waves. The frequency, or cycles per second (cps), is the expression used to describe the action of the instrument. A fork with 512 cps vibrates 512 times per second and is the size of choice for auditory evaluations.

The tines are set into motion by squeezing, stroking, or lightly tapping against your hand. The fork must be held at the handle to prevent interference with the vibration of the tines.

The following tests use a tuning fork heading primarily to evaluate conductive versus perceptive hearing loss. Air conduction (AC) is the transmission of sound through the tympanic membrane to the cochlea and auditory nerve. Bone conduction (BC) is the transmission of sound through the bones of the skull to the cochlea and auditory nerve.

Step 8 *Perform the Rinne test.*

This test compares air and bone conduction.

- Hold the tuning fork by the handle and gently strike the fork on the palm of your hand to set it vibrating.
- Place the base of the fork on the client's mastoid process (Figure 9.36, *A*).
- Ask the client to tell you when the sound is no longer heard.

If the client hears the bone-conducted sound as long as or longer than the air-conducted sound, the client may have some degree of conductive hearing loss.

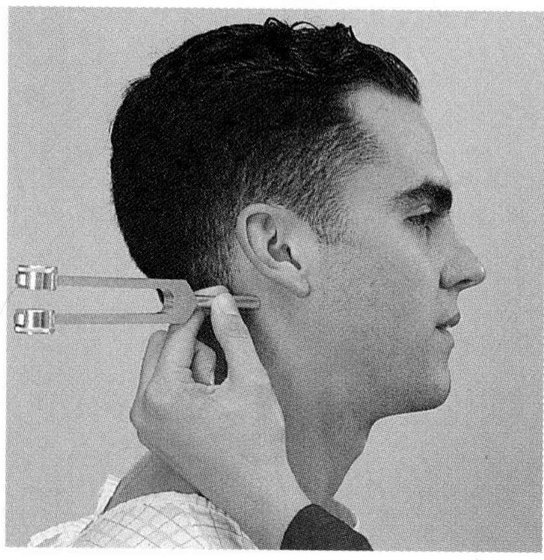

A

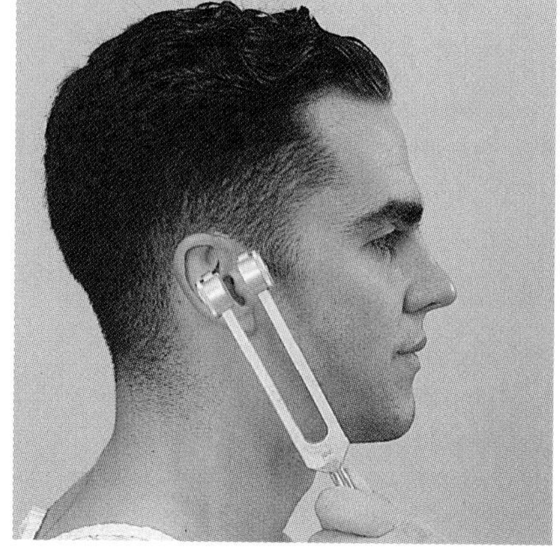

B

Figure 9.36 Rinne test.

ASSESSMENT TECHNIQUE/NORMAL FINDINGS	SPECIAL CONSIDERATIONS

- Note the number of seconds. Then immediately move the tines of the still-vibrating fork in 1 to 2 cm (about ½ inch) in front of the external auditory meatus, and ask the client to tell you again when the sound is no longer heard (Figure 9.36, *B*).
- Again note the number of seconds. Normally the sound is heard twice as long by air conduction than by bone conduction *after bone conduction stops*. For example, a normal finding is AC 30 seconds, BC 15 seconds.

Step 9 ***Perform the Weber test.***

The Weber test uses bone conduction to evaluate hearing in a person who hears better in one ear than in the other.

- Hold the tuning fork by the handle and strike the fork on the palm of the hand.
- Place the base of the vibrating fork against the skull. The midline of the anterior portion of the frontal bone is used. The midline of the forehead is an alternate choice (Figure 9.37).

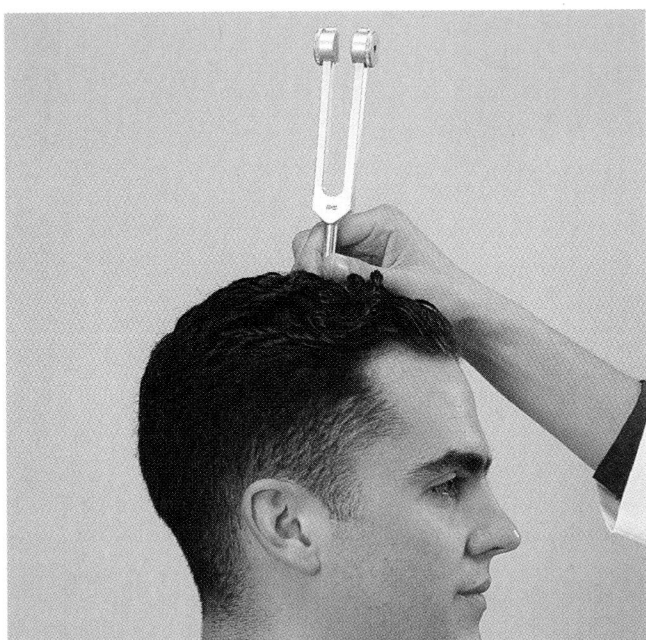

Figure 9.37 Weber test.

- Ask the client if the sound is heard equally on both sides, or better in one ear than the other. The normal response is bilaterally equal sound, which is recorded as "no lateralization." If the sound is lateralized, ask the client to tell you which ear hears the sound better.

If the client hears the sound in one ear better than the other ear, the hearing loss may be due to either poor conduction or nerve damage. If the client has poor conduction in one ear, the sound is heard better in the impaired ear because the sound is being conducted directly through the bone to the ear, and the extraneous sounds in the environment are not being picked up. Conductive loss in one ear may be due to impacted cerumen, infection, or a perforated eardrum. If the client has a hearing loss due to nerve damage, the sound is referred to the better ear, in which the cochlea or auditory nerve is functioning better.

The abnormal findings are recorded as "sound lateralizes to [right or left] ear."

Step 10 ***Perform the Romberg test.***

This test assesses equilibrium.

- Ask the client to stand with feet together, first with eyes opened, and then eyes closed, and arms at sides (Figure 9.38 on page 194).

If the client is unable to maintain balance or needs to have feet farther apart, there may be a problem with functioning of the vestibular apparatus.

ASSESSMENT TECHNIQUE/NORMAL FINDINGS	SPECIAL CONSIDERATIONS

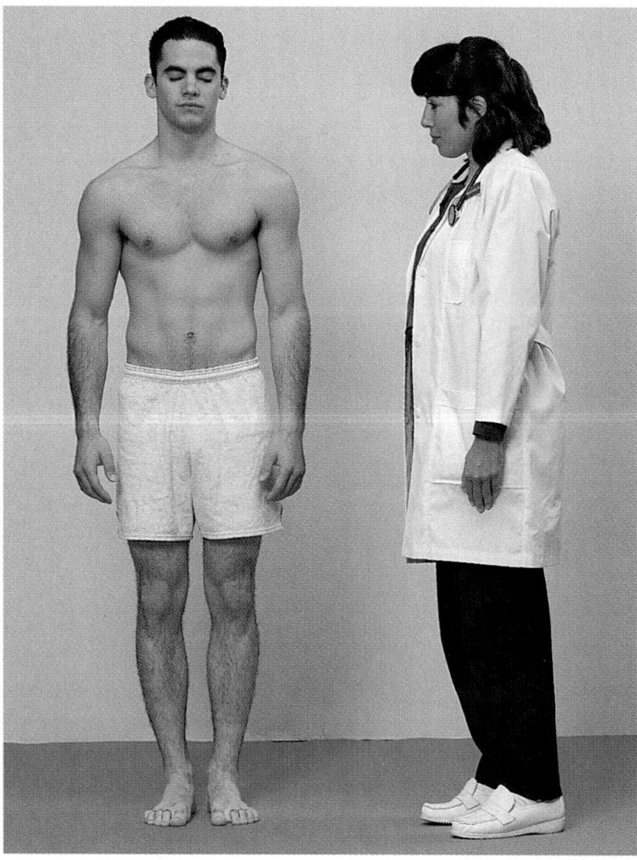

Figure 9.38 Romberg test.

- Wait about 20 seconds. The person should be able to maintain this position, although some mild swaying may occur. It is important to stand nearby in case the client loses balance.

The Nose and Sinuses

The sense of smell and function of cranial nerve I are assessed in Chapter 18.

Step 1 ***Inspect the nose for symmetry, shape, skin lesions, or signs of infection.***

If breathing is noisy or a discharge is present, the client may have an obtruction or an infection.

Step 2 *Test for patency.*

- Press your finger on the client's nostril to occlude one naris, and ask the client to breathe through the opposite side.
- Repeat with other nostril.

The client should be able to breathe through each naris.

If the client cannot breathe through each naris, severe inflammation or an obstruction may be present.

ASSESSMENT TECHNIQUE/NORMAL FINDINGS	SPECIAL CONSIDERATIONS

Step 3 *Palpate the external nose for tenderness, swelling, and stability.*

Ineffective breathing patterns or mouth breathing may be related to nasal swelling.

Step 4 *Inspect the nasal cavity using a nasal speculum.*

- With your nondominant hand, stabilize the client's head. With the speculum in your dominant hand, insert the speculum with blades closed, into the naris. Then separate the blades, dilating the naris (Figure 9.39). The speculum should be in the dominant hand for better control at the time of insertion to avoid hitting the sensitive septum.

If the mucosa is swollen and red, the client may have an upper respiratory infection. If mucosa is pale and boggy or swollen, the client may have chronic allergies. A *deviated septum* appears as an irregular lump in one nasal cavity. Slight deviations do not present problems for most clients. *Nasal polyps* are smooth, pale, benign growths found in many clients with chronic allergies. (See Table 9.5 on page 217 for common alterations in the health of the nose and sinuses.)

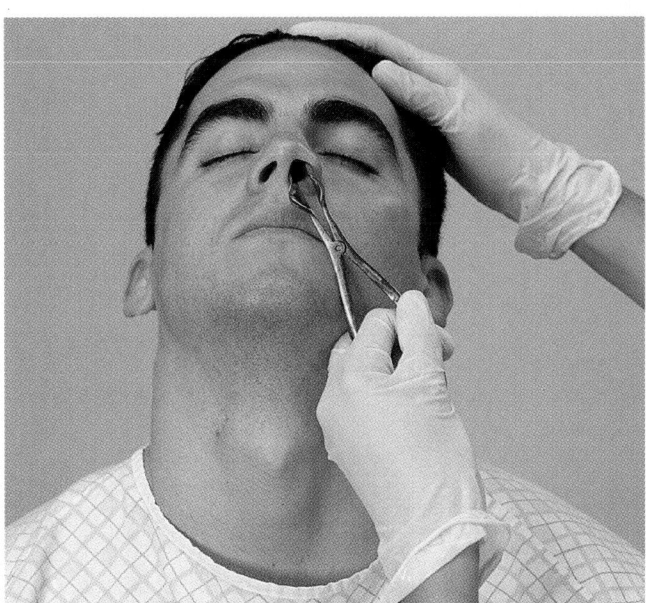

Figure 9.39 Inspecting the nose using a nasal speculum.

- With the client's head erect, inspect the inferior turbinates.
- With the client's head tilted back, inspect the middle meatus and middle turbinates. Mucosa should be dark pink and smooth without swelling, discharge, bleeding, or foreign bodies. The septum should be midline, straight, and intact.
- When finished with inspection, close the blades of the speculum and remove. Again, do not hit the sensitive septum.
- Repeat on other side.

Step 5 *Palpate the sinuses.*

- Begin by pressing your thumbs over the frontal sinuses below the eyebrows and over the maxillary sinuses below the cheekbones.

Tenderness upon palpation may indicate chronic allergies or sinusitis.

Step 6 *Percuss the sinuses.*

To determine if there is pain in the sinuses, percuss the maxillary and frontal sinuses by lightly tapping with one finger.

A dull sound may indicate sinus swelling, fullness, allergies, or infection.

ASSESSMENT TECHNIQUE/NORMAL FINDINGS	SPECIAL CONSIDERATIONS

Step 7 ***Transilluminate the sinuses.***

If you suspect a sinus infecton, the maxillary and frontal sinuses may be transilluminated.

- To transilluminate the frontal sinus, darken the room and hold a penlight under the superior orbit ridge against the frontal sinus area (Figure 9.40, *A*).

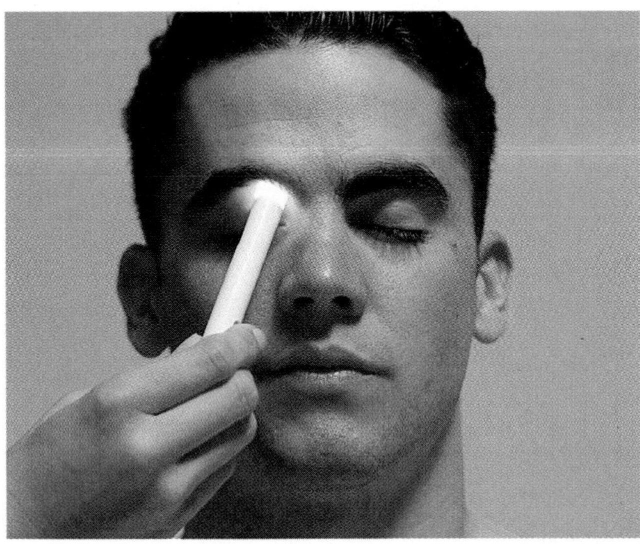

A

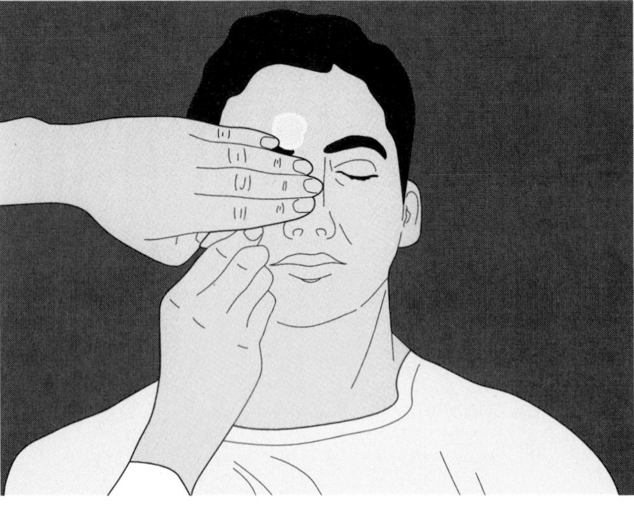

B

Figure 9.40 Transillumination of the frontal sinuses.

- Cover it with your hand. There should be a red glow over the frontal sinus area (Figure 9.40, *B*).

If the sinus is filled with fluid, it will not transilluminate.

- To test the maxillary sinus, place a sterile penlight in the client's mouth and shine the light on one side of the hard palate, then the other (Figure 9.41, *A*). There should be a red glow under the eyes (Figure 9.41, *B*). Make sure you sterilize the penlight before using it again.

If there is no red glow under the eyes, the sinuses may be inflamed.

ASSESSMENT TECHNIQUE/NORMAL FINDINGS | SPECIAL CONSIDERATIONS

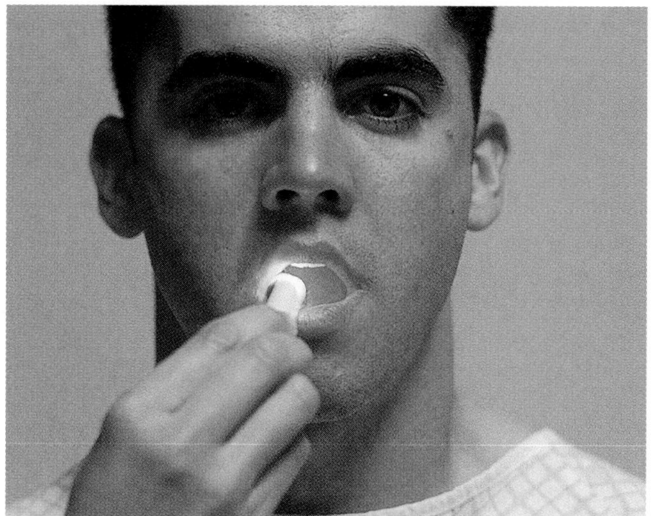

A

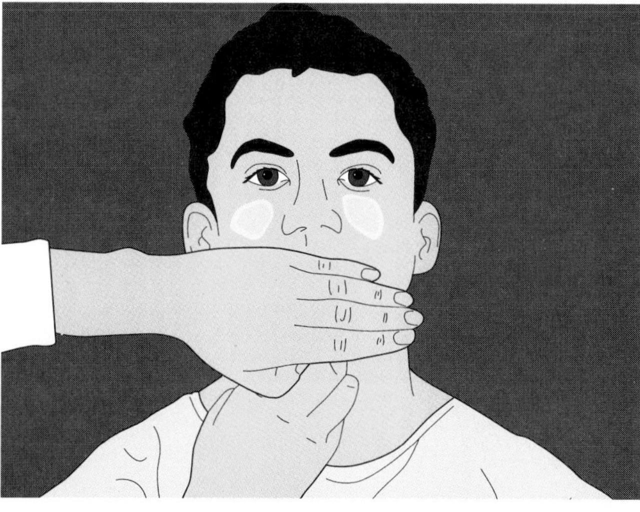

B

Figure 9.41 Transillumination of the maxillary sinuses.

The Mouth and Throat

ALERT!

Make sure you are wearing gloves before proceeding with the following assessments!

Step 1 *Inspect and palpate the lips.*

- Confirm that the lips are symmetric, smooth, pink, moist, and without lesions.

Lesions or blisters on the lips may be caused by the herpes simplex virus. These lesions are also known as *fever blisters* or *cold sores*. However, lesions must be evaluated for cancer, because cancer of the lip is the most common oral cancer. Pallor of the

ASSESSMENT TECHNIQUE/NORMAL FINDINGS | SPECIAL CONSIDERATIONS

lips may indicate cyanosis. (See Table 9.6 on page 217 for common alterations in the health of the mouth and throat.)

Step 2 ***Inspect the teeth.***

- Observe the client's dental hygiene.
- Ask the client to clench the teeth and smile while you observe occlusion.
- Note dentures and caps at this time.

The teeth should be white, with smooth edges, and free of debris. Adults should have 32 permanent teeth (Figure 9.42).

Loose, painful, broken, misaligned teeth, malocclusion, and inflamed gums need further evaluation.

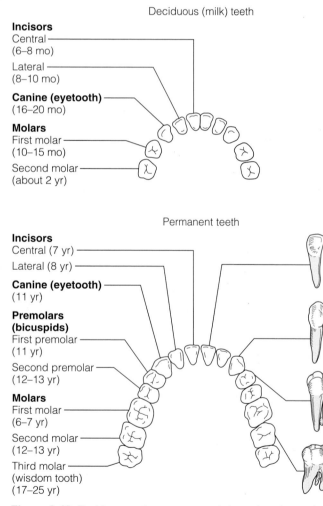

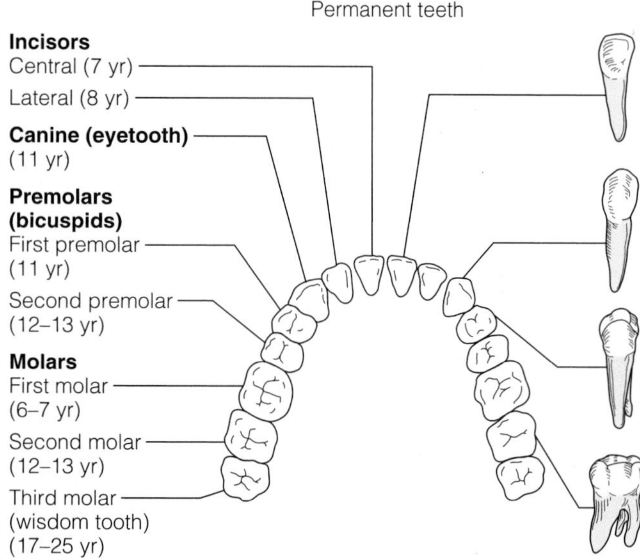

Figure 9.42 Deciduous and permanent teeth, lower jaw. Approximate age at eruption is shown in parentheses.

ASSESSMENT TECHNIQUE/NORMAL FINDINGS

Step 3 ***Inspect and palpate the buccal mucosa, gums, and tongue.***

- Look into the client's mouth under a strong light.
- Confirm that the tongue is pink and moist with papillae on the dorsal surface.
- Ask the client to touch the roof of the mouth with the tip of the tongue. The ventral surface should be smooth and pink.
- Palpate the area under the tongue.
- Check for lesions or nodules. Using a gauze pad, grasp the tongue and inspect for any lumps or nodules (Figure 9.43). The tissue should be smooth.

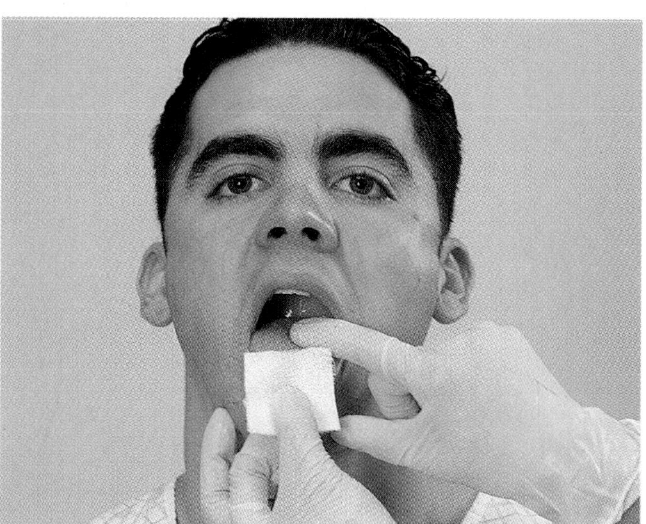

Figure 9.43 Palpating the tongue.

- Use a tongue blade to hold the tongue aside while you inspect the mucous lining of the mouth and the gums.
- Confirm that these areas are pink, moist, smooth, and free of lesions.
- Confirm the integrity of both the soft and the hard palate.

Step 4 ***Inspect the salivary glands.***

The salivary glands open into the mouth. Wharton's duct (submandibular) opens close to the lingual frenulum. Stensen's ducts (parotid) open opposite the second upper molars. Both ducts are visible, whereas the ducts of the sublingual glands are not visible.

- Confirm that all salivary ducts are visible, with no pain, tenderness, swelling, or redness.
- Touch the area close to the ducts with a sterile applicator, and confirm the flow of saliva.

SPECIAL CONSIDERATIONS

A smooth, coated, or hairy tongue is usually related to dehydration or disease. A small tongue may indicate undernutrition. Tremor of the tongue may indicate a dysfunction of the hypoglossal nerve (CN XII). Persistent lesions on the tongue must be evaluated further. Cancerous lesions occur most commonly on the sides or at the base of the tongue. The gums are diseased if there is bleeding, retraction, or overgrowth onto the teeth.

ASSESSMENT TECHNIQUE/NORMAL FINDINGS

SPECIAL CONSIDERATIONS

Step 5 *Inspect the throat.*

Use a tongue blade and a penlight to inspect the throat (Figure 9.44).

Viral pharyngitis may accompany a cold. Tonsils may be bright red, swollen, and may have white spots on them.

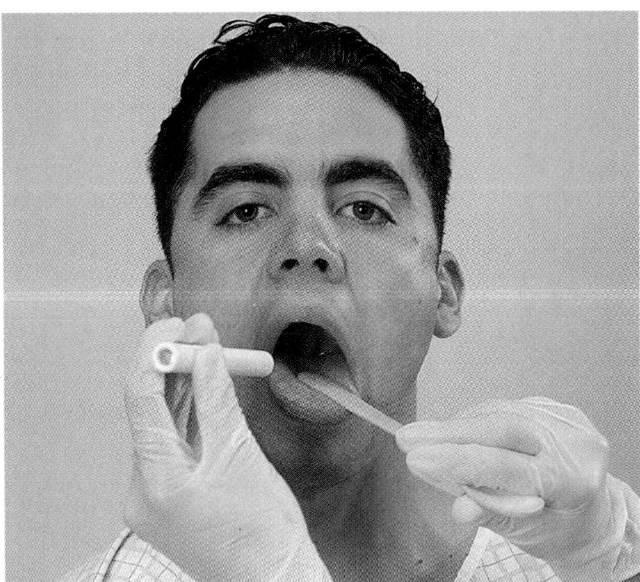

Figure 9.44 Inspecting the oral cavity.

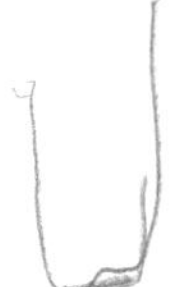

- Ask the client to open the mouth wide, tilt the head back, and say "aah." The uvula should rise in the midline.
- Use the tongue blade to depress the middle of the arched tongue enough so that you can clearly visualize the throat, but not so much that the client gags. Ask the client to say "aah" again.
- Confirm the rising of the soft palate, which is a test for cranial nerve X. (See Chapter 18 for further discussion.)
- Confirm that the tonsils, uvula, and posterior pharynx are pink, and are without inflammation, swelling, or lesions. Observe the tonsils behind the anterior tonsillar pillar. The color should be pink with slight vascularity present. Tonsils may be partially or totally absent.
- As you inspect the throat, note any mouth odors.
- Discard the tongue blade.

Clients with diabetic acidosis have a sweet, fruity breath. The breath of clients with kidney disease smells of ammonia.

The Neck

Step 1 *Inspect the neck for skin color, integrity, shape, and symmetry.*

- Observe for any swelling of the lymph nodes below the angle of the jaw and along the sternocleidomastoid muscle.

The head should be held erect with no tremors.

Excessive rigidity of the neck may indicate arthritis, and inability to hold the neck still may be due to muscle spasms. Swelling of the lymph nodes may indicate infection and requires further assessment (see Step 9).

ASSESSMENT TECHNIQUE/NORMAL FINDINGS	SPECIAL CONSIDERATIONS

Step 2 *Test the range of motion of the neck.*

ALERT!

When assessing range of motion of the neck, do so slowly to prevent dizziness in the client.

- Ask the client to move the chin to the chest, turn head right and left, then touch the left ear to left shoulder and the right ear to right shoulder (without raising the shoulders). Then ask the client to extend head back. (For further discussion, see Chapter 17.)

Any pain or limitation of movement could indicate arthritis, muscle spasm, or inflammation.

There should be no pain and no limitation of movement.

Step 3 *Observe the carotid arteries and jugular veins.*

The carotid artery runs just below the angle of the jaw, and its pulsations can be seen frequently. Assessment of the carotid arteries and jugular veins is discussed fully in Chapter 16.

Any distension or prominence may indicate a vascular disorder.

Step 4 *Palpate the trachea.*

- Palpate the sternal notch. Move the fingerpad of the palpating finger off the notch to the midline of the neck. Lightly palpate the area. You will feel the "C" rings (cricoid cartilages) of the trachea.
- Move the finger laterally, first to the right and then to the left. You have now identified the lateral borders of the trachea.
- The trachea should be midline, and the distance to the sternocleidomastoid muscles on each side should be equal.
- Place your thumb and index finger on each side of the trachea and slide them upward. As the trachea begins to widen, you have identified the thyroid cartilage.
- Continue to slide your thumb and index finger high into the neck. Palpate the hyoid bone. The greater horns of the hyoid bone are most prominent.
- Confirm that the hyoid bone and tracheal cartilages move when the client swallows.

Tracheal displacement is the result of masses in the neck or mediastinum, pneumothorax, or fibrosis.

Step 5 *Inspect the thyroid gland.*

The thyroid is not observable normally until the client swallows.

- Give the client a cup of water.
- Distinguish the thyroid from other structures in the neck by asking the client to drink a sip of water.

The thyroid tissue is attached to the trachea, and, as the client swallows, it moves superiorly. You may want to adjust the lighting in the room if possible so that shadows are cast on the client's neck. This may help you to visualize the thyroid.

If the client has any enlargement of the thyroid or masses near the thyroid, they appear as bulges when the client swallows.

ASSESSMENT TECHNIQUE/NORMAL FINDINGS

Step 6 *Palpate the thyroid gland from behind the client.*

Normally, the thyroid gland is nonpalpable, and so you need to be patient as you learn this technique.

- Stand behind the client.
- Ask the client to sit up straight, lower the chin, and turn the head slightly to the right. This position causes the client's neck muscles to relax.
- Using the fingers of your left hand, push the trachea to the right.
- With the fingers of the right hand, palpate the area between the trachea and the sternocleidomastoid muscle. Slowly and gently retract the sternocleidomastoid muscle, then ask the client to drink a sip of water.
- Palpate as the thyroid gland moves up during swallowing (Figure 9.45). Normally you will not feel the thyroid gland, although in some clients with long, thin necks, you may be able to feel the isthmus. Reverse the procedure for the left side.

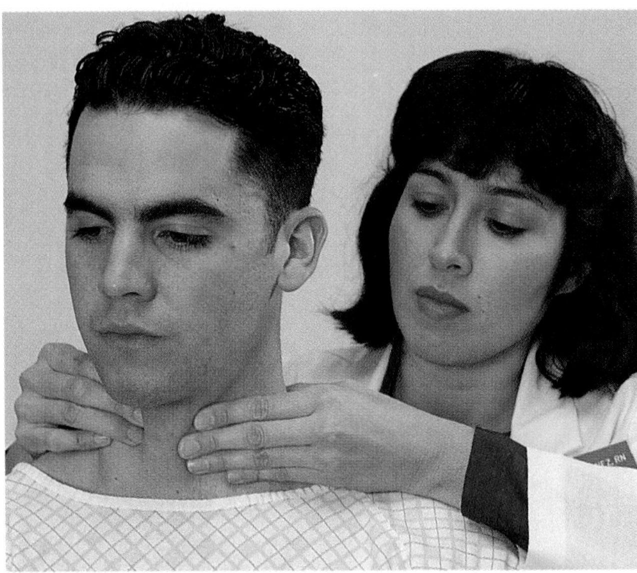

Figure 9.45 Palpating the thyroid: posterior approach.

ALERT!

Never attempt to palpate both lobes of the thyroid gland simultaneously.

Step 7 *Palpate the thyroid gland from in front of the client.*

This is an alternative approach to step 6.

SPECIAL CONSIDERATIONS

An enlarged thyroid gland may be due to a metabolic disorder such as hyperthyroidism. Palpable masses of 5 mm or larger are alterations in health. Their location, size, and shape should be documented, and the client should be evaluated further.

ASSESSMENT TECHNIQUE/NORMAL FINDINGS | SPECIAL CONSIDERATIONS

- Stand in front of the client.
- Ask the client to lower the head and turn slightly to the right.
- Using the thumb of your right hand, push the trachea to the right (Figure 9.46).

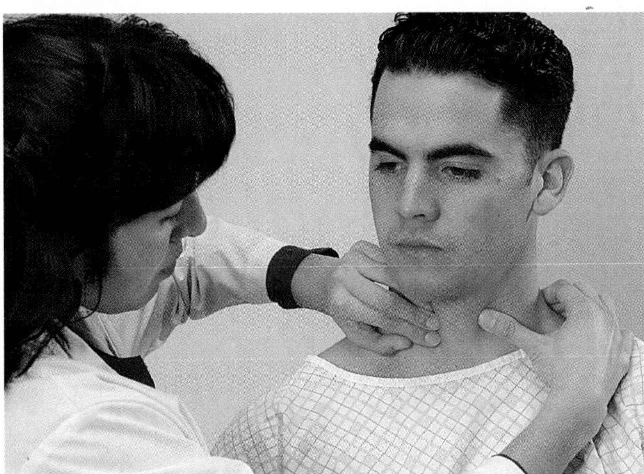

Figure 9.46 Palpating the thyroid: anterior approach.

- Place your left thumb and fingers over the sternocleidomastoid muscle and feel for any enlargement of the right lobe as the client swallows. Have water available to make swallowing easier.
- Reverse the procedure for the left side.

Step 8 ***Auscultate the thyroid.***

If the thyroid is enlarged, the area over the thyroid is auscultated to detect any bruits. In an enlarged thyroid, blood flows through the arteries at an accelerated rate, producing a soft, rushing sound. This sound can best be detected with the bell of the stethoscope.

The presence of a bruit is abnormal and is an indication of increased blood flow.

Step 9 ***Palpate the head and neck lymph nodes.***

- Palpate the lymph nodes by exerting gentle circular pressure with the fingerpads of both hands. It is important to avoid strong pressure, which can push the nodes into the muscle and underlying structures, making them difficult to find. It is also important to establish a routine for examination; otherwise, it is possible to omit one or more of the groups of nodes. One suggested order of examination is (Figure 9.47 on page 204):

  1. Preauricular
  2. Postauricular and occipital
  3. Retropharyngeal and submaxillary
  4. Submental (with one hand)
  5. Superficial cervical chain
  6. Deep cervical chain
  7. Supraclavicular

Enlargement of lymph nodes is called *lymphadenopathy* and can be due to infection, allergies, or a tumor.

ASSESSMENT TECHNIQUE/NORMAL FINDINGS | SPECIAL CONSIDERATIONS

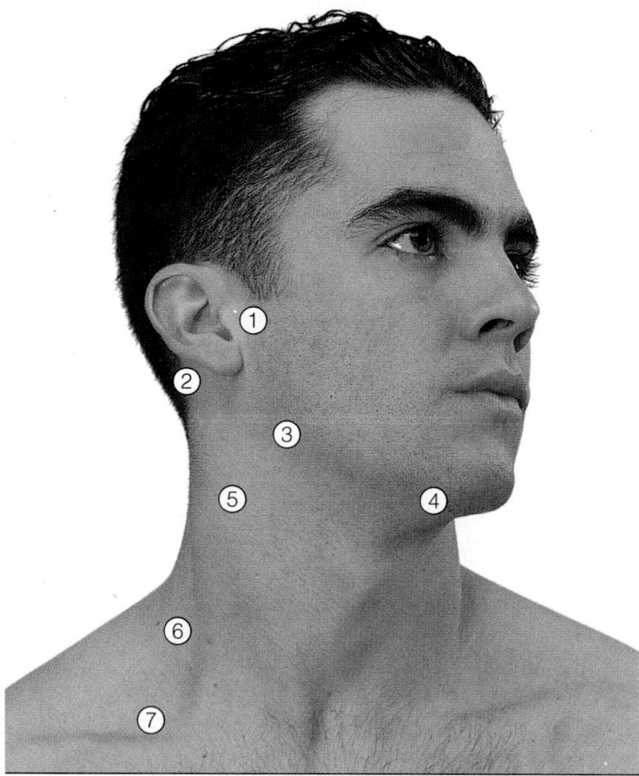

Figure 9.47 Suggested sequence for palpating lymph nodes.

- Ask the client to bend the head toward the side being examined to relax the muscles and make the nodes easier to palpate.
- If any lymph nodes are palpable, make a note of their location, size, shape, fixation or mobility, and tenderness.

Reminders

- In addition to the preceding steps, consider the common variations in physical assessment findings discussed below.
- After completing the physical assessment, answer any questions the client may have, and provide appropriate teaching for health promotion and self-care (see pages 220–222).
- Confirm that the client is comfortable and has no adverse effects from the procedure, then dim the lights and leave the client to rest or to get dressed.
- Document the assessment findings as described in Chapter 1. See pages 208–209 for nursing diagnoses commonly associated with the head and neck.

Developmental Considerations

Infant, Children, and Adolescent Clients

An infant's head should be measured at each visit until the age of 2 years. It should be symmetric from all angles. The head is larger than the chest until the age of 2. Any abnormal increase in head size or failure to grow should be noted. The newborn's skull is shown in Figure 9.48. Suture lines in the skull should be palpable until the age of 6 months. Palpable suture lines in a child older than 6 months of age can indicate hydrocephalus or Down syndrome. Fontanels should be firm and even with the surface of the skull. Slight pulsations of the fontanels are normal. An indented fontanel may indicate dehydration. Bulging fontanels may indicate increased intracranial pressure. It is common to discover bruits when auscultating the skull in children under the age of 4 or 5. After age 5, bruits are an indication of increased intracranial pressure.

At birth, the iris has very little color, and the pupils are small. Infants are born with myopic vision, but peripheral vision is fully developed. By 3 to 4 months of age, the infant can fixate on one visual field with both eyes: this ability is called *binocularity*. The eyes reach adult size by 8 years of age. An ophthalmoscopic examination is difficult in children younger than school age; however, the red reflex should be elicited from birth. Peripheral vision may be assessed by confrontation in children older than 3 years. It is important to assess extraocular muscle function as early as possible in young children because delay can lead to permanent visual damage. The corneal light reflex can be used to determine symmetry of muscle function. Some asymmetry is normal under 6 months of age.

When examining the ears, note the position and alignment. The top of the ear should be even with the inner and outer canthus of the eye (Figure 9.49 on page 206). The child's auditory tube is more horizontal than the adult's, which leads to more frequent infections from the pharynx. The infant's external auditory canal is shorter than the adult's and has an upward curve, which persists until about 3 years of age. Therefore, in children younger than 3, you must grasp the lower portion of the pinna and pull the ear downward and backward to straighten the ear canal before inserting the otoscope (Figure 9.50 on page 206).

A nasal speculum is usually not used to examine the nose of an infant or small child. The preferred method is to push the tip of the child's nose with your thumb, then shine a penlight into the nares. In children younger than 8 years, the sinus area is too small to evaluate by palpation, so it is not necessary to do so.

Both sets of teeth develop before birth. The deciduous teeth begin to erupt between 6 months of age and 2 years of age. Eruption of the permanent teeth begins at about age 6 and continues throughout adolescence. Count the number of teeth the child has and ascertain whether they are appropriate for age. Infants frequently have small white pearly patches on the gums and hard palate. Called *Epstein's pearls,* they are small cysts that disappear a few weeks after birth.

Assess the range of motion of the neck by turning the infant's head from side to side. Then gently flex and extend the neck. When examining older children, ask them to look in different directions. An infant should be able to hold the head at a 90-degreee angle from a prone position by 2 months of age and be able to hold the head up in a seated position by 3 months. The thyroid is difficult to palpate on an infant, but it can be accomplished on a child using two or three fingers. Lymph nodes are usually not palpable in infants, but a child's nodes may be very prominent. Nodes up to 1 cm in size are considered normal, but they should be nontender, movable, and discrete.

Frontal bone
Frontal suture
Anterior fontanel
Coronal suture
Sagittal suture
Parietal bone
Posterior fontanel
Lambdoidal suture
Occipital bone

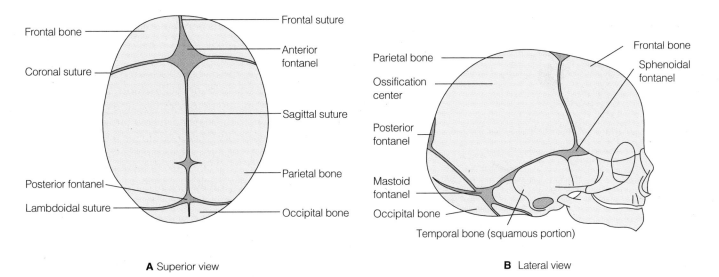

A Superior view

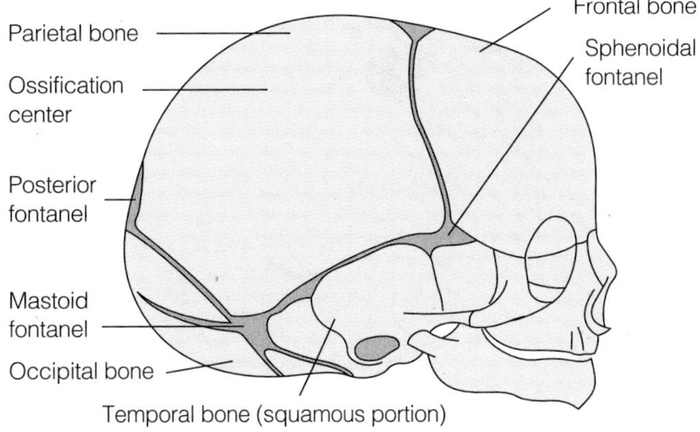

B Lateral view

Figure 9.48 The newborn's skull.

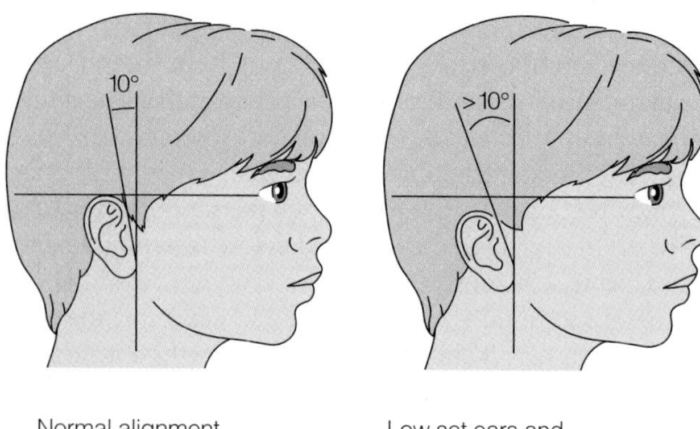

Figure 9.49 Normal alignment of a child's ears.

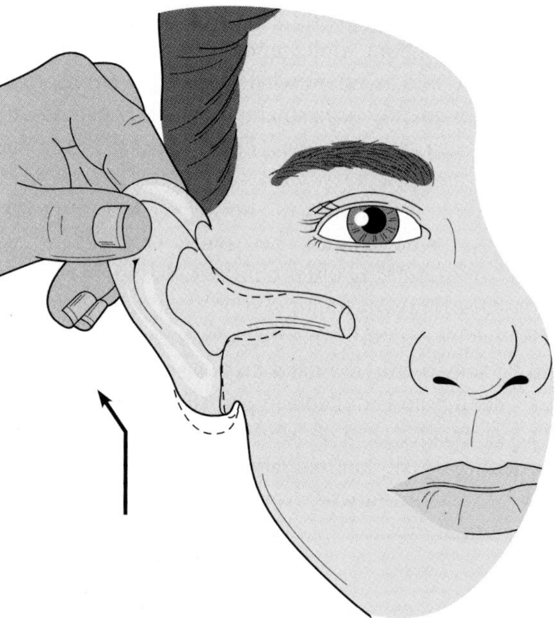

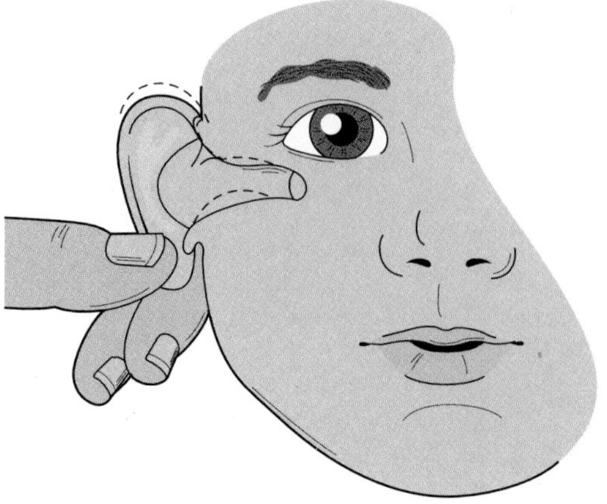

Figure 9.50 Procedure for pulling the pinna before inserting the otoscope in the adult and the child.

Childbearing Clients

The childbearing client may develop blotchy pigmented spots on her face, facial edema, and enlargement of the thyroid. All of these symptoms are considered normal and subside after childbirth. She may also complain of headaches during the first trimester, which may be related to increased hormones, but severe persistent headaches should be evaluated.

The childbearing client may complain of dry eyes and may discontinue wearing contact lenses during her pregnancy. The client may also describe vision changes due to shifting fluid in the cornea. These symptoms are usually not significant and disappear after childbirth. Changes in eyesight, especially blurred or double vision, distorted color perception, or temporary blindness, should be reported to an ophthalmologist.

Nasal congestion and nosebleeds due to increased estrogen levels during pregnancy are common. The client may also become aware of a sense of fullness in the ears, resulting in some degree of hearing loss. This condition is also due to the elevated levels of estrogen, which cause increased vascularity of the upper respiratory tract. Bleeding gums with normal toothbrushing is also related to the increase in estrogen levels, which produces increased vascularity of the gums.

Older Clients

Mild rhythmic nodding of the head due to *senile tremors* is usually a normal finding. Senile tremors may also cause slight protrusion of the tongue.

By age 45, the lens of the eye loses elasticity, and the ciliary muscles become weaker, resulting in a decreased ability of the lens to change shape to accommodate for near vision. This condition is called *presbyopia*. The loss of fat from the orbit of the eye produces a drooping appearance. The lacrimal glands decrease tear production, and the client may complain of a burning sensation in the eyes. The cornea of the eye may appear cloudy, and you may detect a deposit of white-yellow material around the cornea, called *arcus senilis*. This is a deposition of fat, but it is considered normal and has no effect on vision. The pupillary light reflex is slower with age, and the pupils may be smaller in size.

Within the eye, the blood vessels are paler in color, and you may detect small round yellow dots scattered on the retina. They do not interfere with vision. As the client ages, the lens continues to thicken and yellow, forming a dense area that reduces lens clarity. This condition is the beginning of a *cataract* formation. Macular degeneration can occur in the older client, resulting in a loss of central vision. The ophthalmoscopic examination may reveal narrowed blood vessels with a granular pigment in the macula.

The client may have coarse hairs at the opening of the auditory meatus. The ears may appear more prominent, because cartilage formation continues throughout life. The tympanic membrane may be paler in color and thicker in appearance. Assessment of hearing may reveal a loss of high-frequency tones, which is consistent with aging. With time, this loss often progresses to lower-frequency sounds as well. Gradual hearing loss with age is called *presbycusis*.

As the adult ages, many changes occur inside the mouth. The lips and buccal mucosa of the mouth become thinner and less vascular, with a shiny surface. Gums are paler in color. The tongue develops more fissures, and motor function may become impaired, resulting in problems with swallowing. A decreased sense of taste and smell may contribute to a diminished appetite and poor nutrition. There may also be a decrease in saliva production. This decrease may be due to atrophy of the salivary glands, but is often due to side effects from medication. Gums begin to recede, and some tooth loss may occur due to osteoporosis. If teeth are lost, the remaining teeth may drift, causing malocclusion of the maxilla and mandible. This condition can produce headaches and muscle spasms of the jaw. You may notice lesions in the mouth that may be due to ill-fitting dentures, or marked deterioration of old dental restorations. Refer the client to a dentist.

Psychosocial Considerations

A client who is under a great deal of stress may be prone to headaches, including tension headaches, neck pain, and mouth ulcers. Pain in the temporomandibular joint may be due to unconscious clenching of the jaw during stressful situations, such as driving in heavy traffic or taking an exam. Chronic TMJ syndrome may eventually result in a wearing down of the teeth, and the client may need to consult a dentist. Other indications of psychosocial disturbances include tics (involuntary muscle spasms), hair twisting or pulling, biting the lips, and excessive blinking. Relaxation techniques such as meditation and guided imagery may help relieve head and neck symptoms related to stress. If appropriate, refer the client to a mental health professional for assistance.

Self-Care Considerations

It is essential to consider the client's self-care when you assess the head and neck. Most clients spend more time caring for this unique and highly visible region than any other part of the body. The way the client cares for the hair, face, and teeth may afford clues to the client's overall health status or may indicate musculoskeletal problems, neurologic impairments, or psychosocial disturbances.

There may be a link between the client's food consumption and the onset of headaches. Some clients find that eating chocolate or cheese, for example, triggers their headaches. Alchohol ingestion may also lead to headaches.

Helmets are absolutely essential for people riding motorcycles or bicycles, and those participating in certain sports such as hockey or football. The use of seatbelts in automobiles decreases the client's risk of head injury.

Excessive sun exposure without the use of sunglasses may promote cataract formation. A deficiency of vitamin A may cause night blindness. Some medications have side effects that may cause excessive corneal dryness, vision changes, or increased intraocular pressure. When assessing a client who wears contact lenses, ask how long the client wears the lenses each day and evaluate the client's cleansing routine. Sharing eye makeup increases the risk for infection and should be avoided.

Cleaning the ears with invasive instruments can result in trauma. Even cleaning with cotton-tipped swabs may impact cerumen and result in hearing loss. Note that certain medications may cause hearing disturbances such as ringing in the ears.

Clients may have a knowledge deficit related to poor hygiene if teeth have tartar buildup. Some medications, especially if used in childhood, cause permanent discoloration of the teeth. Teeth may also yellow with use of tobacco. Smoking and chewing tobacco increases the risk of oral cancers. Some medications, such as anticholinergics, decrease saliva production and may cause the client's oral mucosa to feel particularly dry. Mouth odors may be due to poor dental hygiene, heavy smoking, or alcohol consumption. Mouth odors may also be affected by the client's diet, especially the use of certain spices.

Family, Cultural, and Environmental Considerations

Asian clients have epicanthic folds (a vertical fold of skin) covering the inner canthus of the eye. Dark-skinned people may have dark pigmented spots on the sclera, and their retinas may be darker. People with light-colored eyes typically have lighter retinas and better night vision but are more sensitive to bright sunlight and artificial light. Dark-skinned clients may also have darker cerumen in the ear, and their oral mucosa may be darker.

People of European ancestry tend to have more tooth decay and tooth loss than people of African ancestry, probably because people of African ancestry tend to have harder and denser tooth enamel. The size of the teeth varies with cultural ancestry, too. People of European descent have the smallest teeth, and Asians, Eskimos, and Australian Aborigines the largest.

A client's occupation may increase the risk for traumatic injury to the eyes or for hearing loss. For example, construction workers, welders, auto mechanics, groundskeepers, farmers, and many others should be evaluated for the use of protective eyewear and/or earplugs. Noise levels in the client's home environment may also need to be evaluated. Clients who live near airports or construction sites and clients who frequently listen to loud music may be at risk for hearing loss.

Remember that a client's socioeconomic status affects the appearance and health of the head and neck. For example, many clients do not have dental insurance and cannot afford regular dental care. Referral to a low-cost dental clinic or a dental school offering free care may be appropriate.

Table 9.1 Nursing Diagnoses Commonly Associated with the Head and Neck

SENSORY/PERCEPTUAL ALTERATION: VISUAL, AUDITORY, OLFACTORY

Definition: A state in which an individual experiences a change in the amount or interpretation of incoming stimuli accompanied by an absent, diminished, exaggerated, or distorted response to such stimuli. These altered responses are a change from the individual's usual response to stimuli and are not a result of mental or personality disorders (NANDA).

DEFINING CHARACTERISTICS

Anxiety
Altered abstraction
Altered conceptualization
Measured change in sensory acuity
Change in usual response to stimuli
Indication of altered body image
Apathy
Disorientation to person, place, time, or situation
Altered communication patterns

RELATED FACTORS

Alcohol/substance abuse (specify), Electrolyte imbalance, Altered sensory reception, transmission and/or integration secondary to CVA, brain trauma, increased intracranial pressure, and so on, Sensory deficit (specify), Sensory overload, Altered environmental stimuli, Others specific to client (specify).

IMPAIRED SWALLOWING

Definition: The state in which an individual has decreased ability to voluntarily pass fluids and/or solids from the mouth to the stomach (NANDA).

DEFINING CHARACTERISTICS

Major

Observed evidence of difficulty in swallowing (eg, stasis of food in oral cavity, coughing/choking)

Minor

Evidence of aspiration

RELATED FACTORS

Altered sensory reception, transmission, and/or integration, Irritated oropharyngeal cavity, Mechanical obstruction, Neuromuscular impairment, Fatigue, Psychologic impairment (specify), Others specific to client (specify).

Table 9.1 Diagnoses Associated with the Head and Neck (continued)

ALTERED ORAL MUCOUS MEMBRANE	
Definition: The state in which an individual experiences disruptions in the tissue layers of the oral cavity (NANDA).	
DEFINING CHARACTERISTICS	
Discomfort with hot or cold foods	Dry, cracked lips
Oral pain/discomfort	Dry mouth
Oral lesions or ulcers	Irritation, inflammation, or ulceration of oral mucosa
Lack of or decreased salivation	Dental caries
Edema	Leukoplakia
Hyperemia	Vesicles
Oral plaque	Hemorrhagic gingivitis
Bad breath	Stomatitis
Coated tongue	
RELATED FACTORS	
Inadequate oral hygiene, Chemotherapy, Lack of or decreased salivation, Medication, Infection, Malnutrition, Radiation to head and neck, Dehydration, NPO for more than 24 hours, Mouth breathing, Trauma (chemical, eg, acidic foods, drugs, noxious agents, alcohol; mechanical, eg, ill-fitting dentures, braces, tubes [nasogastric, endotracheal], surgery in oral cavity), Others specific to client (specify).	

Organizing the Data

After carrying out the focused interview and conducting the physical assessment of the head and neck, group the related data into clusters leading to either nursing diagnoses, which require nursing interventions such as client teaching (discussed on pages 220–222), or alterations in health, which require consultation with other members of the health care team.

Identifying Nursing Diagnoses

Because the head and neck is not a distinct system, but consists of several systems, several nursing diagnoses may be appropriate (Table 9.1). *Sensory/perceptual alterations: visual, auditory, gustatory, or olfactory* may be appropriate if there is an altered response to incoming stimuli from the eyes, ears, mouth, or nose. *Impaired swallowing* may apply if the client has difficulty passing food or fluids from the mouth to the stomach. The client who is experiencing impaired tissue integrity of the oral cavity would probably be given a diagnosis of *altered oral mucous membrane*.

Other nursing diagnoses that may apply include *body image disturbance*; *ineffective individual coping*; *high risk for injury*; *acute or chronic pain*; and *powerlessness*. If the client is unable to maintain a safe home environment because of an alteration in vision or hearing, an appropriate nursing diagnosis is *impaired home maintenance management*.

Common Alterations in the Health of the Head and Neck

Common alterations in the health of the head and neck include headaches, problems related to vision and hearing, oral cancer, and many others. (See Tables 9.2–9.6.)

Table 9.2 Common Alterations in the Health of the Head and Neck

Headaches

Classic migraine A classic migraine is usually preceded by an "aura" during which the client may feel depressed, restless, or irritable; see spots or flashes of light; feel nauseated; or experience numbing or tingling in the face or extremities. The pain of the migraine itself may be mild or debilitating, requiring the client to lie down in the darkness in silence. It is usually a pulsating pain that is localized to the side, front, or back of the head and may be accompanied by nausea, vertigo, tremors, and other symptoms. The acute phase of a classic migraine typically lasts from 4 to 6 hours.

Cluster headache A cluster headache is so named because numerous episodes occur over a period of days or even months and then are followed by a period of remission during which no headaches occur. Cluster headaches have no "aura." Their onset is sudden and may be associated with alcohol consumption, stress, or emotional distress. They often begin suddenly at night with an excrutiating pain on one side of the face spreading upward to behind one eye. The nose and affected eye water, and nasal congestion is common. They may last for only a few minutes or up to a few hours.

Tension headache A tension headache, also known as a muscle contraction headache, is due to sustained contraction of the muscles in the head, neck, or upper back. The onset is gradual, not sudden, and the pain is usually steady, not throbbing. The pain may be unilateral or bilateral and typically ranges from the cervical region to the top of the head. Tension headaches may be associated with stress, overwork, dental problems, premenstrual syndrome, sinus inflammation, and other health problems.

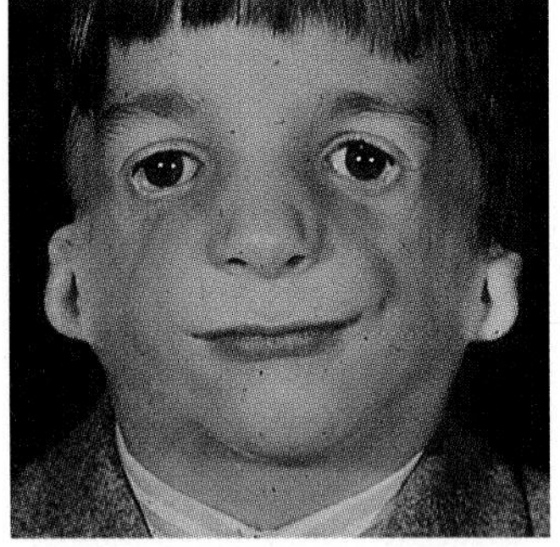

Enlargement of the skull and cranial bones due to increased growth hormone.

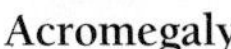

Acromegaly

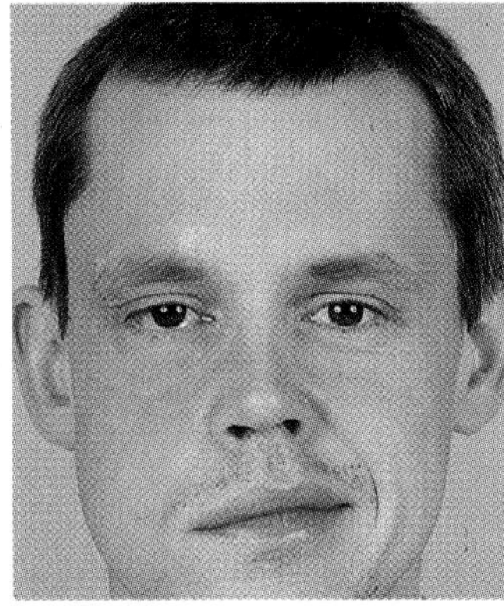

A temporary disorder affecting cranial nerve VII and producing a unilateral facial paralysis. It may be caused by a virus. Its onset is sudden, and it usually resolves spontaneously in a few weeks without residual effects.

Bell's Palsy

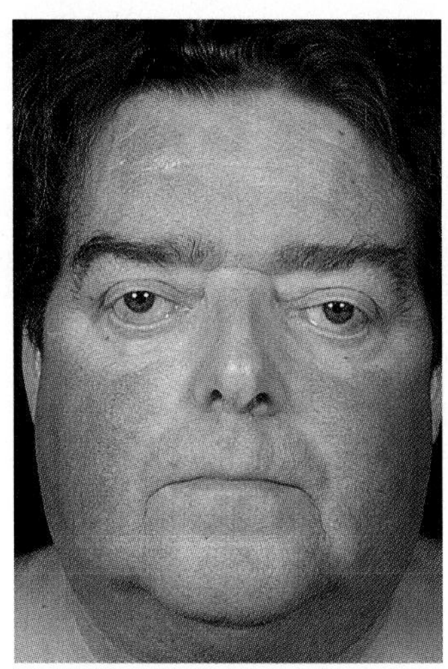

Increased adrenal hormone production leading to a rounded "moon" face, ruddy cheeks, prominent jowls, and excess facial hair.

Cushing's Syndrome

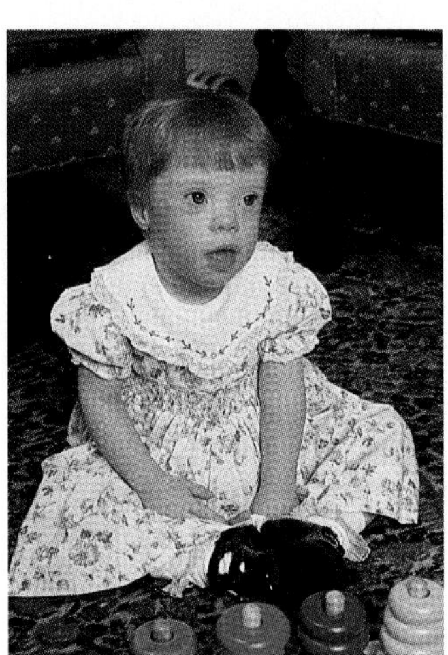

A chromosomal defect causing varying degrees of mental retardation and characteristic facial features such as slanted eyes, a flat nasal bridge, a flat nose, a protruding tongue, and a short, broad neck.

Down Syndrome

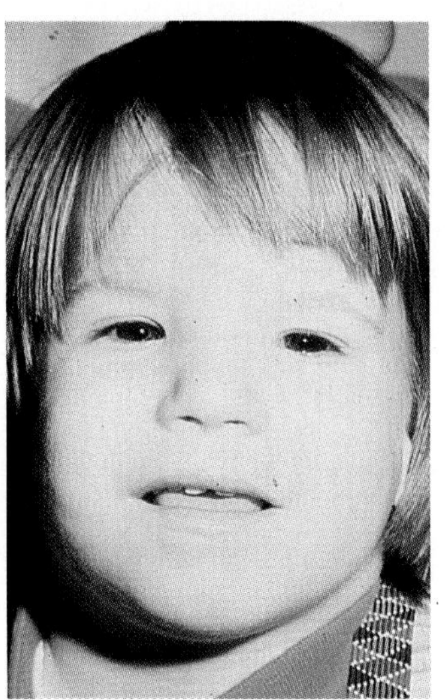

Disorder characterized by epicanthal folds, narrow palpebral fissures, a deformed upper lip below the septum of the nose, and some degree of mental retardation. Fetal alcohol syndrome is seen in infants of mothers whose intake of alcohol during pregnancy was significant.

Fetal Alcohol Syndrome

Table 9.2 Common Alterations in the Health of the Head and Neck (continued)

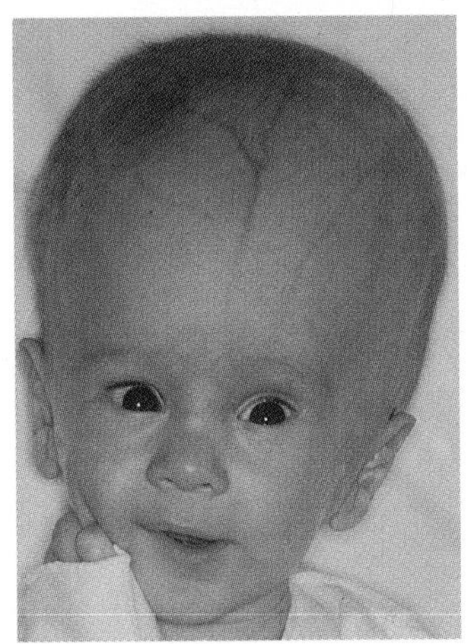

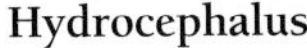

Hydrocephalus

Enlargement of the head caused by inadequate drainage of cerebrospinal fluid resulting in abnormal growth of the skull.

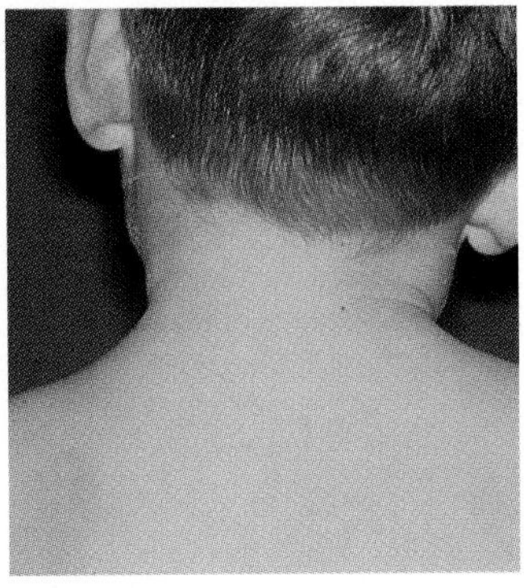

Torticollis

Spasm of the sternocleidomastoid muscle on one side of the body, which often results from birth trauma. If left untreated, the muscle becomes fibrotic and permanently shortened.

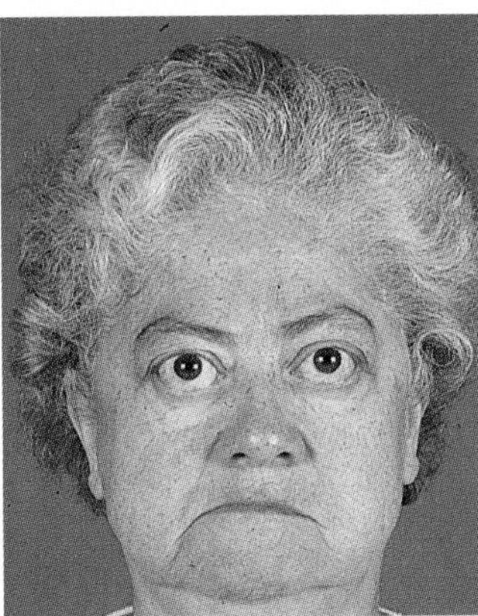

Hyperthyroidism

Excessive secretion of the thyroid gland, causing diffuse enlargement of the gland, exophthalmos (bulging eyes), fine hair, weight loss, diarrhea, and other alterations.

Table 9.3 Common Alterations in the Health of the Eyes

Arcus Senilis

A white ring around the cornea seen in elderly clients. It is caused by fat deposits. This is considered a normal condition and does not interfere with vision.

Diabetic Retinopathy

A vascular complication of diabetes that involves the blood vessels of the retina. Background retinopathy involves seepage of lipids through incompetent capillaries and infarction of the nerve layer. Proliferative retinopathy involves the development of new vessels, which may hemorrhage and cause blindness.

Glaucoma

A condition of increased intraocular pressure that damages the retina and may cause atrophy of the optic nerve. Vision loss is gradual and painless, and the client may be unaware of any alteration in health. Glaucoma is the second most common cause of blindness in the United States.

Pterygium

A triangular patch of mucous membrane growing on the conjunctiva, usually on the nasal side of the eye. It may eventually obstruct the vision as it grows toward the pupil. It occurs as a result of long exposure to the sun.

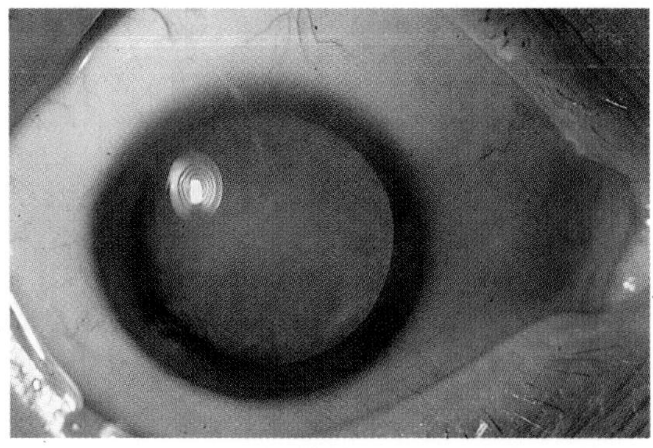

Cataract

A cataract is an opacity of the lens of the eye that is usually associated with advancing age.

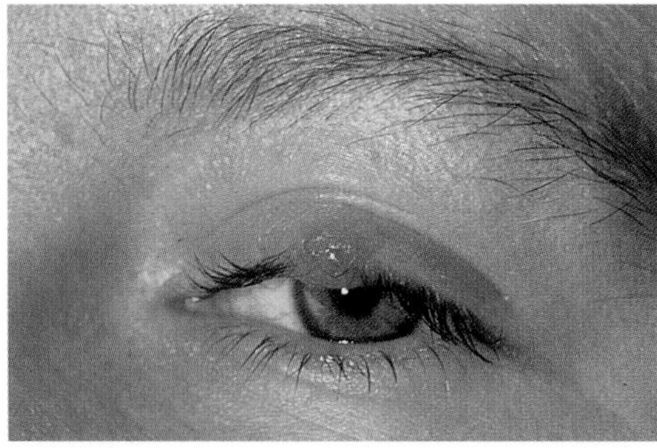

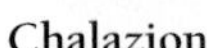

Chalazion

A firm, nontender nodule on the eyelid arising from infection of the meibomian gland rather than a hair follicle (see hordeolum below). It is not painful unless inflamed.

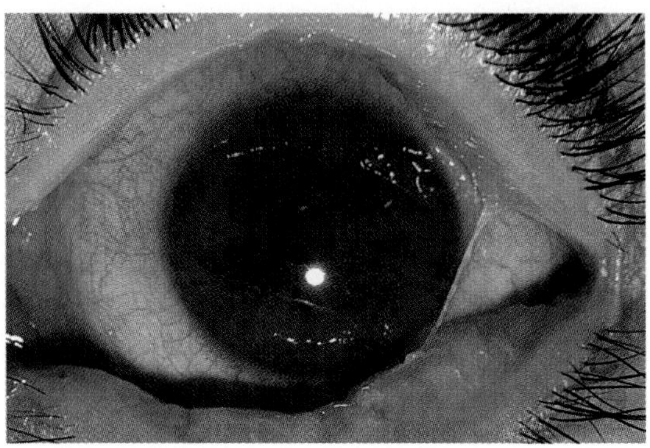

Conjunctivitis

An infection of the conjunctiva usually due to bacterial or viral agent or chemical exposure.

Table 9.3 Common Alterations in the Health of the Eyes (continued)

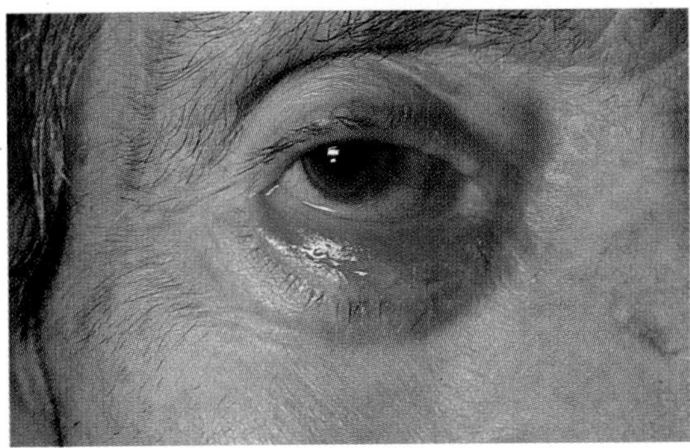

Ectropion

An eversion of the lower eyelid caused by decreased muscle tone. The palpebral conjunctiva is exposed and is thus at increased risk for inflammation.

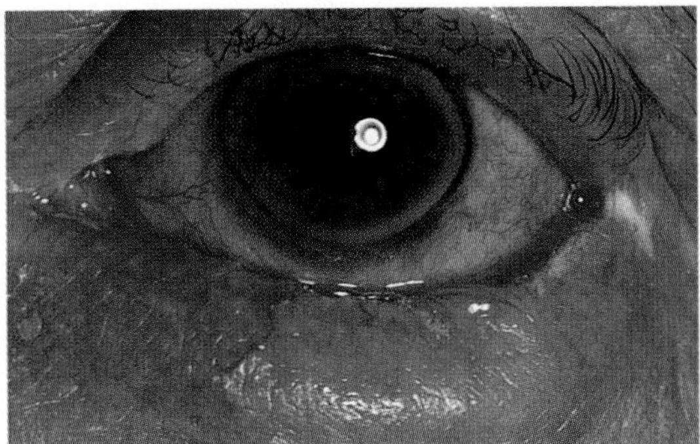

Entropion

An inversion of the lid and lashes caused by muscle spasms of the eyelid. Friction from the lashes may cause corneal irritation.

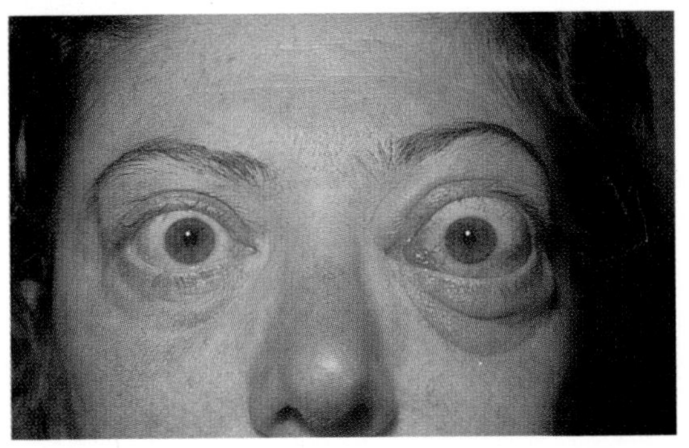

Exophthalmos

A frontal bulging of the eyes associated with hyperthyroidism and caused by deposits of fat and fluids in the retro-orbital tissues, forcing the eyeballs outward. The upper eyelids are usually retracted, and when the eye is open, the sclera above the iris is usually visible.

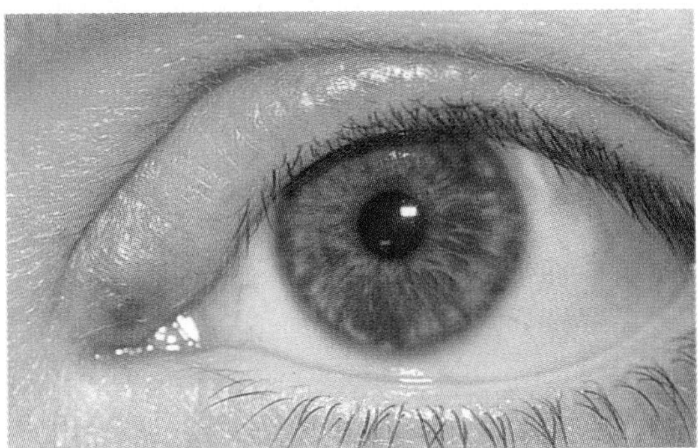

Hordeolum (Sty)

Staphyloccocal infection of hair follicles on the margin of the lids. The affected eye is usually very painful, red, and swollen.

Table 9.3 Common Alterations in the Health of the Eyes (continued)

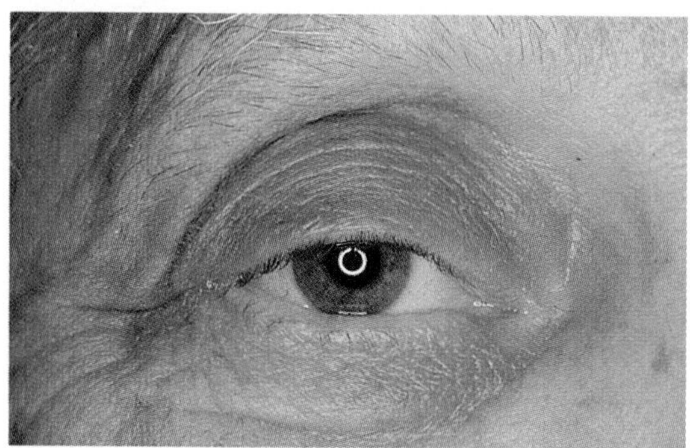
Ptosis

Drooping of the eyelid. This usually occurs with cranial nerve damage or systemic neuromuscular weakness.

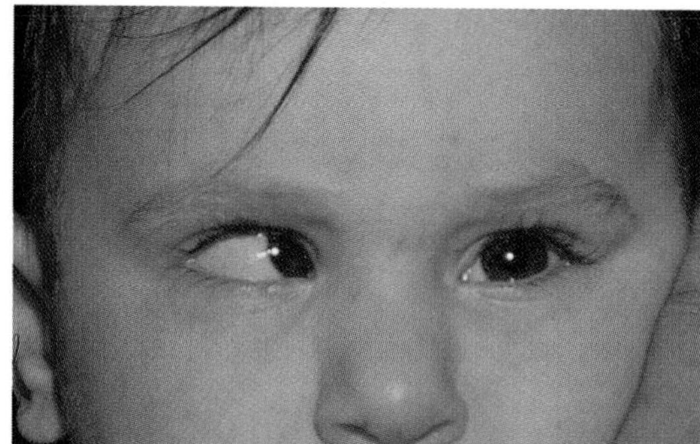
Strabismus

A deviation of the eyes in which the visual axes of the eyes don't meet at the desired point. Strabismus may be caused by an imbalance in muscle tone or by a weakness or paralysis of one or more of the extraocular muscles.

Table 9.4 Common Alterations in the Health of the Ears

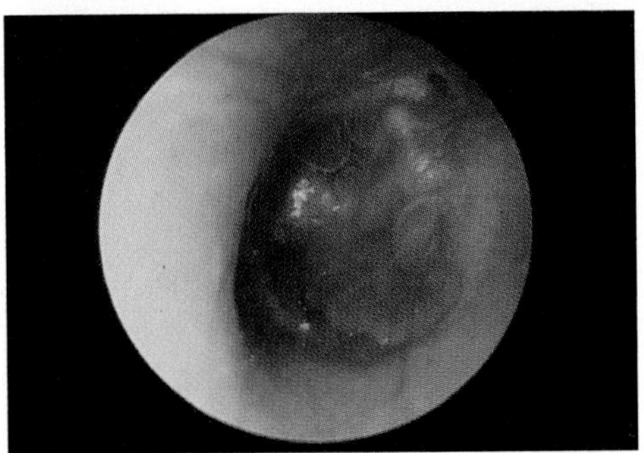

Hemotympanum

A bluish tinge to the tympanic membrane indicating the presence of blood in the middle ear. It is usually caused by head trauma.

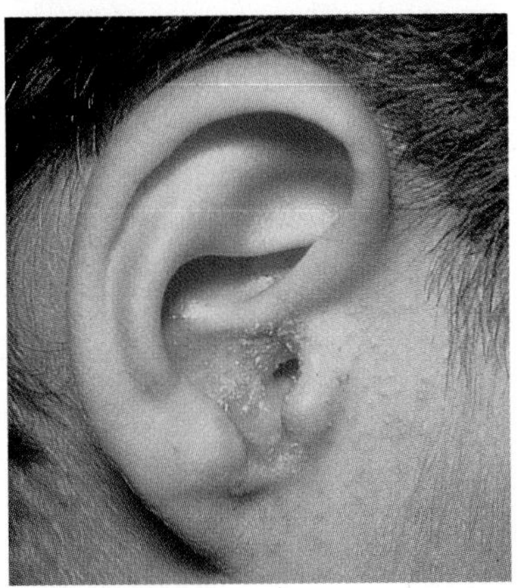

Otitis Externa

Infection of the outer ear, often called "swimmer's ear." Otitis externa causes redness and swelling of the auricle and ear canal. Drainage is usually scanty. It may be accompanied by itching, fever, and enlarged lymph nodes.

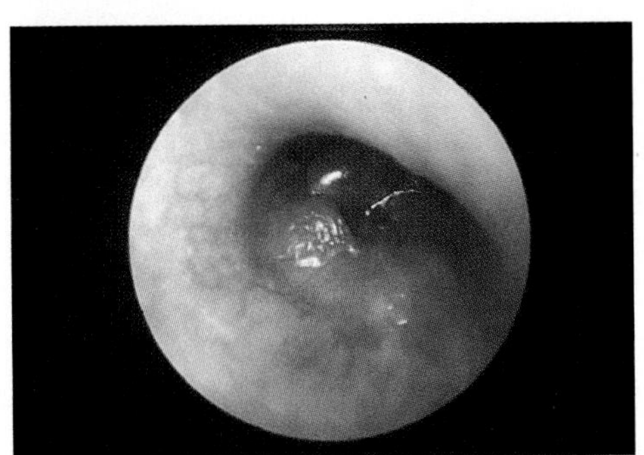

Otitis Media

Infection of the middle ear producing a red, bulging eardrum, fever, and hearing loss. The otoscopic examination reveals absent light reflex. More common in children, whose auditory tubes are wider, shorter, and more horizontal than those of adults and thus allow easier access for infections ascending from the pharynx.

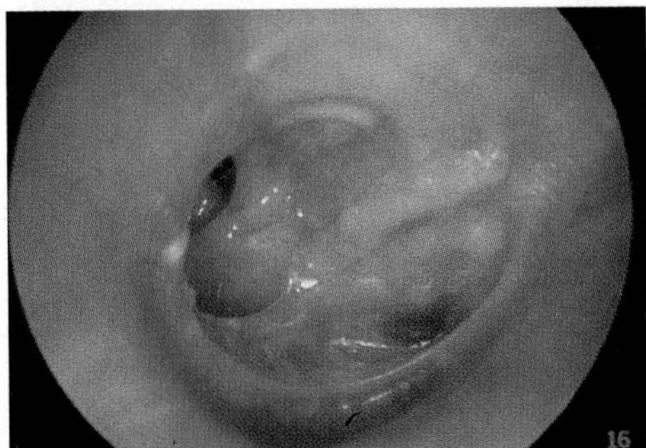

Perforation of Tympanic Membrane

A rupturing of the eardrum due to trauma or infection. During otoscopic inspection, the perforation may be seen as a dark spot on the eardrum.

Table 9.4 Common Alterations in the Health of the Ears (continued)

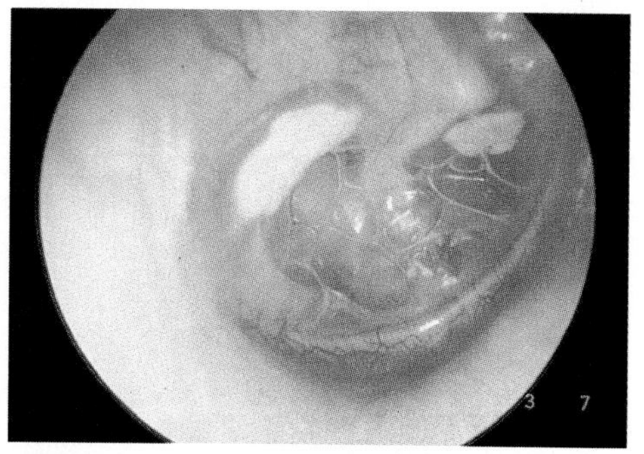

Scarred Tympanic Membrane

A condition in which the eardrum has white patches of scar tissue due to repeated ear infections.

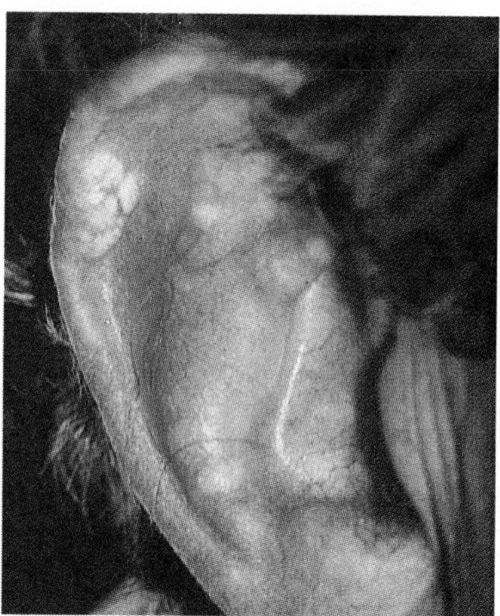

Tophi

Small white nodules on the helix or antihelix. The nodules contain uric acid crystals and are a symptom of gout.

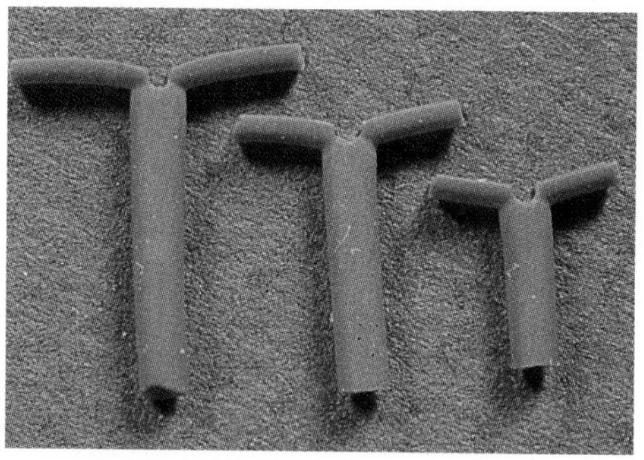

Tympanostomy Tubes

Ear tubes inserted to relieve middle ear pressure and allow drainage from repeated middle-ear infections.

Table 9.5 Common Alterations in the Health of the Nose and Sinuses

Epistaxis

Nosebleed. This may follow trauma, such as a blow to the nose, or it may accompany another alteration in health, such as rhinitis, hypertension, or a blood coagulation disorder.

Rhinitis

Nasal inflammation usually due to a viral infection or allergy. It is accompanied by a watery and often copious discharge, sneezing, and congestion ("stuffy nose"). Acute rhinitis is caused by a virus, whereas allergic rhinitis results from contact with allergens, eg, pollen and dust.

Sinusitis

Inflammation of the sinuses usually following an upper respiratory infection. It causes facial pain, inflammation, and discharge. It may be accompanied by fever, chills, or a dull, pulsating pain in the cheeks or teeth.

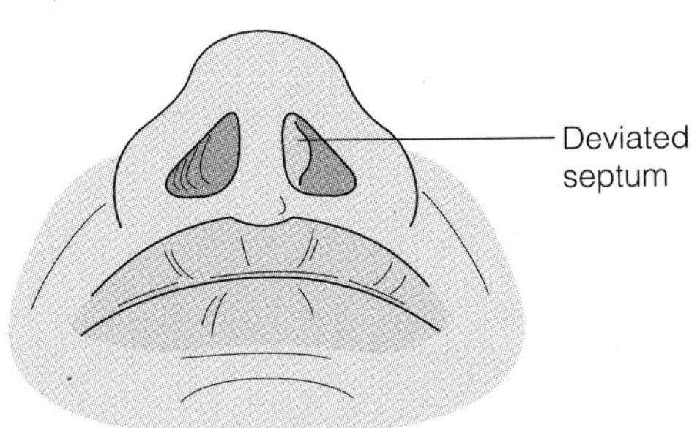

Deviated Septum

A slight ingrowth of the lower nasal septum. When viewed with a nasal speculum, one nasal cavity appears to have an outgrowth or shelf.

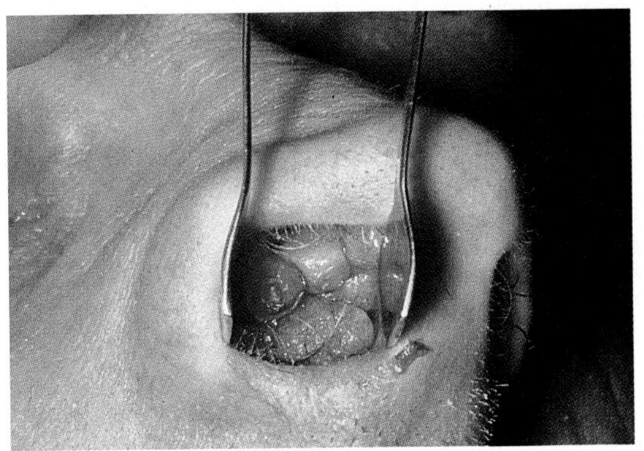

Nasal Polyps

Pale, round, firm, nonpainful overgrowths of nasal mucosa usually caused by chronic allergic rhinitis.

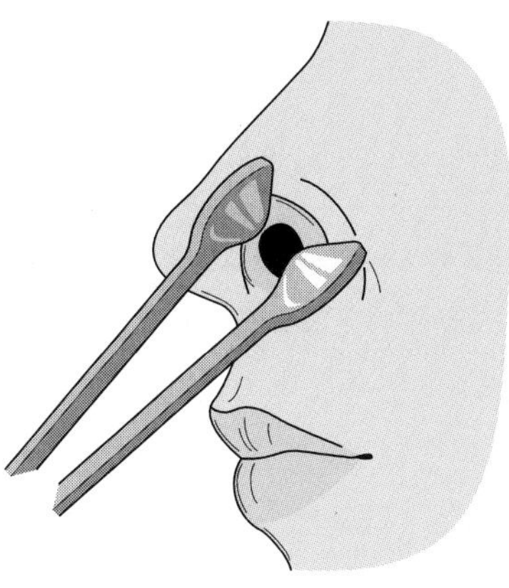

Perforated Septum

A hole in the septum caused by chronic infection, trauma, or sniffing cocaine. It can be detected by shining a penlight through the naris on the other side.

Table 9.6 Common Alterations in the Health of the Mouth and Throat

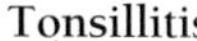

Gingival Hyperplasia

An enlargement of the gums frequently seen in pregnancy, leukemia, or after prolonged use of phenytoin (Dilantin).

Gingivitis

Inflammation of the gums. May be caused by poor dental hygiene or a deficiency of vitamin C. If left untreated, gingivitis may progress to periodontitis and tooth loss.

Tonsillitis

Inflammation of the tonsils. The throat is red and the tonsils are swollen and covered by white or yellow patches or exudate. Lymph nodes in the cervical chain may be enlarged. Tonsillitis may be accompanied by a high fever.

Smooth Tongue

A condition occurring as a result of vitamin B and iron deficiency. The surface of the tongue is smooth and red with a shiny appearance.

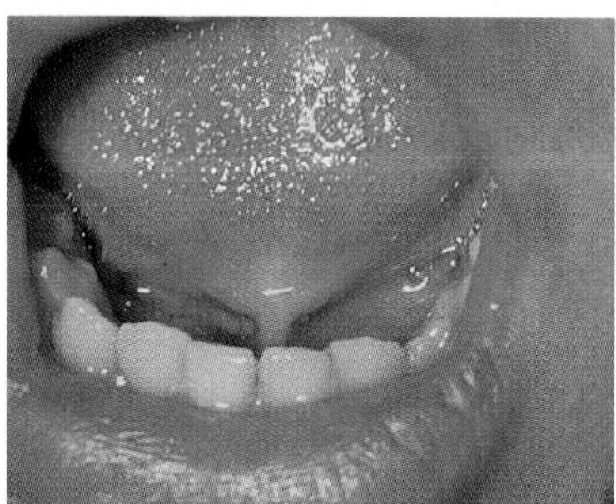

Ankyloglossia

A fixation of the tip of the tongue to the floor of the mouth due to a shortened lingual frenulum. The condition is usually congenital and may be corrected surgically.

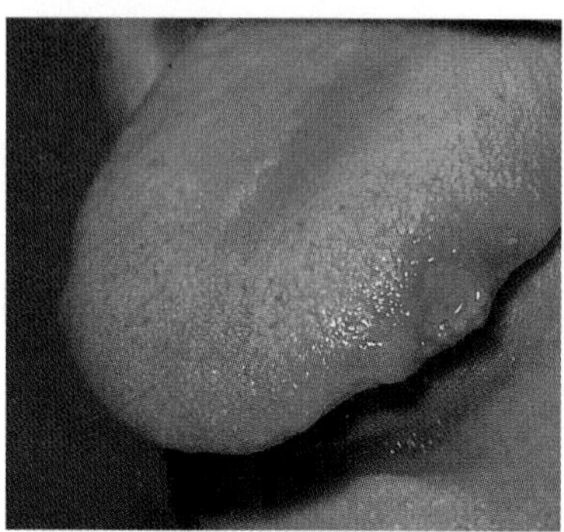

Aphthous Ulcers

Small, round, white lesions occuring singularly or in clusters on the oral mucosa. Commonly called "canker sores." The lesions are acutely painful when they come in contact with the tongue, a toothbrush, or food. They commonly result from oral trauma, such as jabbing the side of the mouth with a toothbrush, but they are also associated with stress, exhaustion, and allergies to certain foods.

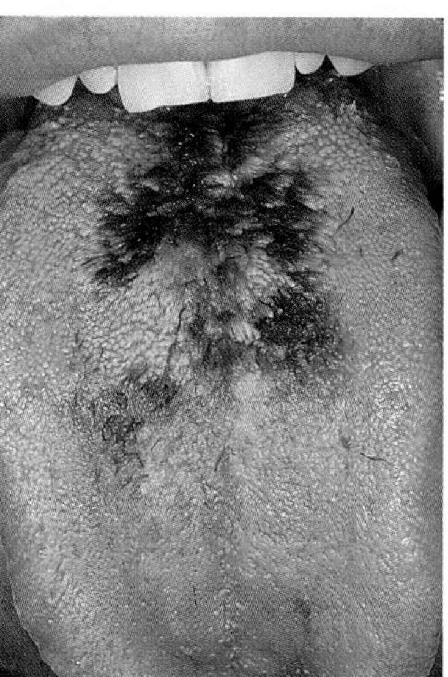

Black Hairy Tongue

A temporary condition caused by the inhibition of normal bacteria and the overgrowth of fungus on the papillae of the tongue. It is usually associated with the use of antibiotics.

Table 9.6 Common Alterations in the Health of the Mouth and Throat (continued)

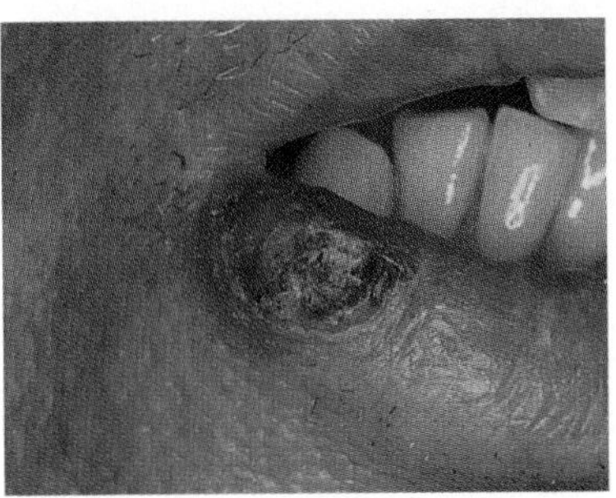

Carcinoma

Oral cancers are most commonly found on the lower lip or the base (underside) of the tongue. Cancer is suspected if a sore or lesion does not heal within a few weeks. Heavy smoking, especially pipe smoking, and chewing tobacco increase the risk of oral cancer, as does chronic heavy use of alcohol.

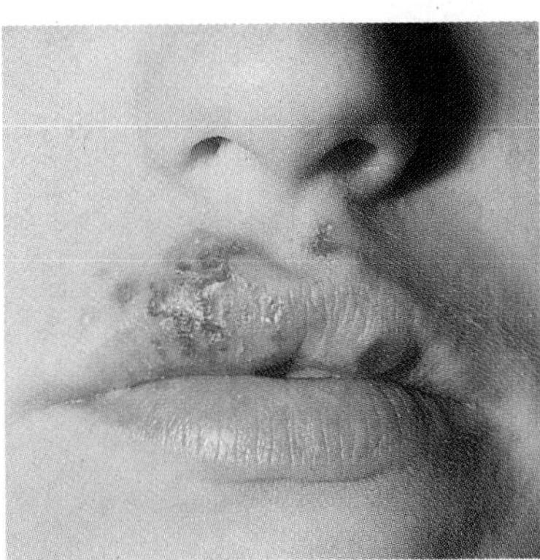

Herpes Simplex

A virus that is often accompanied by clear vesicles commonly called "cold sores" or "fever blisters," usually at the junction of the skin and the lip. The vesicles erupt, then crust and heal within 2 weeks. They usually recur, especially after heavy exposure to bright sunlight, eg, after a day at the beach.

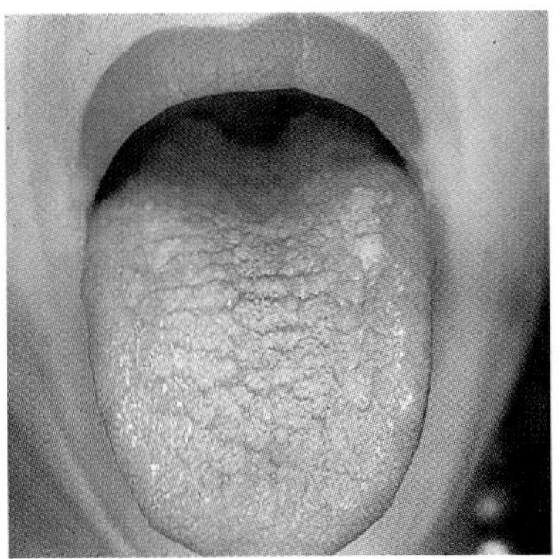

Leukoplakia

A whitish thickening of the mucous membrane in the mouth or tongue. It cannot be scraped off. Most often associated with heavy smoking or drinking, it can be a precancerous condition.

DIAGNOSTIC REASONING IN ACTION

Harold Chandler is a 35-year-old executive in a computer firm who comes to the employees' wellness center complaining of a marked loss of hearing in his left ear. He says that he woke up yesterday with a "feeling of fullness" in his left ear but no pain. He further relates that his 3-year-old daughter has a "bad cold and an earache," and he wonders if he has "the same thing." He denies any other symptoms of infection, has had no discharge from either ear, and is not taking any medicine at this time. He has not had an audiometric examination since his last physical 3 years ago. He further volunteers that he has just returned from a business trip to Europe and wonders whether the pressurized atmosphere of the airplane "created a problem with his hearing."

Nurse Michaela Navarro's focused assessment of Mr. Chandler reveals normal vital signs. His left ear's external canal is of a uniform pink color, with no redness, swelling, lesions, or discharge. The Weber test reveals lateralization to the left ear. The otoscopic examination reveals a left ear impacted with brown-gray cerumen, and the tympanic membrane cannot be visualized. Examination of the right ear shows the external canal is of a uniform pink color with no redness, swelling, lesions, or discharge. During the otoscopic examination the tympanic membrane is easily visualized. It is translucent and pearl-gray with the cone of light at five o'clock. No perforations are noted.

To visualize the tympanic membrane of the left ear, Ms Navarro prepares a solution of mineral oil and hydrogen peroxide and instills the solution into the left ear canal to soften the cerumen. Then she irrigates the canal with warm water using a bulb syringe. After Ms Navarro completes the irrigation, Mr. Chandler is surprised to discover that his hearing has returned in his left ear. Now Ms Navarro completes the otoscopic examination. She is now able to visualize the tympanic membrane, which is translucent and pearl-gray in color with the cone of light at seven o'clock. No perforations are noted.

To be sure that Mr. Chandler's hearing has been restored, Ms Navarro performs a screening evaluation of his auditory function. He is able to hear a low whisper at 2 feet. His Rinne test is positive, and his Weber test indicates equal lateralization.

To cluster the information, Ms Navarro considers the exposure of Mr. Chandler to an infectious disease and the possibility of trauma to the tympanic membrane during recent air travel. She rules out these possibilities because there are no signs of infection or trauma to the ear. The physical examination of the ear reveals normal findings and no interference with auditory function after the cerumen is removed.

Ms Navarro notes that impacted cerumen is a related factor for the diagnosis of sensory/perceptual alteration: reduced hearing, and arrives at the following nursing diagnosis: *sensory/perceptual alteration: reduced hearing related to presence of impacted cerumen.*

Ms Navarro tells Mr. Chandler that his recent air travel may have dislodged the cerumen in his ear just enough to interfere with his hearing. She takes the opportunity to remind Mr. Chandler of the proper method of cleaning the ears: Wash them gently with a cloth, and never insert sharp objects into the ear canal because this action may push cerumen deeper into the canal. Finally, she cautions Mr. Chandler that he may have a tendency to build-up of cerumen and advises him to have them checked frequently.

Health Promotion and Client Education

At the conclusion of the assessment, answer any questions the client may have. All clients need information on promoting the health of the head and neck. Information about the care of chronic disease may also be appropriate, as well as information to prevent any current health problems from progressing. All clients also need information on self-monitoring and reporting of signs and symptoms of cancer of the head and neck.

Promoting the Health of the Head and Neck

The following are the cancer warning signs which apply to the head and neck, as identified by the American Cancer Society:

- Any unexplained lump or thickening
- Changes in the size or color of warts or moles
- Difficulty in swallowing
- Unusual bleeding or discharge
- Any sore that does not heal
- Persistent hoarseness or cough

Caution the client to wear protective head gear during participation in any potentially dangerous activity. Some examples are skateboarding, riding a motorcycle, bicycle riding, rollerskating, or rollerblading, skydiving, bungee jumping, playing football or hockey, and working in construction sites.

When riding in an automobile, make sure that everyone, driver and passengers, is wearing a seat belt. Protect the cervical spine by ensuring that head rests are at the proper height. Be certain that any child under the age of 4 years is secured properly in a carseat each time the child rides in an automobile. Do not use the infant seat in the front seat of a car equipped with a passenger-side air bag, because upon opening the bag can injure the child.

Stress the importance of compliance with any instructions for medications intended to increase cerebral perfusion, or to treat convulsive or thyroid disorders. Teach relaxation techniques as one method of dealing with chronic headaches, jaw pain, or neck pain.

Explain when to seek medical care for any problem of the head, neck, and inclusive structures.

Promoting the Health of the Eyes

Eye examinations for clients without eye disorders should be performed every 5 years. Persons over 40 need eye examinations approximately every 2 years. All clients over the age of 40 need glaucoma screening every 2 years, and every year after the age of 65. This examination is especially important if there is a family history of glaucoma or if the client has a history of eye injury.

Teach clients the warning signs of eye diseases such as excessive tearing, diplopia, halos around lights, loss of any field of vision, flashes of light, dimming or distortion of vision, photophobia, night blindness, change in color vision, and pain.

Clients should always wear protective eye wear during weedwhipping, edging, welding, or any other dangerous activity. When in the sun, clients should wear dark glasses that are ultraviolet-B absorbent to prevent cataracts.

Contact lens wearers should know the signs of keratitis, which is an infection of the cornea. Such symptoms as abnormal sensitivity to light, reduced vision, seeing halos around objects, or acute pain are signs of possible infection. If these symptoms occur, the client should remove the contact lenses and go to an ophthalmologist. Emphasize the importance of disinfecting contact lenses daily to prevent infections of the eye. Contact lens wearers should avoid swimming while wearing lenses because bacteria can get under the lenses and multiply rapidly.

Caution clients not to rub itching or burning eyes. People who have chronically dry eyes should avoid using colored facial tissues near the eyes because they contain dyes that can be irritating. Use plain white tissues which contain no dyes.

Teaching for the vision-impaired includes giving information about social services agencies, eligibility for training and financial assistance, the importance of maintaining a consistent and clutter-free home environment, and the availability of options to enhance daily living, such as clocks with raised numbers, books on tape, and animal companions.

Promoting the Health of the Ears

To preserve hearing, clients should wear ear protectors or ear plugs any time they are around loud noises such as loud music, airplanes or helicopters, explosives, or firearms. Children should be screened for hearing each year; this screening is frequently performed in the school. The elderly should also have their hearing tested at least once a year.

Caution clients never to put foreign objects, including ballpoint pens, pencils, cotton swabs, or hairpins into the ear canal. The external ear may be cleaned with a soft cloth and mild soap.

Tell clients to remember to use sunscreen on the external ears as well as the face and neck to prevent skin cancer. It has recently been discovered that a large number of skin cancers originate on the ear.

If the client has an upper respiratory infection with heavy nasal discharge, advise the client to blow the nose gently. Forcefully blowing the nose may force bacteria from the nose into the ears, contributing to an ear infection.

"Swimmer's ear" or otitis externa is a bacterial infection caused by contaminated water remaining in the outer ear canal. After swimming or showering, clients should always shake the head to remove trapped water and dry the outer ear with a dry towel.

Teaching for the hearing impaired includes discussion of the need for a hearing aid, care of appliances to enhance hearing, and safety measures such as lights on alarm clocks, telephones, doorbells, and burglar alarms. Ask family members and friends to speak to the client in normal tones. Other options to enhance daily living include closed-caption television, telephones for the hearing impaired, keyboard telephones, and animal companions.

Promoting the Health of the Nose and Sinuses

Teach clients the proper use and side effects of prescription medications and nasal sprays. Explain how the overuse of decongestants in spray or pill form leads to tolerance, eventually rendering the medication ineffective.

Teach clients how to care for nosebleeds: Sit up and lean forward to prevent blood from being swallowed. Pinch the anterior nares together. Use ice packs on the bridge of the nose. Have blood pressure monitored if nosebleeds are frequent.

People with colds or nasal congestion should avoid air travel because pressure can back up in the ears, causing severe pain. If air travel is necessary, use a nasal spray or a decongestant an hour before takeoff and an hour before landing to release pressure in the ears.

DIAGNOSTIC REASONING IN ACTION

Ellen Dodson is a 28-year-old banking executive who comes to the wellness clinic for assistance in the management of "tension headaches." She describes her headaches as a dull, bandlike constricting pain in the occipital and temporal area of the head. Her appetite has decreased, and she experiences diarrhea about two times per month when she is especially nervous. Ms Dodson states that she has "been under a lot of pressure at work lately," and her physician has told her that her headaches are related to tension. The physician has suggested that she investigate some stress-management strategies.

The nursing assessment of Ms Dodson reveals a well-developed, well-nourished female in no acute distress at this time. The nursing diagnosis is health-seeking behaviors, stress reduction.

Ed Masters, RN, suggests the following methods for reducing stress:

- Time management: a method for accomplishing work more efficiently
- Regular exercise at least three times a week at the wellness clinic's fitness center
- Guided imagery: a technique in which one concentrates on a relaxing image and visualizes oneself in the image
- Progressive relaxation: a technique in which one learns to constrict and relax muscle groups in a systematic fashion
- Biofeedback: a method by which one learns to influence physiologic responses not usually under voluntary control
- Yoga: a discipline in which prescribed postures and breathing techniques are used to control the body

After considerable discussion, Ms Dodson decides she would like to set up a regular exercise program at the fitness center and also try guided imagery. Mr. Masters and Ms Dodson arrange a time to meet once a week for guided-imagery sessions, and Mr. Masters makes a note to evaluate Ms Dodson's stress level and number of headaches one month from the first session.

Promoting the Health of the Mouth and Throat

Teach oral hygiene to include correct technique for brushing teeth, using dental floss, and cleaning oral appliances. Encourage yearly dental examinations.

Stress the early warning signs of cancer listed earlier. Remind clients to apply sunscreen to the lips when outdoors. The lower lip is a common site for skin cancer. Sunscreen also prevents lip chapping and may help prevent an outbreak of herpes lesions on the lips.

Caution parents of small children against giving toddlers easily aspirated foods that can lodge in the trachea and cause choking. Examples are grapes, nuts, and hard candies. Always cut up solid foods into small pieces and encourage children under 5 years of age to chew vigorously.

Remind parents that safety caps on medicine bottles are child-resistant, not childproof. Young children can often open safety caps; it just takes a little longer. Keep all medicines out of the reach of children, even those with safety caps. Keep the telephone number of the local poison control center on or next to the telephone.

Clients who use smokeless tobacco are at high risk for developing cancer of the mouth, and clients who smoke a pipe are at risk for mouth and lip cancer. Encourage clients who use any form of tobacco to eliminate this habit by referring them to smoking-cessation classes.

Summary

The head and neck provide the protective covering for the brain, which controls the senses of vision, hearing, smell, and taste. Knowledge of the anatomy and physiology of the eyes, ears, nose, and mouth helps you perform the assessment and understand the normal variations that occur in certain client groups. An interview focused on the various parts of the head and neck allows you to consider the client's history, other habits that may affect the head and neck, and cultural and evironmental factors that may influence the health of the head and neck. Physical assessment of the head and neck reveals clues to the status of the body's oxygenation, circulation, fluid balance, hormone balance, and other factors. Nursing diagnoses commonly identified after assessment of the head and neck include sensory/perceptual alteration: visual, olfactory, gustatory, or auditory; impaired swallowing; and altered oral mucous membrane. After performing the health assessment and identifying any appropriate nursing diagnoses, provide the client with the information needed to improve the health of the head and neck region.

Key Points

✓ The head comprises seven bones: two frontal, two parietal, two temporal, and one occipital. The major functions of the eyes are collecting light, transmitting visual images to the brain, and producing tears. The major functions of the ears are collecting and transporting sound to the brain, and providing equilibrium. The major functions of the nose and sinuses are receiving olfactory stimuli and providing warmth and humidity for air flowing to the lungs. The major function of the mouth and throat are saliva production, mastication, taste, and speech production. There are two major muscles in the neck: the sternocleidomastoid and the trapezius. The thyroid gland is found in the middle of the neck and secretes the hormones that influence cellular metabolism.

✓ Conduct a focused interview to gather specific information about the structures of the head and neck, including a history of the health and care of the eyes, ears, nose and sinuses, mouth and throat, and neck; self-care practices; and family, cultural, and environmental factors.

✓ Inspect and palpate the head for size and contour, noting any deformities or tenderness.

✓ Check visual acuity and visual fields, inspect extraocular muscles, and assess corneal reflex. Inspect the external eye structures. Use the ophthalmoscope to inspect internal eye structures such as the retinal vessels and optic disc.

✓ Inspect the external ear for size, shape, position, and any signs of infection. Inspect the external canal. Use the otoscope to inspect the tympanic membrane for color, swelling, or discharge. Test for hearing acuity with the tuning fork and voice test.

✓ Inspect the external nose for symmetry or lesions. Inspect the nasal mucosa, septum, and turbinates. Palpate the sinuses for tenderness.

✓ Inspect the mouth, lips, teeth, gums, and pharynx for color, lesions, or exudate. Palpate structures inside the mouth for lesions or growths.

✓ Inspect and palpate the neck for position of the trachea, and enlargement of the thyroid gland and the cervical lymph nodes. Test range of motion of the neck.

✓ Nursing diagnoses commonly associated with the head and neck include sensory/perceptual alteration: visual, auditory, olfactory, gustatory; impaired swallowing; and altered oral mucous membrane.

✓ Provide the client with information needed to promote health of the head and neck region.

Chapter 10

Assessing the Respiratory System

The respiratory system is responsible for the delicate exchange of gases within the body. The intake of oxygen is required for the metabolic processes, and the carbon dioxide produced by these processes needs to be removed. In addition to performing the exchange of gases essential to body homeostasis, the respiratory system helps maintain the body's fluid and acid-base balance and assists with speech. Thus, an in-depth assessment of the respiratory system provides valuable data regarding the client's overall health status. In turn, respiratory health depends upon the proper functioning of other body systems. For example, the thoracic bones of the musculoskeletal system protect the lungs, and the thoracic muscles enable healthy respiration.

When assessing respiratory health, consider the client's developmental stage, psychosocial factors such as anxiety and stress, self-care factors such as exercise and nutrition, and environmental factors such as pollutants. All of these influence respiratory functioning. Figure 10.1 shows how these factors and other body systems influence respiratory health. Again, respiratory assessment is an integral aspect of the total database assessed by the professional nurse.

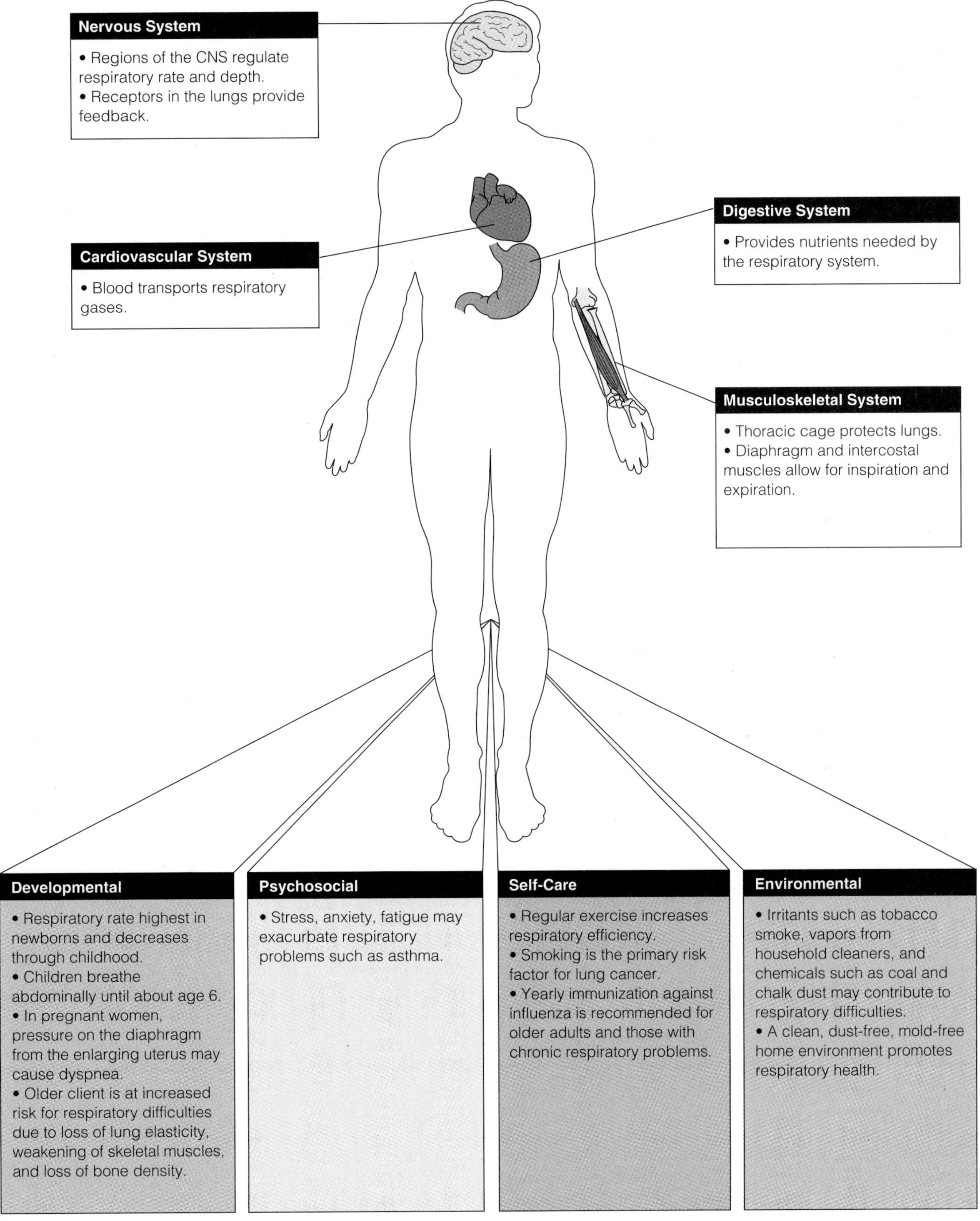

Nervous System
• Regions of the CNS regulate respiratory rate and depth.
• Receptors in the lungs provide feedback.
Cardiovascular System
• Blood transports respiratory gases.
Digestive System
• Provides nutrients needed by the respiratory system.
Musculoskeletal System
• Thoracic cage protects lungs.
• Diaphragm and intercostal muscles allow for inspiration and expiration.
Developmental
• Respiratory rate highest in newborns and decreases through childhood.
• Children breathe abdominally until about age 6.
• In pregnant women, pressure on the diaphragm from the enlarging uterus may cause dyspnea.
• Older client is at increased risk for respiratory difficulties due to loss of lung elasticity, weakening of skeletal muscles, and loss of bone density.
Psychosocial
• Stress, anxiety, fatigue may exacurbate respiratory problems such as asthma.
Self-Care
• Regular exercise increases respiratory efficiency.
• Smoking is the primary risk factor for lung cancer.
• Yearly immunization against influenza is recommended for older adults and those with chronic respiratory problems.
Environmental
• Irritants such as tobacco smoke, vapors from household cleaners, and chemicals such as coal and chalk dust may contribute to respiratory difficulties.
• A clean, dust-free, mold-free home environment promotes respiratory health.

Figure 10.1 An overview of important factors to consider when assessing the respiratory system.

Anatomy and Physiology Review

The respiratory system consists of the upper and lower respiratory tracts. The structures of the upper respiratory tract include the nasal cavity, paranasal sinuses, pharynx, larynx, and the proximal portion of the trachea. The lower respiratory tract involves the distal portion of the trachea, bronchi, and lungs (Figure 10.2). When considering the lower respiratory tract, you must also take into account the pleural membranes, muscles of respirations, and mediastinum.

The anatomy and physiology review and assessment of the upper respiratory tract have been included in Chapter 9 on assessing the head and neck. Before proceeding, you may want to refine your knowledge base by reviewing the information regarding the structures of the upper respiratory tract and other data pertinent to these structures.

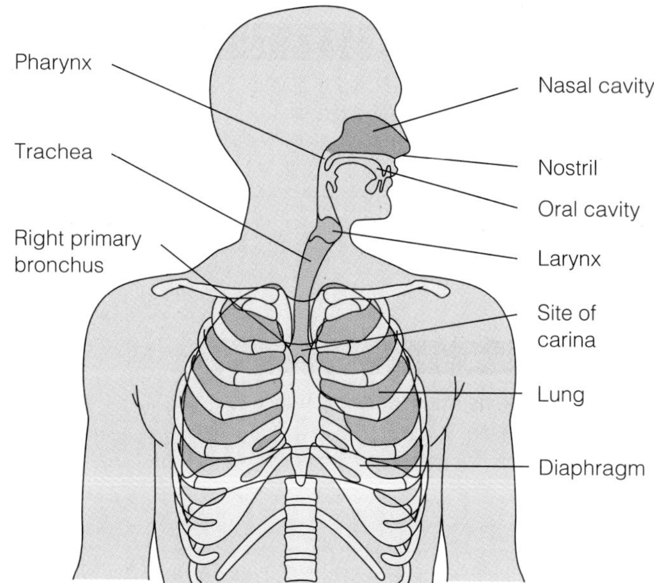

Figure 10.2 Anatomy of the respiratory system.

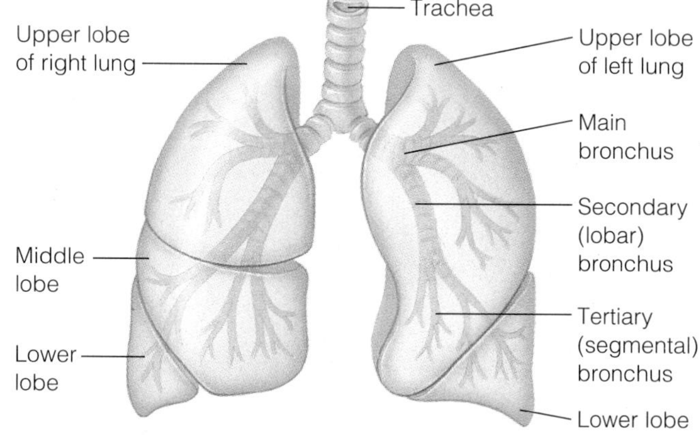

Figure 10.3 Respiratory passages.

Lower Respiratory Tract

Trachea

The **trachea** (or windpipe) is located anterior to the esophagus within the mediastinum. It is approximately 10–12 cm (4 inches) long and 2.5 cm (1 inch) in diameter. It descends from the larynx to its point of bifurcation anteriorly at about the sternal angle and posteriorly at about vertebra T3 to T5. This flexible, tubelike structure is composed of about 16 to 20 rings of hyaline cartilage. These **C**-shaped rings help maintain the shape of the structure and prevent its collapse during inspiration and expiration. Just above the point of bifurcation, the last tracheal cartilage is expanded, and a rounded piece of cartilage called the *carina* projects posteriorly. The trachea, like other structures of the respiratory tract, is lined with a mucus-producing membrane that traps dust, bacteria, and other foreign bodies. The *cilia*, hairlike projections of this mucosal lining, help sweep the debris toward the mouth for removal.

Bronchi

The trachea bifurcates midthorax, forming the right and left primary **bronchi** (Figure 10.3). The main bronchi enter the lungs at the hilus. Both bronchi have an oblique position within the mediastinum. The right bronchus is wider, shorter, and more vertical than the left. For this reason aspirated objects are more likely to enter the right main bronchus than the left. Each bronchus continues to subdivide until the bronchi reach a diameter of less than 1 mm. These terminal points are called *bronchioles*.

Lungs

The **lungs** are two cone-shaped, elastic, spongy, air-filled structures suspended in the pleural cavities on either side of the mediastinum (Figure 10.4). The *apex* of each lung is

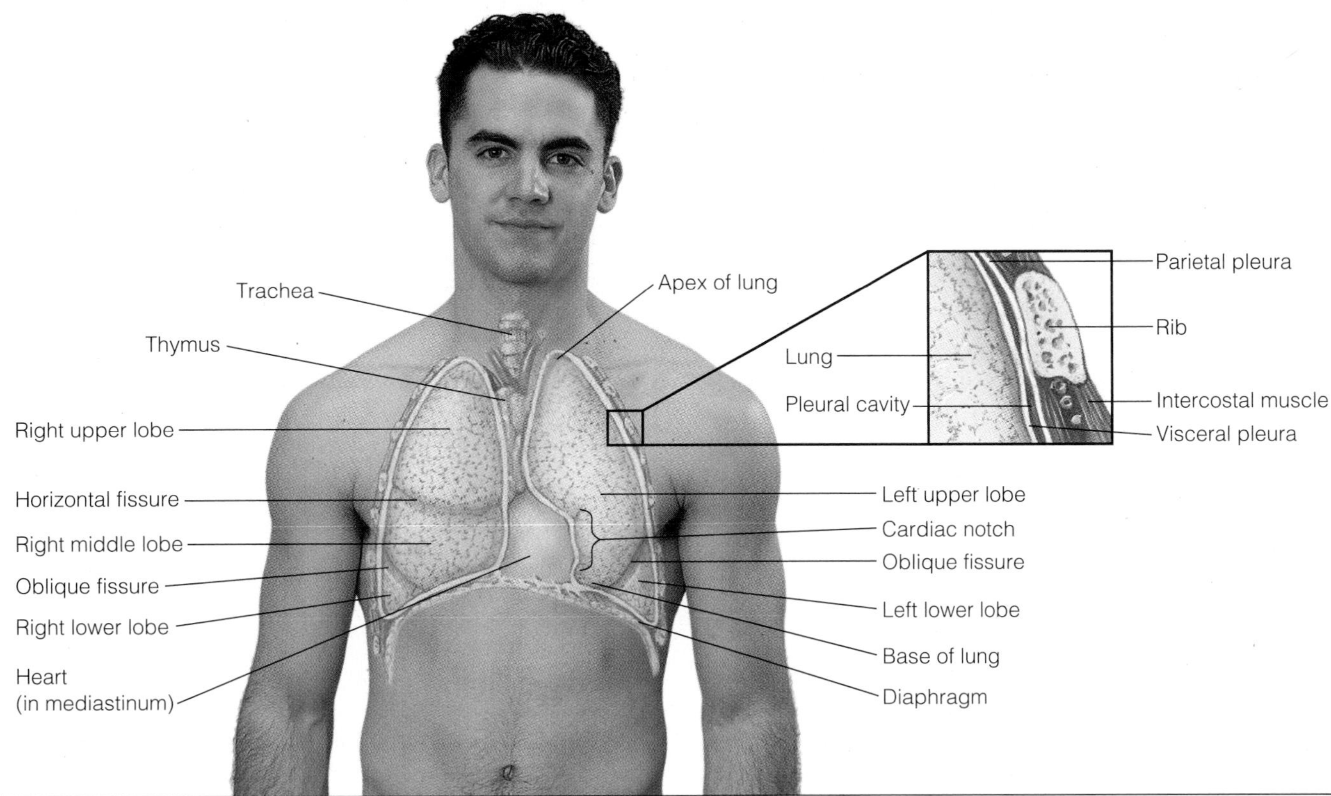

Figure 10.4 Anterior view of the lungs and their relationship to the organs of the mediastinum.

slightly superior to the clavicle, and the *base* is at the level of the diaphragm. The right lung has three lobes (upper, middle, and lower) and is slightly larger, wider, and shorter than the left lung. The left lung has two lobes (upper and lower) and tends to be longer, smaller, and narrower than the right lung. It cradles the heart. The three lobes of the right lung are separated by the oblique and horizontal fissures. The two lobes of the left lung are divided by the oblique fissure. The lung lobes are composed of a myriad of microscopic bronchioles and *alveoli* in which gases (oxygen and carbon dioxide) are exchanged at the capillary level of the cardiovascular system (Figure 10.5 on page 228).

Pleural Membranes

A thin, serous, double-layered membrane called the **pleura** lines the walls of the thoracic cavity (*parietal pleura*) and covers the external surface of the lungs (*visceral pleura*) (Figure 10.4). The membranes produce a lubricating serous secretion that allows the lungs to move easily during the respiratory cycle. Together, the negative pressure between these two membranes and the positive pressure within the lungs keep the lungs from collapsing.

Mediastinum

The medial section of the thoracic cavity is called the **mediastinum** (Figure 10.4). This contains the heart, trachea, esophagus, and great vessels.

Muscles of Respiration

Although not strictly part of the respiratory system, the **thoracic muscles** assist in the breathing process by rhythmically increasing and decreasing the diameters of the chest. With the synchronized contractions and relaxation of the *diaphragm* and the *intercostal muscles*, inspiration and expiration take place. Accessory muscles of the neck (sternocleidomastoids, scalenus, and trapezius), abdomen (rectus), and chest (pectorals) also assist with respirations when necessary.

Thoracic Cage

The **thoracic cage** is another accessory to respiratory health. It consists of ribs, cartilage, and muscles. This sturdy framework surrounds the underlying organs (lungs, heart, blood vessels), providing protection and stability. The anterior portion of the thoracic cage consists of the *sternum* (manubrium, sternal body, and xiphoid process) and the *ribs*. The ribs form

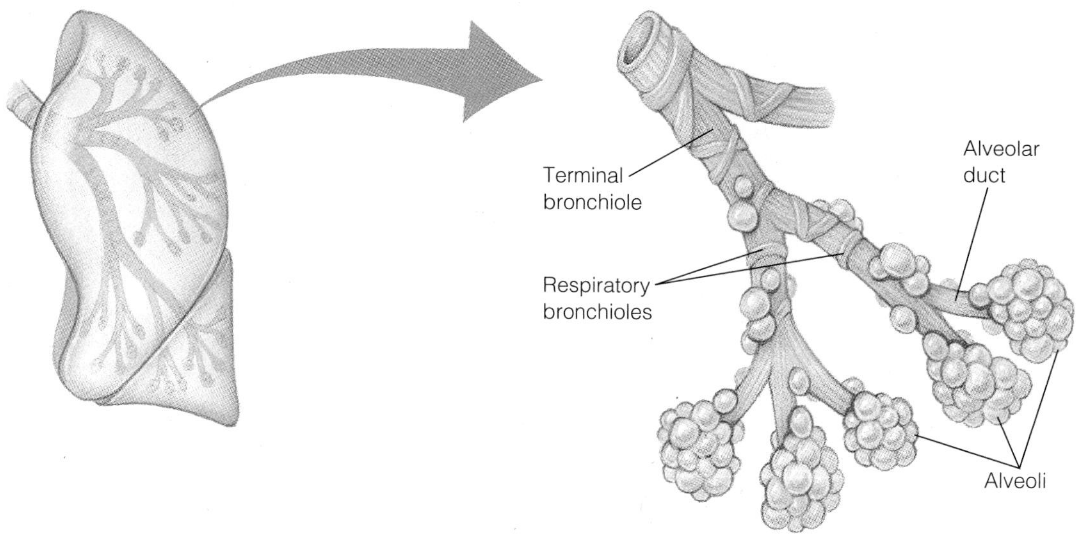

Figure 10.5 Respiratory bronchioles, alveolar ducts, and alveoli.

the lateral and posterior aspects of the thoracic cage as they encircle the body. The twelve pairs of ribs are attached to a vertebral process posteriorly. Anteriorly the first seven pair of ribs articulate directly to the sternum. The cartilage of ribs 8, 9, and 10 articulate with the superior cartilage, whereas pairs 11 and 12 are free, or *floating*, ribs and do not articulate anteriorly.

Functions of the Respiratory System

The major functions of the respiratory system include

- Exchanging of gases between the body and atmosphere
- Warming, moistening, and filtering the air as it enters the body
- Helping to maintain the acid-base balance
- Helping to maintain water balance
- Assisting with speech

Landmarks

Thoracic reference points and anatomical structures are used when performing the physical assessment of the respiratory system (Figure 10.6). **Landmarks** help you identify specific underlying structures by providing an exact location for the assessment findings and an accurate descriptive orientation for documentation.

Generally, landmark identification for the thorax is twofold. First are the horizontal and vertical lines. Second is the division of the thorax. Some professionals see the thoracic cage as having three sections: the anterior, lateral, and posterior sections. Others divide the thorax into anterior and posterior sections. This is usually a professional choice; however, the three aspects will be considered in this discussion.

The twelve pair of **ribs** form the horizontal landmarks and encompass the three aspects of the thorax. Each rib is identified by number, and each intercostal space takes the number of the rib superior to that space. The first rib and first intercostal space are deep to the clavicle and are not palpable. The second rib is the first palpable rib. When assessed anteriorly, ribs 2 to 7 are easiest to count close to the sternal border. When counted posteriorly, ribs are best palpated close to the vertebral column.

The **clavicles** can also be considered a horizontal line on the anterior chest wall. These long, slender, curved bones extend from the manubrium of the sternum to the acromion of the scapula. Lung tissue is assessed above and below each clavicle. Findings above the clavicle are supraclavicular, and findings below are considered infraclavicular.

The **sternum** becomes the first vertical landmark to be considered. Commonly called the breastbone, it is a flat, elongated bone located in the midline of the anterior thoracic cage. The manubrium, body, and xiphoid process are the three parts of the sternum. The *manubrium* articulates laterally with the clavicles and the first two pairs of ribs. The depression or indentation at the superior border is called the *jugular (suprasternal) notch*. As the manubrium joins the body of the sternum, a horizontal ridge is formed at the *sternal angle*

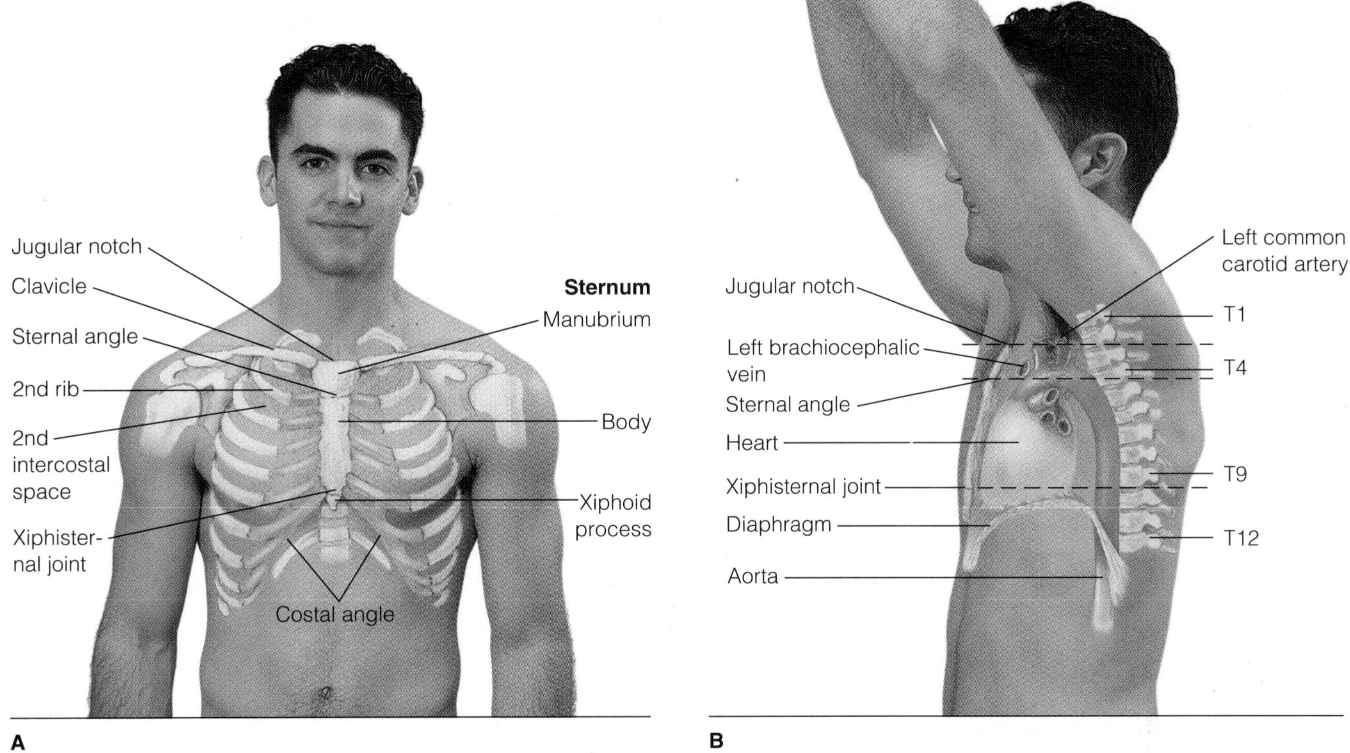

Figure 10.6 Landmarks of the anterior chest *A*, Anterior view. *B*, Left lateral view, showing the relationship of the anterior landmarks to the vertebral column.

(angle of Louis). The second rib and second intercostal space are at this level and become the reference point for counting the ribs and intercostal spaces. The sternum terminates at the inferior edge of the *xiphoid process*. This process and the inferior borders of the seventh ribs form a triangle referred to as the *costal angle*.

The anterior chest is the first division of the thoracic cage. Five imaginary vertical lines divide it. These are the midsternal line, the right and left midclavicular lines, and the right and left anterior axillary lines. The **midsternal line** (or sternal line) is a vertical line that divides the sternum into a right and left half. The **midclavicular line** is parallel to the midsternal line. It is drawn from the middle of the clavicle to the level of the twelfth rib. This line passes close to the nipple of the breast. The **anterior axillary line** is another line drawn parallel to the midsternal line. It falls from the anterior axillary fold along the anteriolateral aspect of the thoracic cage to the level of the twelfth rib. These five lines—the midsternal line, the right and left midclavicular line and the right and left anterior axillary line—form the vertical lines of the anterior chest wall (Figure 10.7 on page 230).

The posterior chest is the second division of the thoracic cage. Five vertical parallel lines are drawn on the posterior aspect of the thoracic cage. The **vertebral line** divides the vertebral column into a right and left half. This line passes through the posterior spinous processes. The **scapular line** is drawn from the inferior angle of the scapula to the level of the twelfth rib. The **posterior axillary line** falls from the posterior axillary fold along the posteriolateral aspect of the thoracic cage also to the level of the twelfth rib. These five lines—the vertebral line, the right and left scapular lines, and the right and left posterior axillary lines—are the vertical lines of the posterior chest wall (Figure 10.8 on page 230).

The third division of the thoracic cage is the lateral aspect. Three parallel vertical lines are drawn through the lateral aspect of the thorax. Two lines, the anterior and posterior axillary lines, have already been identified. Equidistant from the anterior and posterior lines, the **midaxillary line (MAL)** is drawn from the axillae to the level of the twelfth rib. The anterior axillary, posterior axillary, and midaxillary lines provide vertical landmarks to the lateral portion of the thorax (Figure 10.9 on page 231).

Identification of landmarks will help you develop a mental picture of the underlying structure. Recall that the trachea bifurcates, forming the right and left main bronchi. Anteriorly, this bifurcation occurs just inferior to the sternal angle. Posteriorly, it occurs at about the level of the fourth thoracic vertebra (T4).

The apices of the lung extend 2–4 cm above the inner third of the clavicle on the anterior chest wall. On the posterior

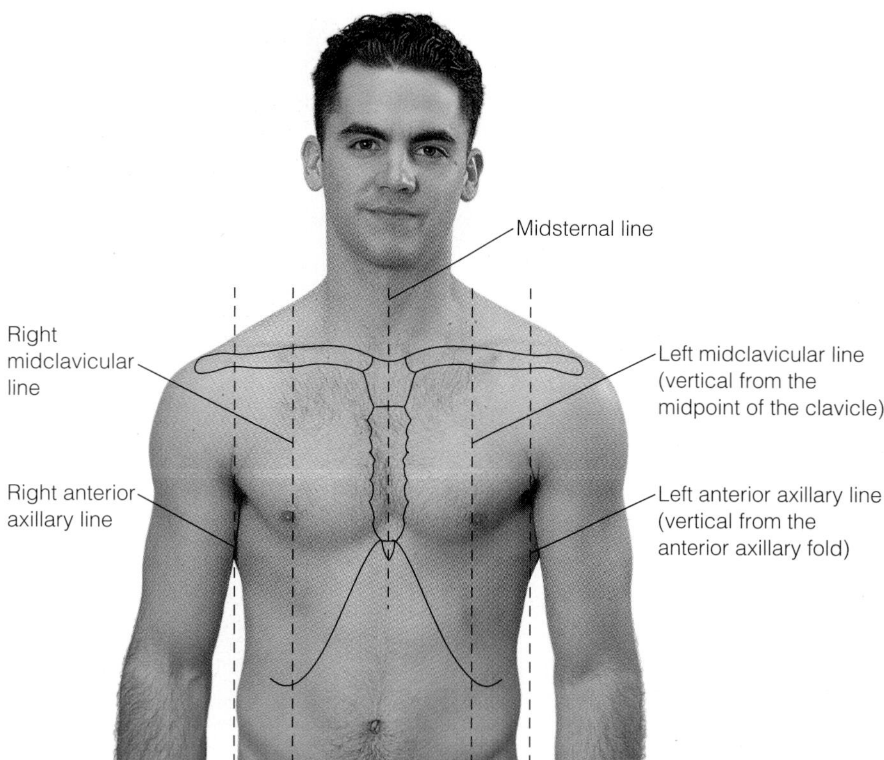

Figure 10.7 Lines of the anterior chest.

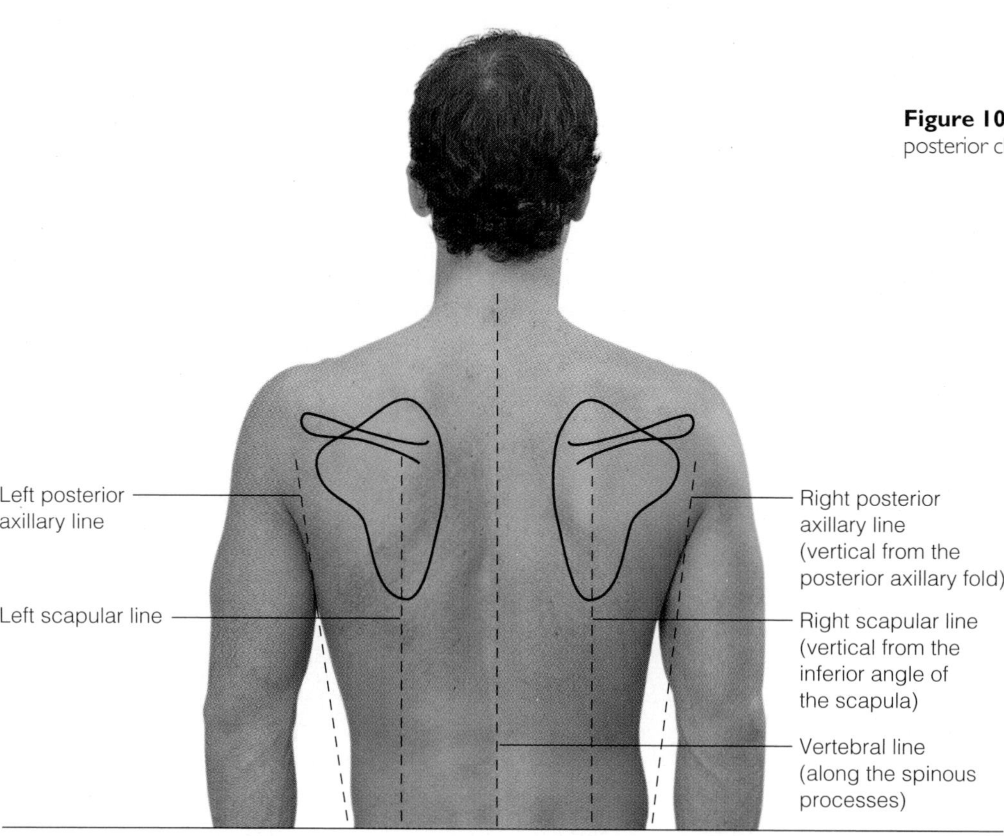

Figure 10.8 Lines of the posterior chest.

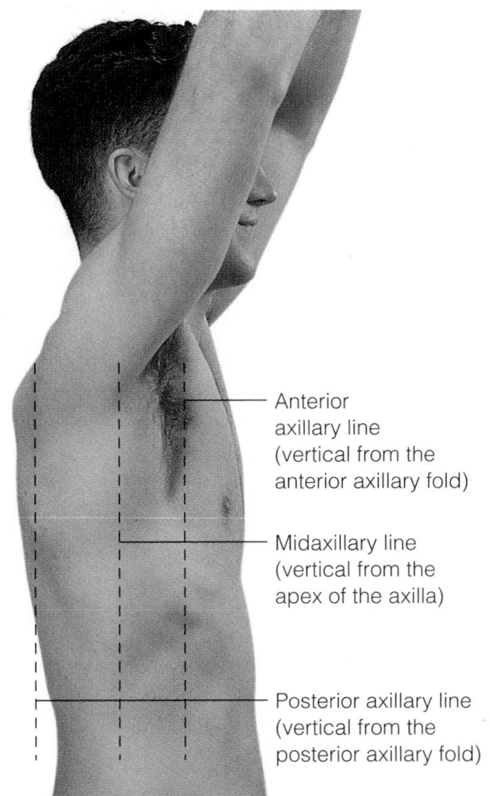

Figure 10.9 Lines of the lateral chest.

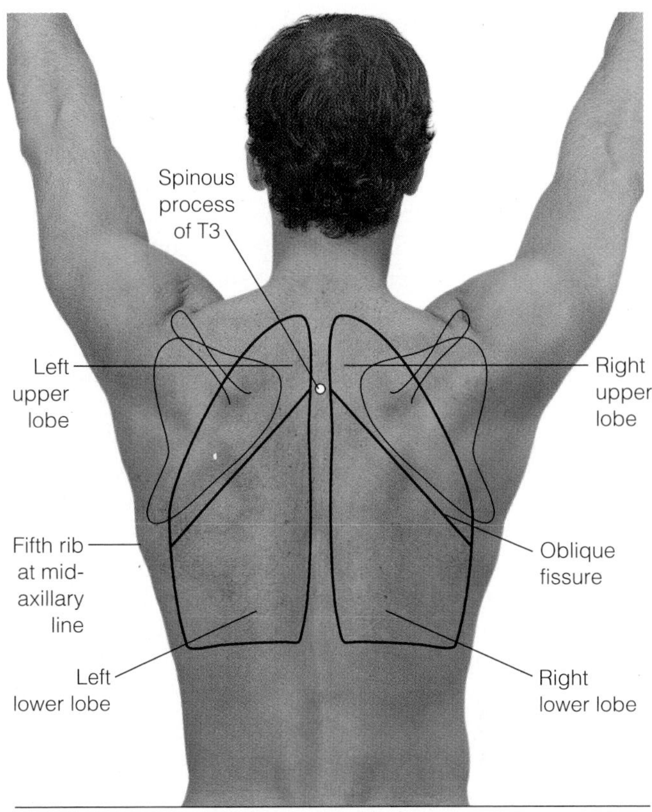

Figure 10.10 Lobes of the lungs, posterior view.

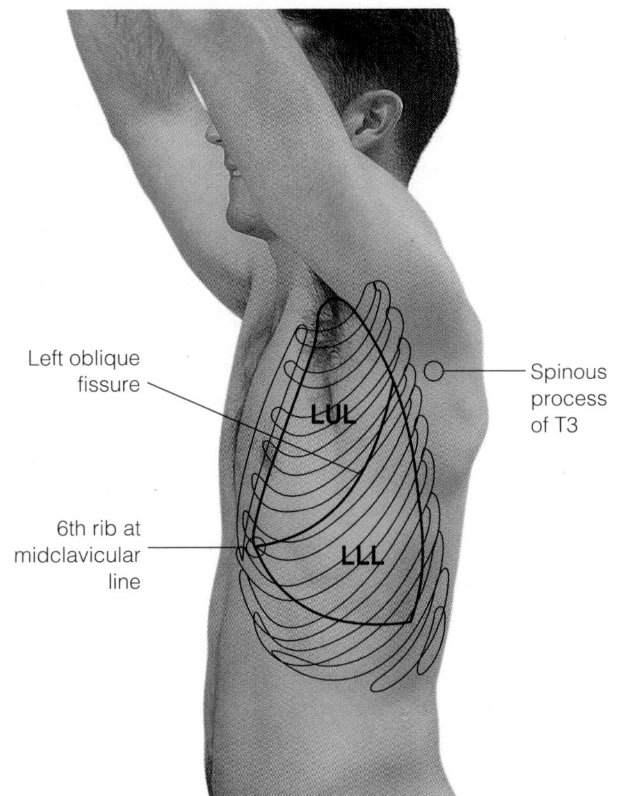

Figure 10.11 Lateral view of lobes of the left lung.

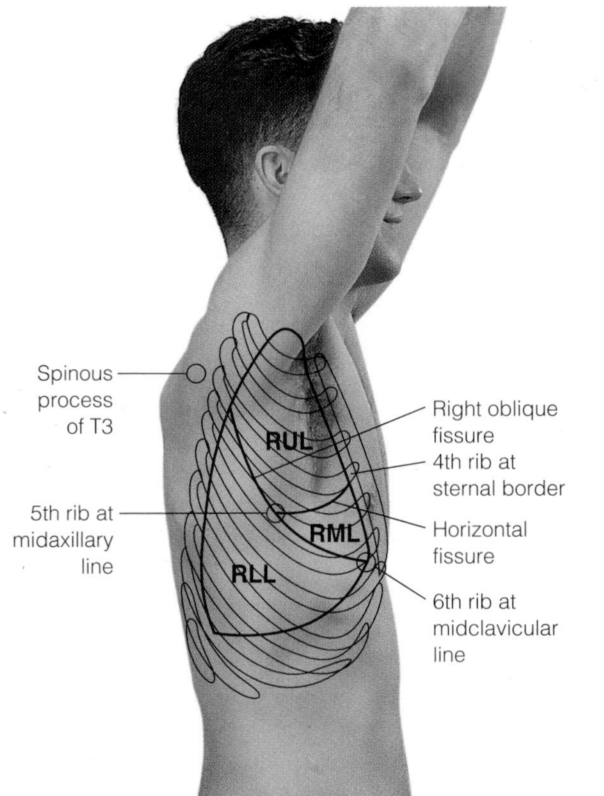

Figure 10.12 Lateral view of lobes of the right lung.

chest wall the apices rise 2–4 cm above the scapula between the scapular and vertebral lines.

The base of the cone-shaped lung has three reference points. Anteriorly at the midclavicular line, the base of the lung is at the sixth rib. Laterally at the midaxillary line, the base is at the eighth rib. Posteriorly at the scapular line, the base of the lung is at about the tenth rib. Forced inspiration and forced expiration alter the horizontal markings.

Imaginary lines are drawn on the skin surface to identify thoracic landmarks. These lines, which correspond to the fissures in the lungs, demarcate the five lobes of the lungs.

The right and left oblique fissure divides the lung into the upper and lower lobes. To find these lobes, draw a line from the third thoracic vertebra (T3) to the fifth rib at the MAL. This line follows the medial border of the scapula when the arms are extended over the head. The line then from T3 to MAL5 reflects the fissure on the posterior chest wall (Figure 10.10).

On the left side, the line continues to the left midclavicular line at the sixth rib. The outline of this fissure is complete, and the two lobes of the left lung have been identified posteriorly, laterally, and anteriorly (Figure 10.11 on page 231).

On the right side the line at MAL5 continues in two directions. One line extends to the sixth rib at the right midclavicular line. Another line extends from MAL5 to the right sternal border following the fourth rib. The outline of the fissures on the right side are complete, and the three lobes of the right lung have been identified (Figure 10.12 on page 231).

Gathering the Data

Before proceeding with the health assessment, think about the data to be obtained from the client. What data is needed, and what skills do you need to acquire this data? Take the time to evaluate your own personal skills and make corrections if any personal deficits exist.

Examine your therapeutic communication skills. Open-ended and some closed statements are most valuable as you begin the focused interview.

Refine your percussion technique. Return to Chapter 7 of this text and review finger placement of the nondominant hand. Accurate tapping with the finger of the dominant hand produces a clear sound. Review the terms used to describe the sounds heard. Remember that both percussion technique and the amount of air in the underlying tissue affect the produced sound.

Focused Interview

Begin by reviewing the database collected during the client's initial interview and information collected during assessment of other body systems. Then determine what additional information you need before beginning the examination of the respiratory system. Review the results of X-ray procedures, blood studies, pulmonary function tests, and any other diagnostic work that has been completed.

The focused interview builds on the health history discussed in Chapter 2 of this text. The focused interview concentrates very specifically on the respiratory system. This data will continue to reflect the state of wellness or illness of the client. To formulate accurate nursing diagnoses, you need to obtain data reflecting both strengths and weaknesses of the client. Before beginning the interview, determine the present respiratory status of the client. Postpone a detailed interview if the client demonstrates dyspnea, cyanosis, difficulty with speech, and accompanying anxiety.

Questions Related to the Respiratory System

1. Describe your breathing of today; 2 months ago; 2 years ago. *This gives the clients the opportunity to share their perception of self and what they consider important regarding this vital function.*
2. Do you consider yourself a nose-breather or mouth-breather? *Follow-up is required if the client's response is "mouth-breather." The air is not filtered, warmed, or moistened as in nose-breathing, and mouth-breathing can also indicate nasal disease.*
3. If you were to stand in front of a mirror with your chest exposed, and breathing naturally (no forced inspirations or expirations) what would you see? *This gives clients the opportunity to share their perception of chest expansion and use of accessory muscles.*
4. Do you smoke? What do you smoke? When did you start smoking? How much do you smoke in 24 hours? Describe your ability to inhale. *Smoking destroys the cilia in the respiratory tract. Certain brands of tobacco may be more irritating than others causing respiratory problems. The American Cancer Society estimates that 80–90% of lung cancer cases are attributed to smoking.*
5. *If the client is a smoker, ask the following:* Have you ever tried to stop smoking? Tell me more about this. How long ago was this? How long did you go without smoking? What did you do to try to stop smoking? Why did you start smoking again? *The response gives the nurse an indication of the tenacity of addiction to nicotine and the strength of the self-concept.*

6. Does anyone living in your home smoke? Does that person smoke in the house? Is one room designated as smoke free? Does the smoker go outside to smoke? *The response gives insight into exposure to secondary smoke. Some research suggests that secondary smoke is more harmful than primary.*
7. Do you have a cough? How often does the coughing occur? What do you think causes the cough? Is the coughing worse at any special time of the day or night? *This data helps to increase your knowledge base regarding the client.*
8. Describe your cough. Is it dry, hacking, hoarse, barking, or wet? *The type of cough may signal the type of lung disease. For example a dry, hacking cough occurs in* pneumocystis carinii *pneumonia, an opportunistic lung infection seen with AIDS. Dry, hacking cough may also indicate irritation from smoking. A barking cough is indicative of tracheal laryngeal edema or throat infection. A wet, moist cough occurs in pneumonia and other lung infections.*
9. Do you cough up sputum? If so, what does the sputum look like? Does the sputum have an odor? *The appearance of the sputum often indicates the underlying cause. For example, yellow or green sputum might signal a lung infection, whereas rust-colored or dark red sputum may indicate tuberculosis or pneumococcal pneumonia. Hemoptysis, blood-streaked sputum, occurs in upper respiratory infection or bronchitis. Larger amounts of blood in the sputum may be related to an* Aspergillus *infection, tuberculosis, carcinoma, or lung abscess.*
10. Has there been a recent change in the amount, color, or consistency of your sputum? How recent? *A recent change in the characteristics of the sputum may indicate underlying disease.*
11. Do you have trouble coughing up sputum? *As a person ages, the muscles of respiration lose tone, and ciliary function becomes less effective. These two factors may impair adequate clearing of the respiratory tract.*
12. Does the coughing hurt? If so, describe the type, severity, and location of the pain. What do you do to decrease the pain? Does it work?
13. Does the coughing wake you up at night? Make you tired?
14. What do you do to stop the coughing? Do you take a prescribed medication? Over-the-counter medication? Use a home remedy? *If so, elicit the name, dose, and frequency.*
15. Do you live in an environment or work in an industry that exposes you to caustic fumes, fungi, or any of the following substances? Asbestos, airplane glue, coal tar, nickel, silver, textile fibers, radon, chloromethyl ethers, chromate, and vinyl chlorides? *All of these substance are known carcinogens.*
16. Do you work in a dust-producing environment, such as a granary or mine? *Large amounts of dust may lead to the development of silicosis. Coal miners are susceptible to coal miner's disease, a form of pneumoconiosis.*
17. *If the client responded yes to questions 15 or 16:* Do you use a protective mask or any device to help keep your lungs clean?
18. Do you experience frequent colds? Have you had a respiratory infection recently? In the past 2 weeks; 2 months; 2 years? If so, describe the symptoms and treatment. *Respiratory infections may be spread by droplet infection, making the client prone to repeated episodes.*
19. Are you having any problems breathing at the present time? In the past? Do you have difficulty breathing when you are eating or drinking fluids? Describe how you feel.
20. When you are having problems, what makes your breathing easier? Worse?
21. Does any position help make breathing easier for you? *A need to sit forward with the hands on the knees (3-point position) and shoulders hunched may indicate respiratory distress.*
22. Do you use a nebulizer, oxygen, humidifier, or any other device to help improve your breathing? Are any of these items used daily if you are not having breathing difficulty?
23. Are you able to sleep flat, or do you need to use additional pillows?
24. Does your breathing problem stop you from doing a specific task: exercising, walking, eating?
25. When you have the breathing problem do you feel dizzy, light-headed, or confused? *This may indicate anoxia or hypoxia of brain tissue.*
26. Have you lost or gained weight recently? If so, how much, and over what length of time? *When a client has a weight loss associated with respiratory problems, lung cancer should be considered. Likewise, when a client has a weight gain associated with respiratory problems, fluid retention related to right-sided congestive heart failure should be considered.*
27. Do any of the members of your family have respiratory disorders? Do you know of any inherited or genetic disorders in your family that affect respiratory function? *Cystic fibrosis is an example of an inherited problem that affects breathing. Alpha$_1$-antitrypsin deficiency, another inherited disorder, leads to emphysema (Finesilver p. 25).*
28. Do you experience wheezing? If so, when does it occur? Is it related to any activity? To any food? To any medication? Does the wheezing happen along with other symptoms such as coughing or chest pain? If so, describe.

29. Does your wheezing happen more often during certain times of the year? *Wheezing may accompany allergic reactions related to seasonal changes.*
30. Do you experience coughing, itching, and runny nose and eyes or other allergic symptoms?
31. Do you have pets? Are you allergic to fur, feathers, or dander? If so, describe your reaction.
32. Have you been tested for allergies? If so, describe the results. *Information concerning the client's allergy history helps the nurse individualize the client's care and reinforce health teaching.*
33. Have you recently traveled to a rural area or foreign country? *The client may have been exposed to a respiratory infection or irritant not common in urban areas or country of origin. For example, histoplasmosis, a fungal infection that causes pneumonia or flulike symptoms, is common in the rural Midwestern United States; blastomycosis, a yeast-like infection that causes pleural pain, dyspnea, and cough, occurs in the Southeast United States, Africa, and South and Central America; and coccidioidomycosis, another yeastlike infection that causes symptoms that mimic flu, pneumonia, or tuberculosis, occurs in the Southwest United States and Mexico (Finesilver, 1992).*

Additional Questions with Infants, Children, and Adolescents

1. How many colds has the child had in the past 12 months? *In early childhood, as many as six uncomplicated upper respiratory infections per year is not unexpected. If the parent reports more than six colds per year, or if the parent reports complications, consider the possibility of chronic respiratory problems such as asthma or chronic bronchitis.*
2. Does your child eat solid food? If so, do you cut it yourself? Does your child seem to have trouble chewing or swallowing food, or keeping food down? *If the child is eating solid foods, there is a possibility of aspiration if the food is not cut properly. Chronic spitting up of food or choking could indicate a gastroesophageal reflux.*
3. Ask the child's parents: Do you smoke? If so, do you smoke in the home? *Children whose parents smoke have more diseases of the respiratory tract than do children of nonsmokers.*

Additional Questions with Childbearing Clients

1. Do you ever feel short-of-breath or have difficulty breathing? *The height of the fundus displaces the abdominal organs and places pressure on the diaphragm, resulting in shortness of breath.*
2. At night, are you able to sleep lying down? Do you need additional pillows, or can you sleep comfortably on your side?

Additional Questions with Older Adults

1. Describe any changes you have noticed in your breathing. Have you had any difficulty performing activities you used to do easily? If so, tell me about this.
2. Would you say that you tire more easily now than a few months ago?
3. Do you take the "flu shot" every year? Explain the reasons for your decision.

Physical Assessment

Preparation

- ☑ **Gather the equipment:**

  examination gown
  drape
  examination gloves
  face mask (optional)
  examination light
  skin marker
  metric ruler
  stethoscope

- ☑ **Wash your hands.**
- ☑ **Ask client to remove all clothing to the waist and put on the examination gown.**
- ☑ **Adjust the room environment; have proper lighting and a warm, draft-free environment.**

Remember

- Ensure the client's privacy.
- Explain the procedure to the client before beginning.
- Be organized in your approach and conserve the client's energy.
- The client may be coughing and sneezing during the examination. Use universal precautions.

ASSESSMENT TECHNIQUE/NORMAL FINDINGS

SPECIAL CONSIDERATIONS

Survey

Step 1 *Survey the client.*

- Make a rapid survey of the client to determine the client's ability to participate in the examination.
- Inspect the general overall appearance and position of the client. Pay special attention to the effort of respiration, facial color and expression, lips, muscles being used, and chest movement in the three divisions of the thorax (anterior, posterior, and lateral).

These observations help you confirm the client's state of eupnea, thereby reinforcing the client's ability to participate in the assessment.

Respirations should be effortless, facial color consistent with the rest of the body, and the facial expression relaxed and not fearful. Breathing should be through the nose, with the lips closed without circumoral pallor. The right and left chest movement should be equal, and no supraclavicular or intercostal retractions should be noted.

Individuals experiencing any degree of dyspnea will not be able to participate or cooperate with you during the assessment process. The client most likely will not sit up unassisted, will use more energy to breathe, and may have an alteration in the level of consciousness.

Referral

Individuals experiencing dyspnea who are restless, anxious, and unable to follow your directions may need *immediate* medical assistance.

Inspect the Thorax

Step 1 *Position the client.*

- Begin the examination with the client in a sitting position with all clothing removed to the waist except for the examination gown and drape (Figure 10.13).

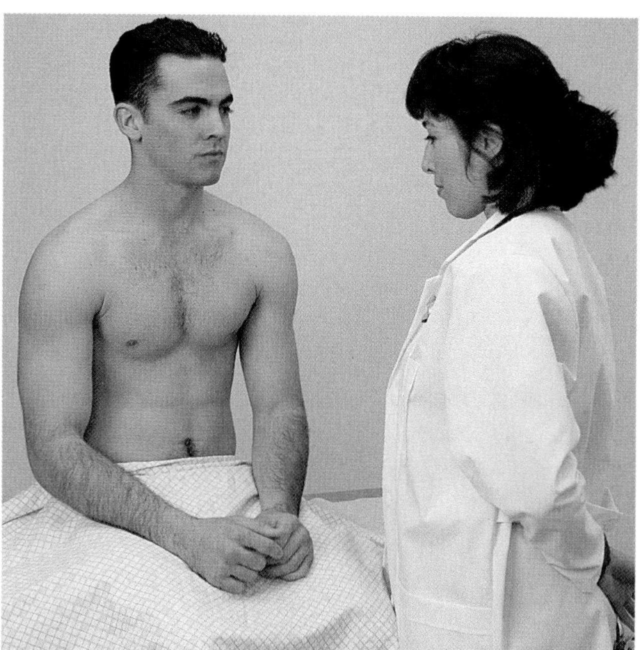

Figure 10.13 Positioning the client.

ASSESSMENT TECHNIQUE/NORMAL FINDINGS

Step 2 *Count the respirations for one full minute.*

- When counting respirations, observe the rate, rhythm, and depth of the respiratory cycle.
- Observe chest movement in the three divisions of the thorax (anterior, posterior, and lateral).
- Confirm respirations as being quiet, symmetric, and effortless.
- Before moving on to the next step, ask the client to take a deep breath and observe muscular involvement. The average adult has 12 to 18 respiratory cycles per minute.

SPECIAL CONSIDERATIONS

The male client tends to breathe abdominally and the female more costally. However, trained athletes and singers tend to breathe abdominally, regardless of gender.

See Table 10.1 on page 247 for altered respiratory patterns.

Step 3 *Inspect skin color.*

- Confirm that the color of the skin of the chest wall (anterior, posterior, and lateral) is consistent with the skin color of rest of the body.

The color of the skin is influenced by pigments of the skin and the oxygen concentration of the blood. Pallor, cyanosis, and a flushed ruddy color call for further evaluation. See Table 8.1 on page 142 for cultural variations in skin tone.

Step 4 *Inspect the configuration of the chest.*

- Compare the transverse diameter to the anteroposterior diameter. This should be approximately a 2:1 ratio in the adult. The infant has a more rounded chest than the adult, and the diameters are more equal.

A change in this ratio may indicate a need for further evaluation. (See Table 10.2 on page 148.)

Step 5 *Determine symmetry of the chest.*

- Stand behind the client and draw an imaginary line across the superior border of the scapulae from the right acromion to the left acromion. This line should be perpendicular to the vertebral line.

One scapula may be higher than the other if the client has had a pneumonectomy. The uneven positions of the scapulae may also be seen with scoliosis and kyphosis (see Chapter 17).

Palpate the Posterior Thorax

Step 1 *Lightly palpate the posterior aspect of the chest.*

- Assess muscle mass and the area directly below the skin for masses.
- Palpate the chest in an organized manner using your finger pads.
- Remember to include the area superior to the scapulae, extend below the twelfth rib, and continue laterally as far as the midaxillary line on both sides.

Muscle mass should be firm, and the skin and subcutaneous area should be free of masses, lesions, and pain.

Painful areas over the posterior thorax may be caused by inflamed fibrous connective tissue. Painful areas overlying intercostal spaces suggest an inflamed pleura.

Crepitus, a crunching feeling like cellophane under the skin, occurs when air escapes into the subcutaneous tissue.

Step 2 *Palpate and count the ribs and intercostal spaces.*

- Ask the client to flex the neck. The seventh cervical spinal process becomes apparent.
- As you move your finger slightly to the left and right of the process, you will feel the first rib.
- As you count the ribs and intercostal spaces, stay close to the vertebral line.

In a thin person, C7 and T1 spinal processes may be visible.

ASSESSMENT TECHNIQUE/NORMAL FINDINGS

SPECIAL CONSIDERATIONS

Step 3 ***Palpate each of the spinal processes in a downward motion.***

- Observe that your finger comes down the column in a straight line.

Deviation indicates a spinal column that is not straight. This can be an indication of scoliosis (see Chapter 17).

Step 4 ***Palpate the posterior thorax for respiratory expansion.***

- Place your hands at about the level of the eighth to tenth ribs. Place your thumbs close to the vertebral line and gently press the skin between your thumbs. Be sure the palm of your hands make contact with the client's back.
- Ask the client to take a deep breath. You should feel equal pressure on your hands, and your thumbs should move evenly away from the vertebral line as the pinched skin becomes relaxed (Figure 10.14).

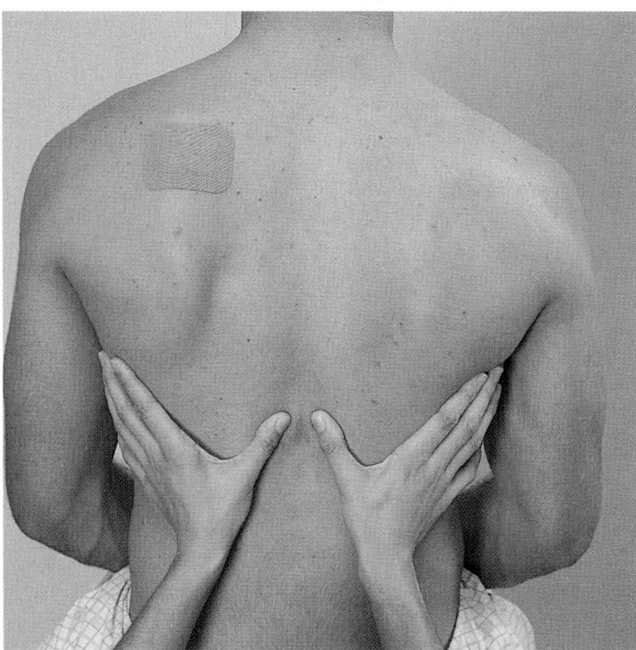

Figure 10.14 Posterior chest expansion.

Decreased chest expansion suggests that the lungs are not expanding to their fullest capacity, gas exchange is reduced, and tissue perfusion is at a minimum. Respiratory expansion decreases in clients with neuromuscular disease or tracheobronchial disease. A decrease in expansion on one side only may result from lung or pleural disease, such as *atelectasis*, tracheobronchial constriction, *pneumonia*, or *pneumothorax* (see Table 10.6 on page 254). It may also be caused by a skeletal problem such as fractured ribs or scoliosis.

Step 5 ***Palpate the posterior chest for tactile fremitus.***

Fremitus is the vibration felt on the outer chest wall as the client speaks. The vibration is greatest over the large diameters of the respiratory system. It should be greatest over trachea, less over bronchi, and almost nonexistent over the alveoli of the lungs.

- Be sure to use only the metacarpophalangeal joint area or the ulnar surface of your hand when palpating for fremitus.
- Ask the client to repeat "ninety-nine" or "one-two-three" as you palpate the areas identified in Figure 10.15.

Diminished vibrations over the trachea or bronchi may indicate simply that the client needs to speak louder. However, diminished vibrations could indicate obstruction of the tracheobronchial tree. Lung consolidation increases the vibrations.

ASSESSMENT TECHNIQUE/NORMAL FINDINGS

SPECIAL CONSIDERATIONS

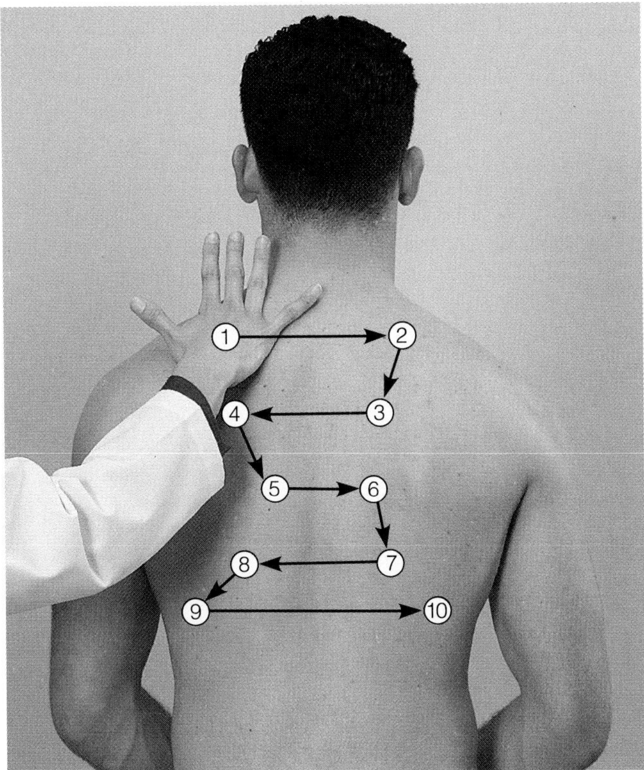

Figure 10.15 Palpating for tactile fremitus on posterior chest.

Percuss the Posterior Thorax

Step 1 *Visualize the thoracic landmarks.*

- Before percussing the posterior thorax, visualize the horizontal lines, vertical lines, level of the diaphragm, and the fissures of the lungs for lobe identification. Also, review the technique of percussion.

Step 2 *Position the client.*

- Help the client lean slightly forward and round the shoulders.

Step 3 *Percuss the lungs.*

- Begin percussion over the apex of the left lung, then move to the apex of the right.
- Move into each intercostal space in a systematic manner. Percuss to the lowest rib and be sure to extend to the left and right midaxillary lines.

Remember not to percuss over the vertebrae, scapulae, or ribs. In the well client, percussion over the lung fields yields a sound of resonance (Figure 10.16 on page 240).

You hear a flat sound when you percuss over bone or solidified tissue.

Hyperresonance over a lung field suggests the possibility of a pneumothorax. However, in some elderly clients, hyperresonance is a normal finding, because the alveoli are overdistended.

ASSESSMENT TECHNIQUE/NORMAL FINDINGS | SPECIAL CONSIDERATIONS

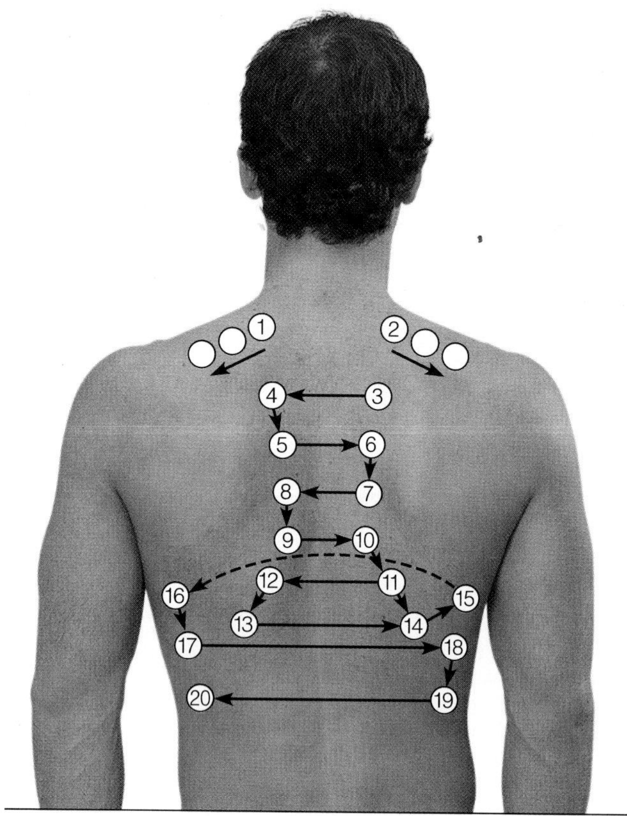

Figure 10.16 Pattern for percussing posterior chest.

Step 4 ***Percuss to determine the movement or excursion of the diaphragm with a forced inspiration and a forced expiration.***

- Beginning at the seventh intercostal space percuss downward along the scapular line to the level of the diaphragm. Resonance should change to dullness.
- Mark the skin using a skin marker.
- Ask the client to take a deep breath and hold it.
- Percuss downward from the skin mark until dullness is again reached.
- Mark the skin for a second time.
- Have the client take several normal breaths.
- Now have the client take one normal breath, exhale as much air as possible, and hold the breath.
- Percuss upward until you hear resonance, mark the skin, and have the client breathe normally. You should have three markings on the skin along the scapular line.
- Repeat the procedure on the other side. The distance between mark number 2 and 3 can be 3 cm to 6 cm in the healthy adult because of diversity in size and body shape (Figure 10.17).
- Return the client to a relaxed sitting position.

A shortened posterior excursion indicates the client is unable or unwilling to take a full breath because of pain, anxiety, abdominal pressure, or phrenic nerve damage. The client with a posterior excursion shorter than 3 cm is not breathing effectively, and exchange of respiratory gases and tissue perfusion may be inadequate.

ASSESSMENT TECHNIQUE/NORMAL FINDINGS | SPECIAL CONSIDERATIONS

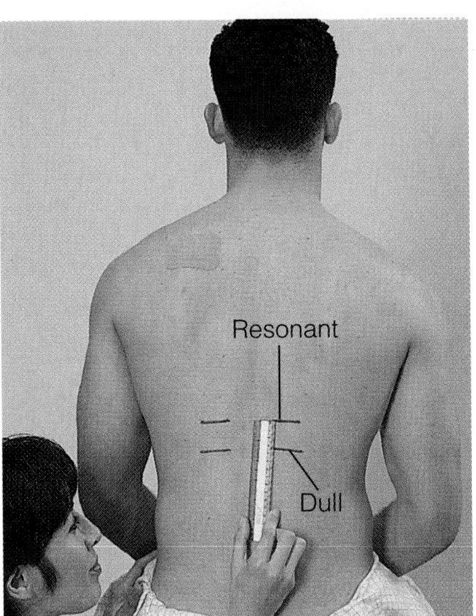

Figure 10.17 Measuring for diaphragmatic excursion on posterior chest.

Auscultate the Posterior Thorax

Step 1 ***Visualize the landmarks.***

- Before auscultating the posterior thorax, visualize the landmarks as before percussion, page 239.

Step 2 ***Auscultate the trachea.***

- Using firm pressure, place the diaphragm of the stethoscope on the chest wall as the client breathes in and out slowly with the mouth open.
- Start at the vertebral line at C7 and work downward to T3. You are auscultating the trachea, and the sound is bronchial.

See Table 10.3 on page 248 for descriptions of normal breath sounds.

Do not confuse static-like sounds with breath sounds. You may hear the sound of the diaphragm rubbing against the client's chest hair, examining gown, pajamas, clothes, or drapes. If the client has thick chest hair, make a tighter contact with the rim of the diaphragm by wetting it down with lotion, water, or water-soluble lubricant.

ALERT!

Make sure to monitor the client's breathing to prevent hyperventilation.

Step 3 ***Auscultate the primary bronchi.***

- Move the stethoscope to the right and left of the vertebral line at the level of T3–T5. Now you are over the right and left primary bronchi, and the sound is bronchovesicular.

A diminished or absent sound may indicate obstruction due to masses, mucous plugs, or even a foreign object.

ASSESSMENT TECHNIQUE/NORMAL FINDINGS

SPECIAL CONSIDERATIONS

Step 4 ***Auscultate the lungs.***

- Auscultate in the same pattern that you used to percuss the lungs, page 239.
- Begin at the apex of the left lung and continue as on page 239. Now you hear a vesicular sound (Figure 10.18).

Clients with emphysema experience diminished lung sounds due to reduced elasticity of lung tissue. Bronchial or bronchovesicular-like sounds heard over the lung periphery usually indicate lung tissue consolidation.

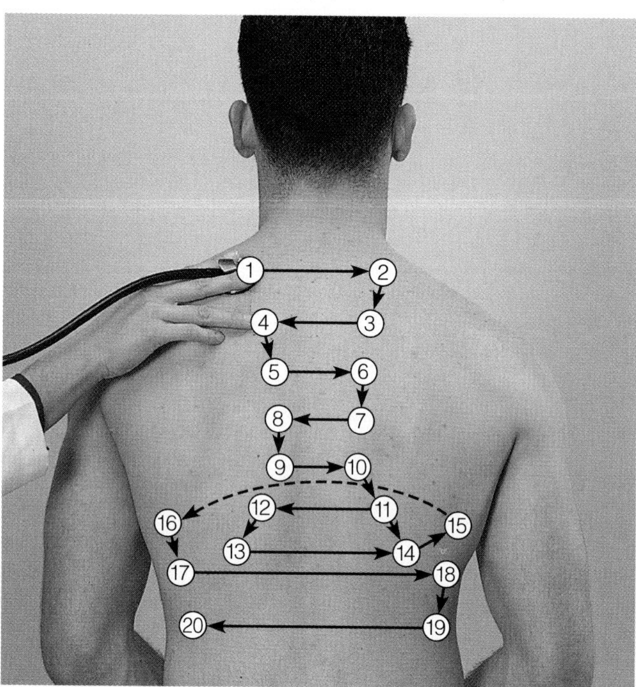

Figure 10.18 Pattern for auscultating posterior chest.

Step 5 ***Listen for adventitious sounds.***

These are sounds superimposed upon the inspiration and expiration of the cycle. When you hear an adventitious sound, note the location, quality, duration, and time of occurrence during the breathing cycle (Table 10.4 on page 249).

Step 6 ***Assess the quality of voice sounds as you auscultate the posterior chest.***

- Ask the client to repeat a phrase such as "ninety-nine" while you listen over the chest wall using the same sequence as step 4, above. The voice transmission is faint, subdued, and indistinguishable.

Bronchophony (words become more clear and distinct) occurs as the lung becomes more dense, as with consolidation or pleural effusion.

- Ask the client to make an "ee-ee-ee-ee" sound while you auscultate again. The "ee-ee-ee-ee" sound is heard clearly through the stethoscope.

Egophony (the "ee-ee-ee" sound becomes "ay" and is less clear) occurs as the lung becomes more dense.

- Ask the client to whisper a phrase such as "a-b-c." The sound is very faint and subdued, almost indistinguishable.

Whispered pectoriloquy (sound becomes more clear and distinct) occurs as the lung becomes more dense.

ASSESSMENT TECHNIQUE/NORMAL FINDINGS | SPECIAL CONSIDERATIONS

Palpate the Anterior Thorax

Step 1 *Position the client.*

The client is usually in a supine position for palpation of the anterior thorax; however, some practitioners prefer the sitting position.

Step 2 *Locate the anterior thoracic landmarks.*

- Locate the jugular (suprasternal) notch with your finger. Palpate downward and identify the ridge of the manubrium at the sternal angle.
- Palpate laterally and find the second rib and the second intercostal space. Count the ribs close to sternal border (see Figure 10.6).

Step 3 *Palpate the muscle mass of the anterior thorax.*

- Palpate the muscle tissue and the tissue directly below the skin.

Muscle mass should be firm and free of pain. The skin should be intact, without masses, and no pain should be elicited.

Step 4 *Palpate the anterior thorax for respiratory expansion.*

- Place your hands on the anterior chest wall just inferior to the costal margins with your thumbs slightly apart at the midsternal line.

As in the posterior chest, decreased chest expansion suggests that the lungs are not expanding to their fullest capacity, gas exchange is reduced, and tissue perfusion is at a minimum.

- Press the skin between your thumbs as you did when palpating the posterior wall, page 238.
- Ask the client to take a deep breath. Observe the movement of your thumbs and the pressure exerted against your hands.

The client with a barrel chest or emphysema will demonstrate little or no movement during this maneuver.

The space between the thumbs should expand evenly and the pressure should be equal (Figure 10.19).

Asymmetric movement occurs when the client splints (guards or holds immobile) one side of the chest because of underlying lung or pleural disease, such as tracheobronchial constriction, pneumonia, or pneumothorax.

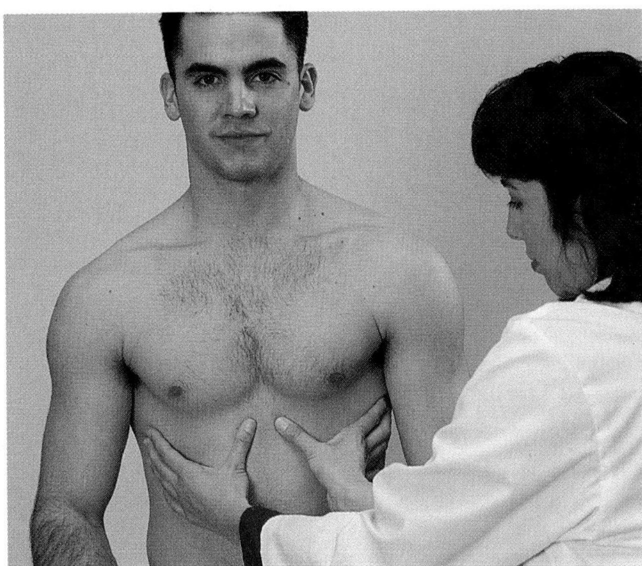

Figure 10.19 Anterior chest expansion.

ASSESSMENT TECHNIQUE/NORMAL FINDINGS	SPECIAL CONSIDERATIONS

Step 5 *Palpate for tactile fremitus on the anterior chest wall.*

Your technique will be similar to that used for the posterior aspect, page 238.

- Using the metacarpophalangeal joint or the ulnar surface of your hand, have the client repeat "ninety-nine" as you palpate the anterior chest wall. Figure 10.20 shows the sequence of palpation.

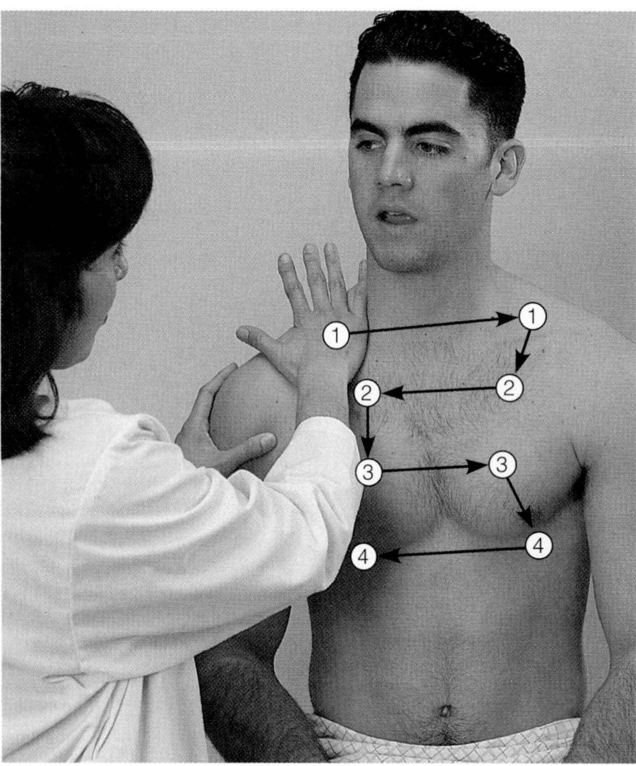

Figure 10.20 Palpating for tactile fremitus on anterior chest.

Percuss the Anterior Thorax

Step 1 *Visualize the anterior thoracic landmarks.*

- Before percussing the anterior chest wall, visualize the vertical and horizontal landmarks. Identify the level of the diaphragm and the lobes of the lungs.

Step 2 *Percuss using an organized pattern.*

- Begin at the apices and continue to the level of the diaphragm. Extend percussion to the midaxillary line on each side. Avoid percussion over the sternum, clavicle, rib and heart.
- Be sure the finger of your nondominant hand is in the intercostal space parallel to the ribs. Before striking this finger, "roll" the finger

ASSESSMENT TECHNIQUE/NORMAL FINDINGS | SPECIAL CONSIDERATIONS

gently on the skin. When you feel the two ribs, your fingers seem to fall into a slight indentation. This is the intercostal space you are looking for (Figure 10.21).

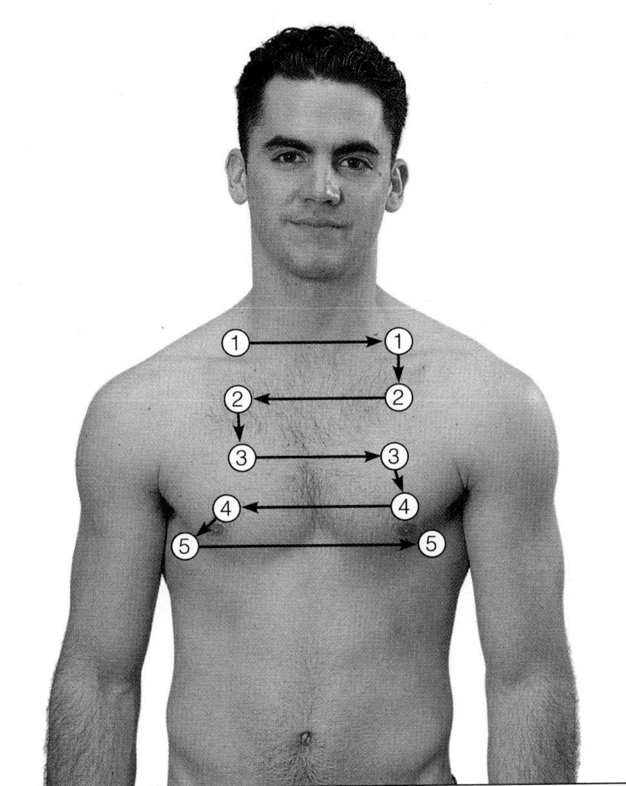

Figure 10.21 Pattern for percussing and auscultating anterior chest.

- If a female client has pendulous breasts, ask her to move the breast during this part of the examination. Percussion over breast tissue in the female will produce a dull sound.

ALERT!

Be sensitive to the client's privacy and limit exposure of body parts.

Auscultate the Anterior Thorax

Step 1 *Visualize the anterior thoracic landmarks.*

Step 2 *Auscultate over the trachea.*

These sounds are best heard in the neck superior to the jugular (suprasternal) notch. The sounds are bronchial (Figure 10.22).

ASSESSMENT TECHNIQUE/NORMAL FINDINGS	SPECIAL CONSIDERATIONS

Step 3 ***Auscultate over the right and left primary bronchi.***

This region is to the right and left of the sternal border at the second and third intercostal spaces. These sounds are bronchovesicular (Figure 10.22).

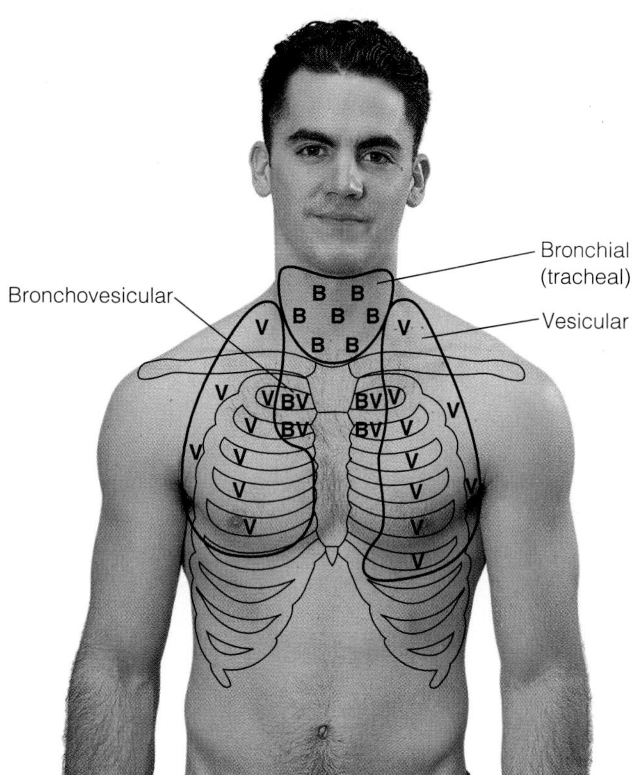

Figure 10.22 Auscultatory sounds.

Step 4 ***Auscultate the lungs.***

- Listen for vesicular sounds. These are heard over lung parenchyma (Figure 10.22).
- Now listen for adventitious sounds. These sounds are superimposed upon the inspiration and expiration of the cycle.
- When you hear an adventitious sound, note the location, quality, and time of occurrence during the respiratory cycle.

Refer to Table 10.4 on page 249 for a description of adventitious sounds.

Reminders

- After completing the respiratory assessment of your client, be sure the client is comfortable and has no adverse effects from the procedure. Assist the client with dressing or returning to a more comfortable position.
- Answer any questions the client has, discuss findings, and provide client teaching to decrease risk factors and promote health and self-care (see page 256).
- In addition to the previous steps of physical assessment, consider common developmental variations for the different client groups discussed on page 250.
- Document the assessment findings as described in Chapter 1. See page 252 for data regarding nursing diagnoses commonly associated with the respiratory system.

Table 10.1 Altered Respiratory Patterns

Type	Pattern	Common Causes
Tachypnea	Rate faster than 24 per minute	Anxiety, pain, or reduced chest expansion caused by enlarged abdominal organs, respiratory insufficiency, pneumonia, pleurisy, and alkalosis
Bradypnea	Rate less than 12 per minute	Upper abdominal or chest pain, electrolyte imbalance, or neurologic damage
Hyperpnea (hyperventilation)	Rapid and deep breathing	Anxiety, exercise, or neurologic or metabolic disease
Kussmaul's respirations	Very deep respirations	Metabolic acidosis
Cheyne-Stokes respirations	Respirations with alternating cycles of deep, rapid breathing followed by periods of apnea	Occur during sleep or with approaching death
Sighing	Frequent sighing	Lack of oxygen or air hunger
Ataxic breathing (Biot's respirations)	Varying depth and rate followed by periods of apnea	Disease of respiratory centers of the brain
Air trapping	Overexpansion of chest and rapid, shallow respirations	Chronic obstructive lung disease: increased bronchial resistance during expiration traps air

Table 10.2 Chest Configurations

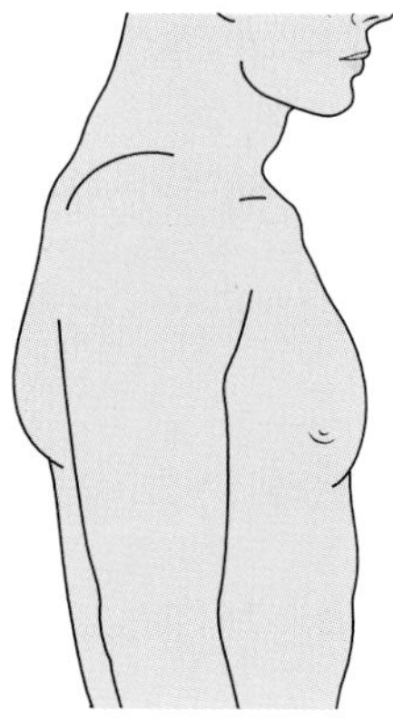

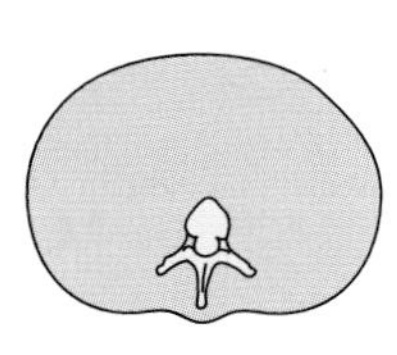

Normal Adult Chest

Ratio of diameters 1:2

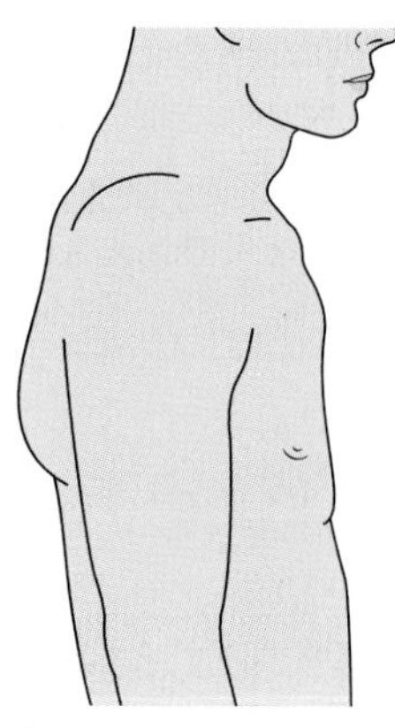

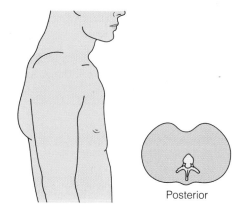

Pectus Excavatum

Also called funnel chest
Sternum and adjacent cartilages appear sunken

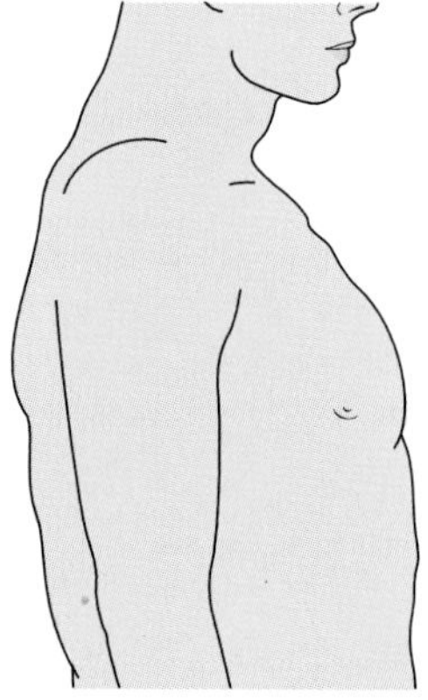

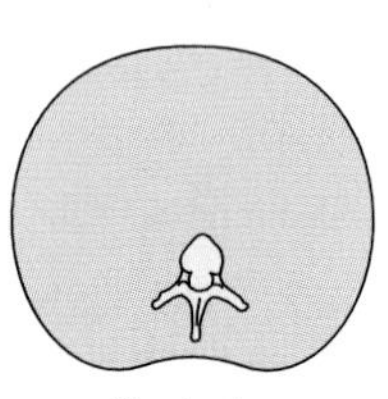

Barrel Chest

Diameters are equal
Ribs more horizontal

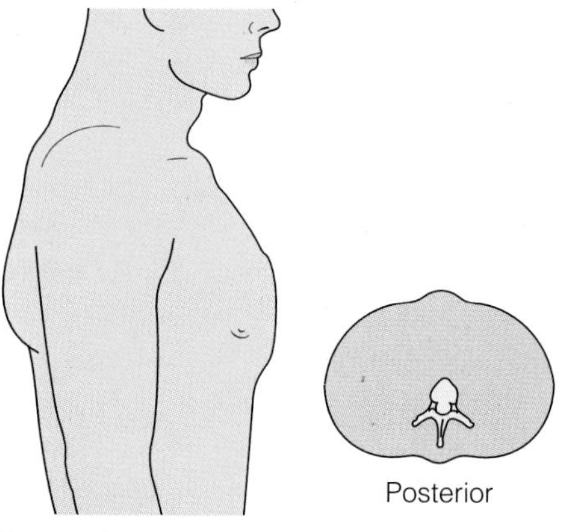

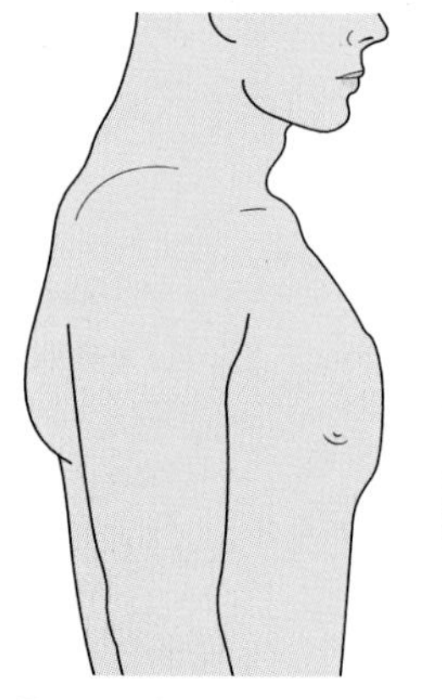

Pectus Carinatum

Also called pigeon breast
Sternum protrudes, ribs slope back

Table 10.3 Normal Breath Sounds

Type	Description	Location	Characteristics
Vesicular	Soft-intensity, low-pitched, "gentle sighing" sounds created by air moving through smaller airways (bronchioles and alveoli)	Over peripheral lung; best heard at base of lungs	Best heard on inspiration, which is about 2.5 times longer than the expiratory phase (5:2 ratio)
Bronchovesicular	Moderate-intensity and moderate-pitched "blowing" sounds created by air moving through larger airways (bronchi)	Between the scapulae and lateral to the sternum at the first and second intercostal spaces	Equal inspiratory and expiratory phases (1:1 ratio)
Bronchial (tubular)	High-pitched, loud, "harsh" sounds created by air moving through the trachea	Anteriorly and posteriorly over the trachea; not normally heard over lung tissue	Louder than vesicular and bronchovesicular sounds; have a short inspiratory phase and long expiratory phase (1:2 ratio)

SOURCE: B Kozier, G Erb, and R Olivieri, *Fundamentals of Nursing*, 4th ed. (Redwood City, Calif.: Addison-Wesley Nursing, 1991), p. 403. Copyright © Addison-Wesley Publishing Co.

Table 10.4 Adventitious Sounds

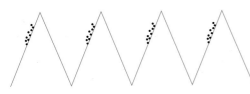

Sound	Characteristics	Occurrence
Crackles or Rales	A series of popping noises similar to a "frying" sound heard in the chest as air coming in suddenly opens the small deflated air passages that are coated and sticky with exudate	Inspiration
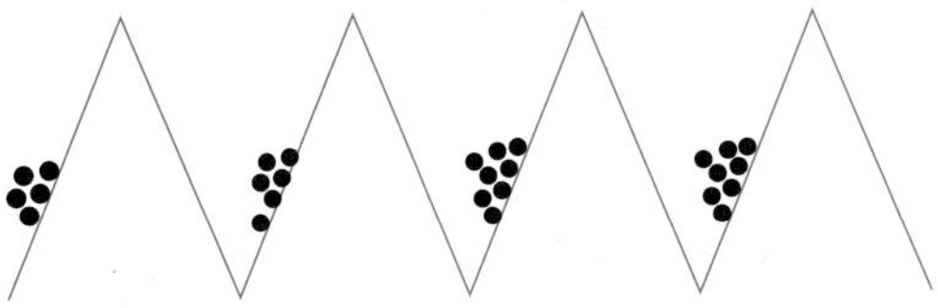 Coarse Rales	Loud, crackling, moist sounds that are low-pitched and bubbling	Inspiration Possible expiration
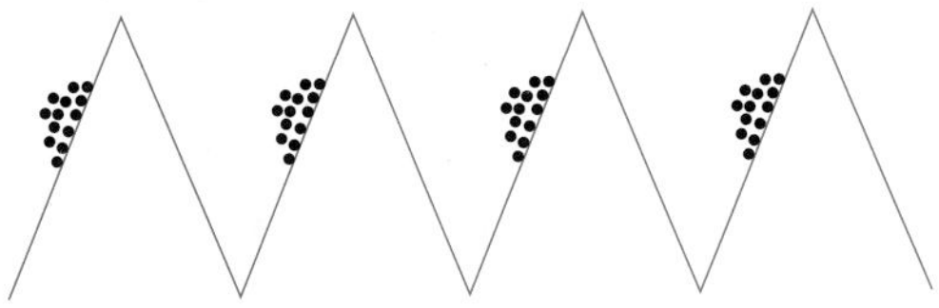 Medium Rales	Similar to but not as loud as course rales	Middle of inspiration
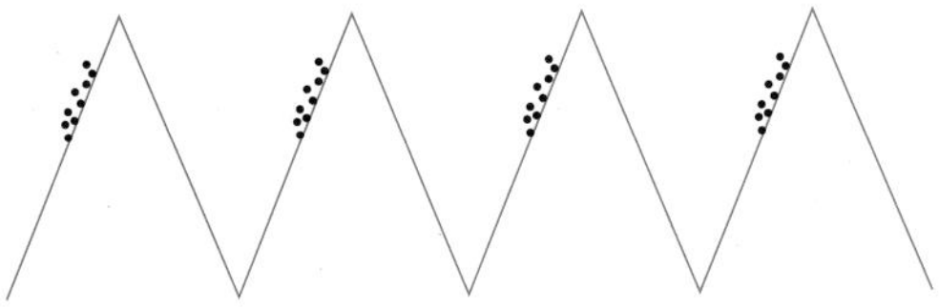 Fine Rales	Noncontinuous popping sound that is high-pitched, short, and crackling	End of inspiration
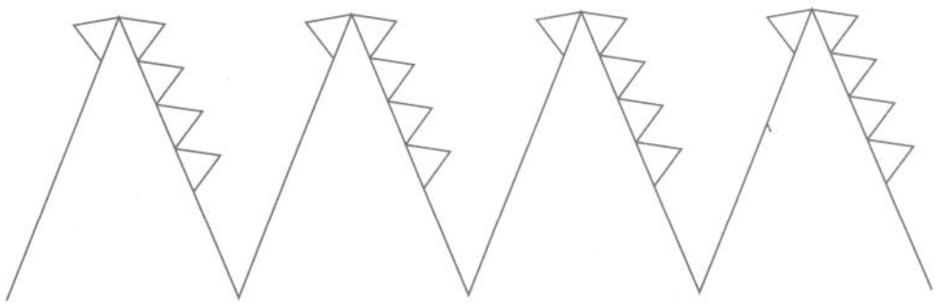 Rhonchi (Sonorous Wheeze)	Continuous, low-pitched, prolonged, deep, and rumbling sound caused by passage of air through trachea or bronchi obstructed by secretions, spasm, or growth	More pronounced during expiration
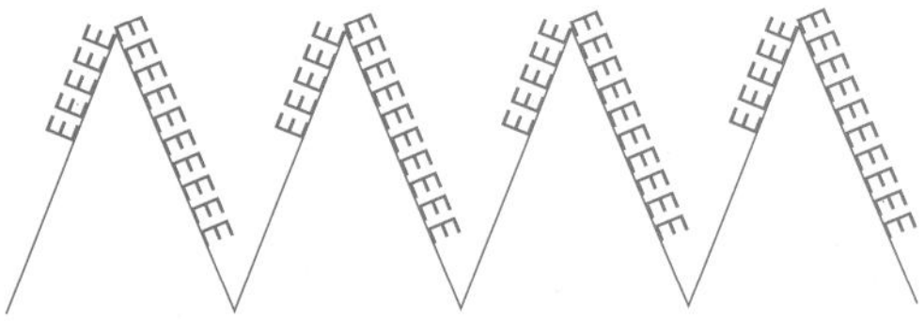 Wheezes (Sibilant Rhonchi)	Continuous, high-pitched, musical sound caused by air forced through narrowed respiratory passages	Inspiration and expiration Louder during expiration
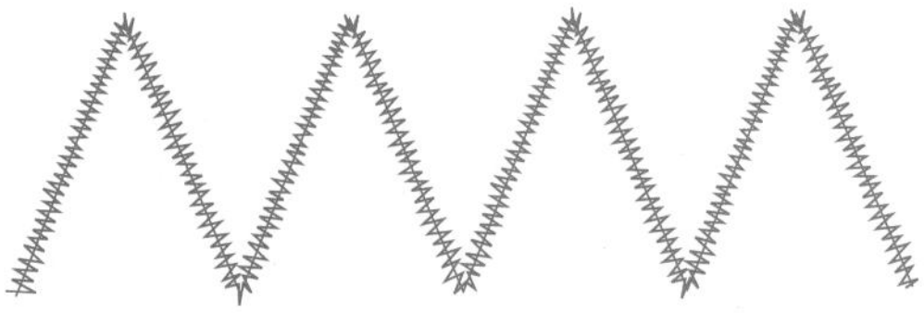 Pleural Friction Rub	Low-pitched, dry, grating sound caused by the rubbing of two inflamed pleural surfaces	Inspiration and expiration

Developmental Considerations

Infant, Children, and Adolescent Clients

A newborn's lungs are not fully inflated until about 2 weeks of age. Respiratory rate is highest in newborns (about 40–80 respirations per minute) and decreases as infancy and childhood progress. Normal respiration at 5 years of age is about 35 breaths per minute. The number of alveoli of the lungs increases throughout infancy and childhood, until a peak in young adulthood.

The infant's chest is round: the anteroposterior diameter roughly equals the transverse diameter. Thus, infants rely on the diaphragm muscle to increase thoracic volume for inspiration, and their characteristic pattern of breathing is diaphragmatic. With growth, the child's chest assumes a more oval shape. Marked disproportions in the chest are checked by measuring the chest size and comparing it with the head size. Generally head and chest circumference are equal at about 1 to 2 years of age. During childhood, chest circumference exceeds head size by about 5–7 cm. The relationship between the two will be altered by abnormal chest shapes such as a barrel chest, which is common with chronic asthma and cystic fibrosis.

Atrophy or hypertrophy of chest muscles should be further evaluated. Asymmetry of the chest may be due to tumors, congenital disorders, pericordial bulging from enlargement of the heart, or poor expansion of one side from a pneumothorax.

If an infant is sleeping, take the opportunity to auscultate lung sounds. But even if the infant is crying, you can easily auscultate breath sounds and palpate for tactile fremitus. Assess an infant's respirations for a full minute, because episodes of irregular respirations are normal in infancy. As noted previously, infants and small children are diaphragmatic breathers. By the age of 6 or 7, costal breathing is the expected pattern. Note that breath sounds in children seem louder than in adults because of the thinness of the chest wall. For a complete physical assessment of infants, children, and adolescents, see Chapter 19.

Childbearing Clients

The increased secretion of estrogen in pregnancy relaxes the ligaments of the thoracic cage, and the horizontal diameter of the thorax expands. At the same time, the enlarging uterus of a childbearing client elevates the diaphragm, and the vertical diameter of the thorax decreases. This increased pressure on the diaphragm, in addition to the increased demand for oxygen placed on the maternal respiratory system by the growing fetus, may lead the woman to experience dyspnea, especially in the later stages of pregnancy. Proper posture throughout pregnancy helps maintain an open thoracic cage. For a complete physical assessment of the childbearing client, see Chapter 20.

Older Clients

As the individual ages, bodily functions change. Many activities of the respiratory system demonstrate a decrease in efficiency. The lungs lose their elasticity, the skeletal muscles begin to weaken, and the bones lose their density. As a result, it becomes more difficult for the older adult to expand the thoracic cage and take a deep breath. The older adult inhales (and thus exhales) smaller amounts of air. As a consequence, there is less oxygen for body use, and more carbon dioxide remains in the body. Weakening of the chest muscles hinders the individual's ability to cough, making clearing of the airways more difficult. Airway clearance is further compromised by the decrease or destruction of cilia in the system.

Many older adults lose subcutaneous adipose tissue, and certain bony thoracic prominences may become more visible. The 2:1 ratio of the chest diameter changes, and a more rounded or barrel chest is observed (see Table 10.2).

Rate of respiration in the older adult is slightly higher than in the middle adult. The older adult has a more shallow respiratory cycle because of the change in the vital capacity. The older adult's normal breath sounds may be difficult to hear because of decreased pulmonary function.

Chronicity is a problem with older adults as changes occur in the lung parenchyma. Upon percussion, the chest may produce hyperresonance rather than resonance, because the alveoli become distended and air becomes trapped in the lungs.

Remember that older adults tire more easily, and it may be necessary to include frequent rest periods during the physical assessment of the respiratory system. Before proceeding, anticipate that you may need more time than usual for assessment, and expect findings to reflect variations of age and history. For a complete physical assessment of the older adult, see Chapter 21.

Psychosocial Considerations

Stress, anxiety, and fatigue may exacerbate respiratory problems such as asthma. Certain drugs, eg, bronchodilators, used in the treatment of respiratory conditions may cause the hands to tremble visibly. Do not confuse this sign with nervousness. Even mild respiratory distress is frightening for the client and family. Proceeding in a calm, reassuring manner helps reduce the client's fear. Parents of young children who have experienced severe asthmatic attacks in the past may be extremely anxious any time the child develops a cold, seasonal allergy, or any other respiratory problem. Again, calm and careful assessment of the child's current health status reduces the parents' anxiety. Many elderly and young children with respiratory ailments may be restricted from participating in pleasurable activities such as shopping, outings, or school sports. Assess these clients for social isolation and low self-esteem.

Self-Care Considerations

Yearly influenza immunization is recommended, especially for older adults and those with chronic respiratory problems.

Regular exercise increases respiratory efficiency. Smoking decreases respiratory efficiency and is the primary risk factor for lung cancer. If smoking is begun in the early teens, the lungs never completely mature, and these additional alveoli are never formed.

Family, Cultural, and Environmental Considerations

Though not always absolute, the chest volume may differ in persons of different races. In some cases, the chest volume of Caucasians and African Americans is greater than that of Asians or Native Americans.

Clients with allergies and/or asthma should be encouraged to explore the possibility of allergens in their work or home environment. For example, pets, dust, and molds are common allergens found in the home. Second-hand smoke in the home or work environment can also lead to respiratory distress, and research has established a link between exposure to second-hand smoke and the development of lung cancer.

Some industries expose workers to substances that are hazardous to their respiratory health, such as caustic fumes, fungi, asbestos, airplane glue, coal tar, nickel, silver, textile fibers, radon, chloromethyl ethers, chromate, and vinyl chlorides. All of these substances are known carcinogens. Exposure to large amounts of dust, eg, in a granary or mine, may lead to the development of silicosis. Coal miners are susceptible to coal miner's disease, a form of pneumoconiosis.

Organizing the Data

After completing the focused interview and the respiratory assessment of the client, review and organize the data collected. Integrate the newly obtained data with previously collected data and then form clusters. The newly formed clusters become the basis for nursing diagnoses. Identify nursing interventions such as client teaching that will help maintain or promote wellness, reduce risk factors, or foster self-care. Collaborative problems may also be identified. Work with other members of the health care team before identifying interventions.

Identifying Nursing Diagnoses

Ineffective airway clearance, *ineffective breathing pattern*, and *impaired gas exchange* are three of the more common nursing diagnoses related to the respiratory system. These three diagnoses have similarities and unique characteristics that are interrelated. For example, the client experiencing ineffective airway clearance may not be able to cough and move the mucus obstructing the passages. This then can lead to impaired gas exchange in which oxygen and carbon dioxide are not exchanged at the alveolar level. See Table 10.5 on page 252 for the related factors and the defining characteristics of these three diagnoses.

Common Alterations in the Health of the Respiratory System

Alterations in the health of the respiratory system include infections, allergic reactions, obstructive processes, and others requiring collaborative care. The most common of these problems are discussed in Table 10.6 on page 254. A comparison of position, precipitating factors, quality, and other descriptors of pain for four common respiratory disorders is provided in Table 10.7 on page 256.

Table 10.5 Nursing Diagnoses Commonly Associated with the Respiratory System

INEFFECTIVE AIRWAY CLEARANCE

Definition: A state in which an individual is unable to clear secretions or obstructions from the respiratory tract to maintain airway patency (NANDA).

DEFINING CHARACTERISTICS

Abnormal breath sounds, such as rales, rhonchi	Cough: effective or ineffective, with or without sputum
Changes in rate or depth of respiration	Cyanosis
Tachypnea	Dyspnea

RELATED FACTORS

Decreased energy/fatique, Trauma, Tracheobronchial infection, Tracheobronchial obstruction, Tracheobronchial secretions, Perceptive/cognitive impairment, Others specific to client (specify).

INEFFECTIVE BREATHING PATTERN

Definition: The state in which an individual's inhalation and/or exhalation pattern does not enable adequate pulmonary inflation or emptying (NANDA).

DEFINING CHARACTERISTICS

Pursed lip breathing/prolonged expiratory phase	Change in depth of respirations
Dyspnea	Abnormal blood gases
Tachypnea	Increased anterioposterior diameter
Cyanosis	Use of accessory muscles
Fremitus	Altered chest excusion
Cough	Premature infant
Assumption of 3-point position	Nasal flaring
Shortness of breath	

RELATED FACTORS

Anxiety, Decreased energy/fatigue, Perception/cognitive impairment, Musculoskeletal impairment, Chronic or acute pain, Neuromuscular paralysis/weakness, Others specific to client (specify).

Table 10.5 Diagnoses Associated with the Respiratory System (continued)

IMPAIRED GAS EXCHANGE	
Definition: The state in which the individual experiences a decreased passage of oxygen and/or carbon dioxide between the alveoli of the lungs and the vascular system (NANDA).	
DEFINING CHARACTERISTICS	
Inability to move secretions	Irritability
Confusion	Hypoxia
Restlessness	Hypercapnia
Somnolence	
RELATED FACTORS	
Decreased pulmonary blood supply secondary to pulmonary hypertension, pulmonary embolus, congestive heart failure, respiratory distress syndrome, anemia; Decreased functional lung tissue secondary to chronic lung disease, pneumonia, thoracotomy, atelectasis, respiratory distress syndrome, mass, diaphragmatic hernia; Ventilation-perfusion imbalance; Others specific to client (specify).	

DIAGNOSTIC REASONING IN ACTION

Mrs. Flower Smith, age 62, is an African-American female who is admitted for an elective lumbar laminectomy.

Following surgery she returns to the nursing unit. Review of the chart reveals she received general anesthetic and underwent endotracheal intubation. She was extubated in the postanesthesia room 5½ hours later.

Postoperatively, Mrs. Smith refuses to be "log-rolled" every 2 hours, indicating her back hurts when she moves. She uses the incentive spirometer; however, she is reluctant to take deep breaths and has not increased her volume to the preoperative level.

By the third postoperative day, her temperature is 39.1C (102.4F), adventitious sounds are auscultated at the base of both lungs, and she is not willing to cough, stating "It hurts my back." Chest radiography confirms bilateral lobe infiltrate, and a postoperative complication of hypostatic pneumonia.

The nursing assessment of Mrs. Smith provides the following subjective and objective data:

- Temperature 39.1C (102.4F), pulse 92
- Respirations 28 and shallow
- Adventitious sounds, bilateral, lower lung fields
- Limited nonproductive cough
- Fatigue
- Lumbar pain
- Immobility
- Ineffective use of the incentive spirometer
- Reluctance to ask for analgesic

To cluster the information the nurse:

- Considers the data regarding vital signs, quality of respirations, adventitious sounds, and nonproductive cough.
- Considers the data regarding immobility and ineffective use of the incentive spirometer.

Jean Sage, RN, arrives at the following nursing diagnoses:

1. *Ineffective airway clearance* related to immobility and pain control
2. *Knowledge deficit* related to ineffective use of the incentive spirometer

Ms Sage reinforces the preoperative teaching regarding pain control and use of the spirometer. She also helps Mrs. Smith with log-rolling at peak medication time.

Table 10.6 Common Alterations in the Health of the Respiratory System

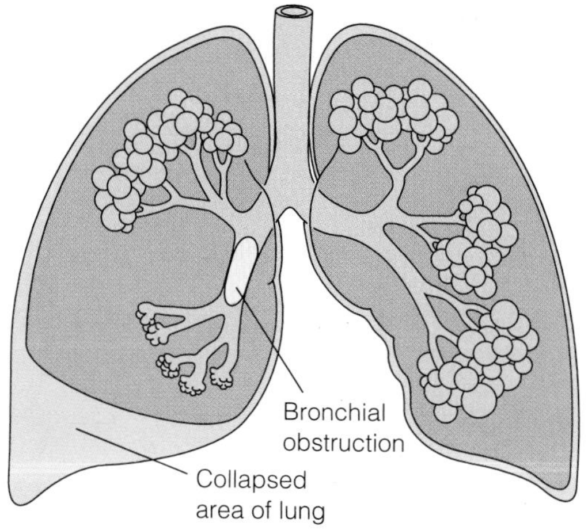

Atelectasis

Collapsing of a section or entire lung. Could be caused by mucous plug, or aspiration of a foreign body.

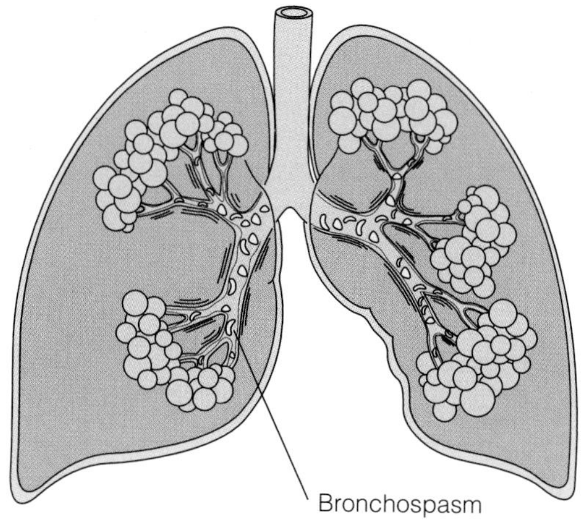

Asthma

Associated with an allergic response, edema, spasms, and irritation to the bronchi. Wheezing on expiration is common.

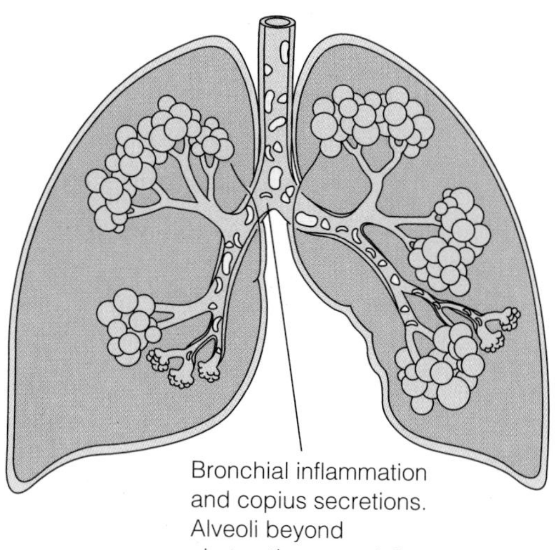

Bronchitis

Inflammation of the bronchi with increased mucus and narrowing of the bronchi. This can spread to the trachea. This is more common in children and is accompanied by a harsh stridorous or "barking" cough.

Table 10.6 Common Alterations in the Health of the Respiratory System

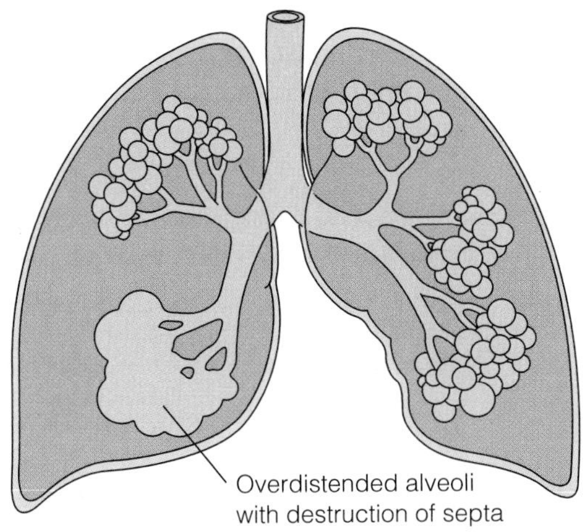

Emphysema

Overdistended alveoli with air trapped in the lung. Diminished breath sounds and pursed lip breathing are common.

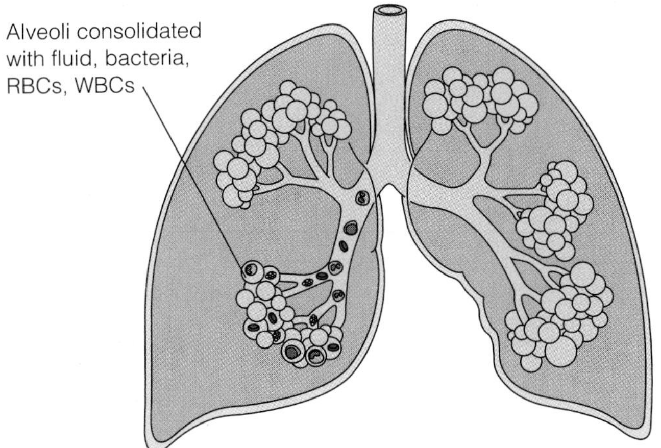

Pneumonia

Infection of the lung tissue with consolidation. Adventitious sounds are auscultated. The client may splint the involved side and have shallow respirations.

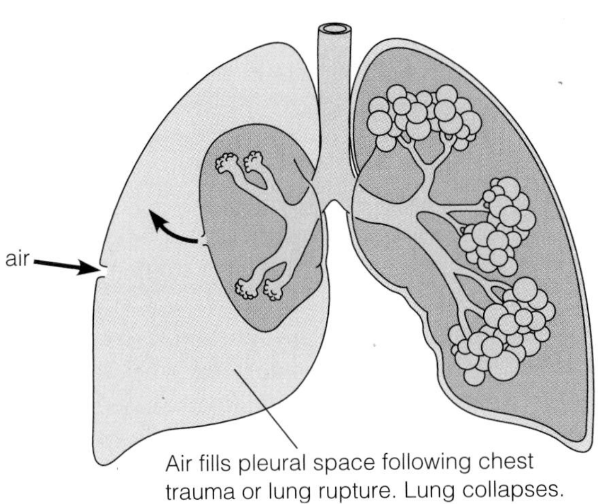

Pneumothorax

Partial or complete collapse of the lung from free air entering the pleural space. Trauma is one cause of a pneumothorax.

Table 10.7 Pain Assessment with Common Respiratory Disorders

	Pulmonary Embolism	Pleurisy	Pneumothorax	Pneumonia
Description	A condition characterized by a blood clot that has traveled to the lungs	An inflammation of both the parietal pleura, which lines the thoracic cavity, and the visceral pleura, which covers the lungs	An accumulation of air or gas in the pleural cavity, between the parietal and visceral pleurae	An inflammation of the tissue of the lungs
Position	Substernal or precordial	Anywhere on the chest, sides, or back	Usually on the sides but may be felt on precordium	Precordium but deep into the chest
Precipitating factors	Virchow's triad precipitators	Deep breath, coughing, twisting of the upper torso	Trauma, coughing, mechanical ventilator, may be spontaneous	Aspiration, ineffective cough effort postsurgery, any condition that contributes to secretion or retention of mucus
Quality	*If massive:* sudden, sharp, crushing chest pain *If acute:* sharp pain that can be stabbing	Stabbing, piercing, can make the client breathe in short breaths	Sharp, stabbing	Sharp, burning, may be described as a punch inside the chest
Radiation	Does not radiate	May radiate to the neck or shoulder	May radiate to shoulder on the same side	Does not radiate
Relief	Sitting upright, may be relieved by administration of thrombolytics	Usually no interventions needed	Analgesia, chest tube insertion, rest	Analgesia, rest, antibiotics
Severity	Variable on the 1–10 scale	Variable on the 1–10 scale, but usually very severe	Variable on the 1–10 scale	Variable on the 1–10 scale
Timing	Usually sudden, without warning	Usually sudden, without warning	Usually sudden, without warning	May be either gradual or sudden
Duration	Minutes to days	Minutes to days	Hours	Days to weeks

Reprinted by permission of Johanna K. Stiesmeyer, RN, MSN.

Health Promotion and Client Education

At the conclusion of the respiratory assessment, answer any questions the client may have and stress the importance of a healthy respiratory system. This could include prevention of problems, limitation of existing problems, or correction of an existing problem to improve health.

Promoting the General Health of the Respiratory System

To maintain the general health of the respiratory system, advise the client of the following:

- Smoking is the primary risk factor for lung cancer. If you smoke, stop. If you don't smoke, don't start. If you live or work with someone who smokes, insist that the person not smoke indoors.
- Exercise daily. If the client has asthma, pretreatment with drugs such as albuterol and theophylline may prevent bronchospasms. Swimming is an excellent exercise for asthmatics, as are activities that require short bursts of energy, such as baseball or gymnastics. Cold-weather events, such as skiing or ice hocky, and nonstop activities, such as basketball or soccer, are more likely to aggravate asthma.
- Eat a balanced diet.
- Consider yearly immunization against influenza.
- Use precautions when with a large group of people or with a person experiencing an upper respiratory infection.
- Avoid pollutants, allergens, and other contaminants. To keep your home free from dust and other allergic irritants, keep surfaces of furniture and floors smooth, uncluttered, and clean. Use low-pile carpeting or keep floors bare of carpeting. Vacuum weekly or more often. If an animal allergy is clearly demonstrated, consider removing pets from the home. Outdoors, eliminate ragweed and wild grasses from yards.

DIAGNOSTIC REASONING IN ACTION

Edwin McInerny is a 42-year-old man who works in the paint shop of a manufacturing company. He reports to the health nurse, Diana Chu, feeling "light-headed, short of breath, and nauseous."

Ms Chu finds that Mr. McInerny's blood pressure is 146/80; his pulse is 88 and thready; and his respirations are 34, labored, and shallow. She also notes an audible wheeze. As he coughs, he produces a tenacious, clear mucus.

The paint shop requires all employees to wear protective face masks, and Mr. McInerny admits to not wearing his mask today. He tells Ms Chu that he usually smokes one pack of cigarettes per day.

Ms Chu reviews all the data, clusters the information, and develops the following nursing diagnoses:

1. *Ineffective breathing pattern* related to environmental pollutants
2. *Impaired gas exchange* related to mucus in bronchial tree

Ms Chu refers Mr. McInerny to the company's physician. She instructs Mr. McInerny in breathing exercises and techniques for productive coughing. She also explains to him the importance of wearing his face mask when working, and gives him information about the company's smoking-cessation program. At the conclusion of their discussion, Ms Chu helps Mr. McInerny to a small private room to rest.

- Avoid irritants that are known to trigger respiratory problems in some people. These include tobacco smoke; strong vapors from household cleaners, paints, and varnishes; chemicals such as coal and chalk dust; air pollution; cold, dry air; and strong winds.
- Use a humidifier and dehumidifier appropriately.
- Routinely change filters in air conditioners and heaters.
- Employ safety features in the workplace such as the use of face masks.
- Avoid anxiety, nervous stress, and fatigue, which may worsen the symptoms of respiratory problems such as asthma.
- Identify personal risk factors and take action.

Summary

The assessment of the client's respiratory system provides valuable data regarding the overall health status of the individual. Knowledge of the anatomy, physiology, and landmarks helps you perform the assessment, identify variations that occur, and perform professional activities. The health history and the focused interview are a strong database for the physical assessment. Physical assessment of the respiratory systems reveals much data concerning the body's ability to take in air, utilize the gases, and then exchange the gases. The ability of the body to transport the gases is influenced by the cardiovascular system. After performing the physical assessment, formulate nursing diagnoses specific to the client. Provide information to the client to maintain a healthy respiratory system, and stop or limit a pathological process in progress. Your actions should be informed, reliable, and reflective of client needs as you implement your professional role.

Key Points

- ✓ The respiratory system consists of the upper and lower tracts. The upper tract includes the nose, sinuses, pharynx, and larynx. The lower tract includes the trachea, bronchi, and lungs. The primary function of the respiratory system is the exchange of gases between the body and the atmosphere.
- ✓ Anatomical landmarks are used to identify underlying structures for assessment, reporting, and recording of the data.
- ✓ Conduct a focused interview to obtain specific data regarding the health status of the respiratory system of the client. The data from the focused interview is added to the health history for a more comprehensive database. The database includes habits, health practices, and cultural and environmental factors.
- ✓ Inspect the client for respiratory rate, quality of the respirations, symmetry of chest movement, color of the skin, and position used in breathing.
- ✓ Palpate the anterior, posterior, and lateral aspects of the thorax for expansion and tactile fremitus.
- ✓ Percuss the anterior, posterior, and lateral aspects of the thorax for diaphragmatic excursion and resonance.
- ✓ Auscultate all aspects of the thorax for bronchial, bronchovesicular, and vesicular sounds. Adventitious sounds superimposed on the respiratory cycle must be evaluated.
- ✓ Nursing diagnoses commonly associated with the respiratory system include ineffective airway clearance, ineffective breathing pattern, and impaired gas exchange.
- ✓ Provide the client with information needed to promote health of the respiratory system.

Chapter 11

Assessing the Cardiovascular System

The cardiovascular system circulates blood continually throughout the body to deliver oxygen and nutrients to the body's organs and tissues and to dispose of their excreted wastes. The health of the cardiovascular system may be promoted throughout the lifespan through self-care habits, such as eating a low-fat diet, exercising, and not smoking. Still, the delicate balance of this system is vulnerable to stress, trauma, and a variety of pathologic mechanisms that may impair its ability to function. Inadequate tissue perfusion results in both a diminished supply of nutrients necessary to carry on routine metabolic functions and a build-up of metabolic wastes. Thus, significant cardiovascular problems may contribute to organ failure.

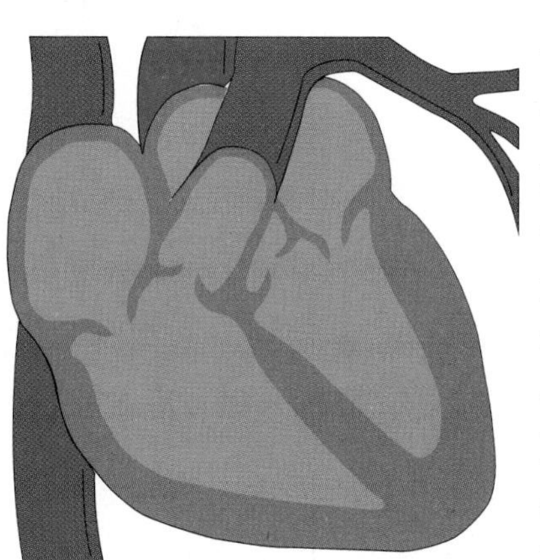

To perform an accurate cardiovascular assessment, you need a solid understanding of cardiovascular anatomy and physiology, reviewed in the next section. By asking appropriate questions during the focused interview, you uncover clues to the client's health status and any cardiovascular problems. Assessment of the client's psychosocial health, self-care habits, family, culture, and environment is an important part of the focused interview; keep these findings in mind as you conduct the physical assessment. Recognize also that the health of the cardiovascular system affects and is affected by the health of all other body sytems. Figure 11.1 summarizes the most significant of these assessment considerations.

During the physical assessment, you assess and evaluate the sometimes ambiguous cues of actual and potential cardiac disease. You then develop nursing diagnoses and a plan of collaborative or independent nursing care. Finally, you play a key role in teaching the healthy client the facts about preventing cardiovascular disease. For the client with cardiovascular disease, you provide teaching to promote optimum health according to the client's individual needs.

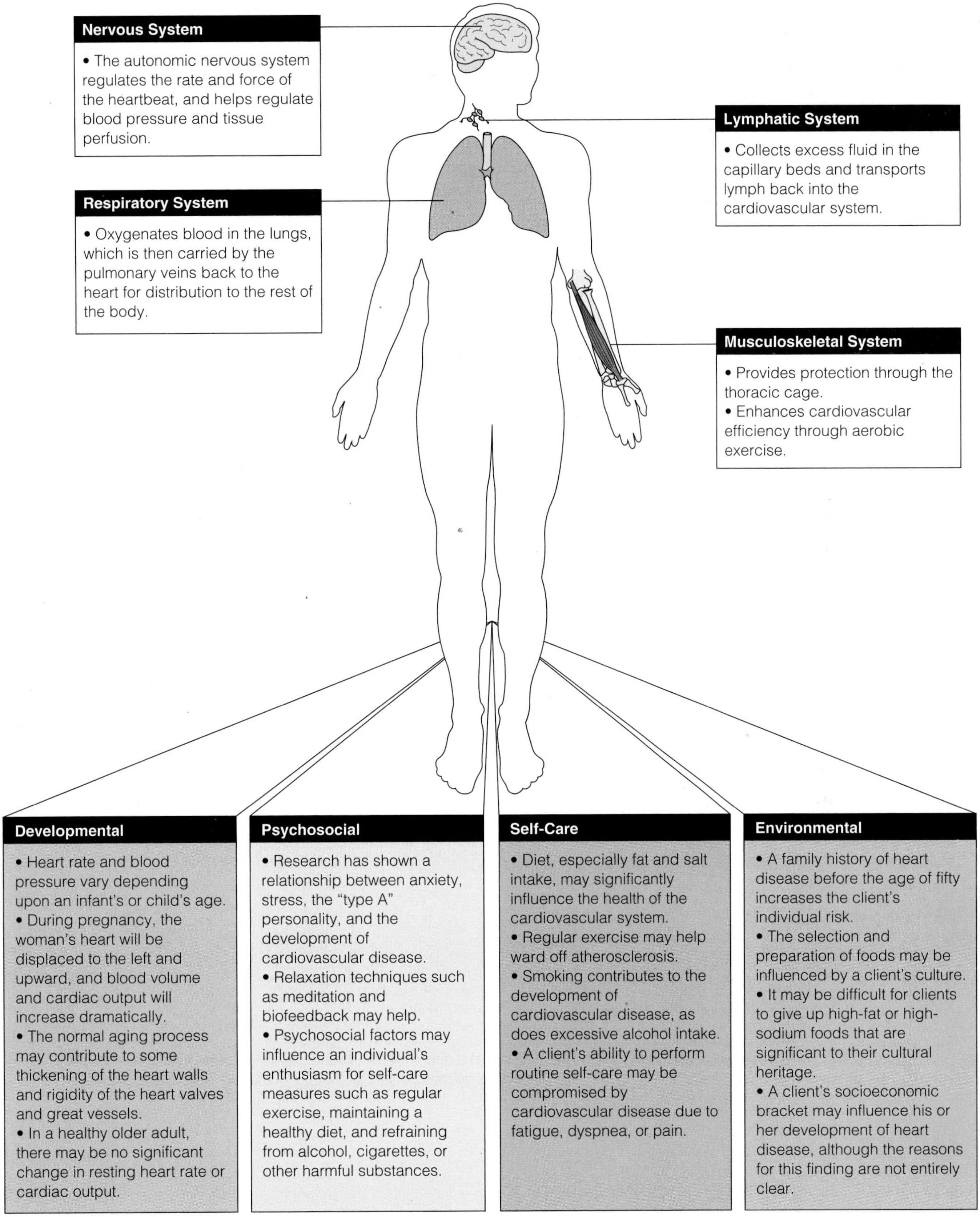

Nervous System
- The autonomic nervous system regulates the rate and force of the heartbeat, and helps regulate blood pressure and tissue perfusion.

Lymphatic System
- Collects excess fluid in the capillary beds and transports lymph back into the cardiovascular system.

Respiratory System
- Oxygenates blood in the lungs, which is then carried by the pulmonary veins back to the heart for distribution to the rest of the body.

Musculoskeletal System
- Provides protection through the thoracic cage.
- Enhances cardiovascular efficiency through aerobic exercise.

Developmental
- Heart rate and blood pressure vary depending upon an infant's or child's age.
- During pregnancy, the woman's heart will be displaced to the left and upward, and blood volume and cardiac output will increase dramatically.
- The normal aging process may contribute to some thickening of the heart walls and rigidity of the heart valves and great vessels.
- In a healthy older adult, there may be no significant change in resting heart rate or cardiac output.

Psychosocial
- Research has shown a relationship between anxiety, stress, the "type A" personality, and the development of cardiovascular disease.
- Relaxation techniques such as meditation and biofeedback may help.
- Psychosocial factors may influence an individual's enthusiasm for self-care measures such as regular exercise, maintaining a healthy diet, and refraining from alcohol, cigarettes, or other harmful substances.

Self-Care
- Diet, especially fat and salt intake, may significantly influence the health of the cardiovascular system.
- Regular exercise may help ward off atherosclerosis.
- Smoking contributes to the development of cardiovascular disease, as does excessive alcohol intake.
- A client's ability to perform routine self-care may be compromised by cardiovascular disease due to fatigue, dyspnea, or pain.

Environmental
- A family history of heart disease before the age of fifty increases the client's individual risk.
- The selection and preparation of foods may be influenced by a client's culture.
- It may be difficult for clients to give up high-fat or high-sodium foods that are significant to their cultural heritage.
- A client's socioeconomic bracket may influence his or her development of heart disease, although the reasons for this finding are not entirely clear.

Figure 11.1 Important factors to consider when assessing the cardiovascular system.

Anatomy and Physiology Review

The cardiovascular system comprises the heart and the vascular system. The heart includes the cardiac muscle, atria, ventricles, valves, coronary arteries, cardiac veins, electrical conducting structures, and cardiac nerves. The vascular system is composed of the blood vessels of the body: the arteries, arterioles, veins, venules, and capillaries. In this chapter, only the coronary blood vessels are considered in detail. The peripheral vascular system is discussed in Chapter 16. The major functions of the cardiovascular system are

- Transporting nutrients and oxygen to the body
- Removing wastes and carbon dioxide
- Maintaining adequate perfusion of organs and tissues

Pericardium

The heart is surrounded by a thin sac composed of a fibroserous material called the **pericardium** (Figure 11.2). Its tougher outer layer, called the *fibrous pericardium*, protects the heart and anchors it to the adjacent structures such as the diaphragm and great vessels. The inner layer is called the *serous pericardium*. It also is composed of two layers: parietal and visceral. The *parietal layer* is the outer layer. The *visceral layer* is the inner layer, which lines the surface of the heart. Fluid between the fibrous and serous pericardium lubricates the layers and allows for a gliding motion between them with each heartbeat.

Heart

The **heart** is an intricately designed pump composed of a meticulous network of synchronized structures. It lies behind the sternum and typically extends from the second rib to the fifth intercostal space (Figure 11.3). It sits obliquely within the thoracic cavity between the lungs and above the diaphragm in an area called mediastinal space. Ventrally, the right side of the heart is more forward than the left. The upper posterior edge of the heart is known as the *base*. The lower edge, or *apex*, is downward, forward, and to the left. The heartbeat is most easily palpated over the apex; thus, this point is referred to as the *point of maximal intensity* (PMI).

The heart is approximately 12.8 cm (5 in) long, 9 cm (3.5 in) across, and 6.4 cm (2.5 in) thick, and slightly larger in size than the client's clenched fist. In the female, the heart typically is smaller and weighs less than the heart of the male.

Heart Wall The **heart wall** is composed of three layers: epicardium, myocardium, and endocardium (see Figure 11.2). The outer layer, called the *epicardium*, is anatomically identical to the visceral pericardium described above. The *myocardium* is the thick, muscular layer. It is mainly responsible for the contraction of the heart. The myocardium is composed of bundles of cardiac muscle fibers reinforced by an interconnecting network of connective tissue fibers called the "fibrous skeleton of the heart." The innermost layer is the *endocardium*, a smooth

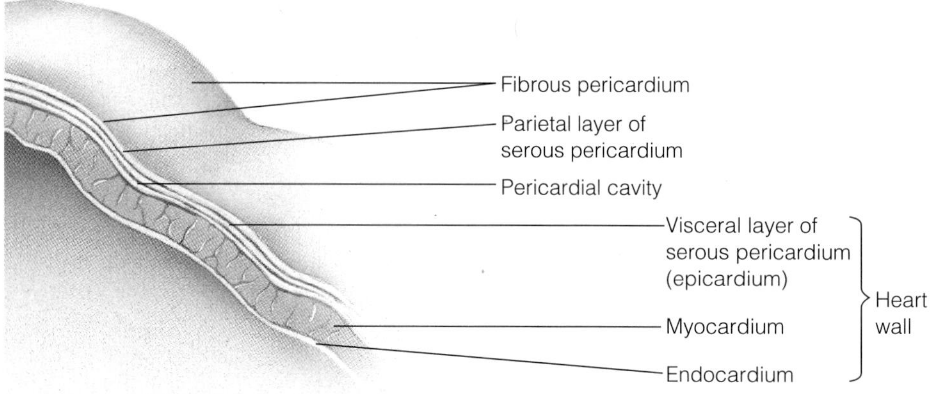

Figure 11.2 The pericardium and the myocardial muscle layers.

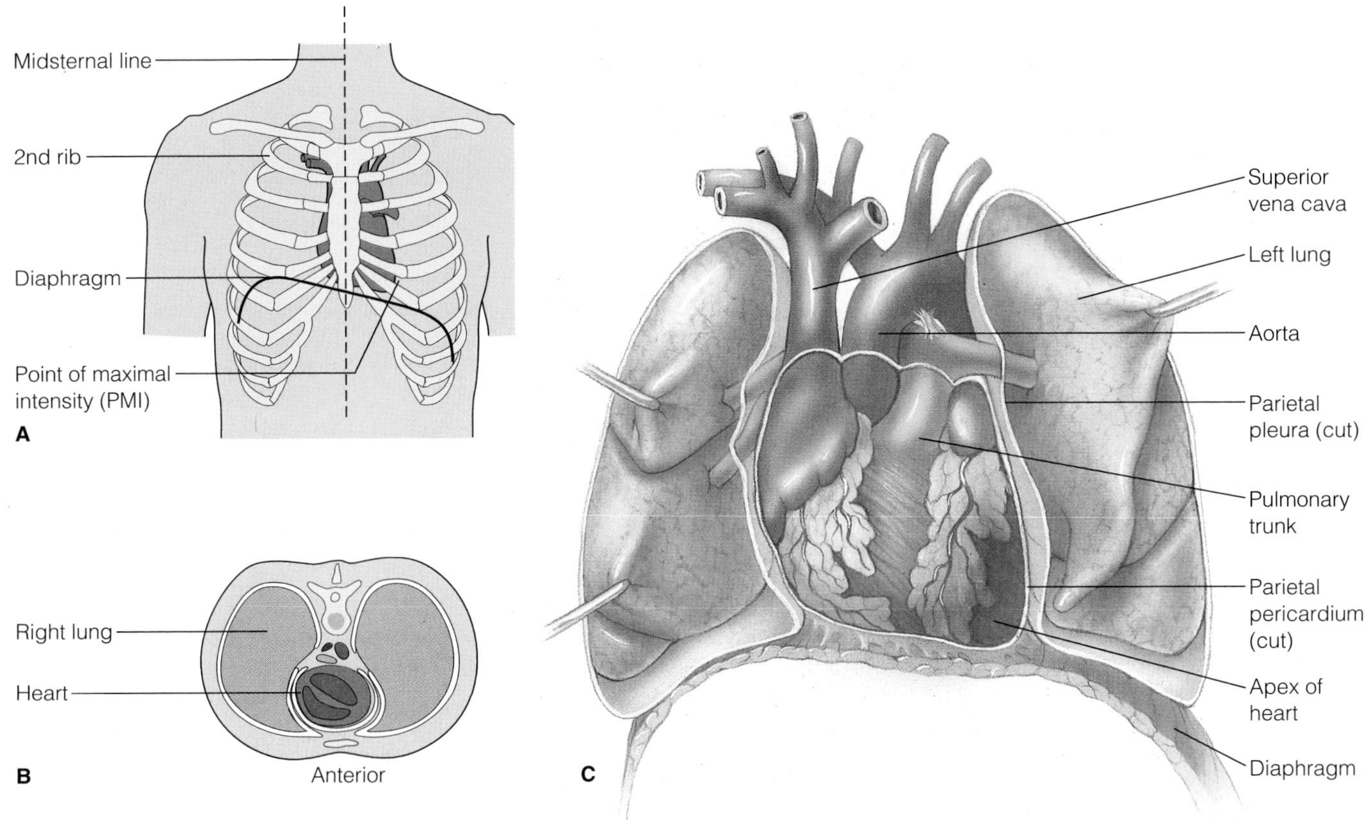

Figure 11.3 Location of the heart in the mediastinum of the thorax. *A*, Relationship of the heart to the sternum, ribs, and diaphragm. *B*, Cross-sectional view showing relative position of the heart in the thorax. *C*, Relationship of the heart and great vessels to the lungs.

layer that provides an inner lining for the chambers of the heart. The endocardium is continuous with the linings of the blood vessels that enter and leave the cardiac chambers.

Cardiac muscle is quite different from skeletal muscle. The muscle cells are shorter, interconnected, branched structures. *Mitochondria*, the cell's energy-producing organelles, compose about 25% of cardiac muscle fibers versus only about 2% in skeletal muscle fibers. This higher ratio is related to the much higher energy requirements of cardiac muscle. Unlike the independently functioning fibers of skeletal muscle, the fibers of cardiac muscle are interconnected by special junctions that provide for the conduction of impulses across the entire myocardium. This property allows the heart to contract as a single unit.

Heart Chambers The heart is composed of four chambers: two smaller, superior chambers called **atria**, and two larger, inferior chambers called **ventricles** (Figure 11.4). One atrium is located on the right side of the heart and one on the left side. These serve as receiving chambers for blood returning to the heart from the major blood vessels of the body. The atria then pump the blood into the right and left ventricles, which lie directly below them. The ventricles also are located on each side of the heart. They eject blood into the vessels leaving the heart. A longitudinal partition separates the heart chambers: the *interatrial septum* separates the two atria, and the *interventricular septum* divides the ventricles.

Right Atrium The right atrium is a thin-walled chamber located above and slightly to the right of the right ventricle. It forms the right border of the heart. Deoxygenated venous blood from the systemic circulation enters into the right atrium via the inferior and superior vena cava and the coronary sinus. The blood is then ejected from the right atrium through the tricuspid valve into the right ventricle. The pressure in the right atrium in the normal adult averages 2–6 mm Hg.

Right Ventricle The right ventricle is formed triangularly and comprises much of the anterior or sternocostal surface of the heart. After receiving deoxygenated blood from the right atrium, the right ventricle ejects it through the trunk of the pulmonary arteries so that the blood may be oxygenated within the lungs. Its wall is much thinner than that of the left

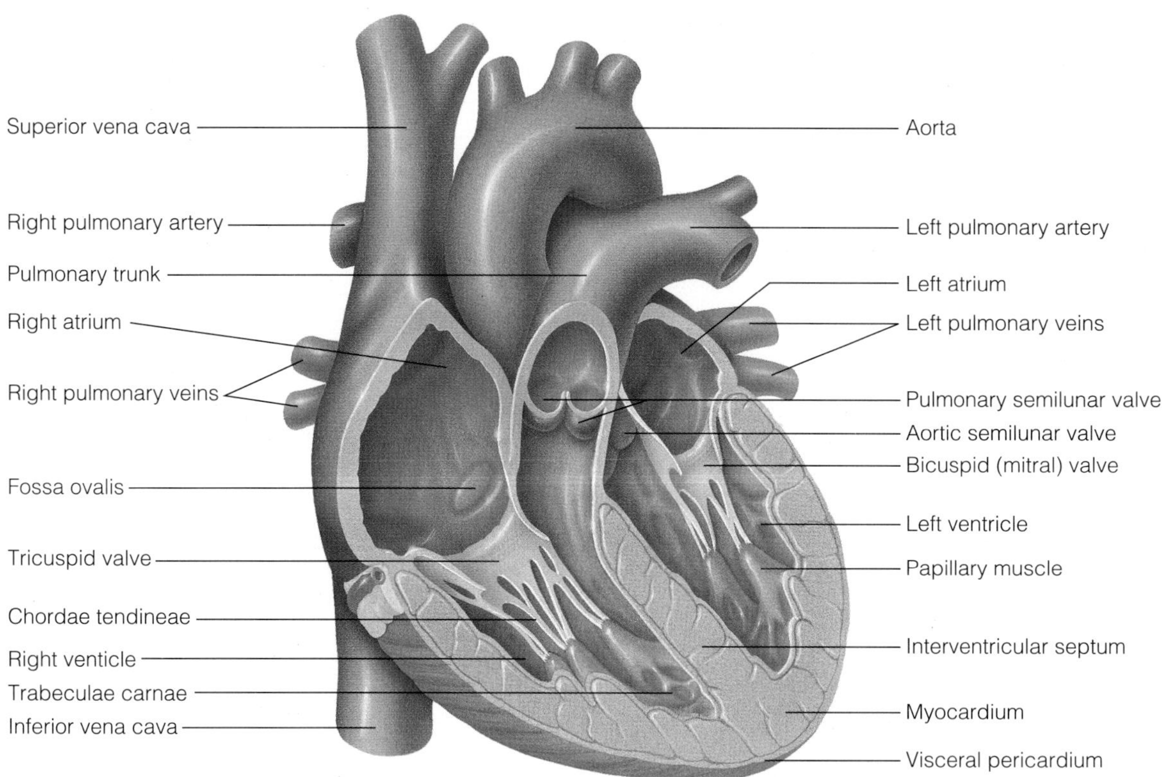

Figure 11.4 Structural components of the heart.

ventricle, reflecting the relatively low vascular pressure in the vessels of the lungs. Normal right ventricular pressure is 20–30/0–5 mm Hg.

Left Atrium The left atrium forms the posterior aspect of the heart. Its muscular structure is slightly thicker than that of the right atrium. It receives oxygenated blood back from the pulmonary vasculature via the pulmonary veins. From here, the blood is pumped into the left ventricle. Normal left atrial pressure is 8–12 mm Hg.

Left Ventricle The left ventricle is located behind the right ventricle and forms the left border of the heart. The left ventricle, which is egg-shaped, is the most muscular chamber of the heart, reflecting its function of propelling blood out into the aorta against high systemic vascular resistance. This work causes the left ventricle to develop more mass than the right ventricle. The left ventricle of a female has about 10% less mass compared to that of a male. Left ventricular function is determined by assessing the pressure in the pulmonary capillary system, which reflects the left ventricular pressure at the end of diastole. The normal value is between 6–12 mm Hg.

Valves The **valves** of the heart are structures through which blood is ejected either from one chamber to another or from a chamber into a blood vessel. The flow of the blood in a healthy individual with competent valves is mostly unidirectional. Valves are classified by their location as either atrioventricular or semilunar.

The **atrioventricular valves** separate the atria from the ventricles: the *tricuspid valve* lies between the right atria and the right ventricle, whereas the thicker *mitral (bicuspid) valve* lies between the left atrium and left ventricle.

The atrioventricular valves open as a direct result of atrial contraction and the concomitant build-up of pressure within the atria. This pressure forces the valvular leaflets to open. Then, when the ventricles contract, the increased ventricular pressure forces the valvular leaflets shut, thus preventing the blood from flowing back into the atria.

The **semilunar valves** separate the ventricles from the vascular system: the *pulmonary semilunar valve* separates the right ventricle from the trunk of the pulmonary arteries, whereas the *aortic semilunar valve* separates the left ventricle from the aorta.

The semilunar valves open in response to rising pressure within the contracting ventricles. When the pressure is great enough, the cusps open, allowing blood to be ejected into either the pulmonary trunk or the aorta. Upon relaxation of the ventricles, the valves close, allowing for ventricular filling and preventing backflow into the chambers.

Heart Sounds Closing of the valvular leaflets causes distinct heart sounds. When auscultated, these sounds provide clues to the health of the client's cardiovascular system. One clue is provided by noting the elapsed time between the closing of the atrioventricular valves and the closing of the semilunar valves—in other words, the contraction phase of the heart. This phase is referred to as **ventricular systole**. The term **diastole** refers to the elapsed time between the closing of the semilunar valves and the closing of the atrioventricular valves—in other words, the relaxation phase of the heart. The closing of the atrioventricular valves causes a heart sound designated as S_1, whereas the closing of the semilunar valves causes a heart sound designated as S_2. Thus, the time between S_1 and S_2 is ventricular systole, and the time between S_2 and S_1 is ventricular diastole (Figure 11.5).

Two other heart sounds that may be present in some healthy individuals are S_3 and S_4. S_3 may be heard in children, young adults, or in pregnant women in their third trimester. It is termed a ventricular gallop. When the atrioventricular valves open, blood flow into the ventricles may cause vibra-

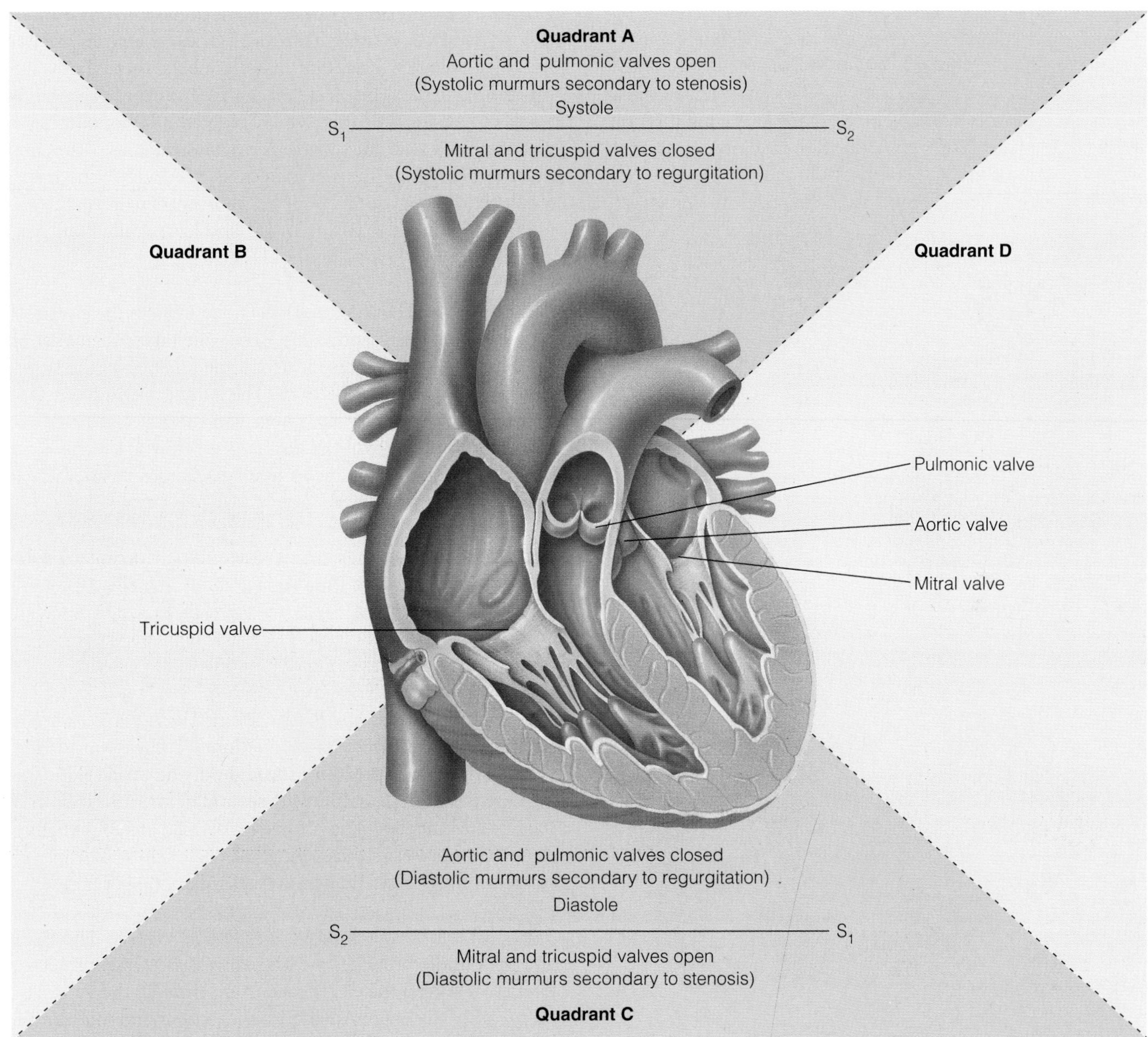

Figure 11.5 Relationship of heart sounds to cardiac mechanical events. Courtesy of Johanna K. Stiesmeyer, RN, MS, CCRN.

tions. These vibrations create the S_3 sound during diastole. The S_4 may also be heard in children, well-conditioned athletes, and even healthy elderly individuals without cardiac disease. It is caused by atrial contraction and ejection of blood into the ventricles in late diastole.

Coronary Arteries The word *coronary* comes from the Latin word meaning "crown," which accurately describes this extensive network of arteries supplying the heart (Figure 11.6). The **coronary arteries** are visible initially on the external surface of the heart but descend deep into the myocardial tissue layers. Their function is to transport blood bringing nutrients and oxygen to the myocardial muscle.

The main coronary arteries are: the *left main coronary artery, right coronary artery, left anterior descending coronary artery*, and *circumflex coronary artery*. These arteries and those that branch from them may vary in size and configuration among individuals. The right and left main coronary arteries originate from the aorta, then diverge to provide blood to different surfaces. Atherosclerotic plaque in these arteries as well as in their branches contributes significantly to the development of ischemic and injury processes and the potential for death.

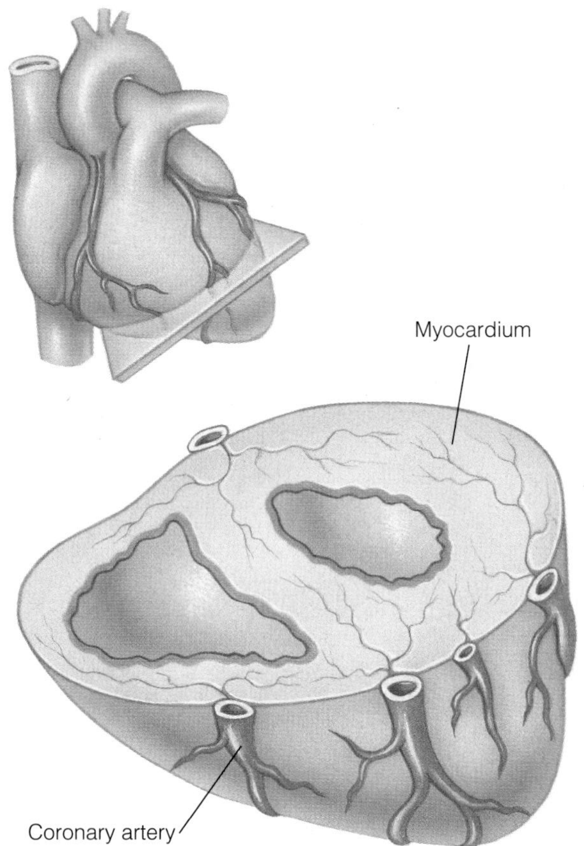

Figure 11.6 Coronary artery network in a transverse section of the ventricles of the heart.

Cardiac Veins The venous system of the heart is composed of the great cardiac vein, oblique vein, anterior cardiac vein, small cardiac vein, middle cardiac vein, cordis minimae veins, and the posterior cardiac vein. The great cardiac vein serves as the tributary for the majority of venous blood drainage and empties into the coronary sinus. Interestingly, the small venae cordis minimae drain into the cardiac chambers.

Cardiac Conduction System The heart has its own conduction system, which can initiate an electrical charge and transmit that charge via cardiac muscle fibers throughout the myocardial tissue. This electrical charge stimulates the heart to contract, causing the propulsion of blood throughout the heart chambers and vascular system. The main structures of the conduction system are the sinoatrial node (SA node), the intra-atrial conducting pathways, the atrioventricular node (AV node), the bundle of His, the right and left bundle branches, and the Purkinje fibers (Figure 11.7).

Sinoatrial Node The sinoatrial (SA) node initiates the electrical impulse. For this reason, it has been called the pacemaker of the heart. The SA node is located at the junction of the superior vena cava and right atrium. The autonomic nervous system feeds into the SA node and can influence it to either speed up or slow down the discharge of electrical current. In the healthy individual, the SA node discharges on an average of 60–100 times a minute.

Intra-Atrial Conduction Network These loosely organized conducting fibers assist in the propagation of the electrical current emitted from the SA node through the right and left atrium (not shown in Figure 11.7). The network is composed of three main pathways: anterior, middle, and posterior.

Atrioventricular Node and Bundle of His These two structures are intricately connected and function to receive the current that has finished spreading throughout the atria. Here the impulse is slowed for about 0.1 second before it passes onto the bundle branches. The AV node is also capable of initiating electrical impulses in the event of SA node failure. The intrinsic rate of firing is slower and averages about 60 per minute.

Right and Left Bundle Branches and Purkinje Fibers The right and left bundle branches are like expressways of conducting fibers that spread the electrical current through the ventricular myocardial tissue. Arising from the right and left bundle branches are the Purkinje fibers. These fibers fan out and penetrate into the myocardial tissue to spread the current into the tissues themselves.

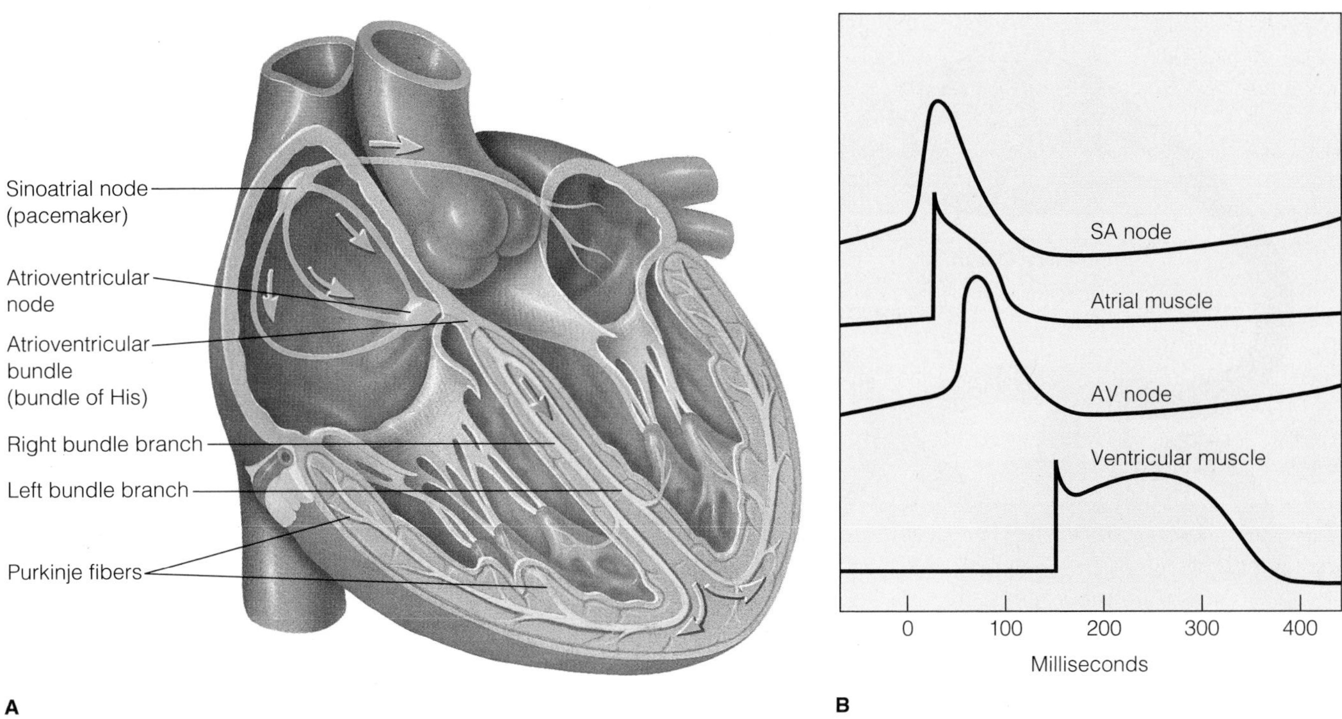

Figure 11.7 *A*, Intrinsic conduction system of the heart; *B*, Succession of the action potential through selected areas of the heart during one heartbeat.

Note that the bundle branches are also capable of initiating electrical charges in case both the SA node and AV node fail. Their intrinsic rate averages 30–40 per minute.

Cardiac Nerves Just as there is an extensive network of vessels transporting oxygen and nutrients to the myocardial tissue and removing waste products, an equally important network of autonomic nerves is present. Both sympathetic nervous fibers and parasympathetic nervous fibers interact with the myocardial tissue. The sympathetic fibers stimulate the heart, increasing the heart rate, force of contraction, and dilation of the coronary arteries. Conversely, the parasympathetic fibers, such as the vagus nerve, exercise the opposite effect. The central nervous system influences the activation and interaction of these nerves through the information supplied by the cardiac plexus.

Pulmonary Circulation

The vessels of the **pulmonary circulation** include arteries, veins, and an expansive network of pulmonary capillaries. This vascular system carries deoxygenated blood to the lungs, where carbon dioxide is exchanged for oxygen. Deoxygenated blood from the veins of the body enters this network by passing into the right atrium. From here it is ejected through the tricuspid valve into the right ventricle and then passes through the pulmonic valve into the pulmonary artery and pulmonary circulation. After going through the pulmonary capillary network, oxygenated blood returns to the left atrium via the pulmonary veins (Figure 11.8). Pressure in the pulmonary capillary system averages 20–30/8–12 mm Hg.

Systemic Circulation

The vessels of the **systemic circulation** also include arteries, veins, and capillaries. This vascular system supplies freshly oxygenated blood to the body's periphery and returns deoxygenated blood to the pulmonary circuit. The arteries of the systemic circulation are composed of elastic tissue and smooth muscle, which allows their walls to stretch during systole. During diastole, the elasticity of the walls propels the blood forward into the systemic circulation. The left ventricle propels freshly oxygenated blood into the aorta. As the blood moves toward the body periphery, the major arteries of the body subdivide into *arterioles*, which carry the nutrients and oxygen to the smallest blood vessels of the body, the *capillaries*. Oxygen and nutrients are exchanged in the capillaries for carbon dioxide and metabolites, which are then carried into the *venules*, then veins, and finally the superior and inferior venae cavae, which carry the deoxygenated blood into the right atrium of the heart (see Figure 11.8). Pressure in the systemic circultion averages 110–120/70–80 mm Hg.

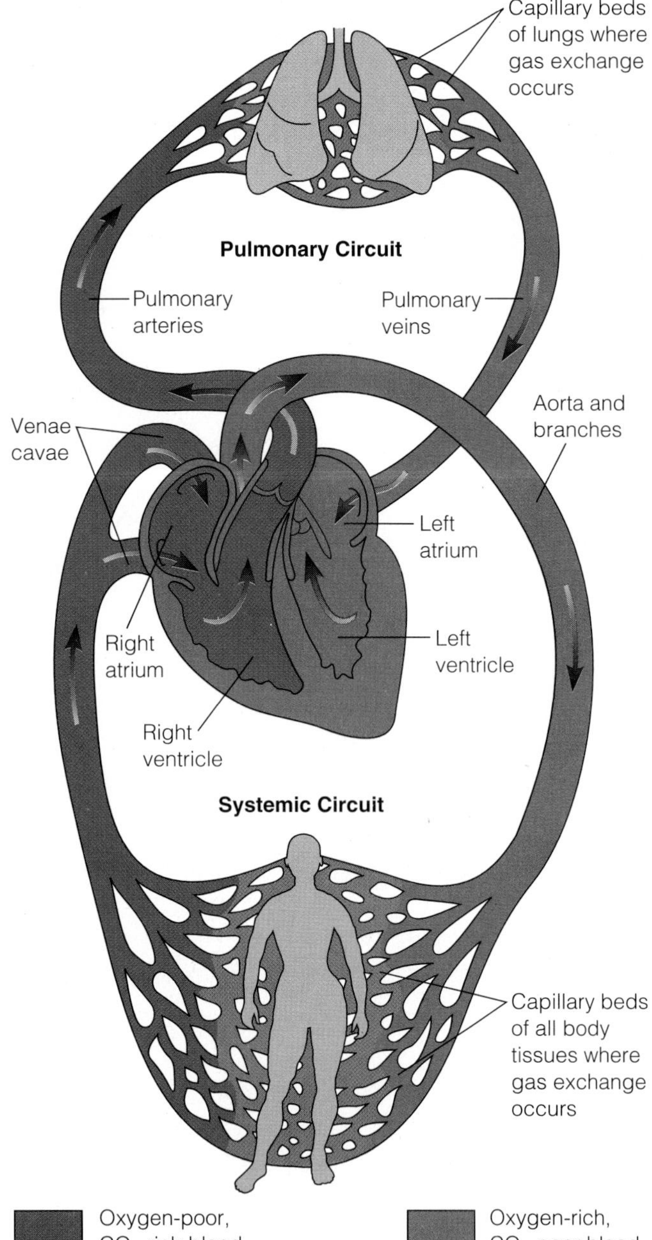

Figure 11.8 Pulmonary and systemic circulation. The left side of the heart pumps oxygenated blood (indicated in red) into the arteries of the systemic circulation, which provides oxygen and nutrients to the cells. Deoxygenated blood (indicated in blue) returns via the venous system into the right side of the heart, where it is transported to the pulmonary arterial system to be reoxygenated.

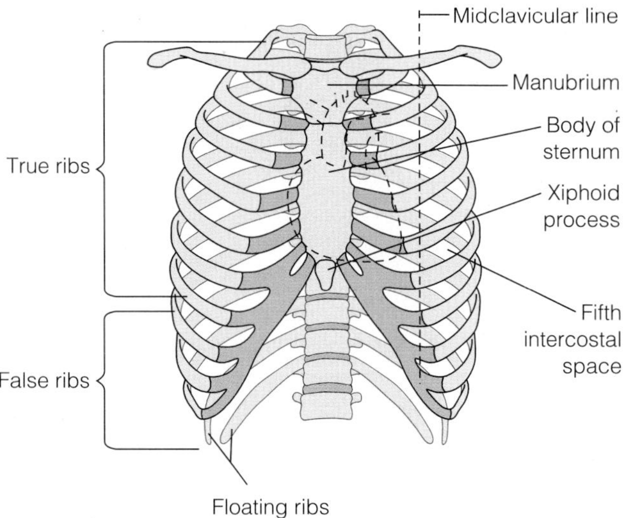

Figure 11.9 The thoracic cavity. The heart is located behind the sternum and extends to the left midclavicular line, 5th intercostal space in the normal adult.

Landmarks for Cardiovascular Assessment

Landmarks for assessing the cardiovascular system include the sternum, clavicle, and ribs. By correlating assessment findings with the overlying body landmarks, you may gain vital information concerning underlying pathologic mechanisms. Many landmarks identified during the respiratory assessment are utilized also when performing a cardiac assessment. Review the landmarks in Chapter 10 before proceeding.

The **sternum** is the flat, narrow center bone of the upper anterior chest (Figure 11.9). There are three portions of the adult sternum. The upper sternum is called the *manubrium*, the middle part is the *body*, and the inferior piece is the *xiphoid process*. The average sternal length in an adult is 18 cm (7 in). During cardiovascular assessment, the sternum is used as a vertical landmark.

The **clavicles** are bones that attach at the top of the manubrium of the sternum above the first rib (Figure 11.9). The *midclavicular line* (MCL) is used as a landmark for cardiovascular assessment.

The **ribs** are flat, arched bones that form the thoracic cage. There are 12 pairs of ribs. Between each rib is an *intercostal space* (ICS). The first ICS lies between the first and the second rib, and each remaining ICS is numbered successively (Figure 11.9). The intercostal spaces are used as horizontal landmarks during cardiovascular assessment. Additional landmarks are identified later in this chapter.

Cardiac Cycle

The **cardiac cycle** decribes the events of one complete heartbeat; that is, the contraction and relaxation of the atria and ventricles. A healthy individual's heart averages about 72 beats per minute; thus, the average time for each cardiac cycle to be completed is 0.8 second. Synchrony between the mechanical and electrical events of the cycle is imperative. Any interruption in this balance affects the ability of the heart

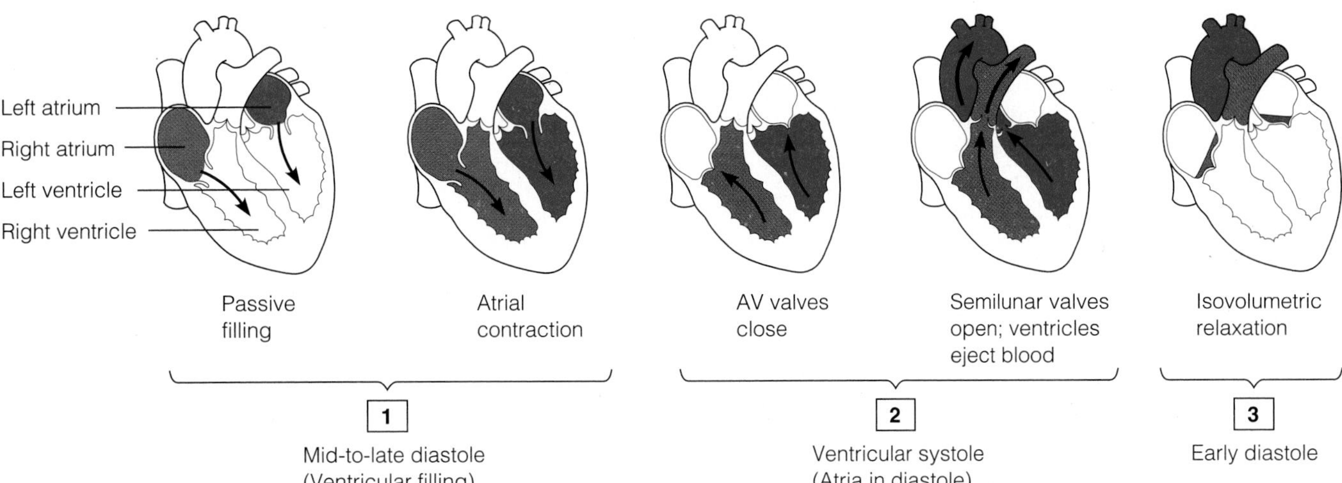

Figure 11.10 The cardiac cycle is composed of three events: ventricular filling in mid-to-late diastole, ventricular systole, and isovolumetric relaxation in early diastole.

to provide oxygen and nutrients to the body. Significant disruptions in synchrony can be fatal.

Electrical and Mechanical Events The cardiac cycle can be divided into three periods (Figure 11.10). These are:

- The period of ventricular filling. This is the start of the cycle. Blood enters passively into the ventricles from the atria. About 70% of the blood that eventually ends up in the ventricles enters at this time. As this blood is entering the ventricles, the atria are stimulated to contract by the electrical current emanating from the SA node. Another 30% volume of blood exits the atria into the ventricles. This extra 30% volume is termed the *atrial kick*.
- Ventricular systole. The electrical current now stimulates the ventricles, and they respond by contracting. The force of contraction increases the pressure within both ventricles. The mitral and tricuspid valves respond to this increased pressure by snapping shut. The ventricular pressure continues to increase until it causes the aortic and pulmonic valves to open. Blood rushes out of the ventricles into the systemic and pulmonary circulation.
- Isovolumetric relaxation. Once the majority of blood is ejected, the aortic and pulmonic valves shut. During ventricular systole, the atria have been filling with blood returning from the systemic and pulmonary circulation. When the pressure in the atria becomes higher than in the ventricles, the mitral and tricuspid valves open, and the cycle begins again.

Electrical Representation of the Cardiac Cycle Electrical representations of the cardiac cycle are documented by deflections on recording paper. A straight horizontal line means the absence of electrical activity. Deflections representing the flow of electrical current toward or away from an electrode record

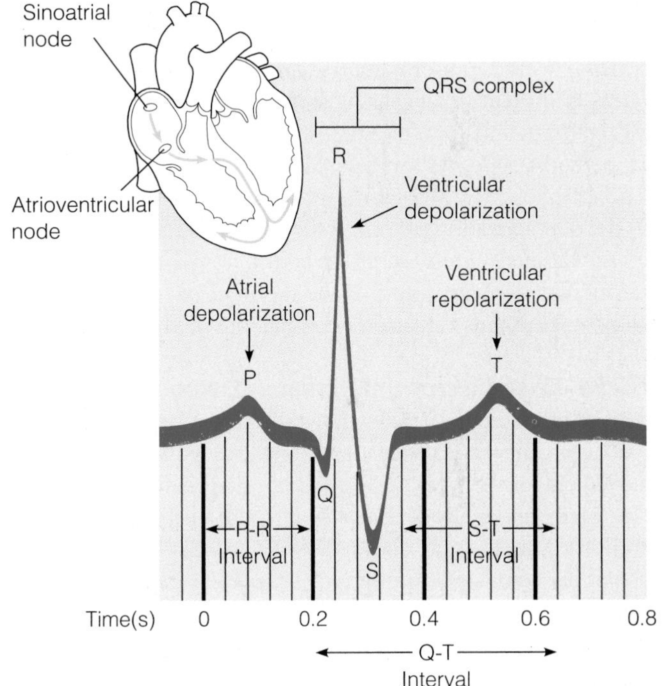

Figure 11.11 Representation of an electrocardiogram tracing showing the three deflection waves typically distinguishable and the important intervals.

the timing of the electrical events in the cardiac cycle. The terms describing the electrical deflections are P wave, PR interval, QRS interval, and T wave (Figure 11.11).

When the cardiac cell is in a resting state, it is more positively charged on the outside of the cell and more negatively charged on the inside of the cell. Depolarization occurs when the electrical current normally initiated in the sinoatrial node spreads across the atria. This spread of electrical current, called *depolarization,* causes the inside of the cardiac cell to become more positively charged. Contraction of the atria follows after the stimulation by the electrical current. After contraction, the cardiac cells experience *repolarization,* during which the inside of the cell returns to its more negatively charged state. The same process occurs in the ventricles.

The P wave represents part of *atrial depolarization.* The pacemaker of the heart, the sinoatrial node (SA node) emits an electrical charge that initially spreads throughout the right and left atria. As a result of the electrical stimulation, the myocardial cells contract. The initial P wave deflection is caused by the initiation of the electrical current and atrial response to the current. It lasts on an average 0.08 second.

The PR interval represents the time needed for the electrical current to travel across both atria and arrive at the AV node. The normal PR interval averages 0.12–0.20 second.

The QRS interval represents *ventricular depolarization.* The ventricular myocardial cells also respond to the spread of electrical current by becoming more positively charged. This change in polarity is ventricular depolarization. The QRS interval should be 0.08–0.11 second.

The T wave represents *ventricular repolarization.* Once the ventricular myocardial cells have been stimulated by the electrical current and contract, they return to their original electrical potential state of about –90 MV. This change in polarity is repolarization. The atria also repolarize, but the wave created by the depolarization process is too small to be recorded.

The QT interval represents the period from the beginning of ventricular depolarization to the moment of repolarization. Thus, it represents ventricular contraction.

Twelve-Lead Electrocardiogram The above representations of electrical flow may be recorded from a variety of perspectives. The 12-lead electrocardiogram (ECG) records the movement of electrical current from 12 different positions. The three standard leads are called I, II, and III. The augmented unipolar limb leads are called aVR, aVL, and aVF. Six unipolar precordial leads—V_1 through V_6—complete the set. Leads 1 and aVL record current flow from the upper lateral surface of the heart; leads 2, 3, and aVF, from the inferior or lower part of the heart; leads V_1–V_4, from the anterior surface; and lead V_{5-6}, from the lateral surface. The 12-lead ECG provides invaluable information about electrical rhythms, conduction disturbances, ischemia, injury, necrosis, and electrolyte disturbances.

Measurements of Cardiac Function When the heart is functioning at optimal level, the synchrony of the events of the cardiac cycle produces an outflow of blood with oxygen and nutrients to every cell in the body. The terms that describe the effectiveness of the action of the cardiac cycle are *stroke volume, cardiac output,* and *cardiac index.*

Stroke volume describes the amount of blood that is ejected with every heartbeat. Normal stroke volume is between 55–100 ml/beat. The formula for calculating stroke volume is

stroke volume = cardiac output / heart rate for 1 minute.

Cardiac output describes the amount of blood ejected from the left ventricle over 1 minute. Normal cardiac output is 4–8 liters/minute. The formula for calculating cardiac output is

cardiac output = stroke volume × heart rate for 1 minute.

The cardiac index is a valuable diagnostic measurement of the effectiveness of the pumping action of the heart. The cardiac index takes into consideration the individual's weight, a significant factor in judging the effectiveness of the pumping action. For example, suppose a cardiac output of 4.0 is obtained for two clients: an elderly female who weighs 60 kg and a middle-aged man who weighs 130 kg. The elderly female's cardiac index is significantly higher than that of the male, whose pumping effectiveness is significantly compromised. Normal cardiac index is 2.5–4.0 liters/minute/meter^2. The formula for calculating cardiac index is

cardiac index = cardiac output / body surface area.

The body surface area (BSA) measurement is obtained and determined from published tables.

There are two strong influences on pumping action: preload and afterload. *Preload* is influenced by the volume of the blood in the ventricles and relates to the length of ventricular fiber stretch at the end of diastole. The *Frank-Starling law* states that an increasingly greater contractile ability is provided with greater stretching of the ventricular muscle fibers.

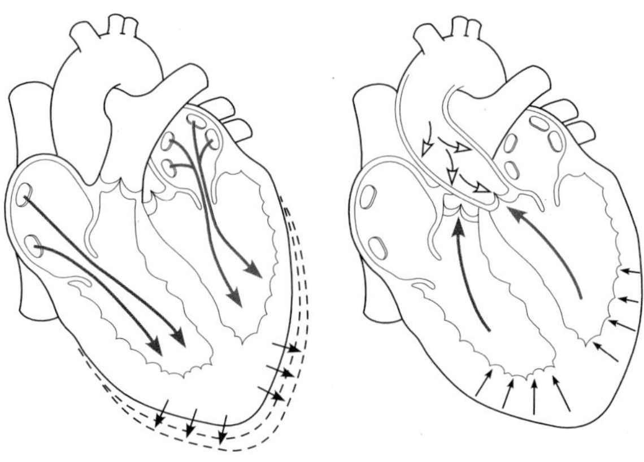

Figure 11.12 *A,* Preload is related to the amount of blood and stretching of the ventricular myocardial fibers. *B,* Afterload is the pressure that the ventricles must overcome in order to open the aortic and pulmonic valvular cusps.

Thus, the greater the stretch, the greater the contractile force, and the greater the volume of blood ejected with each contraction. *Afterload* is the amount of stress or tension present in the ventricular wall during systole. It is interrelated to the pressure in the aorta, because the pressure in the ventricular wall must be greater than that in the aorta and pulmonary trunk for the semilunar valves to open (Figure 11.12).

Influence of Gender on Cardiovascular Health

It is a well-established fact that men have a higher incidence of heart disease and exhibit significantly more heart disease at an earlier age than women. Researchers have assumed that women are protected from heart disease until menopause by their female hormones. Although female hormones do contribute some degree of protection, women with juvenile-onset diabetes, women who experience early menopause, and women who have had their ovaries surgically removed at a young age are at risk of experiencing early development of atherosclerosis.

Diabetes and Cardiovascular Health

Diabetes has devasting effects on the cardiovascular system, because it accelerates the atherosclerotic process. Individuals who have juvenile-onset diabetes are most susceptible to experiencing cardiovascular disease at a younger age. The well-known protective mechanism of female hormones is virtually eliminated in women with juvenile-onset diabetes.

Hypertension and Cardiovascular Health

Hypertension contributes to the atherosclerotic process by increasing the susceptibility of the arterial linings to injury. Thus, hypertension increases the deposition of cholesterol and other minerals. Hypertension also places a greater strain on the heart by increasing (a) the work of the heart in pumping the blood into the vascular system, and (b) the oxygen and nutrient needs of the heart. Hypertension caused by stiffened arterial walls forces the left ventricle to increase its workload to eject the blood against the higher resistance of the elevated systemic pressure.

Disease processes from smoking and hypertension can cause the development of atherosclerotic plaques in the coronary arteries. The plaques may increase in size and diameter in the arteries until ultimately blood flow is partially or totally occluded. Plaques commonly occur at bifurcations, where the turbulence of blood flow is greatest. Clients with unstable angina often have plaques that are associated with the formation of a blood clot, which may ultimately contribute to total occlusion.

Gathering the Data

Focused Interview

The first step in a complete cardiovascular assessment is a focused interview to gather data about the status and extent of the client's wellness and the client's knowledge about maintaining optimal cardiovascular health. The client's history gives you valuable information and insight into the potential influences on the maintenance of cardiovascular health. When disease is present, the interview concentrates on the symptoms identified by the client. The complete health history is discussed in Chapter 2.

You may wish to adopt the following four-step approach for organizing your interview.

- Step 1: First consider the client's current level of wellness. What is the client's present state of wellness? Does the client take health for granted? What lifestyle patterns maintain this level? What are the client's normal patterns of life in relationship to the maintenance of wellness?
- Step 2: Next consider any threats to the maintenance of an optimal level of wellness. What are the client's risk factors for developing cardiovascular disease?
- Step 3: Third, explore what the client can do to prevent the development of cardiovascular pathology and whether the client is willing to do it.
- Step 4: Finally, question the client about the presence of cardiovascular disease. What are the client's symptoms? How are the symptoms being managed? How are they affecting the client's lifestyle? What can the client do to maintain an optimum level of wellness despite the presence of cardiovascular disease?

Questions Related to the Client's Level of Wellness

1. How do you feel? Can you physically and mentally perform all the activities necessary to meet your personal and work-related needs? *Inability to perform the activities of daily living may signal a potential problem. Inquire into the specific nature and extent of the deficit.*
2. Do you exercise?
   a. What type of exercise?
   b. How many times a week?

c. Duration of exercise? Intensity? What is your total exercising time? Is the exercise continuous or interspersed with breaks? What is the amount of aerobic exercise versus nonaerobic? Do you exercise with a partner or alone? Is the exercise pattern regular or sporadic?

d. What is your understanding about the benefits of exercise and the type of exercise selected?

e. What was your reason for choosing the specific exercise routines and patterns?

f. Is your exercise tolerance increasing, staying the same, or decreasing? *(If it is decreasing, examine the characteristics.)* How has the tolerance decreased? What were you able to do before versus now? How rapidly has this change occurred? What symptoms contribute to the decreased tolerance? Do you know the causes?

The benefits of exercise are well documented, yet the type, duration, and frequency of the exercise regime produce variable results. It is important for the client to have a basic understanding of the benefits of aerobic versus nonaerobic exercise. One is not better than the other, and ultimately a blending of routines is invaluable whether the client is a well-conditioned athlete or an individual trying to stay healthy. Studies suggest that both aerobic exercise and resistance or weight training may increase HDL levels in women.

3. Do you monitor your pulse and blood pressure?

   a. If so, demonstrate for me how you monitor your pulse and blood pressure, and describe the type of blood pressure monitor you use. *You may need to validate the accuracy of the blood pressure monitor.*

   b. If so, what is your usual pulse? Your usual blood pressure? When do you check these values, how often, after what activities, any consumption of a particular food or beverages? *It is very important to compare pulse and blood pressure values over time. Single readings may be misleading and not reflective of the usual values for the client. The client may also be nervous about being examined and thus falsely be interpreted as hypertense.*

4. Describe your diet.

   a. What types of food do you eat?

   b. How often, how much?

   c. Do you keep track of the amount of fat, protein, and carbohydrates?

   d. Do you know the difference between saturated versus unsaturated fat?

   e. How much daily fiber do you consume?

   f. Do you add salt or other flavor enhancers to your food? If so, how much and how often? Do you taste the food before adding these flavor enhancers?

   g. Do you eat differently when you travel, when at social functions, when under stress, when on vacation?

   h. Do you diet? If so, describe type, duration of diet, and diet supplements you take. Do you diet under the care of a physician?

   i. Do you supplement your diet with vitamins, protein supplements, or antioxidants?

   j. What type of nonalcoholic liquids do you drink? How much, how often?

Diet is one of the key interventions that a client can control when working to minimize the effects of aging, slow the progression of disease, or maintain optimum health while experiencing cardiac disease. Supplementing the diet with vitamins under proper supervision may be beneficial. Unfortunately, without proper supervision, the poorly informed client may ingest an unbalanced proportion of supplements and compromise a healthy state. Be alert if the client has been dieting to reduce weight. Many diets deplete valuable electrolytes and subject the client to potential complications. Muscle wasting may occur if the diet is deficient in protein. Lack of protein may compromise cardiac function.

5. What is your weight?

   a. Have you gained or lost weight recently? If so, over how much time?

   b. Are you aware of your body composition, such as your percentage of body fat? If you have been keeping track of this information, is it changing? If so, how?

   c. Are you retaining fluid? If so, when did this start and has the retention been slowly progressing or rapidly accelerating?

Many individuals monitor their weight by reading the measurement on a bathroom scale. It is suggested, however, that body-composition testing provides more useful data. A "skinny" individual is not necessary a healthy individual and may actually carry a significant percentage of fat on a thin frame. Weight gain associated with fluid retention may signal the presence of heart failure.

6. How would you describe your personality? How many hours do you work in a typical week? Do you work on weekends? What do you do to unwind? Describe the major stressors in your life. What do you do to relieve stress? *Having a type A versus B personality is often associated with heart disease. It is not so much the behaviors, but the effect of constant sympathetic stimulation upon the cardiovascular system and the constant stress and drain on the rejuvenation process after a stressful event that may contribute to decompensation and vulnerability to disease processes. Excessive stress, no matter what the client's personality type, is a risk factor for cardiovascular disease.*

7. Work
   a. What is your present occupation? *Jobs with long hours, stress, deadlines, and high pressure are thought to contribute to the development of cardiovascular disease.*
   b. What were your previous occupations?
   c. What is your work environment like?
   d. Have you been exposed to passive smoking in your work environment? *Inhalation of second-hand cigarette smoke in a closed environment is currently thought to contribute to the development of coronary artery plaque.*
   e. Have you been exposed to chemicals or other hazardous substances?

Such exposure may correlate to stress, alterations in eating habits and exercise habits, recreational drug use, and alterations in sleep patterns.

8. What is your normal sleeping pattern? Have you experienced any change in this pattern? If so, can you identify any causes of the change in sleep pattern? What have you done to relieve the change? Has it been successful? Do you ever awaken short of breath? If so, describe. *Many factors are potential causes of alterations in sleep patterns: occupational, social, and personal stress; ingestion of foods, drugs, or beverages containing alcohol or caffeine; anatomic structural problems, and heart failure. It is important to explore the client's symptoms and possible causative factors.*
9. What medications do you take?
   a. Describe the medications: Are they prescribed or self-ordered? What are the dose and brand? How often do you take them?
   b. Why do you take these drugs?
   c. Do you take these medications as prescribed?
   d. If you miss a dose, do you double up the next time?
   e. Do you feel that if one is good, two must be better?
   f. Who ordered these medications? If more than one person, do each know what the other(s) have ordered?
   g. Do you know how medications that you are taking react with each other?
   h. Do you know the side effects of the medications?
   i. Are you experiencing any side effects that you think might be related to medications?

It is important to assess the client's knowledge, compliance, and ability to administer medication accurately, whether ordered by a physician or not. Medication actions may vary depending upon the mix of medications, diet, and additional supplementation.

10. Do you smoke or are you frequently exposed to passive smoking? If you smoke, what type of product (cigarette, cigar, pipe), for how long, how many packs per day, and what brand? If you are exposed to passive smoke, where and for how long each day? *Smoking has been linked to hypertension and is strongly suspected of contributing to injury in the walls of arteries, thus accelerating the development of atherosclerotic plaques. It is felt that the chemical contained in the cigarette smoke injures the inner wall of arterial vessels, thus contributing to the subsequent development of a coronary artery plaque.*
11. Do you take any illicit drugs such as cocaine? Do you drink alcohol? If so, describe the type, amount, frequency, and duration of use. *Substance abuse, especially of cocaine, is associated with coronary artery spasm and potential development of ischemia or injury of myocardial tissue.*
12. Do you fear developing cardiovascular disease? *If so, examine the fear and assess the client's willingness to acquire information. If the client knows a family member, friend, or associate with cardiovascular disease, the client may fear developing the same condition. Education about cardiovascular disease and maintaining a healthy lifestyle may help give the client a way of coping and a feeling of control. In families where an individual has died of heart disease at a young age, other family members may experience apprehension as they reach the same age.*
13. Have you recently been tested for cardiovascular wellness? If so, what were the tests? How long ago were they conducted? What were the results? *The client may need coaching for the names of the specific tests such as 12-lead ECG, echocardiography, thallium test, stress test, cardiac catheterization, and laboratory tests such as HDL, LDL, triglyceride, and total cholesterol studies.*

Questions Related to the Client's Risk for Developing Cardiovascular Disease

1. Has any member of your family ever had cardiovascular disease or symptoms that are commonly associated with the presence of cardiovascular disease? *Be sure to identify such conditions as angina, congenital heart disease, diabetes, early menopause, hypercholesterolemia, heart failure, hypertension, myocardial infarction, peripheral vascular disease, valvular disease and symptoms such as bloody sputum, chest pain, collapse, difficulty breathing, fatigue, leg pains after exertion, palpitations, shortness of breath, and syncope.*
   a. If yes, what was it?
   b. How was it treated?

c. At what age did the person develop the disease?

d. Is the person still alive?

e. What is each person's relationship to you?

There is a suspected genetic predisposition toward many cardiac diseases.

2. Do you have a history of cardiovascular disease?
   a. If so, what was it?
   b. When did you develop it?
   c. What were the symptoms?
   d. At what age did you develop it?
   e. How was it treated? Were the interventions repeated?

By examining the client's cardiovascular medical history, you gain information to guide the physical assessment and to assess the need for client education.

3. Have you ever had a history of other medical conditions such as diabetes, neurologic disorders, recent dental work or complications in the past related to dental work, thyroid disorders, and/or venereal disease?
   a. If yes, what was it?
   b. When did you develop it?
   c. What were the symptoms?
   d. At what age did you develop it?
   e. How was it treated? Were the interventions repeated?

Certain medical conditions or procedures may significantly contribute to cardiovascular dysfunction. During dental work, bacterial plaque may be dislodged from the oral area, enter the bloodstream, and become lodged in a defective valve, thus making the client vulnerable to bacterial infection of the heart.

4. Determine the client's risk-factor profile for the development of cardiovascular disease:
   a. Heredity
   b. Sex
   c. Race
   d. Age
   e. Cigarette smoking
   f. Hypertension. *Elevated blood pressure is one of the most significant factors in the development of cardiovascular disease, as demonstrated by the Framingham study. In fact, an increase of 10 mm Hg in a woman's systolic blood pressure has been related to a 20–30% risk of developing fatal coronary heart disease, especially in women of African ancestry.*
   g. Elevated total cholesterol/LDL/triglyceride levels. *The Framingham study suggests that a woman with elevated total cholesterol levels may not have as significant a risk for developing cardiovascular disease as a man, yet it is important to compare the elevated total cholesterol level with the HDL level. If HDL is low, the risk for developing cardiovascular disease increases. A combination of high total cholesterol, low HDL, and high triglyceride levels multiplies the risk of fatality from cardiovascular disease ten times.*
   h. Diabetes. *Juvenile-onset diabetes is just as substantial and devastating a risk factor in the development of cardiovascular disease in women as in men. The contribution of hyperglycemia, hyperlipidemia, hypertension, and hyperinsulinemia to the development of cardiovascular disease is significant. The typical chest discomfort pattern for coronary artery disease may be absent, because neuropathy may inhibit the transmission of pain impulses.*
   i. High body fat composition. *There is a relationship between increased weight and hypertension. Regional distribution of adipose tissue may also play a factor. Current data suggests that clients with adipose distribution in the trunk area, as more commonly seen in men, may be associated with a higher rate of myocardial infarction, stroke, and diabetes. Elevated body fat may be an even more significant contributor to cardiovascular disease in women than in men.*
   j. Sedentary life style
   k. Excessive stress
   l. Diet rich in saturated fats
   m. Type A personality

Questions Related to the Client's Ability to Modify Risk Factors

1. Do you know the risk factors for developing cardiovascular illness?
2. Do you know which of the risk factors you have some control over?
3. State how you think you can realistically modify these risk factors.

Questions Related to the Presence and Management of Cardiovascular Disease

1. Have you experienced any symptoms that may suggest the presence of cardiovascular disease: activity intolerance, anorexia, bloody sputum, changes in sexual practices, confusion or alterations in mental status, chest discomfort, coughing, dizziness, dyspnea (difficulty breathing), fatigue, fever, hoarseness, frequent urination at night, leg pains after activity, sleeping pattern

alteration, syncope (fainting), palpitations, and swelling? *If any of these symptoms is present, gather objective information on the specific characteristics. Have clients describe their own subjective experience. If you prompt them, you may miss valuable clues.*

a. Does a change in position increase, decrease, or do nothing to change the symptoms?
b. Can you identify precipitating factors for the symptoms? *Look for activity, emotion, stress, and drugs as a precipitating factor. However, heart symptoms may have no precipitating factors.*
c. Describe the quality of symptom. Does it feel sharp, dull, like pressure, piercing, or ripping? *The description of the quality offers clues to the potential origin of the disease, especially when chest discomfort is present.*
d. Does the feeling radiate to other parts of the body? *Radiation of pain may occur with chest discomfort.*
e. Where do you feel the symptom on the body? *If the symptom or one of the symptoms is chest discomfort, have the client show you the location on the body. Often, chest discomfort of cardiac origin is identified by a clenched fist over the precordium, whereas pointing with one or more fingers to a limited area on the chest wall is more generally indicative of pain of a pulmonary or muscular origin.*
f. What relieves the symptoms?
g. Rate the severity of the symptoms on a scale of 1 to 10, with 1 being hardly noticeable and 10 being the worst discomfort you have ever experienced. *This technique leaves the nurse's opinion on the degree of discomfort out of the picture.*
h. What is the timing of the symptoms? Is the timing predictable?
i. What is the duration of the symptoms? Is it constant during that time or does it wax and wane?
j. Are the symptoms isolated or do they occur in combinations?

2. If you have any of these symptoms
   a. Have you seen your doctor about these symptoms?
   b. What is being done for these symptoms?
3. If you are currently taking cardiac medications
   a. What are they?
   b. How often do you take them?
   c. What is the dose?
   d. Do you take them as ordered or only when you feel bad?
   e. What side effects have you experienced?
4. What do you do to maintain your health despite the presence of cardiovascular disease? *Assess clients' ability to modify those risk factors over which they have some control, such as smoking, diet, exercise, and stress reduction.*

Questions Related to Women's Cardiovascular Wellness and Risk for Disease

In the past, assessment for the risk of developing cardiovascular disease has not been conducted as thoroughly for women as for men because of the misconception that every woman is "protected" by the presence of female hormones. Less aggressive prevention and treatment have been provided for some women because of this misconception. In addition, there is very little research on, and thus limited data on, women's cardiovascular health and disease. New studies examining women's cardiovascular health are underway.

Most questions relating to cardiovascular disease are equally important for both men and women; however, some important questions address women's cardiovascular wellness specifically. Review the following questions with your client as well as those listed in the previous and following sections.

1. Are you still menstruating? If not, at what age did menopause start? Did you have a hysterectomy? Were your ovaries removed? *It is known that the earlier that menopause starts, the greater the risk for development of heart disease. The use of hormone therapy to protect the client from developing cardiovascular disease is still being investigated. New data suggests that coronary artery disease may be increased eightfold in the client who has had her ovaries removed before menopause.*
2. Do you take oral contraceptives? *If the client is over 40, takes oral contraceptives containing high doses of synthetic estrogen and progesterone, and smokes, the risk of developing cardiovascular disease increases significantly.*
3. What is your age? *The older the woman, especially after the age of 70, the higher the risk of cardiovascular disease. It is significant that women, especially older women who experience cardiovascular disease, suffer a greater degree of disability than men.*

Additional Questions with Infants, Children, and Adolescent Clients

1. What was the pregnancy with this child like? During pregnancy, did you have any complications such as fever? If so, what were they? What was done about them? How was the infant affected? How were the infant's complications treated? Have the interventions helped? *Complications during pregnancy may contribute to malformations in the infant or child.*

2. Did you smoke, take drugs, or drink alcohol during pregnancy? If so, describe substance, frequency, and amount. Did you take the substance early in pregnancy? Did you take it right up to delivery? *Smoking, recreational drugs such as cocaine, and alcohol may have significant effects on the development of the fetal cardiovascular system.*
3. What is the child's energy level? Is the child easily fatigued? Does the child's nap seem to be longer than you would expect? *Reduced energy levels and easy fatigability may suggest underlying cardiovascular abnormalities, such as atrial septal defect and large ventricular septal defect.*
4. Does the child ever become short of breath? If so, what causes it? *Fatigability can be related to congenital heart disease. It is especially noticable during feeding.*
5. Does the infant or child favor squatting rather than sitting up straight? *Squatting is a symptom seen in tetralogy of Fallot. The infant or child will squat when short of breath. It is currently believed that the squatting position decreases venous return to the right atrium from the legs.*
6. Does the child have symptoms of joint pain, headaches, fever, or respiratory infections? *Rheumatic fever may follow a respiratory infection and produce symptoms of fever, swollen and painful joints, and headaches.*
7. Do you feel that your infant or child is gaining weight and growing as normal? *Failure to grow is associated with congenital heart disease, such as ventricular septal defect.*

Additional Questions with Childbearing Clients

1. Do you have any history of heart disease? *The changes of pregnancy can place the client with pre-existing heart disease at risk.*
2. Has hypertension been apparent during this pregnancy? Is there a history of hypertension? *Hypertension is a symptom of eclampsia and places the mother and infant at risk.*
3. Have you observed any swelling in your ankles or legs? Have you experienced headaches or dizziness? *Swelling can indicate an eclamptic condition. Headaches and dizziness are associated with hypertension.*

Additional Questions with Older Clients

All of the questions listed in the general section can offer significant data. In addition to the routine questions, ask the following ones:

1. Have you noticed any change—no matter how subtle—in your ability to concentrate, to remember things, or to perform simple mental tasks such as writing a letter or balancing your checkbook? *In the elderly, a change in mentation suggests inadequate perfusion and can be seen in clients with myocardial ischemia and infarction or increasingly severe congestive heart failure.*
2. Have you experienced any reactions to any medications you are currently taking? These may include palpitations, rashes, vision changes, mentation changes, fatigue, or loss of previous sexual desire or function. *Many cardiovascular medications interact with medications for other diseases and may either potentiate or reduce their effects.*

Physical Assessment

Preparation

☑ **Gather the equipment:**

- appropriate lighting, including a gooseneck lamp
- drape
- two metric rulers
- stethoscope
- Doppler (optional)

☑ **Wash your hands.**

☑ **Explain the examination procedure to the client in a nonthreatening manner. Offer reassurance.**

☑ **Place the client in a comfortable postion with the chest draped.** Examination usually starts with the client sitting upright at a 90-degree angle. You may also want to examine the client in a recumbent position either at a 45-degree angle or flat. Positioning will depend on client's comfort and ability to breathe.

Remember

- ◆ Make sure that the room, the stethoscope, and your hands are warm throughout the examination.
- ◆ Ensure the client's privacy.
- ◆ To conserve the client's energy, walk around the client rather than expecting the client to move from side to side as you proceed with the examination.
- ◆ Observe universal precautions.
- ◆ Remember that many noncardiac disease processes affect the cardiovascular system. Be alert for signs of these processes as well as those indicating the presence of cardiovascular illness.
- ◆ Make sure the room is adequately lit.

ASSESSMENT TECHNIQUE/NORMAL FINDINGS | SPECIAL CONSIDERATIONS

Inspection

Step 1 *Position the client.*

Begin the examination with the client seated upright with the chest undraped (Figure 11.13).

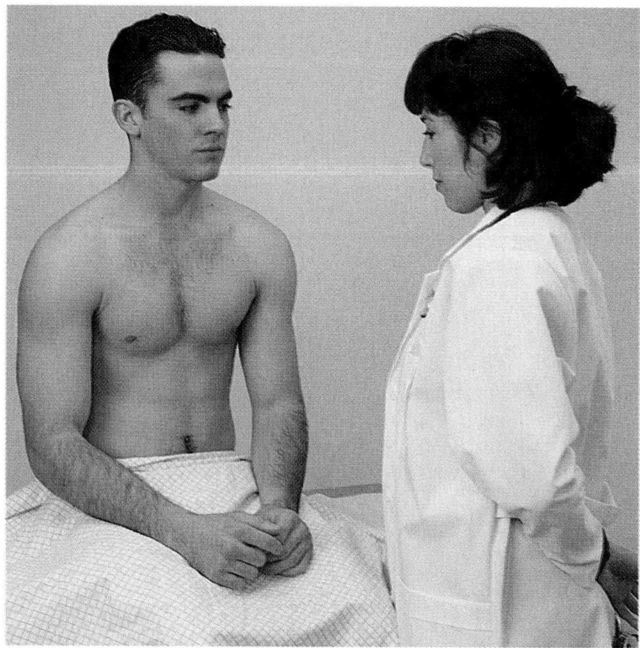

Figure 11.13 Positioning the client.

Step 2 *Inspect the client's face, lips, ears, and scalp.*

These structures can provide valuable clues to the client's cardiovascular health. (Also see Chapter 8.)

- Begin with the facial skin. The skin color should be uniform.

Flushed skin may indicate rheumatic heart disease or presence of a fever. Grayish undertones are often seen in clients with coronary artery disease or those in shock. A ruddy color may indicate *polycythemia*, a condition in which there is a significantly increased number of red blood cells, or *Cushing's syndrome*.

- Examine the eyes and the tissue surrounding the eyes (periorbital area). The eyes should be uniform and not have a protruding appearance.

Protruding eyes are seen in *hyperthyroidism.* High cardiac output states, a tendency toward tachycardias (rapid heart rates), and potential for congestive heart failure accompany this disease.

The periorbital area should be relatively flat. No puffiness should be present.

Periorbital puffiness may result from fluid retention, myxedema, or valvular disease.

ASSESSMENT TECHNIQUE/NORMAL FINDINGS	SPECIAL CONSIDERATIONS
Sclera should be whitish in color. The cornea should be without an *arcus*, which is a ring- like structure.	A blue color in the sclera is often associated with *Marfan's syndrome*, a degenerative disease of the connective tissue, which over time may cause the ascending aorta to either dilate or dissect, leading to abrupt death. An arcus in a young person may indicate hypercholesteremia; however, in people of African descent it may be normal.
The conjunctiva should be pinkish in color. The eyelid should be smooth. For information on how to examine the conjunctiva, see Chapter 9.	*Xanthelasma* are yellowish cholesterol deposits seen on the eyelids and are indicative of premature atherosclerosis.
◆ Inspect the lips. They should be uniform in color without any underlying tinge of blueness.	Blue-tinged lips may indicate cyanosis, which is often a late sign of inadequate tissue perfusion.
◆ Assess the general appearance of the face. It should be relatively uniform and flat.	A child with *Down syndrome* may exhibit large protruding tongue, low-set ears, and an underdeveloped mandible. These children often have congenital heart disease. Wide-set eyes may be seen in a child with *Noonan syndrome,* which is accompanied by pulmonic stensosis (narrowing).
◆ Examine the head. Look first for the ability of the client to hold the head steady. Rhythmic head bobbing should not be present.	Head bobbing up and down in synchrony with heartbeat is characteristic of severe aortic regurgitation. This bobbing is created by the pulsatile waves of regurgitated blood, which reverberate upwards toward the head.
◆ Assess the structure of the skull and the proportion of the skull to the face.	A protruding skull is seen in *Paget's disease*, a rare bone disease characterized by localized loss of calcium from the bone and replacement with a porous bone formation, which leads to distorted, thickened contours. Paget's disease is also characterized by a high cardiac output, which may lead to heart failure.

ASSESSMENT TECHNIQUE/NORMAL FINDINGS

SPECIAL CONSIDERATIONS

- Examine the client's earlobes. The earlobes should be relatively smooth without the presence of creases unless an injury has been sustained.

Bilateral earlobe creases, especially in the young adult, are often associated with coronary artery disease (Figure 11.14).

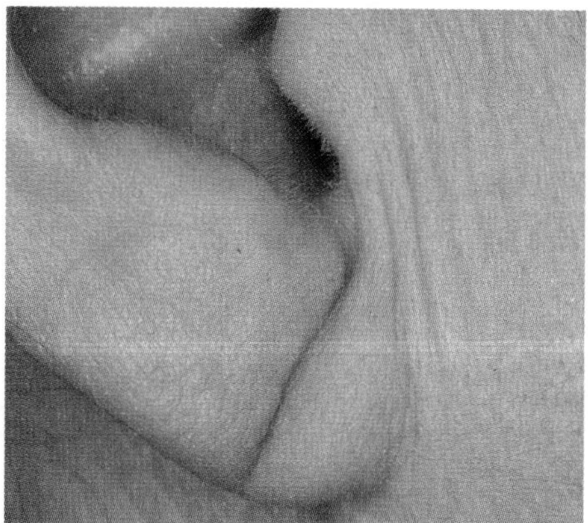

Figure 11.14 Ear lobe crease.

Step 3 *Inspect the jugular veins.*

Examination of the jugular veins can provide essential information about the client's central venous pressure and the heart's pumping efficiency.

- With the client sitting upright, adjust the gooseneck lamp to cast shadows on the client's neck.
- Be sure that the client's head is turned slightly away from the side you are examining.
- Look for the external and internal jugular veins.

Note that the jugular veins are not normally visible when the client sits upright. The external jugular vein is located over the sternocleidomastoid muscle. The internal jugular vein, which is the best indicator of central venous pressure, is located behind this muscle, medial to the external jugular and lateral to the carotid artery.

- If you are able to visualize the jugular veins, measure their distance superior to the clavicle.
- Be sure not to confuse the carotid pulse with pulsations of the jugular veins. The carotid pulse is lateral to the trachea. If jugular vein pulsations are visible, palpate the client's radial pulse and determine if these pulsations coincide with the palpated radial pulse.

Obvious pulsations that are present during inspiration and expiration and coincide with the arterial pulse are commonly seen with severe congestive heart failure.

- Next, have the client lie at a 45-degree angle if the client can tolerate this position without pain and is able to breathe comfortably.
- Place one of the metric rulers vertically at the angle of Louis. Place the other metric ruler horizontally at a 90-degree angle to the first. One end of this ruler should be at the angle of Louis and the other end in the jugular area on the lateral aspect of the neck (Figure 11.15).

ASSESSMENT TECHNIQUE/NORMAL FINDINGS | SPECIAL CONSIDERATIONS

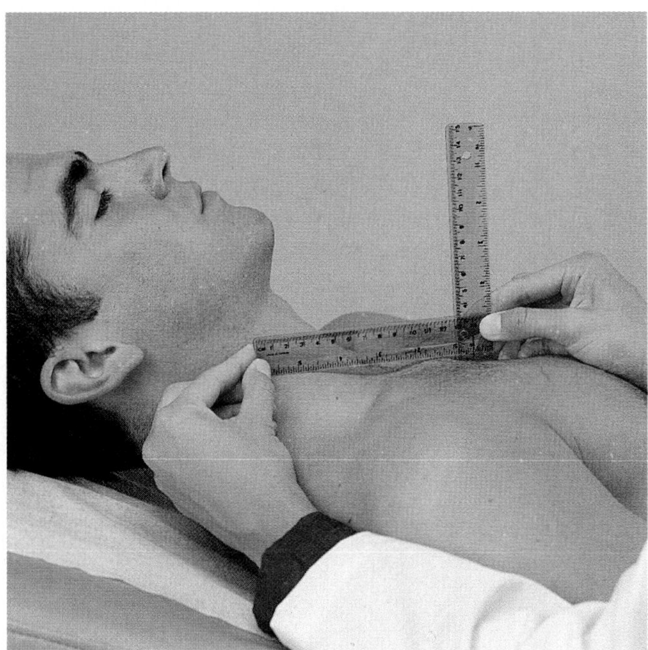

Figure 11.15 Assessment of central venous pressure.

- Inspect the neck for distention of the jugular veins. Raise the lateral portion of the horizontal ruler until it is at the top of the height of the distention and assess the height in centimeters of the elevation from the vertical ruler.

Distention of the neck veins indicates elevation of central venous pressure commonly seen with congestive heart failure, fluid overload, or pressure on the superior vena cava.

The jugular veins normally distend only 3 cm above the sternal angle when the client is lying at a 45-degree angle (Figure 11.15). You need to measure the distention only on one side.

Step 4 *Inspect the carotid arteries.*

The carotid arteries are located lateral to the client's trachea in a groove that is medial to the sternocleidomastoid muscle.

- With the client still lying at a 45-degree angle, inspect the carotid arteries for pulsations. Pulsations should be visible bilaterally.

Bounding pulses are not normal findings and may indicate fever. The absence of a pulsation may indicate an obstruction either internal or external to the artery.

- When you finish, help the client back to an upright position.

Step 5 *Inspect the client's hands and fingers.*

- Help the client to resume a sitting position.

ASSESSMENT TECHNIQUE/NORMAL FINDINGS	SPECIAL CONSIDERATIONS

- Confirm that the fingertips are rounded and even. The fingernails should be relatively flat and pink, with white crescents at the base of each nail.

Fingertips and nails that are clubbed bilaterally are characteristic of congenital heart disease. (Clubbing is described in Chapter 8.) Clubbing may be associated with cyanosis or *infective endocarditis*, a condition caused by bacterial infiltration of the lining of the heart's chambers. Thin red lines or splinter hemorrhages in the nailbeds are also associated with infective endocarditis (Figure 11.16).

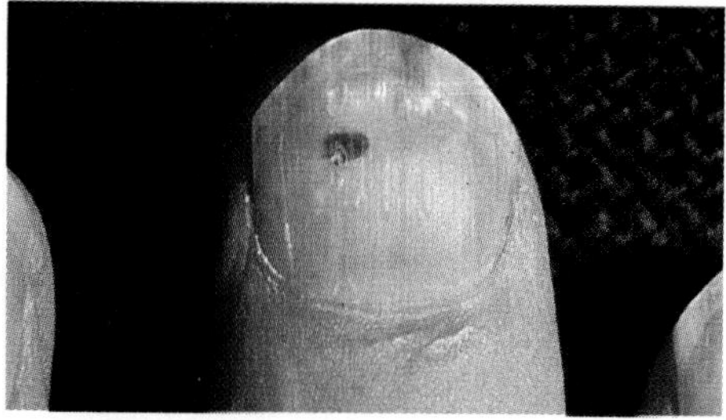

Figure 11.16 Splinter hemorrhage.

Fingernails and tips may be stained yellow when the client is a smoker. Recall that smoking is one of the main contributors to the development of atherosclerosis.

- Assess for Marfan's syndrome. Have the client make a fist by wrapping the fingers over the thumb. You can also assess for this syndrome by having the client wrap the thumb and little finger around the opposite wrist.

If the thumb is readily visible outside of the clenched fist or if the little finger extends at least 1 cm beyond the thumb, suspect Marfan's syndrome.

Step 6 ***Inspect the client's chest.***

- Observe the respiratory pattern, which should be even, regular, and unlabored, with no retractions.

Respiratory distress may be precipitated by various disorders. Pulmonary edema is often a severe complication of cardiovascular disease.

- Observe the veins on the chest, which should be evenly distributed and relatively flat.

Dilated, distended veins on the chest indicate an obstructive process, as seen with obstruction of the superior vena cava.

- Inspect the entire chest for bulges and masses. The intercostal spaces and clavicles should be even.

Bulges are abnormal and may indicate obstructions or aneurysms. Masses may indicate obstructions or presence of tumors.

- Inspect the entire chest for pulsations. Observe the client first in an upright position and then at a 30-degree angle, which is a low- to mid-Fowler's position. In particular, observe for pulsations over the **five key landmarks** (Figure 11.17).

If the entire *precordium* (anterior chest) pulsates and shakes with every heartbeat, extreme valvular regurgitation or shunting may be present.

ASSESSMENT TECHNIQUE/NORMAL FINDINGS	SPECIAL CONSIDERATIONS

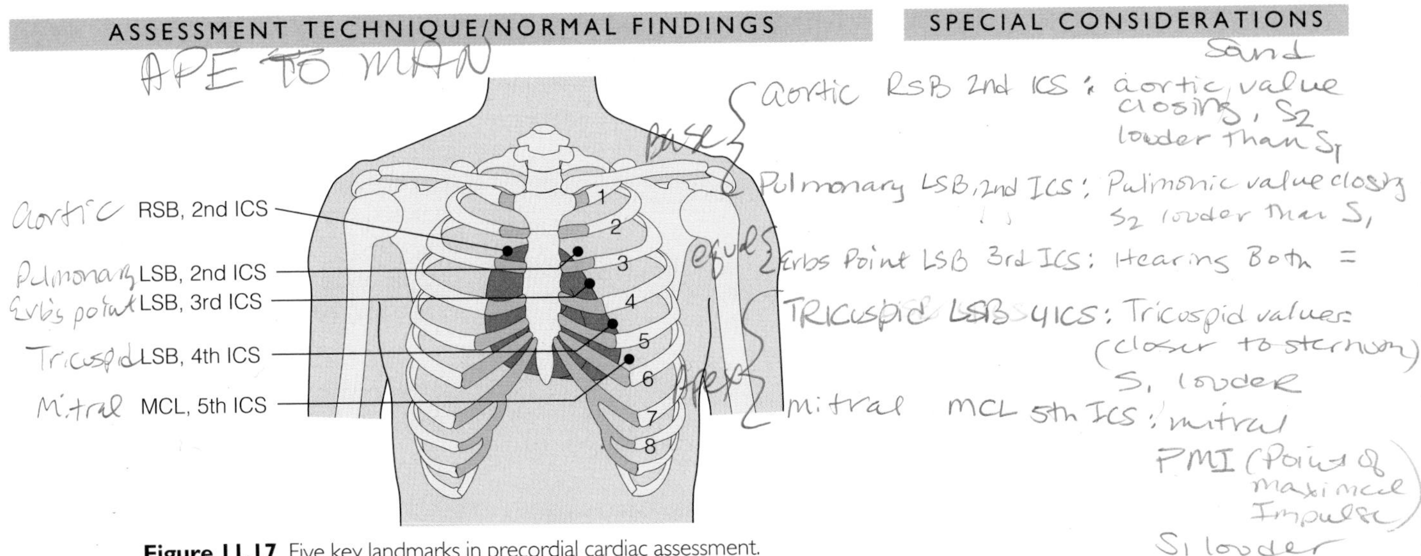

Figure 11.17 Five key landmarks in precordial cardiac assessment.

- Start by observing the right sternal border (RSB), second intercostal space (2nd ICS).
- Next, observe the left sternal border (LSB), 2nd ICS.

Pulsations present in the LSB, 2nd ICS indicate pulmonary artery dilation or excessive blood flow.

- Then observe the LSB, 3rd to 5th ICS.

Pulsations present in LSB, 3rd to 5th ICS may indicate right ventricular overload.

- Move on to the apex: 5th ICS, midclavicular line (MCL).
- Finish with the epigastric area, below the xiphoid process.
- Confirm that the *point of maximum impulse* (PMI) is located at the 5th ICS in the MCL.

If left ventricular hypertrophy is present, the PMI is displaced laterally from the 5th ICS, MCL.

- Inspect the entire chest for heaves or lifts while the client is sitting upright and again with the client at a 30-degree angle.

Heaves or *lifts* are forceful risings of the landmark area.

- In particular, make sure you observe over the five key landmarks listed above.

A heave or lift found in the LSB, 3rd to 5th ICS may indicate right ventricular hypertrophy or respiratory disease, such as pulmonary hypertension.

Step 7 ***Inspect the client's abdomen.***

- Have the client lie flat, if possible.
- Be mindful of any discomfort or difficulty in breathing.

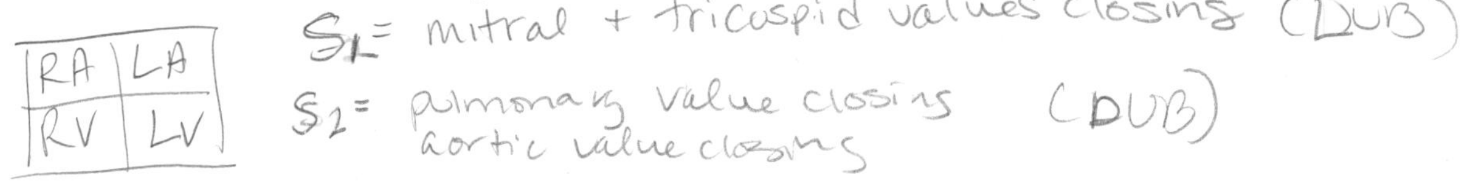

ASSESSMENT TECHNIQUE/NORMAL FINDINGS	SPECIAL CONSIDERATIONS

- Look for pulsations in the abdominal area over the areas where the major arteries are located. (Chapter 13 reviews abdominal arteries.) These sites include:

  The *aorta,* which is located superior to the umbilicus to the left of the midline.

  The *left renal artery,* which is located to the left of the umbilicus in the left upper quadrant. (Chapter 13 reviews abdominal quadrants.)

  The *right renal artery,* which is located to the right of the umbilicus in the right upper quadrant.

  The *right iliac artery,* which is located to the right of the umbilicus in the right lower quadrant.

  The *left iliac artery,* which is located to the left of the umbilicus in the left lower quadrant.

Pulsations may be visible in lean clients. These are usually normal if seen in the epigastric area. Peristalic waves may also be seen in thin individuals. They must not be confused with vascular pulsations. Prominent pulsations that are located in areas outside of the gastric area and are readily visible may be potentially life threatening.

Referral

Abnormal pulsations usually indicate the presence of aortic aneurysm, a ballooning due to a weakness in the walls of arteries. These findings require immediate physician referral.

- Note the pattern of fat distribution.

Males usually deposit fat in the abdominal area. This distribution pattern is thought to be associated with the development of coronary artery disease. Women usually deposit fat in the buttocks and thighs.

Step 8 ***Inspect the client's legs.***

- Help the client to a sitting position.
- Inspect the legs for skin color. The skin color should be even and uniform.

Patches of lighter color may indicate compromised circulation. Mottling indicates severe hemodynamic compromise.

- Inspect the legs for hair distribution. The distribution should be even without bare patches devoid of hair.

Patchy hair distribution is often a sign of circulatory compromise that has occurred over time. Ask the client if the hair distribution on the legs has changed over time.

Step 9 ***Inspect the client's skeletal structure.***

- Ask the client to stand.
- Observe the skeletal structure, which should be free of deformities.

Scoliosis (see Chapter 17) is associated with prolapsed mitral valve.

- Observe the neck and extremities, which should be in proportion to the torso.

A client who is tall and thin with an elongated neck and extremities should be evaluated further for the presence of Marfan's syndrome.

Palpation

You will palpate the chest in the five key landmarks listed in the preceding section and in Table 11.1 on page 289. Palpate each area with the client breathing normally, then breathing out, and finally with the

ASSESSMENT TECHNIQUE/NORMAL FINDINGS	SPECIAL CONSIDERATIONS

client holding the breath if the client is able to do so. Note that palpation may be performed with the client sitting upright, reclining at a 45-degree or 30-degree angle, or lying flat. Start by palpating with the client sitting upright and then in the lowest position that the client can comfortably tolerate.

Step 1 *Palpate the chest in the five key landmarks (Figure 11.18).*

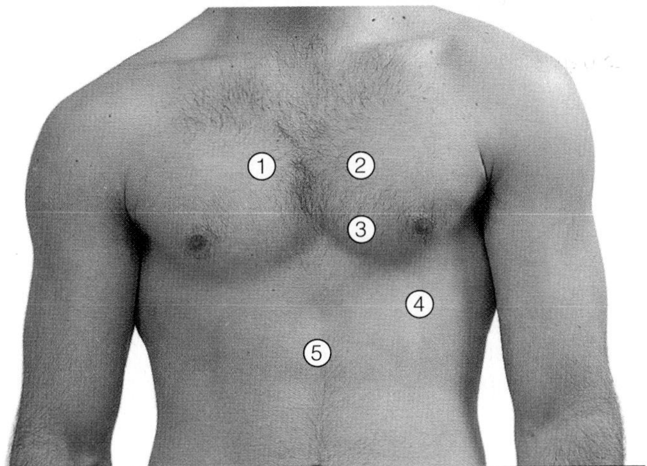

Figure 11.18 Palpating the chest over the five key landmarks.

- Place the palm of your right hand over the RSB, 2nd ICS.

You should not feel any pulsation, heave, or vibratory sensation against your palm in this location.

Pulsations or heaves in the RSB, 2nd ICS indicate the presence of ascending aortic enlargement or aneurysm, aortic stensosis, or systemic hypertension.

- Place your hand on the LSB, 2nd ICS.

You should not feel any pulsation, heave, or vibratory sensation against your palm in this location except in some very thin clients who are nervous about the examination.

Pulsations or heaves in the LSB, 2nd ICS are associated with pulmonary hypertension, pulmonary stenosis, right ventricular enlargement, atrial septal defect, enlarged left atrium, and large posterior left ventricular aneurysm.

- Move your hand to the LSB, 3rd to 5th ICS.

No pulsations, heaves, or vibratory sensations should be felt.

Pulsations or heaves over the LSB, 3rd to 5th ICS may indicate right ventricular enlargement or pressure overload on this ventricle, pulmonary stenosis, or pulmonary hypertension.

- Place your right hand over the apex: MCL, 5th ICS .

When palpating over the MCL, 5th ICS, you should feel a soft vibration, a tapping sensation, with each heartbeat. The vibration felt in this location should be isolated to an area no more than 1 cm in diameter.

The presence of a heave, which is a forceful thrust, over the 5th ICS, MCL indicates the potential presence of increased right ventricular stroke volume or pressure and mild to moderate aortic regurgitation. If you feel a vibration in a downward and lateral position from where the normal PMI should be palpated, or if you can palpate it in an area greater than 1 cm in diameter, these condi-

ASSESSMENT TECHNIQUE/NORMAL FINDINGS	SPECIAL CONSIDERATIONS
	tions may be present: left ventricular hypertrophy, severe left ventricular volume overload, or severe aortic regurgitation.
◆ Palpate the epigastric area, below the xiphoid process.	The presence of heaves or thrills in the subxiphoid area suggests the presence of elevated right ventricular volume or pressure overload. (See Table 11.3 on page 295.) *Thrills* are soft vibratory sensations best assessed with either the fingertips or the palm flattened on the chest.

Step 2 ***Repeat the palpation technique, with the client at either a 30-degree angle or lying flat.***

> **ALERT!**
>
> Some clients are unable to lie flat. Place the client in the lowest angle that is comfortably tolerated. Be alert to any physical distress experienced by the client during examination. Stop activity immediately if distress is experienced.

Palpation with the client lying flat normally reveals either no pulsation or very faint taps in a very localized area. No thrills, heaves, or lifts should be palpated in any of the five locations.

Step 3 ***Palpate the client's carotid pulses.***

The carotid artery is located in the groove between the trachea and sternocleidomastoid muscle.

It is important to palpate carotid pulses to assess their presence, strength, and equality. The client may remain supine, or you may help the client to sit upright.

◆ Ask the client to look straight ahead and keep the neck straight (Figure 11.19).

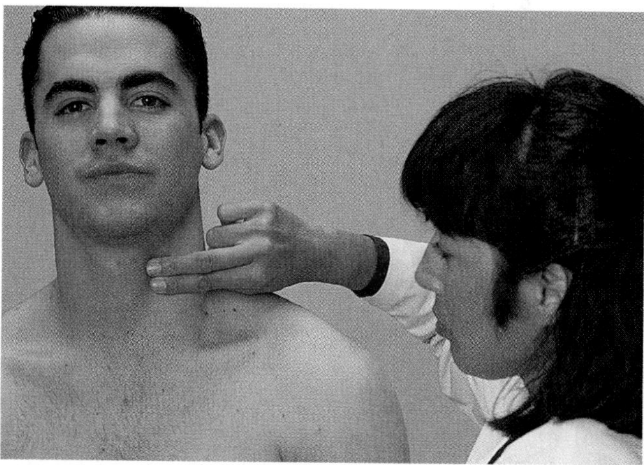

Figure 11.19 Palpating the carotid artery.

ASSESSMENT TECHNIQUE/NORMAL FINDINGS | SPECIAL CONSIDERATIONS

- Palpate each carotid pulse separately (see Chapter 16).

Normal findings bilaterally should demonstrate: equality in intensity and regular pattern. The pulses should be strong but not bounding.

Diminished or absent carotid pulses may be found in clients with carotid disease or dissecting ascending aneurysm. Absence of both pulses indicates *asystole* (absent heart rate). If the client is in critical care and has an arterial line, obtain a printout of the arterial waveform.

ALERT!

Never palpate the carotid pulses simultaneously since this may obstruct blood flow to the brain, resulting in severe *bradycardia* (slow heart rate) or *asystole* (absent heart rate).

Step 4 ***Palpate for hepatojugular reflux.***

- Position the client in the supine or low Fowler's position.
- Observe the level of pulsation of the jugular vein.
- With your right hand flat, press slowly in on the client's abdomen below the right costal margin (Figure 11.20).

This is an important test to perform if you suspect congestive heart failure, because sustained elevated jugular vein distention is suggestive of right-sided ventricular failure. It may also indicate chronic lung disease.

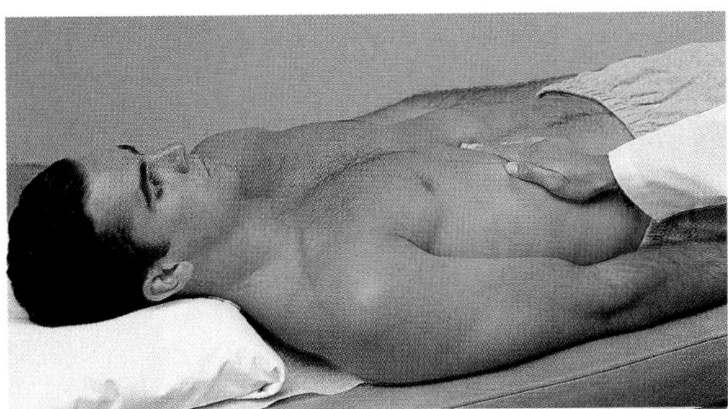

Figure 11.20 Palpating for hepatojugular reflux.

ALERT!

Do not press into the abdomen with a sharp or rapid motion, which may precipitate a *vasovagal response*, a stimulation of the vagus nerve resulting in bradycardia and hypotension.

- Press for 30–60 seconds while you observe for a sustained distention of the jugular vein.

In the client with normal heart function, the distention of the jugular veins should diminish quickly.

In the presence of right-sided heart failure, the distention is sustained.

Percussion

Step 1 ***Percuss the client's chest to determine the cardiac border.***

- Help the client to a reclining position at the lowest angle that the client can tolerate.

An enlarged heart emits a dull sound on percussion over a larger area than a heart of normal size. An X-ray film of the chest provides the most accurate information about the size of the client's heart.

ASSESSMENT TECHNIQUE/NORMAL FINDINGS

- Place the middle finger of your nondominant hand in the 5th ICS at the left anterior axillary line.
- Tap this finger at the distal phalynx, using the fingertip of your index finger or middle finger of your dominant hand (Figure 11.21). You should hear resonance because you are over lung tissue.

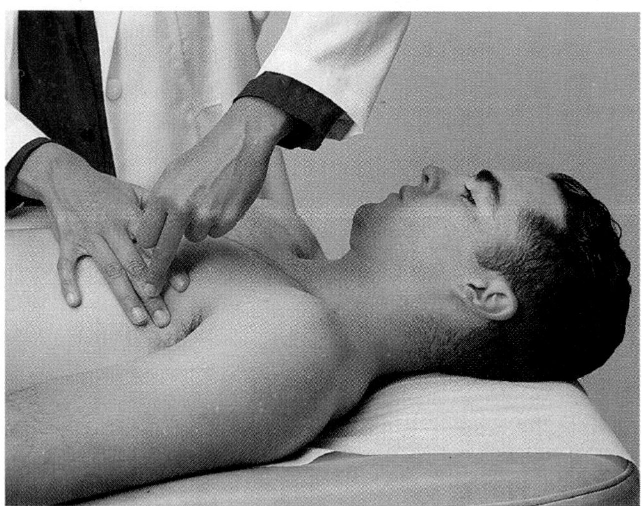

Figure 11.21 Percussing the chest.

- Continue to percuss in the 5th ICS toward the left MCL and the left sternal border. The sound will change to dullness as you percuss over the heart.
- Repeat the above percussion technique in the 3rd ICS and the 2nd ICS on the left side of the thorax. The sound of resonance heard over the lung should change to dullness over the heart.

Auscultation

The position of the client affects data collected from auscultatory examination. A full examination includes aucultation with the client sitting upright, leaning forward when upright, supine, and in the left lateral position. Have the client breathe normally initially. If you recognize the presence of abnormal sounds, have the client slow down the respirations so that you may listen to the effects of inspirations and expiratory efforts on the heart sounds. You may want to have some clients perform a forced expiration.

When preparing to auscultate a child's chest, you may want to let the child listen to the parent's heart sounds with the stethoscope in order to reduce or prevent fear of this unfamiliar object. Use a stethoscope with a smaller bell and diaphragm when you examine a child.

SPECIAL CONSIDERATIONS

ASSESSMENT TECHNIQUE/NORMAL FINDINGS | SPECIAL CONSIDERATIONS

ALERT!

Be sure that your stethoscope and hands are warm, that the stethoscope's connections are tight, and that the rubber tubing is no more than 10 inches long and 3/16 inch in diameter. A good stethoscope should have double tubing and large ear tips. Be sure to assess the client's ability to tolerate position changes and respiratory efforts. Stop if the client expresses discomfort or distress verbally or if posture, facial expression, muscle tightness, or effort of breathing suggests discomfort.

Step 1 ***Auscultate the client's chest with the diaphragm of the stethoscope.***

As you learn this technique, please refer to pages 290–299 for strategies for differentiating and interpreting heart sounds.

- Start the auscultation with the client sitting upright.
- Inch the stethoscope slowly across the chest and listen over each of the five key landmarks (Figure 11.22).

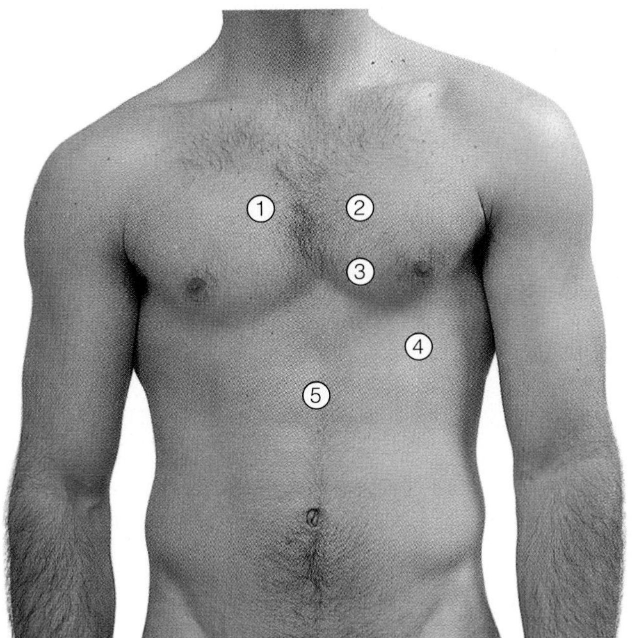

Figure 11.22 Auscultating the chest over the five key landmarks.

- Listen over the RSB, 2nd ICS.

In this location, the S_2 sound should be louder than the S_1 sound, because this site is over the aortic valve.

ASSESSMENT TECHNIQUE/NORMAL FINDINGS	SPECIAL CONSIDERATIONS

- Listen over the LSB, 2nd ICS.

Also in this location the S_2 sound should be louder than the S_1 sound, because this site is over the pulmonic valve.

- Listen over the LSB, 3rd ICS, also called Erb's point.

You should hear both the S_1 and S_2 heart tones, relatively equal in intensity.

- Listen at the LSB at the 4th ICS.

In this location the S_1 sound should be louder than the S_2 sound, because the closure of the tricuspid valve is best ausculated here.

- Listen over the apex: 5th ICS, MCL.

In this location the S_1 sound should also be louder than the S_2 sound, because the closure of the mitral valve is best ausculated here.

Step 2 *Auscultate the client's chest with the bell of the stethoscope.*

- Place the bell of the stethoscope lightly on each of the five key landmark positions shown with Step 1.
- Listen for softer sounds over the five key landmarks. Start with the S_3S_4, and then listen for murmurs.

Low-pitched sounds are best auscultated with light application of the bell. Sounds such as S_3S_4 murmurs (originating from stenotic valves) and gallops are best heard with the bell.

Step 3 *Auscultate the carotid arteries.*

Use a Doppler if you cannot auscultate the pulse with a stethoscope.

- Ask the client to breathe normally.

You will hear the movement of air, tracheal breath sounds, as the client breathes. You should not hear any turbulent sounds like murmurs.

- Have the client hold the breath briefly. You may hear heart tones. This finding is normal.

A *bruit*, a loud blowing sound, is an abnormal finding. It is most often associated with a narrowing or stricture of the carotid artery usually associated with atherosclerotic plaque.

Step 4 *Compare the apical pulse to a carotid pulse.*

- Auscultate the apical pulse.
- Simultaneously palpate a carotid pulse.
- Compare the findings. The two pulses should be synchronous. The carotid artery is used because it is closest to the heart and most accessible.

An apical pulse greater than the carotid rate indicates a pulse deficit. The rate, rhythm, and regularity must be evaluated.

Step 5 *Repeat the auscultation of the client's chest.*

- This time have the client lean forward, then lie supine, and finally lie in the left lateral position. Remember, not all clients will be able to tolerate all positions. In such cases, do not perform the technique.

Reminders

- In addition to the preceding steps, consider the variations in physical assessment findings for the different client groups discussed shortly.
- After completing the physical assessment, answer any questions the client may have, and provide appropriate client teaching for health promotion and self-care (see page 307).
- Confirm that the client is comfortable and has no adverse effects from the procedure. Dim the lights, remove the equipment, and leave the client in a comfortable position to rest or to get dressed.
- Document the assessment findings as described in Chapter 1. See pages 303–304 for information on identifying nursing diagnoses commonly associated with the cardiovascular system.

Table 11.1 Landmarks of the Chest and Findings

Palpation Landmarks	Normal Findings	Abnormal Findings: Heaves and Thrusts Potential Pathologic Mechanisms
RSB, 2nd ICS	Usually nothing palpable	◆ Ascending aorta enlargement or aneurysm ◆ Gross enlargement of right atrium ◆ Severe aortic stenosis ◆ Severe systemic hypertension
LSB, 2nd ICS	Usually nothing palpable	◆ Pulmonary hypertension ◆ Increased pulmonary blood flow ◆ Right ventricular enlargement ◆ Enlarged left atrium ◆ Large posterior left ventricular aneurysm
LSB 3rd to 5th ICS	Usually nothing palpable	◆ Right ventricular enlargement ◆ Severely elevated right ventricular pressure ◆ Pulmonary stenosis ◆ Pulmonary hypertension
MCL, 5th ICS	Soft vibration 1cm or less in diameter	◆ Increased right ventricular stroke volume ◆ Increased right ventricular pressure ◆ Mild to moderate aortic regurgitation *PMI displaced laterally and downward:* ◆ Left ventricular hypertrophy ◆ Severe left ventricular volume overload ◆ Severe aortic regurgitation
Subxiphoid	Usually nothing palpable	◆ Right ventricular volume overload ◆ Right ventricular pressure overload

Strategies for Differentiating and Interpreting Heart Sounds

It is easy to become overwhelmed if abnormal and normal heart sounds are heard together. The following strategies for differentiating and interpreting the sounds will be extremely helpful. You will also want to refer to the tables on distinguishing and interpreting heart sounds and heart murmurs that follow this section. These tables include invaluable information that you will be able to use as you become proficient through time and practice.

Remember: Take your time when auscultating. Listen at all five sites and don't rush. Always follow the same auscultation strategy. You will need absolute quiet. If you hear more than S_1S_2, it is very helpful first to determine which sounds are the S_1S_2 sounds, and then analyze the rest of the sounds. Be sure to use the bell and diaphragm of the stethoscope.

Sequence to Use during Auscultation

Before you begin assessing and interpreting heart sounds, you need to formulate a strategy to guide you. Here is one possible auscultation sequence.

- Use the diaphragm of the stethoscope to listen for the S_1S_2 sounds, then listen for split S_1 and split S_2 sounds.
- Use the bell of the stethoscope to assess for and differentiate the S_3 and S_4 sounds from the split sounds. Listen also for the presence of summation gallop. *Hint:* Apply light pressure on each landmark when using the bell to hear the softer sounds. Using firm pressure causes the bell to act as a diaphragm, and obscures the softer sounds.
- Return to using the diaphragm to assess for other sounds: murmurs originating from regurgitant valves, clicks, ejection sounds, snaps, and pericardial friction rubs.
- Finish by using the bell to assess for murmurs of stenotic valves.

Interpreting Heart Sounds

Refer to Table 11.2 on page 293 for more information on distinguishing heart sounds. Figure 11.23 is an algorithm for differentiating heart sounds in the adult client.

Using the diaphragm in each of the five landmark areas:

- Listen for S_1.

  The S_1 sound is the first sound. It is produced by the closure of the mitral and tricuspid valve leaflets after blood has entered the right and left ventricles. This sound

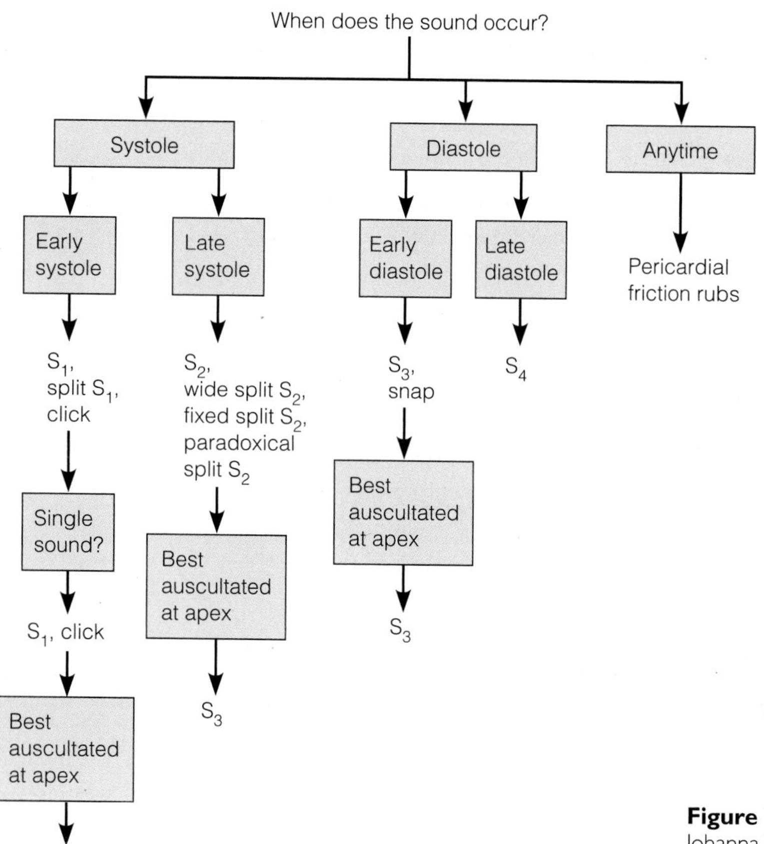

Figure 11.23 Differentiating heart sounds in the adult. Courtesy of Johanna K. Stiesmeyer, RN, MS, CCRN.

is loudest over the apex but may be heard over all five locations.

- Listen for S_2.

  The S_2 sound is the second heart sound. It is produced by the closure of the aortic and pulmonic valvular leaflets after the blood has entered from the ventricles into the aorta and pulmonary artery concomitantly. It is best heard over the base of the heart in the aortic and pulmonic areas.

- Listen for a split S_1.

  A split heart sound consists of two sounds of equal intensity and very close together in sequence. There is only a brief pause between the sounds, unlike the pause between S_1 and S_2.

The degree of split can vary. The narrowly split S_1 is normal when heard at the lower LSB at the tricuspid area. However, when the split is wide and heard over this same area, conditions such as a right bundle branch block and tricuspid stenosis may exist. A client with a pacemaker may also have a widely split S_1. Respirations should not affect the split S_1. The sounds of the split S_1 are equal in intensity. If an S_4 is present, the sounds are not of equal intensity.

Answer these questions if you hear a split S_1 sound:

1. How wide is the split?
2. Is it fixed, or does the respiratory cycle affect the wideness of the split?
3. Are the split S_1 sounds of equal intensity, or is one softer?

Pathologic processes may cause three variations in the split S_1 pattern. These are termed wide splitting, fixed splitting, and paradoxical splitting. *Wide splitting* can occur with delayed closure of the pulmonic valve, early closure of aortic valve, or slowed contraction of the right ventricle and closure of the pulmonic valve secondary to conduction disturbances. In *fixed splitting*, the split is not increased or decreased based upon respiration. In *paradoxical* or *reversed splitting*, the split widens on expiration as opposed to inspiration and is absent on inspiration.

- Listen for a split S_2.

  The split sound is the same as the split S_1 sound, but occurs at the time you expect to hear the S_3 sound. A split S_2 may be either physiologic (normal), or pathologic (abnormal). Physiologic (normal) splitting is best heard in the 2nd or 3rd ICS LSB, at the peak of a slow, deep inspiration, and in the supine position. The splitting is caused by the effect of the normally higher pressure and faster depolarization in the left ventricle versus the right ventricle.

When you hear a double or split sound at the S_2 timing, start by asking the same questions as listed for the split S_1 sound. Some of the most common causes of pathologic (abnormal) splitting S_2 are:

Right bundle branch block
Massive pulmonary embolus
Ventricular septal defect
Mitral regurgitation
Left bundle branch block
Right ventricular ectopy
Hypertension

- Listen for S_3 with the bell of the stethoscope.

  The S_3 is an early diastolic sound occurring shortly after S_2. It is a soft, dull sound best auscultated with the bell of the stethoscope in the apex area. It can be heard with the client placed in any position but is best auscultated with the client in the left lateral position.

The S_3 can be either physiologic or pathologic. In children or younger adults it can be physiologic even up to the age of 40. The pregnant client may develop an S_3 in the last trimester of her pregnancy.

In clients over 40, the S_3 is pathologic and is termed a *ventricular gallop*. It represents decreased ventricular compliance and is one of the earliest signs of the onset of congestive heart failure. It is possible to have both a right-sided and left-sided S_3. Some of the pathologic causes are myocardial infarction and congestive heart failure.

- Listen for S_4 with the bell of the stethoscope.

  The S_4 is a late diastolic sound occurring just before S_1. Like the S_3, the S_4 is best auscultated with the bell at the apex and with the client in the left lateral position. It is also a very soft sound.

The S_4 can also be physiologic or pathologic. It is normally found in children, older adults, and athletes in top condition.

When pathologic, an S_4 reflects decreased ventricular complicance. This is termed an *atrial gallop*. It is also possible to have a right-sided and left-sided S_4.

Conditions that may contribute to the development of an S_4 include

Myocardial infarction
Coronary artery disease
Aortic stenosis
Hypertension

- Listen for a *summation gallop*.

  This is composed of a $S_1S_2S_3S_4$. It sounds like a horse galloping and is associated with a tachycardic rhythm. The presence of this sound is ominous. It is often associated with severe congestive heart failure.

- Listen for clicks, snaps, and rubs.

  Start with systolic sounds, then listen for diastolic sounds.

You may hear these systolic sounds (between S_1 and S_2):

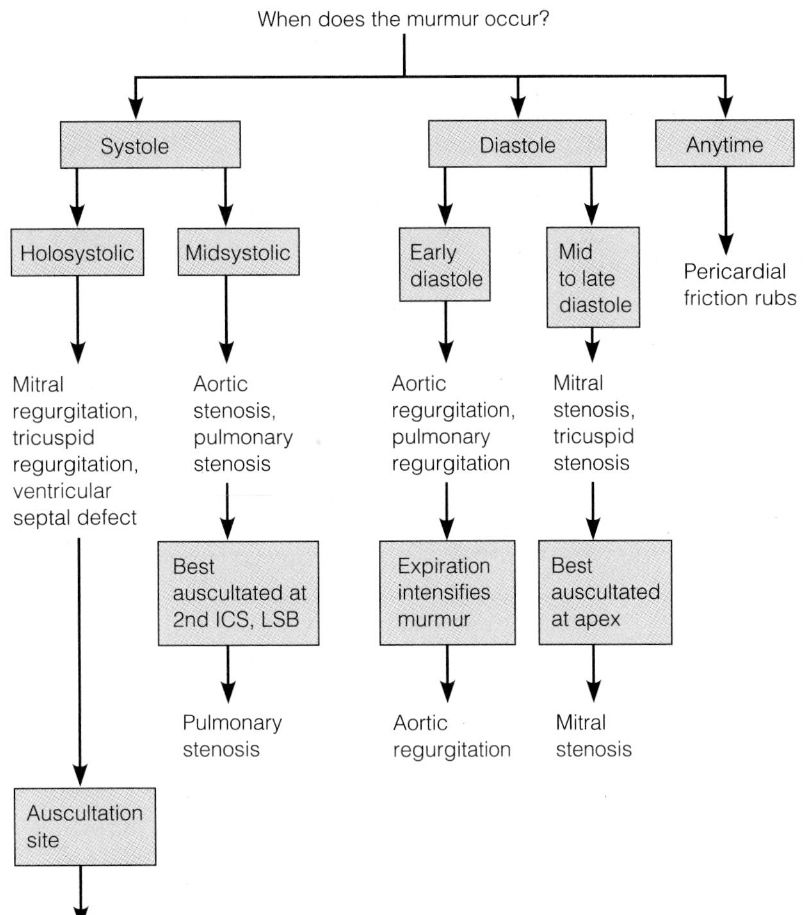

Figure 11.24 Differentiating murmurs in the adult. Courtesy of Johanna K. Stiesmeyer, RN, MS, CCRN.

Ejection click is caused when deformed leaflets of the aortic and/or pulmonic valves open. It imitates a clicking sound. A high-pitched sound of short duration, the aortic ejection click is best auscultated with the diaphragm of the stethoscope. It is best heard over the aortic area and in some cases the apex. The pulmonic ejection click is best heard at the pulmonic area and has the same qualities as the aortic ejection click. Both are auscultated at the start of systole. *Hint:* The pulmonic ejection click becomes softer upon inspiration and louder upon expiration, whereas the aortic ejection click remains unchanged during respiration.

A *systolic click* is associated with the presence of mitral valve prolapse. It may be heard at the beginning of systole or mid-systole. It is best ausculated with the diaphragm at the apex or near the lower LSB. It is a high-pitched, clicking sound.

You may hear these diastolic sounds (between S_2 and S_1):

An *opening snap* is produced by stenosis of the tricuspid or mitral leaflets. Place the diaphragm at the 3rd to 4th ICS LSB or apex to hear a high-pitched sound that is similar to the sound of snapping fingers.

The *pacemaker sound* occurs in clients with permanent pacemakers. It is a high-pitched sound just before S_1. Remember that the pacemaker wire sits in the right ventricle. You might confuse the pacemaker sound with either a split S_1 or an S_4. The pacemaker sound is a higher-pitched, clicking sound. S_4 is a soft sound better heard with the bell. The split S_1 is auscultated better with the bell in the tricuspid area.

- Listen for pericardial friction rub.

  This sound can be very elusive and easily confused with murmurs. It may be found anywhere over the chest and precordium. It may be continuous or sporadic. The distinguishing feature is the grating harshness of the sound. It is usually high-pitched and is variable in loudness. It is caused by an inflammatory process and commonly occurs after open-heart surgery and myocardial infarction, or in renal or metastatic disease.

Hint: To differentiate the pericardial friction rub from the pleural friction rub, have the client hold the breath. If the sound stops, it is pleural in origin because the lungs are no longer in motion; if the sound persists, it is pericardial in origin. If you auscultate a pericardial friction rub, assess for the presence of a *pulsus paradoxus*, described in Chapter 16.

- Listen for murmurs.

  Figure 11.24 is an algorithm for differentiating murmurs in adults. If you detect a murmur, ask yourself the questions listed in Table 11.3 on page 295. Murmurs have many characteristics, which are described fully in Table 11.4 on page 297.

Be concerned if the client develops a new murmur suddenly, or if a pre-existing murmur becomes louder, especially if the client has new physical symptoms of a cardiovascular disorder. Clients with multiple conditions may have a combination of murmurs and heart sounds. Such clients present a challenge even for the most experienced practitioners.

Table 11.2 Distinguishing and Interpreting Heart Sounds

Heart Sound	Cardiac Cycle Timing	Auscultation Site	Position	Pitch
S_1	Start of systole	Best at apex with diaphragm	Position does not affect the sound	High
S_2	End of systole	Both at 2nd ICS; pulmonary component best at LSB; aortic component best at RSB with diaphragm	Sitting or supine	High
Split S_1	Beginning of systole	If normal, at 2nd ICS, LSB; abnormal if heard at apex	Better heard in the supine position	High
Wide Split S_2	End of systole	Both at 2nd ICS, pulmonary component best at LSB; aortic component best at RSB with diaphragm	Better heard in the supine position	High
Fixed Split S_2	End of systole	Both at 2nd ICS; pulmonary component best at LSB; aortic component best at RSB with diaphragm	Better heard in the supine position	High
Paradoxical Split S_2	End of systole	Both at 2nd ICS; pulmonary component best at LSB; aortic component best at RSB with diaphragm	Better heard in the supine position	High
S_3	Early diastole right after S_2	Apex with the bell	Auscultated better in left lateral position or supine	Low
S_4	Late diastole right before S_1	Apex with the bell	Auscultated in almost a left lateral position or supine	Low
Clicks	Early systole	2nd ICS, RSB for aortic click and apex with diaphragm 2nd ICS, LSB for pulmonic click with diaphragm	Sitting or supine position may increase sound	High
Snaps	Early diastole	3-4 ICS, LSB with diaphragm	Sitting or supine position may increase the sound	High
Rubs	Can occur at any time	Best heard with the diaphragm, location variable	May be heard in any position, but best when the client sits forward	High, harsh in sound, grating

Table 11.2 Distinguishing and Interpreting Heart Sounds (continued)

Heart Sound	Effect of Respirations	Other Information
S_1	Less intense with inspiratory effort	◆ Sound caused by the closure of the mitral and tricuspid (atrioventricular valves) ◆ May become softer in sound with barrel chest, myocardial infarction, high body fat, high-grade atrioventricular block
S_2	A physiologic split may occur with inspiratory effort	◆ Sound caused by the closure of the aortic and pulmonic (semilunar valves) ◆ May become softer in sound with barrel chest, myocardial infarction, high body fat, shock state ◆ May be louder in thin individuals
Split S_1	Louder with inspiraton	◆ Rare ◆ May be normal
Wide Split S_2	Louder with inspiration	◆ Persists throughout both inspiration and expiration ◆ Seen in right bundle branch block, pulmonary stenosis, mitral regurgitation
Fixed Split S_2	Louder with inspiration	◆ Inspiration and expiration do not affect split ◆ Can be present in right ventricular failure, atrial septal defect
Paradoxical Split S_2	Heard on inspiration but not on expiration	◆ Causes include left bundle branch block, Wolff-Parkinson-White sydrome Type B (accessory tract on the right side)
S_3	Louder with inspiratory effort	◆ Causes include left ventricular failure; fluid overload; regurgitation of the mitral, aortic, and tricuspid valves ◆ Termed ventricular gallop
S_4	Louder with inspiratory effort	◆ Causes include systemic hypertension, cardiomyopathy, coronary artery disease ◆ Termed atrial gallop ◆ Can hear normally in well-trained athletes and the elderly who do not have cardiovascular heart disease ◆ S_3S_4 in combination with a tachycardic rhythm is associated with severe heart failure and termed gallop rhythm
Clicks	Aortic click sound does not vary with respiratory efforts but pulmonic click is softer with inspiratory effort	◆ Stenosis of aortic or pulmonic valves causes the click sound
Snaps	Respiratory efforts do not affect sound	◆ Stenosis of mitral and tricuspid stenosis causes the snap sound
Rubs	Louder when breath is held	◆ Associated with an inflammatory process ◆ Can be seen after myocardial infarction or coronary artery bypass surgery (CABG) and in chronic renal disease or metastatic cancer

Table 11.3 Distinguishing and Interpreting Heart Murmurs

Ask Yourself	Information
1. How loud is the murmur?	Murmurs are graded on a rather subjective scale of 1–6: ◆ Grade 1: Barely audible with stethoscope, often considered physiologic not pathologic. Requires concentration and a quiet environment. ◆ Grade 2: Very soft but distinctly audible. ◆ Grade 3: Moderately loud; there is no thrill or thrusting motion associated with the murmur. ◆ Grade 4: Distinctly loud, in addition to a palpable thrill. ◆ Grade 5: Very loud, can actually hear with part of the diaphragm of the stethoscope off of the chest; palpable thrust and thrill present. ◆ Grade 6: Loudest, can hear with the diaphragm off of the chest; visible thrill and thrust.
2. Where does it occur in the cardiac cycle: systole, diastole, or both?	Location in cardiac cycle: ◆ Systole: early systole, midsystole, late systole ◆ Diastole: early diastole, mid-diastole, late diastole ◆ Both
3a. Is the sound continuous throughout systole, diastole, or only heard for part of the cycle?	Duration of murmur ◆ Continuous through systole only ◆ Continuous through diastole only ◆ Continuous through systole and diastole *Systolic murmurs* may be of two types: ◆ Midsystolic: Murmur is heard after S_1 and stops before S_2. ◆ Pansystolic/holosystolic: Murmur begins with S_1 and stops at S_2. *Diastolic murmurs* may be one of three types: ◆ Early diastolic: Murmur auscultated immediately after S_2 and then stops. There is a gap where this murmur stops and S_1 is heard. ◆ Middiastolic: Murmur begins a short time after S_2 and stops well before S_1 is auscultated. ◆ Late diastolic: This murmur starts well after S_2 and stops immediately before S_1 is heard.

Table 11.3 Distinguishing and Interpreting Heart Murmurs (continued)

3b. What does the configuration of the sound look like?

Potential configurations:

Pansystolic/holosystolic:

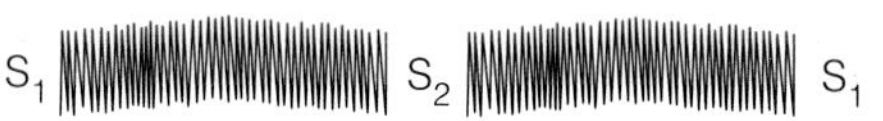

Continuous

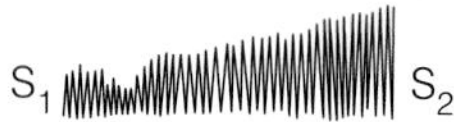

Crescendo (Systolic represented)

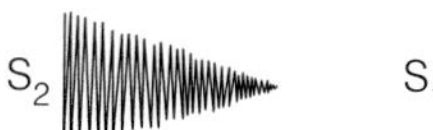

Decrescendo (Diastolic represented)

S_1 S_2

Crescendo-Decrescendo (Systole represented)

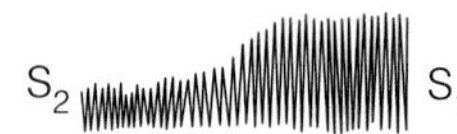

Rumble

4. What is the quality of the sound of the murmur?	◆ Blowing ◆ Harsh ◆ Musical ◆ Raspy ◆ Rumbling
5. What is the pitch or frequency of the sound?	◆ Low ◆ Medium ◆ High
6. In which landmark(s) do you best hear the murmur?	Use the five landmarks for auscultation: ◆ Pulmonic areas 1&2 ◆ Aortic area ◆ Tricuspid area ◆ Mitral area ◆ Apex
7. Does it radiate?	◆ To the throat? ◆ To the axilla ?
8. Is there any change in pattern with respirations?	◆ Increases/decreases with inspiration ◆ Increases/decreases with expiration
9. Is it associated with variations in heart sounds?	◆ Associated with split S_1? ◆ Associated with split S_2? ◆ Associated with S_3? ◆ Associated with S_4? ◆ Associated with a click or ejection sound?
10. Does intensity of murmur change with position?	◆ Increases/decreases with squatting? ◆ Increases/decreases with client in the left lateral position? (Do not have the client perform the Valsalva maneuver or any abrupt positional changes, because some clients do not tolerate position changes well.)

Table 11.4 Classifying Heart Murmurs

Use your assessment data to classify the murmur as follows:

Murmur	Cardiac Cycle Timing	Auscultation Site	Configuration of Sound	Continuity
Aortic stenosis	Midsystolic	RSB, 2nd ICS	S_1 S_2	Crescendo-decrescendo, continuous
Pulmonary stenosis	Midsystolic	LSB, 2nd to 3rd ICS	S_1 S_2	Crescendo-decrescendo, continuous
Mitral regurgitation	Systole	Apex	S_1 S_2	Holosystolic, continuous
Tricuspid regurgitation	Systole	4th ICS, LSB	S_1 S_2	Holosystolic, continuous
Mitral stenosis	Diastole	Apical	S_2 S_1	Rumble that increases in sound towards the end, continuous
Tricuspid stenosis	Diastole	Lower LSB	S_2 S_1	Rumble that increases in sound towards the end, continuous
Ventricular septal defect (left-to-right shunt)	Systole	3rd, 4th, 5th ICS, LSB	S_1 S_2	Holosystolic, continuous
Aortic regurgitation	Diastole (early)	3rd ICS, LSB	S_2 S_1	Decrescendo, continuous
Pulmonic Regurgitation	Diastole (early)	3rd ICS, LSB	S_2 S_1	Decrescendo, continuous

Table 11.4 Classifying Heart Murmurs (continued)

Murmur	Quality	Pitch	Radiation	Changes with Respirations
Aortic stenosis	Usually harsh, coarse	Medium	Most commonly into neck into carotid area and down left sternal border, possibly apex	Expiration may intensify the murmur
Pulmonary stenosis	Usually harsh	Medium	Towards the left upper neck and shoulder areas	Inspiration may intensify the murmur
Mitral regurgitation	Blowing and can be harsh in sound quality	High	Usually to left axilla, LSB, and base	Expiration may intensify the murmur
Tricuspid regurgitation	Blowing	High	May radiate to LSB and MCL but not to axilla	Inspiration may intensify the murmur
Mitral stenosis	Rumbling	Low and best heard with bell	Rare	Expiration may intensify the murmur
Tricuspid stenosis	Rumbling	Low	Rare	Inspiration may intensify the murmur
Ventricular septal defect (Left-to-right shunt)	Harsh	High	May radiate across precordium but not to axilla	Expiration may intensify the murmur
Aortic regurgitation	Blowing	High, best auscultated with diaphragm unless client is sitting up and leaning forward	May radiate to 2nd ICS, RSB and may proceed to apex	Expiration may intensify the murmur if the client leans forward and sits up
Pulmonic regurgitation	Blowing	High, best auscultated with diaphragm	May radiate to 2nd ICS, RSB and may proceed to apex	Inspiration may intensify the murmur

Murmur	Variations in Heart Sounds	Variations with Position Changes	Other Information
Aortic stenosis	Softer S_2, possible paradoxical split S_2, possible S_4, may hear an ejection click	Decreased when sitting upright	◆ Thrill may be palpated in right side of neck and RSB, 2nd to 3rd ICS ◆ Thrust felt to the left of the apex with left ventricular hypertrophy ◆ Auscultatory gap ◆ Caused by calcific process to cusps ◆ Seen in infective processes that include cardiac involvement, rheumatic fever
Pulmonary stenosis	Wide split S_2, possible S_4, ejection click	Sudden lying down from a sitting position intensifies murmur (perform any sudden moves cautiously and avoid in the elderly)	◆ May be associated with right ventricular hypertrophy ◆ Thrill may be palpated at apex ◆ Is often associated with mitral regurgitation ◆ Caused by calcific process to valvular leaflets ◆ Seen in rheumatic fever
Mitral regurgitation	S_3, soft S_1, and in later disease an S_3-S_4 gallop may be auscultated	Increased intensity when sitting upright	◆ Can be associated with fatigue and orthopnea ◆ A thrill maybe palpated at apex ◆ Caused by incompetent valvular leaflets
Tricuspid regurgitation	May have S_3	Sudden lying down from a sitting position intensifies murmur (perform any sudden moves cautiously and avoid in the elderly)	◆ Neck veins can be distended severely, even pulsating ◆ Thrill at lower LSB ◆ If right ventricular hypertrophy is present, a thrust may be palpated ◆ Commonly seen with pulmonary hypertension ◆ Caused by incompetent valvular leaflets

Table 11.4 Classifying Heart Murmurs (continued)

Murmur	Variations in Heart Sounds	Variations with Position Changes	Other Information
Mitral stenosis	Opening snap after S_2	None known	
Tricuspid stenosis	Split S_2 may be present with inspiration	None known	◆ Can see prominent jugular venous pulsations ◆ Thrill may be palpated over right ventricle during diastole ◆ Is caused by stenosis of tricuspid leaflets ◆ Pathologic processes such as rheumatic fever and congenital defects may contribute to the development of this murmur.
Ventricular septal defect (Left-to-right shunt)	May have S_3 and/or S_4 if congestive heart failure is present	Sudden lying down from a sitting position intensifies murmur (perform any sudden moves cautiously and avoid in the elderly) Louder when sitting upright	◆ Thrill may be present ◆ Can be seen with congenital heart defect or as a complication of a myocardial infarction ◆ Occurs because of an opening between the right and left ventricles
Aortic regurgitation	S_3, S_4, ejection click in 2nd ICS	Murmur becomes louder if client sits up and leans forward and is best heard with the bell when the client is in this position Murmur if client is not in above position is best heard with the diaphragm	◆ May be associated with bounding carotid and femoral pulses (Called water-hammer pulse) ◆ Apical impulse thrusts and is displaced in a left lateral direction secondary to left ventricular hypertrophy ◆ Wide pulse pressure ◆ Can be associated with a crescendo-decrescendo shaped systolic murmur ◆ Caused by incompetent valvular leaflets, rheumatic heart disease ◆ Can be seen in Marfan's syndrome
Pulmonic regurgitation	S_3	Murmur becomes louder if client sits up and leans forward	Very difficult to differentiate from the murmur of aortic regurgitation

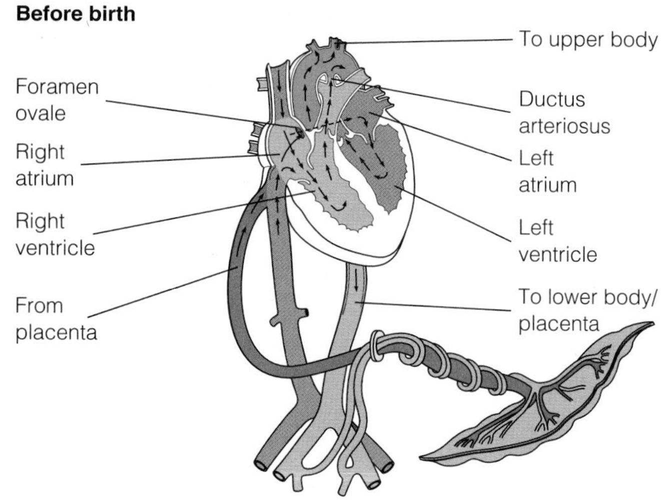

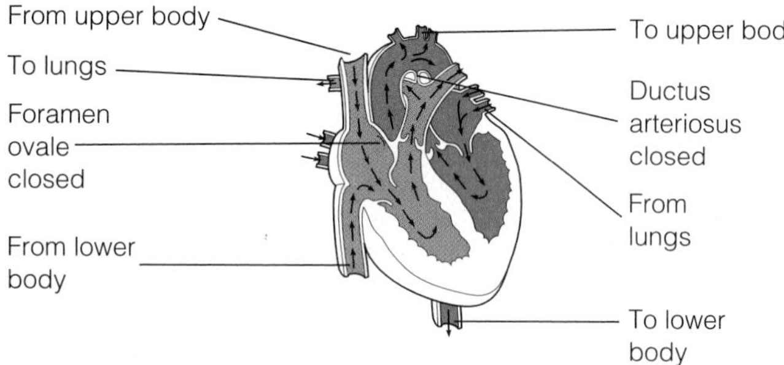

Figure 11.25 Location of the main structures and vessels present in the fetal and post-partal cardiovascular anatomy.

Developmental Considerations

Infants, Children, and Adolescent Clients

During development, the fetus receives its nutrients and oxygen from its mother. The lungs are nonfunctional, and oxygen is carried in blood from the placenta to the right side of the heart. The majority of this blood passes through the *foramen ovale* to the left side of the heart, then into the aorta to enter the systemic circulation. The foramen ovale is a passageway for blood between the right and left atria. The rest of the blood passes through the pulmonary artery and *ductus arteriosus* and enters the aorta (Figure 11.25). The ductus arteriosus is an opening between the pulmonary artery and the descending aorta.

Inflation of the lungs at birth causes the pulmonary vasculature to dilate. Oxygenation now occurs for the first time within the newborn's lungs. The foramen ovale closes shortly after birth because of increased pulmonary vascular return and decreased pressures in the right side of the heart. The ductus arteriosus closes within 24–46 hours in response to multiple physiologic events, including decreased pulmonary resistance and decreased pressure in the right atrium versus increased pressure in the left atrium. Murmurs may be auscultated if these openings remain patent. However, if a ventricular septal defect is present, the murmur it causes may not be auscultated until the 4th to 6th week after delivery.

The infant's arterial pressure rises at birth, and the systemic vascular resistance increases significantly when the umbilicus is cut. Over time, the left ventricle increases in size and mass as it works to pump blood into the aorta against increasingly elevating systemic vascular resistance. The blood pressure of the full-term infant may average 70/50 mm Hg, and 10 mm Hg less in both systolic and diastolic readings in the preterm newborn. Weight significantly influences blood pressure.

The heart rate of the newborn initially may be as high as 175–180 beats per minute. Over the first 6–8 hours, it gradually decreases to an average of 115–120 beats per minute. Stimulation that causes crying, screaming, or coughing may cause the heart rate to rise temporarily to 180 beats per minute.

A newborn's cardiovascular system thus undergoes tremendous changes at birth and in the next several days of life. The infant should be easily aroused and alert. The skin should demonstrate perfusion with pink quality in the nailbeds, mucous membranes, and conjunctiva no matter what the baby's race. Precordial bulging and chest deformities such as pigeon chest and barrel chest are of concern.

There are six landmark sites for auscultating infants' and children's heart sounds. These are

- Aortic area, RSB, 2nd ICS
- Pulmonic area, LSB, 2nd ICS
- Tricuspid area, LSB, 4th ICS
- Mitral area, MCL, 5th ICS (also called the apical area)
- Erb's Point: LSB, 3rd to 5th ICS
- Sternoclavicular area: upper LSB and RSB

Normal findings for infants and children are

- S_1, S_2, and S_3 sounds are present.
- The presence of S_4 may be normal but might also indicate a pathologic process.
- A split S_2 may be normal if it widens with inspiration. This sound should be absent when the child holds the breath.
- Innocent systolic murmurs are normal. These are low-pitched sounds of short duration, grade 1–3 (see Table 11.3). They are nonradiating and originate in the lower LSB.
- Sinus arrhythmia is very common. Be sure to perform simultaneous observation of the respiratory pattern and the heart sounds. The heart rate accelerates upon inspiration and slows upon expiration.
- Heart rate and blood pressure vary depending upon the infant's and child's age.

Be concerned with these findings:

- Gallop rhythm, tachycardia, pulsus alternans
- Displacement of the PMI laterally to the left
- Bulges, heaves
- Fixed, split S_2
- Diastolic murmurs
- Loud murmurs of long duration, grade 4–6
- Clicks, snaps, rubs

Be sure to use a small diaphragm and bell with an infant or child for optimal auscultation of heart sounds. Murmurs of a congenital cause include patent ductus arteriosus, tetralogy of Fallot, septal defects, and coarctation of the aorta (see page 307).

A complete assessment of infants, children, and adolescents is provided in Chapter 19.

Childbearing Clients

During pregnancy, a woman's body undergoes phenomenal adaptations, especially in the cardiovascular system. Usually these adaptations do not place her life at risk; however, if preexisting cardiovascular or other disease is present, her health may be significantly compromised.

The heart is displaced to the left and upward, and the apex is pushed laterally and to the left. This anatomic shift may be seen when examining the electrical axis on the woman's 12-lead ECG. The axis is rotated to the left. The extent of this shift is influenced by the physical strength of the woman's abdominal muscles, the shape of the fetus, the gestational age, and the structural anatomy of the uterus.

The cardiovascular system undergoes many physiologic changes during pregnancy. Blood volume may increase as much as 40–50%. Red blood cell genesis is dramatically stimulated, and plasma volume increases by as much as 50%. Plasma albumin, conversely, decreases. Cardiac output increases 30–50% in just the first trimester. Dilation of surface veins, together with the low resistance of the uteroplacental circulation, increases the venous return to the heart. Stroke volume increases 30%. Because of the substantial increase in volume and the resultant increased workload, the heart may appear as much as 10% larger on chest radiography. Interestingly, systolic blood pressure may decrease by 2–3 mm Hg and diastolic blood pressure by 5–10 mm Hg during the first half of the woman's pregnancy. As the pregnancy progresses, these values return to their previous levels. Last, the great vessels may become more tortuous in appearance.

These are some common assessment findings during pregnancy:

- Slight increase in resting pulse 10–15 beats/min
- Systolic and diastolic murmurs, very soft, grade 1–2
- Split S_1
- S_3

There may be a slight increase in resting pulse by about 10–15 beats per minute, although not every client experiences this increase. Because of the increased volume, preexisting murmurs may become louder. Murmurs may even be auscultated for the first time. Systolic murmurs are the most common (90% incidence), whereas diastolic murmurs occur less frequently (20% incidence). Heart tones may also change. The S_1 may split, and a prominent S_3 may be heard.

The position of the client may influence the cardiovascular dynamic state. Cardiac output may decrease when she lies on her back because of compression of the vena cava and aorta. The brachial pressure is highest when the client is sitting, then decreases when she is supine. Pressure is lowest when she is in the lateral recumbent position. Monitoring a client's blood pressure and pattern of the pressures is crucial. A rise of 30 mm Hg in systolic pressure or 15 mm Hg in diastolic pressure may signal a critical situation.

A complete assessment of the childbearing client is provided in Chapter 20.

Older Clients

There is limited data on the effects of aging on the cardiovascular system. The reasons for this lack of information are:

- Many older individuals experience cardiovascular disease. To determine the effects of aging, researchers need to test individuals who are free of cardiovascular disease.
- Little research has focused on the geriatric population. It is imperative to design research studies examining the anatomic and physiologic changes in the geriatric population. The most recent information available highlights essential features that alter cardiovascular wellness and function.

The heart may stay the same size, enlarge, or atrophy. During normal aging in the absence of disease, the heart walls may thicken to some extent. The left atrium may increase in size over time. Significant enlargement of the left ventricle can be attributed to the influence of hypertension. Atrophy is associated with wasting diseases. Aging can also contribute to the loss of ventricular compliance as the cardiac valves and large vessels become more rigid. The aorta may dilate and lengthen.

Physiologically, systolic blood pressure may increase; however, there may be no significant change in resting heart rate. Diastolic filling time and pressure may increase to maintain a cardiac output adequate for physiologic needs. Upon auscultation, the elderly client may have an S_4. The presence of an S_4 may be either physiologic in individuals free of cardiovascular disease or may reflect cardiovascular disease. Last, the electrical conduction system may experience a loss of automaticity when the SA node and conducting pathways become fibrotic and lose cellular integrity.

In the healthy geriatric client, cardiac output may remain stable. Stroke volume may increase just slightly when the client is at rest. The healthy client may tolerate exercise well. The healthy client may actually show a decreased heart rate, maximum oxygen consumption, and an increase in stroke volume during exercise. A client who has been physically active may have twice the work capacity than a client who has not.

Be sure to assess the older client in a position that is comfortable. Do not have the client make any sudden movements such as suddenly sitting or standing up, or lying down suddenly after standing or sitting. Systolic murmurs become more common as people age, especially because of aortic stenosis. These murmurs are usually best auscultated in the aortic area or base. Nonphysiologic murmurs are not normal findings. However, an S_4 sound is a common finding in older adults who do not have identified cardiovascular disease. In individuals with pre-existing heart disease, however, an S_4 is a pathologic finding. Be mindful of the presence of any other heart sounds beyond S_1 and S_2 or any change in characteristics of pre-exisiting heart sounds. Inform the physician of any significant findings.

Chapter 21 describes a complete assessment of the older client.

Psychosocial Considerations

Stress causes an individual to experience longer periods of sympathetic stimulation, which increases the workload on the heart. Systemic vascular resistance may be elevated for longer periods of time, especially in situations of excessive stress. Counseling, relaxation, meditation, and biofeedback techniques are usually helpful.

"Workaholic, driven to succeed, driven to excel and to be the best regardless of the cost" describes an individual who exhibits type A behavior, which for many years has been thought to contribute to the development of heart disease. Again, counseling, relaxation, meditation, and biofeedback techniques may be helpful.

Self-Care Considerations

Self-care considerations in the development of cardiovascular disease include diet, activity level, obesity, smoking, use of recreational drugs, and alcohol consumption.

Diet is one factor that may significantly influence the development of cardiovascular disease. Intake of fat, especially saturated fat, contributes significantly to cardiovascular disease. Consumption of animal fat elevates total cholesterol in the blood, but total blood cholesterol can also be elevated when the liver converts saturated fat to cholesterol (Ornish 1990). Low-density lipoproteins (LDL) have been shown to contribute to atherosclerosis, whereas high-density lipoproteins (HDL) assist in the removal of LDL. Salt and monosodium glutamate (MSG), which are often hidden ingredients of processed foods, have been shown to contribute to hypertension. Processed sugar contributes to elevated triglycerides, which directly influence the development of atherosclerosis.

"Couch potato" is a popular term that describes a lifestyle of inactivity. Studies on individuals who perform continuous aerobic exercise for at least 30–45 minutes at least three times a week have shown a significant correlation to a slower progression of atherosclerosis. Exercise also helps to diffuse the effects of stress and, in most individuals, provides a feeling of relaxation.

It is common to find a significantly lower resting heart rate in well-conditioned competitive athletes. Often, left ventricular enlargement is found upon examination, as well as S_3 and S_4 heart sounds. Various benign dysrhythmias related to increased vagal tone may be found in athletes during exercise. The 12-lead ECG may demonstrate left ventricular hypertrophy and elevated QRS voltage related to increased ventricular mass that accompanies extended periods of intensive physical exercise. ST segment elevation associated with T wave abnormalites are common, especially among athletes of African origin. These may be normal findings, or they may indicate disease. The death of several athletes who have experienced fatal dysrhythmias and syncopal episodes in the last few years have been well publicized.

A client's weight and appearance may not be indicative of overall percentage of body fat. Research that focuses on the "overweight" as stipulated by height/weight charts is increasingly being replaced by research on the "overfat" as determined by body composition (Bailey 1991). It has been suggested that ideal body-fat percentage for men is 15% and for women is 22%. Overfat contributes to the development of hypertension and increases workload of the heart.

Smoking is a well-known contributor to the development of cardiovascular disease. In fact, it is one of the most devasting. The chemicals inhaled in cigarette smoke alter and injure the linings of the arteries, especially in areas of bifurcation (division into branches). Inhalation of passive smoke is also detrimental to the cardiovascular system.

Cocaine, especially crack cocaine, causes increased oxygen demands on the heart. *Ventricular ectopy*, electrical impulses that originate in the ventricles and cause early contraction of the ventricles, has been linked to cocaine use. Coronary artery spasm, myocardial infarction, malignant hypertension, and ruptured aorta also have been attributed to cocaine. Many of these health problems are discussed later in the chapter.

Alcoholism is associated with the development of many cardiovascular complications, such as cardiomyopathy (discussed later in the chapter). Alcohol consumption may also cause ventricular ectopy, which contributes to decreased cardiac output and may be life-threatening.

Family, Cultural, and Environmental Considerations

Individuals whose blood-related parents, aunts, uncles, and/or siblings demonstrate atherosclerotic heart disease before the age of 50 are considered at risk.

In some cultures, "overfat" individuals are considered healthier than those who are leaner. The selection and preparation of food may also reflect cultural influences. The use of lard and other forms of saturated fat is common in some cultures and may contribute to the development of hypertension and diabetes. African-Americans have a significantly higher percentage of hypertension than Caucasians. Cardiovascular disease is the leading cause of death among African-American women in their 30s and contributes to a significant percentage of deaths in individuals from varied cultural backgrounds. Individuals of Cuban, Filipino, and Mexican heritage have a higher incidence of hypertension. The correlation of diet and heritage is also significant, as demonstrated by the low incidence of heart disease in Japanese individuals adhering to a traditional Japanese diet and the increasing incidence of heart disease in Japanese who have adopted the "western" diet of red meat and saturated fats.

Some data suggests that low socioeconomic bracket is correlated with a higher incidence of hypertension, especially among women. There may be a correlation between this situation and the effect of stress related to lower incomes, limited exercise, diets containing saturated fats, or lack of access to quality health care.

Organizing the Data

To develop a care plan that reflects the specific need of the client with cardiovascular pathology, you begin with the information obtained from the interview and physical assessment. NANDA has developed specific diagnoses for cardiovascular illness, but several other nursing diagnoses may be applicable for this same client.

Identifying Nursing Diagnoses

NANDA lists six nursing diagnoses that relate specifically to the cardiovascular system: *Decreased cardiac output; Denial; Impaired gas exchange; Fluid volume excess; Acute pain;* and *Altered tissue perfusion.* In addition, other nursing diagnoses may be appropriate for the client.

Cardiac output, decreased is the inability of the heart to pump efficiently to provide oxygenated blood to the cells of the body. This condition may be seen in the acute setting after myocardial infarction or in a chronic state when a condition such as heart failure exists (Table 11.5).

Denial, ineffective: This behavior is usually a protective mechanism utilized by a client and/or the client's support group in response to a stressful situation. It is commonly seen as one of the initial reactions to a myocardial infarction. Although it is a protective mechanism, it can contribute to detrimental outcomes if the client delays seeking medical attention. (See Table 11.5.)

Fluid volume excess can be a significant outcome of cardiovascular ischemia or injury caused by myocardial infarction. It may also be a sequella of chronic conditions such as heart failure or hepatic and renal disease.

Gas exchange, impaired describes the state in which the individual experiences a decreased passage of oxygen and/or carbon dioxide between the alveoli of the lungs and the vascular septum (NANDA). The heart may weaken or fail and be unable to pump blood to the pulmonary septum for oxygenation. This is seen in pulmonary hypertension. When the left ventricle fails as a pump, blood will back up into the pulmonary vascular septum, also contributing to the inability to oxygenate blood.

Pain, acute is usually seen in the emergent situation as a result of conditions such as myocardial ischemia, injury, pericarditis, and cardiac trauma. Acute pain is a very subjective experience. Often, the client will not describe the sensation as pain but as discomfort. Having the client rate the pain on a scale of 1 to 10 helps you interpret the client's subjective analysis of the experience. Acute pain may also vary greatly among individuals. (See Table 11.5.)

Altered tissue perfusion: cardiovascular: The inability to provide adequate oxygen and nutrients to the myocardial tissue significantly affects the function and viability of the heart.

Other nursing diagnoses that may be appropriate for clients with cardiovascular disease or who are susceptible for developing cardiovascular disease are: *Activity intolerance, Impaired adjustment, Anxiety, Body image disturbance, Ineffective breathing pattern, Constipation, Ineffective individual coping, Dysfunctional ventilatory weaning response, Altered family process, Fatigue, Fluid volume deficit, Altered health maintanence, Hopelessness, Knowledge deficit, Noncompliance, Altered nutrition: less than body requirements, Altered parenting, High risk for injury, Powerlessness, Altered role performance, Self-care deficit, Self-esteem disturbance, Altered sexuality patterns, Impaired skin integrity, Sleep pattern disturbance,* and *Altered tissue perfusion.*

Table 11.5 Nursing Diagnoses Commonly Associated with the Cardiovascular System

CARDIAC OUTPUT, DECREASED

Definition: A state in which the blood pumped by an individual's heart is sufficiently reduced that it is inadequate to meet the needs of the body's tissues (NANDA).

RELATED FACTORS

Cardiac anomaly (specify), Drug toxicity, Dysfunctional electrical conduction, Hypovolemia, Increased ventricular workload, Ventricular ischemia, Ventricular damage, Ventricular restriction, Others specific to client (specify).

DEFINING CHARACTERISTICS

Major	Minor
Color changes in skin and mucous membranes	Change in mental status
Restlessness	Shortness of breath
Dyspnea	Syncope
Decreased peripheral pulses	Vertigo
Cold, clammy skin	Edema
Jugular vein distention	Cough
Rales	Frothy sputum
Oliguria	Gallop rhythm
Orthopnea	Weakness
Variations in blood pressure readings	
Arrhythmias	
Fatigue	

INEFFECTIVE DENIAL

Definition: The state of a conscious or unconscious attempt to disavow the knowledge or meaning of an event to reduce anxiety/fear to the detriment of health (NANDA).

RELATED FACTORS

Specific to client.

DEFINING CHARACTERISTICS

Major	Minor
Delay in seeking or refusal of health care attention to the detriment to health	Minimizing symptoms
Failure to perceive personal relevance of symptoms or danger	Displacing source of symptoms to other organs
	Inappropriate affect
	Failure to admit fear of death or invalidism
	Inability to admit impact of disease in life pattern
	Displacing fear of impact of the condition
	Making dismissive gestures or comments when speaking of distressing events

Table 11.5 Nursing Diagnoses Commonly Associated with the Cardiovascular System (continued)

PAIN (ACUTE)	
Definition: A state in which an individual reports discomfort or an uncomfortable sensation (adapted from NANDA). This discomfort is whatever the experiencing person says it is, existing whenever he/she says it does.	
RELATED FACTORS	
Injury, Recent surgery, Noxious stimulus (specify), Others specific to client (specify).	
DEFINING CHARACTERISTICS	
Communication of pain descriptors, eg, pain, discomfort, nausea, night sweats, muscle cramps, itching skin, numbness, tingling of extremities Increased blood pressure Increased/decreased pulse rate Increased respiratory rate Diaphoresis, pallor Crying Grimacing	Restlessness Limited attention span Withdrawal/focus on self Guarding, protective behavior Moaning Pacing Facial mask of pain Alteration in muscle tone

DIAGNOSTIC REASONING IN ACTION

Jason Tibbs, a 56-year-old African-American male, presents to the emergency room with a history of hypertension and juvenile-onset diabetes, which he has controlled with diet and insulin injections. Today, when taking his morning walk, he fatigued quickly, had difficulty catching his breath, felt a little nauseated, and experienced some unusual tingling in his left arm. He states that his wife noticed that he was back from his walk early and saw that he did not look right. He felt it was not something to worry about, "It will go away if I rest," he said. His wife insisted that he go to the hospital.

The ED nurse, Janet Frazier, notes that Mr. Tibbs is diaphoretic and his skin has a grayish tinge, especially under his eyes and along his cheek bones. His blood pressure is 89/52, pulse 42, respirations are 34/min. He is nauseated. After administering atropine, Ms Frazier notes that Mr. Tibbs's blood pressure increases to 110/70 and his heart rate to 70. He occasionally rubs his hand across his chest and shakes his left arm, but emphatically denies that he is having pain. He belches sporadically, and states "It was probably something I ate, or maybe I'm having an insulin reaction. I feel silly. I just want to go home."

Mr. Tibbs's physical presentation indicates that an insult to his cardiovascular system is present. The diaphoretic, gray-tinged skin color is suggestive of altered tissue perfusion. His fatigue state is increasing, and he is having difficulty breathing. His vital signs reveal hypotension. All these symptoms suggest the presence of a cardiovascular problem. His history of diabetes, his obesity, and his heredity favor the development of cardiovascular illness. His denial is a protective mechanism that he is using to suppress his fear.

Nursing diagnoses appropriate for Mr. Tibbs include:

1. *Decreased cardiac output* related to hypotension
2. *Ineffective denial* related to Mr. Tibbs's statement that he does not need health care although he exhibits dramatic physical signs of cardiovascular disease
3. *Fatigue* related to disease process, decreased energy, and state of discomfort
4. *Impaired gas exchange* related to decreased pulmonary blood supply

Common Alterations in the Health of the Cardiovascular System

Common alterations in the health of the cardiovascular system include myocardial infarction (heart attack), congestive heart disease, valvular heart disease, congenital problems, and many others. Table 11.6 provides information on the variety of characteristics that are associated with four of the most common cardiovascular conditions: unstable angina, myocardial infarction, pericarditis, and dissecting aneurysm.

Myocardial Ischemia

Ischemia is a common problem where the oxygen needs of the body are heightened, thus increasing the work of the heart. Unfortunately, the oxygen needs of the heart are not met as it works harder, and an ischemic process ensues. Ischemia is usually due to the presence of an atherosclerotic plaque. A blood clot may be associated with the plaque.

Myocardial Infarction

During infarction, there is complete disruption of oxygen and nutrient flow to the myocardial tissue in the area below a total occlusion. Infarction leads to the death of the myocardial tissue unless flow of blood is reestablished.

Valvular Heart Disease

Disease of the valves denotes either narrowing (stenosis) of the valve leaflets, or incompetence (regurgitation) of these same leaflets. Valvular disease may be caused by rheumatic fever, congenital defects, myocardial infarction, and normal aging.

Congestive Heart Disease

This condition is the inability of the heart to produce a sufficient pumping effort. Most commonly, both right-sided and left-sided heart failure are present. Left-sided heart failure causes blood to back up into the pulmonary system and results in pulmonary edema. Right-sided heart failure causes backup of the blood into the systemic circulation and leads to distended neck veins, liver congestion, and peripheral edema.

Ventricular Hypertrophy

This condition occurs in response to pumping against high pressures. Right ventricular hypertrophy occurs with pulmonary hypertension, congenital heart disease, pulmonary disease, pulmonary stenosis, and right ventricular infarction. Left ventricular hypertrophy occurs in the presence of systemic hypertension, congenital heart disease, aortic stenosis, or myocardial infarction to the left ventricle.

Septal Defects

An atrial septal defect is an opening between the right and left atria, whereas a ventricular septal defect is an opening between the right and left ventricles. Both of these septal defects may result from congenital heart disease and myocardial infarction.

Congenital Heart Disease

There are many forms of congenital heart disease, which is related to developmental defects. Most often valves and septal structures are affected.

Coarctation of the Aorta In this condition, the aorta is severely narrowed in the region inferior to the left subclavian artery. The narrowing restricts blood flow from the left ventricle into the aorta and out into the systemic circulation, thus contributing to the development of congestive heart failure in the newborn. It can be surgically treated.

Patent Ductus Arteriosus The ductus arteriosus is an opening between the aorta and pulmonary artery that is present in the fetus. This opening should spontaneously close permanently between 24–48 hours after delivery. If this closure does not occur completely, a condition called patent ductus arteriosus exists. It may be treated medically, through pharmacologic therapy, and surgically.

Tetralogy of Fallot The condition involves four cardiac defects: dextraposition of the aorta, pulmonary stenosis, right ventricular hypertrophy, and ventricular septal defect. This condition is life-threatening for the newborn but can be treated surgically.

Electrical Rhythm Disturbances

Rhythm disturbances are a very common occurrence. Lethal dysrhythmias, such as ventricular tachycardia and ventricular fibrillation, are common complications of myocardial ischemia, myocardial infarction, and cardiomegaly. Heart blocks, such as first-degree atrioventricular block and second-degree atrioventricular heart block type 1, rarely compromise hemodynamic stability, but second-degree atrioventricular heart block type 2 and third-degree atrioventricular heart block can significantly compromise hemodynamic stability especially in the presence of myocardial infarction. Young individuals, mostly males, may suffer from tachycardias when extraconducting structures are present, as in Wolff-Parkinson-White syndrome. These may be fatal in some cases.

Table 11.6 Pain Assessment with Common Cardiovascular Disorder

	Unstable Angina	Myocardial Infarction	Pericarditis	Dissecting Aneurysm
Description	Narrowing of the luminal wall of a coronary artery due to atherosclerotic plaque. Sign of coronary artery disease.	Death of the oxygen-deprived cardiac muscle cells. Also called a heart attack.	Inflammation of the sac that surrounds the heart.	A longitudinal separation of the vascular wall of an artery, which causes ballooning and susceptibility to rupture.
Position	Substernal and/or precordial: Client brings clenched fist or open hand to chest. Atypical: Burning in both elbows, little fingers of both hands, toothache.	Substernal and/or precordial: Same as for angina.	Substernal: May radiate to shoulders. May point to location with one or more fingers.	Chest, back, shoulders.
Precipitating Factors	If stable angina, predictable: activity, emotion. If unstable angina, unpredictable: can happen at any time; can also be related to cold weather, emotion, and stress.	Same as for angina; may awaken from sleep with symptoms.	Any movement that causes chest movement and expansion.	Unpredictable; may occur after activity that involves severe physical exertion.
Quality	Squeezing, burning pressure like a belt being tightened around the chest; like indigestion; like an elephant standing on the chest; heaviness.	Same as for angina.	Sharp, piercing, stabbing.	Tearing, searing, ripping.
Radiation	Typical: To neck, jaw, left arm, elbow, hand, shoulder. Atypical: To back, right arm, elbow, hand, last two fingers, scrotum.	Same as for angina.	If Dressler's syndrome: radiate to back. Otherwise: may be felt in left shoulder, arm, neck, back.	Back; may also radiate to abdomen.
Relief	If unrelated to specific activity: stop precipitator; administer nitrates, possibly calcium channel blockers, beta blockers.	Morphine, nitrates. Potentially: thrombolytics, PCTA, athrectomy, etc.	Sitting upright; aspirin, Indocin.	Narcotics; surgical intervention.
Severity	Variable on the 1 to 10 scale.	Variable on the 1 to 10 scale.	Variable on the 1 to 10 scale.	Excrutiating, severe.
Timing	May or may not be predictable; see "Precipitators." Onset may be sudden or gradual.	May occur at any time; can cause client to awaken. Onset may be sudden or gradual.	If Dressler's syndrome: Occurs from 2–3 days to 10 days post MI, or may be of sudden onset if MI is not origin.	Sudden onset.
Duration	Variable, usually minutes.	Variable; hours or until thrombolytics and/or interventional therapy available; discomfort may come and go.	Persistent.	Persistent.

Health Promotion and Client Education

After the cardiovascular assessment is completed, answer any questions the client has about cardiovascular health. Use this opportunity to give clients information to promote, maintain, and optimize their cardiovascular health.

Promote the general health of the cardiovascular system in two phases:

1. Promote cardiovascular health before the development of cardiovascular disease.
2. Optimize and maintain present level of cardiovascular health when cardiovascular disease is present.

Strategies to optimize cardiovascular health center on clients knowing their unmodifiable and modifiable risk factors. Thus, you should provide information on modifying risk factors over which the client has control, as well as strategies for successfully incorporating permanent lifestyle changes. You may teach this information yourself, provide literature, or refer the client to programs that specialize in helping clients attain optimal cardiovascular health.

Promoting Cardiovascular Health by Modifying Risk Factors

Hyperlipidemia and Diet To help the client reduce or eliminate saturated fat from the diet:

- Provide information that defines saturated fat, discusses its detrimental effects, and lists foods that contain saturated fat.
- Provide information on how to determine the fat content of processed foods.
- Help the client identify the sources of hidden fat.
- Review with the client how to identify menu items that contain saturated fat.

To help the client reduce or eliminate salt and MSG from the diet:

- Provide information that describes the effect of salt and MSG and lists foods that contain one or both.
- Provide information on salt alternatives and their correct use.
- Review with the client how to identify menu items that contain salt and MSG.
- Discuss the need for including daily fiber in the client's diet.
- Provide information that defines dietary fiber, describes its beneficial effects, and lists foods high in dietary fiber. These include vegetables such as sweet corn, carrots, lentils, peanuts, salad, and broccoli and fruits such as raisins, pears, bananas, apples, peaches, and oranges. Even popcorn is good (remember to watch the butter and salt).
- Explain to the client that it is better to eat fiber in its natural, raw form. The client does not have to eat bran or cereal products to receive the daily requirement.

Make sure that clients understand that they do not need to eliminate their favorite foods from their diets forever. A client can wisely choose when to eat moderately and when to "splurge." Encourage clients to try new recipes and new spices to enhance the pleasure of eating. You can recommend recipe books, such as the *American Heart Association Cookbook*.

Inactive Lifestyle A person does not need to become a world-class athlete to achieve optimum cardiovascular health. Help the client to define a well-balanced program that includes aerobic activity of a duration and intensity that stimulate the heart without causing injury. Clients stop exercising if they experience pain or extreme fatigue after sessions. The exercise intensity should not exceed the client's ability to hold a conversation while performing the activity. Supervision in developing an individualized program helps clients avoid injury and promotes compliance. Finally, help the client to see the value of a regular exercise program.

Individuals with Body Compositions of Elevated Fat Percentage Although it seems impossible that thin clients may be "overfat," research indicates otherwise. Dietary changes and exercise are important in reducing total body fat. Here are a few guidelines for individuals attempting fat (weight) reduction (Bailey 1991, Colgan 1993, Ornish 1990):

- Be sure to have lab work to assess electrolytes, kidney function, cholesterol levels (total, LDL, HDL, triglycerides), and uric acid before you begin the exercise and diet program. A 12-lead ECG is also important. Repeat these tests throughout the program.
- Have a body composition analysis done every 2 months to assess progress.
- Be a smart shopper: look for hidden fat, salt, and processed sugar.
- Start the day with a healthy breakfast. Research suggests that people are more prone to deposit fat when they consume food toward the end of the day than at the start of the day.
- Cut out all saturated fats.
- Avoid crash or fad diets.
- Do not take any drugs advertised to suppress appetite or decrease fatigue.
- Don't lose more than ½ pound of fat per week.
- Do not judge the success of the program by your bathroom scale. Use body composition testing, reduction in

inches, tone of muscles, and increased energy and endurance as measures of success.

Smoking If clients don't smoke, encourage them not to start. If clients do smoke, encourage them to quit. Ensure that the client understands that all types of smoking are harmful to the cardiovascular system. Ensure that the use of nicotine patches for smoking cessation is supervised.

Stress Examine the causes of stress for the client. Provide information on techniques for stress reduction. Help the client explore which technique will be most beneficial and most easily incorporated into the daily routine.

Type A Behavior Explain Type A behavior, and explore whether the client demonstrates these behaviors. Determine with the client what behaviors the client feels able to modify.

Promoting Cardiovascular Health in the Healthy Client

Make information available to help healthy clients optimize cardiovascular health. Remember, it is extremely important for clients to take charge of attaining and maintaining cardiovascular wellness.

- Advise clients to inform dentists of the presence of murmurs and any cardiovascular problems.
- Inform clients of the signs of a potential heart attack. Give information about when and how to contact emergency medical services (911). Classic signs of a heart attack include

  Chest discomfort/pain

  Syncope

  Shortness of breath

  Nausea/vomiting

  Radiation of discomfort to jaw, back, left arm

  Diaphoresis

  Fatigue

  Pallor

  Flulike feeling

  Atypical signs of a heart attack include:

- Radiation of pain to right arm
- No discomfort/pain
- Discomfort/pain in elbows/fingers
- Toothache
- Persistent sore throat with no identifiable cause
- Sore jaw, as if the client had been chewing gum for days
- Mentation changes
- Pulmonary edema as a late sign when the client has had a heart attack without pain

It is important to realize and teach the client that not all of the above classic or atypical signs will be present. Every client is an individual, and each person experiences individual symptoms related to cardiovascular disease. Review with diabetics the fact that, because of neuropathy, chest discomfort may not be a presenting symptom.

Inform the client to seek medical attention if these signs of cardiovascular disorders develop:

Sudden weight gain or loss

Palpitations

Difficulty breathing with or without effort

Peripheral swelling

New chronic headache *(may indicate presence of severe hypertension)*

Ringing in the ears *(may indicate presence of severe hypertension)*

Some individuals and their family members will be interested in learning adult, child and/or infant cardiopulmonary resuscitation (CPR). Classes are available from the American Heart Association, American Red Cross, and other community programs. Individuals with heart disease should be cautioned against taking a vigorous class, but their family members should be encouraged to attend, after consulting the client's physician.

There is a popular belief, supported to some extent by research, that aspirin prevents myocardial infarction by preventing the formation of a clot. The risk/benefit analysis of this practice is still a subject of controversy. Without proper guidance, a client may take more aspirin than is currently recommended (½–1 aspirin every other day). These individuals are at greater risk of suffering from gastrointestinal side effects, bleeding of the GI tract, hemorrhagic stroke, and prolonged bleeding after an injury. As a measure to prevent myocardial infarction, aspirin should be taken only under the supervision of a physician.

Some clients will ask about herbs and spices for the treatment of cardiovascular disorders. Garlic can lower cholesterol levels, as can alfalfa (Ornish 1990). However, the most important factor in reducing cholesterol levels is reducing consumption of saturated fats and cholesterol. Clients cannot reduce cholesterol levels by placing herbs in foods rich in cholesterol.

Considerations for the Client with Cardiovascular Disease

- Review the signs of cardiovascular disease, both classic and atypical, with the client. Symptoms in the elderly are atypical, and a change in mentation may be the first sign that a cardiovascular problem exists.

DIAGNOSTIC REASONING IN ACTION

Sally Devlin arrives at the Community Urgent Care Center in obvious distress. The paramedics state that Ms Devlin is a 44-year-old Caucasian female who collapsed after playing two vigorous sets of tennis. She is complaining of chest discomfort, which she rates as 2 on a scale of 10. She is short of breath, her blood pressure is 155/100, and she is tachycardic (122). The paramedics state that she was having frequent premature ventricular contractions (PVCs), which were multifocal in origin. She received a bolus of lidocaine and was started on a lidocaine infusion, which has decreased the ectopy. She is also receiving supplemental oxygen, which has significantly reduced her shortness of breath. The paramedics state that she has no known history of heart disease. She did not hit her head as she fell.

Ms Devlin tells the admitting nurse, Rajeev Rao, that she works full time as the vice-president of marketing of a start-up computer company. She is married and states she works 10–12 hours a day, six days a week, plus works out.

Mr. Rao observes that she is perspiring; her lips are dry; her facial expression shows anxiety and fear. She reports that the chest discomfort is still present; She describes it as "tight, like someone is squeezing my heart. It seems to be pounding." She reveals that both of her parents died of a myocardial infarction, her father at age 48 and her mother at 56. Four months ago her sister was hospitalized with an MI at the age of 52. "I couldn't let the same thing happen to me. I decided to change my life. I joined a health club, started exercising every day, and went on an 800-calorie-a-day diet." Mr. Rao asks Ms Devlin whether or not she has consulted a physician about her diet or exercise regimen. "I'm young," she answers, "why do I need a doctor?"

A 12-lead ECG demonstrates the beginning of an ischemic process in the lateral leads. The laboratory work indicates a dehydrated state. Ms Devlin's potassium and magnesium levels are slightly lower than normal. Her cardiac assessment demonstrates no abnormal heart sounds. Her heartbeat is fast but regular, and no murmurs are present.

Ms Devlin demonstrates a variety of signs that Mr. Rao clusters to identify nursing diagnoses. The first cluster centers on the dehydrated state as demonstrated by the dry mucous membranes, the lab work, and the low levels of magnesium and potassium. When Ms Devlin is hydrated, these levels will probably be even lower. It is well established that low levels of magnesium and potassium contribute significantly to ventricular ectopy and may lead to repeated loss of consciousness or contribute to cardiac arrest if not replaced. The ventricular ectopy, especially if sustained, will contribute to decreased tissue perfusion as well as cardiac output. Thus, the potential for Ms Devlin to experience injury, decreased tissue perfusion, and cardiac output is present. Ms Devlin is also experiencing discomfort suggestive of a cardiac origin. Her ECG suggests the presence of myocardial ischemia. *Acute pain* is an appropriate nursing diagnosis. The significance of these findings plus her family history point to the urgent need for a complete cardiovascular workup. Ms Devlin exhibits *Anxiety* and *Fear* related to her own wellbeing. Both of these nursing diagnoses are significant for Ms Devlin because she is demonstrating behaviors that focus on her fear of sustaining a myocardial infarction.

Mr. Rao identifies the following nursing diagnoses for Ms Devlin:

1. *Knowledge deficit* related to lack of information on how to alter lifestyle to decrease the risk or slow the progression of coronary heart disease
2. *Pain* related to the potential myocardial ischemic process
3. *Fear* and *Anxiety* related to her fear of sustaining a myocardial infarction

Other appropriate nursing diagnoses include *High risk for injury, Altered cardiovascular tissue perfusion,* and *Decreased cardiac output* related to the low potassium and magesium levels.

In addition to medical intervention for her ischemic process, Ms Devlin needs information to help her to take control of her life. Supervised exercise and fitness, diet management, and analysis with modification of her type A behaviors are some of the areas in which Ms Devlin needs counseling.

- .If the client has coronary heart disease, review the use of nitroglycerin. Review what dose is usually required to relieve/reduce symptoms. Advise the client to inform the physician (preferably cardiologist) and to contact emergency medical services if symptoms are not relieved with the usual dosage.
- If the client takes digitalis, review the early signs of digitalis toxicity: nausea, vision changes such as blurring, loss of vision clarity (yellow, green, or brown halos are a later sign), loss of appetite, mentation changes. Advise the client to inform the physician if these symptoms appear. Inform the client that some medications, such as amiodarone, quinidine, verapamil, and diltiazem potentiate the effects

of digitalis. Clients taking these drugs should be aware of the danger of digitalis toxicity and watch for its signs.

- It is important to instruct clients taking diuretics to increase their intake of foods rich in potassium and to follow a potassium-replacement regimen. Low serum levels of potassium can lead to ventricular ectopy. Additionally, low potassium levels actually potentiate the effect of digitalis.
- After a diagnosis of cardiovascular disease, many clients need information on resuming sexual relations. Valuable information is available through the American Heart Association and other sources. Women who have experienced myocardial infarctions are usually very reluctant to ask for information about sexual relations. It is therefore very important for you to assess this need.
- The American Heart Association and the American Red Cross provide a wealth of information for both health care professionals and the general public.

Summary

Cardiovascular disease is one of the most extensive and devasting diseases prevalent in this country. The nurse plays a role in preventing disease, providing care during an acute episode of disease, and facilitating rehabilitation. Based upon a foundation of an understanding of normal anatomy and physiology, you can help the client to identify risk factors for developing cardiovascular disease. By examining the client's risk factors, eliciting pertinent facts from the client's history, and evaluating present lifestyle and present symptoms, you gain information that you can use to initiate physical assessment and direct client teaching. Once you have the facts about the client's cardiovascular background, you can focus on the client's cardiovascular status by reviewing the physical findings gained after observation, palpation, percussion, and auscultation. You cluster this information and identify appropriate nursing diagnoses. It is so important to encourage the client's involvement in optimizing cardiovascular wellness, whether cardiovascular disease is present or not. There is a wealth of informational resources available to help the client make lifestyle adjustments.

Key Points

- ✓ Assessing the cardiovascular system requires a sound knowledge of the anatomy and physiology of the heart, heart chambers, heart valves, coronary arteries, cardiac conduction system, and associated vascular structures.
- ✓ During the focused interview, perform a general survey of the cardiovascular system, family history, lifestyle patterns as they relate to cardiovascular wellness, health problems (cardiovascular and otherwise), and environmental factors that may have contributed to cardiovascular problems.
- ✓ Begin the physical assessment by observing the client's general appearance, orientation, and level of consciousness.
- ✓ Observe the chest and neck for unusual shape, heaves, and thrills.
- ✓ Palpate the chest in the five key landmark locations to assess the presence of heaves and thrills. Palpate the carotid arteries unilaterally. Never palpate the carotid arteries bilaterally simultaneously.
- ✓ Blunt percussion provides limited information but may be done to determine the presence of an enlarged heart when chest radiography is not available, as in the home setting.
- ✓ Auscultate in the five key landmark areas. Listen for S_1, S_2, split S_1, split S_2, S_3, S_4, clicks, snaps, rubs, and murmurs.
- ✓ Nursing diagnoses commonly associated with the cardiovascular system include *Decreased cardiac output, Ineffective denial, Fluid volume excess, Acute pain, and Altered tissue perfusion: cardiovascular.*
- ✓ Encourage clients to know their risk factors for developing cardiovascular disease. Help clients formulate strategies for modifying those factors that clients can control and for incorporating lifestyle changes to optimize cardiovascular health.
- ✓ For those clients who do not have known coronary heart disease, review the signs of a heart attack and the way to access emergency medical services. For those who do have known coronary heart disease, review how to assess signs of angina, how to comply with the pharmacologic treatment scheme, and when to access emergency medical services for persistent discomfort and other symptoms.
- ✓ There are myths regarding women's susceptibility to cardiovascular disease. Just like men, women suffer from cardiovascular conditions. The "protection factor" from female hormones does not keep all women from experiencing life-threatening cardiovascular episodes at younger ages than commonly expected. Factors that contribute significantly to early disease are smoking, high percentage of fat in body composition, significant family history, early menses, and surgical removal of ovaries at a young age. Stress, a diet of saturated fats, type A pesonality, and sedentary lifestyle, may also contribute to significant cardiovascular illness at a younger age.

Chapter 12

Assessing the Breasts and Axillae

Statistics compiled by the American Cancer Society (1992) indicate that 1 in every 9 women in the United States will develop breast cancer. In fact, breast cancer is the second most common cause of cancer deaths in women. Breast cancer incidence rates have increased about 3% a year since 1980. In part, this increased incidence may reflect increasing use of screening programs that detect tumors before they become clinically apparent. A thorough breast examination is a part of that screening process.

Begin the assessment of the breast and axillae with a thorough health history. Then, during the focused interview, gather additional information by asking pertinent questions relating to the client's general health and breast and lymph nodes in particular. The physical examination of the breasts may be incorporated into the total body assessment along with the heart and lung assessment when the client is sitting and again when supine. Note that although the majority of the material in this chapter assumes that the client is female, it is important that you incorporate assessment of the male client's breasts during the physical assessment, usually when assessing the thorax.

To carry out the assessment activities related to the breasts and axillae, you need accurate knowledge of the structure and function of the breasts and lymphatic system. You must also understand the interrelationships of the various body systems that contribute to this region, eg, the musculoskeletal supports, the nerves, the blood vessels, the overlying integument, and as mentioned, the lymphatic system that drains the region. In addition, while performing the assessment, keep in mind the normal variations for the client's developmental stage. An understanding and acceptance of different individuals' feelings, beliefs, and practices regarding the breasts and breast care are also essential. Figure 12.1 shows how these many factors influence the health of the breasts and axillae.

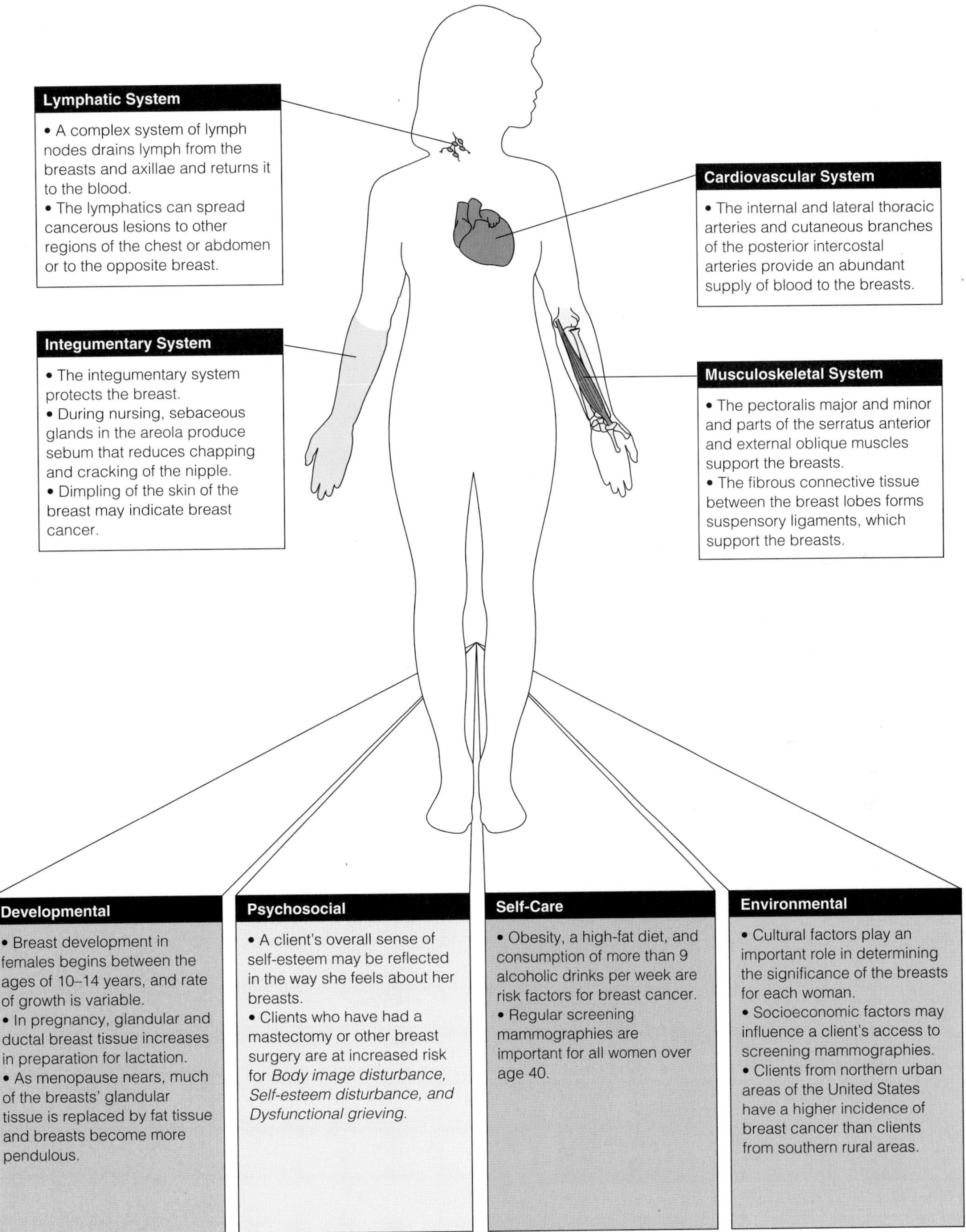

Lymphatic System
• A complex system of lymph nodes drains lymph from the breasts and axillae and returns it to the blood.
• The lymphatics can spread cancerous lesions to other regions of the chest or abdomen or to the opposite breast.
Cardiovascular System
• The internal and lateral thoracic arteries and cutaneous branches of the posterior intercostal arteries provide an abundant supply of blood to the breasts.
Integumentary System
• The integumentary system protects the breast.
• During nursing, sebaceous glands in the areola produce sebum that reduces chapping and cracking of the nipple.
• Dimpling of the skin of the breast may indicate breast cancer.
Musculoskeletal System
• The pectoralis major and minor and parts of the serratus anterior and external oblique muscles support the breasts.
• The fibrous connective tissue between the breast lobes forms suspensory ligaments, which support the breasts.
Developmental
• Breast development in females begins between the ages of 10–14 years, and rate of growth is variable.
• In pregnancy, glandular and ductal breast tissue increases in preparation for lactation.
• As menopause nears, much of the breasts' glandular tissue is replaced by fat tissue and breasts become more pendulous.
Psychosocial
• A client's overall sense of self-esteem may be reflected in the way she feels about her breasts.
• Clients who have had a mastectomy or other breast surgery are at increased risk for Body image disturbance, Self-esteem disturbance, and Dysfunctional grieving.
Self-Care
• Obesity, a high-fat diet, and consumption of more than 9 alcoholic drinks per week are risk factors for breast cancer.
• Regular screening mammographies are important for all women over age 40.
Environmental
• Cultural factors play an important role in determining the significance of the breasts for each woman.
• Socioeconomic factors may influence a client's access to screening mammographies.
• Clients from northern urban areas of the United States have a higher incidence of breast cancer than clients from southern rural areas.

Figure 12.1 Important factors to consider when assessing the breasts and axillae.

Anatomy and Physiology Review

Breasts

The **breasts** are paired mammary glands located on the anterior chest wall. Breast tissue extends from the second or third rib to the sixth or seventh rib and from the sternal margin to the midaxillary line, depending on body shape and size (Figure 12.2). The breasts lie anterior to the *pectoralis major* and *serratus anterior* muscles. The nipple is centrally located within a circular pigmented field of wrinkled skin called the **areola**. The surface of the areola is speckled with tiny sebaceous glands known as *Montgomery's glands* (or *Montgomery's tubercles*). Hair follicles are normally seen around the periphery of the areola. Commonly, breast tissue extends superiolaterally into the axilla as the *axillary tail* (or *tail of Spence*). The internal and lateral thoracic arteries and cutaneous branches of the posterior intercostal arteries provide an abundant supply of blood to the breasts.

Breasts are composed of glandular, fibrous, and adipose (fat) tissue: The *glandular tissue* is arranged into 15 to 20 **lobes** per breast that radiate from the nipple (Figure 12.3). Each lobe is composed of 20–40 *lobules* that contain the *acini cells* (or alveoli) that produce milk. These cells empty into the *lactiferous ducts,* which carry milk from each lobe to the nipple. The *fibrous tissue* provides support for the glandular tissue. *Suspensory ligaments* (also called *Cooper's ligaments*) extend from the connective tissue layer, through the breast, and attach to the fascia underlying the breast. Subcutaneous and retromammary *adipose tissue* makes up the remainder of the breast. The proportions of these three components vary with age, the general state of the client's health, the point in the female client's menstrual cycle, pregnancy, lactation, and other factors.

Supernumerary nipples or breast tissue may be present along the *mammary ridge* (or "milk line"), which extends from each axilla to the groin (Figure 12.4). Usually this tissue atrophies during development, but occasionally a nipple persists and is visible. It needs to be differentiated from a mole.

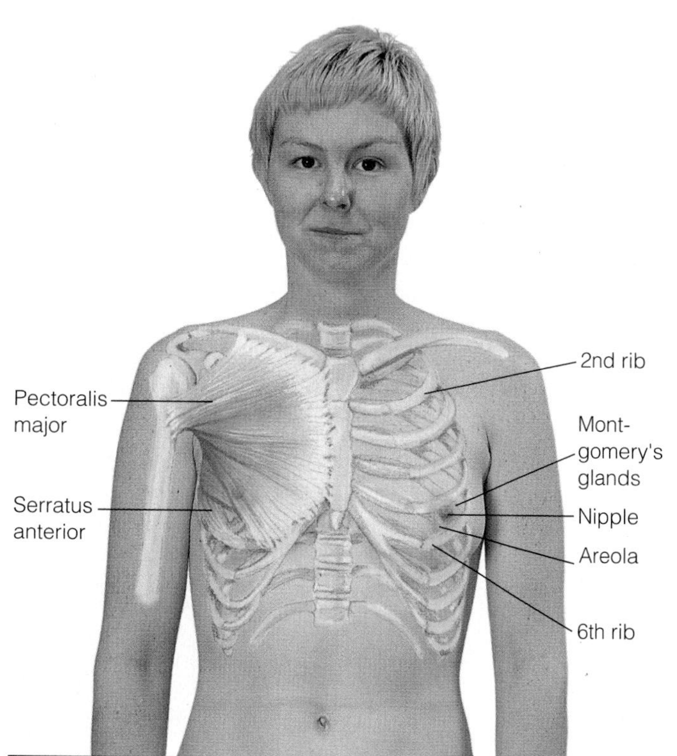

Figure 12.2 Anterior view of the breasts, showing underlying muscles and bones.

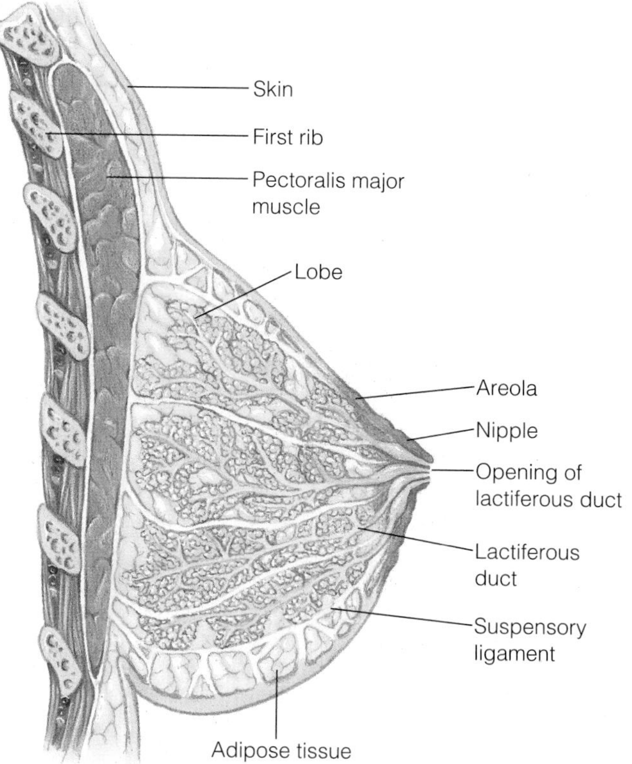

Figure 12.3 Structure of lactating mammary glands.

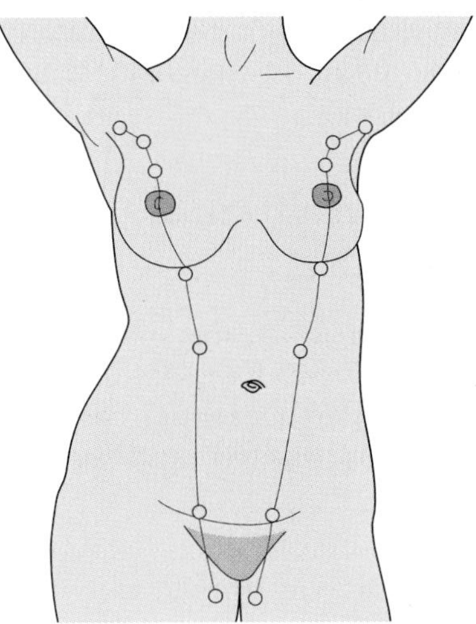

Figure 12.4 Mammary ridge.

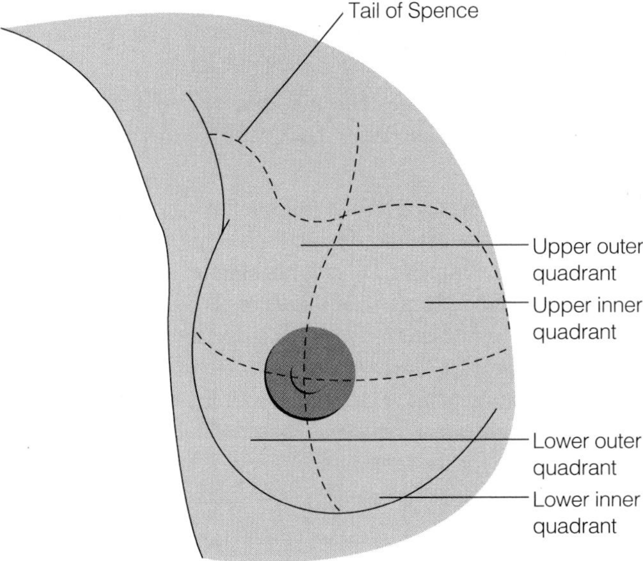

Figure 12.5 Quadrant and face-of-clock method of recording breast findings.

For the purpose of documenting assessment findings, the breast is divided into four quadrants defined by a vertical and horizontal line that intersect at the nipple (Figure 12.5). The location of clinical findings may be described also according to "clock" positions, eg, at two o'clock, 5 cm from nipple.

The male breast is composed of a small nipple and flat areola. These are superior to a thin disc of undeveloped breast tissue that may not be distinguishable from the surrounding tissues.

The major functions of the breasts are

- Providing a mechanism for producing, storing, and supplying milk
- Providing a mechanism for sexual arousal

Axillae and Lymph Nodes

A complex system of **lymph nodes** drains lymph from the breast and axillae and returns it to the blood. Superficial lymph nodes drain the skin, and deep lymph nodes drain the mammary lobules. Figure 12.6 shows the groups of nodes that drain the breasts and axillae. These are the nodes that you palpate during the assessment. They include

1. Internal mammary nodes
2. Supraclavicular nodes
3. Subclavicular nodes
4. Interpectoral nodes
5. Central axillary nodes
6. Brachial (lateral axillary) nodes
7. Subscapular (posterior axillary) nodes
8. Pectoral (anterior axillary) nodes

The internal mammary nodes drain toward the abdomen and the opposite breast. Most of the lymph from the rest of the breast drains toward the axillae and subclavian region. Thus, a cancerous lesion can spread via the lymphatic system to the subclavian nodes, into deep channels within the chest or

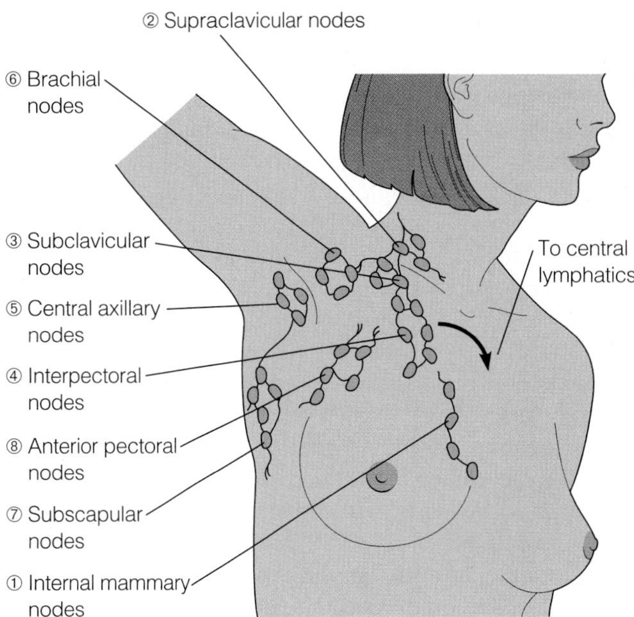

Figure 12.6 Lymphatic drainage of the breast.

abdomen, and even to the opposite breast. The male breast has the same potential and needs to be examined as well.

The major functions of the lymphatic system are

- Returning water and proteins from the interstitial spaces to the blood, thus helping to maintain blood osmotic pressure and body fluid balance
- Filtering out microorganisms and other body debris

Muscles of the Chest Wall

The major muscles of the chest wall, which support the breast and give it its shape, are the **pectoralis major** and **serratus anterior** muscles (see Figure 12.2). The overall contour of the breasts is determined by the **suspensory ligaments** (see Figure 12.3), which provide support.

The major function of the muscles of the chest wall is

- Supporting breast and lymphatic tissue

Gathering the Data

Focused Interview

During the focused interview, the nurse gathers information not only about the health of the breasts, but also about how the client perceives her breasts and how this perception affects her body image. A complex interaction of cultural and psychosocial factors determines the significance of the breasts for each woman. For instance, North American culture, especially through its advertising, puts a disproportionate value on the "perfect" female figure. Because people develop their body images in part via external feedback, the disproportionate glorification of the breasts may have profound effects on a woman's body image. Some women are willing to undergo potentially disfiguring surgeries to improve the appearance of their breasts. Some women even choose loss of life over the loss of a breast by delaying or refusing to seek medical care for a breast lump (Olds et al 1992). Be sensitive to these issues when asking questions regarding perceived variations from normal, the effect on the client's relationships, and the client's self-care practices.

As mentioned earlier, although most of the information in this chapter assumes a female client, assessment of the male breasts and axillae is also important.

General Survey of the Breasts and Axillae

1. Describe your breasts today. How do they differ, if at all, from 3 months ago? Three years ago? *This question gives the client the opportunity to share her perception of her breasts and any changes she has experienced that may be related to breast health.*
2. Are you still menstruating? If so, have you noticed any changes in your breasts that seem to be related to your normal menstrual cycle, such as tenderness, swelling, pain, or enlarged nodes? Please describe them. *These changes may occur with changing hormone levels, or they may be related to the use of oral contraceptives. "Lumpy breasts" occurring monthly prior to the onset of menses and resolving at the end of menstruation may be due to a benign condition called fibrocystic breast disease.*
3. What was the date of your last menstrual period? *This information, if applicable, helps correlate current status of breasts to cycle.*
4. Have you noticed any changes in breast characteristics, such as size, symmetry, shape, thickening, lumps, swelling, temperature, color of skin or vessels, or sensations such as tingling or tenderness? If so, how long have you had them? Please describe them. *Pain and tenderness can be caused by fibrocystic breast disease, cancer, or other disorders. A lump may indicate a benign cyst, a fibroadenoma, or a malignant tumor. Skin irritation may be due to friction from a bra or to pendulous breasts. In older clients, decreased estrogen levels may cause the breasts to sag.*
5. Have you noticed any changes in nipple and areola characteristics, such as size, shape, open sores, lumps, pain, tenderness, discharge, skin changes, or retractions? If so, how long have you had them? Please describe them. *Nipple discharge resulting from medication is usually clear. A bloody drainage is always a concern and needs to be further evaluated, especially in the presence of a lump. Eczematous changes of the skin of the nipples and areola may indicate Paget's disease, a rare form of breast cancer. Dimpling of skin or retraction of the nipple also suggests cancer.*
6. Have you ever experienced any trauma to your breasts? *Contact sports, automobile accidents, and physical abuse can cause bruising of the breast and tissue changes.*
7. Do you exercise? If so, describe your routine. What kind of bra do you wear when you exercise? *Firm sup-*

port is recommended during exercise to prevent loss of tissue elasticity.

8. What medications are you presently taking? *Oral contraceptives and other hormones may affect breast tissue and are associated with an increased risk of cancer. Women taking these drugs need to be monitored.*
9. How do you feel about your breasts? *Answers to this question may reveal a body image disturbance, self-esteem disturbance, dysfunctional grieving (in a woman who has had a mastectomy), or ineffective breast-feeding (in a lactating woman).*

History

1. Have you ever had any breast disease such as cancer, fibrocystic breast disease, or fibroadenoma? *A history of breast cancer poses the risk of recurrence. Both fibroadenoma and the general lumpiness of fibrocystic breast disease need to be differentiated from cancer.*
2. Have you ever had breast surgery? If so, what type and when? How do you feel about it? How has it affected you? Has it affected your sex life? If so, how? *Previous breast surgery has implications for how you teach the client to perform a breast self-exam. Answers may also indicate a need for psychologic counseling. Much is still unknown about the psychologic effects of mastectomy, breast reconstruction, breast reduction, and breast augmentation.*
3. How old were you when you started to menstruate? *Clients with a history of menarche before age 12 are at greater risk for breast cancer.*
4. Do you have children? How old were you when they were born? *Women who have never had children or who had their first child after the age of 30 are at greater risk for breast cancer.*
5. Have you gone through menopause? If so, at what age? Were there any residual problems? *Women who undergo menopause after the age of 55 are at greater risk for breast cancer. Postmenopausal weight gain may increase risk of breast cancer. After menopause, decreased estrogen levels may result in decreased firmness of breast tissue. Reassure the client that this is normal.*
6. Have you ever had a mammogram? If so, when was your most recent one? *Mammography can detect a cancer as much as 2 years before it is detectable by palpation. The American Cancer Society's (1992) recommendations for women ages 20–40 are: a manual examination by a physician every 3 years, a self-exam every month,and a baseline mammogram between the ages of 35 and 39. For women ages 40 and over: a professional exam every year, a self-exam every month, and a mammogram every 1 or 2 years for those 40–49 and every year for those 50 and over.*
7. Have you had cancer in any other region of your body such as the endometrium, ovaries, or colon? *A history of these cancers increases the risk for breast cancer.*
8. Have you been treated with hormone therapy during or since menopause? *Estrogen replacement therapy places client at increased risk for breast cancer.*
9. Do you see your doctor regularly for a physical exam? *Clients from lower socioeconomic brackets may have reduced access to health care.*
10. Have you been exposed to any environmental carcinogens such as benzene or asbestos, or to excessive radiation such as frequent repeated X-rays? *Such exposure increases risk of breast cancer.*

Family History

1. Has your mother or sister had breast cancer? *If so, the client is at greater risk, especially if the relative's cancer occurred before menopause.*
2. Has one of your grandmothers or an aunt had breast cancer? *If so, the client is at slightly greater risk.*

Practice of Breast Self-Examination

- Do you perform breast self-exam? If so, how often? At what time of your menstrual cycle do you perform this exam? *The answer indicates the client's knowledge level and the importance placed on it. You may use this opportunity to share information about the importance of breast self-exam, but waiting until after the physical examination is completed for actual demonstration and teaching may allow for better learning. When your examination is completed, you can proceed to assess the client's technique and enhance teaching.* *(See information on teaching breast self-examination on page 335.)*

Additional Questions with Preadolescent Clients

1. Have you noticed any changes in the size or shape of your breasts? If so, tell me about these changes. *Growth of the breasts is not necessarily steady or symmetric. This may be frustrating or embarrassing to some girls. Reassure the client that her breast development is normal.*
2. How do you feel about your breasts and the way they are changing? *Breast development provides visual confirmation that the adolescent is becoming a woman. For the developing adolescent, her breasts are a visible symbol of her feminine identity and an important part of her body image and self-esteem (Olds et al 1992). Reassure girls that the rate of growth of breast tissue depends on changing hor-*

mone levels and is uniquely individual, as are the eventual size and shape of the breasts.

Additional Questions with Childbearing Clients

- What changes in your breasts have you noticed since your last exam? *The breasts continue to change throughout pregnancy. Some expected changes are increased size, sense of fullness or tingling, prominent veins, darkened areolae, and a more erect nipple. A thick, yellowish discharge called colostrum may be expressed from the breasts in the final weeks of pregnancy. Reassure the client that all of these signs are normal.*

Additional Questions with Older Clients

Most of the preceding questions apply to the menopausal and postmenopausal client.

Physical Assessment

Preparation

- ☑ **Gather the equipment.**
  small pillow or folded towel
  gown
  gloves (in case of drainage)
  ruler marked in centimeters
- ☑ **Wash hands with warm water. Make sure your hands are warm.**
- ☑ **Explain the examination procedure to the client to allay any fears or apprehensions.**
- ☑ **Make sure that the room is warm and that the client is given privacy.**
- ☑ **Observe universal precautions.**

Remember

Many women are embarrassed to have their breasts examined. Use a friendly yet matter-of-fact approach.

ASSESSMENT TECHNIQUE/NORMAL FINDINGS

SPECIAL CONSIDERATIONS

Inspection

Step 1 ***Have the client assume a sitting position.***

- Instruct the client to sit comfortably and erect with arms at the side; gown should be around the waist so that both breasts are exposed (Figure 12.7).

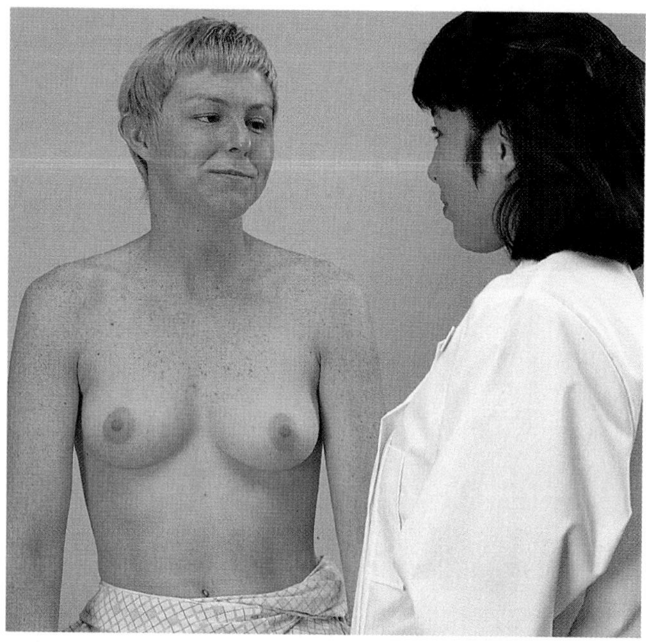

Figure 12.7 The client is seated at the beginning of the exam.

Step 2 ***Inspect and compare size and symmetry bilaterally.***

It is normal for one breast to be slightly larger than the other.

Obvious masses, flattening of the breast in one area, dimpling of the skin, or recent increase in the size of one breast may indicate abnormal growth or inflammation.

Step 3 ***Inspect for skin color.***

- Look for thickening, tautness, redness, rash, or ulceration.

Inflamed skin is red and feels warm. Edema caused by blocked lymphatic drainage in advanced cancer causes an "orange-peel" appearance called *peau d'orange* (Figure 12.8).

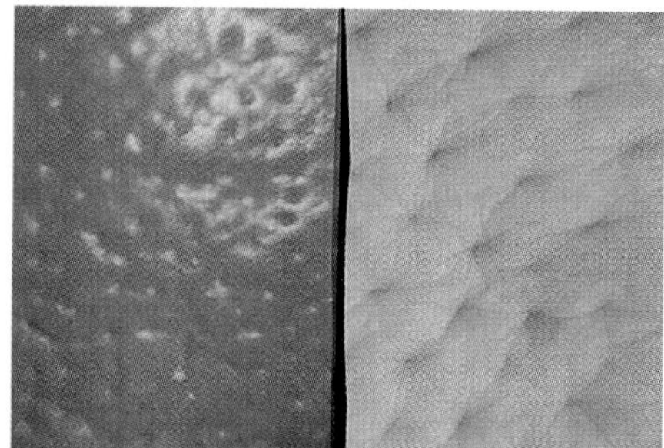

Figure 12.8 Left, Orange peel; Right, Peau d'orange sign.

ASSESSMENT TECHNIQUE/NORMAL FINDINGS	SPECIAL CONSIDERATIONS

Step 4 ***Inspect for venous patterns.***

Normally, venous patterns are much the same bilaterally. They may be more visible in the pregnant or obese client.

Pronounced venous patterns that are unilateral may indicate increased blood flow to a malignancy.

Step 5 ***Inspect for moles and other markings.***

If moles are unchanged, nontender, and of long standing, they are of no concern. Striations may be purple in pregnant clients and clients who have recently lost or gained weight. These fade and turn silver-white over time.

Moles that have appeared recently or changed suddenly must be evaluated further.

Step 6 ***Inspect the areolae for size, shape, and surface characteristics.***

The areolae should be round or oval and nearly equal in size. They are pink in light-skinned people and brown in dark-skinned people. Pregnancy usually darkens the areolae and Montgomery's tubercles are present.

Peau d'orange associated with cancer may be seen first on the areolae. Redness and/or fissures may develop as a result of breast-feeding.

Step 7 ***Inspect the nipples for size, shape, color, direction, surface characteristics, and discharge.***

ALERT!

If any drainage is observed, use universal precautions and wear gloves.

Nipples should be almost equal in size and shape and of the same color as the areolae. They are generally everted but may be flat or inverted. The nipples should point in the same direction: outward and slightly upward. They should be free of cracks, crust, erosions, ulcerations, pigment changes, or discharge.

Recent retraction or inversion of a nipple is suggestive of malignancy, as is a recent change in the direction of a nipple. Bloody discharge from a nipple always warrants further investigation, especially when accompanied by a mass. Any discharge should be saved for cytological examination. A red, scaly, eczemalike area over the nipple could indicate *Paget's disease of the nipple,* a rare type of breast cancer, especially if the nipple changes persist beyond a few weeks. The area may exude fluid, scale, or crust (Figure 12.9).

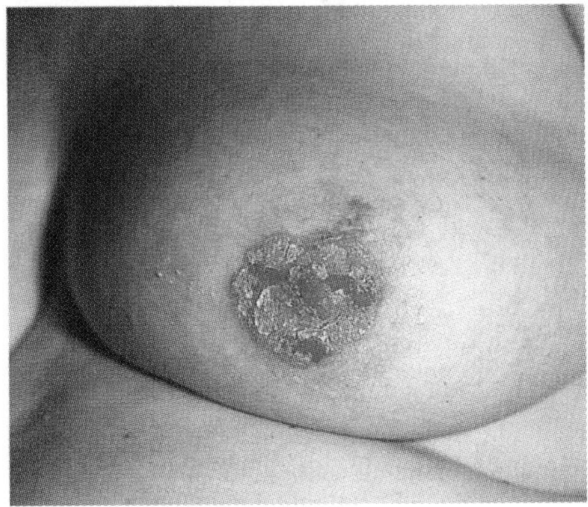

Figure 12.9 Paget's disease of the nipple.

Step 8 ***Observe the breasts for size, shape, symmetry, surface characteristics, and bilateral pull on suspensory ligaments.***

Ask the client to assume the following positions while you continue to inspect the breasts:

Dimpling of the skin over a mass is usually a visible sign of breast cancer. Dimpling is accentuated in this position. Variations in contour and symmetry may also indicate breast cancer.

ASSESSMENT TECHNIQUE/NORMAL FINDINGS

SPECIAL CONSIDERATIONS

- Inspect the breasts with the client's arms extended above the head (Figure 12.10).

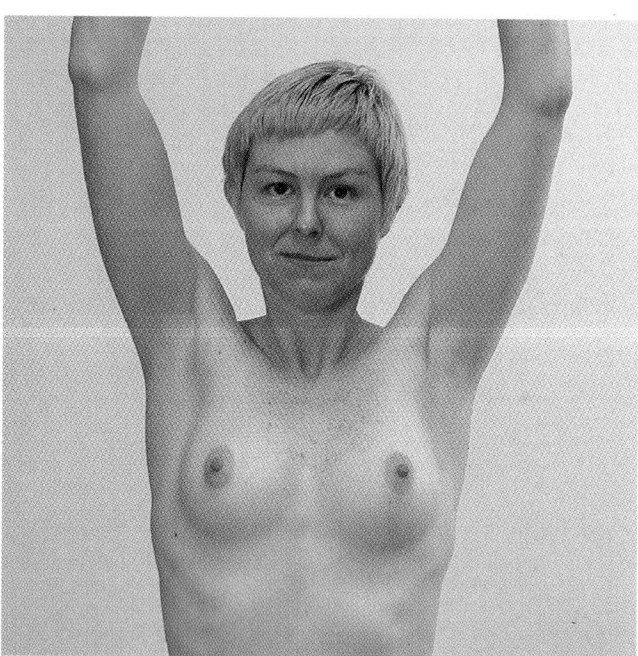

Figure 12.10 Inspection of the breasts with the client's arms above her head.

- Inspect the breasts with the client's hands pressed against her hips (Figure 12.11).

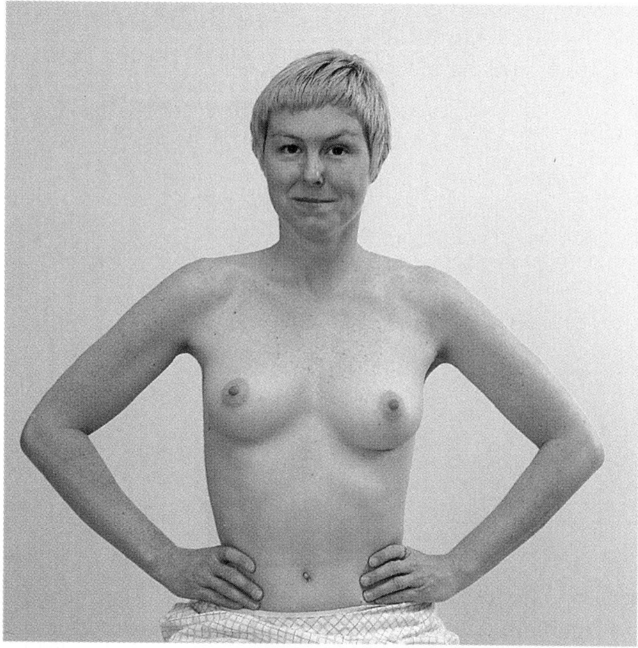

Figure 12.11 Inspection of the breasts with the client's hands pressed against her waist.

ASSESSMENT TECHNIQUE/NORMAL FINDINGS | SPECIAL CONSIDERATIONS

- Inspect the breasts with the client pushing hands together at the level of her waist (Figure 12.12).
- Inspect the breasts with the client leaning forward from the waist (Figure 12.13).

This position allows you to assess whether the breasts fall freely and evenly from the chest.

Suspect breast cancer if the breasts do not fall freely and evenly.

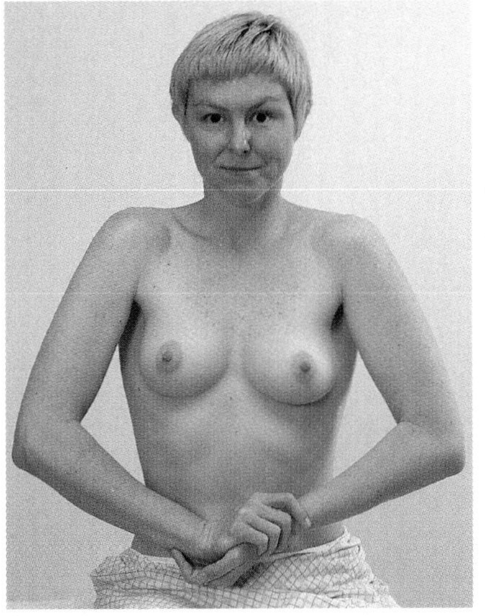

Figure 12.12 Inspection of the breasts with the client's hands pressed together at the level of her waist.

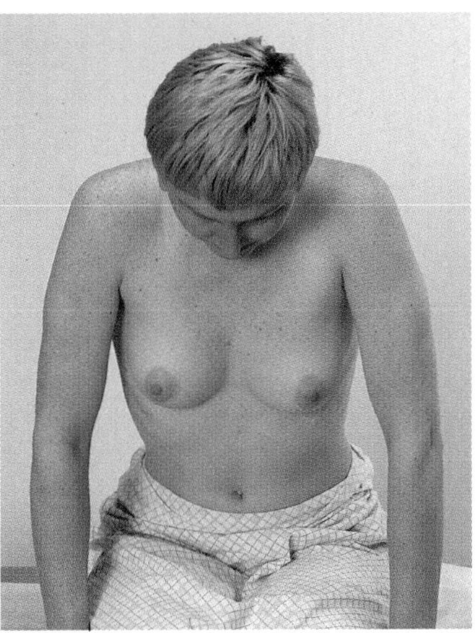

Figure 12.13 Inspection of the breasts with the client leaning forward from the waist.

Palpation

Step 1 *Position the client.*

- Ask client to lie supine.
- Cover the breast that is not being palpated to ensure the woman's comfort.
- Place a small pillow or folded towel under the side to be palpated and position the client's arm over her head. This flattens the breast tissue more evenly over the chest wall.

Step 2 *Palpate skin texture of the breast.*

Skin texture shoud be smooth and the contour uninterrupted.

Thickening of the skin suggests an underlying carcinoma.

Step 3 *Palpate the breast.*

- Use the pads of your first three fingers and a slightly rotary motion to press the breast tissue against the chest wall. Note your starting point and end at the same point so that no area is missed.

The incidence of breast cancers is highest (48%) in the upper outer quadrant, including the axillary tail. Masses in the axillary tail must be distinguished from enlarged axillary lymph nodes.

ASSESSMENT TECHNIQUE/NORMAL FINDINGS

SPECIAL CONSIDERATIONS

There are at least half a dozen different patterns used in palpating breast tissue, but the most common is the *concentric-circle pattern* (Figure 12.14).

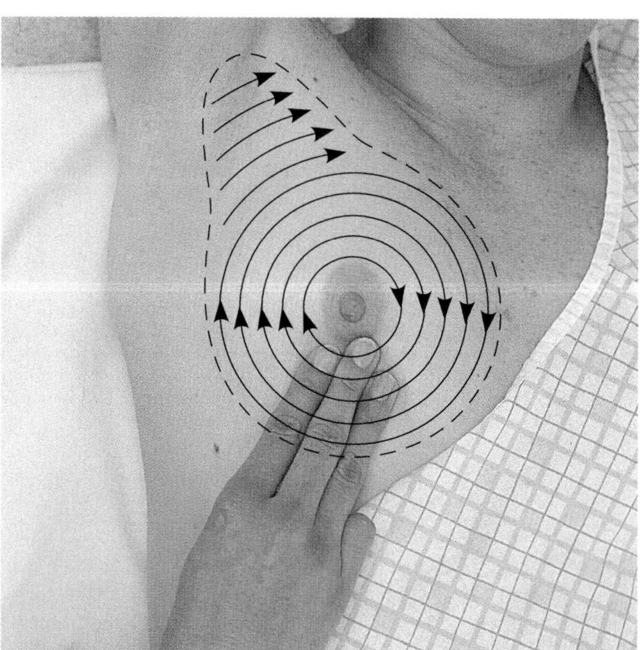

Figure 12.14 Palpating the breast.

- Starting at the periphery of the breast, palpate in large circles, proceeding to smaller circles until you reach the center of the breast at the nipple. Try not to lift your fingers off the breast as you move from one area to another to ensure that you palpate every part of the breast, including the axillary tail.
- If the client's breasts are pendulous, palpate with one hand under the breast to support it and the other hand pushing against the breast tissue in a downward motion (Figure 12.15).

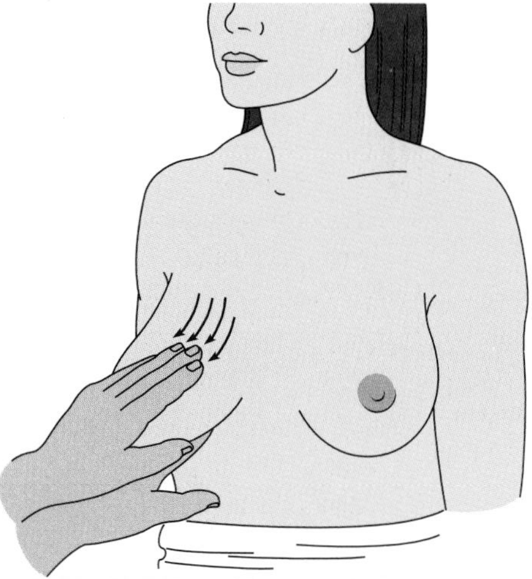

Figure 12.15 Palpating a pendulous breast.

ASSESSMENT TECHNIQUE/NORMAL FINDINGS

SPECIAL CONSIDERATIONS

- Regardless of which method you use, palpate lightly at first, and then a little deeper, using a firm yet gentle touch.

Breast tissue feels slightly granular, and there is a firm transverse ridge along the lower edge of the breast.

Expect variations such as the lobular feel of glandular tissue or the fine granular feel of breast tissue of older women. Be aware of where the client is in her menstrual cycle so that changes such as tenderness can be properly interpreted.

> ***Referral***
>
> **Any hard, irregular, poorly circumscribed nodule fixed to the skin or to underlying tissues suggests cancer and must be investigated further.**

Step 4 ***Palpate the nipple and areola.***

- Compress the tissue between your thumb and forefinger (Figure 12.16). Observe for discharge.

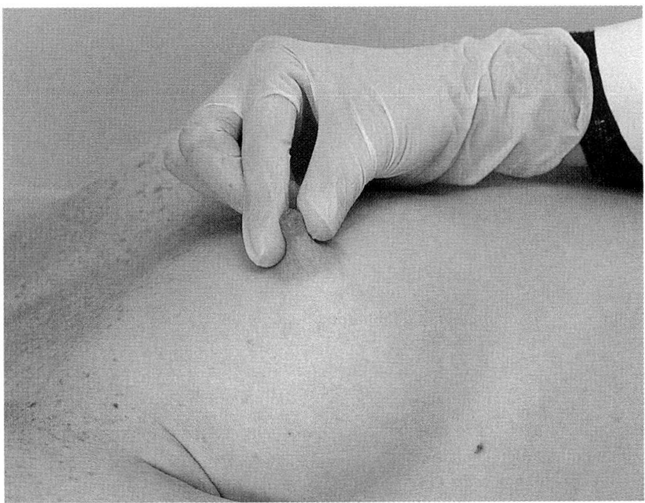

Figure 12.16 Palpating the nipple.

- Confirm that the nipple is free of discharge and is not tender, and that the areola is free of masses.
- Repeat steps 1 through 4 on the other breast.

Lactation not associated with childbearing is called *galactorrhea.* It is most commonly caused by endocrine disorders or medications, including tricyclic antidepressants, antihypertensive drugs, and estrogen. Unilateral discharge from one nipple or duct suggests a local lesion such as may occur with *fibrocystic breast disease,* an *intraductal papilloma* (see page 333), or possibly cancer.

Step 5 ***Inspect and palpate each axilla.***

- Ask the client to assume a sitting position. Help her to flex her arm at the elbow and support it on your arm. Explain to her that you are doing this to promote relaxation of her muscles.
- Note the presence of axillary hair.
- Confirm that the axilla is free of redness, lumps, or rashes.
- With the palmar surface of your fingers, reach deep into the axilla (Figure 12.17 on page 326). Gently palpate the tissue against the chest wall and underlying muscles of axilla. Be sure to palpate the anterior border of the axilla, the central or medial aspect along the rib cage, the posterior border, and along the inner aspect of the upper arm.

Infections of the breast, arm, and hand cause the axillary lymph nodes to enlarge and become tender, as do some disease processes. Hard, fixed nodes may suggest metastatic cancer or lymphoma.

Note that clients who have had a *wide local excision* (removal of the tumor and a narrow margin of normal tissue) and/or *mastectomy* (removal of the tumor and an extensive amount of surrounding tissue) need to be examined carefully as well. Palpate the remaining tissue on the chest wall using the same technique as for clients without previous surgery. Do not assume that remaining tissue is free of disease

ASSESSMENT TECHNIQUE/NORMAL FINDINGS | SPECIAL CONSIDERATIONS

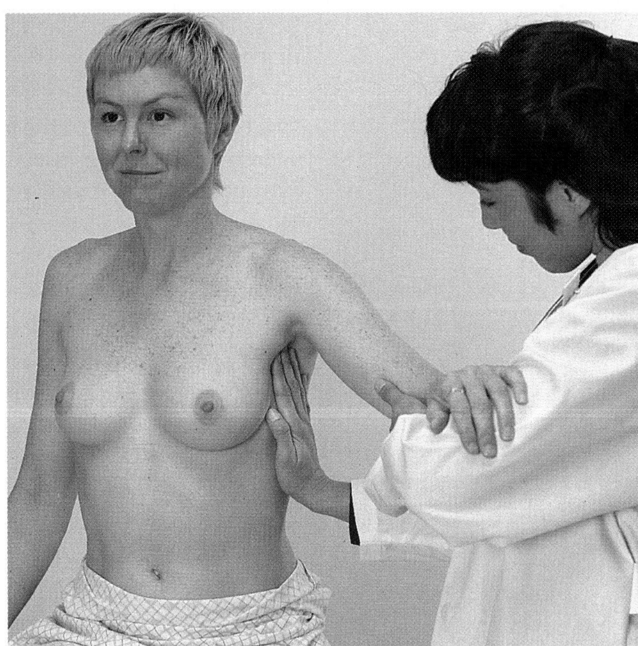

Figure 12.17 Palpating the axilla. Note that the nurse is supporting the woman's arm with her own nondominant arm.

because a lump or breast has been removed. The box below describes surgical treatments for breast cancer.

Surgical Treatments for Breast Cancer

Radical mastectomy: Removal of the entire breast, pectoralis major and minor muscles, axillary lymph nodes, and surrounding adipose tissue.

Modified radical mastectomy: As for radical mastectomy, but the pectoralis major muscle is preserved.

Total (or simple) mastectomy: Removal of the breast.

Subcutaneous mastectomy: Removal of the internal breast tissue. The skin of the breast remains, and an implant is inserted.

Partial mastectomy: Removal of the tumor and 2 to 3 cm of surrounding tissue and, commonly, at least a portion of the axillary nodes.

Wide local excision (tylectomy or lumpectomy): Removal of the tumor and a narrow margin of normal tissue surrounding the mass.

Adapted from Olds S, London M, Ladewig P, *Maternal-Newborn Nursing*, 4th ed. Redwood City, CA: Addison-Wesley Nursing 1992.

Examination of the Male Breast

Examination of the male breast is simpler but still essential.

Even though breast cancer in the male is rare, it does occur, and incidence increases after age 65.

Step 1 *Inspect the breasts.*

Inspection can take place during the anterior chest examination. Confirm that the breasts are flat and free of lumps and rashes.

Step 2 *Palpate the breasts.*

- Place the client in supine position.
- The male breast feels like a thin disc of tissue under a flat nipple and areola.

Gynecomastia (breast enlargement in males) is a temporary condition seen in some adolescents. It also occurs as the result of some hormonal medications and diseases. Breast cancer in the male is identified as a hard, irregular nodule often fixed to the nipple

ASSESSMENT TECHNIQUE/NORMAL FINDINGS	SPECIAL CONSIDERATIONS
◆ Compress the nipple between your fingers to check for discharge. ◆ Palpate the axilla for nodes in the same manner as in the female.	and underlying tissue. Nipple discharge may also be present. Swelling of the axillary lymph nodes suggests infection.

Reminders

- When the examination is complete, assess the client's knowledge of breast self-examination. Have the client tell you when she performs the exam, how often, and what she looks and palpates for. Then have her demonstrate her technique to you. Often the client will ask questions or otherwise demonstrate uncertainty at this point. Give positive feedback as you teach. It is also a good idea to provide pamphlets or handouts for the client to refer to at home. (For a full description of breast self-examination, see page 335.)
- In addition to the preceding steps, consider the common variations in physical assessment findings for the different client groups discussed below.
- Confirm that the client is comfortable and has no adverse effects from the procedure, then dim the lights and leave the client to rest or to get dressed.
- Document the assessment findings. If a mass is detected, document all of the following information:

  Location. Describe the location of each lump found, using quadrants or face-of-clock method. Drawing a picture may be helpful. State distance from nipple.

  Size. State in centimeters.

  Shape. Describe as round, oval, regular, or irregular.

  Consistency. State if soft, firm, or hard.

  Tenderness. Describe the degree.

  Mobility. Does the lump move, or is it fixed to skin or underlying tissue?

  Borders. Are the borders discrete or poorly defined?

  Presence or absence of dimpling or retraction.

  Are any adjacent lymph nodes palpable?

Developmental Considerations

Infant, Children, and Adolescent Clients

The breast tissue of newborns is sometimes swollen because of the hyperestrogenism of pregnancy. Some infants may produce a thin discharge called "witch's milk." This secretion subsides as the infant's body eliminates maternal hormones.

Breast tissue starts to enlarge in females with the onset of adolescence, usually between the ages of 10 and 14. At first there is only a bud around the nipple and areola, which may be tender initially. The ductile system matures, extensive fat deposits occur, and the areola and nipples grow and become pigmented. These changes are correlated with an increased level of estrogen and progesterone in the body as sexual maturity progresses.

Growth of the breasts is not necessarily steady or symmetrical. This may be frustrating or embarrassing to some girls. Because a female's primary sexual organs cannot be observed, breast development provides visual confirmation that the adolescent is becoming a woman. For the developing adolescent, her breasts are a visible symbol of her feminine identity and an important part of her body image and self-esteem (Olds et al 1992). Reassure girls that the rate of growth of breast tissue is dependent upon changing hormone levels and is uniquely individual, as are the eventual size and shape of the breasts. See Chapter 19 for a discussion of the stages of growth and development of the breasts in adolescent girls.

Benign fibroadenomas (see page 332) in adolescent girls are not uncommon. Reassure the girl and her parents or caregivers that no correlation has been established between fibroadenomas and malignant cancers. Although the American Cancer Society recommends that women begin breast self-examination at age 20, teaching the adolescent girl how to examine her breasts can help her to establish an important self-care practice that will last for her lifetime.

Adolescent boys may experience temporary breast enlargement, called gynecomastia, in one or both breasts. It is usually self-limiting and resolves spontaneously. Another concern to adolescent males are transient masses beneath one areola or both. These "breast buds" usually disappear within a year of onset.

For a comprehensive health assessment of infants, children, and adolescents, see Chapter 19.

Childbearing Clients

During pregnancy, breast tissue enlarges as glandular and ductal tissue increases in preparation for lactation. During the second month of pregnancy, nipples and areolae darken in color and enlarge. The degree of pigmentation varies with complexion. Nipples may leak colostrum in the month prior to childbirth. As breast tissue enlarges, venous networks may be more pronounced.

Breast self-examination needs to be done during pregnancy as well as at other times. The procedure is the same, even though the breast tissue will be firmer, larger, and possibly more tender. The lobules are more distinct. The areolae and nipples are usually darker. Cancer of the breast during pregnancy needs to be identified as soon as possible and is treated on an individual basis.

For a comprehensive health assessment of childbearing clients, see Chapter 20.

Older Clients

Devote a little more time to the focused interview of an older client. Many people have a difficult time talking about something as private as the breasts, and older adults may be even less comfortable with this discussion. They may be modest and self-conscious, or they may feel that you are too young to understand. There may also be cultural taboos about such private matters. Acknowledge that talking about their breasts may be somewhat uncomfortable for them, but tell them that sharing this information will promote their health.

Older adults may have limitated range of motion. If so, ask the client to raise her arms to a height that does not cause discomfort. Because the older adult may have failing eyesight, you may want to provide large mirrors, additional lighting, and a magnifying glass for close inspection when teaching breast self-examination. You may also provide pamphlets and handouts with large print.

As menopause approaches, there is a decrease in glandular tissue, which is replaced by fatty tissue. The lobular feel of glandular tissue is replaced by a finer, granular feeling. Breasts are less firm and tend to be more pendulous: as the suspensory ligaments relax, breast tissue hangs more loosely from the chest wall. The nipples become smaller and flatter and lose some erectile ability. The inframammary ridge thickens and can be palpated more easily.

Gynecomastia may occur in older adult males as a result of hormonal changes due to disease or medication. Be sensitive to possible embarrassment during the exam.

Breast cancer becomes increasingly more common as the population ages; therefore, breast self-examination is extremely important. The older client needs reinforcement that even though she no longer menstruates, she still needs to examine her breasts at the same time each month.

For a comprehensive health assessment of older clients, see Chapter 21.

Psychosocial Considerations

A client's overall sense of self-esteem may be reflected in the way she feels about her breasts. In fact, some women may view their breasts as a badge of their femininity. Media portrayal of idealized images of "perfect" breasts, especially by advertisers, may further this feeling (Olds et al 1992). Thus, clients whose breasts are smaller or larger than average, clients with asymmetric breasts, and clients who have had a mastectomy or other breast surgery or trauma are at an increased risk for body image disturbance, self-esteem disturbance, and dysfunctional grieving.

You should be aware that many women do not perform breast self-examination even after receiving instruction in the procedure. In addition, many women do not seek medical attention after discovering a breast lump. These behaviors may be related to anxiety and fear, eg, fear of cancer or surgery, a body image change, or a change in significant relationships. Other factors may include denial, feelings of powerlessness, or a lack of knowledge about breast disorders. During the assessment of the breasts and axillae, you need to encourage the client to share her fears and concerns.

Self-Care Considerations

As breasts develop, a supportive garment minimizes pull on suspensory ligaments, especially during strenuous exercise. Pregnant and lactating women, in particular, should wear supportive garments.

Some women experience tenderness and feelings of fullness premenstrually. Applying ice packs to tender areas of the breast may help. Limiting salt intake is also a useful self-care measure.

Monthly breast self-examination (BSE) is the best method for detecting breast masses early. A woman who knows the texture and feel of her own breasts is far more likely to detect any changes. Include teaching of routine BSE during the nursing assessment, and ask the client to perform the technique for you to observe. (The technique for BSE is described later in this chapter.) In addition, regular screening mammograms are important for all women from age 40 on.

Research indicates that a high-fat diet may increase a woman's risk of developing breast cancer. Alcohol intake in excess of nine drinks a week has also been implicated.

Family, Culture, and Environmental Considerations

You need to be aware of variations in breast development related to ethnicity. For example, girls of African ancestry may develop secondary sexual characteristics earlier than girls of European ancestry. The time of appearance, texture, and distribution of axillary and pubic hair also varies according to race. Feelings of embarrassment may differ among clients of different cultural or religious groups.

Breast cancer rates vary across different cultural groups, but this variation may be due partly to differences in diet or alcohol consumption.

Socioeconomic factors may influence a client's access to screening mammography and regular physical examinations.

Clients from urban northern areas of the United States have a higher incidence of breast cancer than clients from rural southern areas.

Organizing the Data

After carrying out the focused interview and conducting the physical assessment of the breasts and axillae, group the related data into clusters leading either to nursing diagnoses that require interventions such as client teaching or to the identification of alterations in health that require you to work with other members of the health care team.

Identifying Nursing Diagnoses

NANDA lists several nursing diagnoses that can be used with clients experiencing physical and/or psychologic concerns related to the health and/or appearance of the breasts. Making a complete diagnostic statement guides the care plan.

Because cancer of the breast is the most common cancer in American women, and because of the importance many cultures place on the female breast, *Body image disturbance* is frequently an appropriate diagnosis, especially for women who have had a mastectomy. Body image disturbance is defined as "viewing oneself differently as a result of actual or perceived changes in body structure or function" (NANDA). Treatment of breast cancer frequently alters both. (See Table 12.1 on page 330.)

Dysfunctional grieving is another nursing diagnosis that may be appropriate. It is defined as "a state in which an individual reacts to an actual, anticipated, or perceived loss of a significant person, ideal, status, object, or body part with an absent, delayed, exaggerated, or prolonged response" (NANDA). Clients who cannot adjust to changes brought on by the disease process may experience dysfunctional grieving (Table 12.1).

Some of the other nursing diagnoses that may be appropriate following assessment of the breasts and axillae include: ineffective breast-feeding, ineffective individual coping, knowledge deficit related to lack of information about breast self-examination, anxiety related to the diagnosis of cancer, and pain related to metastasis.

Table 12.1 Nursing Diagnoses Commonly Associated with the Breasts and Axillae

BODY IMAGE DISTURBANCE

Definition: Viewing oneself differently as a result of actual or perceived changes in body structure or function.

DEFINING CHARACTERISTICS

A verbal response to actual or perceived change in structure or function must be present to justify the diagnosis. This response may include:

Expressing negative feelings about the body

Expressing feelings of helplessness, hopelessness, or powerlessness

Reporting changes in lifestyle

Refusing to accept change

Preoccupation with change or loss

Verbalizing fear of rejection by or reaction of others

Focusing on past strengths, function, or appearance

Extension of body boundary to incorporate environmental objects

Personalization of body part or loss by name

Emphasis on remaining strengths and heightened achievement

Depersonalization of part or loss by impersonal pronouns

In addition, a nonverbal response to actual or perceived change in structure or function must be present. This may include:

Not touching body part

Showing reluctance to touch or look at affected body part

Actual change in structure or function

Missing body part

Hiding or overexposing body part (intentional or unintentional)

Change in ability to estimate spatial relationship of body to environment

Trauma to nonfunctioning part

Change in social involvement

Not looking at body part

RELATED FACTORS

Cultural or spiritual beliefs, Eating disorders, Surgery, Pregnancy, Situational crisis, Psychologic impairment, Chronic illness, Chronic pain, Treatment side effects, Congenital defects, Others specific to client (specify).

DYSFUNCTIONAL GRIEVING

Definition: A state in which an individual reacts to an actual, anticipated, or perceived loss of a significant person, ideal, status, object, or body part with an absent, delayed, exaggerated, or prolonged response.

Table 12.1 Nursing Diagnoses Commonly Associated with the Breasts and Axillae (continued)

DYSFUNCTIONAL GRIEVING	
DEFINING CHARACTERISTICS	
Expressing distress at loss	Developmental regression
Denial of loss	Labile affect
Expressing guilt	Alteration in concentration and/or pursuit of tasks
Expressing unresolved issues	Difficulty in expressing loss
Anger	Alteration in dream patterns
Sadness	Alteration in libido
Crying	Idealization of lost object
Alteration in eating habits	Reliving past experiences
Alteration in sleep patterns	Interference with life functioning
Alteration in activity level	
RELATED FACTORS	
Actual loss, Anticipated loss, Chronic illness, Perceived loss, Terminal illness, Others specific to client (specify).	

DIAGNOSTIC REASONING IN ACTION

Mrs. Ingrid Heller is a 46-year-old woman of German ancestry who first noted a lump on her right breast one day while taking a shower. She stated she thought it would go away, and so she delayed seeking medical advice for 3 months until she noticed that it felt larger and harder and that her breast had a dimple over the area of the lump.

Physical assessment revealed the following: Left breast round and pendulous, without lumps or changes in skin texture. Nipple everted, no discharge. Firm mass felt in right upper outer quadrant of right breast, 3 cm from the nipple, approximately 2 cm by 2 cm by 1 cm. Nontender, nonmovable, irregular to touch. Dimpling of skin over area of mass. Nipple everted, no discharge. No lymphadenopathy bilaterally.

The diagnostic cues Mrs. Heller presented were quite typical of the shock and horror women feel when they find a breast lump. First, she tried to ignore it, hoping that it would go away. When it became evident that the lump not only did not go away but was actually larger and now caused dimpling over the area, she expressed a fear of surgery, chemotherapy, and disfigurement.

Several nursing diagnoses could apply to Mrs. Heller. The following demonstrates how one nursing diagnosis was determined:

The factors contributing to Mrs. Heller's problems include

- Cultural beliefs
- Possibility of surgery
- Possibility of experiencing side effects

The diagnostic cues demonstrated by Mrs. Heller include

- Expressing negative feelings about her body
- Expressing feelings of hopelessness and powerlessness

The nurse identified the nursing diagnosis of *Body image disturbance* related to a lump in the right breast as evidenced by Mrs. Heller's expressed negative feeling about her body and her expression of feelings of hopelessness and powerlessness. The nurse facilitated an appointment with the surgeon and a follow-up appointment for counseling regarding Mrs. Heller's feelings and perceptions related to body image disturbance.

Common Alterations in the Health of the Breasts and Axillae

Some of the problems identified during the physical assessment are entirely within the realm of nursing and are addressed with appropriate nursing interventions. Some problems, however, require collaborative management. Fibrocystic breast disease, fibroadenoma, intraductal papilloma, mammary duct ectasia, and breast cancer are the most common breast conditions that will challenge you and the rest of the health care team. These common problems are discussed in this section; Table 12.2 summarizes their distinguishing characteristics.

Fibrocystic Breast Disease One of the most common benign breast problems is **fibrocystic breast disease** (also called *mammary dysplasia*). It is typically first seen in women in their twenties and is characterized by lumps, breast pain or tenderness, and nipple discharge. These symptoms are a result of *fibrosis*, a thickening of the normal breast tissue, which may be accompanied by cyst formation. Usually located in the upper outer quadrant, the cysts probably are a result of fluctuating hormones in the body that cause excessive cell growth in the ducts and lobules and inhibit the draining of normal secretions. The breasts usually become painful just prior to the onset of menses, and pain resolves at the end of menstruation. Upon palpation, the masses feel soft, well demarcated, and freely movable; they are almost always bilateral (Figure 12.18). Discharge from the nipples may be clear, straw colored, milky, or green. This is a disease of the reproductive years, and symptoms usually resolve after menopause because of a lack of estrogen.

Fibrocystic breast disease is not usually clinically significant, and there is no direct link between fibrocystic tissue changes and the incidence of cancer. In some cases, however, it may result in ductal hyperplasia and dysplasia, which may eventually develop into noninvasive intraductal, lobular, or intraepithelial carcinoma. This can be a potential focus for invasive carcinoma. Additionally, the presence of nodular tissue in the breast makes the early detection of malignant nodules more challenging. The physician monitors fibrocystic breast disease through periodic mammography or xeroradiography and determines if an aspiration or biopsy is necessary.

Pharmacologic hormones and diuretics are used in the medical management to relieve symptoms. Some studies suggest that limiting caffeine may help relieve symptoms, but the evidence is inconclusive. The nurse might suggest that the woman try eliminating caffeine, especially in the premenstrual period, and determine for herself if she feels this action brings relief. The nurse may also suggest decreasing salt intake and taking mild analgesics. Wearing a supportive bra decreases discomfort. The nurse reinforces the need for regular breast self-examination as well as regular mammography and physical examination.

Fibroadenoma A **fibroadenoma** is a common benign tumor of the glandular tissue of the breast. It is most common in women in their teens and early twenties. Its development in

Table 12.2 Summary of Common Breast Disorders

Condition	Age	Pain	Nipple discharge	Location	Consistency and mobility
Fibrocystic breast disease	20–49 years; median age 30 (may subside with menopause)	Yes	No	Upper outer quadrant	Bilateral multiple lumps influenced by the menstrual cycle
Fibroadenoma	15–39 years; median age 20	No	No	No specific location	Mobile, firm, smooth, well delineated
Intraductal papilloma	35–55 years; median age 40	Yes	Serous or serosanguineous; usually unilateral from one duct	No specific location	Usually soft, poorly delineated
Duct ectasia	35–55 years; median age 40	Burning around nipple	Sticky, multicolored; usually bilateral	No specific location	Retroareolar mass with advanced disease
Carcinoma of the breast	30–90; more common after age 50	Usually none	May be bloody or clear, if present	48% occur in upper outer quadrant, but may occur in any part of breast or axillary tail	Firm to stony mass that is fixed to skin or underlying tissues

Modified from Fogel CI, Woods NF, editors. *Health care of women: A nursing perspective*. St. Louis: Mosby, 1981, p 337.

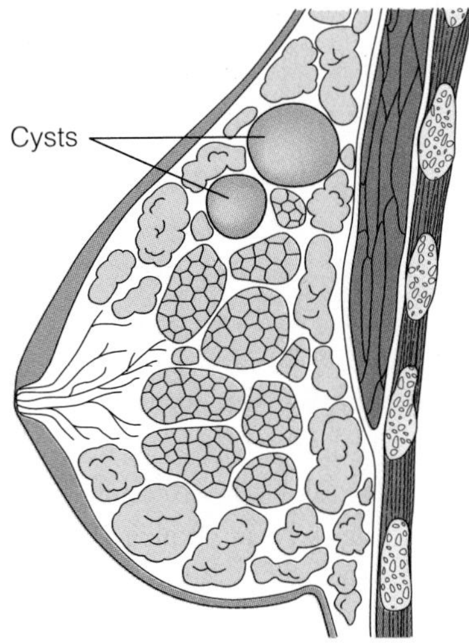

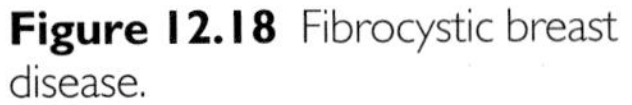
Figure 12.18 Fibrocystic breast disease.

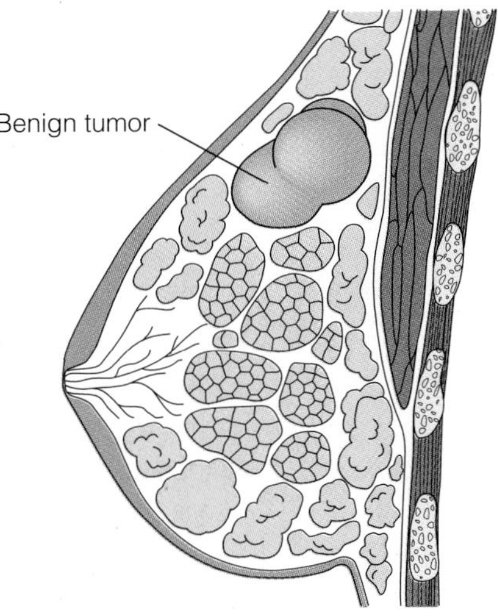

Figure 12.19 Fibroadenoma.

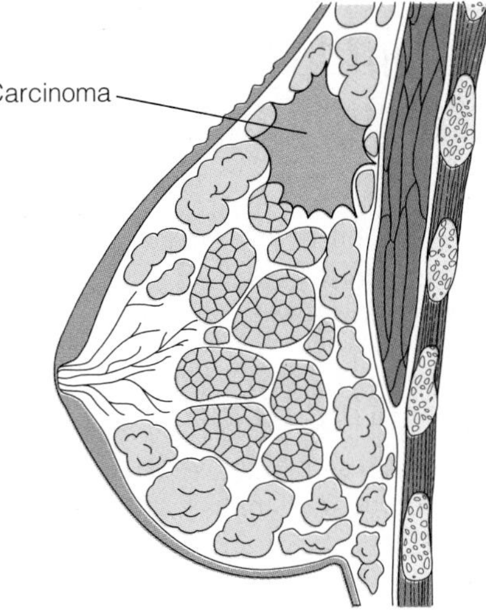

Figure 12.20 Breast cancer.

adolescents appears to be linked to breast hypertrophy, which may occur during the growth spurt of puberty. Fibroadenomas are well-defined, round, firm tumors, about 1 cm to 5 cm in diameter, that can be moved freely within the breast tissue (Figure 12.19). They usually occur singly near the nipple or in the upper outer quadrant. Because they are asymptomatic, they are often not discovered until breast self-examination or examination by a physician. Careful observation over time is the usual treatment. Biopsy or excision of the lump, performed on an outpatient basis, is indicated if the findings are inconclusive. No relationship has been established between fibroadenomas and malignant neoplasms.

Intraductal Papilloma **Intraductal papillomas** are tiny growths of epithelial cells that project into the lumen of the lactiferous ducts. These growths are fragile, and even minimal trauma causes leakage of blood or serum into the involved duct and subsequent discharge. Intraductal papillomas are the primary cause of nipple discharge in women who are not pregnant or lactating. They are more commonly found in menopausal women but may occur in women of any age.

Mammary Duct Ectasia **Mammary duct ectasia** is an inflammation of the lactiferous ducts behind the nipple. As cellular debris and fluid collect in the involved ducts, they become enlarged and form a palpable, painful mass. A thick, sticky discharge from the nipple is common. Because there may be some nipple retraction, a careful assessment is required to distinguish the condition from breast cancer. Although the disorder is painful, it is not associated with cancer and usually resolves spontaneously.

Carcinoma of the Breast The common visible signs of **carcinoma of the breast** (Figure 12.20) include

- *Dimpling* of the skin over the tumor caused by a retraction or pulling inward of breast tissue, which results primarily from tissue fibrosis. Retraction is also caused by fat necrosis and mammary duct ectasia (described in the previous section).
- *Deviation* of the breast or nipple from its normal alignment. Deviation is also caused by retraction. The nipple typically deviates toward the underlying cancer.
- *Nipple retraction.* The nipple flattens or even turns inward. Retraction is also caused by tissue fibrosis.
- *Irregular shape* of one breast as compared to the other, such as a flattening of one quadrant. Irregularity of shape is also caused by retraction.
- *Edema,* which may result in a peau d'orange appearance, especially near the nipple. Edema is caused by blockage of the lymphatic ducts that normally drain the breast.
- *Discharge,* which may be bloody or clear.

The diagnosis of cancer is made by a combination of tests including physical examination and mammography. A positive diagnosis is made by histologic examination following an open or closed biopsy. The tumor is then staged to determine characteristics of the tumor, nodal involvement, and the presence or absence of distant metastasis. The outcome of this staging determines which protocol is used for treatment. Treatment may consist of a surgical treatment, radiation therapy, chemotherapy, or a combination of these. All treatment protocols for breast cancer have side effects. The various surgical approaches to breast cancer treatment are described briefly in the box on page 326.

Throughout diagnosis and treatment of breast cancer, there is a potential for multiple physiologic and psychosocial nursing diagnoses.

Health Promotion and Client Education

When the breast and axillary assessment is completed, answer any questions and take this opportunity to do client teaching to promote wellness.

Promoting Healthy Breasts

All women should know that they are at risk for breast cancer and should be familiar with the risk factors (Table 12.3). Some risk factors, such as age and sex, cannot be changed, but others can be monitored, and self-care practices can be changed to promote wellness. Early detection and treatment of breast cancers have greatly increased survival rates, and clients need to be aware of screening and detection measures. As a health professional, you can be instrumental in teaching the client how to take charge of her health. Below is a list of specific tips for promoting healthy breasts.

- Identify risk factors for breast cancer (Table 12.3).
- Identify the self-care practices that reduce the risk of breast cancer:

  Perform breast self-examination once every month after age 20.

  Avoid obesity.

  Reduce dietary fat.

  Reduce alcohol intake.

  Ensure that oral contraceptive use is monitored by physician.

  Ensure that supplemental estrogen use is monitored by physician.
- Obtain a physical examination every 3 years (women 20–40 years of age) and every year (women over 40 years).
- Obtain a baseline mammogram between 35–39 years of age. For women 40–49 years of age who are not at risk for breast cancer, obtain a mammogram every 2 years. For women 40–49 years of age who are at risk for breast cancer, and for all women over age 50, obtain a yearly mammogram.
- Wear a supportive garment when exercising.
- Report to a physician any changes in the breasts or axillae that deviate from normal patterns. These include lumps, dimpling, deviation, recent nipple retraction, irregular shape, edema, or discharge.
- Utilize the resources of the American Cancer Society for information and answers to your questions about breast cancer.

Table 12.3 Summary of Risk Factors for Breast Cancer

Factor	Higher risk	Lower risk
Age	≥40	<40
History of cancer in one breast	Yes	No
Family history of premenopausal bilateral breast cancer	Yes	No
Country of residence	North America Northern Europe	Asia Africa
Any first-degree relative with breast cancer	Yes	No
History of fibrocystic condition with atypical hyperplasia	Yes	No
Alcohol consumption	>9 drinks/wk	<9 drinks/wk
History of primary cancer in ovary or endometrium	Yes	No
Radiation to chest	Large doses	Minimal exposure
Socioeconomic class	Upper	Lower
Age at first full-term pregnancy	>30	<20
Oophorectomy	Yes	No
Postmenopausal body build	Obese	Thin
Race	White	Black
Marital status	Never married	Married
Age at menarche	Early	Late
Age at menopause	Late	Early
U.S. place of residence	Urban northern	Rural southern

Teaching Breast Self-Examination (BSE)

Step 1 Teach the client to observe her breasts in front of a mirror and in good lighting. Tell her to observe her breasts in four positions:

With her arms relaxed and at her sides

With her arms lifted over her head.

With her hands pressed against her hips

With her hands pressed together at waist, leaning forward

Instruct her to look at each breast individually, and then to compare them. She should observe for any visible abnormalities, such as lumps, dimpling, deviation, recent nipple retraction, irregular shape, edema, discharge, or asymmetry.

Step 2 Teach the client to palpate both breasts while standing or sitting, with one hand behind her head (Figure 12.21, *A*). Tell her that many women palpate their breasts in the shower because water and soap make the skin slippery and easier to palpate. Show the woman how to use the pads of her fingers to palpate all areas of her breast, using the concentric circles technique (Figure 12.21, *B*). Tell her to press the breast tissue gently against the chest wall, and to be sure to palpate the axillary tail.

Step 3 Instruct the client to palpate her breasts again while lying down, as described in step 2. Suggest that she place a folded towel under the shoulder and back on the side to be palpated. The arm on the examining side should be over the head, with the hand under the head (Figure 12.21, *C*).

Step 4 Teach the client to palpate the areola and nipples next. Show her how to compress the nipple to check for discharge (Figure 12.21, *D*).

Step 5 Remind the client to use a calendar to keep a record of when she performs BSE. Teach her to perform BSE at the same time each month, usually 5 days after the onset of menses, when there is less hormonal influence on tissues.

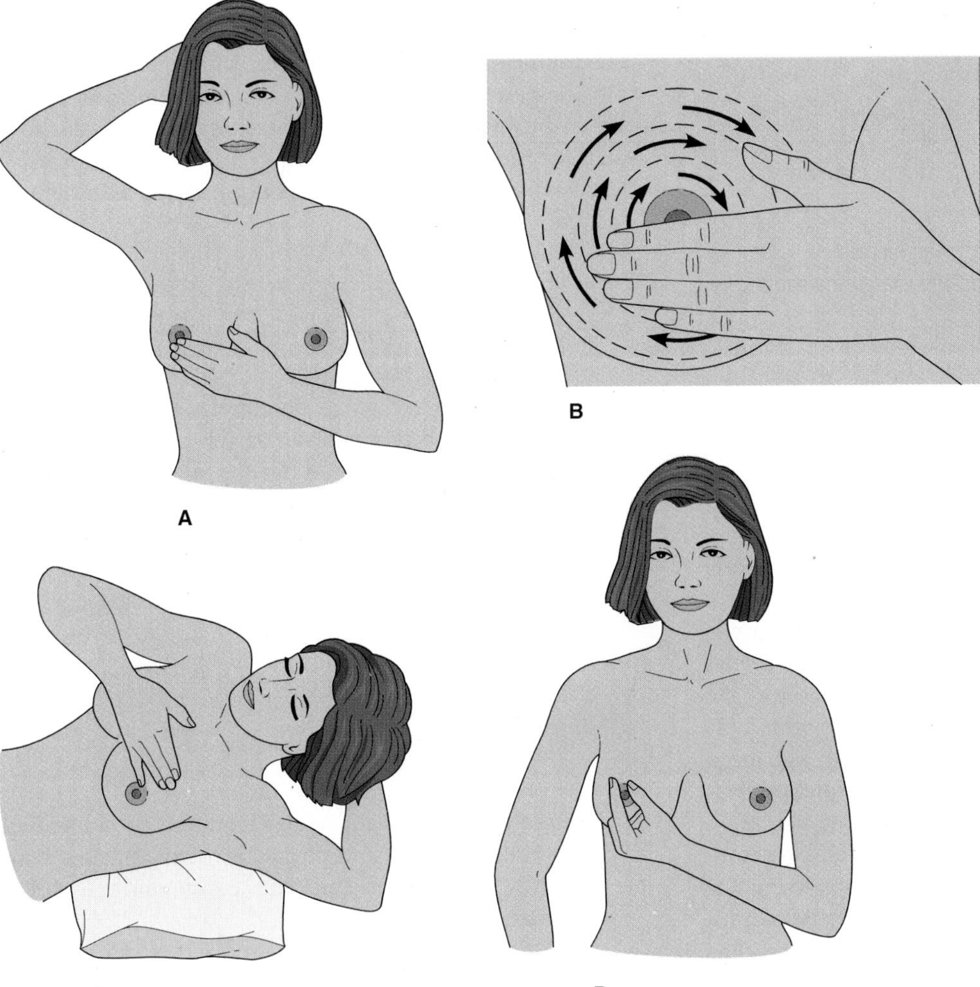

Figure 12.21 Breast self-examination. *A*, The woman palpates her breasts while standing or sitting upright. *B*, The concentric-circles approach. *C*, The woman palpates her breasts while lying down. *D*, The woman palpates her nipples.

DIAGNOSTIC REASONING IN ACTION

Kate Saunders is a 22-year-old student in apparent good health. She presents herself to the university clinic because of information she learned in a health class she is taking. She tells the nurse that she heard there may be some familial tendencies toward breast cancer. Both her mother and aunt have undergone mastectomy, and she wants to know what her chances are.

The nurse, Letitia Baum, asks Ms Saunders about other risk factors and learns that she has never been pregnant, started menarche at age 12, and has had regular 28-day cycles since age 13. She is not sexually active and states she eats a well-balanced diet. She takes vitamin C daily to prevent colds and ibuprofen as needed for occasional menstrual cramps. She drinks an occasional beer on weekends with her friends. She does not know how to do breast self-examination.

The nursing assessment reveals that her breasts and nipples are symmetrically shaped, with the right breast slightly larger than the left. There are no rashes, skin lesions, dimpling, retractions, nodules, inflammation, or tenderness. Both nipples point outward. There is no discharge, and the axillary nodes are not palpable.

The nursing assessment of Ms. Saunders provides the following subjective and objective data:

- Lacks information about cancer risk factors
- Does not know how to perform breast self-examination
- Uses vitamin C and ibuprofen
- Occasionally drinks alcohol
- Has never been pregnant, started menarche at age 12, has had a normal 28-day cycle since age 13
- Eats a well-balanced diet
- Physical examination unremarkable

To cluster the information, Ms Baum:

- Considers the data regarding Ms Saunder's menstrual history but it does not require action as it is within normal limits.
- Considers the data regarding Ms Saunder's self-care practices but disregards it because these are not high-risk behaviors.
- Notes that Ms Saunders does not know cancer risk factors.
- Notes that Ms Saunders does not perform breast self-examination.

Ms Baum arrives at the following nursing diagnosis: *Knowledge deficit* related to lack of information about cancer risk factors and breast self-examination. The nurse tells Ms Saunders why she is at risk for developing breast cancer and teaches her how to perform breast self-examination.

Summary

Conduct a thorough breast examination not only to ensure and maintain health but also to facilitate prevention and early detection of breast cancer. The focused interview includes a general survey of the breasts and axillae, past history, family history, and assessment of risk factors. Also assess the client's knowledge of breast self-examination. Inspect and palpate the breasts and axillae to determine if structures are within normal limits. To perform a successful assessment, you need knowledge of the anatomy and physiology of the breasts, lymphatic system, and muscles of the chest wall, as well as an understanding of the influence of self-care, cultural, environmental, and developmental factors. Upon completing the assessment, provide information the client can use to promote, protect, and maintain her own breast health. The process of breast self-examination is taught or reinforced. In addition, explain the risk factors for breast cancer and teach the client how to recognize conditions that need to be reported to a health professional. At the completion of the assessment, document the findings for other health professionals that will care for the client. Throughout the assessment process, use the diagnostic reasoning process to identify and validate appropriate nursing diagnoses, and when indicated, identify problems that are collaborative in scope.

Key Points

- ✓ Assessing the breasts and axillae requires a sound knowledge of the anatomy and physiology of the breasts, lymphatic system of the breasts and axillae, and muscles of the chest wall.
- ✓ During the focused interview, conduct a general survey of the breasts and axillae, past history, family history, and assessment of risk factors.

- ✓ Ensure privacy before beginning the examination, and be sensitive to the client's potential embarassment regarding exposure of the breasts.
- ✓ During the physical examination, inspect the breasts and axillae as well as general appearance of chest wall. Perform palpation of breast tissue and axillary lymph nodes using one of several acceptable techniques.
- ✓ Assess the client's knowledge of breast self-examination, and teach the proper technique as indicated. Instruct the client to perform breast self-examination once every month after age 20.
- ✓ The American Cancer Society recommends that all individuals perform breast self-examination monthly; have a breast examination by a physician every 3 years prior to age 40 and every year after age 40; have a baseline mammogram between the ages of 35 and 39; have a mammogram every 2 years between age 40 and 49 if not at high risk, once every year after age 40 if at high risk, and once every year after age 50.
- ✓ Nursing diagnoses most commonly associated with the breasts and axillae are: body image disturbance, dysfunctional grieving, ineffective breast-feeding, ineffective individual coping, knowledge deficit related to lack of information about breast self-examination, anxiety related to the diagnosis of cancer, and pain related to metastasis.
- ✓ When assessing the client's breasts and axillae, you may encounter findings suggestive of common alterations in health that are collaborative in scope. These include fibrocystic breast disease, fibroadenoma, intraductal papilloma, mammary duct ectasia, and carcinoma of the breast.

Chapter 13

Assessing the Abdomen

The abdomen houses the digestive organs, which are essential for taking in, breaking down, and absorbing nutrients to fuel all of the body's cells and ensure optimal functioning. Thus, assessment of the abdomen is an important component of the complete physical assessment, and it is essential in helping clients to promote and maintain their overall health.

The abdominal cavity is inferior to the diaphragm and superior to the pelvic floor. The anterior borders of the abdomen are formed by the abdominal muscles, the intercostal margins, and the pelvis. The posterior borders of the abdomen are formed by the vertebral column and the lumbar muscles. A large cavity, the abdomen contains organs of many systems, including the gastrointestinal, urinary, reproductive, and vascular systems. Although this chapter focuses primarily on the gastrointestinal system, it addresses organs of other systems as appropriate.

The gastrointestinal system processes food—its ingestion, its digestion, and the elimination of waste products after its processing. The ability to perform these functions is influenced by the health of many other body systems. In addition, the client's developmental stage, self-care practices, cultural and environmental variations, and the psychosocial implications of food are all important parameters for you to assess during the focused interview. The integration of these factors is depicted in Figure 13.1.

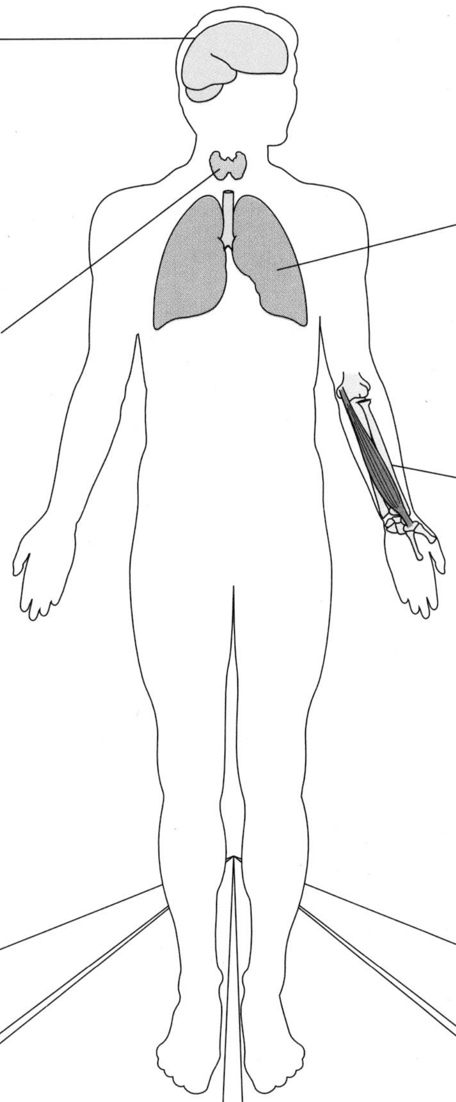

Nervous System

- The parasympathetic fibers promote digestion, and the sympathetic fibers inhibit digestion.
- The gastrointestinal system provides nutrients needed for healthy neural function.

Endocrine System

- Hormones of the endocrine system help regulate digestion.
- The liver removes hormones from the blood, thereby ceasing their activity.

Respiratory System

- The respiratory system provides oxygen and removes carbon dioxide produced by the abdominal organs.
- The gastrointestinal system provides nutrients needed for healthy respiratory function.

Musculoskeletal System

- Portions of the rib cage protect various abdominal organs.
- Musculoskeletal activity increases the motility of the gastrointestinal tract.
- The gastrointestinal system provides nutrients for musculoskeletal activity, growth, and repair.

Developmental

- During infancy and childhood, food allergies are common.
- During pregnancy, the uterus enlarges and moves into the abdominal cavity, often causing compression and displacement of many abdominal structures. This may result in constipation, flatulence, and hemorroids.
- The older adult experiences a gradual decrease in digestive enzymes, peristalsis, and intestinal absorption, resulting in possible indigestion, constipation, and gastroesophageal reflux.

Psychosocial

- A high level of stress may cause or aggravate gastritis, gastric and duodenal ulcers, ulcerative colitis, and irritable colon.
- Gastrointestinal surgery may result in a colostomy, which often causes clients embarrassment and anxiety, and may lead to withdrawn behavior.

Self-Care

- Abdominal and gastrointestinal self-care focuses on diet, exercise, and safety measures to reduce traumatic injury.
- Clients should avoid harmful substances such as alcohol, caffeine, and certain medications, such as aspirin and ibuprofin, that irritate the gastric lining.

Environmental

- Culture, customs, religious practices, and financial considerations influence food choice and thus gastrointestinal health.
- Homeless clients are at increased risk for malnutrition and food poisoning.

Figure 13.1 Important factors to consider when assessing the gastrointestinal system.

Anatomy and Physiology Review

The abdomen contains structures of many systems. The anatomy and physiology review of the abdomen has a two-point focus. The primary focus is the gastrointestinal system, and the secondary focus is abdominal structures of other systems.

The gastrointestinal system consists of the alimentary canal and the accessory digestive organs. The alimentary canal, a continuous, hollow, muscular tube, begins at the mouth and terminates at the anus. The mouth, pharynx, esophagus, stomach, small intestines, and large intestines form the canal. The accessory organs include the teeth, salivary glands, liver, gallbladder, and pancreas (Figure 13.2).

The anatomy, physiology, and assessment of the mouth, teeth, tongue, salivary glands, and pharynx are discussed in Chapter 9, "Assessing the Head and Neck." Before proceeding with the gastrointestinal assessment, you may want to review the information in that chapter to strengthen your knowledge base.

The Alimentary Canal

Esophagus

The **esophagus**, a collapsible tube, connects the pharynx to the stomach. Approximately 25 cm (10 inches) in length, it passes through the mediastinum and diaphragm to meet the stomach at the cardiac sphincter. The primary function of the esophagus is

- Propelling food and fluid from the mouth to the stomach

Stomach

The **stomach** extends from the esophagus at the cardiac sphincter to the duodenum at the pyloric sphincter. Located

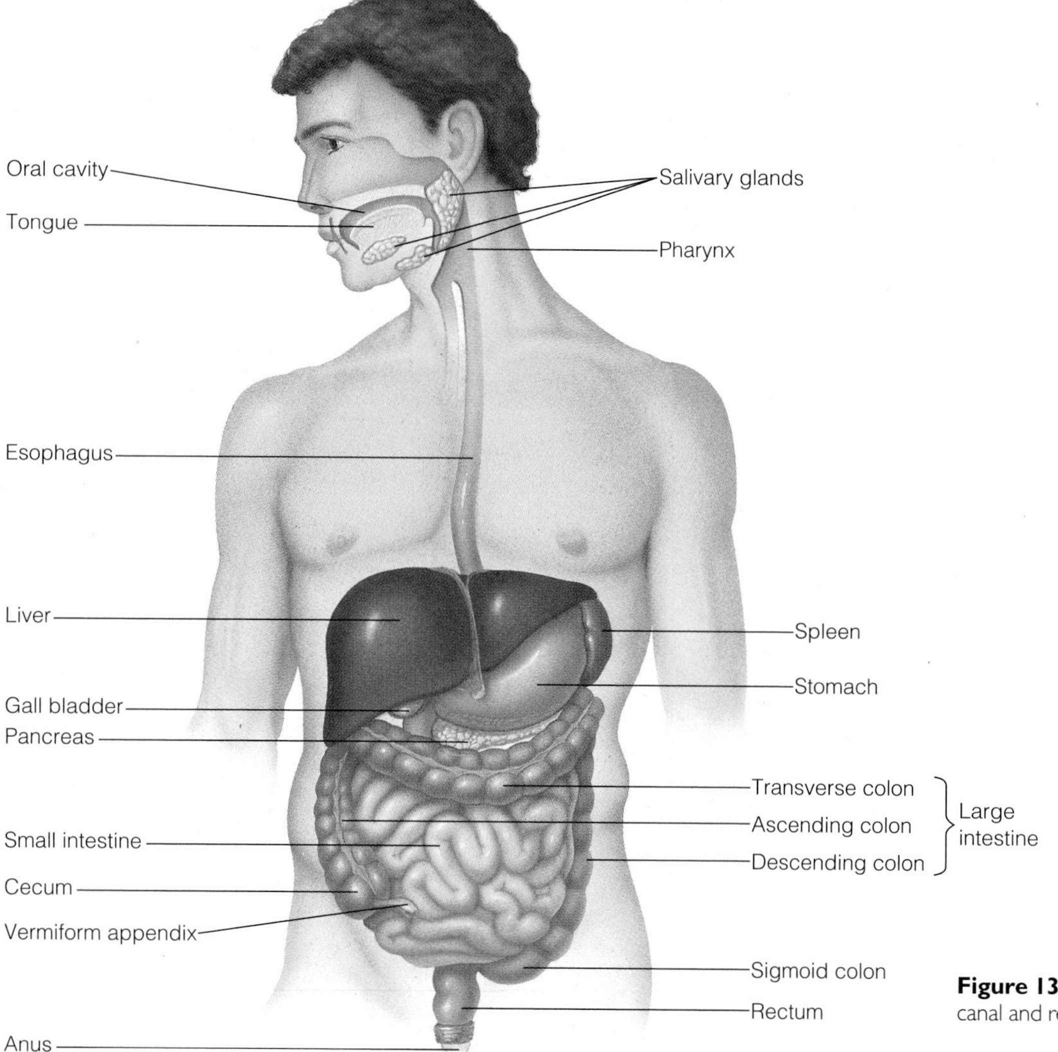

Figure 13.2 Organs of the alimentary canal and related accessory organs.

in the left side of the upper abdomen, the stomach is directly inferior to the diaphragm. The diameter and volume of the stomach are directly related to the food it contains. Food mixes with digestive juices in the stomach and becomes *chyme* before entering the small intestines. The primary function of the stomach is

- Chemical and mechanical breakdown of food

Small Intestine

The **small intestine** is the body's primary digestive and absorptive organ. Approximately 2 m (6 ft) in length, it has three subdivisions. The first segment, the *duodenum*, meets the stomach at the pyloric sphincter and extends to the middle region, called the *jejunum*. The *ileum* extends from the jejunum to the ileocecal valve at the cecum of the large intestines. Intestinal juices, bile from the liver and gallbladder, and pancreatic enzymes mix with the chyme to promote digestion and facilitate the absorption of nutrients. The primary functions of the small intestine are

- Continuing chemical breakdown of food
- Absorbing digested foodstuffs

Large Intestine

The last portion of the alimentary canal is the **large intestine,** which extends from the ileocecal valve to the anus. It consists of the cecum, ascending colon, transverse colon, descending colon, sigmoid colon, rectum, and anus. The vermiform *appendix* is attached to the large intestines at the cecum. The appendix contains masses of lymphoid tissue that make only a minor contribution to immunity; however, when inflamed, the appendix causes significant health problems. The large intestine is wider and shorter than the small intestine. It is on the periphery of the abdominal cavity, surrounding the small intestine and other structures. The main functions of the large intestine are

- Absorbing water from indigestible food residue
- Eliminating the residue in the form of feces

Accessory Digestive Organs

Liver

The largest gland of the body, the **liver** is located in the right upper portion of the abdominal cavity directly inferior to the diaphragm and extends into the left side of the abdomen. The rib cage protects the liver, making only its lower border palpable. The liver has many metabolic and regulatory functions in the body. The only digestive function of the liver is

- Producting and secreting bile for fat emulsification

Gallbladder

Chiefly a storage organ for bile, the **gallbladder**, a thin-walled sac, is nestled in a shallow depression on the ventral surface of the liver. The gallbladder releases stored bile into the duodenum when stimulated and thus promotes the emulsification of fats. The main functions of the gallbladder are

- Storing bile
- Assisting in the digestion of fats

Pancreas

An accessory digestive organ, the **pancreas** is a triangular-shaped gland located in the left upper portion of the abdomen. The head of the pancreas is nestled in the C curve of the duodenum, and the body and the tail of the pancreas lie deep to the left of the stomach and extend toward the spleen at the lateral aspect of the abdomen. Pancreatic juice, which contains a broad spectrum of enzymes, mixes with bile in the duodenum. The main function of the pancreas is

- Assisting with the digestion of proteins, fats, and carbohydrates

Other Related Structures

Peritoneum

The **peritoneum** is a thin double layer of serous membrane in the abdominal cavity. The visceral peritoneum covers the external surface of most digestive organs. The parietal peritoneum lines the walls of the abdominal cavity. The serous fluid secreted by the membranes helps lubricate the surface of the organs, allowing motion without friction.

Muscles of the Abdominal Wall

Having no bony reinforcements, the anterior and lateral abdominal walls depend upon the musculature for support and protection. The four pairs of **abdominal muscles**, when well toned, support and protect the abdominal viscera most effectively. The muscle groups are the rectus abdominis, external oblique, internal oblique, and transverse abdominis (Fig-

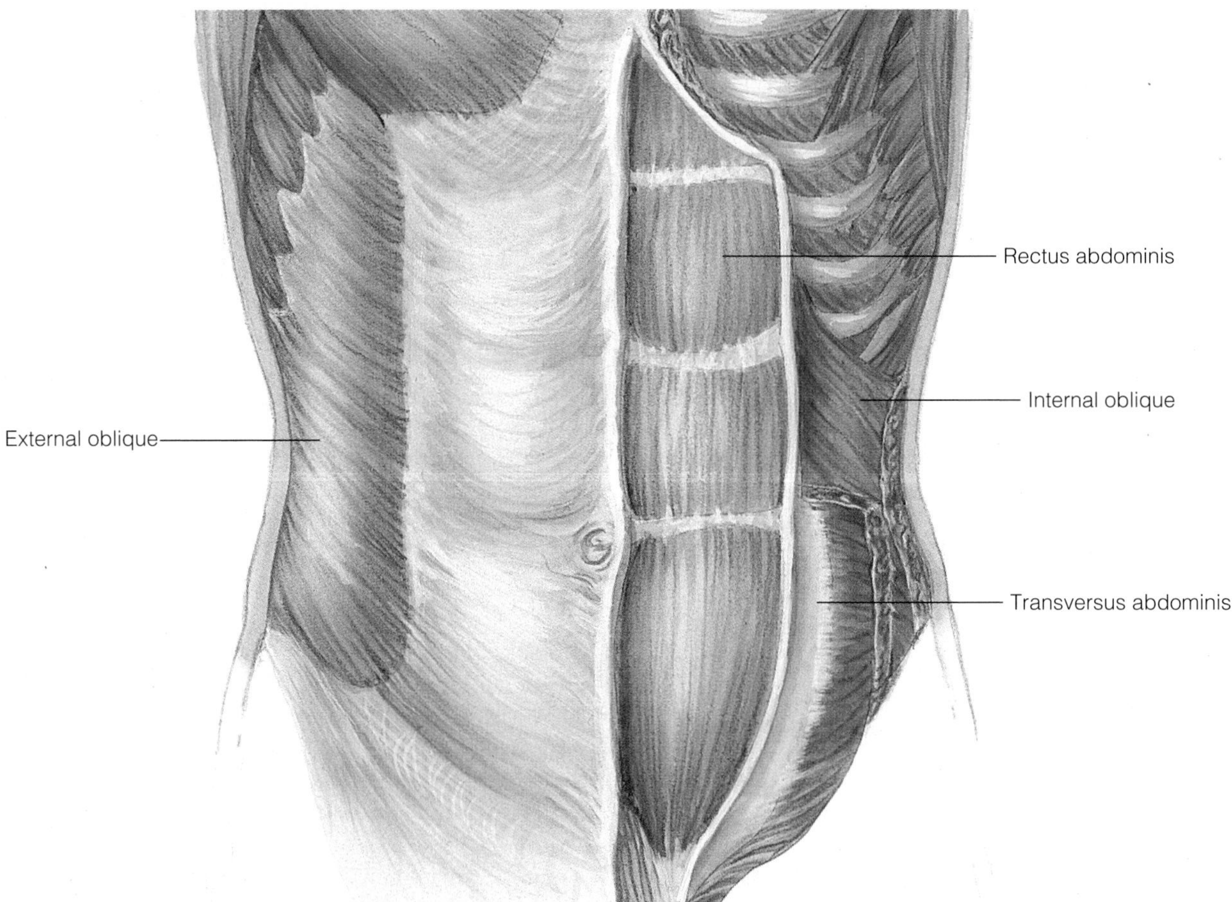

Figure 13.3 Muscles of the abdominal wall.

ure 13.3). Secondary functions of these muscle groups include lateral flexion, rotation, and anterior flexion of the trunk. Simultaneous contraction of the muscle groups increases intra-abdominal pressure by compressing the abdominal wall.

Aorta

As the descending aorta passes through the diaphragm and enters the abdominal cavity, it becomes the **abdominal aorta**. This penetration occurs at the T12 level of the vertebral column. The abdominal aorta continues to the L4 level of the vertebral column, where it bifurcates to form the right and left common iliac arteries. The many branches of the abdominal aorta serve all the parietal and visceral structures.

Kidneys, Ureters, and Bladder

The *kidneys* lie within the abdomen behind the peritoneum. Responsible for the filtration of nitrogenous wastes and the production of urine, the kidneys are protected by the lower ribs. The slender tubelike structures that carry the urine from the kidneys to the bladder are the *ureters*. The *urinary bladder*, a smooth, collapsible muscular sac, is located in the pelvis of the abdominal cavity. The primary function of the bladder is to store urine until it can be released. As the bladder fills with urine, it may rise above the symphysis pubis into the abdominal cavity. Assessment of the kidneys, ureters, and bladder is discussed in Chapter 14.

Spleen

The largest of the lymphoid organs, the **spleen** is located in the left upper portion of the abdomen directly inferior to the diaphragm. Surrounded by a fibrous capsule, the spleen provides a site for lymphocyte proliferation and immune surveillance and response. It filters and cleanses blood, destroying worn-out red blood cells and returning their breakdown products to the liver.

Reproductive Organs

In the female, the uterus, uterine tubes, and ovaries are in the pelvic portion of the abdominal cavity. In the male, the prostate gland surrounds the urethra just below the bladder. The reproductive organs of the male and female are discussed in Chapter 15.

Landmarks

You need to identify reference points and anatomic structures when assessing the abdomen. Defined landmarks help you identify specific underlying structures and provide a source for description and recording of findings. Landmarks for the abdomen include the xiphoid process, umbilicus, costal margin, iliac crests, and pubic bone.

Mapping is the process of dividing the abdomen into quadrants or regions for the purpose of examination. To obtain the four abdominal quadrants, extend the midsternal line from the xiphoid process through the umbilicus to the pubic bone. Then draw a horizontal line perpendicular to the first, through the umbilicus. These two perpendicular lines form four equal quadrants of the abdomen. The quadrants are simply named right upper quadrant (RUQ), right lower quadrant (RLQ), left upper quadrant (LUQ), and left lower quadrant (LLQ) (Figure 13.4).

The second mapping method divides the abdomen into nine regions. To obtain these abdominal regions, extend the right and left midclavicular lines to the groin. Then draw a horizontal line across the lowest edge of the costal margin. Draw another horizontal line at the level of the iliac crests. You have now divided the abdomen into nine regions. The names of the regions are right hypochondriac, epigastric, left hypochondriac, right lumbar, umbilical, left lumbar, right inguinal, hypogastric or pubic, and left inguinal (Figure 13.5).

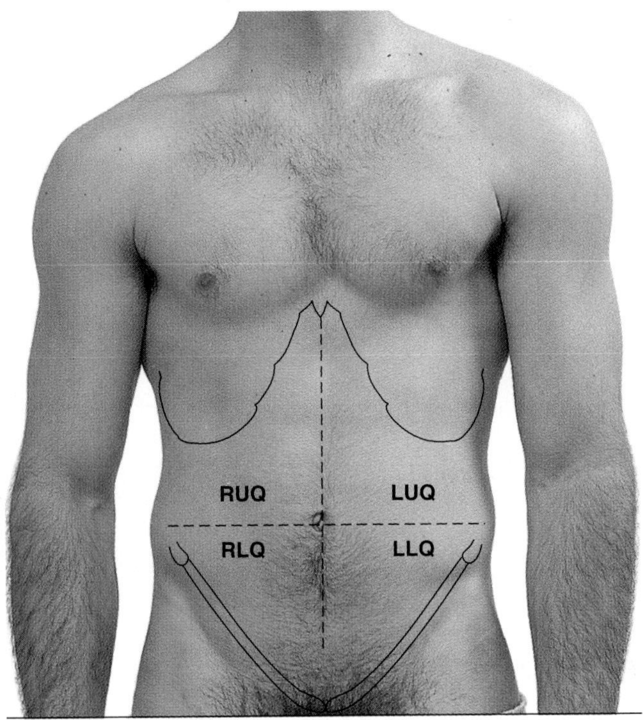

Figure 13.4 Mapping of the abdomen into four quadrants.

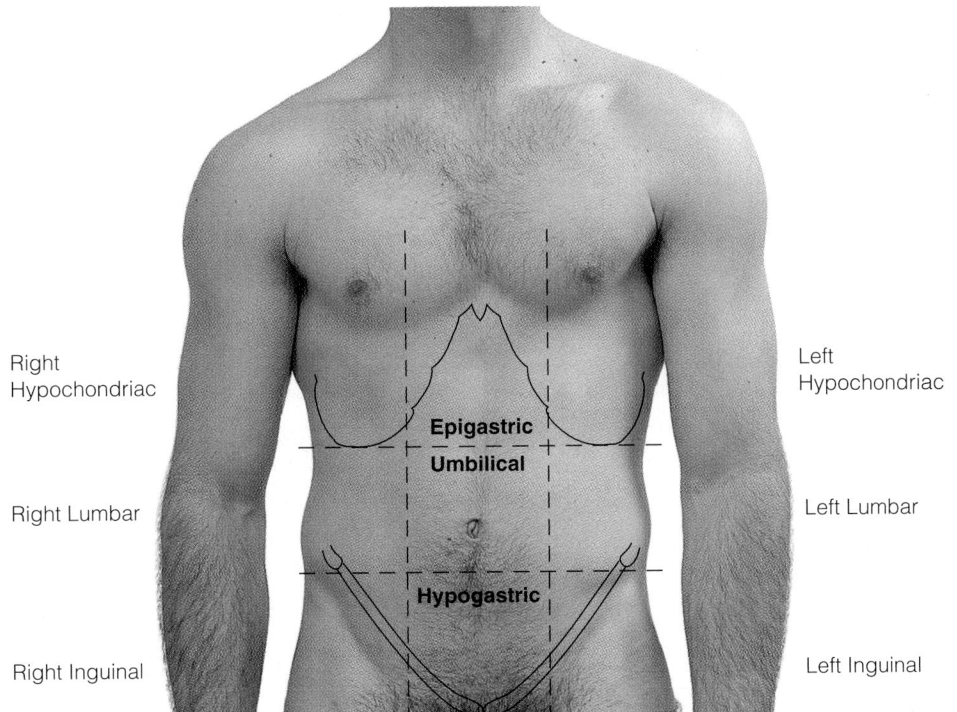

Figure 13.5 Mapping of the abdomen into nine regions.

Of the two methods described, the quadrant method is more commonly used. When using the quadrant method, remember to pay attention to the structures that are in the midline of the abdomen and do not belong to any specific quadrant. These structures include the abdominal aorta, the urinary bladder, and the uterus.

Choose one mapping method and use it consistently. Once you have selected a method, you need to visualize the underlying structures before proceeding (Figure 13.6).

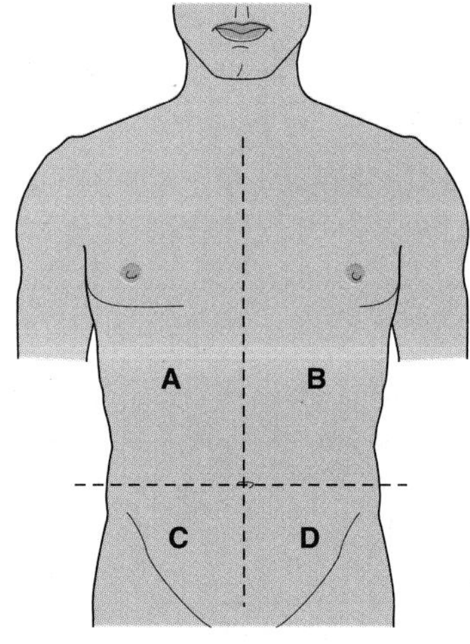

Midline
Aorta
Bladder
Uterus

A ○ = Umbilicus

A ***Right Upper Quadrant***	B ***Left Upper Quadrant***
Liver and gallbladder Pyloric sphincter Duodenum Head of pancreas Right adrenal gland Portion of right kidney Hepatic flexure of colon Portions of ascending and transverse colon	Left lobe of liver Spleen Stomach Body of pancreas Left adrenal gland Portion of left kidney Splenic flexure of colon Portions of transverse and descending colon
C ***Right Lower Quadrant*** Lower pole of right kidney Cecum and appendix Portion of ascending colon Ovary and uterine tube Right spermatic cord Right ureter	D ***Left Lower Quadrant*** Lower pole of left kidney Sigmoid colon Portion of descending colon Ovary and uterine tube Left spermatic cord Left ureter

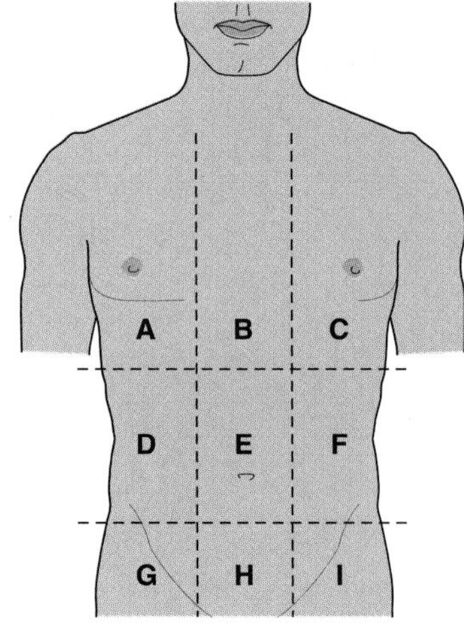

A ***Right Hypochondriac***	B ***Epigastric***	C ***Left Hypochondriac***
Right lobe of liver Gallbladder Portion of duodenum Hepatic flexure of colon Portion of right kidney Right adrenal gland	Pyloric sphincter Duodenum Pancreas Portion of liver Aorta	Stomach Spleen Tail of pancreas Splenic flexure of colon Upper pole of left kidney Left adrenal gland
D ***Right Lumbar*** Ascending colon Lower half of right kidney Portion of duodenum and jejunum	E ***Umbilical*** Lower part of duodenum Jejunum and ileum	F ***Left Lumbar*** Descending colon Lower half of left kidney Portions of jejunum and ileum
G ***Right Inguinal*** Cecum Appendix Lower end of ileum Right ureter Right spermatic cord Right ovary and uterine tube	H ***Hypogastric (Pubic)*** Ileum Bladder Uterus (in pregnancy)	I ***Left Inguinal*** Sigmoid colon Left ureter Left spermatic cord Left ovary and uterine tube

B

Figure 13.6 *A*, Organs of the four abdominal quadrants. *B*, Organs of the nine abdominal regions.

Gathering the Data

Assessment of the client's abdomen provides detailed data about the client's overall health status and placement of the client on the health-illness continuum. Assessment of the abdomen also provides data regarding self-care practices, especially those related to nutrition.

Before beginning the focused interview, review the data obtained in the health history. Be sure to review data regarding the nutritional status of the client. You need to consider the client's religion, because religion may influence dietary practices. Review pertinent laboratory, radiology and endoscopy reports. Remember that the focused interview builds on all previously collected data. You may want to review the discussions of the health history and nutritional assessment in Chapters 2 and 5, respectively.

Physical assessment is the second source for data, and you must perform it systematically. You use the usual four assessment techniques but in a different sequence. First, you inspect, as for all other systems. Next, you auscultate in all quadrants using the bell and diaphragm of the stethoscope. Postpone percussion and palpation, because these techniques may disturb the client's natural bowel sounds. During auscultation, listen for both bowel and vascular sounds. Next percuss all areas. The amount of air in the underlying structure influences the produced sound. Perform palpation last, using both light and deep palpation. Always determine the client's level of comfort before proceeding. If the client reports pain in any area, palpate this area last. If palpation increases the client's pain, end the assessment at that time.

You may want to review the discussion of percussion, description of produced sounds, and palpation in Chapter 7.

Focused Interview

Use open-ended statements to begin the focused interview. The data you collect now builds on the health history. Review data from the health history regarding family history of gastrointestinal disease and abdominal surgery.

Questions Related to the Gastrointestinal System

1. Describe your appetite. Has it changed in the last 24 hours? In the last month? In the last year? Has your weight changed? Tell me what you have had to eat and drink in the last 24 hours. Be sure to include snacks. How much of each item did you consume? Is this a typical eating pattern for you? *You are building on the nutritional data already collected. You are establishing the client's dietary patterns, paying special attention to overconsumption and underconsumption.*
2. How much coffee, tea, cola, alcoholic beverages, or chocolate do you eat in a 24-hour period? *Caffeine and alcohol irritate the gastrointestinal system and can contribute to ulcers and irritable-bowel syndrome.*
3. Do you associate any foods with problems such as indigestion, pain, nausea, vomiting, constipation, diarrhea, belching, or gas? Do you avoid these foods? *You are assessing self-care practices, the client's knowledge base, and food intolerance.*
4. Do you experience nausea or vomiting? If so, when did you last experience them? What was the cause, in your opinion? How frequently do you have this experience? What do you do to relieve the symptoms? When you vomit, describe what comes up and the amount. *Any of these symptoms can be related to a variety of pathologic conditions, eg, food poisoning, ulcers, varices of the esophagus, hepatitis, and beginning of an intestinal obstruction.*
5. Do you have any difficulty chewing or swallowing your food? Do you wear dentures? Do you have any crowns? Do your gums bleed easily? *Ill-fitting dentures, failure to wear them, and missing or diseased teeth make chewing and swallowing difficult. Disorders of the throat and esophagus can also make swallowing difficult.*
6. Describe your bowel habits. Describe the color and consistency of your stool. Do you have pain? Do you notice any blood? Do you suffer from diarrhea or constipation? What do you think is the cause? What have you done to correct the situation? Have these measures helped the situation? Do you experience any rectal itching or bleeding? *Dark, tarry stool indicates bleeding, usually in the upper or middle part of the intestinal tract. Bright red (frank) blood usually indicates lower tract bleeding. A gray or clay-colored stool indicates lack of bile in the intestinal tract.*
7. Do you work with any chemical irritants? *Exposure to benzol, lead, and nickel may lead to gastric irritation. Excessive exposure to chemical hepatotoxins such as carbon tetrachloride may lead to postnecrotic cirrhosis.*
8. Have you recently done any traveling? Where did you travel? *Water purification and food storage methods vary in different regions and different countries. Exposure to food- or water-borne microorganisms can lead to gastroenteritis, hepatitis, diarrhea, or parasite infestation.*
9. How would you describe your stress level? Do you think you are coping well? Could your coping be better? *Prolonged stress is linked to gastrointestinal disease.*

10. Are you having any abdominal pain at this time? Where is it? Is it constant? Does it radiate? What do you think is causing the pain? What do you do to relieve the pain? *Pain could indicate cardiac disease, ulcers, cholecystitis (inflammation of the gallbladder), renal calculi, diverticulitis, labor, urinary cystitis, or ectopic pregnancy. To determine proper action, obtain as much data as possible regarding the pain.*

Additional Questions with Infants, Children, and Adolescents

1. Is the baby breast-fed or bottle-fed? Does the baby tolerate the feeding? How frequently does the baby eat? Have you recently started the baby on any new foods? Is the baby colicky? What do you do to relieve the colic? How much water does the baby drink? *Evaluate gastrointestinal function by the baby's ability to take in nutrients, digest them, and eliminate waste products. The types of formula and food consumed influence color, consistency, amount, and frequency of the stool.*
2. Does the toddler eat at regular times? What and how much? Is the toddler able to feed himself or herself? What type of snacks does the toddler eat? *Eating habits, patterns, and preferences established in the early years of life are likely to have a lasting effect.*
3. Is the child toilet-trained? Describe how you toilet-trained your child. Have there been any lapses in toilet training? If so, how frequently? How recently? How do you typically respond to this? *As the nervous system matures, the child gradually achieves control of the anal sphincter. Explore the developmental level and readiness of the child.*
4. What does the child eat? Does the child bring a lunch and snack to school or buy it at school? When at home, how often does the child snack, and what are the snacks? Does the family have one meal a day together? What kind of food do you eat at this meal? Describe the atmosphere at this meal. *The quality of the food is more important than the quantity of food. Mealtime should be enjoyable. Often this is the only time the family is together.*

Additional Questions with Childbearing Women

1. Are you experiencing any nausea and/or vomiting? *Nausea is common during early pregnancy and may be due to changing hormone levels and changes in carbohydrate metabolism. Fatigue is also a factor. Vomiting is less common. If it occurs more than once a day or for a prolonged period, refer the client to a physician.*
2. Are you experiencing any elimination problems such as constipation? *A number of factors increase the likelihood of constipation during pregnancy. Among these are displacement of the intestines by the growing uterus, bowel sluggishness caused by increased progesterone and steroid metabolism, and the use of oral iron supplements, which are prescribed for many women during pregnancy.*
3. Are you experiencing heartburn or flatulence? *Heartburn (regurgitation of gastric contents into the esophagus) is primarily caused by displacement of the stomach by the enlarging uterus. Flatulence results from the decreased gastrointestinal motility, common during pregnancy, and pressure on the large intestine from the growing uterus.*

Additional Questions with Older Clients

1. Are you ever incontinent of urine or feces? *Muscle tone decreases with age, and the older adult may lose sphincter control.*
2. How often are you constipated? Do you take laxatives? How often? Which one? *Constipation is a common problem with older adults. Influencing factors include decreased peristaltic activity, decreased desire to eat, and self-limited fluid intake. To help relieve the problem, some older clients take over-the-counter laxatives. With prolonged use, laxatives can become habit-forming.*
3. How many foods containing fiber or roughage do you eat during a typical day? *Older adults tend to have diets low in fiber or roughage. Loss of natural teeth and ill-fitting dentures make chewing difficult.*
4. Are you able to get to the store for groceries?
5. Do you eat alone? With someone? *Responses to questions 4 and 5 help determine mobility patterns, availability of food, and social isolation at mealtimes.*

Physical Assessment

Preparation

- ☑ **Gather the equipment.**

examination gown
drape
examination light
gloves
stethoscope
skin-marking pen
ruler
tape measure

- ☑ **Wash your hands.**
- ☑ **Explain the procedure to the client.**
- ☑ **Ask the client to void.**
- ☑ **Be sure the room is warm and draft free with the proper lighting.**

Remember

- Ensure client privacy.
- Use universal precautions.
- Determine if abdominal pain is present before proceeding, and examine the painful area last.
- Vary the usual sequence of techniques. Follow this order: inspection, auscultation, percussion, and palpation.
- Visualize the underlying structures before proceeding.
- Have the client relax the abdominal muscles by taking several deep breaths.
- Observe the client for nonverbal signs of pain or discomfort, including facial grimaces, legs flexed at knees and hips, and abdominal guarding with hands.
- Stand on the right side of the client unless otherwise indicated. This conserves the nurse's energy, because the liver, spleen, and right kidney are assessed from the client's right side.

ASSESSMENT TECHNIQUE/NORMAL FINDINGS

SPECIAL CONSIDERATIONS

Inspection

Step 1 *Position the client.*

- Place the client in a supine position.
- Place a small pillow under the client's head and knees.
- Drape the examination gown over the chest, exposing the abdomen. Place the drape at the symphisis pubis, covering the client's pelvic area and legs (Figure 13.7).

These measures relax the abdominal musculature and prevent unnecessary exposure of the client.

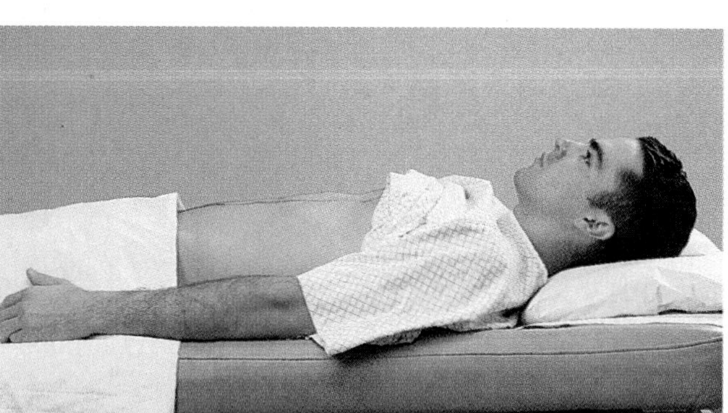

Figure 13.7 Client positioned and draped.

Step 2 *Map the abdomen.*

- Visualize the imaginary horizontal and vertical lines delineating either the abdominal quadrants or regions.
- Visualize the underlying structures.

Step 3 *Determine the contour of the abdomen.*

- Observe the profile of the abdomen between the costal margins and the symphysis pubis.

You may need to assume a sitting or kneeling position, because the abdominal profile should be at eye level.

Normal findings include the flat, rounded, or scaphoid abdomen. See the box on page 349 for description of these terms.

A protuberant abdomen is normal in pregnancy. It may indicate obesity or ascites in a nonpregnant client (see the box on page 349).

ASSESSMENT TECHNIQUE/NORMAL FINDINGS | SPECIAL CONSIDERATIONS

Contour of the Abdomen

Flat. A straight horizontal line is observed from the costal margin to the symphysis pubis.
This contour is common in a thin person.

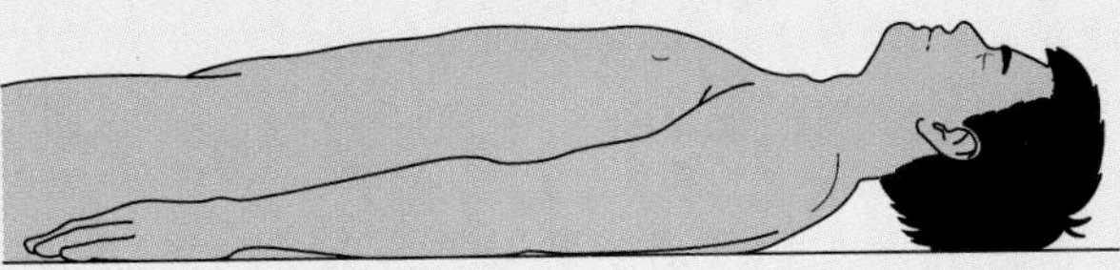

Flat

Scaphoid. Sometimes called a concave abdomen.
The horizontal line now curves inward toward the vertebral column, giving the abdomen a sunken appearance. In the adult, this contour is seen in the very thin person.

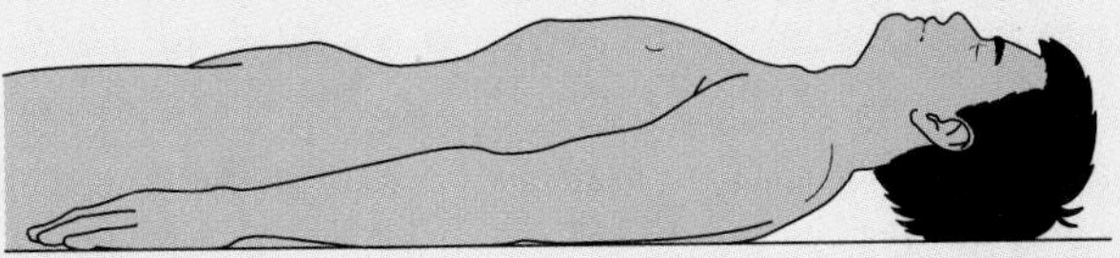

Scaphoid

Rounded. Sometimes called a convex abdomen.
The horizontal line now curves outward, indicating an increase in abdominal fat or a decrease in muscle tone.
This contour is considered a normal variation in the toddler and the pregnant female.

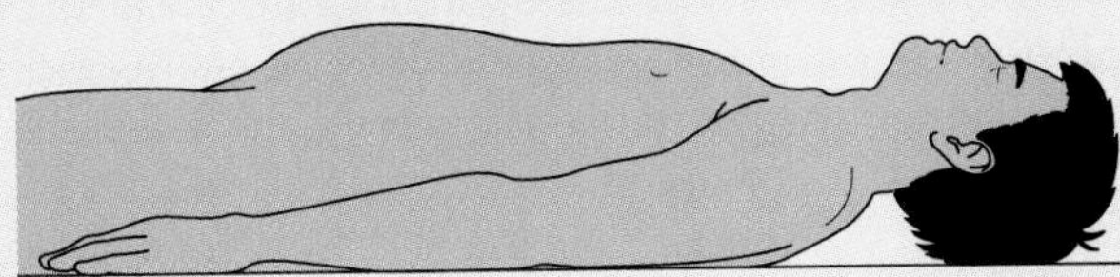

Rounded

Protuberant. Similar to the rounded abdomen, only greater. This contour is anticipated in pregnancy. It is also seen in the adult with obesity, ascites, and other conditions.

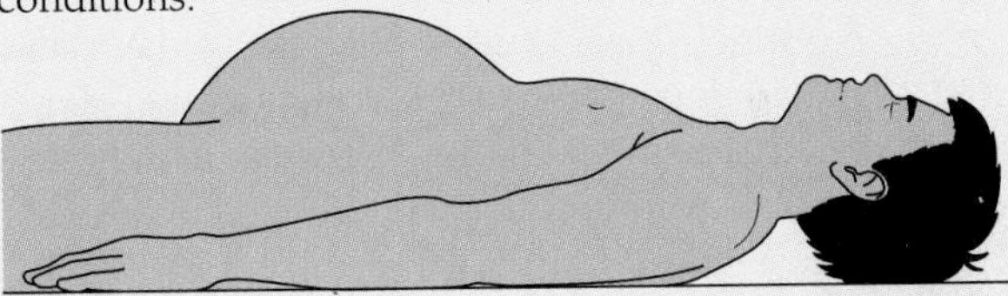

Protuberant

Step 4 ***Observe the location of the umbilicus.***

The umbilicus is normally in the center of the abdomen, inverted or protruding. It should be clean and free of drainage or inflammation.

A protruding or displaced umbilicus is considered a normal variation in the pregnant woman. In the nonpregnant adult, it could indicate an abdominal mass or distended urinary bladder. Accompanying drainage or inflammation could indicate an infectious process or a complication of recent laparoscopic surgery. In a child, a protruding or displaced umbilicus could indicate a hernia.

Referral

A client with drainage from the umbilicus following laparoscopic surgery should be referred to the physician immediately.

Step 5 ***Observe the skin of the abdomen.***

The abdominal skin should be consistent in color and luster with the skin of the rest of the body.

- Observe the location and characteristics of scars.

Taut, glistening skin may indicate abdominal ascites.

Striae, commonly called stretch marks, are silvery, shiny, irregular markings on the skin. These are common in obesity, pregnancy, and ascites (see Chapter 8).

Scars indicate previous surgery and the possibility of underlying adhesions.

ASSESSMENT TECHNIQUE/NORMAL FINDINGS	SPECIAL CONSIDERATIONS

Step 6 ***Observe the abdomen for symmetry, bulging, or masses.***

- First observe the abdomen while standing at the client's side.
- Now observe the abdomen while standing at the foot of the bed or table, comparing the right and left sides.
- Return to the client's side and shine your light across the client's abdomen.

The light produces a shadow on small bulges or masses.

- Place yourself in a sitting or kneeling position, and continue to shine the light and observe the abdomen.
- Look for symmetry. Check for bulging or masses.

A bulge could indicate a tumor, cyst, or hernia.

- You may repeat the above procedure asking the client to take a deep breath and to raise the head off the pillow.

Deep breathing and head raising accentuate masses.

Step 7 ***Observe the abdominal wall for movement.***

The movements could be pulsations or peristaltic waves. In a thin adult, it is common to observe a pulsation of the abdominal aorta below the xiphoid process. Peristaltic waves are also a normal finding in the thin adult with a well-relaxed muscle wall. They produce a rippling motion.

Although these findings are considered normal, you must also rule out disease. Marked pulsations could indicate aortic aneurysm or increased pulse pressure. Increased peristaltic activity could indicate gastroenteritis or an obstructive process.

Auscultation

Use the diaphragm of the stethoscope to listen for bowel sounds and the bell to listen for vascular sounds. See the box below for a summary of abdominal sounds heard with auscultation.

Bowel sounds are relatively high in pitch and are heard better with the diaphragm.

ALERT!

Remember to auscultate before percussing and palpating, because the latter techniques could alter peristaltic action.

Abdominal Sounds Heard upon Auscultation

Bowel sounds. Movement of the gastrointestinal tract produces irregular, gurgling, high-pitched sounds.

Borborygmi. Similar to bowel sounds, but more frequent. Borborygmi signals increased movement of the gastrointestinal tract and produces loud, high-pitched, gurgling sounds. Commonly heard with hunger and diarrhea.

Bruit. A blowing or swishing sound indicating an obstruction in the vessel.

Venous hum. A soft, low-pitched, vibrating sound. This bruit-like sound is an indication of liver or splenic disease.

Friction rub. A rough, grating sound indicating irritation of the peritoneum. near spleen

ASSESSMENT TECHNIQUE/NORMAL FINDINGS | SPECIAL CONSIDERATIONS

Step 1 ***Ausculate for bowel sounds.***

- Use the diaphragm of the stethoscope.
- Begin auscultation in the right lower quadrant (RLQ) over the ileocecal junction of the intestines (Figure 13.8).

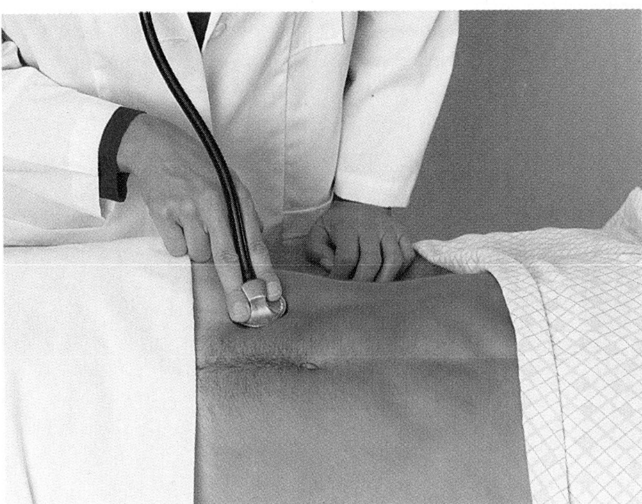

Figure 13.8 Auscultating the abdomen for bowel sounds.

- Note the character and frequency of sounds.
- Count sounds for at least 60 seconds.

Bowel sounds travel throughout the abdominal cavity. Nevertheless, it is a good idea to auscultate in all four quadrants. Normal sounds are irregular, gurgling, and high in pitch. They occur from 5 to 30 times per minute. You may hear *borborygmi* (commonly called stomach growling) in a client who has not eaten in a few hours.

Hyperactive sounds are loud, high-pitched, and rushing. They are common with gastroenteritis or diarrhea.

Hypoactive sounds are common following abdominal surgery or end-stage obstruction.

Absent sounds may be indicative of a paralytic ileus.

ALERT!

It may be difficult for the beginning practitioner to hear bowel sounds in some clients. Always auscultate all four quadrants for a total of *at least 5 minutes* before documenting absent bowel sounds.

Referral

Clients with intestinal obstruction or paralytic ileus require immediate medical attention.

Step 2 ***Auscultate for vascular sounds.***

- Use the bell of the stethoscope.
- Listen over the abdominal aorta and renal, iliac, and femoral arteries (Figure 13.9 on page 352).

Bruits are vascular sounds that are pulsatile and blowing. They sound similar to heart murmurs (see Chapter 11). When heard during systole and diastole, they may be indicative of partial arterial occlusion.

A *venous hum* (soft, continuous, and low-pitched) in the abdomen usually indicates increased portal tension.

ASSESSMENT TECHNIQUE/NORMAL FINDINGS	SPECIAL CONSIDERATIONS

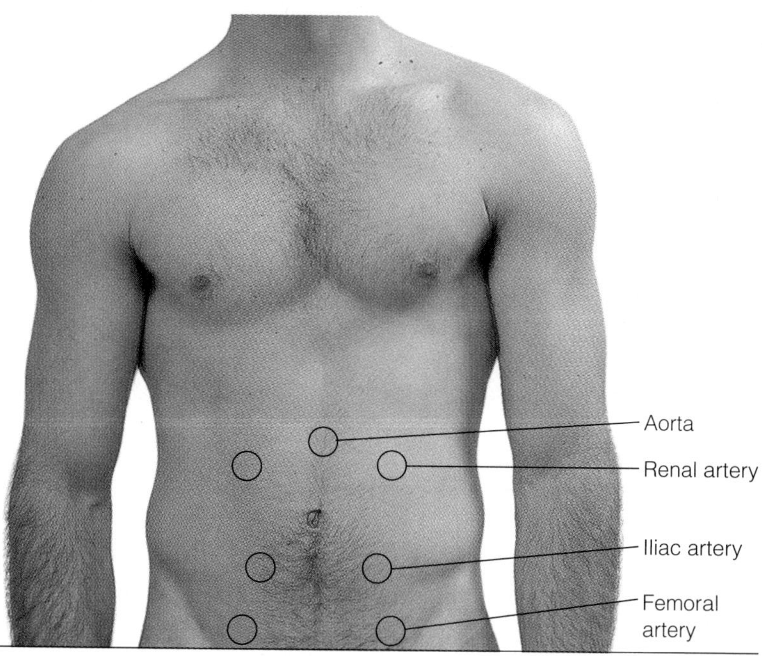

Figure 13.9 Auscultatory areas for vascular sounds.

Step 3 ***Auscultate for a friction rub.***

- Auscultate the abdomen, listening for a coarse, grating sound.
- Listen carefully over the liver and spleen.

Friction rubs are not normally heard.

Friction rubs are caused by two organs rubbing together or by an organ rubbing against the peritoneum (peritoneal friction rub). A friction rub in the abdomen usually indicates tumor, infection, infarct, or peritonitis and requires further medical evaluation.

Percussion

The accompanying box provides a summary of abdominal sounds heard with percussion.

Abdominal Sounds Heard upon Percussion

Tympany. A loud hollow sound should be obtained in the four quadrants. They are loudest over the gastric bubble and intestines.

Dullness. A short, high-pitched sound heard over liver, spleen, and distended bladder.

Hyperresonance. Louder than tympany. Heard over air-filled or distended intestines.

Flat. A very soft, short, abrupt sound. This is heard when no air is present in the structure, as over muscle, bone, or tumor mass.

ASSESSMENT TECHNIQUE/NORMAL FINDINGS

SPECIAL CONSIDERATIONS

Step 1 *Percuss the four quadrants of the abdomen to determine the amount of tympany and dullness* (Figure 13.10).

Dullness may indicate an enlarged uterus, distended urinary bladder, or ascites.

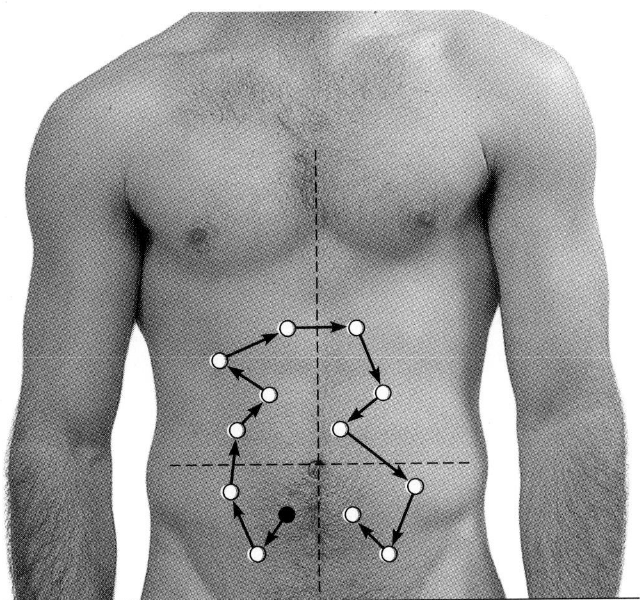

Figure 13.10 Percussion pattern for abdomen.

Normally, you hear tympany because of the air in the underlying structures.

Percussion over the liver and spleen produces a dull sound.

Step 2 *Percuss the liver.*

- Percuss the abdomen to determine the upper and lower borders or the height of the liver.
- Begin percussion at the level of the umbilicus and move toward the rib cage along the extended right midclavicular line (Figure 13.11).

Dullness below the costal margin suggests liver enlargement or downward displacement due to respiratory disease.

Dullness above the fifth or sixth intercostal space could indicate an enlarged liver, upward displacement due to ascites, or an abdominal mass.

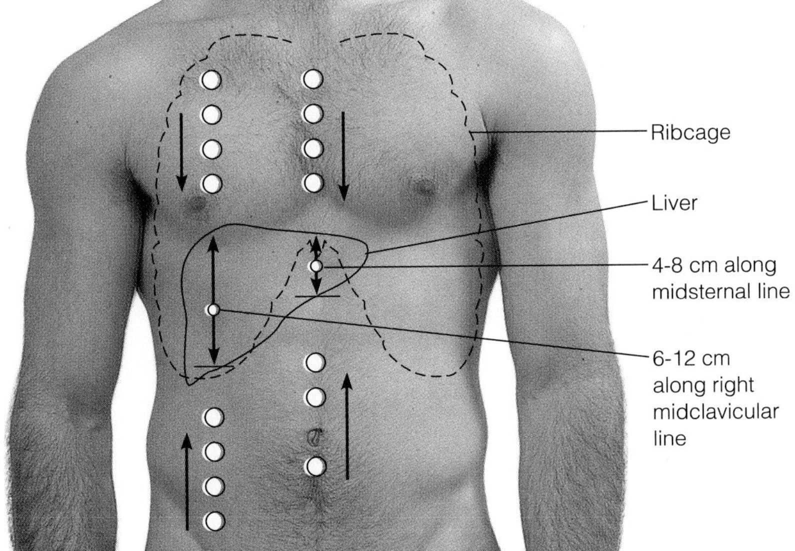

Figure 13.11 Percussion pattern for liver.

ASSESSMENT TECHNIQUE/NORMAL FINDINGS	SPECIAL CONSIDERATIONS

The first sound you should hear is tympany. When the sound changes to dullness, you have identified the lower border of the liver.

- Mark the point with the skin-marking pen. This is usually at the costal margin.
- Percuss downward from the fourth intercostal space along the right midclavicular line.

The first sound should be resonance, because you are percussing over the lung.

- Continue to percuss downward until you hear dullness. This is the upper border of the liver.
- Mark the point.

The upper border will most likely be at the level of the sixth intercostal space. The distance between the two points should be approximately 5 to 10 centimeters (2 to 4 inches).

- Percuss along the midsternal line using the same technique as before.

The liver size at the midsternal line should be about 4 to 9 centimeters (1½ to 3 inches).

- To determine movement of liver with breathing, ask the client to take a deep breath and hold it. Percuss upward along the extended right midclavicular line.

Movement of the liver is diminished in the presence of an atelectasis or pneumothorax of the right lung.

The lower liver border should descend about 1 inch. Remember that liver size is influenced by age, gender, height, and disease processes.

Step 3 *Percuss to determine the size and location of the spleen.*

- Percuss the left side of abdomen posterior to the midaxillary line (Figure 13.12).

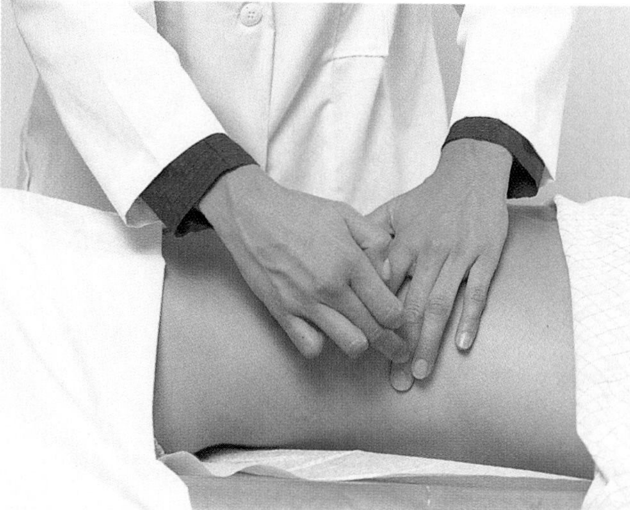

Figure 13.12 Percussing the spleen.

Splenic dullness at the left anterior axillary line indicates *splenomegaly*, an enlarged spleen (Figure 13.13). The dull percussion sound is identifiable before an enlarged spleen is palpable. The spleen enlarges anteriorly and inferiorly.

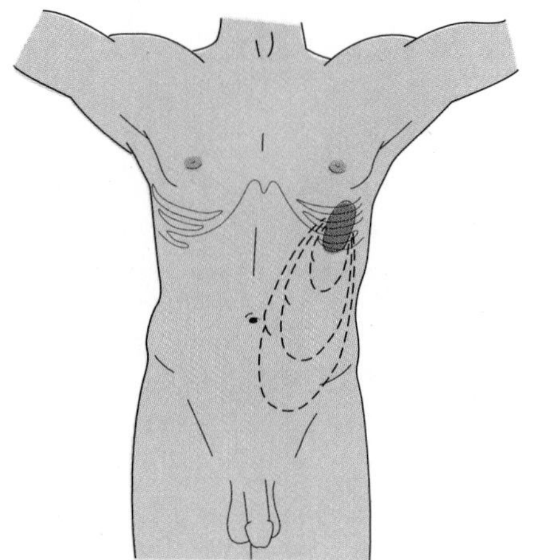

Figure 13.13 Splenic enlargement.

ASSESSMENT TECHNIQUE/NORMAL FINDINGS

A small area of splenic dullness will most likely be heard from the sixth to tenth intercostal space.

The contents of the stomach and intestines influence the sound percussed.

Step 4 ***Percuss the gastric bubble.***

The gastric bubble is located in the area between the left costal margin and the midsternal line extended below the xiphoid process.

- Listen for a low-pitched sound of tympany to determine the area occupied by the stomach. This sound is influenced by the contents of the stomach.

SPECIAL CONSIDERATIONS

A dull percussion sound in this area suggests a mass of the stomach.

A very loud sound and an increased area suggest gastric dilation.

Palpation

Palpate the abdomen to determine organ size and placement, muscle tightness or guarding, masses, tenderness, and presence of fluid. Identify painful areas before proceeding, and palpate these areas last. You use both light and deep palpation. Your hands must be warm. The client must be as relaxed as possible. For a discussion of palpation of the kidneys, see Chapter 14.

Step 1 ***Lightly palpate the abdomen.***

- Place the palmar surface of your hand on the abdomen and extend your fingers.
- Lightly press into the abdomen with your fingers (Figure 13.14).

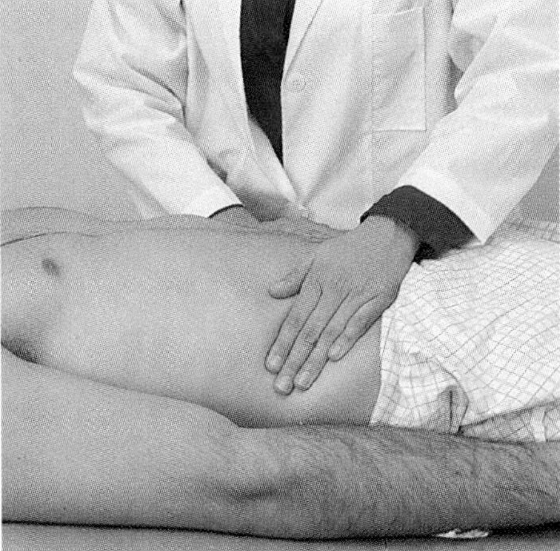

Figure 13.14 Light palpation of abdomen.

- Move your hand over the four quadrants by lifting the hand and then placing it in another area. *Do not* drag or slide your hand across the skin surface.

The abdomen should be soft, smooth, nontender, and pain free.

SPECIAL CONSIDERATIONS

Muscle tightness or guarding may indicate abdominal pain.

Abdominal pain from an organ is often referred to the surface of the abdomen or back (Figure 13.15 on page 356).

ASSESSMENT TECHNIQUE/NORMAL FINDINGS

SPECIAL CONSIDERATIONS

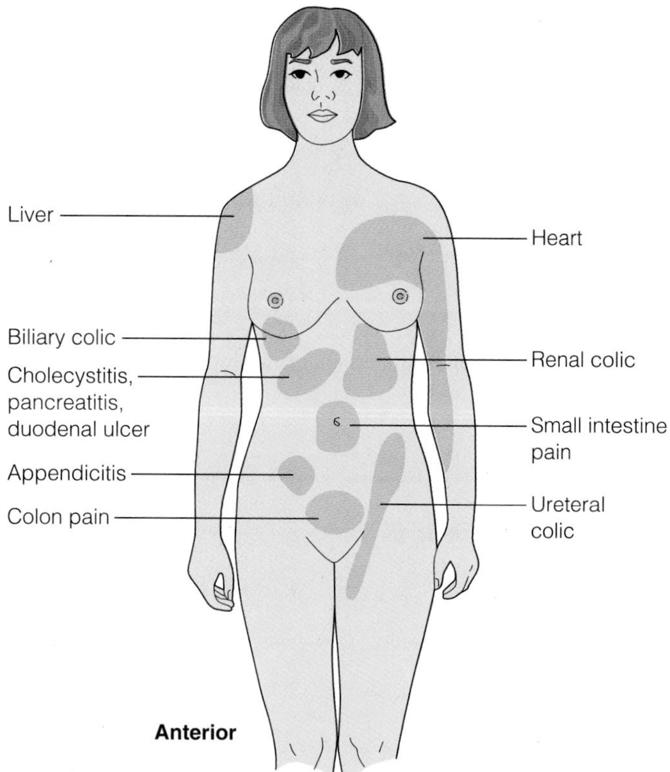

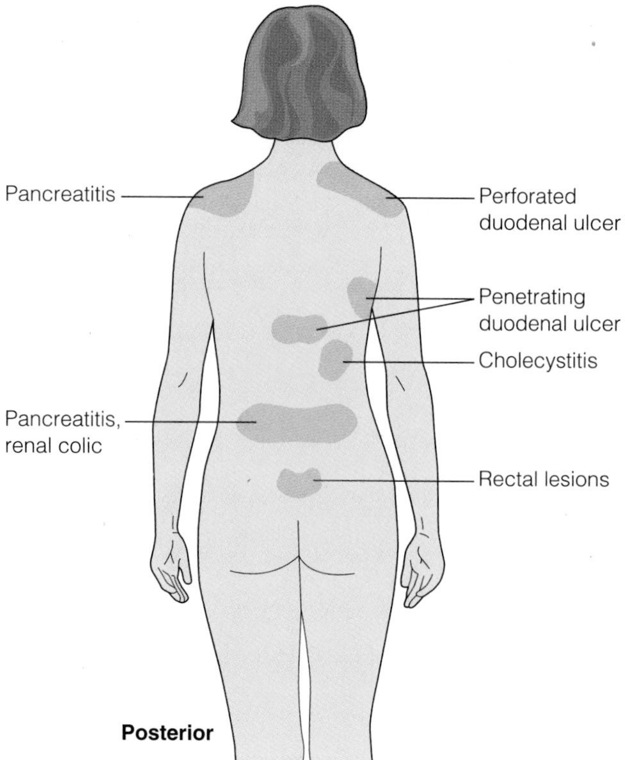

Figure 13.15 Referred cutaneous pain areas: *A*, Anterior; *B*, Posterior.

ASSESSMENT TECHNIQUE/NORMAL FINDINGS	SPECIAL CONSIDERATIONS

Step 2 ***Palpate the abdomen using a moderate amount of pressure.***

- Proceed as for light palpation, described in the previous step.
- Exert pressure with your hand to depress the abdomen about 2 inches.

Masses, tumors, or intestinal obstructions may be palpated.

A distended urinary bladder is palpable above the symphysis pubis as a smooth, tense mass.

- Be sure to palpate in the four quadrants in an organized sequence.
- For the obese client or client with an enlarged abdomen, use a bimanual technique: place the fingers of your nondominant hand over your dominant hand (Figure 13.16).

In the pregnant woman, the uterus is palpable. The height or placement of the fundus varies according to the week of gestation.

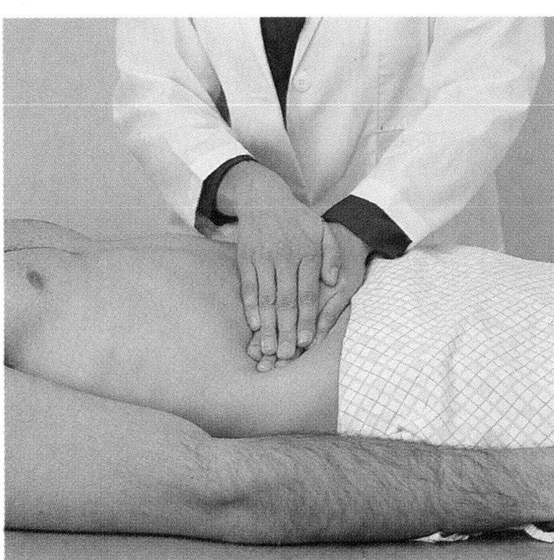

Figure 13.16 Deep palpation of abdomen.

- Identify the size of the underlying organs, any tenderness or masses.

Note that the pancreas is nonpalpable because of its small size and deep location.

A mass in the LLQ may be feces in the colon.

A vaguely palpable sensation of fullness in the epigastric region may be of pancreatic origin.

Step 3 ***Attempt to palpate the liver.***

- Stand on the client's right side.
- Place your left hand under the lower portion of the rib cage (ribs 11 and 12).
- Instruct the client to relax into your left hand.
- Lift the rib cage with your left hand.
- Place your right hand gently but firmly into the abdomen, using an upward and inward thrust along the costal margin (Figure 13.17).

ASSESSMENT TECHNIQUE/NORMAL FINDINGS

SPECIAL CONSIDERATIONS

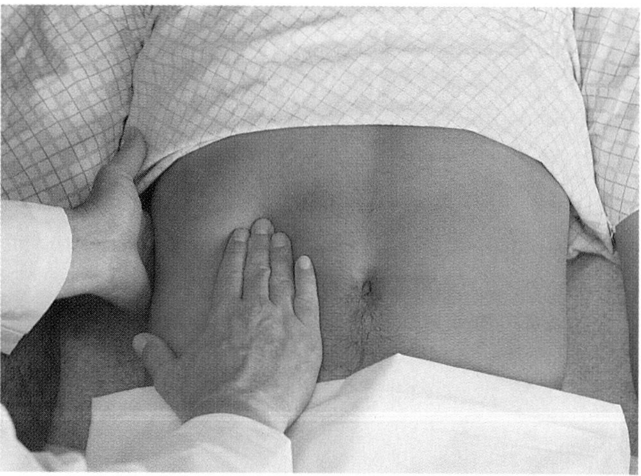

Figure 13.17 Palpating the liver.

- Ask the client to take a deep breath. The diaphragm will descend, causing the lower edge of the liver to meet your right hand.

Normally the liver is nonpalpable, except in some thin clients. The lower edge, if you can feel it, should be smooth, firm, and nontender.

The client should not have pain during this procedure.

Pain on palpation indicates gallbladder disease, acute hepatitis, or enlarged liver associated with congestive heart failure.

If you feel nodules, suspect metastatic carcinoma or cirrhosis. All of these conditions require further medical evaluation.

Step 5 *Attempt to palpate the spleen.*

- Stand on the client's right side.
- Place your left hand beneath the left lower rib cage and elevate the cage. This maneuver moves the spleen anteriorly.
- Press the fingertips of your right hand into the left costal margin area of the client (Figure 13.18).

Splenomegaly occurs with acute infections such as mononucleosis. Be gentle when palpating an enlarged spleen, because it is very sensitive and fragile.

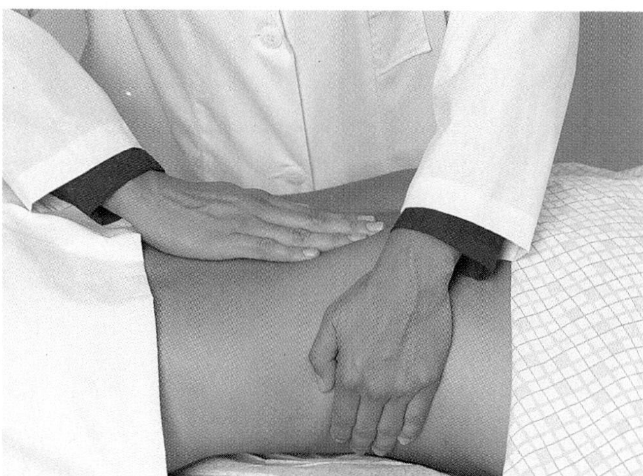

Figure 13.18 Palpating the spleen.

ASSESSMENT TECHNIQUE/NORMAL FINDINGS | SPECIAL CONSIDERATIONS

- Ask the client to take a slow deep breath through the mouth.

As the diaphragm descends, the spleen moves toward the fingertips of your right hand.

However, the spleen is usually not palpable unless it is greatly enlarged.

Additional Procedures

Step 1 *Palpate the aorta for pulsations.*

- Using your fingertips, press firmly and deeply in the upper abdomen to the left of the midline below the xiphoid process.

The average normal adult aortic width is 3 cm.

Obesity and abdominal masses make aortic palpation difficult.

A widened aorta may suggest an aneurysm.

> **ALERT!**
>
> If you see a strong, wide, abdominal pulsation, do not palpate.

Step 2 *Palpate for rebound tenderness.*

- With the client in a supine position, hold your hand at a 90-degree angle to the abdominal wall in an area of no pain or discomfort.
- Press deeply into the abdomen, moving your fingers in a slow, steady manner (Figure 13.19, *A*).
- Rapidly remove your fingers from the abdomen (Figure 13.19, *B*).

The client with peritoneal irritation experiences a sharp, stabbing pain as the compressed structures return to a precompressed state. This is a positive *Blumberg sign*.

Rovsing's sign is positive when the client experiences pain in the lower-right quadrant when you exert pressure in the lower-left quadrant. This pain may be due to peritoneal irritation or appendicitis.

> ***Referral***
>
> Clients with positive Blumberg or Rovsing's signs should be referred to a physician immediately.

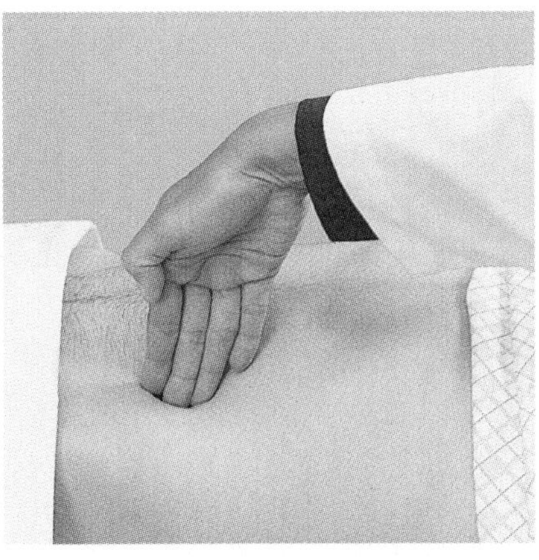

A

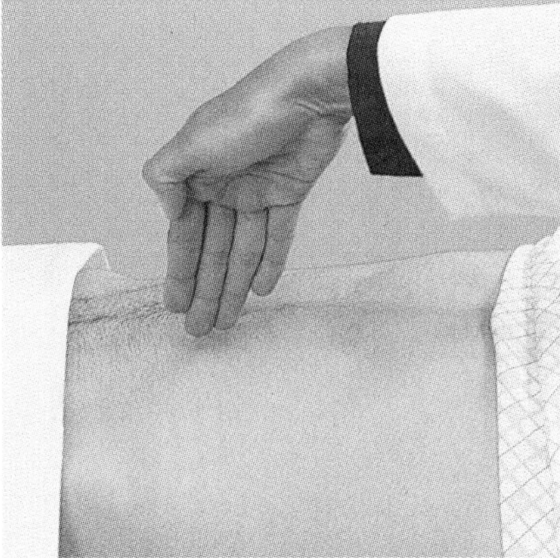

B

Figure 13.19 Palpating for rebound tenderness.

Step 3 *Percuss the abdomen for ascites.*

Ascites is an abnormal collection of serous fluid in the peritoneal cavity.

Remember that gravity causes fluid to be dependent (settle) at the lowest possible level.

Ascites is a common finding in clients with congestive heart failure, cirrhosis of the liver, or renal disease.

ASSESSMENT TECHNIQUE/NORMAL FINDINGS

SPECIAL CONSIDERATIONS

- Start with the client in a supine position and draped as previously described.
- Percuss at the midline and determine a sound of tympany (Figure 13.20).
- Continue to percuss toward lateral aspects and listen for dullness (Figure 13.20).

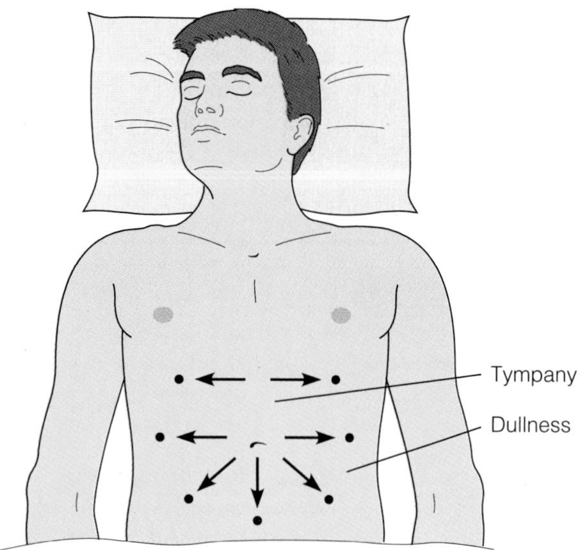

Figure 13.20 Percussion pattern for ascites.

- Mark the skin, identifying possible levels of fluid.

Here is an alternative technique:

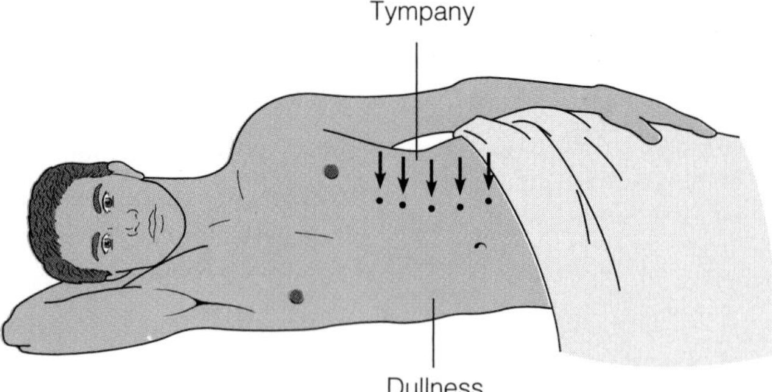

Figure 13.21 Alternate percussion pattern for ascites.

- Position the client on his or her right side (Figure 13.21).
- Percuss the abdomen.
- Because fluid settles, anticipate tympany at a superior level and dullness at an inferior level.

ASSESSMENT TECHNIQUE/NORMAL FINDINGS

SPECIAL CONSIDERATIONS

When you suspect ascites, you may wish to measure the abdominal girth with a tape measure.

Step 4 *Test for the psoas sign.*

Perform this test when lower abdominal pain is present and you suspect appendicitis.

- Assist the client to a supine position.
- Place your right hand just above the level of the client's right knee.
- Ask the client to raise the right leg to meet your hand.

During this maneuver, an inflamed appendix causes pain by irritating the psoas muscle during contraction.

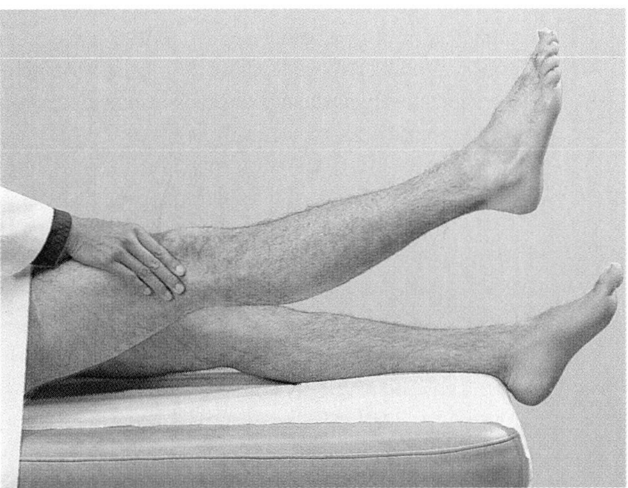

Figure 13.22 Psoas sign.

Flexion of the hip causes contraction of the psoas muscle (Figure 13.22).

Step 5 *Test for Murphy's sign.*

In a normal client, palpation of the liver causes no pain. The client might complain of pressure from the examiner's hand; however, pain is not present.

- While palpating the liver, ask the client to take a deep breath.

The diaphragm descends, pushing the liver and gallbladder toward your fingers.

Murphy's sign is positive if the client experiences sharp abdominal pain and immediately halts the inspiration. It is typically present in the client with cholecystitis (inflammation of the gallbladder).

Many practitioners conclude the abdominal assessment with an assessment of the rectum. This is discussed in Chapter 15.

Reminders

- After completing the assessment of the abdomen, assist the client to a comfortable position. Be sure the client has no adverse effects from the procedures.
- Assist the client with dressing if needed.
- Answer any questions the client has, discuss your findings, and provide client teaching to decrease risk factors and promote health and self-care.
- In addition to the previous steps of physical assessment, consider variations for the different client groups discussed in the following section.
- Document the assessment findings as described in Chapter 1. See pages 364–366 for data regarding nursing diagnoses commonly associated with the abdomen.

Developmental Considerations

Infants, Children, and Adolescent Clients

Use the same assessment techniques with younger clients as with adults. You may need to alter your routine to gather the necessary data. Employ the help of the parent or caregiver to gain the cooperation of the child.

The abdomen of the newborn and infant is round. The toddler has a characteristic "potbelly" appearance, which persists until about the fifth year (Figure 13.23). The respirations of toddlers are abdominal; therefore, anticipate abdominal movement with respirations. This breathing pattern is evident until about the sixth year, at which age respirations become thoracic.

The size of the abdomen at all ages is an indication of the nutritional state of the child. For children of all ages, ascertain feeding habits and tolerance of the feeding. Determine the symptoms and the actions taken by the parent or caregiver.

In infants, inspect the umbilical stump. The stump has two arteries and one vein and should be clean and dry. A protrusion around the umbilicus at any age is suggestive of an umbilical hernia and needs further evaluation (Figure 13.24). Be sure to determine any home remedies the parents or caregivers may be using.

Peristaltic waves are usually more visible in infants and children than in adults. Use tangential lighting and keep the abdominal wall at eye level during inspection. This inspection is especially important if the parent or caregiver has reported frequent episodes of vomiting.

Auscultation of the abdomen should reveal bowel sounds. Bruits are indicative of vascular stenosis.

Tympany is a more common percussion finding in children than in adults because children tend to swallow more air when eating.

With children, you follow the same principles of palpation as with adults. Use both light and deep palpation, and make sure that the child relaxes the musculature of the abdomen before proceeding. Tenderness or pain may be difficult to detect. Any mass that is palpated needs further assessment.

Congenital defects such as cleft lip, cleft palate, esophageal atresia, tracheoesophageal fistula, pyloric stenosis, and hernias influence the nutritional status, growth, and development of the child and must be assessed with care.

When assessing the adolescent, employ the same techniques used for adults. See Chapter 19 for a complete assessment of infants, children, and adolescents.

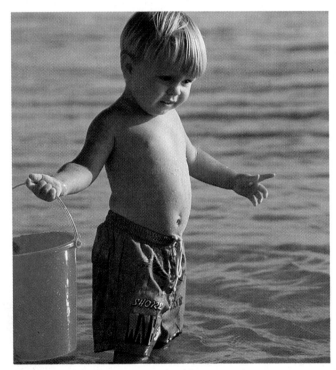

Figure 13.23 Potbelly stance of toddler.

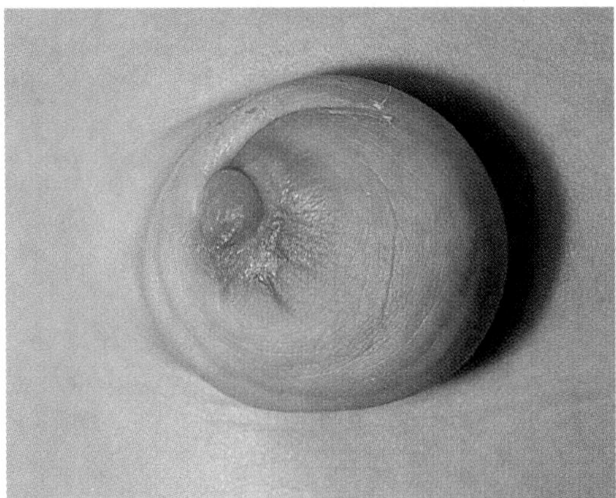

Figure 13.24 Umbilical hernia.

Childbearing Clients

During pregnancy, the abdomen undergoes many changes. As the pregnancy progresses, the uterus enlarges and moves into the abdominal cavity. Measure the height of the fundus and compare it against predictable levels based on the gestational week. By the 14th week of the pregnancy, the fundus should be above the pubic bone and easily palpable. By the 36th week, the fundus is high in the abdomen, close to the diaphragm, and compresses many abdominal structures. Constipation, flatulence, and hemorrhoids are common problems resulting from the displacement of abdominal organs and pressure from the uterus.

Changing levels of hormones decrease peristaltic activity, leading to a decrease in bowel sounds. The decrease in motility may cause nausea, vomiting, and constipation.

The skin of the abdomen undergoes some characteristic changes. *Striae gravidarum* (stretch marks) become most visible during the second half of the pregnancy. You may see a *linea nigra*, a dark line extending from the pubic bone to the umbilicus along the midline.

The muscles of the abdominal wall are stretched and may lose tone. Exercise restores tone following birth. See Chapter 20 for a complete assessment of the childbearing client.

Older Clients

The digestive system of the older adult undergoes characteristic changes; however, these may not be as pronounced as changes in other systems. There is a gradual decrease in secretion of digestive enzymes, peristalsis, intestinal absorption, and intestinal activity. These changes may lead to indigestion, constipation, and gastroesophageal reflux and could exacerbate any pre-existing changes or disease.

The loss of teeth makes chewing and swallowing of food difficult. Ill-fitting, broken, or lost dentures also prejudice nutritional status.

Constipation is a common problem with older adults. Many factors contribute to the problem of constipation. Periodontal disease with the subsequent loss of natural teeth is one such factor. Lack of fruits and vegetables or other sources of bulk or fiber contributes to the pattern of constipation. Other factors include self-limiting the daily fluid intake, especially of water, and leading a more sedentary lifestyle. Some older clients rely on the use of laxatives or enemas to achieve regular bowel movements. Explore this practice carefully with the client.

Abdominal assessment of the older adult is similar to that of the younger adult. Begin with a focused interview that explores dietary habits and history of gastrointestinal problems. The client may present a long history of previous diseases and abdominal surgeries; however, it is imperative to assess the present implications of this data.

As the client advances in age, the size of the liver decreases, and the liver borders determined during percussion change accordingly. The liver may also descend below the costal margin as a direct result of pulmonary disease.

When performing the physical assessment, modify your procedures to accommodate the physiologic changes that occur in the older adult. Inspection of the abdomen of the older adult may reveal a rounded or protuberant profile due to increased adipose tissue distribution and decreased muscle tone of the abdominal wall. Because of decreased muscle tone and reduced fibro-connective tissue, the abdomen tends to be softer and more relaxed than in the younger adult, requiring less pressure during palpation. Because of their increased pain threshold, older adults do not experience or exhibit painful responses to assessment maneuvers as readily as a younger person, making it more difficult for you to identify problems. Other age-related changes predispose the older adult to obstruction, reflux, carcinoma, hernias, and perforations of the gastrointestinal tract. A complete assessment of the older client is found in Chapter 21.

Psychosocial Considerations

A client's self-perception may have a subtle influence on the client's weight. Clients who perceive themselves as naturally thin may show greater dedication to restricting their calorie intake and exercising to maintain that self-image. Conversely, clients who perceive themselves as naturally fat may overeat and avoid exercise, feeling that there is nothing they can do to alter their weight.

Surgical scars may alter a client's body image. Many times gastrointestinal surgery ends with a colostomy, which might be a temporary or permanent change. Many adults consider "wearing a bag" a significant limitation. They may withdraw socially, becoming depressed and unable to function.

Abdominal problems that may be either caused or aggravated by stress include gastritis, gastric and duodenal ulcers, ulcerative colitis, and irritable colon. Relaxation techniques such as meditation, guided imagery, and biofeedback have been shown to help some clients reduce stress.

Self-Care Considerations

Self-care considerations need to focus on diet, weight control, and exercise. Diet, the amount and type of food consumed, influences gastrointestinal activity as well as the client's weight. It is important to eat a well-balanced diet. See Chapter 5 for more information. Exercise helps tone the abdominal muscles and promotes gastrointestinal motility.

Aspirin and ibuprofen may irritate the lining of the stomach. Monitor clients who take aspirin frequently (such as clients with rheumatoid arthritis or chronic headaches) for gastric upset and gastric ulcers. Many other drugs, including caffeine, alcohol, and some prescription drugs may cause gastric irritation in some individuals. Prolonged alcohol intake may lead to chronic gastritis. Heavy drinking over a number of years frequently results in cirrhosis of the liver.

Most smokers usually swallow a certain amount of smoke. Thus, the esophagus and other portions of the gastrointestinal tract are at increased risk from cancer in clients who smoke.

Many abdominal injuries are caused by trauma from automobile accidents. Trauma is reduced greatly in clients who wear seat belts and in children restrained in car seats. Other safety considerations include keeping medications, household chemicals, alcohol, and other products out of the reach of children.

Family, Cultural, and Environmental Considerations

Family and family structure have an important influence on the client's food choices. Clients used to a diet of meat and potatoes may not fully appreciate the value of fresh fruits and vegetables to gastrointestinal health. Culture, customs, and religious practices also influence the foods clients choose to eat. Certain foods may be proscribed in certain cultures or religions; however, a healthy diet usually can be achieved even in cultures with significant food restrictions.

The financial security of the client also has an impact on eating habits. In some areas, certain foods may not be available year-round or may be much more costly than in other areas. For example, fresh fruits and vegetables typically increase in price in many regions in winter months. Unfortunately, highly processed foods are often lower in fiber than their fresh counterparts, and sometimes the financial saving is not significant. The homeless population is at greater risk for undernutrition because of underavailability of food. Additionally, some homeless clients may regularly eat discarded food, which may be spoiled, increasing their risk for gastrointestinal distress.

Organizing the Data

Review and cluster all the data you have gathered. Use your newly developed clusters to identify nursing diagnoses and plan the client's care. You will identify nursing interventions to maintain wellness, promote self-care, reduce risk factors, and limit disease. To ensure consistency and promote continuity of care, all members of the health care team may need to confer.

Identifying Nursing Diagnoses

The first step of the nursing process is data collection. Through the health history, focused interview, and physical assessment, you have gathered data. Now you analyze the data to develop nursing diagnoses. The nursing care plan you develop should reflect client strengths and weaknesses, wellness as well as illness states.

One nursing diagnosis commonly applicable to clients experiencing gastrointestinal problems is *Bowel incontinence*. Bowel incontinence is a state in which an individual experiences a change in normal bowel habits characterized by involuntary passage of stool (NANDA). The involuntary passage of feces may occur at specific times during the day or it may occur at regular intervals. Incontinence is associated with decreased control of the anal sphincter, a change in the neurologic impulse to the lower colon, and other pathologic conditions such as spinal cord injury. Regardless of the cause, incontinence lowers the individual's self-esteem and may lead to *Social isolation*. Many clients view the use of adult disposable undergarments (diapers) as regressive behavior, and their use can further lower self-esteem and deepen the social isolation. See Table 13.1 for further information on bowel incontinence.

Constipation is a state in which an individual experiences a change in normal bowel habits characterized by a decrease in frequency and/or passage of hard, dry stool (NANDA). Aging and a decrease in fluid intake, fiber in the diet, daily activity, or exercise all contribute to the problem of constipation. Medications such as ferrous sulfate (Feosol) also contribute to constipation. It is imperative to gather accurate data regarding the regular defecation habits of the client. Because patterns of defecation are highly individual, you need to conduct a thorough assessment before you make a diagnosis of constipation. Table 13.1 provides defining characteristics and related factors.

Diarrhea is a state in which an individual experiences a change in normal bowel habits characterized by the frequent passage of loose, fluid, unformed stools (NANDA). The rapid movement of the chyme through the intestines decreases the ability of large intestines to resorb water and electrolytes, resulting in loose, watery, unformed stool. The individual also experiences lower abdominal pain and cramping with a strong urgency to defecate. The causes of diarrhea are numerous and include, but are not limited to, gastroenteritis, food poisoning, antibiotic therapy, food allergies, and inflammatory bowel disease (Crohn's disease). Lack of complete control of bodily function can lower self-esteem, and the individual may retreat into *Social isolation*. See Table 13.1 for additional information on this nursing diagnosis.

The diagnosis *Altered nutrition: more or less than body requirements* applies to clients who have a weight problem. The weight problem may be due to the client's inability to follow a nutritional plan. *Noncompliance* may be appropriate for

Table 13.1 Nursing Diagnoses Commonly Associated with the GI System

BOWEL INCONTINENCE

Definition: A state in which an individual experiences a change in normal bowel habits characterized by involuntary passage of stool (NANDA).

RELATED FACTORS

Decreased awareness of need to defecate, Loss of sphincter control, Others specific to client (specify).

DEFINING CHARACTERISTICS

Involuntary passage of stool

CONSTIPATION

Definition: A state in which an individual experiences a change in normal bowel habits characterized by a decrease in frequency and/or passage of hard, dry stools (NANDA).

RELATED FACTORS

Decreased motility (secondary to aging, Multiple sclerosis, Hirschsprung's disease, and so on), Decreased activity, Decreased fluid intake, Dietary changes, Medications (specify), Painful defecation, Others specific to client.

DEFINING CHARACTERISTICS

Major	Minor
Decreased frequency of defecation	Abdominal pain
Hard, forced stools	Appetite impairment
Palpable mass	Back pain
Reported feeling of rectal fullness	Headache
Straining at stool	Interference with daily living
	Use of laxatives

DIARRHEA

Definition: A state in which an individual experiences a change in normal bowel habits characterized by the frequent passage of loose, fluid, unformed stools (NANDA).

RELATED FACTORS

Dietary changes, Increased intestinal motility secondary to _____, Excessive alcohol intake, Impaction, Medications (specify), Stress, Food intolerance, Others specific to client (specify).

DEFINING CHARACTERISTICS

Abdominal cramping
Abdominal pain
Urgency to defecate
Change in usual consistency, frequency, and volume of stool
Loose/liquid stool
Change in color of stool

DIAGNOSTIC REASONING IN ACTION

Mr. Ronald Todd, age 54, is employed at County Bank as a senior vice-president. Mr. Todd is married and has three adult children and one grandchild. Two years ago he was diagnosed as having a peptic ulcer and has been asymptomatic using diet, medications, and relaxation.

He now reports to his physician that he is no longer following his diet or taking his medication because he was feeling better and had no symptoms. He has a burning pain "in the pit of the stomach" that seems to get worse after meals, especially mid-morning and mid-afternoon. Because of the pain, he has the tendency to eat less and has lost 10 lb in the last several weeks. He continues to smoke about one pack of filtered cigarettes a day.

He notices an increase in belching and nausea; however, he is not vomiting. Since the increase in symptoms, he is irritable at home and work. He attributes some of his irritability to lack of sleep, because pain often keeps him awake. Lack of sleep often leaves him with a headache for which he takes two aspirin every 4 hours. A survey of his diet reveals a preference for food low in protein and high in fats and carbohydrates. He usually has one or two martinis, wine, and an after-dinner drink a least twice a week.

Peggy Steineman, RN, gathers the following objective and subjective data:

- Epigastric pain and burning
- Pain worse after meals
- Bowel sounds all 4 quadrants
- Complains of feeling of fullness in stomach
- BP 162/84, P 84, R 24
- Lung sounds clear in all lobes
- Recent weight loss
- Decreased appetite
- Smoking
- Use of alcohol
- Use of aspirin
- No medications for 3 weeks
- Tired, irritable
- Stool negative for blood

To cluster the data, Ms Steineman considers

1. Pain, burning, feeling of fullness, nausea
2. Diet, weight loss, anorexia
3. Smoking, use of alcohol, noncompliance with diet, use of aspirin

Ms Steineman identifies the following nursing diagnoses:

1. *Pain* related to changes in gastric mucosa
2. *Altered nutrition: less than body requirements* related to decreased food intake
3. *Noncompliance* related to knowledge deficit regarding self-care

Ms Steineman counsels Mr. Todd about the importance of following his prescribed diet, medications, and relaxation techniques. She also discusses with him the harmful effects of smoking, alcohol, and aspirin on the stomach lining and gives him a pamphlet listing things he can do to care for and reduce the symptoms of his peptic ulcer.

clients who are unwilling or refuse to follow a nutritional plan. *Knowledge deficit* applies to clients who do not have sufficient information to maintain a sound nutritional status.

Related diagnoses include: *Fluid volume deficit* related to decreased fluid intake, vomiting, or diarrhea; *Ineffective breathing pattern* related to abdominal pain, ascites, or increased abdominal pressure; and *Body image disturbance* related to colostomy, malodor, or inability to control bodily function.

Common Alterations in the Health of the Gastrointestinal Tract

Problems commonly associated with the abdominal assessment include nutritional imbalances, eating disorders, ulcers, inflammatory processes, abdominal hernias, and cancer. These are described below. Also see Table 13.2, a pain-assessment tool for four common gastrointestinal disorders.

Nutritional Imbalances

Malnutrition Malnutrition is an imbalance—whether a deficit or excess—of the required nutrients of a balanced diet. *Undernutrition* denotes inadequate intake of the nutrients needed to maintain optimal body functioning. *Overnutrition* is an excessive intake of nutrients, either as food or as food supplements. For example, overnutrition of vitamin A can lead to toxicity symptoms such as nausea and vomiting. Both undernutrition and overnutrition are forms of malnutrition.

Obesity Obesity is defined as a weight of 20% or more above recommended body weight. Severe obesity signifies an excess of 100% or 100 pounds above recommended body weight.

Table 13.2 Pain Assessment with Common Gastrointestinal Disorders

	Esophageal Reflux	Esophageal Spasm	Esophageal Rupture	Gastric Dysfunction
Definitions	Regurgitation of stomach and duodenal contents into the esophagus	Nonpropulsive, intermittent contraction with swallowing	Refers to a tear through the wall of the esophagus. Food, fluids or gastrointestinal contents enter the mediastinum or pleural cavity.	Abnormal gastric muscle tone with noncoordination of the emptying mechanism of the stomach
Position	Epigastric area, and/or behind the sternum	Behind the sternum, and sometimes across the chest	Epigastric area, and/or behind the sternum	Epigastric area, and/or behind the sternum
Precipitating factors	Food (spicy), aspirin, coffee, alcohol, smoking, straining, lying flat after a meal	May not have an identifiable cause; exercise and ingestion of cold fluids may precipitate spasm	Alcohol, heavy meal, vigorous coughing, swallowing, vomiting	Heavy meal, bubbly fluids, paralytic ileus
Quality	Burning, heartburn, may be squeezing in nature	Crushing, dull pressure; burning pressure	Crushing, tearing	Bloated, sharp, burning
Radiation	Usually does not radiate	Like angina: left arm, jaw, back	Lower spine	Left shoulder
Relief	Bland food, antacids	Nitroglycerin	Surgery	Belching
Severity	Variable on a scale of 1 to 10	Variable on a scale of 1 to 10	Upper end of the scale of 1 to 10	Variable on a scale of 1 to 10
Timing	During or right after a meal	Sudden, no warning or predictable pattern	Sudden, no warning or predictable pattern	Sudden, no warning or predictable pattern
Duration	Minutes to an hour	Seconds to minutes	Persistent	Depends upon individual, gets worse as the day progresses

Obesity has been linked to an increased risk for a number of gastrointestinal problems, such as cancers of the gallbladder and colon. In addition, research suggests that obese people experience a variety of psychosocial problems, such as job discrimination and social isolation.

Overweight Overweight is defined as a weight of 10–20% in excess of recommended body weight. The likelihood of developing significant health problems is lower in those who are overweight than in those who are obese.

Eating Disorders

An eating disorder is a condition in which a person's current intake of food differs significantly from that person's normal intake. Eating disorders typically result from an attempt to lose weight; however, the attempt to lose weight may be a misguided response to psychosocial problems.

Anorexia Nervosa Anorexia nervosa is a complex psychosocial problem characterized by a severely restricted intake of nutrients and a low body weight (Figure 13.25 on page 368). The anorexic typically experiences intense fear of gaining weight or becoming fat, feels fat even when emaciated, and refuses to maintain body weight over a minimal normal weight for age and height (DSM-IIIR 1987). Many anorexics experience constipation, gastrointestinal bloating, nausea, and abdominal pain.

Bulimia Nervosa Bulimia nervosa is an eating disorder characterized by binge eating and purging or another compensatory mechanism to prevent weight gain. Typically, the bulimic consumes large portions of high-calorie food, typically about 4000 calories at one time. The individual then tries to force the food out of the body by vomiting or using laxatives, enemas, diuretics, or diet pills. Many bulimics experience tooth decay, dehydration, laxative dependence, and rectal bleeding.

Ulcers

An ulcer is an erosion or wearing away of the mucosal lining of an organ (Figure 13.26 on page 368). In the gastrointestinal tract, digestive juices cause the erosion.

Peptic Ulcer A peptic ulcer is an ulcer located in the esophagus, stomach, or duodenum. It is a general term used to describe ulcerations in the mucosa of the gastrointestinal tract. Because it was believed that gastric and duodenal ulcers were caused by the same factors, the term has been used to describe both. Because gastric and duodenal ulcers now are thought to have different causes, the more specific terms *gastric ulcer* and *duodenal ulcer* are preferred.

Gastric Ulcer A gastric ulcer is an erosion of the mucosal lining of the stomach. The distal half, the lesser curvature, and the pyloric area of the stomach are most susceptible to the ulcer formation. It is believed that an increase in hydrochloric acid and a breakdown in the gastric barriers contribute to the ulcer

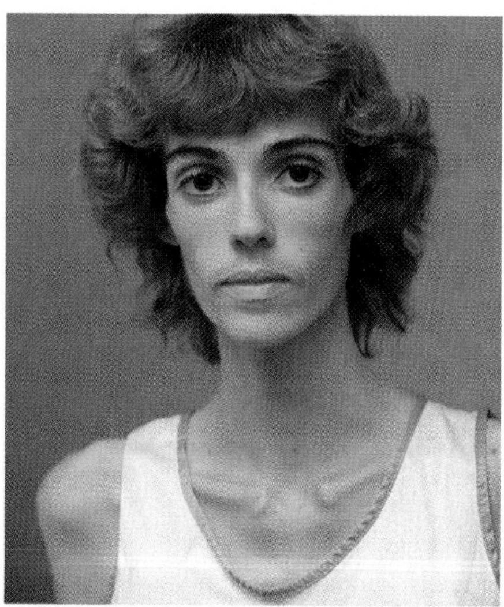

Figure 13.25 Individual with anorexia nervosa.

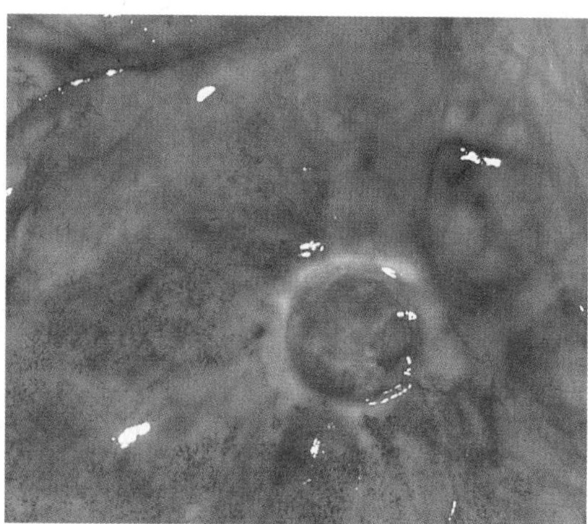

Figure 13.26 A gastric ulcer.

formation. As the pyloric area becomes irritated, duodenal reflux further aggravates the condition. Bleeding occurs more frequently with this type of ulcer.

Duodenal Ulcer A duodenal ulcer is a loss of tissue in the duodenum of the small intestines. Many of these ulcers are located at the junction of the pyloric and duodenal mucosa. This location suggests the early emptying of the stomach contents into the duodenum. People with duodenal ulcers typically have a high acid content level in their gastric secretions and a decreased buffering ability to neutralize the acid. Perforation is common.

Ulcerative Colitis Ulcerative colitis is a recurrent inflammatory process causing ulcer formation in the lower portions of the large intestines and rectum. The condition is common in adolescents and young adults. The distribution of the inflammatory process is diffuse. The ulcerative areas abscess and later become necrotic. Diarrhea, abdominal pain, and cramping with weight loss are common symptoms of the disease process.

Inflammatory Processes

Esophagitis Esophagitis is an inflammatory process of the esophagus. It is caused by a variety of irritants. The more common causes include smoking, alcohol abuse, reflux of gastric contents, and ingestion of extremely hot or cold foods and liquids.

Gastritis Gastritis is an inflammatory process of the stomach. This process may be acute or chronic. Acute gastritis is commonly linked to alcohol abuse and use of certain drugs (aspirin, nonsteroidal antiinflammatory agents). It is a side effect of certain drugs (antibiotics, digitalis). It is also associated with systemic diseases such as renal failure, cirrhosis, or respiratory infections.

The causes of chronic gastritis are unknown. It is classified according to the changes in the mucosal lining and segment of the stomach involved. It is common in clients with pernicious anemia.

Enteritis Enteritis is an inflammatory process of the intestines, specifically the small intestines. Causes are the same as for gastritis. Many times, enteritis is caused by gastritis.

Cholecystitis Cholecystitis is an acute or chronic inflammation of the gallbladder. Stones in the gallbladder (cholelithiasis) account for more than 90% of the cases. Bacterial invasion of the gallbladder is responsible for a small percentage. Incidence is higher among women than men. Obesity, pregnancy, and use of birth control pills are also associated with increased incidence.

Peritonitis Peritonitis is a local or generalized inflammatory process of the peritoneal membrane of the abdomen. The precipitant can be an infectious process (pelvic inflammatory disease), perforation of an organ (ruptured duodenal ulcer), internal bleeding (ruptured ectopic pregnancy), or trauma (stab wound to abdomen). Symptoms include abdominal pain, abdominal distention, abdominal rigidity, decreased bowel sounds, nausea, vomiting, chills, and fever.

Hepatitis Hepatitis is an inflammatory process of the liver. Its causes include viruses, bacteria, chemicals, and drugs. Hepatitis is common in clients of all ages. Viral hepatitis A is the most commonly reported form. Previously called infectious hepatitis, it is transmitted by contaminated food or water, eg, because of poor sanitation, inadequate disposal of sewage, poor hygiene practices of individuals handling food, and eating raw shellfish from contaminated water.

Hepatitis B, formerly called serum hepatitis, is transmitted by contaminated blood or blood products, instruments, or needles. Hepatitis B may be transmitted by direct contact with infected body fluids or contaminated objects. The basic signs and symptoms are the same.

Pancreatitis Pancreatitis is a nonbacterial inflammatory process of the pancreas. Alcoholism and biliary tract disease are common predisposing factors. The pancreatic enzymes are unable to reach the small intestines. An autodigestive process ensues.

Crohn's Disease Crohn's disease is a chronic inflammatory process of the ileum. It is sometimes called *regional ileitis*, which is a misnomer, because it can involve any part of the lower intestinal tract. Crohn's disease is characterized by "skipped" sections of involvement. It is most common in young adults and usually has an insidious onset. The inflammation involves all layers of the intestinal mucosa. Transverse fissures develop in the bowel, producing a characteristic cobblestone appearance.

Abdominal Hernias

A hernia, commonly called a rupture, is a protrusion of an organ or structure through an abnormal opening or weakened area in a body wall. The abdominal wall is the most common site of hernias. This weakening could be congenital or acquired. An umbilical hernia is caused by an overstretched muscle with weakened fascia. An incisional hernia is an example of an acquired type.

If the protruding or displaced abdominal contents return to their normal position when the individual relaxes, the hernia is said to be reducible or reduced. When the displaced or protruding structures do not return to their normal position, the hernia is said to be incarcerated or nonreducible. An incarcerated hernia can become strangulated. In strangulated hernias, the blood supply to the displaced abdominal contents is compromised. The strangulated visceral contents can become gangrenous.

Umbilical Hernia An umbilical hernia occurs at the umbilicus (see Figure 13.24). The abdominal rectus muscle separates or weakens, allowing abdominal structures, usually the intestines, to push through and come closer to the skin. Umbilical hernias are more common in children than in adults.

Ventral (Incisional) Hernia A ventral hernia is also known as an incisional hernia, because it occurs at the site of an incision (Figure 13.27). The incision weakens the muscle, and the abdominal structures move closer to the skin. Causes include obesity, repeated surgeries, infection during the postoperative period, impaired wound healing, and poor nutrition.

Hiatal Hernia A hiatal hernia is due to a weakening in the diaphragm that allows a portion of the stomach and the esophagus to move into the thoracic cavity (Figure 13.28 on page 370). This hernia is classified as sliding or rolling and is more common in adults than children.

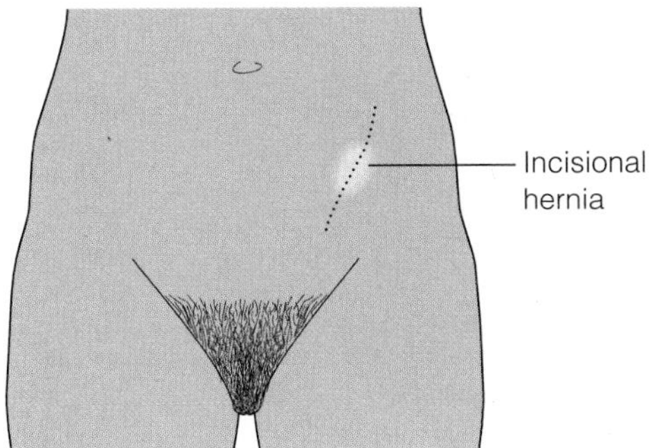

Figure 13.27 Incisional hernia.

Cancers

Cancer of the Esophagus Cancer of the esophagus is a malignant growth of the esophagus, most common in males over 50 years of age. The lower third of the esophagus is most commonly involved. Clients commonly complain of weight loss, dysphagia (difficulty swallowing), and odynophagia (pain on swallowing). Alcohol abuse, smoking, and poor oral hygiene appear to be predisposing factors.

Cancer of the Stomach Cancer of the stomach is a malignant growth of the stomach. The cancerous lesions are found most frequently in the distal third of the stomach. The disease is often in the advanced stages before a diagnosis is made. Dietary habits seem to be an influencing factor. Weight loss, nausea, vomiting, abdominal pain, abdominal distention, and some bleeding are the common complaints of the client.

Colorectal Cancer Colorectal cancer is a malignant lesion involving any part of the large intestines, sigmoid colon, or rectum. Predisposing factors include poor dietary habits and chronic constipation. Signs and symptoms vary according to the location of the growth. A change in bowel habits or patterns is a characteristic with any location. In many cases, an intestinal obstruction occurs, surgery is required, and the client has a permanent colostomy.

Health Promotion and Client Education

At the conclusion of the physical assessment, answer the client's questions. If family members are present, answer their questions. Stress the importance of abdominal health, including good dietary habits and other preventive measures.

Promoting the Health of the Gastrointestinal System

The client's position on the health/illness continuum is influenced by the health and functioning of the gastrointestinal

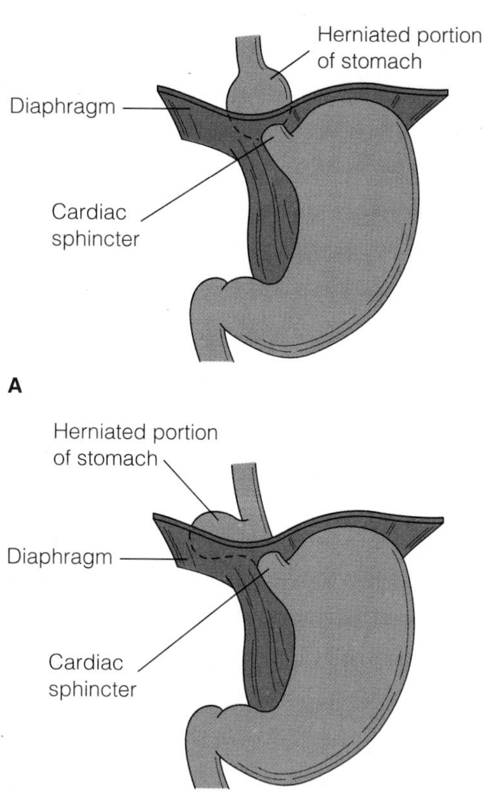

Figure 13.28 *A*, Sliding hiatal hernia; *B*, Rolling hiatal hernia.

system. It is imperative for the individual to take an active role in maintaining gastrointestinal health. Many health problems of the gastrointestinal tract relate to the misuse of food. After analyzing the data regarding dietary habits, quality and quantity of food consumed, and the atmosphere at mealtime, help the client adopt health-maintaining interventions. Teach the client the essentials of a balanced diet, including proteins, fats and carbohydrates. Encourage the client to eat fresh fruit and vegetables, a good source of fiber and natural sugar. For more information, see Chapter 5.

Including fiber-rich foods in the diet promotes peristaltic activity and prevents constipation. Drinking six to eight glasses of water per day also helps prevent constipation, as does exercising on a daily basis. A healthy diet promotes regular bowel habits, which decrease the need for and misuse of laxatives and enemas. Because enemas and laxatives decrease the natural muscle activity of the bowel, the client's dependency on them increases with increasing usage.

Food poisoning can be prevented by proper storage, refrigeration, and preparation of food.

Individuals need to identify foods that are irritating to their gastrointestinal systems. Adverse reactions to food include constipation, diarrhea, flatus, belching, and nausea. Clients need to decrease consumption of these foods or eliminate them from the diet to prevent symptoms.

The American Cancer Society has identified seven early warning signs of cancer. Three are specific to the gastrointestinal system. These three signs are

- Changes in bowel or bladder habits

DIAGNOSTIC REASONING IN ACTION

Mrs. Rita Flores is a 46-year-old Cuban immigrant who has been living in Florida with her three children for 6 years. She returned to the clinic today for her first postoperative visit following a laparoscopic cholecystectomy a week ago. She is accompanied by her 18-year-old daughter, Maria, who interprets for her mother.

Through Maria, Mrs. Flores says that she has minimal abdominal pain. She has taken acetaminophen on three occasions for the discomfort. She comments that her preoperative nausea and belching are gone. Further assessment reveals three abdominal incisions are approximated with no redness or drainage. Bowel sounds are auscultated in all quadrants. The abdomen is soft and nontender.

With the help of her daughter, Mrs. Flores tells the nurse, Jim O'Neill, that she is voiding "light yellow" urine and has one soft brown bowel movement every other day. She says that she is eating a bland, low-fat diet and is having no problems. Maria questions Mr. O'Neill about the diet, because the discharge papers indicate regular diet as tolerated. The bland, low-fat diet is Mrs. Flores's own choice. Maria tells Mr. O'Neill Mrs. Flores is "afraid of the pain coming back to her belly" if she eats high-fat foods.

Mr. O'Neill reassures Mrs. Flores and her daughter that progress is being made, recovery is uncomplicated, and the diet at this time is not a problem. Mr. O'Neill does identify the following nursing diagnosis: *High risk for constipation* related to a bland, low-fat diet. He informs Maria that her mother will most likely introduce foods with higher fat content in the near future. He reminds her that this limited use of low-fat foods gives the body an opportunity to adjust to the inability to store bile. He takes the opportunity to instruct Mrs. Flores and Maria on the need to increase fiber in the diet, thereby preventing constipation. He lists some foods that contain fiber. The increase of fiber in the diet and the avoidance of constipation will be evaluated at the next clinic visit.

Mrs. Flores's next visit is scheduled in 2 weeks. Mr. O'Neill reminds Mrs. Flores to call if she has abdominal pain, drainage from the incisions, nausea or vomiting, change in skin color, change in color of urine, changes in color and consistency of stool, or itching of the skin.

- Unusual bleeding or discharge
- Indigestion or difficulty swallowing

Research and data analysis closely correlate cancer of the gastrointestinal system to poor diet. Although the research results are not conclusive, clients may be able to reduce their risk by following these recommendations:

- Avoid obesity.
- Reduce consumption of saturated and unsaturated fats.
- Eat fruits and vegetables.
- Increase fiber in the diet.
- Use alcohol only in moderation.
- Decrease intake of smoked, salt-cured, or nitrate-cured foods.

Research has shown a link between high levels of stress and ulcer formation. Stress is part of daily life and needs to be controlled using healthy strategies. People often turn to smoking, food, drugs, and alcohol to deal with stress. The individual must identify the problems and limitations of these strategies and seek alternative coping mechanisms.

Many medications have gastrointestinal side effects. Stress the importance of using medications correctly and knowing their side effects.

Summary

Abdominal assessment provides in-depth data regarding the gastrointestinal tract, accessory organs of digestion, and organs of other systems located in the abdominal cavity. Position, size, and density of the organs are determined through the appropriate assessment techniques. Dietary habits and the psychologic implications of food play a major role in the health of the individual. Many health-inhibiting changes originate in the gastrointestinal system as a direct result of the poor diet. Diarrhea, constipation, ulcers, and heartburn are a few examples of preventable health-inhibiting changes.

Cancer prevention and early detection through screening are most important. Teach clients the warning signs of cancer and recommended risk-reduction strategies. With client input, identify interventions to maintain wellness, enhance self-care, reduce risk factors, and limit any pathologic process in progress.

Key Points

- ✓ The abdomen is a cavity situated below the diaphragm. It contains most of the alimentary canal, the accessory digestive organs, and organs of other systems.
- ✓ Mapping the abdomen into four equal quadrants or nine regions provides landmarks for identification of underlying structures during assessment, recording, and reporting of data.
- ✓ Conduct the focused interview to obtain specific information regarding digestive functions and functions of other structures of the abdomen. Integrate this data with that in the health history for a comprehensive database. This database includes information on diet, health practices, habits, self-care practices, and cultural and environmental factors.
- ✓ You use all four techniques of assessment in the physical assessment of the abdomen, but you vary the usual sequence as follows: inspection first, then auscultation, then percussion, and finally palpation.
- ✓ Inpect the abdomen for skin characteristics (pigmentation, scars, lesions), contour, and pulsations.
- ✓ Perform auscultation of the abdomen to ascertain vascular and bowel sounds.
- ✓ Percuss the abdomen to determine the presence of air, fluid, and masses and the density of underlying structures.
- ✓ Palpate the abdomen using light and moderate pressure to determine the size, shape, position, and consistency of the underlying structures and muscle guarding.
- ✓ Nursing diagnoses commonly associated with the digestive system include *Bowel incontinence, Constipation, Diarrhea, Altered nutrition,* and others.
- ✓ Common alterations in the health of the abdomen include nutritional imbalances, eating disorders, ulcers, inflammatory processes, hernias, and cancer.
- ✓ After the physical assessment, provide the client with information to promote wellness and health of the digestive tract and abdomen.

Chapter 14

Assessing the Urinary System

The urinary sytem includes the kidneys, ureters, bladder, and urethra. Of these organs, the "major players" are the kidneys, which are responsible for filtering the blood. Like a giant sieve, the glomeruli of the kidneys filter approximately 1000–1200 ml of fluid each minute, removing wastes, toxins, and other foreign matter, and keeping the body in homeostasis and in health. Without the filtering function of the kidneys, dangerous levels of nitrogenous wastes and toxins build up, fluid and electrolyte levels become imbalanced, blood pressure rises, and production of red blood cells is decreased. Thus, the health of the urinary system is essential to the health of the whole body. While conducting the assessment of the urinary system, be aware of its interrelationship with other body systems. Consider also the client's developmental stage. Pscyhosocial factors such as stress play a role in urinary function, as do the client's self-care practices, such as alcohol intake, smoking, and hygiene. You must also consider various environmental factors when assessing the urinary system. These factors are summarized in Figure 14.1.

Because the organs of the urinary system are distributed among the retroperitoneal space, abdomen, and genitals, the examination of the urinary system is incorporated into other segments of the physical assessment. For example, you examine the kidneys during the assessment of the posterior thorax, back, and abdomen; the urinary bladder during the assessment of the lower abdomen; and the urinary meatus during the assessment of the genitals.

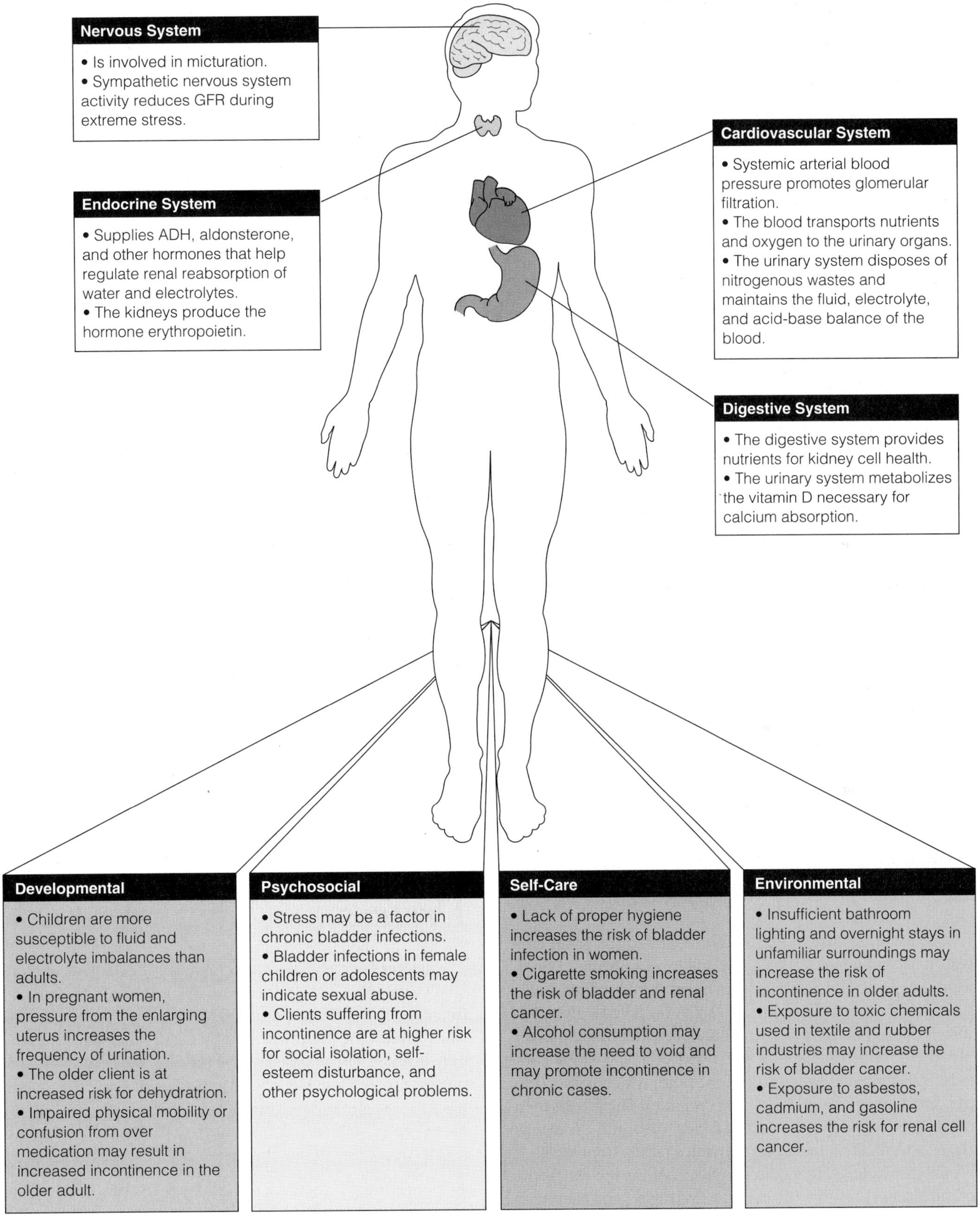

Nervous System
- Is involved in micturation.
- Sympathetic nervous system activity reduces GFR during extreme stress.

Endocrine System
- Supplies ADH, aldonsterone, and other hormones that help regulate renal reabsorption of water and electrolytes.
- The kidneys produce the hormone erythropoietin.

Cardiovascular System
- Systemic arterial blood pressure promotes glomerular filtration.
- The blood transports nutrients and oxygen to the urinary organs.
- The urinary system disposes of nitrogenous wastes and maintains the fluid, electrolyte, and acid-base balance of the blood.

Digestive System
- The digestive system provides nutrients for kidney cell health.
- The urinary system metabolizes the vitamin D necessary for calcium absorption.

Developmental
- Children are more susceptible to fluid and electrolyte imbalances than adults.
- In pregnant women, pressure from the enlarging uterus increases the frequency of urination.
- The older client is at increased risk for dehydratrion.
- Impaired physical mobility or confusion from over medication may result in increased incontinence in the older adult.

Psychosocial
- Stress may be a factor in chronic bladder infections.
- Bladder infections in female children or adolescents may indicate sexual abuse.
- Clients suffering from incontinence are at higher risk for social isolation, self-esteem disturbance, and other psychological problems.

Self-Care
- Lack of proper hygiene increases the risk of bladder infection in women.
- Cigarette smoking increases the risk of bladder and renal cancer.
- Alcohol consumption may increase the need to void and may promote incontinence in chronic cases.

Environmental
- Insufficient bathroom lighting and overnight stays in unfamiliar surroundings may increase the risk of incontinence in older adults.
- Exposure to toxic chemicals used in textile and rubber industries may increase the risk of bladder cancer.
- Exposure to asbestos, cadmium, and gasoline increases the risk for renal cell cancer.

Figure 14.1 An overview of important factors to consider when assessing the urinary system.

Anatomy and Physiology Review

Kidneys

The **kidneys** are bean-shaped organs located in the retroperitoneal space on either side of the vertebral column (Figure 14.2). Extending from the level of the twelfth thoracic vertebra to the third lumbar vertebra, the upper portion of the kidneys is protected by the lower rib cage. The right kidney is displaced downward by the liver and sits slightly lower than the left. Each kidney is cushioned by a layer of fat, and the kidney itself is surrounded by tissue called the *renal capsule* (Figure 14.3 on page 376). The *renal fascia* connects the kidney and fatty layer to the posterior wall of the abdomen. Each adult kidney weighs approximately 150 g (5 oz), is 11–13 cm (4–5 in) long, 5–7 cm (2 to 3 in) wide, and 2.5–3 cm (1 in) thick. The lateral surface of the kidney is convex. The medial surface is concave and contains the **hilus**, a vertical cleft that opens into a space within the kidney referred to as the *renal sinus*. The ureters, renal blood vessels, nerves, and lymphatic vessels pass through the hilus into the renal sinus. The superior part of the kidney is referred to as the upper pole, whereas the inferior surface is called the lower pole.

The inner portion of the kidney is called the **renal medulla**. The renal medulla is composed of structures called pyramids and calyces. The *pyramids* are wedgelike structures made up of bundles of urine-collecting tubules. At their apex, the pyramids have papillae that are enclosed by cuplike structures called *calyces*. The calyces collect urine and transport it into the **renal pelvis**, which is the funnel-shaped superior end of the ureter.

The outer portion of each kidney is called the **renal cortex.** It is composed of over one million **nephrons,** which form the urine. The first part of each nephron is the renal corpuscle, which consists of a tuft of capillaries called a **glomerulus**. These glomeruli begin the filtration of the blood. Larger blood components, such as red blood cells and larger proteins, are separated from most of the fluid, which passes into the *glomerular capsule* (or *Bowman's capsule*). The filtrate then moves into a *proximal convoluted tubule,* then into the *loop of Henle*, and finally into a *distal convoluted tubule*, from which it is collected as urine by a *collecting tubule*. Along the way, some of the filtrate is resorbed along with electrolytes and chemicals such as glucose, potassium, phosphate, and sodium. Each collecting tubule guides the urine from several nephrons out into the renal pyramids and calyces, and from there through the renal pelvis and into the ureters.

The major functions of the kidneys are

- Eliminating nitrogenous waste products, toxins, excess ions, and drugs through urine
- Regulating volume and chemical makeup of the blood
- Maintaining balance between water and salts, and acids and bases
- Producing renin, an enzyme that assists in the regulation of blood pressure
- Producing the hormone erythropoietin, which stimulates production of red blood cells in the bone marrow
- Assisting in the metabolism of vitamin D

Renal Arteries

The kidneys require a tremendous amount of oxygen and nutrients and receive about 25% of the cardiac output. Although not part of the urinary system, an extensive network of arteries intertwines within the renal network. These arteries include renal arteries, arcuate arteries, interlobular arteries, afferent arteries, and efferent arterioles. The vasa recta are looping capillaries that connect with the juxtamedullary nephrons and continue into the medulla alongside the loops of Henle. They help to concentrate urine.

The major function of the renal arteries is

- Providing a rich supply of blood (approximately 1200 ml per minute when an individual is at rest) to the kidneys

Ureters

The **ureters** are mucus-lined narrow tubes approximately 25–30 cm (10–12 in) in length and 6–12 mm (0.25–0.50 in) in diameter. As the ureter leaves the kidney, it travels downward behind the peritoneum to the posterior wall of the urinary bladder. The middle layer of the ureters contains smooth muscle that is stimulated by transmission of electric impulses from the autonomic nervous system. Their peristaltic action propels urine downward to the urinary bladder.

The major function of the ureters is

- Transporting urine from the kidney to the urinary bladder

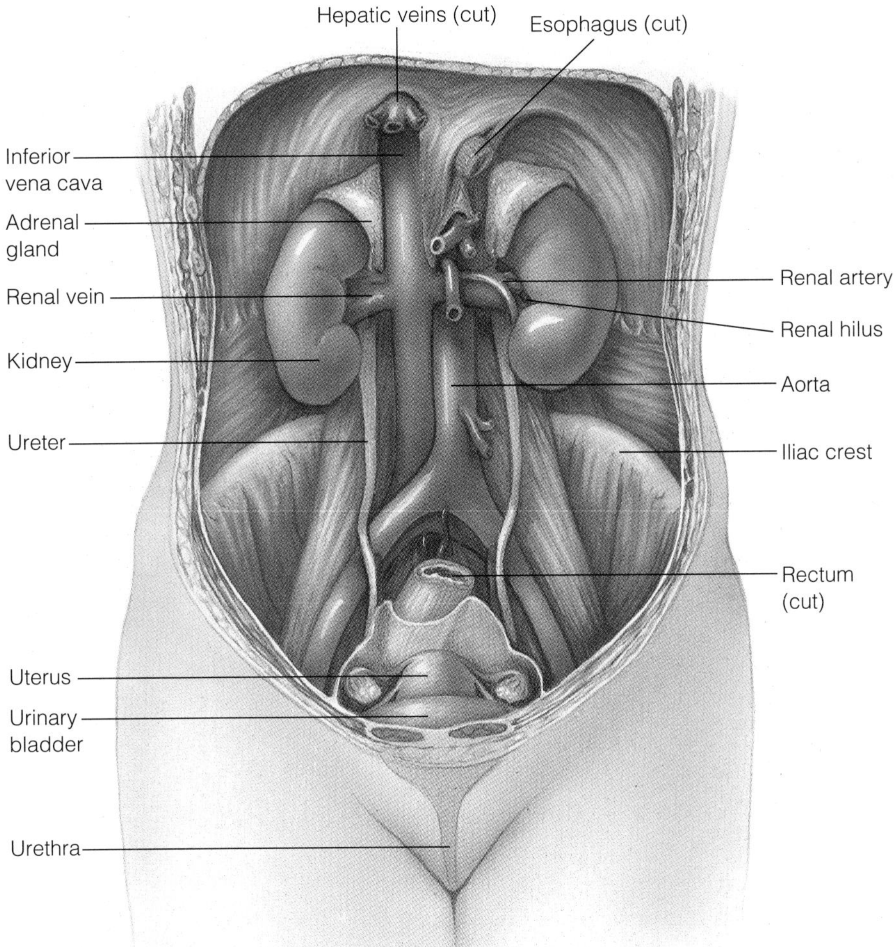

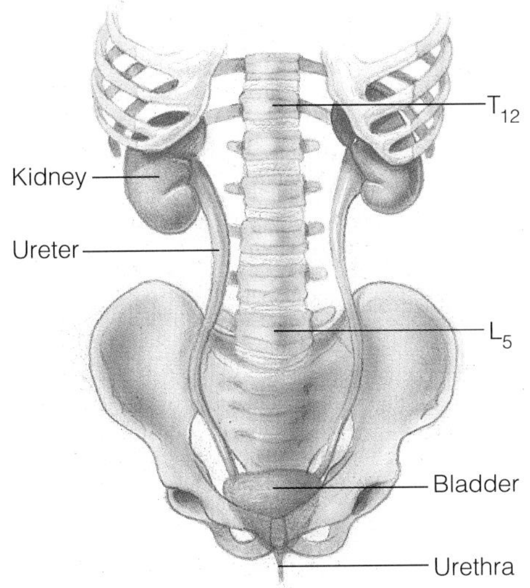

Figure 14.2 The urinary system. *A*, Anterior view of the urinary organs of a female. *B*, Relationship of the kidneys to the vertebrae and lower ribs.

Urinary Bladder

The **urinary bladder** is a hollow, muscular, collapsible pouch that acts as a reservoir for urine. It lies on the pelvic floor in the retroperitoneal space. The bladder is composed of two parts; the rounded muscular sac made up of the *detrusor muscle*, and the portion between the body of the bladder and the urethra known as the *neck*. In males, the bladder lies anterior to the rectum, and the neck of the bladder is encircled by the prostate gland of the male reproductive system. In females, the bladder lies anterior to the vagina and uterus. The detrusor muscle allows the bladder to expand as it fills with urine, and to contract to release urine to the outside of the body during *micturition* (voiding). When empty, the bladder collapses upon itself forming a thick-walled, pyramidal organ that lies low in the pelvis behind the symphysis pubis. As urine accumulates, the *fundus*, the superior wall of the bladder, ascends in the abdominal cavity and assumes a rounded shape that is

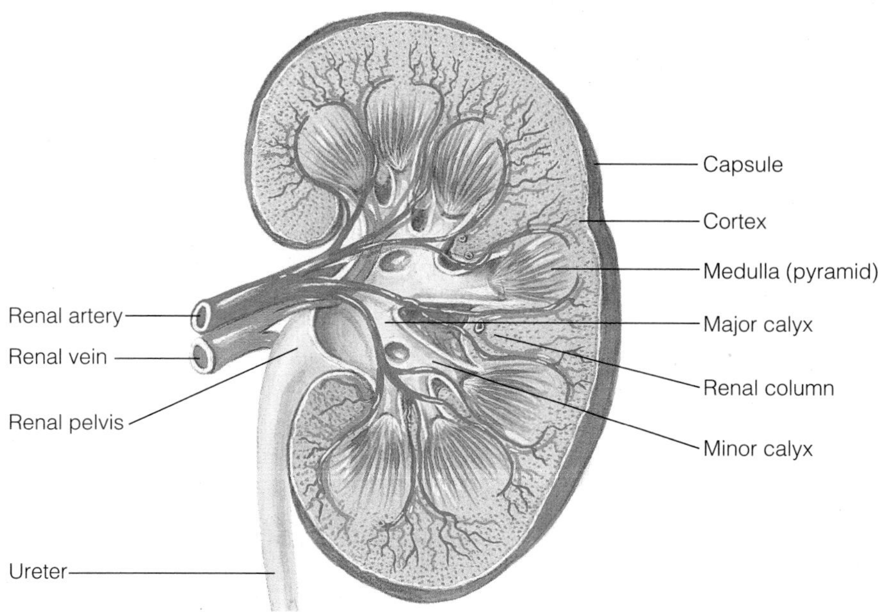

Figure 14.3 Internal anatomy of the kidney.

palpable. When moderately filled (500 ml), the bladder is approximately 12.5 cm (5 in) long. When larger amounts of urine are present, the bladder becomes distended and rises above the symphysis pubis.

The major functions of the urinary bladder are

- Storing urine temporarily
- Contracting to release urine during micturition

Urethra

The **urethra** is a mucus-lined tube that transports urine from the urinary bladder to the exterior. In females, the urethra is approximately 3–4 cm (1.5 in) long and lies along the anterior wall of the vagina. The female urethra terminates in the *external urethral orifice* or *meatus,* which lies between the clitoris and the vagina. The male urethra is approximately 20 cm (8 in) long and runs the length of the penis. It terminates in the external urethral orifice in the glans penis. In addition to providing a passageway for urine, the male urethra also carries semen outside of the body. Because the female urethra is short and its meatus lies close to the anus, it can become contaminated with bacteria more readily than the male urethra. A more detailed review of the penis, prostate gland, and male and female external genitalia is presented in Chapter 15.

The major function of the urethra is

- Providing a passage for the elimination of urine

Locating Landmarks

During the assessment of the urinary system, you use three landmarks to locate and palpate the kidneys and urinary bladder. These landmarks are the costovertebral angle, the rectus abdominis muscle, and the symphysis pubis. The *costovertebral angle* is the area on the lower back formed by the vertebral column and the downward curve of the last posterior rib (Figure 14.4, *A*). It is an important anatomical landmark because the lower poles of the kidney and ureter lie below this surface. The *rectus abdominis muscles* are a longitudinal pair of muscles that extend from the pubis to the rib cage on either side of the midline (Figure 14.4,*B*). Use these muscles as guidelines for positioning your hands when palpating the kidneys through the abdominal wall. The *symphysis pubis* is the joint formed by the union of the two pubic bones by cartilage at the midline of the body (Figure 14.4,*B*). The bladder is cradled under the symphysis pubis. When the bladder is full, you will be able to palpate it as it rises above the symphysis pubis.

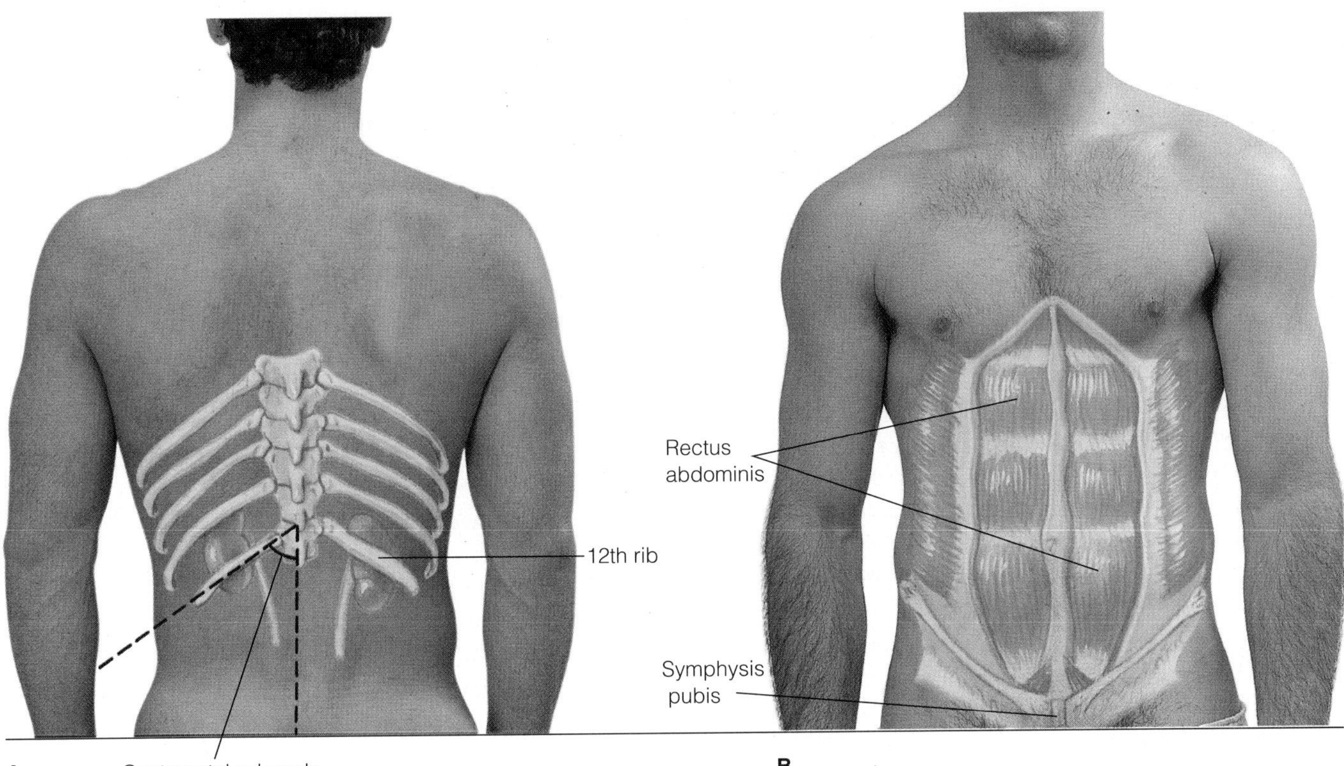

Figure 14.4 Landmarks for urinary assessment. *A,* The costovertebral angle. *B,* The rectus abdominis muscles and the symphysis pubis.

Gathering the Data

Focused Interview

Before initiating the focused interview and carrying out the physical assessment of the urinary system, review the information you already have gathered from the initial interview and health history, medical records, family members, diagnostic tests, and other sources. The focused interview adds specific information about the urinary system not obtained during the initial interview and health history. For example, encourage the client to provide both general and specific information about family history, urinary elimination patterns, fluid intake, and environmental factors that may contribute to urinary problems. By gathering information in this manner you can see patterns or clusters of characteristics that highlight strengths and problems specific to the urinary system. Be sure to start with the client's normal patterns and then focus on any deviations from normal. Throughout the focused interview, be aware that client may be reluctant to answer questions regarding the urinary system, because many people regard this topic as private and personal. Acknowledge that it may be difficult for the client to provide this information, but stress the importance of answering the questions honestly and accurately.

Questions Related to the General Health of the Urinary System

1. What are your normal patterns when you void? How often do you urinate each day? How much do you void each time you urinate? *Many factors influence the number of times and amount that a client voids. Among these are size of the bladder, amount of fluid intake, type of fluid or solid intake, medications, amount of perspiration, and the client's temperature. The normal adult may void 5 or 6 times per day in amounts averaging 100 to 400 ml. Average adults may urinate as much as 2 liters of fluid. The child may void more frequently in smaller amounts. The key point is to determine the client's normal patterns.*
2. Have you noticed any change from your normal voiding patterns? Have you noticed any changes in your pattern recently? Have you had any of these changes: urinating more often, urinating less often, urinating more fluid, or urinating less fluid? *Changes in urinary elimination patterns signal fluid retention, which may indicate heart failure, kidney failure, or improper nutritional intake. Other consideration include obstructions, infections, and endocrine alterations.*

3. Have you noticed any changes in the quality of the urine? If so, describe the change. Has your urine been cloudy? Does it have an odor? Has the color changed? If there has been a color change, what is it? Is the color change happening each time you urinate? Is there a pattern? Can you predict the color change? *Color changes offer clues to the presence of infection, kidney stones, or neoplasm. The quantity of urine may indicate the presence of renal failure or may reflect hydration status.*
4. *If the urine is bloody (hematuria), ask these questions:* Have you fallen recently? Do you experience burning when the blood is present? Have you seen clots in the urine? Have you noticed any stones or other material in the urine? Have you noticed any granular material on the toilet paper after you wipe? *The client may offer valuable information about the source and characteristics of bleeding, because this symptom is present in a wide variety of conditions. Hematuria is a serious finding and warrants additional follow-up.*
5. Have you noticed any pain or discomfort when your urine is bloody? If so describe the type, location, and timing of the discomfort. *Hematuria without pain is often associated with cancer.*
6. Is your urine foamy and amber in color? *This finding may indicate the presence of hepatic illness.*
7. Have you had any weight gain recently? If so, describe it. Are you retaining fluid? Are your rings, clothing, or shoes becoming tighter? Has this change been gradual or did it come on suddenly? *This may alert you to the presence of hypertension, associated heart failure or endocrine problems. These ultimately affect the renal circulation and function of the kidneys.*
8. Has anyone in your family had a kidney disease or urinary problem? If so, when did they have it? How was it treated? Do they still have it? *A family history of kidney disease may signify a genetic predisposition to the development of renal disorders in some individuals.*
9. Do you have a history of kidney disease or urinary problems? If so, when did you have it? How was it treated? Do you still have it?
10. Have you ever had surgery on the urinary system? If so, describe the procedure. How long ago did you have it done? Is the problem corrected? If not, describe it. Has anyone in your family ever had surgery on the urinary system? If so, please describe the procedures. How long ago was the surgery? Is the problem corrected? If not, describe it.
11. Do you have any of these problems: high blood pressure, diabetes, frequent bladder infections, kidney stones? If so, how was the problem treated? Describe any associated symptoms. Do you still have problems with this condition? Do you have any idea what causes this problem? *High blood pressure may contribute to the development of renal disease. Diabetes may significantly contribute to the development of renal disease. Infections may be caused by inadequate fluid intake, inadequate hygiene, and structural anomalies. In some clients this is an infrequent situation; in others it is a common malady. Kidney stones may be an isolated event or a recurring condition. Parathyroid disorders and any condition that causes an increase in calcium may contribute to the formation of kidney stones.*
12. Do you have any of these neurologic diseases: multiple sclerosis, Parkinson's disease, spinal cord injury, stroke? If so, which one? When was it diagnosed? How are you being treated? *These conditions contribute to the retention and stasis of urine, thus placing the client at risk for chronic urinary infections.*
13. Do you have any cardiovascular disease? If so, what was the diagnosis? When was it diagnosed? How are you being treated? *Hypertension in particular may significantly contribute to the development of renal failure.*
14. What medications do you currently take? What medications have you been taking in the last several months? Describe the type, the dose, and the reason why you are taking the medication. How often do you take it? Every day, as needed, or only when you remember? *It is important to know the client's compliance with the medication regimen. If the client has not completed a regimen of antibiotic therapy to clear a urinary tract infection, kidney infection, or sexually transmitted disease, the infection and may persist.*
15. Do you use any recreational drugs? If so, describe the type, amount, and frequency. How long have you been using these drugs? *Substance abuse over time may lead to kidney failure, potential for inadequate nutrition and hydration, and susceptibility to infection.*
16. Do you take any vitamins, protein powders, or dietary supplements ? If so, which ones? How much do you take? How many days a week do you take it? How many times a day? Why do you take it? *Excessive ingestion may contribute to the development of renal disorders.*
17. Describe your diet. Describe what you have eaten and drunk over the last week. How is your appetite? On a typical day, how much do you eat and drink? Do you drink alcoholic beverages? How many glasses of water do you drink a day? Are there any foods or beverages that bother you? Do any foods or beverages cause you discomfort either before or upon urination? Do any foods or beverages cause you to feel bloated or gassy? Do any foods or beverages affect the color, clarity, or smell of your urine? How much salt do you use? Do you retain fluid after consuming certain foods or beverages? *Questions such as these may provide information regarding the client's hydration status, potential allergic reaction to foods, and retention of fluid.*

18. Do you smoke or are you exposed to passive smoke? If so, what type of smoking (cigarette, cigar, pipe), for how long, how many packs per day? *Smoking has been linked to hypertension, which over time may contribute to the development of renal failure.*
19. Have you had any shortness of breath or difficulty breathing lately? If so, describe it. *This may alert you to the presence of hypertension and associated heart failure. These ultimately affect the renal circulation and function of the kidneys.*
20. Have you had influenza, a skin infection, a respiratory tract infection, or other infection recently? If so, what was it? What medication did the physician prescribe? Did you take all of the medication? Is this a recurrent problem? *If the infection was untreated, the client may be at risk for developing a renal infection.*
21. Have you recently had nausea, vomiting, diarrhea, or chills? If so, which one? Describe it. How was it treated? Has it recurred? *These conditions may indicate the presence of infection or recurring infection.*
22. Do you have any pain or discomfort in your back, sides, or abdomen? If so, show me where the pain or discomfort is located. Describe the pain. What aggravates or alleviates the symptoms?

    Here are some key factors to assess regarding the characteristics of the discomfort:

- *Quality*
- *Severity* (Rate the pain on a 1 to 10 scale.)
- *Location* (Is it on one side only?)
- *Duration* (Is it present all the time? How long does it last?)
- *Predictability* (Is it predictable?)
- *Onset* (When did it start?)
- *Relief* (Does anything relieve it?)
- *Radiation* (Does it radiate to another part of your body?)

23. Have you noticed any discharge from the urethral area or penis? If so, describe the color, odor, amount, and frequency. When did it start? Is this a recurrent problem? If so, what was the diagnosis, and how did the physician treat it? Did you follow the treatment as prescribed by the physician? *Discharge signals the potential presence of an infective process.*
24. Have you noticed any redness or other discoloration in the urethral area or penis? If so, describe the characteristics. *Redness may indicate the presence of inflammation, irritation, or infection.*
25. *If the client is a male:* Do you have prostate problems? If so, describe the symptoms and treatment. When was your last prostate exam?
26. *If the patient is a female:* How many children have you had? How do you cleanse yourself after urination, bowel movement? Do you use bubble bath? *Cleansing materials such as bubble bath may increase the incidence of urinary tract infections. Improper cleasing methods after elimination may also lead to infection.*
27. How often do you have intercourse? Do you urinate after intercourse? Are you aware of any sexual partners who may have sexually transmitted diseases? *Some clients may have a tendency to develop urinary tract infections if they do not urinate after intercourse.*
28. Has your skin changed recently? Describe the change. Has the color changed? Is it itchy all the time? *Clients with chronic renal failure have itchy skin (pruritus), and a uremic frost may develop on the skin as an adaptive response to renal failure.*
29. Have you had a recent urine analysis or blood work evaluating your kidneys? Do you know the results? *It is valuable for clients to know the results of their lab work and to provide the health care professional with their impression of the results.*
30. Do you live in an environment or work in an industry that exposes you to toxic chemicals? *These may contribute to the development of cancer of the urinary system.*
31. Have you traveled recently to a foreign country or any unfamiliar place? *The client may have been exposed to bacterial, viral, or fungal agents that affect renal function.*
32. Do you have difficulty concentrating, reading, or remembering things? *Difficulty remembering may be associated with renal dysfunction. Remember that there are many conditions that contribute to memory disturbances.*
33. If you have urinary problems, have they caused you embarrassment or anxiety? Have your urinary problems affected your social, personal, or sexual relationships? *These are important considerations, because they may affect clients' ability to function in other parts of their lives.*

Questions Related to Urinary Elimination Patterns

1. When you void, do you feel you are able to empty your bladder completely? If not, describe your feeling. *The feeling of being unable to empty the bladder may indicate the client is retaining urine or developing increased residual urine, which may contribute to the development of infection.*
2. Are you always able to control when you are going to urinate? If not, do you have to hurry to the bathroom as soon as you feel the urge to urinate? When you feel the urge to urinate, are you able to get to the toilet? Have you had an "accident" and wet yourself? Have you ever

urinated by accident when you've coughed, sneezed, lifted a heavy object? *Urgency and stress incontinence may be caused by an infection, inflammatory process, or the loss of muscle control over urination.*

3. Do you ever have to get up at night to urinate? If so, can you describe why? Is there any predictable pattern? How many times per night? *Nocturia may indicate the presence of aging changes in the older adult, cardiovascular changes, diuretic therapy, or habit.*
4. Do you have difficulty starting the flow of the stream? Does the stream flow continuously, or does it start and stop? Do you need to strain or push during urination to empty your bladder completely? *Difficulties of this sort may signify the presence of prostate disease.*
5. Do you ever have pain, burning, or other discomfort before, during, or after urination? If so, describe the discomfort, location, and timing. Do you have symptoms all of the time or some of the time? Is the discomfort predictable? For instance, is it related to time of the day, certain foods or beverages? Do you feel it after sexual intercourse? *Painful urination may indicate the presence of an infective process.*

Additional Questions with Infants, Children, and Adolescent Clients

Many of the preceding are appropriate for younger clients. In addition, you will gather information regarding functional status, presence of any congenital disorders, anatomic anomalies, and involuntary urination.

1. Have you ever been told that your child has a kidney that has failed to grow? *Renal agenesis may involve one or both kidneys. A genetic factor may be associated with the development of this condition in some cases.*
2. Has your child ever been diagnosed with a kidney disorder? If so, what is it called, what were the symptoms, and how was (is) it treated? *Some disorders, such as infections, are easily treated and do not recur, whereas others, such as glomerulonephritis, may be chronic.*
3. Have you ever observed any unusual shape or structure in your child's private anatomy? *Parents may report abnormally shaped external genitals, as seen in hypospadias and epispadias. In children with exstrophy of the bladder, the lower urinary tract is visible .*
4. Has your child ever had problems with involuntary urination? If so, what are the characteristics? What was the diagnosis? How was it treated? Is it still occurring? *Enuresis is the medical term for involuntary urination. If it occurs at night, it is termed nocturnal enuresis. This condition may have extensive impact on the social, mental, and physical well-being of the family and child.*
5. Have you started toilet training with your child? If yes, how successful has it been? Are there any current problems with toilet training?
6. Has you child decreased play activity? *Loss of interest in play may signal fatigue, which may be associated with renal failure.*
7. Are you changing the baby's diaper more or less than you were? *There are a variety of contributors to changes in elimation patterns, but renal failure, dehydration, overhydration, diet changes, obstruction, and stress may contribute to a change in normal pattern.*

Additional Questions with Childbearing Clients

The same questions that apply to adults apply in general to childbearing clients. The key indicators for this client are the presence of peripheral edema, swelling, hypertension, and headache. You should ask the childbearing client if she has experienced any of these symptoms, because they are often associated with the presence of pre-eclampsia, a potentially life-threatening condition.

1. Have you noticed any changes in your urinary pattern? *Often, the developing fetus places increasing pressure on the mother's bladder, causing urinary urgency. As a result, the client voids more often, in smaller amounts.*
2. Have you noticed unusual swelling in your ankles, feet, fingers, or wrists? Have you noticed any headaches? *These signs may be associated with pregnancy-induced hypertension and pre-eclampsia.*

Additional Questions with Older Clients

Questions for adults in general also apply to the older adult. The key considerations are the assessment of the presence of heart failure, hypertension, weight gain, difficulty voiding, urine characteristics, and changes in elimination patterns. Be sure to ask questions from the previous section that highlight these conditions and symptoms.

1. Have you noticed any unusual swelling in your ankles, feet, fingers, or wrists? *Swelling may be indicative of congestive heart failure. Associated with the swelling can be weight gain, fatigue, activity intolerance, and shortness of breath.*
2. *For males:* Have you noticed difficulty initiating the stream of urine, voiding in small amounts, and feeling the need to void more frequently than in the past? *These symptoms may be due to an enlarged prostate.*

Physical Assessment

Preparation

☑ **Gather the equipment.**

examination gown	examination light
gloves	stethoscope
drape	specimen container

☑ **Wash your hands.**

☑ **Explain the examination procedure to the client to allay any apprehension.**

☑ **Warm your hands and stethoscope to ensure the comfort of the client.**

☑ **Have the client empty the bladder, and send the urine to the laboratory for analysis. Explain proper collection of the specimen to the client. Be sure to allow the client privacy during the sample collection.**

☑ **If the client is a child, it may be important to have a parent in the exam room with you. In some cases, however, the parent's presence in the room may disturb the child. Determine the proper course of action.**

☑ **When examining a child, use a calm, reassuring approach. Because the examination includes assessment of intimate body parts, the child may be apprehensive, embarrassed, and fearful, especially if there is a history of abuse.**

Remember

- Provide a warm, comfortable environment.
- Ensure the client's privacy.
- To conserve the client's energy, walk around the client rather than having the client move from side to side as you proceed with the examination.
- Observe universal precautions.

ASSESSMENT TECHNIQUE/NORMAL FINDINGS | SPECIAL CONSIDERATIONS

General Appearance

Step 1 *Position the client.*

- Begin the examination with the client in a supine position with the abdomen exposed from the nipple line to the pubis (Figure 14.5).

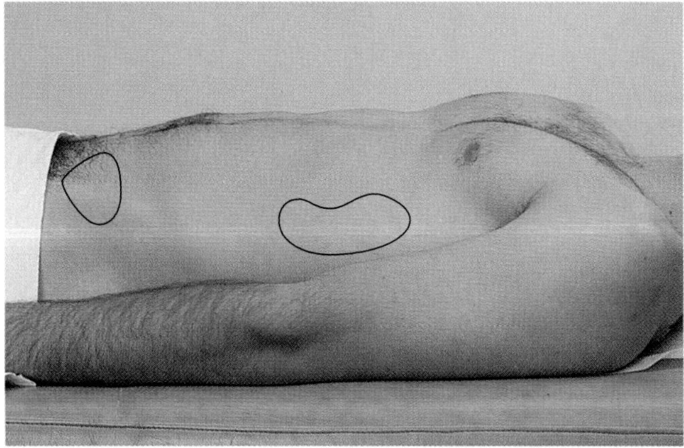

Figure 14.5 The client is supine at the beginning of the exam.

Step 2 *Assess the client's general appearance.*

- In addition, inspect the patient's skin for color, hydration status, scales, masses, indentations, or scars.

The client should not show signs of acute distress and should be mentally alert and oriented.

Clients with kidney disorders frequently look tired and complain of fatigue. If you suspect that the client has a kidney disorder, look for signs of circulatory overload (pulmonary edema) or peripheral edema (puffy face or fingers), or indications of pruritus (scratch marks on the skin).

Elevated nitrogenous wastes (azotemia) in the blood contribute to mental confusion.

The Abdomen and Renal Arteries

Step 1 *Inspect the abdomen for color, contour, symmetry, and distention.*

It may be helpful to stand at the client's side and inspect the abdomen under tangential light. You should also inspect the abdomen from the foot of the exam table (Figure 14.6).

A distended bladder may be visible in the suprapubic area, indicating the need to void and perhaps the inability to do so.

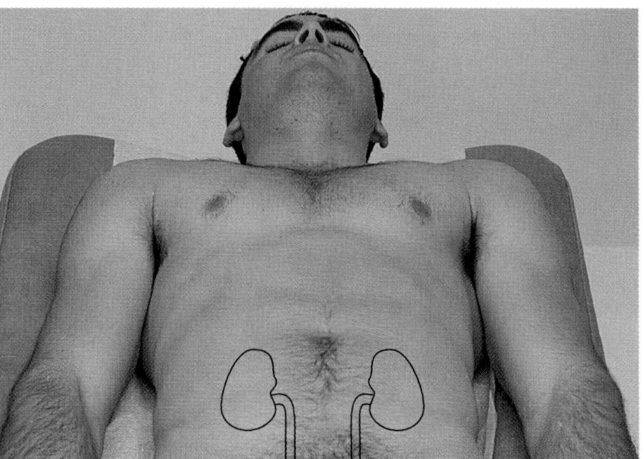

Figure 14.6 Inspecting the abdomen from the foot of the exam table.

ASSESSMENT TECHNIQUE/NORMAL FINDINGS	SPECIAL CONSIDERATIONS

Note that visual inspection of the suprapubic area may confirm the presence or absence of a distended bladder.

Normally, the client's abdomen is not distended, is relatively symmetric, and is free of bruises, masses, and swellings. (A complete discussion of abdominal assessment is provided in Chapter 13).

Many diseases may contribute to abdominal distention. These include renal conditions such as polycystic kidney disease; enlarged kidneys, as seen in acute pyelonephritis; ascites (accumulation of fluid) due to hepatic disease; and displacement of abdominal organs. Pressure from the abdominal contents on the diaphragm may alter the client's breathing pattern.

Step 2 ***Auscultate the right and left renal arteries to assess circulatory sounds.***

- Gently place the bell of the stethoscope over the extended midclavicular line on either side of the abdominal aorta, which is located above the level of the umbilicus (Figure 14.7).

Listen for a renal *bruit,* a swishing or blowing sound over the renal arteries. A renal bruit signals narrowing of the renal artery (renal stenosis). Stenosis of the artery or increased blood flow through the artery causes turbulent blood flow. Bruits heard over the epigastric area in the hypertensive client may also indicate the presence of renal arterial stenosis.

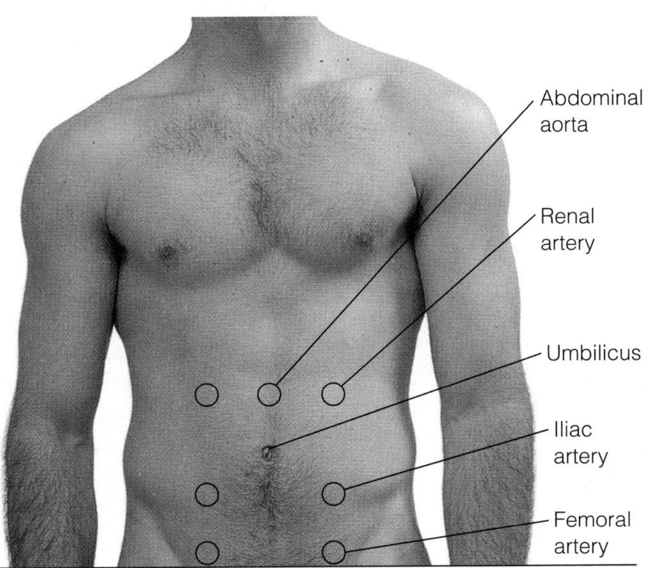

Figure 14.7 Auscultating the renal arteries.

- Be sure to auscultate both the right and left sides, and over the epigastric and umbilical areas.

In most cases, no sounds are heard; however, an upper abdominal bruit is occasionally heard in young adults and is considered normal. On a thin adult, renal artery pulsation may be auscultated.

The Kidneys and Flanks

Step 1 ***Position the client.***

- Place the client in a sitting position facing away from you with the back exposed.

ASSESSMENT TECHNIQUE/NORMAL FINDINGS	SPECIAL CONSIDERATIONS

Step 2 ***Inspect the left and right costovertebral angles for color and symmetry.***

A protrusion or elevation over a costovertebral angle occurs when the kidney is grossly enlarged or when a mass is present.

Step 3 ***Inspect the flanks (the side areas between the hips and the ribs) for color and symmetry.***

The costovertebral angles and flanks should be symmetric and even in color.

Carefully correlate this finding to other diagnostic cues as you proceed with the assessment. If ecchymosis is present (Grey Turner Sign), look for other signs of trauma such as blunt, penetrating wounds or lacerations.

ALERT!

Do not percuss or palpate the client who reports pain or discomfort in the pelvic region. Do not percuss or palpate the kidney if you suspect a tumor of the kidney, such as a neuroblastoma or Wilms' tumor. Palpation increases intra-abdominal pressure, which may contribute to intraperitoneal spreading of this nephroblastoma. Deep palpation should be performed only by experienced practitioners.

Step 4 ***Gently palpate the area over the left costovertebral angle*** (Figure 14.8).

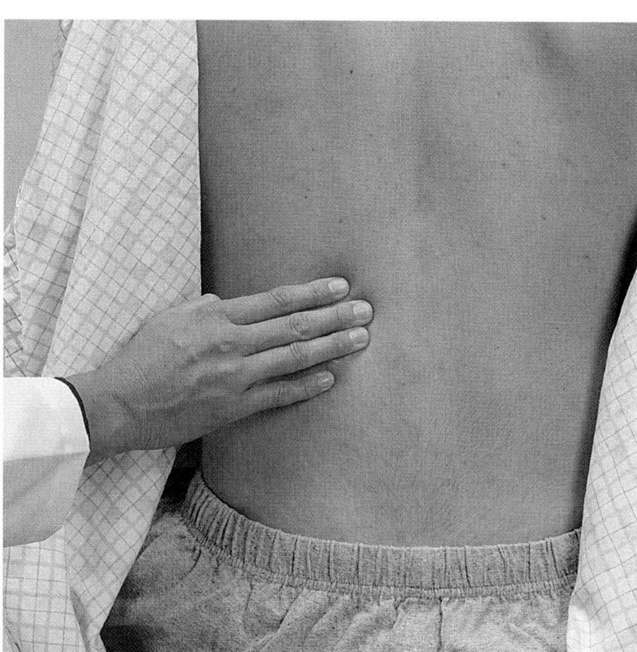

Figure 14.8 Palpating the left costovertebral angle.

- Watch the reaction and ask the client to describe any sensation the palpation causes. Normally, the client expresses no discomfort.
- Repeat over the right costovertebral angle.

Pain, discomfort, or tenderness from an enlarged or diseased kidney may occur over the costovertebral angle, flank, and abdomen. When questioned, the client complains of a dull, steady ache. This type of pain is associated with polycystic formation, pyelonephritis, and other disorders that cause kidney enlargement. In the client with polycystic kidney disease, sharp, sudden, intermittent pain may mean that a cyst in the kidney has ruptured. If the costovertebral angle is tender, red, and warm, and the client is experiencing chills, fever, nausea, and vomiting, the underlying kidney could be inflamed or infected.

The pain caused by *calculi* (stones) in the kidney or upper ureter is unique and different in character, severity, and duration than that caused by kidney enlargement. This pain occurs as calculi travel from the kidney to the ureters and the urinary bladder. Some clients experience no pain, and others feel excruciating pain. A stationary stone causes a dull, aching pain. As stones travel down the urinary tract, spasms occur. These spasms produce sharp, intermittent, colicky pain (often accompanied by chills, fever, nausea, and vomiting) that radiates from the flanks to the lower quadrants of the abdomen, and in some cases, the upper thigh and scrotum or labium.

ASSESSMENT TECHNIQUE/NORMAL FINDINGS | SPECIAL CONSIDERATIONS

Referral

If the client reports severe pain, hematuria (blood in the urine) or oliguria (diminished volume of urine), and nausea and vomiting, be alert for hydroureter, a frequent complication that occurs when a renal calculus moves into a ureter. The calculus blocks and dilates the ureter, causing spasms and severe pain. Hydroureter can lead to shock, infection, and impaired renal function. If you suspect hydroureter or obstruction at any point in the urinary tract, seek medical collaboration immediately.

Step 5 *Use blunt or indirect percussion to further assess the kidneys.*

ALERT!

Do **not** proceed with blunt percussion over the costovertebral angle if the client complains of pain, discomfort, or tenderness.

Pain or discomfort during and after blunt percussion suggests kidney disease. Correlate this finding with other assessment findings.

- Place your left palm flat over the left costovertebral angle.
- Thump the back of your left hand with the ulnar surface of your right fist, causing a gentle thud over the costovertebral angle (Figure 14.9).

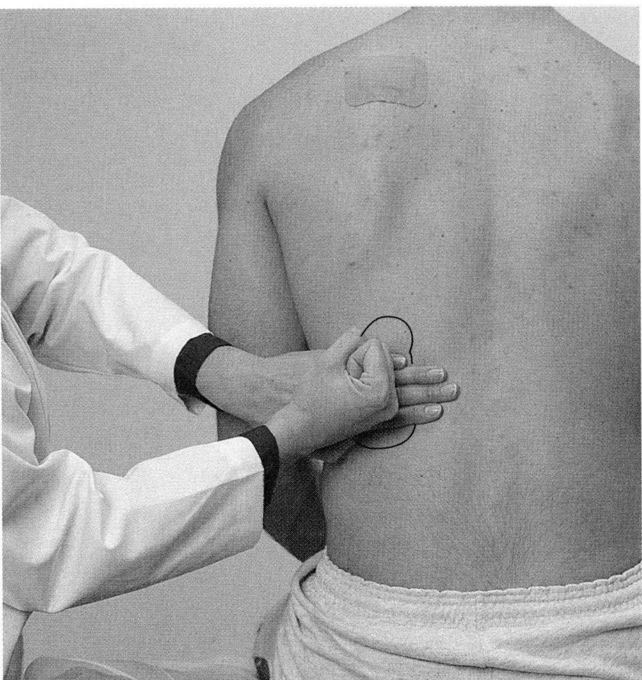

Figure 14.9 Blunt percussion over the left costovertebral angle.

ASSESSMENT TECHNIQUE/NORMAL FINDINGS

SPECIAL CONSIDERATIONS

- Repeat the procedure on the right side. Ask the client to describe the sensation as you examine each side.

The client should feel no pain or tenderness with pressure or percussion.

The Left Kidney

Step 1 *Attempt to palpate the lower pole of the left kidney.*

- Although it is not usually palpable, attempt to palpate the lower pole of the kidney for size, contour, consistency, and sensation. Note that the rib cage obscures the upper poles.

When enlargement occurs in the presence of conditions such as neoplasms and polycystic disease, the kidneys may be palpable. Otherwise, they are rarely palpable.

ALERT!

Because deep kidney palpation can cause tissue trauma, beginning practitioners should not attempt either deep palpation or "capture" of the kidney unless supervised by an experienced nurse practitioner. Deep kidney palpation should not be done in clients who have had a recent kidney transplant or an abdominal aortic aneurysm.

- Position the client in the supine position. All palpation should be performed from the client's right side.
- While standing on the client's right side, reach over the client and place your left hand between the posterior rib cage and the iliac crest (the left flank).
- Place your right hand on the left upper quadrant of the abdomen lateral and parallel to the left rectus muscle just below the costal margin.
- Instruct the client to take a deep breath. As the client inhales, lift the client's left flank with your left hand and press deeply with your right hand (approximately 4 cm) to attempt to palpate the lower pole of the kidney (Figure 14.10).

Be careful not to mistake an enlarged spleen for an enlarged left kidney. An enlarged kidney feels smooth and rounded, whereas an enlarged spleen feels sharper, with a more delineated edge.

ASSESSMENT TECHNIQUE/NORMAL FINDINGS | SPECIAL CONSIDERATIONS

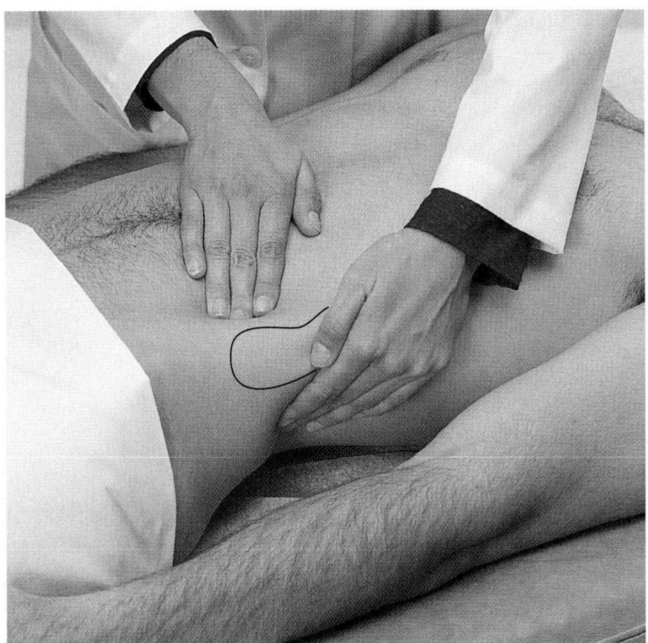

Figure 14.10 Palpating the lower poles of the left kidney.

Step 2 *Attempt to "capture" the left kidney.*

Because of its position deep in the retroperitoneal space, the left kidney is not normally palpable. The "capture" maneuver may enable you to palpate it. This maneuver is possible because the kidneys descend during inspiration and slide back into their normal position during exhalation.

- Standing on the client's right side, place your left hand under the client's back to elevate the flank as before. Place your right hand on the left upper quadrant of the abdomen lateral and parallel to the left rectus muscle with the fingertips just below the left costal margin.
- Instruct the client to take a deep breath and hold it. As the client inhales, attempt to "capture" the kidney between your two hands.
- Ask the client to exhale slowly, then briefly hold the breath. At the same time, slowly release the pressure of your fingers.
- As the client exhales, you will feel the captured kidney move back into its previous position.

ASSESSMENT TECHNIQUE/NORMAL FINDINGS	SPECIAL CONSIDERATIONS

The kidney surface should be rounded, smooth, firm, and nontender.

An enlarged palpable kidney could be painful for the client. This suggests tumor, cyst, or hydrodnephrosis.

The Right Kidney

Step 1 ***Attempt to palpate the lower pole of the right kidney.***

- Standing on the client's right side, place your left hand under the back parallel to the right twelfth rib (about halfway between the costal margin and iliac crest) with your fingertips reaching for the costovertebral angle.
- Place your right hand on the right upper quadrant of the abdomen lateral to the right rectus muscle and just below the right costal margin.
- Instruct the client to take a deep breath.
- As the client inhales, lift the flank with your left hand and use deep palpation to feel for the lower pole of the kidney.

Step 2 ***Attempt to "capture" the right kidney.***

- Place your left hand under the client's right flank.
- Place your right hand on the right upper quadrant of the abdomen with the fingertips lateral and parallel to the right rectus muscle just below the right costal margin.
- Instruct the client to take a deep breath and hold it. As the client inhales, attempt to "capture" the kidney between your two hands.
- Ask the client to exhale slowly, then briefly hold the breath. At the same time, slowly release the pressure of your fingers.
- As the client exhales you will feel the captured kidney move back into its previous position.

The kidney surface should be rounded, smooth, firm, and nontender.

The lower pole of the right kidney is palpable in some individuals, especially in thin, relaxed females. If palpable, the lower pole of the kidney has a smooth, firm, uninterrupted surface.

During the capture maneuver, some clients describe a nonpainful sensation as the kidney slides between the nurse's fingers back into its normal position.

Be careful not to mistake an enlarged liver for an enlarged right kidney. An enlarged kidney feels smooth and rounded, whereas an enlarged liver is closer to the midline and has a more distinct border. Suspect polycystic kidney disease or carcinoma when there is gross enlargement of the kidney. The kidneys may be twice or three times their normal size in clients with polycystic disease.

The Urinary Bladder

Step 1 ***Palpate the bladder to determine symmetry, location, size, and sensation.***

A distended bladder feels smooth, round, and taut. An asymmetric contour or nodular surface suggests abnormal growth that should be correlated with other findings. In males with urethral obstruction due to hypertrophy or hyperplasia of the prostate, the bladder is enlarged.

ASSESSMENT TECHNIQUE/NORMAL FINDINGS | SPECIAL CONSIDERATIONS

ALERT!

Deep palpation should be done only with caution. Palpate gently, because this technique may cause discomfort.

- Use deep palpation to locate the fundus of the bladder, approximately 5 to 7 cm (2 to 3 in) below the umbilicus in the lower abdomen.
- Once you have located the fundus of the bladder, continue to palpate, outlining the shape and contour (Figure 14.11).

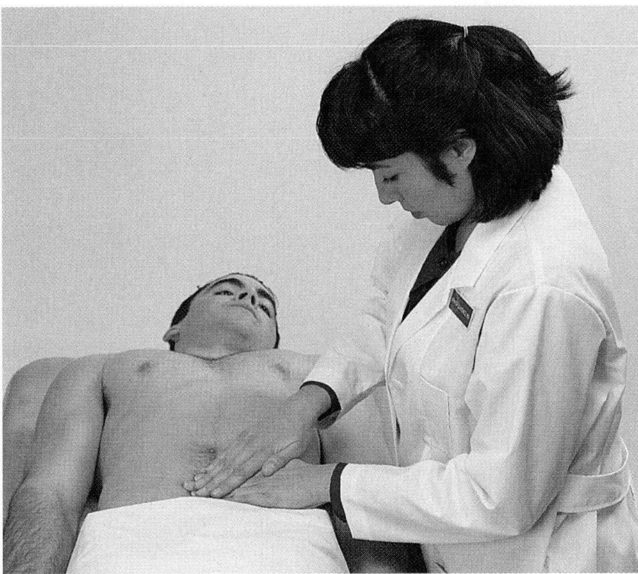

Figure 14.11 Palpating the bladder.

- Slide your fingers over the surface of the bladder and continue palpating to determine smoothness and continuity.

The surface of the bladder should feel smooth and uninterrupted. An empty bladder is usually not palpable. When the bladder is moderately full, it should be firm, smooth, symmetric, and nontender. As the bladder fills, the fundus can reach the level of the umbilicus. A full bladder is firm and buoyant.

Step 2 ***Percuss the bladder to determine its location and degree of fullness.***

ALERT!

If the bladder is distended with urine and the client is unable to void, obtain an order to catheterize the client. Reduce the contents of a distended bladder *slowly* to prevent atony of the bladder wall.

ASSESSMENT TECHNIQUE/NORMAL FINDINGS | SPECIAL CONSIDERATIONS

- Begin with direct percussion of the bladder over the suprapubic area.
- Move your fingers upward toward the umbilicus as you continue to percuss. A full bladder produces a dull tone upon percussion.
- Continue percussing upward toward the umbilicus until no more dull tones are heard (Figure 14.12). The point at which dull tones cease is the upper margin of the bladder.

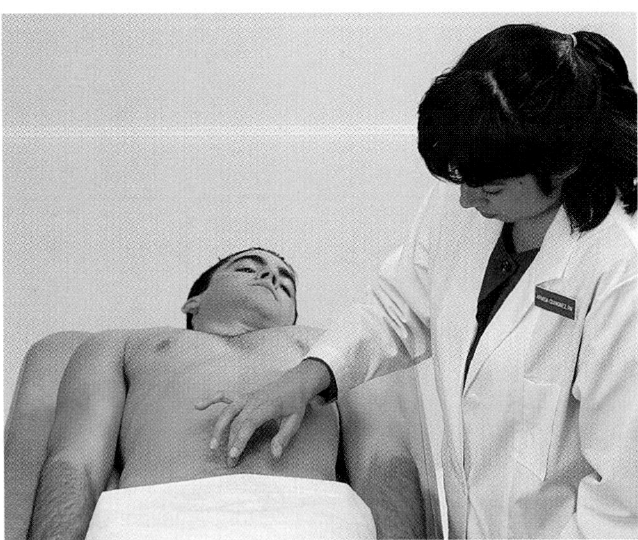

Figure 14.12 Indirect percussion of the bladder.

Some practitioners conclude the assessment of the urinary system with the inspection and palpation of the penis and urethral meatus in the male client or the inspection of the urethral meatus in the female client. Other practitioners consider these structures with the assessment of the genitalia. These techniques are discussed in Chapter 15.

Reminders

- In addition to the above steps, consider the common variations in physical assessment findings for the different client groups discussed in the following sections.
- After completing the physical assessment, answer any questions the client has, and provide appropriate client teaching for health promotion and self-care (see page 395).
- Confirm that the client is comfortable and has no adverse effects from the procedure. Dim the lights, remove the equipment, and leave the client in a comfortable position to rest or to get dressed.
- Document the assessment findings as described in Chapter 1. See pages 393–395 for information on identifying nursing diagnoses commonly associated with the urinary system.

Developmental Considerations

Infant, Children, and Adolescent Clients

At birth, renal blood flow increases, with a significant allotment to the renal medulla. The glomerular filtration rate also increases at birth compared to the fetal filtration rate and continues to increase until the first or second year of life. The fluid and electrolyte balance in an infant or child is fragile. Illnesses that cause dehydration, loss of fluids, or lack of fluid intake may rapidly lead to metabolic acidosis and fluid imbalance. Serious, chronic dysfunction of this system may impair the child's growth and development.

It is important to consider the health practices of the family when the genital areas are unclean in infants or children of any age. Presence of a diaper rash is a clue that you should explore the family's hygiene practices; however, diaper rash is often difficult to control, and patient, supportive client teaching is indicated. (See Chapter 8.)

Examine infants for anomalies such as scrotal edema, undescended testes, and noncentral placement of the urinary meatus. Bed-wetting is a difficult problem for both the child and the family and may influence the child's relationship with the family. The child's confidence and social development may also be affected by bed-wetting.

A reduction in the child's play activity may be an indicator of renal dysfunction. Renal disease can contribute to fatigue.

Sexual relations are not limited to adults. Potential signs that a child or adolescent is sexually active are perineal inflammation, rash, warts, abnormal discharge, urinary tract infection, and vaginal plaques. When these are present, explore the possibility that the child or adolescent is sexually active. Consider that the child or adolescent may be in an abusive situation and not a willing participant in this activity.

For a comprehensive health assessment of infants, children, and adolescents, see Chapter 19.

Childbearing Clients

During the first trimester, the enlarging uterus presses against the bladder, increasing the frequency of urination. Frequency decreases during the second trimester, then recurs during the third trimester as the presenting part of the fetus descends into the pelvis and again presses on the bladder.

During pregnancy, the amount of urine a woman produces increases, causing the childbearing client to feel the need to urinate more frequently. There is also a tendency for the urine to test positive for sugar. In the postpartum period, edema and hyperemia of the bladder mucosa cause decreased sensation and contribute to overdistention of the bladder. Incomplete emptying of the bladder often accompanies this condition, increasing the client's susceptibility to urinary tract infection.

For a comprehensive health assessment of childbearing clients, see Chapter 20.

Older Clients

The effects of aging certainly take their toll on the kidneys. The weight of the kidneys may drop by as much as 30%, particularly in the renal cortex. Renal blood flow and perfusion gradually decrease. The capillary system in the glomeruli atrophies. Although the vasculature in the renal medulla remains relatively well preserved, the arcuate and interlobular arteries may become distorted, resulting in a tortuous configuration. All structures of both the renal cortex and renal medulla experience some degree of decline, especially the nephrons. About 30–50% of the glomeruli degenerate because of fibrosis, hyalinization, and fat deposition. All of these factors contribute to the loss of filtration surface area in the glomerular capillary tufts by the age of 75. Creatinine clearance decreases slowly after 40 years of age, as does the ability to concentrate and dilute urine.

The older client's decreased sensation of thirst and resultant decreased intake of water relates directly to the body's compensatory response of concentrating urine. Yet, antidiuretic hormone is not as effective as in a younger client; thus, concentrations and activity of renin and aldosterone are reduced with advanced age by as much as 30–50%. This combination of circumstances places the older client at risk for hyperkalemia.

The older client also has a reduced capacity to produce ammonia, which interacts with acids. Reduced ability to clear medications and acids, along with reduced ability to resorb bicarbonate and glucose, makes the older client more susceptible to (1) toxicity related to medications, (2) the effects of respiratory and/or metabolic acidosis, (3) increased concentrations of glucose in the urine, and (4) the loss of fluids.

Urinary elimination becomes a major concern as an individual advances in age and significant changes in urinary and bladder function begin to occur. Major changes in both men and women include urinary retention leading to increased urinary infections; involuntary bladder contractions resulting in urgency, frequency, and incontinence; decreased bladder capacity causing frequent voiding; and weakening of the urinary sphincters causing urgency and incontinence.

Nocturia is another major concern of older persons, especially men. When an older person is at rest in a horizontal position, the heart is able to pump blood through the kidneys more efficiently, facilitating the excretion of urine. This factor, combined with weakened bladder and urethral muscles, contributes to nocturnal micturition. Other causes of nocturia, such as urinary infection, hyperglycemia, medication use, and stool impactions, should not be ruled out.

Benign prostatic hypertrophy (hyperplasia) is a common cause of urinary retention and obstruction in men. As men age, the prostate gland enlarges, encroaching upon the urethra. Unrecognized urinary tract obstruction from an enlarged prostate results in damage to the upper urinary tract.

Postmenopausal women experience a decrease in estrogen that may lead to urine leakage, reduced acidity in the lower urinary tract, and urinary tract infections.

Allow older clients with urinary tract problems extra time to explain their concerns. Quite often, older people have difficulty talking about bladder or bowel concerns because they consider discussion of one's "privates" too personal. Additionally, some clients may find it distasteful to discuss elimination with anyone of the opposite sex. Make an effort to use the terms with which the client is familiar. For example, some older clients still use the term "dropsy" to describe a kidney disorder, or "Bright's disease" to describe glomerulonephritis.

When you assess an individual who experiences incontinence, ask about the client's ability to get to the bathroom. Many clients who are diagnosed as incontinent simply cannot get to the bathroom on time because of other age-related conditions such as arthritis, strokes, or blindness. Whenever possible, observe clients in their own settings to determine what disabilities or environmental barriers (eg, stairs, distance) hinder the client's ability to function.

The physical assessment of the older person is similar to that of any other adult; however, use special caution when palpating the kidneys through the abdominal wall. Because the abdominal musculature of older persons tends to be more flaccid than that of younger adults, use less pressure during deep palpation. Be aware that the kidneys of the older client are more difficult to palpate abdominally because the mass of the adrenal cortex decreases with age. Omit blunt percussion in a frail older person; instead, rely on palpation of the costovertebral angles and flanks to reveal any pain or tenderness. A digital examination of the prostate gland is always included as part of the urinary assessment in older men (see Chapter 15), and palpation of the urethra through the anterior vaginal wall is recommended for all older women.

For a comprehensive health assessment of older clients, see Chapter 21.

Psychosocial Considerations

Clients suffering from incontinence are at increased risk for social isolation, self-esteem disturbance, and other psychosocial problems. A stressful lifestyle may contribute to chronic urinary tract infections. Stasis of urine, and resultant infection, may occur when a client feels "too busy" to empty the bladder as needed. Urinary tract infections in females may also result from sexual trauma or sexual intercourse with a new partner. Consider the possibility of sexual abuse in a child or adolescent who presents with a urinary tract infection.

Self-Care Considerations

Inhalation of cigarette smoke significantly increases the risk for renal cell carcinoma. Cigarette smokers have been shown to develop bladder cancer four times more often than nonsmokers; however, the incidence is related to the number of cigarettes smoked, the age at which smoking began, and degree of inhalation. Also, although not consistently demonstrated, it has been suggested that coffee and tea consumption may contribute to the development of bladder cancer.

Consumption of alcohol may cause an increase in the need to void and lead, in some cases, to incontinence. Men who are chronic abusers of alcohol may experience testicular atrophy and impotence. Women may experience amenorrhea. Diets high in fats may lead to the development of atherosclerosis, which may affect the renal arteries and vasculature, potentially resulting in renal failure.

Lack of proper hygiene may make the client susceptible to infective processes. This is especially true for women because their urethra is shorter than that of men. Some people do not bathe daily, thus increasing the potential for infective processes. Some individuals use bubble baths or baking-soda baths, which have been implicated in an increased incidence of urinary tract infections.

Family, Cultural, and Environmental Considerations

When considering the culture's influence on a client's health care practices, be open-minded and sensitive to the specific values and beliefs of the client without passing judgment. Also, remember that not all individuals adhere to the norms, values, and practices of their culture.

When you question a client regarding urinary elimination patterns, examine private areas, or obtain a sample of urine, consideration for the client's privacy and modesty is essential. Though not every client is embarrassed by these components of assessment, many individuals experience considerable uneasiness. It is essential to afford the client as much privacy and dignity as possible. Some individuals will not disrobe or allow a physical examination by anyone of the opposite sex. Some will not allow a sample of their body fluids to be taken and examined by strangers.

Clients with hypertension or diabetes mellitus are especially vulnerable to kidney damage if they do not follow a strict medication and diet regimen. Hispanic and African Americans experience higher rates of hypertension and diabetes mellitus; however, these conditions are not limited to these populations. You can help all clients maintain optimal health by providing information on diet, prevention of hypertension, and the importance of compliance with medication regimens.

People from certain cultures ingest more calcium than usual from sources such as milk products, leafy vegetables, and seafood. As a result, they may be more susceptible to renal calculi. Also, people who live in the southwestern United States or other areas where the mineral content of water is high are more susceptible to renal calculi.

Information obtained during the focused interview may identify whether the client is taking herbs prescribed by a healer. Obtain as complete information about the herbs as possible.

Organizing the Data

Based upon the information obtained from the interview and physical assessment, identify nursing diagnoses to guide an individualized plan of care. Certain nursing diagnoses apply specifically to the urinary system; however, a wide variety of nursing diagnoses may be appropriate for the client.

Identifying Nursing Diagnoses

NANDA lists eight nursing diagnoses that relate specifically to the urinary system: *Altered urinary elimination, Dysreflexia, Incontinence* (functional, stress, urge, reflex, and total), and *Urinary retention.* In addition, other nursing diagnoses may be appropriate for the client.

Altered urinary elimination may be precipitated by a wide variety of factors. It reflects any significant change in a client's urinary elimination pattern. (See Table 14.1 on page 394.)

Dysreflexia affects clients with spinal cord injuries at level T7 or higher. Bladder distention causes a sympathetic response that can trigger a potentially life-threatening hypertensive crisis.

If *Incontinence*, the inability to retain urine, is the client's problem, determine which of the five types of incontinence is present. *Functional incontinence* occurs when the client is unable to reach the toilet in time because of environmental, psychosocial, or physical factors. *Reflex incontinence* occurs in clients with spinal cord damage when urine is involuntarily lost. In *Stress incontinence*, involuntary urination occurs when intra-abdominal pressure is increased during coughing, sneezing, or straining. Aging changes may also contribute to stress incontinence. *Urge incontinence* may be caused by con-

DIAGNOSTIC REASONING IN ACTION

Ms Sadie Basset is a 52-year-old African American female who arrives at the Metropolitan Women's Clinic complaining of itching, burning, and frequency of urination. She tells Louise Lo, RN, "I feel like I have to go to the bathroom every 10 minutes. I'm just miserable. I'm burning all the time, and I have tenderness here." She is pointing to her lower abdominal area. Ms Basset states that sometimes she feels a sharp abdominal pain and a sudden urge to urinate. On a few of these occasions, she has difficulty getting to the bathroom on time and even has a few "accidents." Ms Lo asks if Ms Basset has any illnesses. Ms Basset reports that she was diagnosed with diabetes mellitus a few weeks ago.

After the interview, Ms Lo performs a physical examination. Blood pressure is 106/82; pulse 68, respirations 20, and temperature 101.2F. Abdomen is flat and soft. Bowel sounds are active and present in all four quadrants. Client complains of tenderness over the suprapubic area on palpation. The urinary meatus is red and edematous with no apparent discharge. Induration of the urinary meatus is noted on palpation of the anterior vaginal wall. The urinary stream is strong and steady. The urine is dark yellow with a hint of blood. It is cloudy and has a strong, foul odor.

Many pieces of information have been provided that, when clustered, will guide Ms Lo to select appropriate nursing diagnoses. The combination of urgency, frequency, inability to retain urine, and lower abdominal tenderness alerts her to the potential problem of infection. The sudden sharp abdominal pain and sudden urge to void relate to the clinical sign of bladder spasms, which may accompany an infective process and contribute to incontinence. Ms Bassett also has been diagnosed with diabetes mellitus. The elevated blood sugar provides a rich medium for bacteria to grow.

The nursing diagnoses appropriate for Ms Bassett are:

1. *Urge incontinence* related to elevated blood sugar and reduced estrogen blood levels
2. *Pain* related to bladder spasms
3. *Altered body temperature* related to bacterial infection
4. *Knowledge deficit* related to lack of information about diabetes mellitus and the increased risk of infection

Ms Lo explains that diabetes mellitus can make a client more susceptible to infection. She explains the clinical signs and what they mean. Then she reviews how to prevent urinary tract infections.

Table 14.1 Nursing Diagnoses Commonly Associated with the Urinary System

ALTERED URINARY ELIMINATION

Definition: The state in which the individual experiences a disturbance in urine elimination (NANDA).

DEFINING CHARACTERISTICS

Dysuria	Nocturia
Frequency	Retention
Hesitancy	Urgency
Incontinence	

RELATED FACTORS

Multiple causality including anatomic obstruction; Sensory; Motor impairment; Urinary tract infection.

STRESS URINARY INCONTINENCE

Definition: The state in which an individual experiences a loss of urine of less than 50 ml occurring with increased abdominal pressure (NANDA).

DEFINING CHARACTERISTICS

Major	*Minor*
Reported or observed dribbling with increased abdominal pressure	Urinary urgency; urinary frequency (more often than every 2 hours)

RELATED FACTORS

Degenerative changes in pelvic muscles and structural supports associated with increased age; High intra-abdominal pressure; Incompetent bladder outlet; Overdistention between voidings; Weak pelvic muscles and structural supports.

URINARY RETENTION

Definition: The state in which the individual experiences incomplete emptying of the bladder (NANDA).

DEFINING CHARACTERISTICS

Major:	*Minor:*
Bladder distention; small, frequent voiding or absence of urine output	Sensation of bladder fullness, dribbling, residual urine, overflow incontinence

RELATED FACTORS

High urethral pressure caused by weak detrusor; Inhibition of reflex arc; Strong sphincter; Blockage.

suming a significant volume of fluids over a relatively short period. Urge incontinence may also be due to diminished bladder capacity. *Total incontinence* is related to a neurologic condition. A variety of physiologic, psychologic, environmental, developmental, medical, and self-care factors may be related to incontinence. (See Table 14.1.)

Urinary retention is a chronic state in which the client cannot empty the bladder. (See Table 14.1.) In most cases the client voids small amounts of overflow urine when the bladder reaches its greatest capacity. After determining whether the client has the defining characteristics of urinary retention, identify pathophysiologic, situational, maturational, and treatment-related factors that contributed to the development of this problem.

Other nursing diagnoses that are often associated with conditions affecting the urinary system are: anxiety, pain, fatigue, altered family processes, fluid volume excess, altered growth and development, noncompliance, altered nutrition (less than body requirements), toileting self-care deficit, body image disturbance, situational low self-esteem, and impaired skin integrity.

Common Alterations in the Health of the Urinary System

Problems commonly associated with the urinary system include:

Bladder Cancer Seen later in life, bladder cancer is more frequently seen in men than women. Smoking has been linked to this disease. The patient may be totally asymptomatic or have hematuria, flank pain, and frequent urination.

Glomerulonephritis This entity is an inflammation of the glomerulus. The key clinical manifestations are hematuria with red blood cell casts and proteinuria.

Renal Calculi Calculi are stones that block the urinary tract. They are usually composed of calcium, struvite, or a combination of magnesium, ammonium, phosphate, and uric acid. Pain is the primary symptom. The pain may radiate and is variable in location and severity. Other symptoms include spasms, nausea, vomiting, pain on urination, frequency and urgency of urination, and gross hematuria.

Renal Tumor Tumors may be either benign or malignant, with malignant being more common. There is an association with smoking. The key manifestations are hematuria, flank pain, weight loss, and palpable mass in the flank.

Renal Failure Renal failure may be either acute or progress to a chronic state. Acute renal failure that does not progress to a chronic state includes three stages: oliguria, diuresis, and recovery. Other symptoms include fluid retention, hyperkalemia, hyperphosphatemia, nausea, and vomiting. Uremia is the classic hallmark of chronic renal failure. Anorexia, nausea, vomiting, mentation changes, uremic frost, pruritus, weight loss, fatigue, and edema are common symptoms of uremia.

Urinary Tract Infection Bacteria are the cause of urinary tract infections. The bladder is the most common site of the infection, which results in inflammation of the bladder called cystitis; however, infection may include the kidneys. Clients may be asymptomatic, but the classic symptoms include urgency, frequency, dribbling, pain upon urination, and suprapubic or lower back pain. Hematuria, as well as cloudy and foul-smelling urine, may accompany the other signs.

Health Promotion and Client Education

When the urinary assessment is ended, answer questions the client has about urinary health. Use this opportunity to give clients information to promote, maintain, and protect the health of their urinary system.

Promoting the General Health of the Urinary System

To promote the general health of the urinary system

- Drink at least eight glasses of water or other fluids each day.
- Consume coffee, alcohol, and cola drinks in moderation. These fluids are associated with urinary tract disorders.
- Drink carbonated beverages in moderation, and eat foods that contain caffeine, baking powder, or baking soda in moderation.
- Avoid cigarettes. Smoking causes bladder irritation and is associated with the development of bladder carcinoma.
- Use over-the-counter drugs that contain phenacetin in moderation.
- Maintain an active lifestyle.
- Use protective devices to prevent chemical contamination in the workplace.

- Report to a health professional any of the following: changes in urinary elimination patterns as well as any changes in the appearance of the urine, including blood, pus, excessive mucus, or color change.
- Seek assistance from a health professional for any problems associated with urinary elimination such as an elevated temperature, chills, painful or burning urination, urgency, frequency, lower back pain or flank pain, urinary retention, or any other abnormal signs.

Preventing Bladder Infections

To prevent bladder infections

- Drink plenty of water.
- Maintain the proper acid pH of the urine by including meat, eggs, cheese, whole grains, cranberries, prunes, and plums in the diet.
- Avoid urethral irritants such as bubble bath, scented tissue, and perfumed soap.
- Always clean the perineum from front to back to avoid contamination of the urethra.
- Wear cotton underwear for adequate ventilation.
- If using a diaphragm for contraception, switch to another method.
- Urinate immediately after sexual intercourse.

Preventing Cancer of the Urinary Tract

All clients should know if they are at risk for urinary tract cancer so that they can make lifestyle changes if necessary. The American Cancer Society states that the incidence of bladder cancer is three times higher in men than in women, and the age-adjusted bladder cancer rate is two times higher in European Americans than in persons of African ancestry.

To prevent cancer of the urinary tract, you should know that the etiologic factors associated with bladder cancer include

- Cigarette smoking
- Exposure to chemicals used in the textile and rubber industries
- Exposure to *Schistosoma haemotobium,* a parasite common in Asia, Africa, and South America

The risk factors for renal cell carcinoma are:

- Most frequently seen in males over the age of 35 who smoke
- Use of analgesics containing phenacetin
- Exposure to asbestos, cadmium, and gasoline

Clients should be cautioned to seek professional assistance for the following changes: weight loss (10–20 pounds in recent months); a change in normal urinary elimination patterns; hematuria; or persistent lower back or flank pain. An abdominal mass or distended abdomen should be reported immediately.

DIAGNOSTIC REASONING IN ACTION

A 35-year-old female, Ms Toni Jackson, checks in to the emergency room. She has recently been diagnosed with parathyroid adenoma. Her serum calcium is elevated. She is scheduled to undergo surgery in 2 weeks. She states that today while driving to work she experienced a sudden, sharp pain in her right flank. She needed to pull off the road because the pain was so severe. After several minutes, it subsided to a dull ache. She proceeded to go to work, where the pain recurred and was so severe that it caused her to double over. It radiated to her back and into the groin area. She became nauseated, vomited, and could not straighten up. The situation was further complicated by a frequent urgency to void. When she did void, she produced only small amounts. Initially the urine was clear yellow, but blood began to appear. The blood was first seen to tinge the urine pink, but after several voidings her urine demonstrates frank bleeding. Ms Jackson is writhing on the exam table and moaning. Physical examination reveals blood pressure 160/90; pulse 110, respirations 32, and temperature 98 F.

Jonathan Green, RN, clusters and critically analyzes this information to determine appropriate nursing diagnoses. He considers the client's inability to straighten up, her nausea and vomiting, and her moaning and writhing. It is known that pain is the paramount symptom of renal calculi. A renal calculus that is stationary or lodged may cause either no pain or dull pain. When the calculus is moving, the pain may be excruciating. The size and shape of the calculus can contribute to the intensity of the pain. Nausea and vomiting are commonly associated symptoms. If the calculus cuts into the tissue, blood will be mixed with the urine and cause both burning upon urination and contribute to the urinary frequency.

One of several nursing diagnoses that applies to Ms Jackson in this situation is *Pain*. Because of her parathyroid adenoma, Ms Jackson's serum calcium is elevated and can lead to the development of renal calculi. Ms Jackson's report of pain radiating to the back and groin, frank bleeding, urgency and burning, hypertension, tachycardia, and agitated state all are diagnostic cues suggestive of pain.

Other nursing diagnoses that may apply to Ms Jackson include *Altered urinary elimination, Fluid volume deficit* related to nausea and vomiting, and *Anxiety*.

Summary

The urinary system is crucial to total health. Every organ in the body depends upon the kidneys to remove metabolic wastes and toxins. When assessing the urinary system, gather data about the client's family and past history, urinary elimination patterns, exposure to substances that are hazardous to the urinary system, and psychosocial factors that may plague the client with a urinary problem. By inspecting, auscultating, percussing, and palpating the abdomen, costovertebral angles, and the urinary meatus, you can determine whether the client's urinary system is functioning properly and whether nursing interventions need to be instituted. To perform a successful assessment, you need a knowledge of the anatomy and physiology of the urinary system as well as an understanding of pertinent cultural, ethnic, and developmental factors. Upon completing the assessment, provide information the client can use to promote, protect, and maintain urinary health. In addition, teach the client how to assess urinary problems that should be reported to a health professional. At the completion of the assessment, document the findings for other health professionals who will care for the client. Throughout the assessment process, use the diagnostic reasoning process to identify and validate appropriate nursing diagnoses.

Key Points

- ✓ Assessing the urinary system requires a sound knowledge of the anatomy and physiology of the kidneys, renal arteries, ureters, urinary bladder, and urethra.
- ✓ During the focused interview, perform a complete review of the urinary system, investigate the chief complaint, family history, urinary patterns, health problems, and environmental factors that may have contributed to urinary problems.
- ✓ Begin the physical assessment with a general survey, observing the client's general appearance, orientation, and level of consciousness.
- ✓ Use the costovertebral angle, the rectus abdominis muscle, and the symphysis pubis as landmarks when you locate and palpate the kidneys and urinary bladder.
- ✓ During the physical examination, inspect the abdominal wall; auscultate the renal arteries; inspect, palpate, and percuss the kidneys and flanks; percuss and palpate the urinary bladder.
- ✓ Blunt percussion is not used if the client has lower back pain, a recent kidney transplant, or tenderness on palpation of the costovertebral angles.
- ✓ Deep abdominal palpation is done only by an experienced practitioner or under the supervision of an experienced practitioner.
- ✓ Nursing diagnoses commonly associated with the urinary system include altered urinary elimination, dysreflexia, incontinence, and urinary retention.
- ✓ Encourage clients to drink at least eight glasses of water or other fluids each day; consume coffee, alcohol, and carbonated drinks in moderation; use baking powder or baking soda in moderation; and include meat, eggs, cheese, whole grains, cranberries, prunes, and plums in the diet. Also encourage clients to avoid cigarettes.
- ✓ Women should clean the perineum from front to back to avoid contamination of the urethra; wear cotton underwear for adequate ventilation; and avoid urethral irritants such as bubble bath, scented tissue, and perfumed soap.

Chapter 15

Assessing the Reproductive System

The reproductive system is one of the most dynamic and fascinating systems of the human body. A healthy reproductive system is essential for the overall well-being of the client, as it is the means and outlet for both sexual gratification and human reproduction. Many factors influence the client's reproductive health on physiologic and psychologic levels. Recognition of these factors and their potential effects is an essential skill to incorporate into your practice. Assessment of the client's psychosocial health, self-care habits, family, culture, and environment is an important part of the focused interview, and you should keep these findings in mind as you conduct the physical assessment. You also must have a thorough understanding of the constituents of a healthy reproductive system, and you must be able to consider the relationship of other body systems to the reproductive system. The factors to consider when assessing the reproductive system are depicted in Figure 15.1.

During the physical assessment, you will assess and evaluate the sometimes ambiguous cues of actual and potential reproductive disease and the variety of contributors to the development of pathology. You will then document and communicate your findings to the other members of the health care team, and you will develop nursing diagnoses and a plan of collaborative or independent nursing care. Additionally, remember that you play a key role in teaching the client how to establish and maintain reproductive wellness, indicators of disease, and effects of the disease process. The goal of client education is the promotion of optimum health according to the client's individual needs.

Protocols for the performance of some aspects of examination of the reproductive system will vary greatly from agency to agency. For example, some agencies require that when a male (including students) examines a female client, another female must accompany him during the examination. Many agencies only allow advanced practitioners to perform certain maneuvers, such as the female speculum and bimanual examinations. Therefore, always review agency protocols before performing a detailed examination.

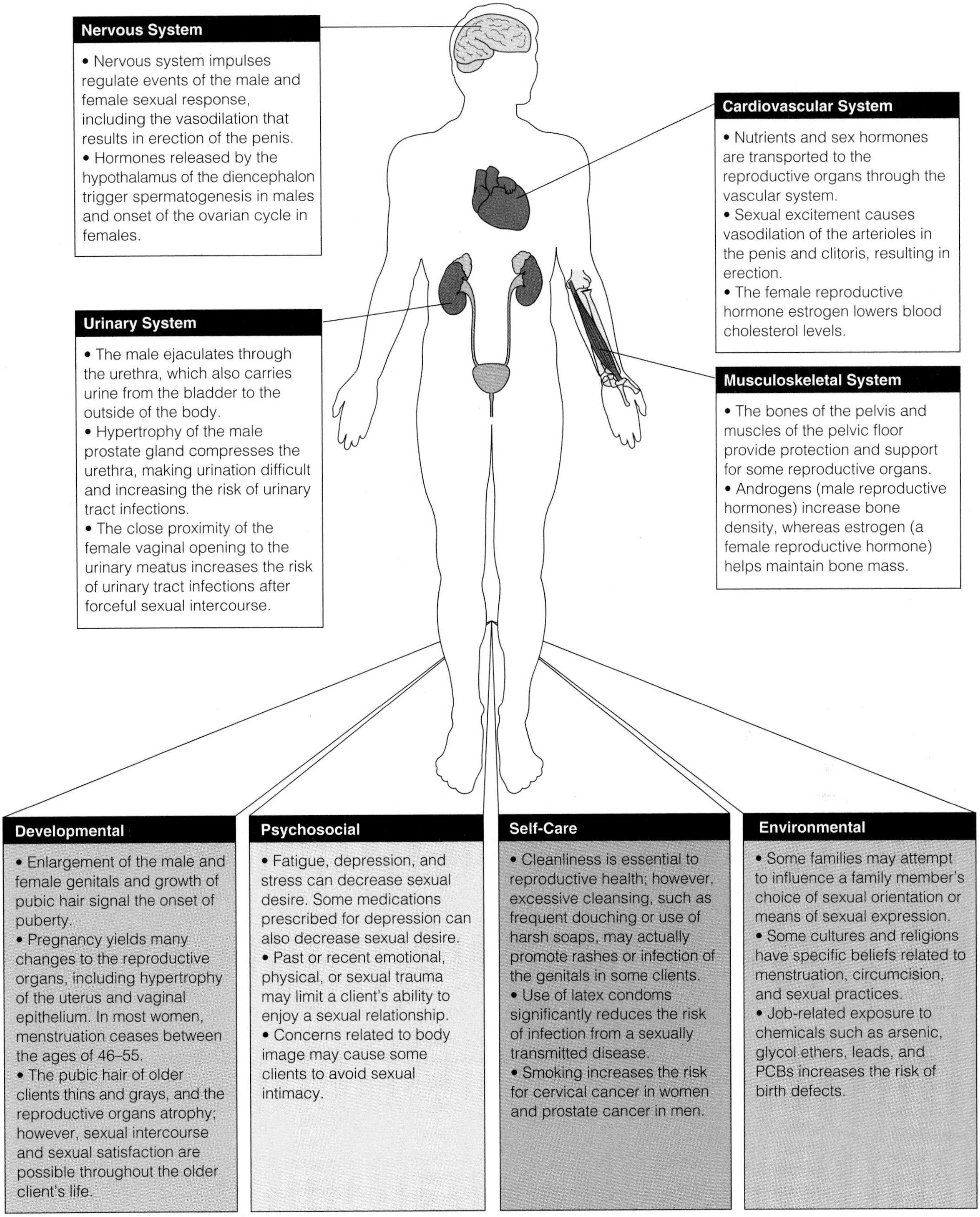

Nervous System

- Nervous system impulses regulate events of the male and female sexual response, including the vasodilation that results in erection of the penis.
- Hormones released by the hypothalamus of the diencephalon trigger spermatogenesis in males and onset of the ovarian cycle in females.

Cardiovascular System

- Nutrients and sex hormones are transported to the reproductive organs through the vascular system.
- Sexual excitement causes vasodilation of the arterioles in the penis and clitoris, resulting in erection.
- The female reproductive hormone estrogen lowers blood cholesterol levels.

Urinary System

- The male ejaculates through the urethra, which also carries urine from the bladder to the outside of the body.
- Hypertrophy of the male prostate gland compresses the urethra, making urination difficult and increasing the risk of urinary tract infections.
- The close proximity of the female vaginal opening to the urinary meatus increases the risk of urinary tract infections after forceful sexual intercourse.

Musculoskeletal System

- The bones of the pelvis and muscles of the pelvic floor provide protection and support for some reproductive organs.
- Androgens (male reproductive hormones) increase bone density, whereas estrogen (a female reproductive hormone) helps maintain bone mass.

Developmental

- Enlargement of the male and female genitals and growth of pubic hair signal the onset of puberty.
- Pregnancy yields many changes to the reproductive organs, including hypertrophy of the uterus and vaginal epithelium. In most women, menstruation ceases between the ages of 46–55.
- The pubic hair of older clients thins and grays, and the reproductive organs atrophy; however, sexual intercourse and sexual satisfaction are possible throughout the older client's life.

Psychosocial

- Fatigue, depression, and stress can decrease sexual desire. Some medications prescribed for depression can also decrease sexual desire.
- Past or recent emotional, physical, or sexual trauma may limit a client's ability to enjoy a sexual relationship.
- Concerns related to body image may cause some clients to avoid sexual intimacy.

Self-Care

- Cleanliness is essential to reproductive health; however, excessive cleansing, such as frequent douching or use of harsh soaps, may actually promote rashes or infection of the genitals in some clients.
- Use of latex condoms significantly reduces the risk of infection from a sexually transmitted disease.
- Smoking increases the risk for cervical cancer in women and prostate cancer in men.

Environmental

- Some families may attempt to influence a family member's choice of sexual orientation or means of sexual expression.
- Some cultures and religions have specific beliefs related to menstruation, circumcision, and sexual practices.
- Job-related exposure to chemicals such as arsenic, glycol ethers, leads, and PCBs increases the risk of birth defects.

Figure 15.1 An overview of important factors to consider when assessing the reproductive system.

Anatomy and Physiology Review

The Male Reproductive System

The male reproductive system is divided anatomically into external and internal genital organs. The penis and scrotum, the two external organs, are easily inspected and palpated. Only some of the internal structures are palpable; however, a basic understanding of anatomic structure and function is fundamental to performing assessment techniques correctly and safely. Figure 15.2 pictures the gross anatomy of the male reproductive system.

Some of the male reproductive organs serve dual roles as part of the reproductive system and the urinary system. As part of the urinary system, the male genitals serve as a passageway for expelling urine (see the previous chapter). The functions of the male reproductive system are

- Manufacturing and protecting sperm for fertilization
- Transporting sperm to the vagina
- Regulating hormonal production of and secretion of male sex hormones
- Providing sexual pleasure

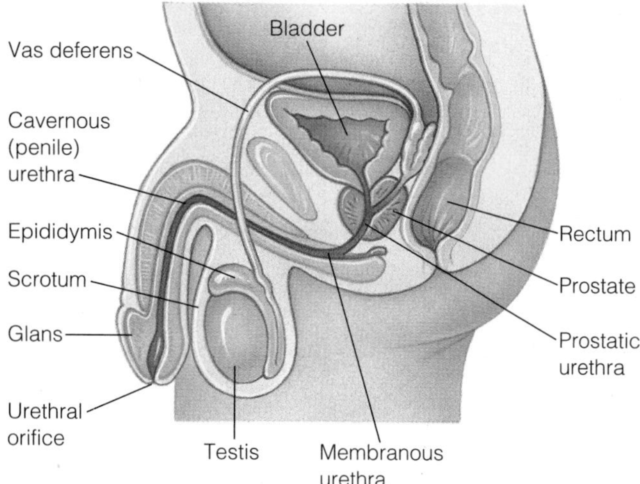

Figure 15.2 Gross anatomy of the male reproductive organs.

Scrotum

The **scrotum** is a loosely hanging, pliable, pear-shaped pouch of darkly pigmented skin that is located behind the penis. It houses the *testes*, which produce sperm. *Spermatogenesis* (sperm production) requires an environment in which the temperature is slightly lower than core body temperature; thus, the scrotum hangs outside of the abdominopelvic cavity, and is usually about 37.4F (3C) cooler than core body temperature. A vertical septum within the scrotum divides it into two sections, each containing a *testis, epididymis, vas deferens,* and *spermatic cord*, as well as other functional structures (Figures 15.2 and 15.3). Pubic hair scantily covers the scrotum. It is visibly asymmetric, with the left side extending lower than the right, because the left spermatic cord is longer.

Below the scrotal surface lie two muscles, the *cremaster muscle* and the *dartos muscle,* which play a protective role in sperm production and viability. In cold temperatures, the dartos muscle wrinkles the scrotal skin, whereas the cremaster muscle contracts, causing the testes to elevate towards the body. Warmer temperatures cause the reverse reaction. The testes also become more wrinkled and contract toward the body during sexual arousal.

The major functions of the scrotum are

- Protecting the testes, epididymides, and part of the spermatic cord
- Protecting sperm production and viability through the maintenance of an appropriate surface temperature

Testes

The **testes** are two firm, rubbery, olive-shaped structures that measure 4 to 5 cm long and 2 to 2.5 cm wide. They manufacture sperm, and are thus the primary male sex organs. Each testis has two coats, the outer *tunica vaginalis* and the inner *tunica albuginea*, that separate it from the scrotal wall. Within each testis are the *seminiferous tubules* that produce sperm and *Leydig's cells* that produce testosterone. The latter plays a significant role in sperm production and the development of male sexual characteristics. The testes receive their blood supply from the *testicular arteries*. The *testicular veins* not only remove deoxygenated blood from the testes, but also form a network called the *pampiniform plexus* (Figure 15.3), which plays a crucial supportive role in regulating the temperature in the testes by cooling arterial blood before it passes into the testes.

The major functions of the testes are

- Producing spermatozoa
- Secreting testosterone

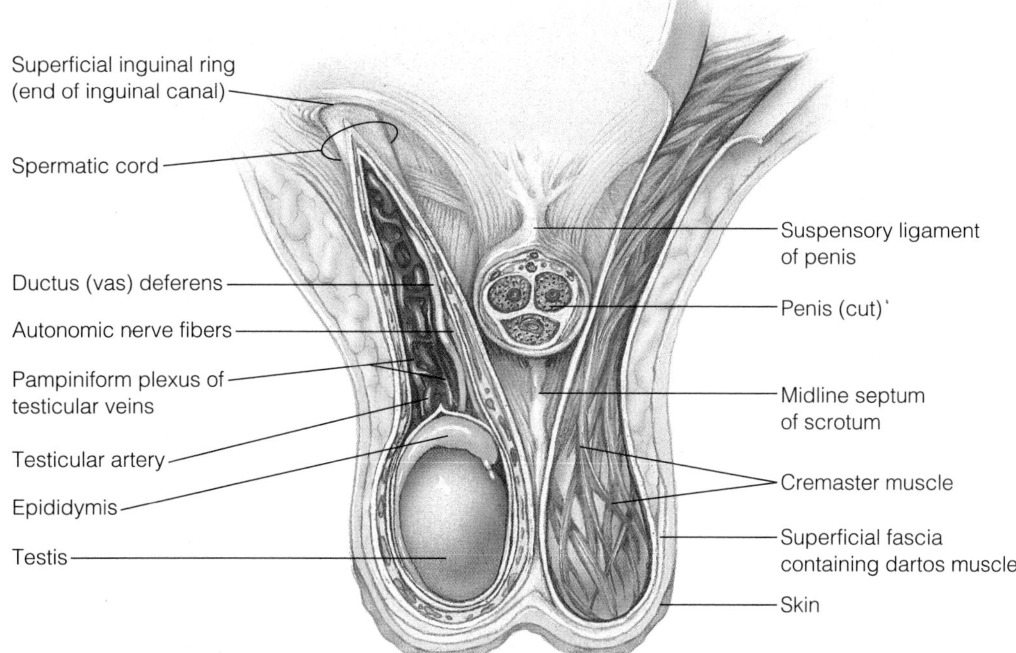

Figure 15.3 Contents of the scrotum, anterior view.

Spermatic Cord

The **spermatic cord** is composed of fibrous connective tissue. Its purpose is to form a protective sheath around the nerves, blood vessels, lymphatic structures, and muscle fibers associated with the scrotum (Figure 15.3).

The Duct System

The *duct system* plays a crucial role in the transportation of sperm. The three structures comprising the duct system are the *epididymis*, the *ductus deferens*, and the *urethera* (Figures 15.2 and 15.3).

Epididymis Positioned on top of and just posterior to each testicle is a comma- or crescent-shaped **epididymis,** which is palpable upon physical examination. It is actually a long, coiled tube, about 18 to 20 feet in length, which forms the beginning of the male duct system. Once the immature sperm have been produced in the testes, they are transported into the epididymis where they mature and become mobile. During orgasm, forceful contraction of muscles in this structure drive the sperm into the ductus deferens.

The major functions of the epididymis are

- Storing sperm as they mature
- Transporting sperm to the ductus deferens

Ductus Deferens Also known as the *vas deferens*, this tubular structure stretches from the end of the epididymis to the *ejaculatory duct*. Extending about 46.15 cm (18 inches) long, the tube runs through the *inguinal canal*, on the back side of the bladder, and to the ejaculatory duct as it enters into the prostate gland. Mature sperm remain in the ductus deferens until ready for transport.

The major functions of the ductus deferens are

- Serving as an excretory duct in the transport of sperm
- Serving as a reservoir for mature sperm

Urethra The *urethra* serves as a conduit for the transportation of both urine and semen to the outside of the body. It is composed of three sections: the *prostatic urethra*, the *membranous urethra*, and the *spongy (penile) urethra* (Figure 15.4).

Accessory Glands

The accessory glands play a crucial role in the formation of semen.

The Seminal Vesicles The **seminal vesicles** are a pair of saclike glands, 7.5 cm long, located between the bladder and rectum. These vesicles are the source of 60% of the semen produced. *Semen*, a thick yellow fluid, is composed of a high concentration of fructose, amino acids, prostaglandins, ascorbic acid, and fibrinogen. It is secreted into the *ejaculatory duct*, where it mixes with sperm which has been propelled from the ductus deferens. Semen nourishes and dilutes the sperm, enhancing its motility. Seminal fluid is propelled from the ejaculatory duct into the prostatic urethra.

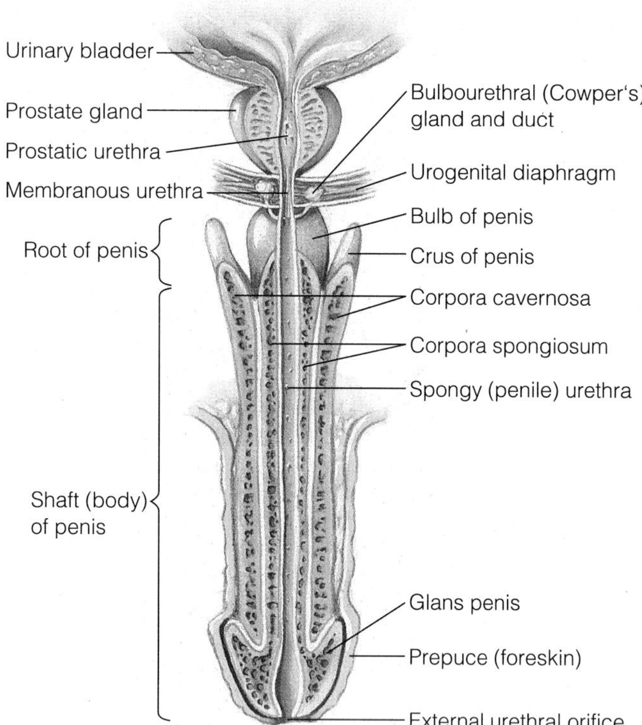

Figure 15.4 Structure of the penis.

Prostate Gland The **prostate gland** borders the urethra near the lower part of the bladder. About the size of a chestnut (2 cm), it is partially palpable through the front wall of the rectum because it lies just anterior to the rectum (Figure 15.2). The prostate is composed of glandular structures that continuously secrete a milky, alkaline solution. During sexual intercourse, glandular activity increases, and the alkaline secretions flow into the urethra. Because sperm motility is reduced in an acidic environment, these secretions aid sperm transport. Additionally, the prostate gland produces about one third of all semen.

Bulbourethral Glands Also referred to as *Cowper's glands*, the **bulbourethral glands** are located below the prostate within the urethral sphincter (Figure 15.2). These glands are small (4.5 to 5 mm) and round. Just before ejaculation, the bulbourethral glands secrete a clear mucus into the urethra that lubricates the urethra and increases its alkaline environment.

Penis

The **penis** is centrally located between the left and right groin areas and lies directly in front of the scrotum. Internally, the penile shaft consists of the penile urethra and three columns of highly vascular, erectile tissue: the two dorsolateral columns (*corpora cavernosa*) and the midventral column surrounding or encasing the urethra (Figure 15.4). The penis contracts and elongates during sexual arousal when its vasculature dilates as it fills with blood. This process allows the penis to become firm and erect so that it can deposit sperm in the female vagina. The distal end of the urethra (the external meatus) appears as a small opening centrally located on the *glans* of the penis, the cone-shaped distal end of the organ. In uncircumcised males, the glans is covered by a layer of skin called the *foreskin*.

The major functions of the penis are

- Serving as a passageway for sperm to exit and be deposited into the vagina during sexual intercourse
- Serving as an exit for urine

Inguinal Areas

These areas are located laterally to the pubic region over the iliac region or the upper part of the hip bone. Within this area is the *inguinal ligament* and the *inguinal canal,* which lies above the inguinal ligament. The inguinal canals are associated with the abdominal muscles and actually represent a potential weak link in the abdominopelvic wall. When a separation of the abdominal muscle exists, the weak points of these canals afford an area for the protrusion of the intestine into the groin region. This is called an *inguinal hernia*.

The Female Reproductive System

The female reproductive system is unique in that it undergoes cyclical changes in direct response to hormonal levels of estrogen and progesterone during the childbearing years. The uterus undergoes an ovarian cycle during which the ova (eggs) are prepared for fertilization with sperm. During the menstrual cycle, the uterine lining is prepared for the development of a fetus. The onset of menopause represents the end of the childbearing years.

Unlike the male reproductive system, the female reproductive tract is completely separate from the urinary tract. However, structures of the two tracts lie within close proximity. The functions of the female reproductive system are

- Manufacturing and protecting ova for fertilization
- Transporting the fertilized ovum for implantation and embryonic/fetal development
- Regulating hormonal production and secretion of several sex hormones
- Providing sexual stimulation and pleasure

External Genitals

Mons pubis The **mons pubis** is the rounded mound of adipose tissue overlying the symphysis pubis (Figure 15.5). In the mature woman, it is thickly covered with hair.

It provides protection to the underlying reproductive structures.

Labia majora and labia minora The *labia* are a dual set of liplike structures lying on either side of the vagina (Figure 15.5). The exterior **labia majora** are two thick, elongated pads of tissue that become fuller towards the center. An extension of the external skin surface, the labia majora are covered with coarse hair extending from the mons pubis. The enclosed **labia minora** are two thin, elongated pads of tissue that overlie the vaginal and urethral openings, as well as several glandular openings. Anteriorly, the labia minora join to form the *prepuce*, which covers the clitoris. Posteriorly, they join to form the fourchette.

The labia minora border an almond-shaped area of tissue known as the *vestibule*. It extends from the clitoris to the fourchette. The urethral meatus, vaginal opening (*introitus*), Skene's glands, and Bartholin's glands lie within the vestibule.

The major function of the labia is

- Providing protection from infection and physical injury to the urethra and vagina, and ultimately other urinary and reproductive structures

Skene's and Bartholin's glands The **Skene's glands**, also called *paraurethral glands*, are located just posterior to the urethra (Figure 15.5). They open into the urethra and secrete a fluid that lubricates the vaginal vestibule during sexual intercourse. The **Bartholin's glands** or *greater vestibular glands*, are located posteriorally at the base of the vestibule and produce mucus, which is released into the vestibule (Figure 15.5). This mucus actively promotes sperm motility and viability.

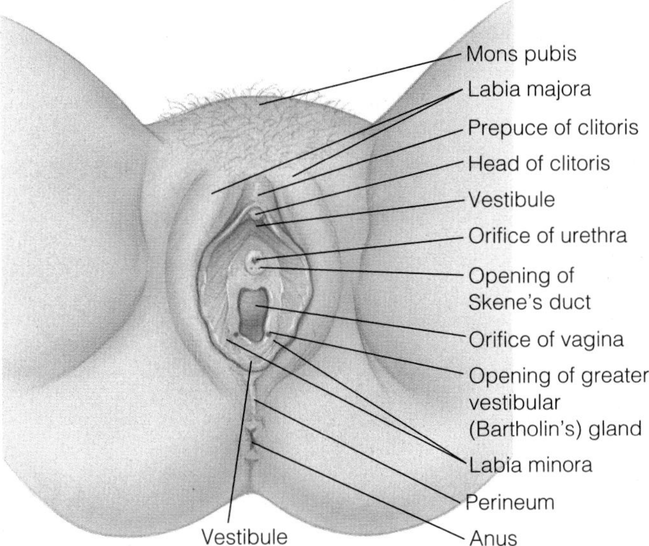

Figure 15.5 External genitals of the female.

Clitoris Located at the anterior of the vestibule is the **clitoris**, a small, elongated mound of erectile tissue (Figure 15.5). As the labia minora merge together anteriorly, a small hoodlike covering is formed that lies over the top of the clitoris. The clitoris is homologous with the penis. It is permeated with numerous nerve fibers responsive to touch. When stimulated, the clitoris becomes erect as its underlying corpus cavernosa become vasocongested.

The major function of the clitoris is

- Serving as the primary organ of sexual stimulation

Perineum The **perineum** is the area bordered anteriorly by the top of the labial folds, laterally by the ischial tuberosities, and posteriorally by the anus (Figure 15.5).

Internal Reproductive Organs

Vagina The **vagina** is a long, tubular, muscular canal (approximately 9 to 15 cm in length) that extends from the vestibule to the cervix at the inferior end of the uterus (Figure 15.6). The muscularity of the vaginal wall, and its thick, transverse *rugae* (ridges) allow it to dilate widely to accommodate the erect penis and, during childbirth, the head of the fetus. At the point of juncture with the cervix, a continuous circular cleft called the *fornix* is formed.

The major functions of the vagina are

- Serving as the female organ of copulation
- Serving as the birth canal
- Serving as a channel through which menstrual flow can exit

Uterus The **uterus** is a pear-shaped, hollow, muscular organ that is located centrally in the pelvis between the neck of the bladder and the rectal wall (Figure 15.6). The body of the uterus is about 4 cm wide and 6 to 8 cm in length. Its walls are 2 to 2.5 cm thick and are composed of serosal, muscular, and mucosal layers. Anatomically, the uterus is divided into three segments. The *fundus* forms the top of the uterus; the *corpus*, the body; and the *cervix*, the lower part, or neck. The cervix projects into the vagina about 2.5 cm and is about 2.5 cm round. A small central canal, called the cervical *os*, connects the vaginal canal to the inside of the uterus. The *external cervi-*

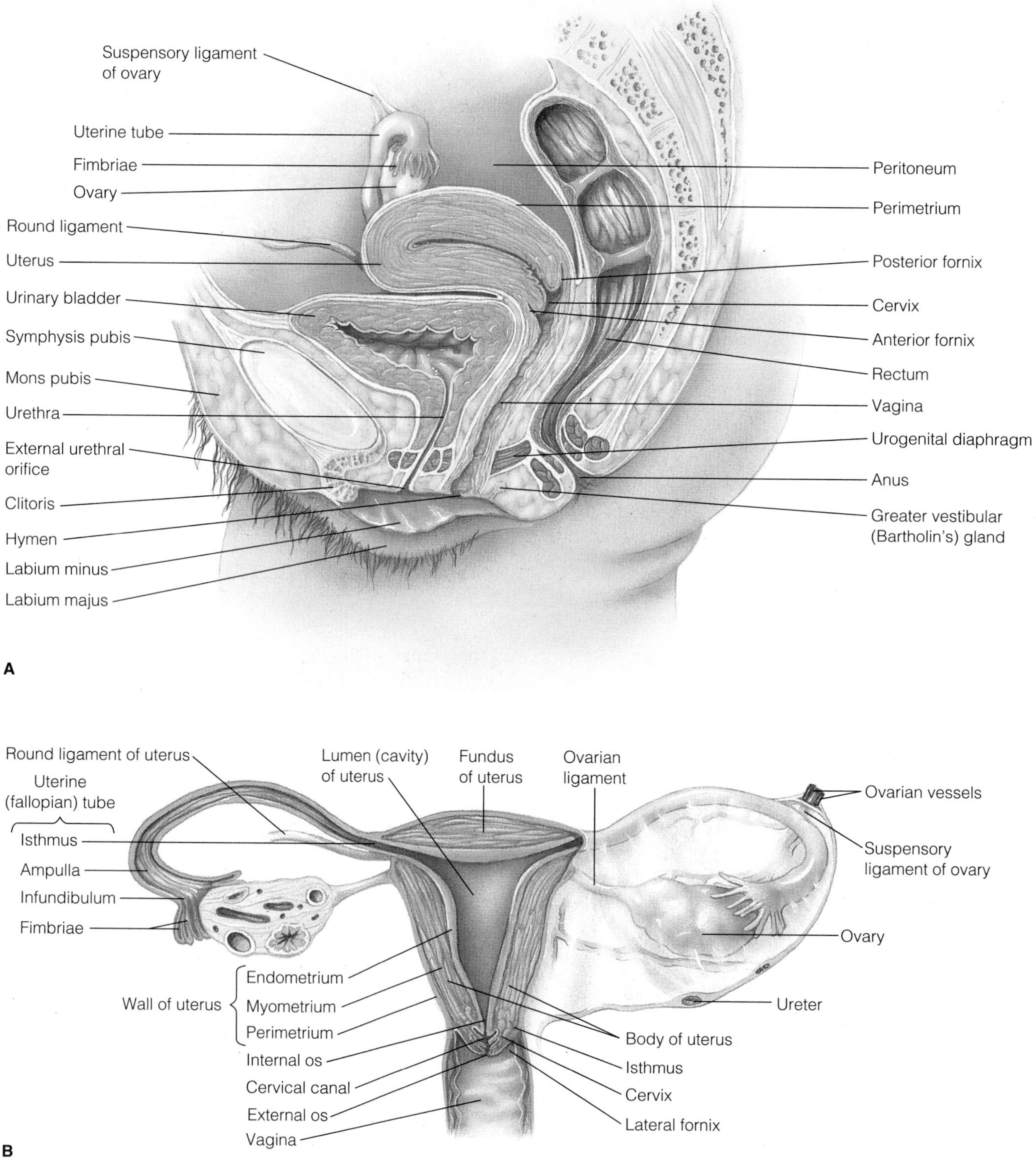

Suspensory ligament of ovary
Uterine tube
Fimbriae
Ovary
Round ligament
Uterus
Urinary bladder
Symphysis pubis
Mons pubis
Urethra
External urethral orifice
Clitoris
Hymen
Labium minus
Labium majus
Peritoneum
Perimetrium
Posterior fornix
Cervix
Anterior fornix
Rectum
Vagina
Urogenital diaphragm
Anus
Greater vestibular (Bartholin's) gland
A
Round ligament of uterus
Uterine (fallopian) tube
Isthmus
Ampulla
Infundibulum
Fimbriae
Lumen (cavity) of uterus
Fundus of uterus
Ovarian ligament
Ovarian vessels
Suspensory ligament of ovary
Ovary
Wall of uterus
Endometrium
Myometrium
Perimetrium
Internal os
Cervical canal
External os
Vagina
Ureter
Body of uterus
Isthmus
Cervix
Lateral fornix
B

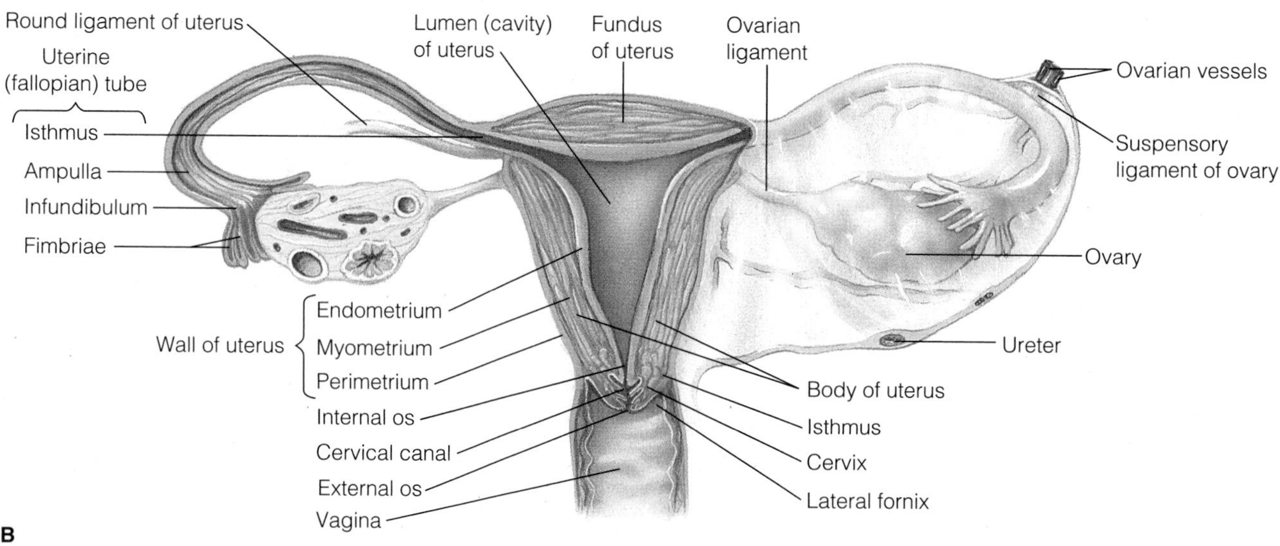

Figure 15.6 *A*, Internal organs of the female reproductive system. *B*, Structures of the female pelvis.

cal os is the inferior opening (the vaginal end), and the *internal cervical os* opens directly into the uterine chamber.

The uterus is easily moved within the pelvic cavity, but its basic position is secured with several ligaments that attach it to the pelvic floor. The ligaments also prevent the uterus from dropping into the vaginal canal.

The major functions of the uterus are

- Serving as the site of implantation of the fertilized ovum
- Serving as a protective sac for the developing embryo and fetus

Uterine Tubes The **uterine tubes** (or *fallopian tubes*) are two ducts on either side of the fundus of the uterus (Figure 15.6). They are about 7 to 10 cm in length and extend from the uterus almost to the ovaries. An ovum released by an ovary travels to the uterus within the uterine tubes. Normally fertilization takes places within the uterine tubes.

The major functions of the fallopian tubes are

- Serving as the site of fertilization
- Providing a passageway for unfertilized and fertilized ova to travel to the uterus

Ovaries Lying close to the distal end of either side of the uterine tubes are the **ovaries** (Figure 15.6). These almond-shaped glandular structures produce ova, as well as estrogen and progesterone. They are about 3 cm long and 2 cm wide. The *ovarian ligaments* and *suspensory ligaments* hold the ovaries in place. The ovaries become fully developed after puberty and atrophy after menopause.

The major functions of the ovaries are

- Producing ova for fertilization by sperm
- Producing estrogen and progesterone

Gathering the Data

After completing the database and comparing this information with data gathered during assessment of other body systems, elicit additional information concerning problems uncovered during the initial interview related to reproductive function. It is essential to assess not only the function of the reproductive system but also the client's sexual fulfillment on both a physical and psychologic basis.

To be efficient in gathering data, you need to understand your own feelings and comfort about various aspects of sexuality. It is essential to put aside your personal beliefs and values about sexual practices and focus in a nonjudgmental manner on gathering data to determine the health status of the client.

Keep in mind that during the focused interview you need to create an atmosphere that facilitates open communication and comfort for the client. Clients commonly feel anxiety, fear, and embarrassment when you request information about a topic that, in most clients' minds, is very personal. These emotions may be expressed either verbally or nonverbally. With this in mind, approach the client in as nonthreatening a manner as possible. Assure the client that the information that is provided and the results of the physical examination will remain confidential. Furthermore, be aware of your own behaviors that may serve as a communication block. Sit down with clients to convey that you have time to spend discussing their concerns. Your verbal and nonverbal communication should convey that you are being nonjudgmental and are requesting only the information needed to assess the client's health status. Because the information you gather may reveal some abnormality that may threaten sexual activity and health, begin with questions that are least threatening and have the least sexual connotation. Especially with adolescents, a conversational approach with the use of open-ended statements may be helpful. As the client provides information, allow the client's choice of terminology to guide you in deciding which terms would be most appropriate for you to use. When discussing any sensitive or controversial topic, it is always best to start with a general statement that opens the door for clients to express their thoughts. For example, if you suspect sexual abuse of a female client, you might initiate a discussion by commenting, "Some women have said that it is hard to discuss abusive relationships. How do you feel about this?"

The Focused Interview

Questions for Male Clients

Because of the dual functions of some of the male reproductive structures, some of the data gathered during the focused interview will relate to the status of the urinary system as well as the reproductive system. Some commonly reported problems are those related to altered patterns of voiding, the presence of masses or lesions, unusual discharge, pain and tenderness, changes in sexual functioning, suspected contact with a sexual partner who may have a sexually transmitted disease, and infertility. See the previous chapter for information on the focused interview for the urinary system.

Questions Related to Reproductive Health

1. Do you now or have you in the past had concerns about your reproductive health? If so, please tell me about those concerns. *This question may prompt the client to discuss any concerns about reproductive health.*
2. Have you noticed any blisters, ulcers, sores, warts, or rashes on your penis, scrotum, or surrounding areas? If so, describe them. When did you notice this? *There are two main sources for these signs: infective processes and*

cancer. Many infections, including sexually transmitted diseases, are characterized by lesions, some of which have specific features. Of the major sexually transmitted diseases, only gonorrhea lacks ulceration as a prominent feature. Carcinoma of the penis is usually manifested as a nontender ulcer or small lump.

3. Have you felt any lumps or masses on your penis, scrotum, or surrounding areas? If so, describe the mass. Exactly where is it? About what size? Is it soft or hard? Is it movable? When did you first notice the mass? Is it painful? Has there been any pattern to the swelling: an increase, decrease, or unchanged pattern? Any treatments that you have tried? *This information helps you to understand the nature of the mass or lump.*
4. Have you noticed any swelling of your scrotum, penis, or surrounding areas? If so, when did it start? Is it painful? Has there been any pattern to the swelling: an increase, decrease, or unchanged pattern? What treatment have you tried? *This information could help identify problems of rapid onset, which sometimes have the potential to be more detrimental. Swelling in the inguinal area may signal the presence of a hernia. Sources of swelling in the scrotal area include an acute or chronic inflammatory process, a hydrocele, scrotal edema, or scrotal hernia.*
5. Have you noticed any unusual discharge from your penis? If so, of what color? Is there any odor to the discharge? Is it a small, moderate, or large amount? When did you first notice the discharge? Any burning or pain with the discharge? *Discharge characteristics may indicate whether an infectious process is occurring.*
6. Have you noticed any change in color of your penis or scrotum? If so, describe the change and the location. *Inflammatory processes may cause redness in the affected area.*
7. Have you noticed any pain, tenderness, or soreness in the areas of your penis or scrotum? If so, describe the pain. Is it dull? Sharp? Radiating? Intermittent? Continuous? Does anything make the pain better or worse? *Testicular torsion may cause excruciating pain in the testicular area. A dull, aching pain is a common symptom of epididymitis, a common infection in males.*
8. Are you having any pain in the area now? *This question helps you determine if the problem is current, experienced in the past only, or chronic.*
9. Have you had any unusual itching in your genital area? If so, where? Have you noticed any rash, scaling, or lumps? *Causes may include environment allergens, soaps, or lotions. Treatment usually includes topical creams.*
10. Do you know if your mother received DES (diethylstilbestrol) treatment during pregnancy? *Some reports indicate that sons of DES women have higher than average rates of genitourinary problems such as hypospadias, infertility, and undescended or enlarged testicles. They may be at risk for testicular cancer and have low sperm counts. Physician referral is indicated if the client's response is yes.*
11. Have you had surgery on any of your reproductive organs? If so, what was the surgery? *Some surgeries, such as penile implants, require periodic follow-up for problems such as possible infection. Some surgeries may have bearing on sexual function, as well as attitude about oneself in relation to sexuality.*

Questions Related to Sexual Function

You may want to introduce this section by saying, "Now I would like to ask you some questions regarding sexual function."

1. Are you able to be sexually aroused? Has this ability changed over time or recently? *A variety of factors may influence an individual's ability to become sexually aroused. These include use of prescribed and/or illicit drugs, disorders of the nervous system, diabetes, stress, and fear (eg, of intimacy, inability to satisfy a partner, or acquiring a sexually transmitted disease).*
2. Are you able to achieve and maintain an erection? Have any aspects in your ability to achieve an erection changed? Are you satisfied with the length of time it takes to achieve and maintain an erection? *The ability to achieve an erection depends on both physiologic factors and state of mind.*
3. When you have an erection, is the shaft of the penis straight or crooked? *Peyronie's disease causes the shaft of the penis to be crooked during an erection.*
4. Are you able to achieve orgasm? Are you satisfied with your ability to control the timing of your orgasms? *Premature ejaculation is defined by some researchers as orgasm immediately after, or even before, penetration. It may also be defined as ejaculation before the man's sexual partner reaches orgasm in more than half of the man's sexual experiences. It is often a devastating disorder that may severely compromise sexual relationships. The client can learn techniques to delay ejaculation.*

Questions for Female Clients

Because of the close proximity of some of the female reproductive structures to the urethra, data gathered during the focused interview will relate to the status of the urinary system as well. Questions related to the health and function of the female urinary system are covered in the previous chapter. Abnormal vaginal discharge, pelvic pain, inflammation, infection, and suspicion of contracting a sexually transmitted disease are some of the more frequent problems that the female reports.

Questions Related to Reproductive Health

1. What brings you in today?
2. Do you now, or have you in the past, had concerns about your reproductive health? If so, please tell me about those concerns. *This question may prompt the client to discuss any concerns about reproductive health.*
3. Have you noticed any rashes, blisters, ulcers, sores, or warts on your genital area or surrounding areas? *Rashes are common with yeast infections, which is the most common female genital infection. Herpes infection causes small painful ulcerations, whereas syphilitic chancres are not painful. In the older client, a raised reddened lesion may indicate carcinoma of the vulva. Contact dermatitis is characterized by reddened lesions that eventually weep and form crusts. Venereal warts are cauliflower shaped.*
4. Have you felt any lumps or masses in any of these areas? If so, describe the mass. Exactly where is it? About what size? Is it soft or hard? Is it movable? When did you first notice the mass? Is it painful? Have you noticed any change in it since it developed? Have you used any remedies such as ice, heat, or creams? *Sebaceous cysts can be noted in the labial area. A lump created by an abscess of the Bartholin's gland causes localized pain. An abscess of the Bartholin's gland may indicate the presence of gonorrhea.*
5. Have you noticed any swelling or redness of your genitals? *Vulvovaginitis may cause edema in the area, including the vulva. Redness and swelling may indicate an alteration in health such as an abscess of the Bartholin's gland, which may be caused by gonorrhea. Bruising may indicate sexual trauma.*
6. Do you have any structures extruding from your vagina? Have you felt any pressure from the vagina or feeling of bulging or masses from within the vagina? *Uterine prolapse may be so severe that the uterus protrudes into and at times out of the vagina.*
7. Have you experienced any itching in your labia or vaginal area? If so, when did it start? Has it been treated and, if so, how? Have there been any associated urinary symptoms? *Crab lice, atrophic vaginitis, candidiasis, and contact dermatitis may cause intense itching.*
8. Have you noticed any discharge from your vagina? If so, what color is it? Is there any odor to it? Is it a small, moderate, or large amount? When did you first notice the discharge? *Vaginal discharge is a typical complaint of clients with vaginitis. The most common presenting symptom in females with sexually transmitted diseases is vaginal discharge; however, the client may have no symptoms.*
9. Have you had any vaginal bleeding outside the time of your normal menstrual period? *Abnormal bleeding may be related to hormonal influences and be easily corrected. Conditions such as cervical cancer or endometrial cancer can also cause abnormal bleeding patterns. If the client answers yes:* When did it occur? How much bleeding was there? *Obtain quantitative data by asking whether panties were saturated or how many pads or tampons were saturated in 24 hours. Use a calendar to determine the number of days since her last menstrual period.*
10. Do you have any pain, tenderness, or soreness in your pelvic area? If so, describe the pain. Is it dull? Sharp? Radiating? Intermittent? Continuous? When did it start? Are you having any pain in the area now? What makes the pain better or worse? Do you have associated symptoms of headache, vomiting, or diarrhea? *Common causes of gynecologic pain include infection, menstrual difficulties, endometriosis (abnormal condition involving the endometrial lining of the uterus), ectopic pregnancy (fetus implanted in abnormal location), threatened abortion, or pelvic masses.*
11. Have you ever had any surgery of the reproductive system? If so, what was it? When? Where?
12. Have you ever had an abnormal Pap smear? If so, how long ago was this? What treatment, if any, did you receive? Have you had follow up Pap smears? When? What were the results?
13. Do you know if your mother received DES (diethylstilbestrol) treatment during pregnancy with you? *Studies indicate that daughters of women who received DES during pregnancy have a significantly higher number of reproductive tract problems, including cervical cancer, infertility, and ectopic pregnancy. This may have some bearing on the current problem. If the client answers yes to this question, refer her to the physician.*

Questions Related to Sexual Function

You may want to introduce this section by saying, "Now I would like to ask you some questions regarding sexual function."

1. Are you able to be sexually aroused? Has this ability changed over time or recently? *A variety of factors may interfere with a woman's ability to be sexually aroused. These are prescribed and/or illicit drug use, disorders of the nervous or endocrine systems, stress, and fear (eg, of intimacy, inability to satisfy a partner, acquiring a sexually transmitted disease, becoming pregnant).*
2. Are you satisfied with your sexual experiences? *If the client expresses dissatisfaction, then ask:* Are you able to achieve orgasm? *A variety of factors may interfere with a woman's ability to experience orgasm.*
3. Have you noticed a change in your ability to have an orgasm?

Questions for the Menstruating Woman

1. How old were you when you had your first menstrual period?
2. What was the first day of your last menstrual period?
3. How many days does your cycle usually run? *A cycle may be defined as the first day of one period to the first day of the next.* Is this consistent from month to month?
4. How many days does bleeding occur?
5. Describe your menstrual flow. Is this consistent each month? How many tampons or pads do you use each day? For how many days? *Clotting and excessive bleeding warrant additional follow-up. Any uterine bleeding that the client views as unusual is considered abnormal. The client's assessment of her flow is subjective. Generally, an excessively heavy flow is characterized by use of more than one pad or tampon per hour.*
6. How do you usually feel during your period? Is this a pattern for you? *This may provide some clue as to whether excessive discomfort is occurring, indicating some underlying disease. Dysmenorrhea (painful or difficult menstruation) is the most common gynecologic disorder.*
7. How do you usually feel just before your period? Has this gotten worse or better? Do you use any self-care remedies? *Premenstrual syndrome (PMS) presents with a variety of signs and symptoms and usually occurs a few days before menstruation. Typically, sudden relief occurs with the onset of full menstrual flow.*
8. Do you take any medications for cramps? If so, what do you take and how much? If not, how do you relieve your cramps? *This helps to determine if the woman is able to continue with daily routines.*
9. Do you use tampons? If so, how frequently do you change the tampons? Are you aware of the risk for toxic shock syndrome with the use of tampons? Are you aware of the signs of toxic shock?

Questions for the Menopausal Woman

1. When did menopause begin for you?
2. Tell me about physical changes you have noticed since menopause. *It is common for women to experience a variety of symptoms, including mood changes and "hot flashes." Vaginal dryness causes dyspareunia.*
3. Are you on estrogen therapy?
4. Have you had any vaginal bleeding since starting menopause? *Some women assume that postmenopausal bleeding is normal and tend to ignore it. Postmenopausal bleeding may be suggestive of inadequate estrogen therapy and endometrial cancer. It could also be indicative of serious problems such as genital tract cancer.*

Questions Related to Pregnancy

1. Have you ever been pregnant? If so, how many times?
2. Did you have any problems during pregnancy, delivery, or postpartum? *If the client answers yes:* Describe the problem(s).
3. Was delivery vaginal or by cesarean section?
4. Have you ever had a miscarriage? What were you told was the cause? Was surgery required? Have you ever had an abortion? At how many weeks, and by what method? *Strong emotions often accompany the issue of termination of a pregnancy by either spontaneous or surgical abortion. You might want to follow up with this question:* How has it been for you emotionally since the abortion/miscarriage?

Questions for Both Male and Female Clients

Questions Related to Fertility

1. Do you have children? If so, how many? *If the client answers no:* Have you tried to have children? *If the client answers yes:* How long have you been trying to have a child? *The couple is not considered potentially "infertile" unless they have been unable to conceive for a year.*
2. *If the client indicates inability to conceive after 1 year:* How often do you and your partner have intercourse? *For couples attempting to have a child, it is important to engage in intercourse routinely, two to three times a week. Although nurses do not treat infertility, you may be involved in teaching the client about certain measures that may be helpful, such as temperature tracking to determine the optimal time for intercourse. Concerns about infertility can produce great anxiety for many.*
3. *Ask males:* Have you ever had mumps? *Mumps occurring after puberty has been linked to sterility in men .*
4. Have you ever sought professional help for fertility problems? If so, describe this experience.
5. Has an inability to conceive placed a strain on your relationship with your partner? How has this problem affected your relationship? How are you feeling about this?

Questions Related to Sexual Satisfaction

1. How would you describe your sexual relationship?
2. Are you sexually active? *The client may feel pressured to be in a sexual relationship. These pressures may be external (expectations of family, friends, or work associates) or internal (fear of being viewed by others as less than desirable or*

not of an accepted sexual orientation, fear of being alone, and fear of not being loved or accepted).

3. Are there any obstacles to your ability to achieve sexual satisfaction? *Causes of inability to achieve sexual satisfaction include fear of acquiring a sexually transmitted disease, fear of being unable to satisfy the partner, fear of pregnancy, confusion regarding sexual preference, unwillingness to participate in sexual activities enjoyed by the partner, job stress, financial considerations, crowded living conditions, loss of partner, attraction to or sexual involvement with individuals that the partner does not know about, criticism of sexual performance by partner, or history of sexual trauma.*
4. Have you noticed a change in your sex drive recently? *This may be indicative of some physical or psychologic problems that need follow-up. If the client answers yes:* Can you associate the change with anything in particular? *Often clients can relate a decrease in sex drive with stress, illness, drug therapy, or some other factor.*
5. *If the client is sexually active, ask:* What type of contraception do you use?
6. Do your family and friends support your relationship with your sexual partner? *The client's family and friends can influence the client's sexual relationship in a variety of ways. The client may feel tension if the partner is not accepted.*
7. Are you able to talk to your partner about your sexual needs? Does your partner accept your needs and help you fulfill them? Are you able to do the same for your partner?
8. *Tell the client:* Some clients come to me to discuss sexual abuse. Have you ever been forced to have sexual intercourse or other sexual contact against your will? Have you ever been molested or raped? *If the client answers yes:* When was this? Who abused you, what was the experience, and what was done about the situation and for you?

Questions Related to Sexual Practices

1. *If the client is sexually active, ask:* Are you in a mutually monogamous relationship? If not, how many sexual partners have you or your partner had over the last year? *Sexual activity with many different partners increases the risk of acquiring sexually transmitted diseases and possibly certain gynecologic cancers.*
2. Have you ever had a sexually transmitted disease (such as herpes, gonorrhea, syphilis, or chlamydia)? *If the client answers yes:* Was it treated? Did you inform your partner? Did you have sexual relations with your partner while you were infected? *If the client answers yes:* Did you use condoms? What treatment did you receive? *Serious, sometimes fatal, complications can develop if treatment is delayed. For example, untreated syphilis can eventually involve the cardiovascular and central nervous systems.*
3. Are you aware of having had any exposure to HIV? *If the client answers yes:* Describe the situation and how you feel you were exposed. What are your views on sexual relations and the potential for acquiring HIV? *The incidence of HIV is still on the rise. Despite the wide availability of information on the risk and methods of protection for sexually active individuals, many people continue to have unprotected sex.*
4. Have you ever been tested for HIV? *If the client answers yes:* On one occasion or routinely?

Questions Related to Self-Care

1. Do you check your genitals on a routine basis? *If the client answers yes:* How often? *Ask males:* Do you know how to perform testicular self-exam? How often do you perform this exam? What technique do you use? *Self-examination of the genitals should be performed at least monthly for early detection of changes that need follow-up. Teaching may be indicated if the client is not performing self-examination.*
2. How often do you get physical examinations? *Screening for problems such as prostate or testicular cancer, or cervical or endometrial cancer, usually is performed during routine physical or gynecologic examinations.*
3. *Ask males:* Are you circumcised? Have you had any difficulty keeping this area clean? *If the client is having problems with maintaining hygiene of the area, client teaching may be necessary.*
4. Are you using contraception? If so, what kind? Are you using it consistently?
5. Would you like to know more about the use of birth control? *This is a very important question to ask adolescents who shy away from talking about sexual practices but have verbalized that they are sexually active.*
6. How do you protect yourself from sexually transmitted diseases, including HIV? *Abstinence is the only 100% effective protection against sexually transmitted diseases. Latex condoms offer significant protection, especially when treated with spermicide; however, they are not 100% effective.*
7. Do you drink alcohol? How many drinks per week? *Chronic alcoholism has been linked to impotence. Additionally, intake of alcoholic beverages can contribute to an individual "taking chances," such as failing to use condoms.*
8. Do you use illicit drugs? If so, what type and how much? *Taken in sufficient amounts, some drugs, such as marijuana and opiates, may decrease libido and lead to impotence. Drug use may also contribute to failure to use protection against sexually transmitted diseases.*

Additional Questions with Infants and Children

Ask the parent these questions:

1. Have you noticed any redness, swelling, or discharge that is discolored or foul-smelling in your child's genital areas? *These may indicate inflammatory processes or infection.*
2. Have you noticed any asymmetry, lumps, or masses in the infant's genitals? *If the parent answers yes:* Where are they? Are they movable? Hard or soft? Does touching the mass elicit a pain response from the child? *These symptoms may indicate the development of an obstructive process.*
3. Has your child complained of itching, burning, or swelling in the genital area? *These symptoms may indicate the presence of pinworms or infections such as yeast infections.*

Ask the preschool or school-age child:

- Has anyone ever touched you when you didn't want them to? Where? *(You may want to have the child point to a picture.)* Has anyone ever asked you to touch them when you didn't want to? Where did they ask you to touch them? *If the child answers yes, the child may be experiencing sexual abuse. Try to obtain additional information but remember to be sensitive. Ask:* Who touched you? How many times did this happen? Who knows about this? *Try to determine exactly what the person did to the child. Has there been more than touching? Has any other form of sexual contact occurred? The child may feel responsible for the situation and not wish to discuss it. The abuser may be a parent or relative. Assure the child that she or he has not been bad and that it helps to talk to an adult about it. Referral should be made to a specialist immediately.*

Additional Questions with Adolescents

Many of the questions you ask adolescents are similar to those you ask adults. Be sure to explore adolescents' feelings and concerns regarding their sexual development, for instance, concerns about wet dreams. Reassure the adolescent that these changes are normal. Some adolescents may be confused about their feelings of sexual attraction to the opposite or same sex. Ask open-ended questions and, again, assure the adolescent that such feelings are normal.

Whether or not an adolescent admits to being sexually active, offer information on teenage pregnancy, birth control, and protection against sexually transmitted diseases. Some teenagers may be fearful that you will relay this information to their parents. Be sure to reinforce that all information is confidential.

Additional Questions with Childbearing Clients

Chapter 20 provides a comprehensive interview of the childbearing client.

Additional Questions with Older Adults

The questions for aging adults are the same as those for younger adults. In addition, you should explore whether older clients perceive any changes in their sexuality related to advancing age. For example, an older male may find he needs more time to achieve erection, or an older female may notice a decrease in vaginal lubrication even when she is fully aroused. Reassure the older adult that these changes are normal and do not indicate disease.

Physical Assessment of the Male

Preparation

- ☑ **Gather the equipment:**

  disposable examination gloves
  drape
  examination gown
  lubricant
  culturette set for obtaining specimen of any abnormal discharge

- ☑ **Alleviate discomfort and embarrassment before and during the examination by using the following strategies:**
  - Have the client empty his bladder and bowels before the exam.
  - Explain that the client can help with the exam by relaxing and focusing on your instructions.
  - Maintain eye contact.
  - Reassure the client that anxiety and embarrassment are normal.
  - Humor may alleviate stress; however, it must be used only in good taste and appropriately.
  - Explain to the client what you are doing and why as you proceed through the exam. Explain what you see that is normal. You may also describe any abnormality, but be sure not to alarm the client.
  - Touch the client firmly but gently, avoiding ambiguity.
  - Use an unhurried, deliberate manner.
  - If the client experiences an erection during the examination, explain that this is normal and has no sexual connotation, then continue with a professional demeanor.

- ☑ **Ensure that the room is warm and the client has privacy. Double-check that the "in use" sign is on the examination room door.**

- ☑ **Ask the client to remove any clothing below the waist. He may leave his T-shirt and socks on. Leave the room while he undresses.**

- ☑ **Wash your hands and put on the examination gloves. Change the gloves as needed during the exam to prevent cross-contamination and exposure to body fluids.**

- ☑ **Remember to culture any abnormal discharge.**

ASSESSMENT TECHNIQUE/NORMAL FINDINGS | SPECIAL CONSIDERATIONS

Inspection

Step 1 *Position the client.*

- Position yourself on a stool sitting in front of the client (Figure 15.7).

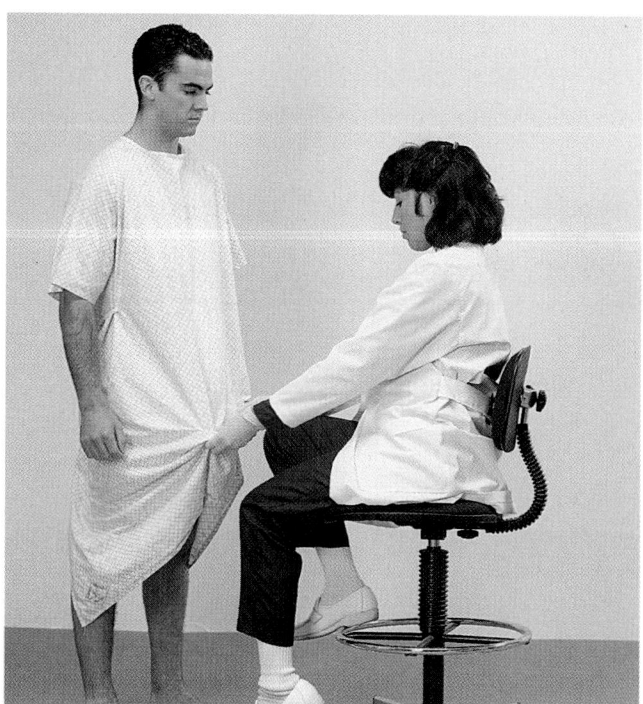

Figure 15.7 Positioning the client.

- Begin the examination with the client in a standing position.

Step 2 *Inspect the pubic hair.*

- Observe the pubic hair for normal distribution, amount, texture, and cleanliness (Figure 15.8).

The amount, distribution, and texture of pubic hair vary according to the client's age and race. Absent or extremely sparse hair in the pubic area may be indicative of sexual underdevelopment. The pubic hair of elderly males may be gray and thinning.

Table 15.1 on page 425 depicts normal pubic hair characteristics for the client's stage of development.

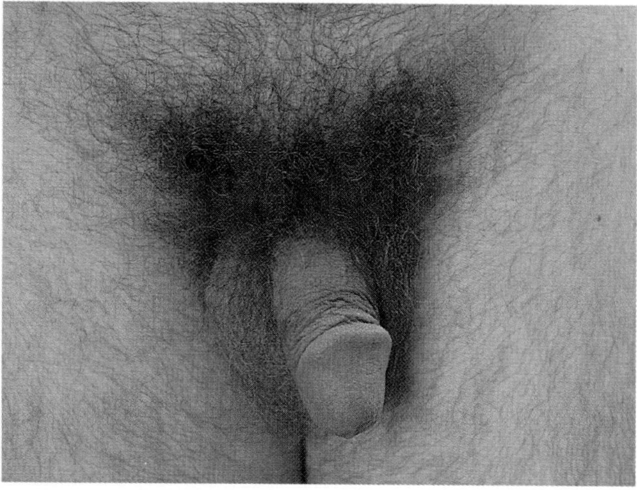

Figure 15.8 Inspecting the pubic hair.

ASSESSMENT TECHNIQUE/NORMAL FINDINGS	SPECIAL CONSIDERATIONS

- Confirm that pubic hair is distributed heavily at the symphysis pubis in a diamond or triangular-shaped pattern, thinning out as it extends toward the umbilicus. The hair will thin as it reaches the inner thigh area and over the scrotum. Hair should be absent on the penis.
- If the client has complained of itching in the pubic area, comb through the pubic hair with two or three fingers.
- Confirm the absence of small bluish gray spots, or nits (eggs) at the base of the pubic hairs.

These signs indicate the presence of crab lice. You may see marks from persistent scratching to relieve the intense itching crab lice cause.

Step 3 ***Inspect the penis.***

Inspect the penis size, pigmentation, glans, location of the dorsal vein, and the urethral meatus.

- Start by confirming that the penis size is appropriate for the stage of development of the client. In adult males, penis size varies.

Penis size varies according to the developmental stage of the client. See Table 15.1 on page 425.

- Note the pigmentation of the penis. Pigmentation should be evenly distributed over the penis. The color depends on the client's race but will be slightly darker than the color of the skin over the rest of his body.

Pigmentation of the penis of males with lighter complexions ranges from pink to light brown. In dark-skinned clients, the penis is light to dark brown.

- Assess the looseness of the skin over the shaft of the penis. The skin should be loose over the flaccid penis.
- Confirm that the dorsal vein is midline on the shaft.
- Inspect the glans penis. It should be smooth, and free of lesions or discharge. No redness or inflammation should be present. *Smegma*, a white, cheesy substance may be present. This finding is considered normal.

Discharge or lesions may indicate the presence of infective diseases such as *herpes*, *genital warts*, or *syphilis* (see Table 15.4 on page 450) or may indicate cancer. If discharge is present, culture the substance. Note consistency, color, and odor.

> **ALERT!**
>
> **Remember to change the gloves as needed during the exam to prevent cross-contamination. Also remember to culture any abnormal discharge.**

- If the client is uncircumcised, either ask the client to pull the foreskin back or do so yourself. To retract the foreskin, gently pull the skin down over the penile shaft from the side of the glans using the thumb and first two fingers or forefinger (Figure 15.9).

Phimosis is a condition in which the foreskin is so tight that it cannot be retracted.

Paraphimosis describes a condition in which the foreskin, once retracted, becomes so tight that it cannot be moved back over the glans.

ASSESSMENT TECHNIQUE/NORMAL FINDINGS

SPECIAL CONSIDERATIONS

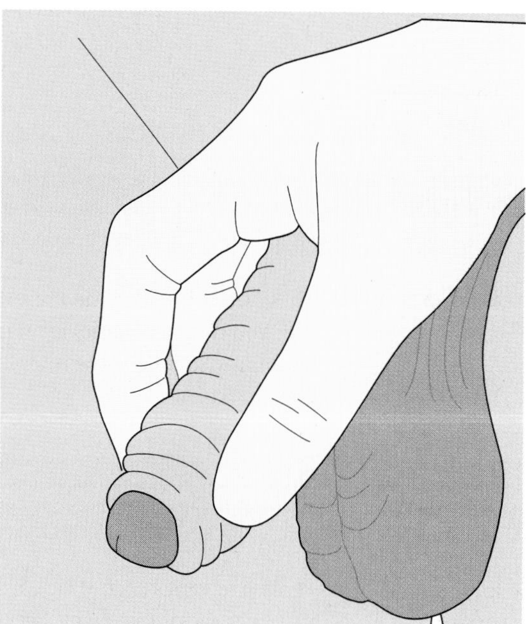

Figure 15.9 Retracting the foreskin.

- Gently move the foreskin back into place over the glans. The foreskin should move smoothly.

> ***Referral***
>
> **Seek immediate assistance if the foreskin cannot be retracted. Prolonged constriction of the vessels can obstruct blood flow and lead to tissue damage or necrosis.**

- Assess the position of the urinary meatus. The meatus should be located in the center of the tip of the penis (Figure 15.10).

In rare cases, the urinary meatus is located on the upper side of the glans (*epispadias*) or the underside of the glans (*hypospadias*). These conditions are usually corrected surgically shortly after birth.

A pinpoint appearance of the urinary meatus is indicative of *urethral stricture*.

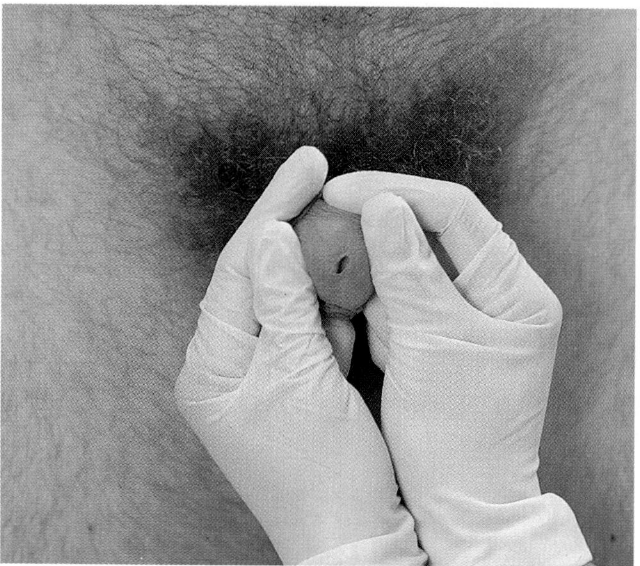

Figure 15.10 Assessing the position of the urinary meatus.

ASSESSMENT TECHNIQUE/NORMAL FINDINGS	SPECIAL CONSIDERATIONS

Step 4 *Inspect the scrotum.*

- Ask the client to hold his penis up so that the scrotum is fully exposed (Figure 15.11). Optionally, you may hold the penis up by letting it rest on the back of your nondominant hand.

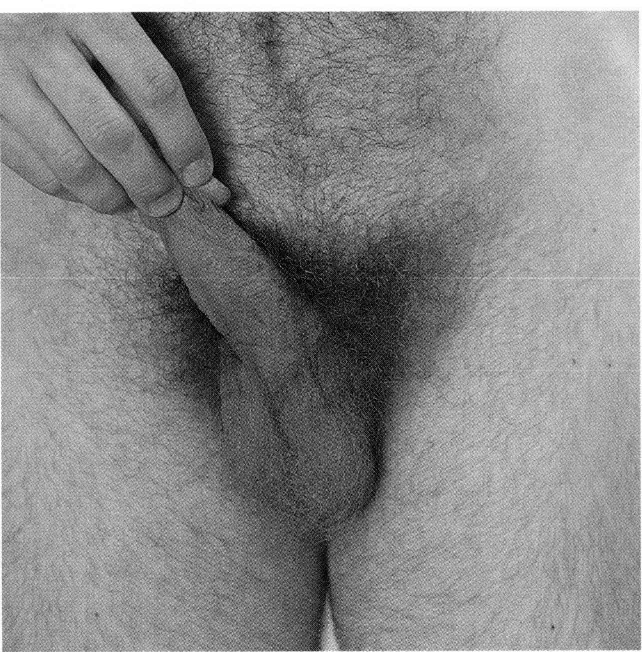

Figure 15.11 Inspecting the scrotum.

- Observe the shape of the scrotum and how it hangs. It should be pear-shaped, with the left side hanging lower than the right.

An appearance of flatness could suggest testicular abnormality. Elderly males may have a pendulous, sagging scrotal sac.

- Inspect the front and the back of the scrotum. The skin should be wrinkled, loosely fitting over its internal structures. Note any swelling, redness, distended veins, and lesions. If swelling is present, note if it is unilateral or bilateral.

Scrotal swelling and inflammation could suggest problems such as *orchitis* (inflammation of the testicles), *epididymitis* (inflammation of the epididymis), *scrotal edema* (an accumulation of fluid in the scrotum), a *scrotal hernia,* or *testicular torsion*. Swelling and inflammation may also be seen in renal, cardiovascular, and other systemic disorders.

If you detect a mass, you may want to perform transillumination.

- In a darkened room, place a lighted flashlight behind the area in which the abnormal mass was palpated (Figure 15.12).

Note any area where the light does not transilluminate. Light will not penetrate a mass. Masses may indicate *testicular tumor*, *spermatocele* (a cyst located in the epididymis), and other conditions.

ASSESSMENT TECHNIQUE/NORMAL FINDINGS | SPECIAL CONSIDERATIONS

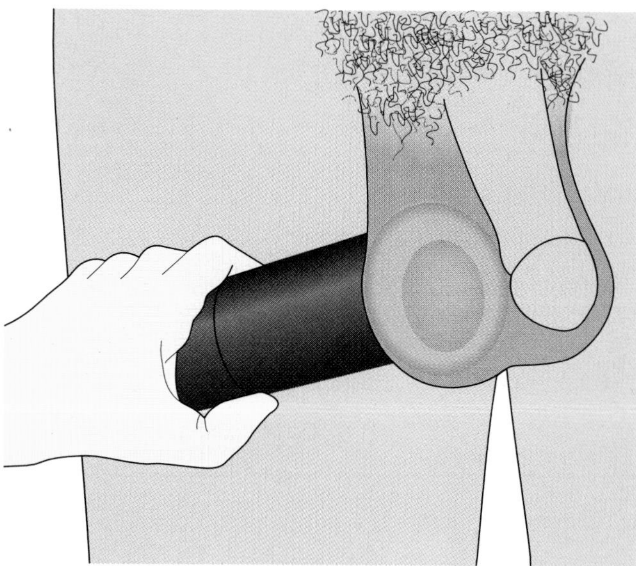

Figure 15.12 Transilluminating the scrotum.

- Note that the light shines through the scrotum with a red glow. The testicle shows up as a nontransparent oval structure.
- Repeat these steps on the other side and compare the results.

Step 5 ***Inspect the inguinal area.***

The inguinal area should be flat. This may be difficult to confirm if the client is overweight. But even in the presence of adipose tissue, the contour of the inguinal area should be consistent with the rest of the body. Lymph nodes are present in this location.

- Inspect both the right and left inguinal areas with the client breathing normally.
- Have the client hold his breath and bear down as if having a bowel movement.
- Observe for any evidence of lumps or masses. The contour of the inguinal areas should remain even.

Masses or lumps may be related to the presence of an inguinal hernia or cancer.

ALERT!

Some clients may not tolerate bearing down for more than a few seconds. Do not have hypertensive clients perform this maneuver. Observe for discomfort and lightheadedness. Have the client breathe normally after 15–20 seconds.

ASSESSMENT TECHNIQUE/NORMAL FINDINGS | SPECIAL CONSIDERATIONS

Palpation

Step 1 *Palpate the penis.*

- Place the glans between your thumb and forefinger.

Be aware that the client may be hesitant to verbalize pain when you perform palpation. Watch for nonverbal facial and body gestures.

- Gently compress the glans, allowing the meatus to gape open (Figure 15.13). The meatus should be pink, patent, and free of discharge.

Suspect a *urethral stricture* if the meatus is only about the size of a pinpoint.

Signs of *urethritis* include redness and edemaround the glans and foreskin, eversion of urethral mucosa, and drainage. If you suspect urethritis, ask the client if he experiences itching and tenderness around the meatus and painful urination. If drainage is present, observe for color, consistency, odor, and amount. Obtain a specimen if indicated. Suspect a gonococcal infection (gonorrhea) if the drainage is profuse and thick, purulent, and greenish yellow in color. Consider inflammation or infection higher up in the urinary tract if you see redness, edema, and discharge around the urethral opening, because the mucous membrane in the urethra is continuous with the mucous membrane in the rest of the tract.

Be alert for any lesions, masses, swelling, or nodules.

Note characteristics of any abnormal findings. Culture any discharge.

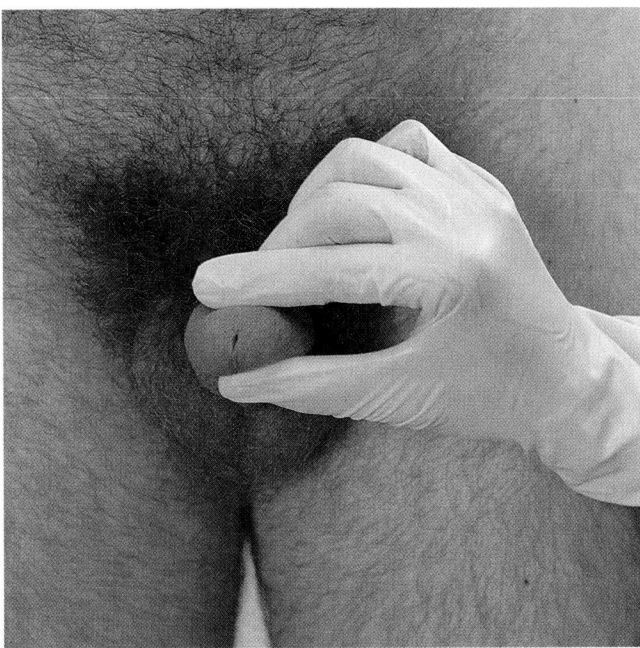

Figure 15.13 Palpating the penis.

- Note any discharge or tenderness.
- Continue gentle palpation and compression up the entire shaft of the penis.

Step 2 *Palpate the scrotum.*

- Ask the client to hold his penis up to expose the scrotum.
- Gently palpate the left and then the right scrotal sacs (Figure 15.14). Each scrotal sac should be nontender, soft, and boggy. The structures within the sacs should move easily with your palpation.

Assess shape, size, consistency, location, and mobility of any masses. If the client expresses pain, lift the scrotum. If the pain is relieved, the client may have *epididymitis*, inflammation of the epididymis.

ASSESSMENT TECHNIQUE/NORMAL FINDINGS	SPECIAL CONSIDERATIONS

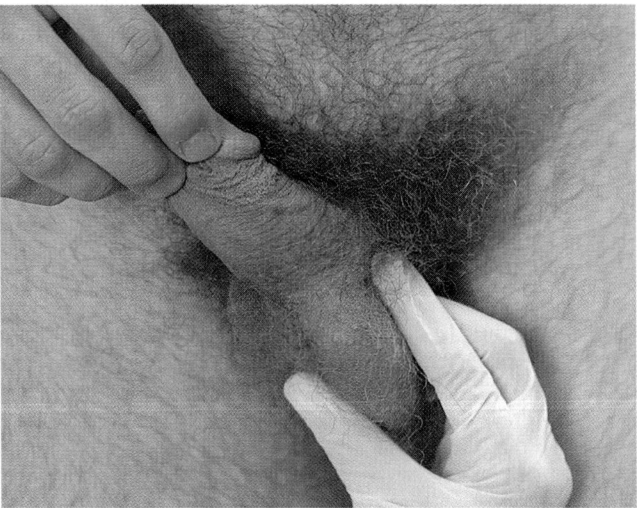

Figure 15.14 Palpating the scrotum.

- Note any tenderness, swelling, masses, lesions, or nodules.

ALERT!

Do not pinch or squeeze any mass, lesion, or other structure.

Step 3 *Palpate the testes.*

- Be sure that your hands are warm.
- Approach each testis from the bottom of the scrotal sac and gently rotate it between your thumb and fingertips (Figure 15.15). Each testis should be nontender, oval-shaped, walnut-sized, smooth, elastic, and solid.

The *cremasteric reflex* may cause the testicles to migrate upward temporarily. Cold hands, a cold room, or the stimulus of touch could cause this response.

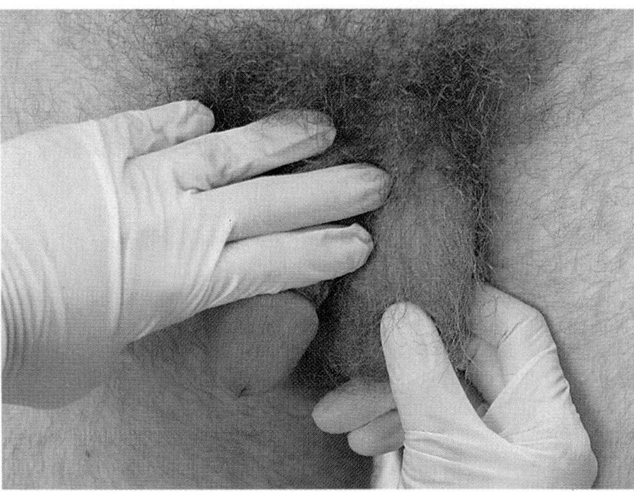

Figure 15.15 Palpating the testes.

ASSESSMENT TECHNIQUE/NORMAL FINDINGS	SPECIAL CONSIDERATIONS

Step 4 *Palpate the epididymes.*

- Slide your fingertips around to the posterior side of each testicle to find the epididymis, a small, crescent-shaped structure.
- Palpate gently. Gentle palpation should not elicit a painful response.

In some clients, the epididymis may be palpated on the front surface of each testis.

Step 5 *Palpate the spermatic cord.*

- Slide your fingers up just above the testicle, feeling for a vertical, ropelike structure about 3 mm wide.
- Gently grasp the cord between your thumb and index finger (Figure 15.16).

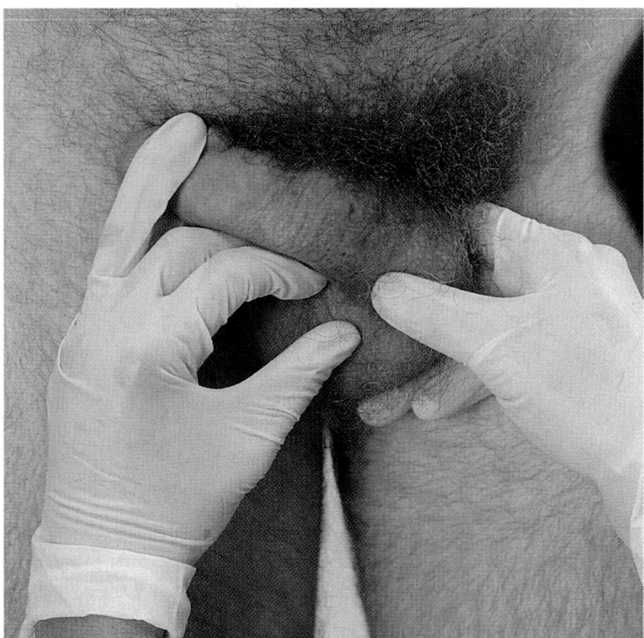

Figure 15.16 Palpating the spermatic cord.

- Do not squeeze or pinch.
- Trace the cord up to the external inguinal ring using a gentle rotating motion.

The cord should feel thin, smooth, nontender to palpation, and resilient.

A cord that is hard, beaded, or nodular could indicate the presence of a varicosity or varicocele. A *varicocele* is a distended cord and is a common cause of male infertility. Upon palpation, it may feel like a "bag of worms."

Step 6 *Palpate the inguinal region.*

ALERT!

This is a very sensitive area. Instruct the client to inform you of any pain or discomfort. This area is also very ticklish. Use firm, deliberate movements.

An *inguinal hernia* feels like a bulge or mass. A *direct inguinal hernia* can be palpated in the area of the external ring of the inguinal ligament. You will feel it either right at the external ring opening or just behind it.

An *indirect inguinal hernia* is more common, especially in younger males. It is located deeper in the inguinal canal than

ASSESSMENT TECHNIQUE/NORMAL FINDINGS

- Start by preparing the client for palpation in the right inguinal area.
- Ask the client to shift his balance so that his weight is on his left leg.
- Place your right index finder in the upper corner of the right scrotum.
- Slowly palpate the spermatic cord up and slightly to the client's left.
- Allow the client's scrotal skin to fold over your index finger as you palpate.
- Proceed until you feel an opening that feels like a triangular slit. This is the external ring of the inguinal canal.
- Attempt to gently glide your finger into this opening (Figure 15.17).

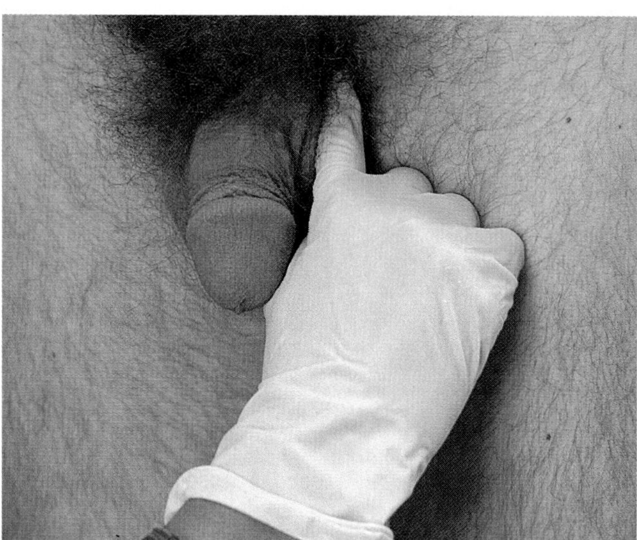

Figure 15.17 Palpating the inguinal canal.

- If it has admitted your finger, ask the client to either cough or bear down.
- Palpate for masses or lumps.

ALERT!

If you cannot insert your finger with gentle pressure, do not force your finger into the opening.

- Repeat this procedure by palpating the client's left inguinal area. Use your left index finger when performing the palpation.

SPECIAL CONSIDERATIONS

the direct inguinal hernia. However, it can pass into the scrotum, whereas a direct inguinal hernia rarely protrudes into the scrotum.

It is also possible that a *femoral hernia* may be present. It is more commonly found in the right inguinal area and near the inguinal ligament. Table 15.6 on page 454 illustrates these three types of hernias.

Referral

If the client displays an acute bulge with tenderness, pain, nausea, or vomiting, he may have a strangulated hernia. Help him to lie down and request immediate medical assistance.

Step 7 ***Palpate the inguinal lymph chain.***

- Using the pads of your first three fingers, palpate the inguinal lymph nodes.

It is important to assess if a node is larger than 0.5 cm or if multiple nodes are present. Tenderness in this area suggests infection of the scrotum, penis, or groin area.

ASSESSMENT TECHNIQUE/NORMAL FINDINGS | SPECIAL CONSIDERATIONS

- Confirm that nodes are nonpalpable and the area is nontender (Figure 15.18).

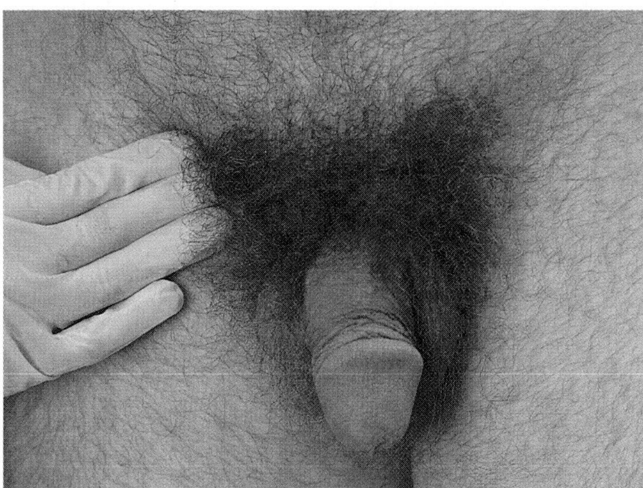

Figure 15.18 Palpating the inguinal lymph nodes.

Occasionally some of the inguinal lymph nodes are palpable. They are usually less than 0.5 cm in size, spongy, movable, and nontender.

Step 8 ***Palpate the bulbourethral gland and the prostate gland.***

- Reposition the client. Ask the client to turn and face the table and bend over at the waist. The client can rest his arms on the table (Figure 15.19).

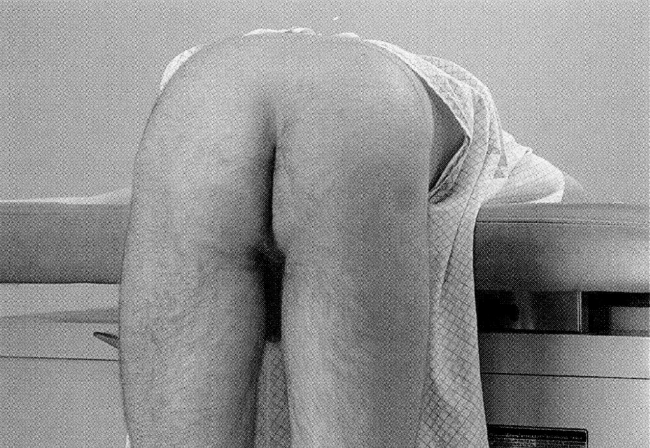

Figure 15.19 Positioning the client for palpation of internal structures.

- If the client is unable to tolerate this position, he may lie on his left side on the examination table with both knees flexed.
- Lubricate your right index finger with lubricating gel.
- Tell the client that you are going to insert your finger into his rectum in order to palpate his prostate gland. Explain that the insertion may cause him to feel as if he needs to have a bowel movement. Tell him that this technique shouldn't cause pain but to inform you immediately if it does.

ASSESSMENT TECHNIQUE/NORMAL FINDINGS

SPECIAL CONSIDERATIONS

- Place the index finger of your dominant hand against the anal opening (Figure 15.20). Be sure that your finger is slightly bent and not forming a right angle to the buttocks. If you insert your index finger at a right angle to the buttocks, the client may experience pain.

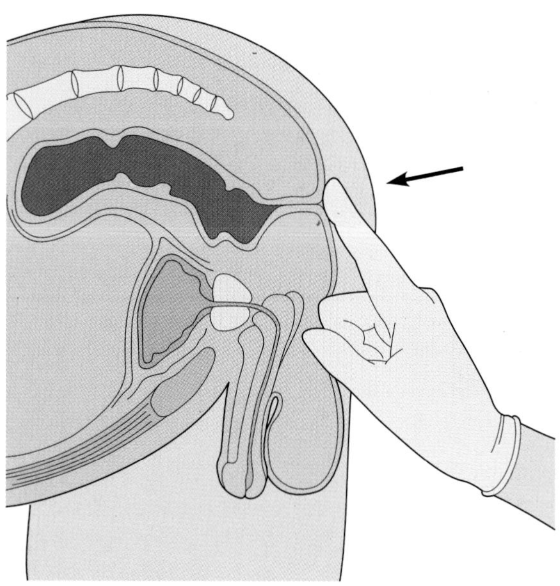

Figure 15.20 Placing the finger against the anal opening.

- Apply gentle pressure as you insert your bent finger into the anus (Figure 15.21).

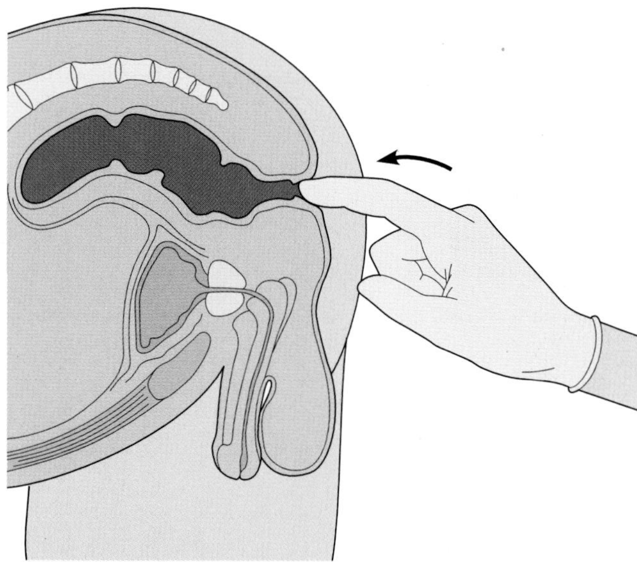

Figure 15.21 Inserting the finger into the anus.

ASSESSMENT TECHNIQUE/NORMAL FINDINGS	SPECIAL CONSIDERATIONS

- As the sphincter muscle tightens, stop inserting your finger.
- Resume as the sphincter muscle relaxes.
- Press your right thumb gently against the perianal area.
- Palpate the bulbourethral gland by pressing your index finger gently toward your thumb (Figure 15.22). This should not cause the client to feel pain or tenderness. No swelling or masses should be felt.

If the bulbourethral gland is inflamed, the client may feel pain upon palpation.

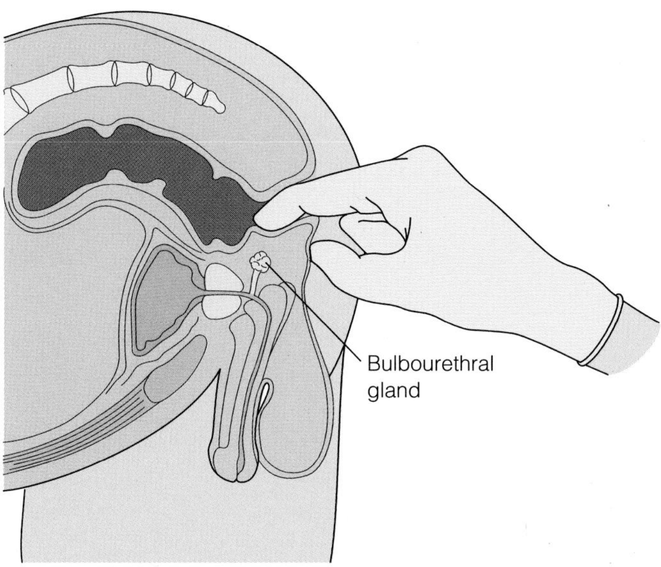

Figure 15.22 Palpating the bulbourethral gland.

- Release the pressure between your index finger and thumb. Continue to insert your index finger gently (Figure 15.23).
- Palpate the posterior surface of the prostate gland.

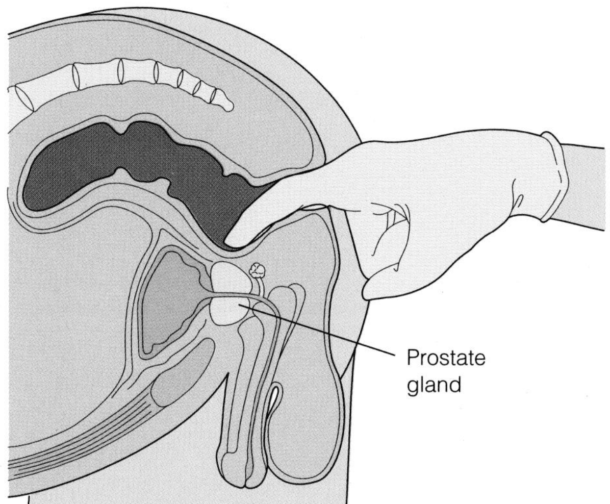

Figure 15.23 Palpating the prostate gland.

ASSESSMENT TECHNIQUE/NORMAL FINDINGS	SPECIAL CONSIDERATIONS
◆ Confirm that it is smooth, firm, even somewhat rubbery, nontender, and extends out no more than 1 cm into the rectal area.	Note tenderness, masses, nodules, hardness, or softness. Nodules are characteristic of *prostate cancer* (see Table 15.5 on page 452). Tenderness indicates inflammation.

- ◆ Remove your finger slowly and gently.
- ◆ Remove your gloves.
- ◆ Help the client to a standing position.
- ◆ Wash your hands.
- ◆ Give the client tissues to wipe the perianal area.
- ◆ Review the reminders on page 442.

Table 15.1 Maturation Stages in the Male

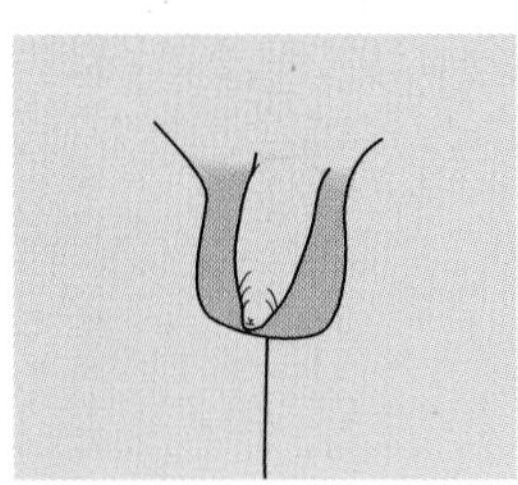

Stage 1.

No pubic hair. Penis is small. Scrotum looks large in comparison to penis.

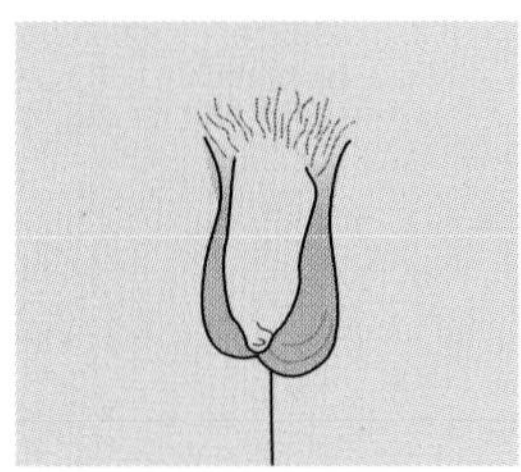

Stage 2.

Sparse pubic hair at base of penis. Penis is small. Scrotum begins to grow.

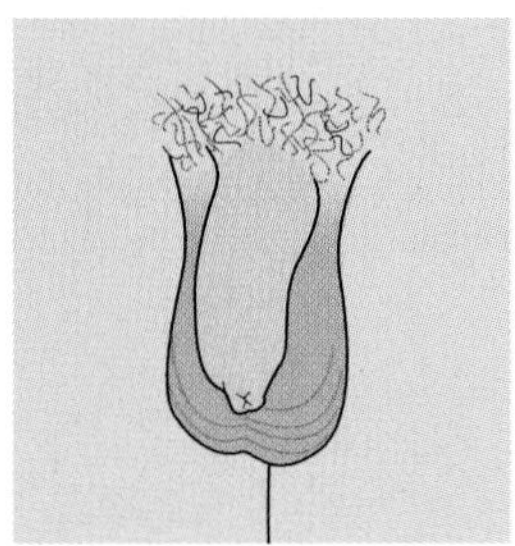

Stage 3.

Penis begins to enlongate. Scrotum also continues to enlarge, and pubis covered with curly hair.

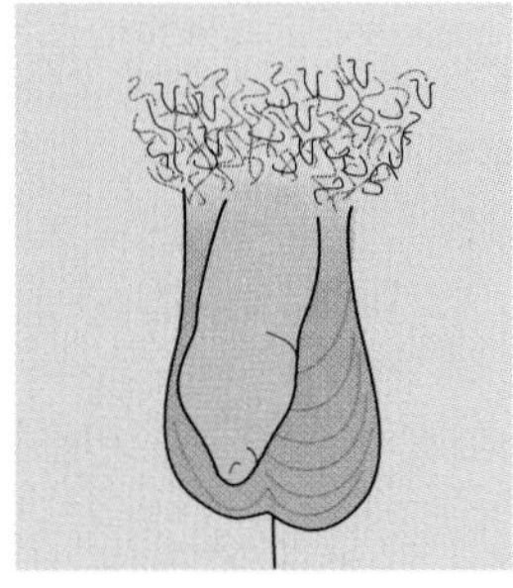

Stage 4.

Continued elongation and thickening of penis. Pubic hair coarse and thickening.

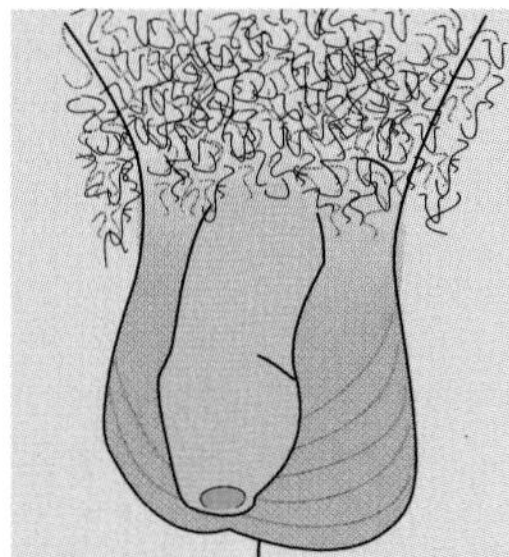

Stage 5.

Adult size penis and scrotum, with thick, curly pubic hair.

Physical Assessment of the Female

Preparation

☑ **Gather the equipment:**

examination gloves
examination gown
drape
gooseneck lamp
lubricating jelly
appropriate-sized speculum
culturette set
cotton-tipped applicators or cytobrush
bifid spatula
prelabeled glass slides for specimens
cytologic fixative for specimens
Thayer-Martin culture plate labeled "cervical"
sterile saline solution
receptacle for used speculum
hand-held mirror

☑ **Alleviate discomfort and embarrassment before and during the examination by using the following strategies:**

- Have the client empty her bladder and bowels before the exam.
- Explain that the client can help with the exam by relaxing and focusing on your instructions.
- Maintain eye contact.
- Reassure the client that anxiety and embarrassment are normal.
- Humor may alleviate stress; however, it must be used only in good taste and appropriately.
- Before starting, determine if the client has had this type of examination before. If not, you may want to use a booklet with diagrams of the examination, especially if the client is an adolescent. Show pictures of the equipment, slides for specimens, and the bimanual examination. Explain what you will do and why.
- As you proceed through the exam, explain to the client what you are doing and why. Explain what you see that is normal. You may also describe any abnormality, but be sure not to alarm the client.
- Touch the client firmly but gently, avoiding ambiguity.
- Use an unhurried, deliberate manner.
- Ask the client throughout the examination how she is doing.

☑ **Ensure that the room is warm and the client has privacy. Double-check that the "in use" sign is on the examination room door.**

☑ **Ask the client to remove her clothing and put on the examination gown. She may leave her socks on. Leave the room while she undresses.**

☑ **Wash your hands and put on the examination gloves. Change the gloves as needed during the exam to prevent cross-contamination and exposure to body fluids.**

☑ **Remember to culture any abnormal discharge.**

ASSESSMENT TECHNIQUE/NORMAL FINDINGS | SPECIAL CONSIDERATIONS

Inspection

Step 1 *Position the client.*

- Ask the client to lie down on the examination table.
- Assist her into the lithotomy position (supine with legs and hips flexed so that feet rest flat on the examination table), then have her slide her hips as close to the end of the table as possible.
- Place her feet in the stirrups (Figure 15.24).

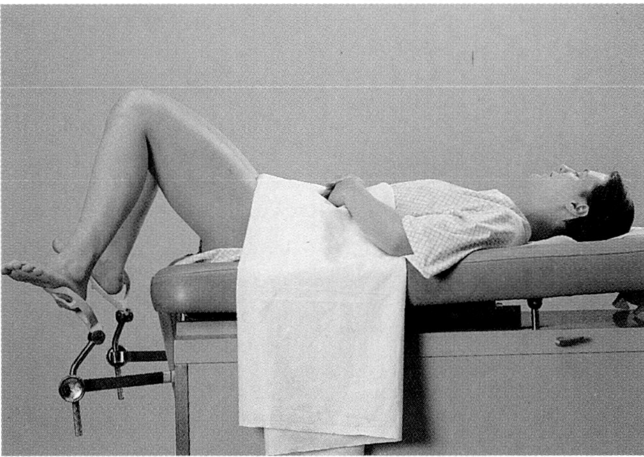

Figure 15.24 Positioning the client.

Step 2 *Inspect the pubic hair.*

- Confirm that the hair grows in an inverted triangle and is scattered heavily over the mons pubis. It should become sparse over the labia majora, perineum, and inner thighs (Figure 15.25).

A sparse hair pattern may be indicative of delayed puberty. It is also a common normal finding in people of Asian ancestry. The elderly client's pubic hair will become sparse, scattered, and gray. Table 15.2 on page 443 depicts normal pubic hair characteristics according to developmental stage.

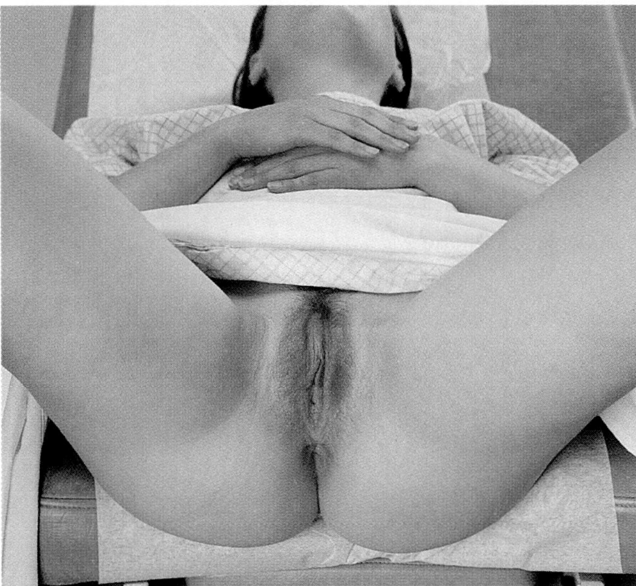

Figure 15.25 Inspecting the pubic hair.

ASSESSMENT TECHNIQUE/NORMAL FINDINGS	SPECIAL CONSIDERATIONS

- If the client has complained of itching in the pubic area, comb through the pubic hair with two or three fingers.
- Confirm the absence of small bluish gray spots, or nits (eggs) at the base of the pubic hairs.

These signs indicate crab lice. You may see marks from persistent scratching to relieve the intense itching caused by the lice.

Step 3 *Inspect the labia majora.*

The labia majora of elderly females may be thinner and wrinkled.

- Confirm that the labia majora are fuller and rounder in the center of the structure, and that the skin is smooth and intact.
- Compare the right and left labia majora for symmetry.
- Observe for any lesions, warts, vesicles, rashes, or ulcerations. If you notice drainage, note the color, distribution, location, and characteristics.

These findings may signal a variety of conditions. *Contact dermatitis* appears as a red rash with associated lesions that are weepy and crusty. There often are scratches due to intense itching.

Genital warts are raised, moist, cauliflower-shaped papules.

Red, painful vesicles accompanied by localized swelling are seen in *herpes* infection. See Table 15.4 on page 000 for a discussion of sexually transmitted infections.

ALERT!

Remember to change the gloves as needed during the exam to prevent cross-contamination. Also remember to culture any abnormal discharge.

- Confirm the absence of any swelling or inflammation in the area of the labia majora.

Swelling over red, inflamed skin that is tender and warm to palpation may indicate an abscess in the Bartholin's gland. The abscess may be caused by gonorrhea.

Step 4 *Inspect the labia minora.*

The elderly female may have drier, thinner labia minora.

- Confirm that the labia minora are smooth, pink, and moist.
- Observe for any redness or swelling. Note any bruising or tearing of the skin.

Redness and swelling indicate the presence of an infective or inflammatory process. Bruising or tearing of the skin may suggest forceful intercourse or sexual abuse, especially in the case of adolescents and children.

Step 5 *Inspect the clitoris.*

- Place your right or left hand over the labia majora and separate these structures with your thumb and index finger.
- The clitoris should be midline, about 1 cm in length, with more fullness in the center. It should be smooth.

An elongated clitoris may signal elevated levels of testosterone and warrants further investigation and referral to a physician.

- Observe for any redness, lesions, or tears in the tissue.

Step 6 *Inspect the urethral orifice.*

- Confirm that the urethral opening is midline, pink, smooth, slitlike, and patent.
- Have the woman cough. No urine should leak from the urethral opening.

Urine leakage indicates stress incontinence and weakening of the pelvic musculature.

ASSESSMENT TECHNIQUE/NORMAL FINDINGS | SPECIAL CONSIDERATIONS

- Inspect for any redness, inflammation, or discharge.

These symptoms indicate urinary tract infection. See the previous chapter.

Step 7 ***Inspect the vaginal opening and perineum.***

- Confirm that the vaginal opening or *introitus* is pink and round. It may be either smooth or irregular.
- Locate the *hymen* which is a thin layer of skin within the vagina. It may be present in women who have never had sexual intercourse.
- Inspect for tears, bruising, or lacerations.

Tears, bruising, or lacerations could be due to forceful consensual sex or to rape. Additional follow-up is needed after examination. Do not ask any questions that the client may interpret as probing or threatening during the physical assessment.

- Scars from episiotomy procedures may be observed. These are normal.
- Have the client bear down.
- Inspect for any protrusions from the vagina.

A *prolapsed uterus* may protrude right at the vaginal wall with straining, or it may hang outside of the vaginal wall without any straining (Figure 15.26).

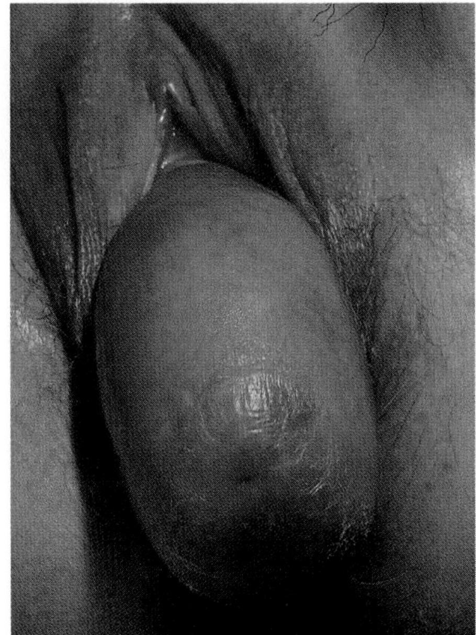

Figure 15.26 Prolapsed uterus.

A *cystocele* is a hernia that is formed when the urinary bladder is pushed into the vaginal opening.

A *rectocele* is a hernia that is formed when the rectum pushes into the vaginal opening.

ASSESSMENT TECHNIQUE/NORMAL FINDINGS | SPECIAL CONSIDERATIONS

Palpation

Step 1 ***Palpate the vaginal walls.***

- Explain to the client that you are going to palpate the vaginal walls. Tell her that she will feel you insert your finger into her vagina.
- Place your left hand above the labia majora and spread the labia minora apart with your thumb and index finger.
- With your right palm facing toward the ceiling, gently place your right index finger at the vaginal opening.
- Insert your right index finger gently into the vagina (Figure 15.27).

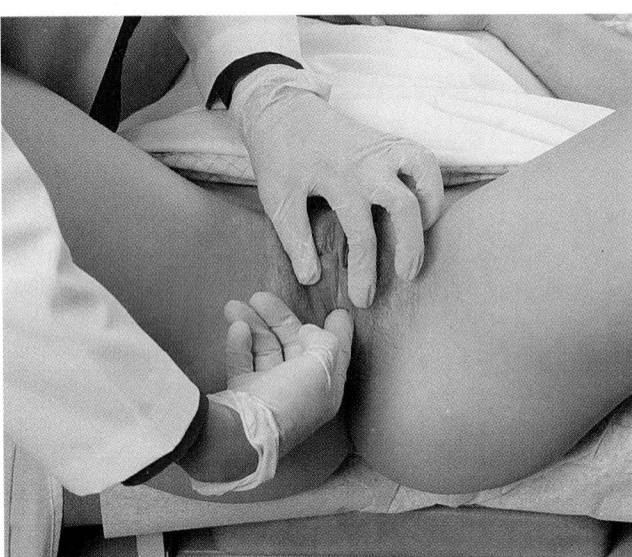

Figure 15.27 Palpating the vaginal walls.

- Gently rotate the right index finger counterclockwise. The vaginal wall should feel rugated, consistent in texture, and soft.
- Ask the patient to bear down or cough.
- Note any bulging in this area.

Bulging may occur with uterine prolapse, cystocele, or rectal prolapse (rectocele).

Step 2 ***Palpate the urethra and Skene's glands.***

- Explain to the client that you are going to palpate her urethra. Tell her that she will again feel pressure against her vaginal wall.
- Your left hand should still be above the labia majora and you should still be spreading the labia minora apart with your thumb and index finger.
- Your right index finger should still be inserted in the client's vagina.
- With your right index finger, apply very gentle pressure upward against the vaginal wall.
- Milk the Skene's glands by stroking outward (Figure 15.28).

ASSESSMENT TECHNIQUE/NORMAL FINDINGS | SPECIAL CONSIDERATIONS

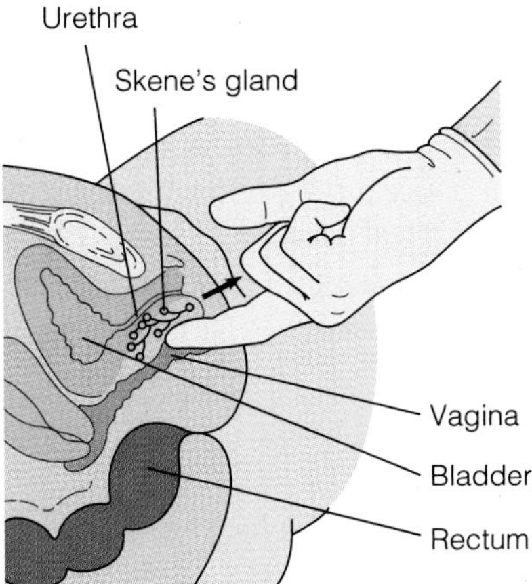

Figure 15.28 Palpating Skene's glands.

- Now apply the same upward and outward pressure on both sides of the urethra.

No pain or discharge should be elicited.

Discharge from the urethra or Skene's glands may indicate an infection such as gonorrhea. Obtain a culture.

Step 3 ***Palpate the Bartholin's glands.***

- With your right index finger still inserted in the client's vagina, gently squeeze the posterior region of the labia majora between your right index finger and right thumb (Figure 15.29).

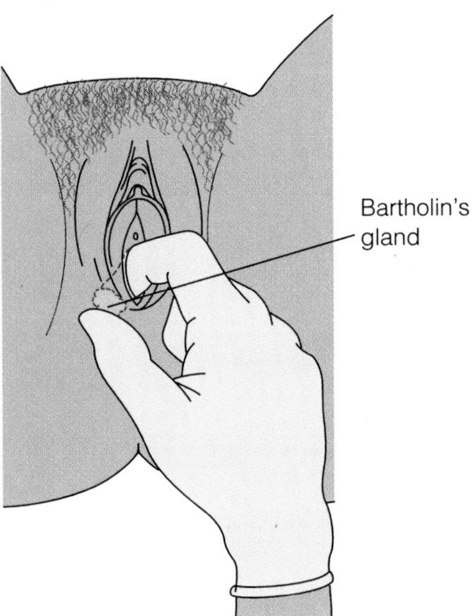

Figure 15.29 Palpating Bartholin's glands.

ASSESSMENT TECHNIQUE/NORMAL FINDINGS | SPECIAL CONSIDERATIONS

- Perform this maneuver bilaterally, palpating both Bartholin's glands.

No lump or hardness should be felt. No pain response should be elicited. No discharge should be produced.

Lumps, hardness, pain, or discharge suggest the presence of an abscess and infective process. Often the source is a gonorrheal infection. Obtain a culture of any discharge.

Inspection with a Speculum

ALERT!

Be sure that the client has not douched within 24 hours before obtaining cervical and vaginal specimens. Otherwise, the results of the test may not be accurate.

If the client has vaginitis, delay the speculum examination until the problem has been treated unless this is the client's chief complaint and the reason for her visit.

Step 1 *Select the speculum.*

The speculum should be the proper size for the client.

Use a speculum that has been prewarmed with a heating pad. Do not prewarm a speculum with warm water, because it is not desirable to introduce water into the vagina. Do not use gel lubricant, as it may distort the cells in your specimens.

Step 2 *Hold the speculum in your dominant hand.*

- Place the index finger on top of the blades, the third finger on the bottom of the blades, and the thumb just underneath the thumbscrew (Figure 15.30).

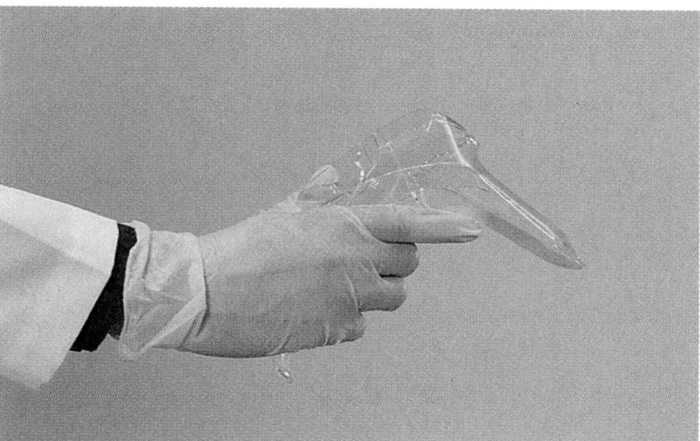

Figure 15.30 Holding the speculum.

Step 3 *Insert the speculum.*

- Tell the client that you are going to examine her cervix, and that to do so, you are going to insert a speculum. If this is the client's first such examination, show her the speculum and briefly demonstrate how you will use it to visualize her cervix. Have a mirror available

ASSESSMENT TECHNIQUE/NORMAL FINDINGS

SPECIAL CONSIDERATIONS

to share findings with the client. Also explain that she will feel pressure, first of your fingers, and then of the speculum. You may also want to show her a booklet with a picture demonstrating the technique.

- With your nondominant hand, place your index and middle fingers on the posterior vaginal opening and apply pressure gently downward.
- Turn the speculum blades obliquely.
- Place the blades over your fingers at the vaginal opening and slowly insert the closed speculum at a 45-degree downward angle (Figure 15.31). This angle matches the downward slope of the vagina when the client is in the lithotomy position.
- Ask the client to bear down as you insert. It is normal for the client to tense as the speculum is inserted, and bearing down helps to relax the muscles.

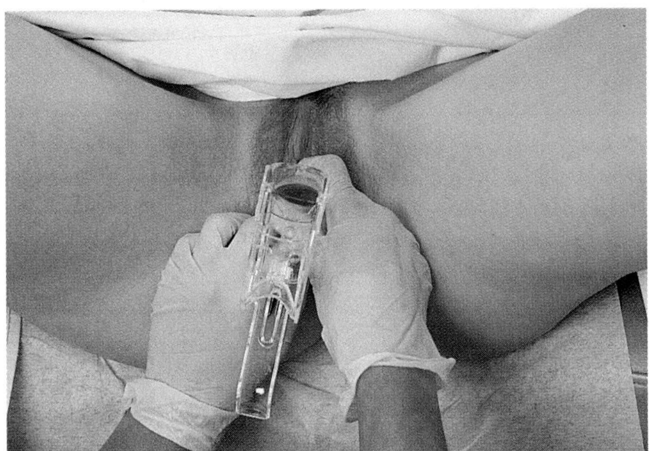

Figure 15.31 Inserting the speculum at a 45-degree angle downward.

- Once the speculum is inserted, withdraw your fingers and turn the speculum clockwise until the blades are in a horizontal plane.
- Advance the blades at a downward 45-degree angle until they are completely inserted. This maneuver should not cause the client pain.

ALERT!

Avoid pinching the labia or pulling on the client's pubic hair. If insertion of the speculum causes the client pain, stop immediately and reevaluate your technique.

- To open the speculum blades, squeeze the speculum handle.

ASSESSMENT TECHNIQUE/NORMAL FINDINGS	SPECIAL CONSIDERATIONS

- Sweep the speculum blades upward until the cervix comes into view.
- Adjust the speculum blades as needed until the cervix is fully exposed between them (Figure 15.32).

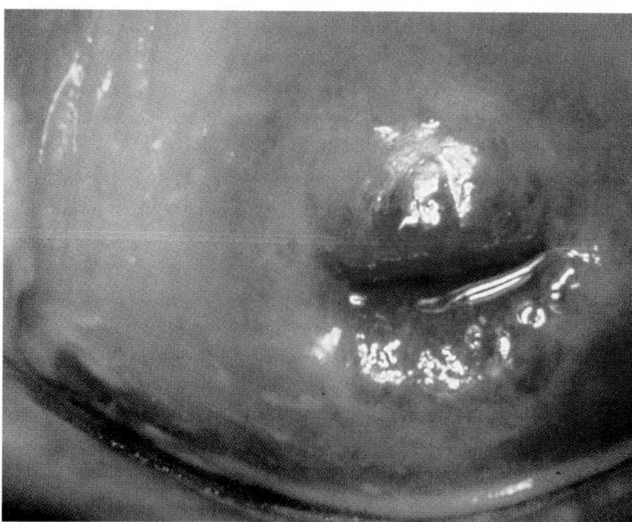

Figure 15.32 A close-up view of the fully exposed cervix.

- Tighten the thumbscrew to stabilize the spread of the blades.

Step 4 *Visualize the cervix.*

- Confirm that the cervix is pink, moist, round, centrally positioned and has a small opening in the center.
- Note any bluish coloring.

A bluish coloring is seen during the second month of pregnancy and is called *Chadwick's sign*. Otherwise, a bluish color is indicative of cyanosis.

- Confirm that any secretions are clear and without odor.

Green discharge that has a foul smell is associated with gonorrhea. White discharge is seen in candidiasis. Frothy yellow-green discharge is seen in *trichomoniasis*. A yellow discharge can also be visualized in chlamydial infection. Bacterial vaginosis presents with a creamy-gray to white discharge that has a fishy odor. See Table 15.4 on page 450.

- Confirm that the cervix is free from erosions, ulcerations, lacerations, and polyps.

Erosions are associated with carcinoma or infections. Ulcerations can be due to carcinoma, syphilis, and tuberculosis. Yellow cysts or nodules are *nabothian cysts,* benign cysts that may appear after childbirth.

ASSESSMENT TECHNIQUE/NORMAL FINDINGS | SPECIAL CONSIDERATIONS

Obtaining the Pap Smear and Gonorrhea Culture

The Pap (Papanicolaou) smear consists of three specimens: an endocervical swab, a cervical scrape, and a vaginal pool sample.

Have ready prelabeled glass slides for specimens, either (a) one labeled "endocervical," one labeled "vaginal," and one labeled "cervical" or (b) one slide that has sections for each sample.

Step 1 ***Perform an endocervical swab.***

- Carefully insert a saline-moistened, cotton-tipped applicator or cytobrush into the vagina and into the cervical os.

Moistening the applicator with saline prevents the cells from being absorbed into the cotton. The cytobrush is recommended over the cotton-tipped applicator because more endocervical cells adhere to it, and it thus yields more accurate results.

- Do not use force to insert the applicator.

If you cannot slip the applicator into the cervical os, a tumor may be blocking the opening.

- Rotate the applicator in a complete circle (Figure 15.33).
- Roll a thin coat across the slide labeled "endocervical."

A thin coat is preferred because a thick coat may be difficult to assess under the microscope.

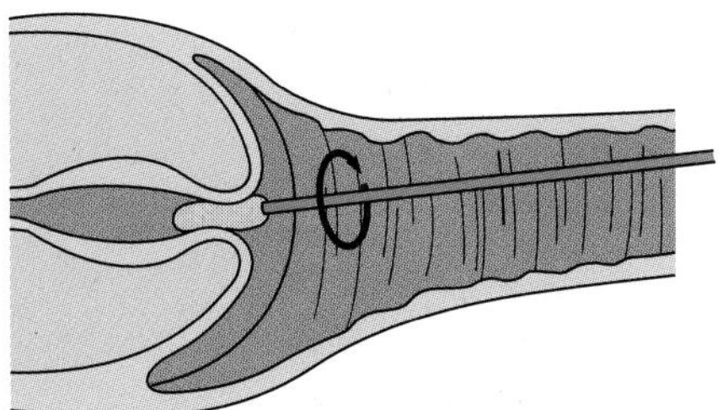

Figure 15.33 The endocervical swab.

- Spray fixative on the slide immediately or place it in a container filled with fixative.

Step 2 ***Obtain a cervical scrape.***

If the client has had a hysterectomy, obtain the scrape from the surgical stump.

- Insert the bifid end of a bifid spatula into the client's vagina.
- Advance the fingerlike projection of the bifid end gently into the cervical os.
- Allow the shorter end to rest on the outer ridge of the cervix.
- Rotate the applicator one full 360-degree turn clockwise to scrape cells from the cervix (Figure 15.34).

ASSESSMENT TECHNIQUE/NORMAL FINDINGS | SPECIAL CONSIDERATIONS

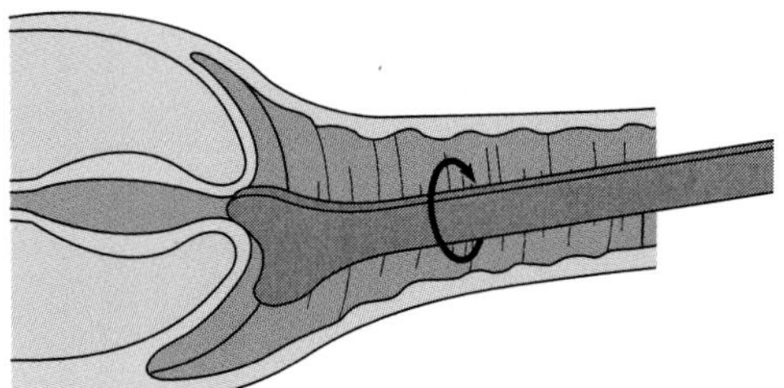

Figure 15.34 The cervical scrape.

- Do not rotate the applicator more than once or turn it in a counterclockwise manner.
- Spread a thin smear across the slide labeled "cervical" from each side of the applicator.
- Spray fixative on the slide immediately or place in a container filled with fixative.

Step 3 ***Obtain a vaginal pool sample.***

- Insert the paddle end of the spatula into the vaginal recess area (fornix). Alternatively, you may use a saline-moistened cotton applicator.
- Gently rotate the spatula back and forth to obtain a sample (Figure 15.35).

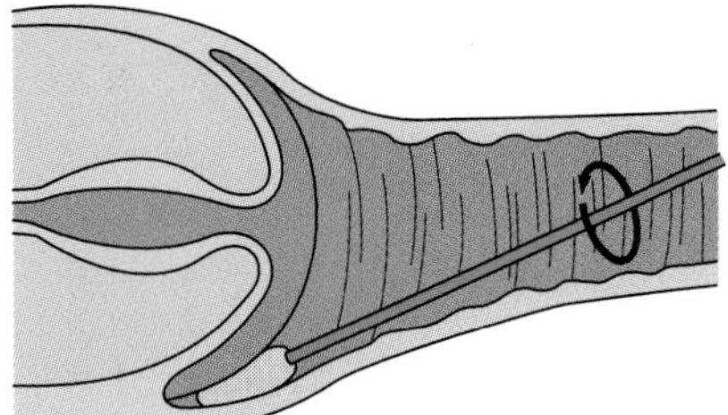

Figure 15.35 The vaginal pool sample.

- Apply the specimen to the slide labeled "vaginal."
- Spray fixative on the slide immediately.

Step 4 ***Obtain a gonorrhea culture.***

- Obtain a gonorrhea culture if the assessment findings indicate.
- Insert a saline-moistened cotton applicator into the cervical os.

Be sure to check with the laboratory in your institution, because techniques and protocols may differ.

ASSESSMENT TECHNIQUE/NORMAL FINDINGS	SPECIAL CONSIDERATIONS

- Leave the applicator in place for 20 seconds to allow full saturation of the cotton.
- Using a **Z**-shaped pattern, roll a thin coat of the secretions onto the Thayer-Martin (TM) culture plate labeled "cervical."

Step 5 ***Remove the speculum.***

- Gently loosen the thumbscrew on the speculum while holding the handles securely.
- Slant the speculum from side to side as you slide it from the vaginal canal.
- While you withdraw the speculum, note that the vaginal mucosa is pink, consistent in texture, rugated, and nontender, and discharge is thin or stringy, clear or opaque.
- Close the speculum blades before complete removal.

The infections that contribute to the development of discolored or foul-smelling vaginal discharge are the same as those listed in the previous section on identifying cervical discharge.

Bimanual Palpation

Stand at the end of the examination table. The client remains in the lithotomy position.

Step 1 ***Palpate the cervix.***

- Lubricate the index and middle fingers of your gloved dominant hand.
- Inform the client that you are going to palpate her cervix.
- Place your nondominant hand against the client's thigh, then insert your lubricated index and middle fingers into her vaginal opening.
- Proceed downward at a 45-degree angle until you reach the cervix.
- Keep the other fingers of that hand rounded inward towards the palm and put the thumb against the mons pubis away from the clitoris (Figure 15.36).

Pressure on the clitoris may be painful for the client.

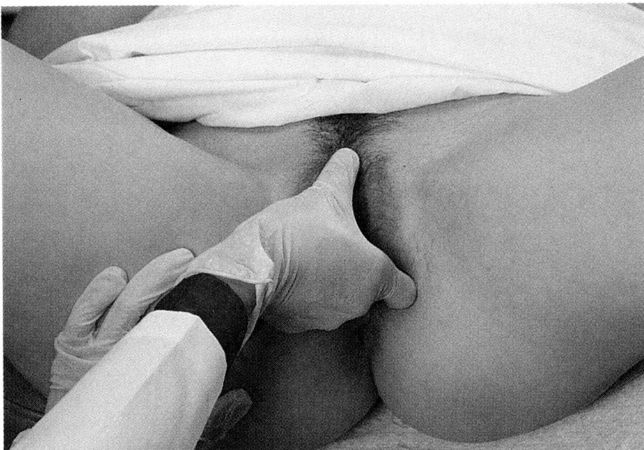

Figure 15.36 Palpating the cervix.

ASSESSMENT TECHNIQUE/NORMAL FINDINGS	SPECIAL CONSIDERATIONS
◆ Palpate the cervix. It should feel firm and smooth, somewhat like the tip of a nose.	Nodules, hardness, or lack of mobility suggests a tumor.
◆ Gently try to move it. It should move easily about 1–2 cm in either direction.	If the woman is pregnant, the cervix will be soft. This is a normal finding and is called *Goodell's sign*.

Step 2 *Palpate the fornices.*

- ◆ Slip your fingers into the vaginal recess areas, called the fornices.
- ◆ Palpate around the grooves.
- ◆ Confirm that the mucosa of the vagina and cervix in these areas is smooth and nontender.
- ◆ Leave your fingers in the anterior fornix when you have checked all sides.

Step 3 *Palpate the uterus.*

ASSESSMENT TECHNIQUE/NORMAL FINDINGS	SPECIAL CONSIDERATIONS
◆ Place the fingers of your nondominant hand on the client's abdomen.	Note any tenderness, which could be indicative of inflammation.
◆ Invaginate the abdomen midway between the umbilicus and the symphysis pubis by pushing with your fingertips downward toward the cervix (Figure 15.37).	Note tenderness, masses, nodules, or bulging. These findings may indicate inflammation, infection, cysts, tumors, or wall prolapse. Note size, shape, consistency, and mobility of nodules and masses. In the obese woman, it may be difficult to clearly differentiate the uterine structures, and an ultrasound study may be needed. When palpating uterine structures, beginning practitioners may have difficulty differentiating normal from abnormal findings. If a variation cannot be clearly identified, refer the client for additional follow-up.

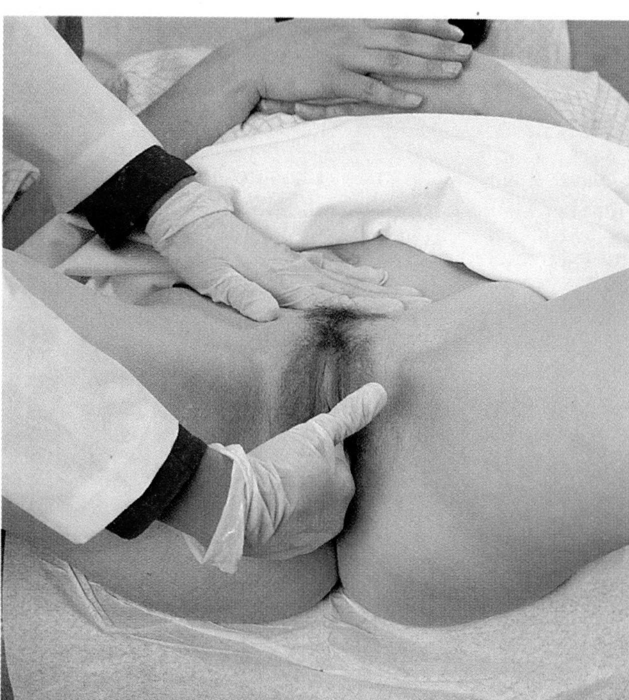

Figure 15.37 Palpating the uterus.

ASSESSMENT TECHNIQUE/NORMAL FINDINGS

- Palpate the front wall of the uterus with the hand that is inside the vagina, and the back wall of the uterus with your other hand.
- As you palpate, note the position of the cervix in relation to the position of the uterine body to determine that the uterus is in a normal position. When in a normal position, the uterus is tilted slightly upward above the bladder, and the cervix is tilted slightly forward.

Normal variations of uterine position are

Anteversion (uterus tilted forward, cervix tilted downward; Figure 15.38, A)

Midposition (uterus lies parallel to tailbone, cervix pointed straight; Figure 15.38, B)

Retroversion (uterus tilted backward, cervix tilted upward (Figure 15.38, C)

SPECIAL CONSIDERATIONS

Abnormal variations of uterine position are

Anteflexion (uterus folded forward at about a 90-degree angle, and cervix tilted downward; Figure 15.38, D)

Retroflexion (uterus folded backward at about a 90-degree angle, cervix tilted upward (Figure 15.38; Figure 15.38, E)

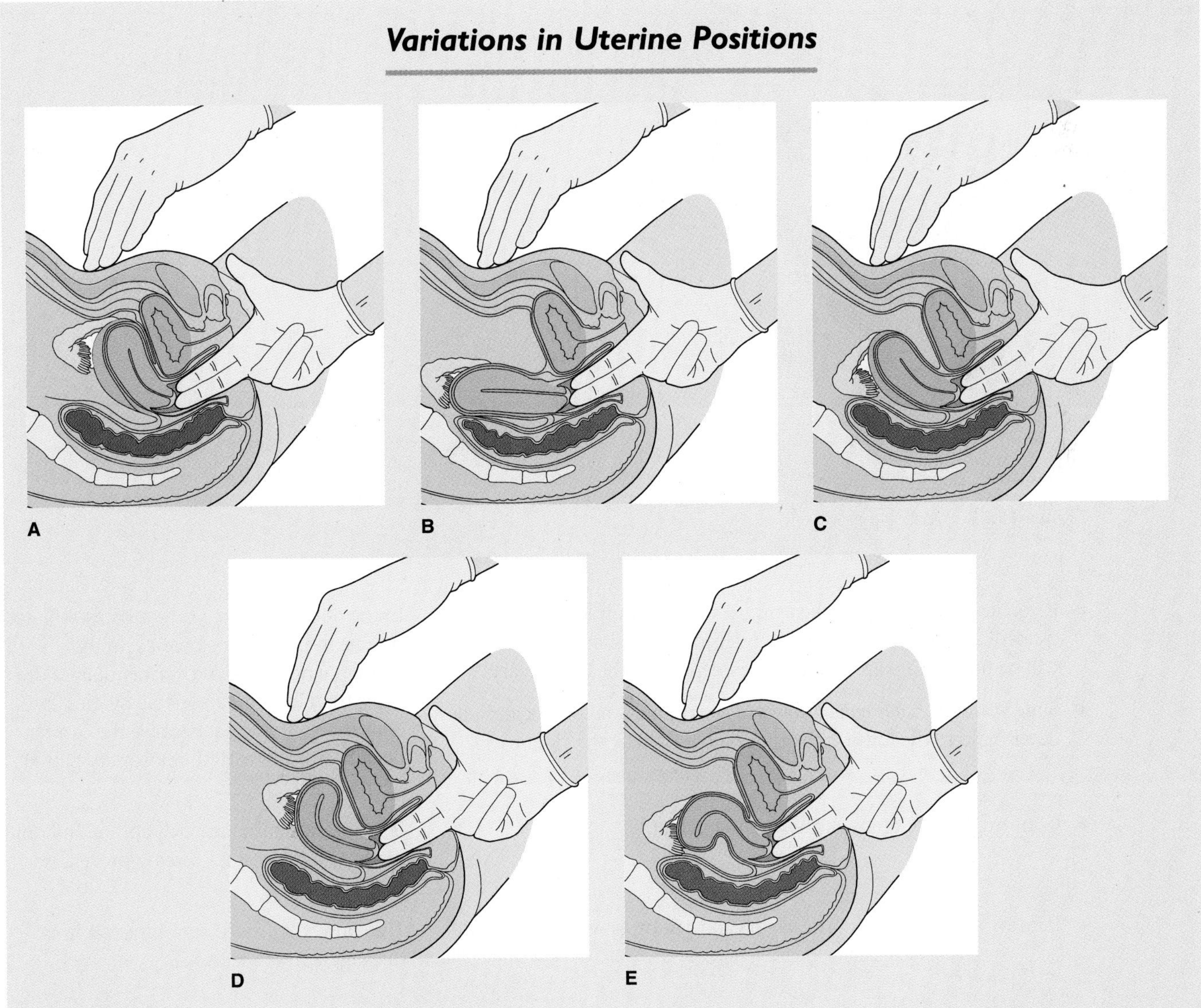

Figure 15.38 Variations in uterine position. *A*, Anteversion. *B*, Midposition. *C*, Retroversion. *D*, Anteflexion. *E*, Retroflexion.

ASSESSMENT TECHNIQUE/NORMAL FINDINGS	SPECIAL CONSIDERATIONS
◆ Move the inner fingers to the posterior fornix, and gently raise the cervix up toward your outer hand. ◆ Palpate the front and back walls of the uterus as it is sandwiched between the two hands.	Masses, tenderness, nodules, or bulging require further evaluation.
Step 4 *Palpate the ovaries.* ◆ While positioning the outer hand on the left lower abdominal quadrant, slip the vaginal fingers into the left lateral fornix. ◆ Push the opposing fingers and hand toward one another, then use small circular motions to palpate the left ovary with your intravaginal fingers (Figure 15.39).	Extreme tenderness, nodularity, and masses are suggestive of inflammation, infection, cysts, malignancies, or tubal pregnancy.

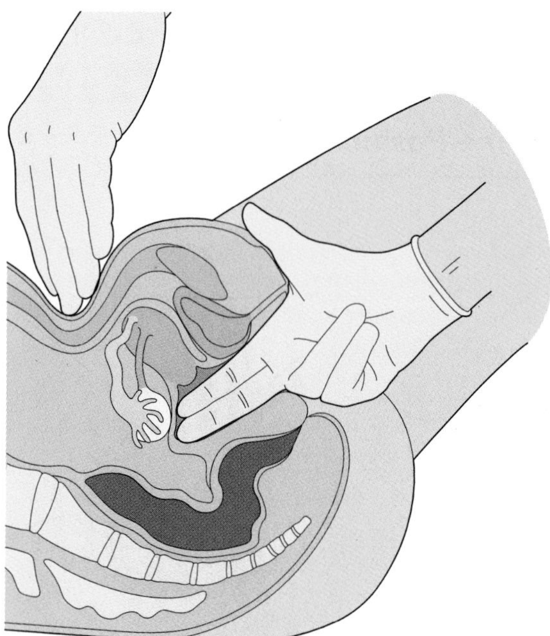

Figure 15.39 Palpating the ovaries.

◆ If you are able to palpate the ovary, it will feel mobile, almond-shaped, smooth, firm, and nontender to slightly tender. Often you will be unable to palpate the ovaries, especially the right ovary. ◆ Slide your vaginal fingers around to the right lateral fornix and your outer hand to the lower right quadrant to palpate the right ovary.	In the obese woman, you probably will not be able to palpate the ovaries. In the woman who has been postmenopausal for more than 2½ years, palpable ovaries are considered abnormal because the ovaries usually atrophy with the postmenopausal decrease in estrogen.
◆ Confirm that the uterine tubes are not palpable.	If the uterine tubes are palpable, an inflammation or some other disease process may be present.
◆ Remove your hand from the vagina and put on new gloves.	This prevents cross-contamination from the vagina to the rectum.

ASSESSMENT TECHNIQUE/NORMAL FINDINGS	SPECIAL CONSIDERATIONS

Step 5 ***Perform the rectovaginal exam.***

- Tell the client that you are going to insert one finger into her vagina and one finger into her rectum in order to perform a rectovaginal exam. Tell her that this maneuver may make her feel as though she needs to have a bowel movement.
- Lubricate the gloved index and middle fingers of the dominant hand.
- Ask the client to bear down.
- Touch the client's thigh with your nondominant hand to prepare her for the insertion.
- Insert the index finger into the vagina (at a 45-degree downard slope) and the middle finger into the rectum.
- Compress the rectovaginal septum between your index and middle fingers.
- Confirm that it is thin, smooth, and nontender.
- Place your nondominant hand on the client's abdomen.
- While maintaining the position of your intravaginal hand, press your outer hand inward and downward on the abdomen over the symphysis pubis.
- Palpate the posterior side of the uterus with the pad of the rectal finger while continuing to press down on the abdomen (Figure 15.40).

Note tenderness, masses, nodules, bulging, and thickened areas.

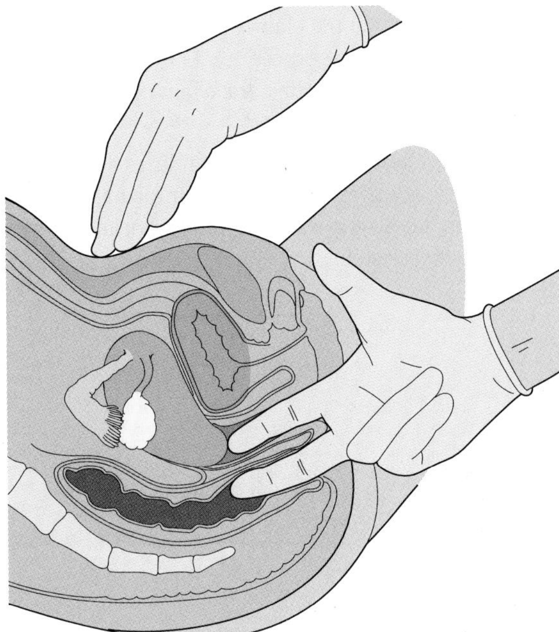

Figure 15.40 Rectovaginal palpation.

- Confirm that the uterine wall is smooth and nontender.

Tenderness, masses, nodules, bulging, or thickened areas require further evaluation.

ASSESSMENT TECHNIQUE/NORMAL FINDINGS	SPECIAL CONSIDERATIONS
◆ If the ovaries are palpable, note that they are normal in size and contour. ◆ Remove your fingers from the vagina and rectum slowly and gently. ◆ Remove your gloves. ◆ Assist the client into a comfortable position. ◆ Wash your hands. ◆ Give the client tissues to wipe the perineal area. Some clients may need a perineal pad. ◆ Inform the client that she may have a small amount of spotting for a few hours after the speculum examination.	

Reminders

- In addition to the above steps, consider the common variations in physical assessment findings for the different client groups discussed on pages 444–446.
- After completing the physical assessment, answer any questions the client may have, and provide appropriate client teaching for health promotion and self-care (see page 454).
- Confirm that the client is comfortable and has no adverse effects from the procedure. Dim the lights, remove the equipment, and leave the client in a comfortable position to rest or to get dressed.
- Document the assessment findings as described in Chapter 1. See pages 447–449 for information on identifying nursing diagnoses commonly associated with the reproductive system.

Table 15.2 Maturation Stages in the Female

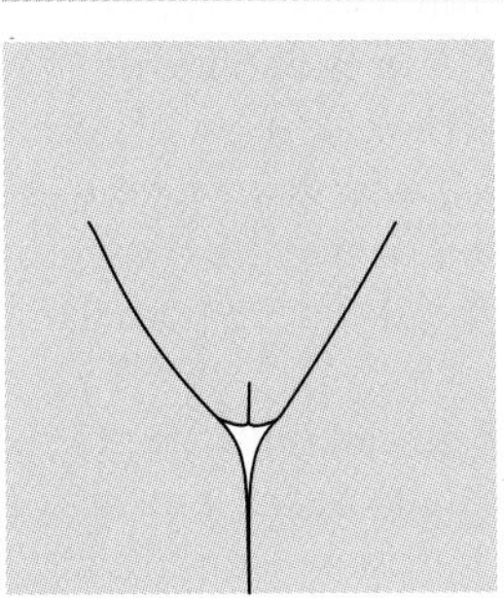

Stage 1.

No pubic hair.

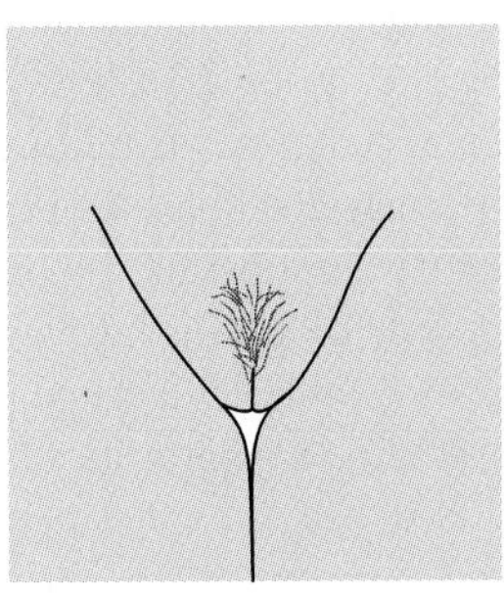

Stage 2.

Fine, sparse pubic hair on labia.

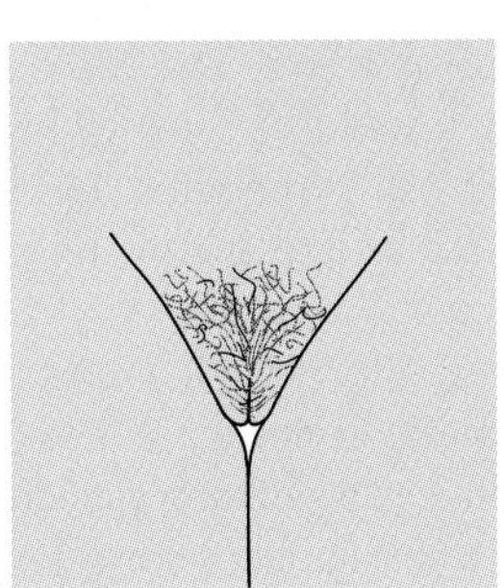

Stage 3.

Pubic hair fine and rising up pubis.

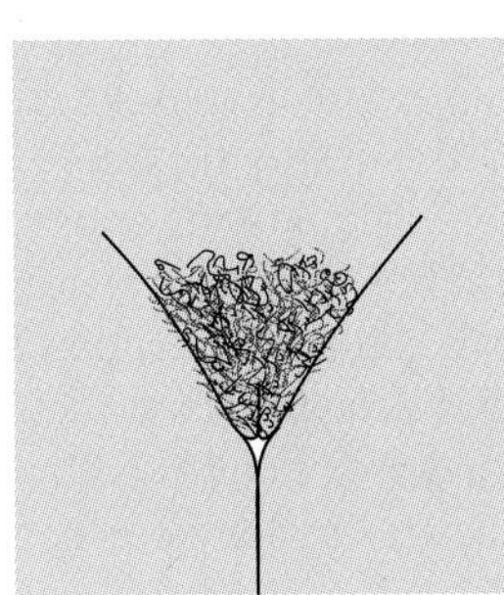

Stage 4.

Pubic hair thickening and beginning to cover pubis.

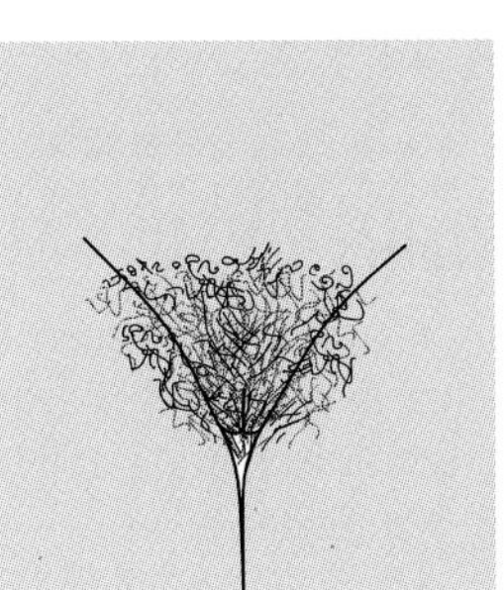

Stage 5.

Pubic hair coarse and thick, covering pubis and extending to thighs.

Developmental Considerations

Infants

The male newborn's genitals should be clearly evident and not ambiguous. If there is ambiguity, referral for genetic counseling is indicated. The penis may vary in size but averages about 2.5 cm in length and is slender. The urethral meatus should be in the center of the glans. If the opening is located on the underside of the glans, *hypospadias* is present. If the opening is on the superior aspect of the glans, *epispadias* exists. The foreskin may be somewhat tight for the first 2 or 3 months. If it is still tight after this time, *phimosis* exists. Cultural values and religious beliefs determine whether the family circumcises the child. The family requires teaching either about maintaining the cleanliness of the uncircumcised penis or caring for the penis in the days following a circumcision.

The male infant's scrotum should not be discolored. It should seem oversized in comparison with the penis. This proportion changes as the infant grows. If the scrotum is enlarged and filled with fluid, a *hydrocele* may be present. The testes should be palpable and are about 2 cm at birth. Undescended testes, called *cryptorchidism*, is a common finding, especially if the infant is preterm. The testes should descend spontaneously within the first year of life. If they do not descend, the male will be infertile and will be at a greater risk for the development of testicular cancer. Enlargement of the testes indicates the presence of a tumor. Testes smaller than 1.5 to 2.0 cm may indicate adrenal hyperplasia.

The female infant's genitals will be enlarged at birth in response to maternal estrogen. The labia majora should cover the labia minora. The urinary meatus and vaginal orifice should be visible. No inflammation or discharge should be present.

Children and Adolescents

The onset of puberty in the male child occurs between 10 to 15 years of age. At this time, under the influence of elevating levels of testosterone, the boy begins to develop adult sexual charactertistics. The testes and scrotum enlarge. Pubic, facial, and axillary hair develops. The penis begins to elongate, and the testes begin to produce mature sperm. The child will experience unexpected erections and nocturnal emissions ("wet dreams"). Open, supportive communication is essential at this time. You can show these children pictures of the sexual maturation of genitals to demonstrate that their development is normal. Table 15.1 on page 425 gives a scale for evaluating sexual maturity.

The child often displays a fascination with his genitals. Masturbation and exploration of the genitals are usual practices. Males may express curiosity in comparing their genitals with those of other children, both male and female.

Precocious puberty is an endocrine disorder characterized by an early onset of the development of adult male characteristics, including dense pubic hair, penile enlargement, and enlargement of the testes. It may be caused by a genetic trait, lesions in the pituitary gland or hypothalamus, or testicular tumors.

It is important to assess not only the physical development of the male child's sexual organs but also the presence of abnormalities such as infection, tumors, and hernias. Assessment is completed using the same methods as described for the adult male.

The female child reaches puberty a few years before the male. Changes begin to occur at any time from 8 to 13 years of age, most commonly at age 11. Release of estrogen initiates the changes, which are first demonstrated in the development of breast buds and growth of pubic hair, followed several years later by menstruation. Table 15.2 on page 443 describes growth of pubic hair according to maturational stage in girls.

The female child may also experience a precocious puberty. These children develop at an early age the adult female sex characteristics of dense pubic and axillary hair, breasts, and menstrual bleeding. The early development of sexual characteristics allows for pregnancy before the child is intellectually or emotionally prepared for the experience. Early maturation can also lead to anemia related to menstrual bleeding and to emotional difficulties.

It is essential to assess for sexual molestation with both female and male children. Some signs of sexual molestation are trauma, depression, eating disorders, bruising, swelling, and inflammation in the vaginal, perineal, and anal areas. Additionally, the child may appear withdrawn. Often the child will deny the experience.

Adolescents often express interest in the changes related to puberty in both sexes. The desire to explore sexual relationships and sexual contact, from kissing and fondling to intercourse, may be intense. Thus, adolescents need counseling on relationship issues, birth control, protection against sexually transmitted diseases, and delaying sexual activity. An adolescent may be concerned about or confused by an attraction to individuals of the same sex. Provide open communication so that the adolescent may express concerns.

For more information on assessing infants, children, and adolescents, see Chapter 19.

Childbearing Clients

Pregnancy brings a multitude of changes to the woman's reproductive organs. The uterus, cervix, ovaries, and vagina undergo significant structural changes related to the pregnancy and the influence of hormones.

The uterus becomes hypertrophied and weighs about 1 kg (2.2 lbs) by the end of pregnancy. Its capacity increases to about 5 liters. The growth of the uterus during pregnancy causes it to push up into the abdominal cavity and displace the liver and intestines from their normal positions. Contractions of the uterus occur. Throughout the pregnancy, the woman may have irregular *Braxton Hicks contractions,* which are usually not painful. However, by the end of the pregnancy, these contractions may become more intense and cause pain.

During pregnancy, the vascularity of the cervix increases and contributes to the softening of the cervix. This softening is called *Goodell's sign*. The vascular congestion creates a blue-purple blemish or change in cervical coloration. This change is considered normal and is referred to as *Chadwick's sign*. Estrogen causes the glandular cervical tissue to produce a thick mucus, which builds up and forms a mucous plug at the endocervical canal. The mucous plug prevents the introduction of any foreign matter into the uterus. At the initiation of labor, this plug is expelled. This expulsion is called the "bloody show."

During pregnancy, the vagina undergoes changes similar to those of the uterus. Hypertrophy of the vaginal epithelium occurs. The vaginal wall softens and relaxes to accommodate the movement of the infant during birth. The vagina also displays Chadwick's sign.

For more information on assessing the childbearing client, see Chapter 20.

Older Clients

The male client experiences the following changes to the external genitals: Pubic hair thins and grays, the prostate gland enlarges, the size of the penis and testes may diminish, the scrotum hangs lower, and the testes are softer to palpation. Sperm production decreases in middle age, but the male may remain able to contribute viable sperm and father children throughout the lifespan.

Sexual function and ability change as well. Testosterone production decreases, resulting in diminished libido. Sexual response is often slower and not as intense. The man may be slower to achieve erection, yet may be able to maintain the erection longer. Ejaculation can be less forceful and last for a shorter time; less semen may be ejaculated.

Reproductive ability in the woman usually peaks in the late 20s. Over time, estrogen levels begin to decline and, in response, around the age of 46–55, menstrual periods become shorter and less frequent until they stop entirely. *Menopause* is said to have occurred when the woman has not experienced a menstrual period in over a year. Other symptoms of menopause include mood changes and unpredictable episodes of sweating or hot flashes.

As the woman progresses into older age, her sexual organs atrophy. Vaginal secretions are not as plentiful, and the woman may experience pain during intercourse. Intercourse may produce vaginal infections. The clitoris becomes smaller.

Even though older adults can achieve sexual gratification and participate in a satisfying sexual relationship, a decrease in sexual drive may contribute to the client's withdrawing from sexual experiences and relationships. These factors are known to influence sexual drive:

- Chronic or acute diseases
- Certain medications
- Loss of spouse or significant other
- Loss of privacy
- Depression
- Fatigue
- Any stressful situation
- Use of alcohol or illicit drugs

For more information on assessing the older client, see Chapter 21.

Psychosocial Considerations

Fatigue, depression, and stress can decrease sexual desire in a client of any age. Grief over the loss of a relationship, whether because of separation, divorce, or death, can have long-term effects on a client's willingness to seek new relationships. Feelings of betrayal, for example when a partner becomes intimate with another person, can have the same effect.

Past or recent trauma, as from childhood abuse, physical assault, and sexual assault, whether or not penetration occurred, may have a significant impact on a client's ability to enjoy a sexual relationship. This may be true even if the trauma is unremembered.

A male's body image may be affected by his perception of his penis size in relation to that of other men. Some men fear that they are "too small" to satisfy a woman sexually. Caring and sensitive teaching is needed to help the client understand that variations in penis size are normal, and that there is little correlation between penis size and a partner's sexual satisfaction. Similarly, some women may fear sexual intimacy because of an altered body image related to their weight, body type, breast size, or other factors. Reproductive surgeries can affect a male or female client's self-image and sexual expression. For example, men and women who have had a surgical sterilization procedure may feel suddenly freed from the worry of unwanted pregnancy and experience an increase in sexual desire, or they may suddenly feel less masculine or feminine than before the surgery and withdraw from sexual relationships.

Self-Care Considerations

Maintaining the cleanliness of the genitals requires daily washing and changing of underclothes. For women, douching is not only unnecessary but may even be harmful. Douching has been shown to promote irritation, rashes, and infection in some women. Keeping the genitals dry, eg, by changing sweaty underclothes after physical exercise, changing into dry clothes immediately after bathing or swimming, and changing an infant's diaper immediately after it is wet, reduces the likelihood of rashes or infections.

Although research has shown that infections can be transmitted sexually even when the partners are using a latex condom, its use significantly lowers the incidence of transmission. A history of sexually transmitted diseases increases a female client's risk for cervical cancer. A history of sexually transmitted diseases in a child or adolescent may indicate sexual abuse.

Smoking increases the risk for cervical cancer, as does early (before age 18) and frequent sexual activity and a history of many sexual partners. Obesity is a risk factor for uterine cancer. Testicular cancer is the most common type of cancer in men between the ages of 20 and 35; thus, even adolescent males should perform a monthly testicular self-examination. Prostate cancer is the second leading cause of cancer-related deaths in men. An annual prostate exam after the age of 40 is essential. Prostate cancer is more common in males of African ancestry. The signs of the condition are not usually noticeable until the prostatic cancer is advanced. These signs are dribbling, retention of urine, difficulty initiating the urinary stream, and cystitis. Risk factors include a family history of prostatic cancer and smoking. (See Table 15.5 on page 453 for more information.)

Family, Cultural, and Environmental Considerations

Families living in overcrowded conditions may feel that their lack of privacy inhibits their ability to experience sexual gratification. Today, one or more grandparents or older relatives may live with their adult child, and sexual expression and gratification may be compromised for all of the adults in the family.

Sexual, physical, or verbal abuse among family members may cause significant sexual dysfunction. Some family members may be aware of the experience but be unwilling or unable to stop the perpetrators or help the victims.

Although sexual orientation is not determined by family wishes, negative family reactions to an individual's lifestyle choices can constrain a person's ability and willingness to find a sexual partner and maintain a satisfying sexual relationship. The family's influence may be so strong that individuals may choose partners acceptable to the family who do not meet their own needs or desires. This can have a negative emotional and physical impact on the individuals, especially among adolescents.

Some cultures and religions have specific beliefs or encourage specific behaviors related to menstruation, circumcision, and sexual practices. For example, many religions forbid premarital sex. When assessing clients, never assume that they share all of the beliefs or follow all the practices of their religious or cultural group.

People who work in the microelectronics industry may be exposed to arsenic, glycol ethers, lead, and radiation. These substances have been linked to birth defects and spontaneous abortions. Lead is also still present in some homes. Men who have been exposed to lead may experience decreased libido, diminished sperm count, and abnormal sperm morphology. Exposure to vinyl chloride may increase the risk for stillbirths, premature births, and chromosomal changes in the male germ cells. Exposure to high concentrations of halogenated hydrocardons (PCBs), found in plastics manufacturing and in the electrical industries, is associated with low birth weight, spontaneous abortion, hyperpigmentation of infants, and microcephaly (abnormally small head size). Oncology nurses exposed to antineoplastic drugs may have spontaneous abortions, fetal anomalies, changes in the regularity of their menstrual cycle, or even cessation of the menstrual cycle.

Organizing the Data

Use the information obtained from the interview and physical assessment to help you identify nursing diagnoses and develop an individualized plan of care to help the client reach a higher level of wellness. A wide variety of nursing diagnoses may be appropriate for the client with an alteration in reproductive health.

Identifying Nursing Diagnoses

NANDA lists a number nursing diagnoses that relate specifically to a client's sexuality, including three types of *Rape-trauma syndrome*, *Sexual dysfunction*, and *Altered sexuality patterns*. A number of other diagnoses may be appropriate for clients with actual or potential alterations in the health of the reproductive system, such as *High risk for infection, Altered growth and development, Body image disturbance, Knowledge deficit, Altered family processes, Fear,* and others.

Rape-trauma syndrome is an appropriate nursing diagnosis for an individual who has experienced a rape whether or not sexual penetration occurred. This syndrome describes the physical and psychologic responses of the victim immediately following the rape as well as the responses experienced and demonstrated over time (Table 15.3). *Rape-trauma syndrome: compound reaction* may be identified in an individual who has a history of psychiatric or medical conditions that become active again after the individual has been the victim of a rape or attempted rape. The physical and psychologic reactions to the rape experience are compounded by the symptoms of the

Table 15.3 Nursing Diagnoses Commonly Associated with the Reproductive System

RAPE-TRAUMA SYNDROME

Definition: The stress response pattern that occurs as a result of forcible or attempted forcible sexual penetration against the victim's will and consent. It includes an acute phase of disorganization of the victim's lifestyle and a long-term process of reorganization of lifestyle (adapted from NANDA).

RELATED FACTORS

Client's biopsychosocial response to event.

DEFINING CHARACTERISTICS

Acute Phase (several weeks)

Emotional reactions
- Anger
- Embarrassment
- Fear of physical violence and death
- Self-blame
- Fear of pregnancy, sexually transmitted diseases
- Humiliation
- Revenge
- Suicidal/homicidal behavior
- Psychotic states
- Confusion
- Memory disturbance
- Inability to make decisions

Multiple physical symptoms
- GI irritability (eg, stomach pains, appetite disturbance, nausea)
- GU disturbance (eg, vaginal discharge, itching, burning on urination, generalized pain)
- Muscle tension (eg, tension headaches and fatigue)
- Sleep pattern disturbance (eg, hyperalertness, edginess, nervousness)
- Physical trauma (eg, general soreness, bruises, lesions, trauma to mouth and rectum)

Reorganization Phase

Lifestyle changes
- Changing residences
- Taking trips
- Seeking out family, friends for support
- Initiating period of celibacy

Emotional reactions
- Suicidal/homicidal behavior
- Psychotic states
- Promiscuity
- Use of alcohol/drugs
- Body image disturbance

Recurrent dreams and nightmares
- Reliving rape and victimization
- Symbolic dreams related to the rape
- Mastery dreams (indicate recovering)

Fears and phobias
- Fear of environment (location of rape/attempted rape)
- Fear of being alone
- Fear of crowds
- Sexual fears
- Fear of initiating/continuing relationships that may lead to intimacy

Table 15.3 Nursing Diagnoses Commonly Associated with the Reproductive System (continued)

SEXUAL DYSFUNCTION

Definition: The state in which an individual experiences a change in sexual function that is viewed as unsatisfying, unrewarding, or inadequate (NANDA).

RELATED FACTORS

Drugs, Surgery, Pain, Disease, Health-related transitions, Altered body function or structure, Illness/medical treatment, Trauma, Lack of significant other, Lack of privacy, Pregnancy, Recent childbirth, Physical/emotional abuse, Sexual trauma/exploitation, Hormonal changes, Body image disturbance, Impaired relationship, Unrealistic expectations of self and partner, Disturbance in self-esteem, Others specific to patient (specify).

DEFINING CHARACTERISTICS

Verbalization of problem	Alteration in orgasm/ejaculation
Conflicts involving values	Impotence
Seeking confirmation of desirability	Vaginal dryness
Decreased interest in others	Painful coitus
Concern over adequacy in meeting sexual desire of partner	Change in sexual desire
	Phobic avoidance of sexual experience

ALTERED SEXUALITY PATTERNS

Definition: The state in which an individual expresses concern regarding his or her sexuality patterns (adapted from NANDA).

RELATED FACTORS

Knowledge/skill deficit, Lack of privacy, Lack of significant other, Ineffective or absent role models, Conflicts with sexual orientation or variant preferences, Fear of pregnancy or acquiring sexually transmitted disease, Impaired relationship with significant other, Body image disturbance, Disturbance in self-esteem, Others specific to patient (specify).

DEFINING CHARACTERISTICS

Reported difficulties, limitations, or changes in sexual behaviors or activities

previous psychiatric or medical conditions. When an individual experiences rape or attempted rape and does not report the assault, the nursing diagnosis of *Rape-trauma syndrome: silent reaction* is appropriate.

Sexual dysfunction is applicable for clients who perceive their sexual ability, function, or satisfaction as insufficient, unsuitable, or unfulfilling. A variety of precipitating factors may be related to sexual dysfunction, including medications, illness, changes related to aging, and psychologic factors such as loss of self-esteem. See Table 15.3.

In individuals who express distress and anxiety related to their pattern of sexual activity, the nursing diagnosis of *Altered sexuality patterns* may be appropriate. Some cues that indicate the appropriateness of this diagnosis are concerns or conflict over sexual orientation, lack of a significant other, and fear of acquiring a sexually transmitted disease (see Table 15.3).

DIAGNOSTIC REASONING IN ACTION

Jennifer Hernandez arrives at the Women's Health Center. She is a petite, 29-year-old financial analyst for an investment firm. Her husband, Carlos, has accompanied her. He tells the nurse, Claudine Baker, RN, that his wife has not been herself lately. "Her moods keep changing. She will snap at me one minute, cry the next, then get very quiet and not talk to anyone at all. She doesn't let me touch her anymore. It has been weeks since we've been intimate." He also states that Jennifer seems afraid to leave the house, and her career is suffering.

Jennifer follows Ms Baker to the examination room in silence. She sits down, gazes at the floor, and is reluctant to make eye contact. When Ms Baker asks her what she is feeling, she says that she is confused. "I can't understand what's going on with me. I keep trying to get on with my life, but I don't seem to be able to. I can't even sleep without nightmares." Ms Baker continues to ask Jennifer open-ended questions, and after several minutes, Jennifer bursts into tears. Ms Baker holds her hand as Jennifer cries. Eventually, she begins to speak. "Two months ago, I was working late. When I walked out to my car, a man approached me and demanded my purse. I gave it to him. But that wasn't enough. He grabbed my car keys out of my hand, threw me in my car, and raped me. I tried to scream, but nothing came out of my mouth. I'm so humiliated. I feel so dirty. No matter how many times I bathe, I can't get rid of the dirty feeling. I don't have the courage to report it to the police. What if I had to testify? Everyone would find out, including my husband. I couldn't bear it if he knew. But I can't bear to be intimate with him. The thought of having sex makes me sick. I just can't go on any more. I want to die."

Ms Baker clusters the data from this preliminary interview and develops the following nursing diagnoses:

1. *Rape-trauma syndrome* related to the actual sexual assault
2. *Body image disturbance* related to perception that she is "dirty"
3. *Ineffective individual coping* related to the rape and demonstrated by the withdrawing of the client from her husband, social interactions, and job
4. *Hopelessness* related to the rape and demonstrated by the verbalization that she can't see any resolution to her situation and wants to die
5. *Social isolation* characterized by the withdrawal from social interactions with husband, friends, and co-workers

Ms Baker recommends that Jennifer remain at the clinic for a complete physical examination. She explains that Jennifer should be tested immediately for sexually transmitted diseases. Jennifer agrees, and Ms Baker schedules an appointment for that morning. She also asks Jennifer if she has any reason to suspect that she is pregnant. Jennifer replies that she uses birth control pills and has had her period since the attack. Finally, Ms Baker asks Jennifer if she would like to talk with one of the center's counselors, and an appointment is made for the early afternoon.

Common Alterations in the Health of the Reproductive System

Common alterations of the reproductive system include sexually acquired diseases, cancer, and hernias. These conditions are described in Tables 15.4, 15.5, and 15.6.

Table 15.4 Sexually Transmitted Diseases

Disease	Characteristics	Signs and Symptoms	Treatment
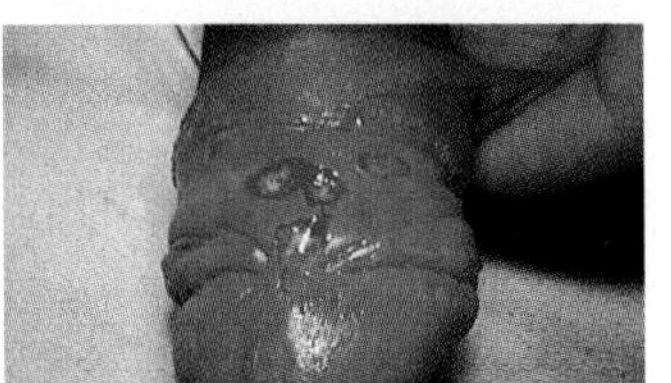 Chancroid	◆ Incubation period of 3–5 days. ◆ More common in males, especially if uncircumcised.	◆ Painful. ◆ May ulcerate. ◆ Shape is irregular, gray color, up to 1 inch in size. ◆ May appear on genitals, thigh, oral area, breasts. ◆ May have associated pus.	◆ Antibiotics such as erythromycin. ◆ Aspiration of lesions filled with fluid. ◆ Client teaching: Complete antibiotic therapy. Cleanliness. Advise against sexual contact for 2 weeks after initiation of therapy. Inform partners and advise treatment. ◆ Prevention: Cleanliness. Use of condom. Avoid sex with anyone infected.
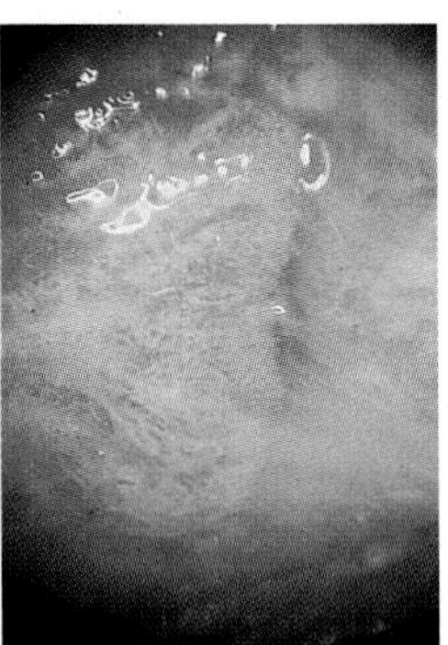 Chlamydia	◆ Can lead to sterility and/or spontaneous abortions. ◆ One of the most common sexually transmitted diseases.	◆ Symptoms can vary among individuals. ◆ Primary lesion is painless. ◆ May appear as a vesicle or ulcer. ◆ Size averages 2–3 mm. ◆ Can lead to swollen lymphatic nodes in the inguinal area. ◆ Men may develop inguinal masses, scrotal swelling, diarrhea, bloody, mucosal discharge from rectum, lower back pain, painful ejaculations. ◆ Women may develop cervical erosion, signs of pelvic inflammatory disease, breakthrough bleeding, bleeding during or after sexual intercourse.	◆ Antibiotics such as doxycycline, erythromycin, or tetracycline. ◆ Client teaching: Complete antibiotic therapy. Cleanliness. Advise against sexual contact until cultures are negative. Inform partners and advise treatment. ◆ Prevention: Cleanliness. Use of condom. Avoid sex with anyone infected.
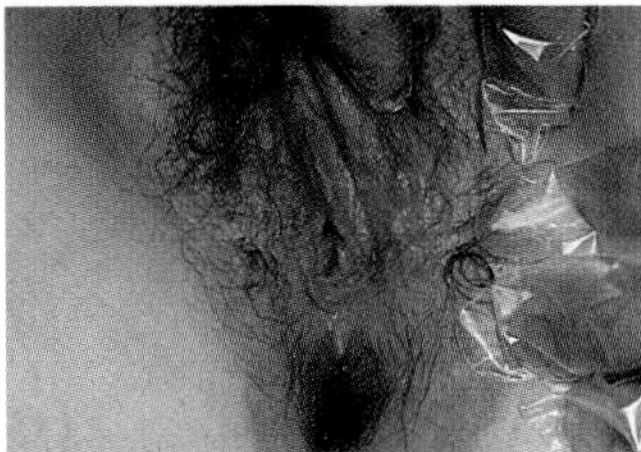 Genital herpes	◆ Is spread by physical contact including sexual intercourse, kissing, and oral-genital contact. ◆ Incubation of 3–7 days. ◆ May become dormant with recurring infections.	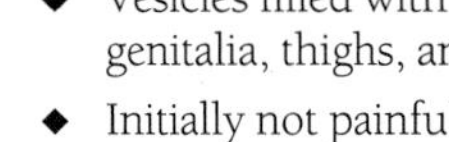 ◆ Vesicles filled with fluid on or near genitalia, thighs, and possibly mouth. ◆ Initially not painful but may elicit a tingly sensation and become painful. ◆ May see redness, edema, ulcerations, and yellow pus from center of lesion. ◆ Associated signs of fever, fatigue.	◆ Treated with Acyclovir ointment or oral acyclovir. ◆ Client teaching: Proper use of medication. Cleanliness. Advise against sexual contact until cultures are negative. Pap smear every 6 months. Inform partners and advise treatment. ◆ Prevention: Cleanliness. Use of condom. Avoid sex with anyone infected.
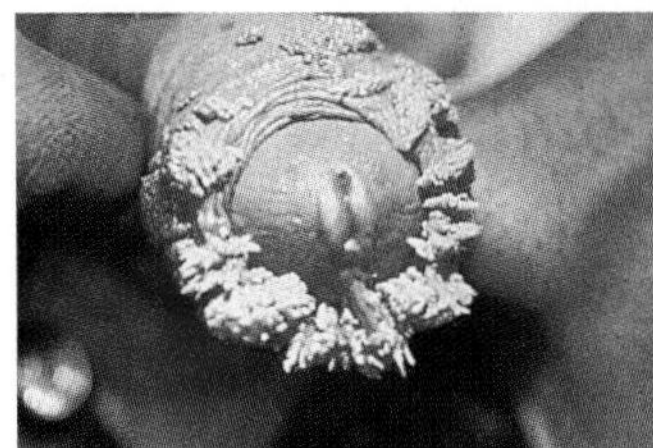 Genital warts	◆ Rapidly growing lesion. ◆ Least prevalent before puberty. ◆ Incubation period 1–6 months with an average of 2 months.	◆ Occur on or around genitals. ◆ Appearance is wartlike, pink to red in coloration, rapidly growing, may look like a cauliflower.	◆ Medications such as trichloroacetic acid, podophyllum in nonpregnant women. ◆ Larger lesions removed by electrical excision, carbon dioxide, laser. ◆ Client teaching: Cleanliness. Inform partners and advise treatment. ◆ Prevention: Cleanliness. Use of condom. Avoid sex with anyone infected.

Table 15.4 Sexually Transmitted Diseases (continued)

Disease	Characteristics	Signs and Symptoms	Treatment
Gonorrhea	◆ Common STD. ◆ Higher incidence in individuals with multiple sexual partners. ◆ Incubation period 3–6 days.	◆ Redness and swelling at infection site. ◆ Females may develop a green to yellow discharge in the cervical area. ◆ Males may have signs of urethritis. ◆ Signs of polyarthritis. ◆ Abdominal pain. ◆ Painful lesions which may be present on extremities.	◆ Antibiotics such as ceftriaxone, doxycycline, and erythromycin, possibly IV penicillin G. ◆ Client teaching: Complete antibiotic therapy. Cleanliness. Advise against sexual contact until cultures are negative. Inform partners and advise treatment. ◆ Prevention: Cleanliness. Use of condom. Avoid sex with anyone infected.
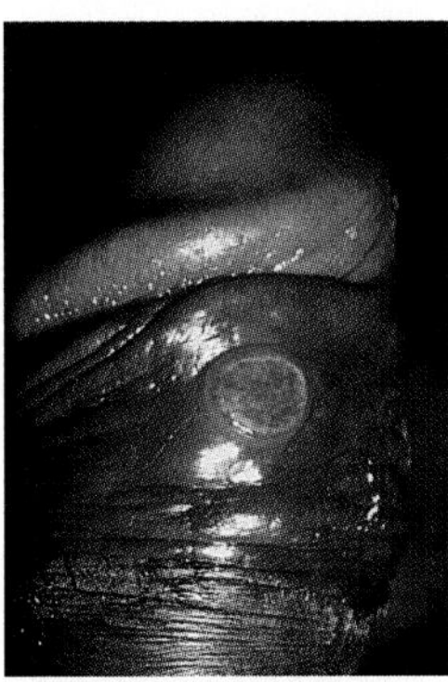 Syphilis	◆ Caused by *Treponema pallidum,* a spirochete. ◆ Incubation period about 3 weeks. ◆ Associated with 3 stages. ◆ If not treated, can lead to death.	◆ Primary period: Lesions are small, painless, silver. May be filled with fluid. Located on genitals, thighs, oral area, nipples, eyelids. You may see regional lymphadenopathy. ◆ Secondary period: Symptoms occur within days up to several months after initial symptoms. Rash and/or pink to gray lesions may appear on the genitals, trunk, head, or extremities. Associated with fever, fatigue, and weight loss. ◆ Tertiary period: Lesions may develop from 1 year to a decade after initial infection. These lesions affect the cardiac, respiratory, skeletal, and nervous systems.	◆ Penicillin is the primary initial treatment. Tetracycline in nonpregnant women, or erythromycin may be used instead. ◆ Client teaching: Complete antibiotic therapy. Cleanliness. Advise against sexual contact until cultures are negative. Inform partners and advise treatment. ◆ Prevention: Cleanliness. Use of condom. Avoid sex with anyone infected.
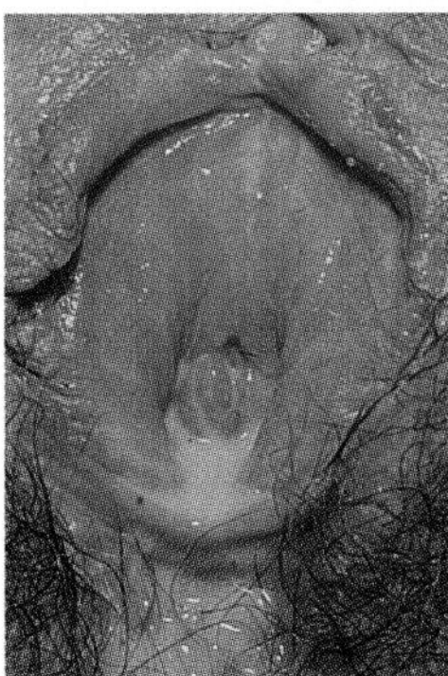 Trichomoniasis	◆ Caused by *Trichomonas vaginalis,* a protozoan.	◆ May be asymptomatic. ◆ Vaginal discharge that is green or gray and frothy. ◆ May cause itching, urinary frequency, swelling.	◆ Medication such as metronidazole. ◆ Client teaching: Recommended that partner take medication as well. Avoid alcohol during treatment with metronidazole. Do not use douches. Cleanliness. ◆ Prevention: Cleanliness. Use of condom. Avoid sex with anyone infected.

Table 15.5 Abnormal Cell Growth in Reproductive Organs

Disease	Characteristics	Signs and Symptoms	Treatment
Female			
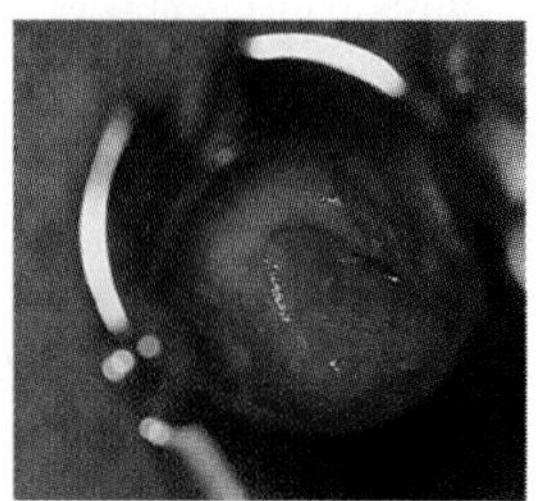 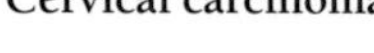 Cervical carcinoma	◆ Incidence is higher in women who have a history of multiple sexual partners, exposure to sexually transmitted disease, intercourse at an early age, or smoking.	◆ Asymptomatic in early stage. ◆ With invasive process, unexpected vaginal bleeding, vaginal discharge beyond normal characteristics, and ulceration. ◆ Later, pain in pelvic area, discharge of urine and/or feces from vagina.	◆ Biopsy, surgery, and/or laser treatment in early stages. ◆ Hysterectomy and radiation in late stages.
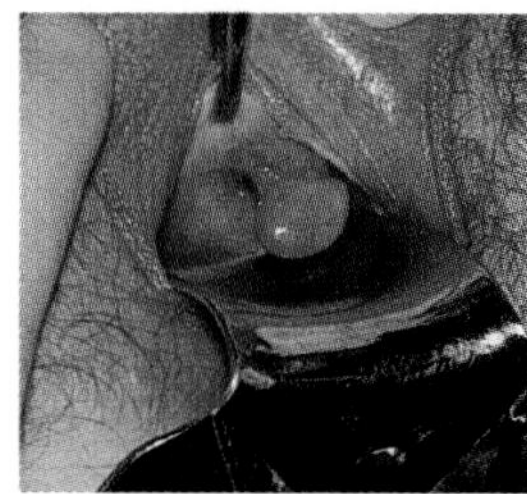 Cervical polyps	◆ Majority originate in the endocervix.	◆ Vaginal discharge beyond normal is a key indicator. ◆ May be accompanied by bleeding.	◆ Surgery or cautery may be indicated.
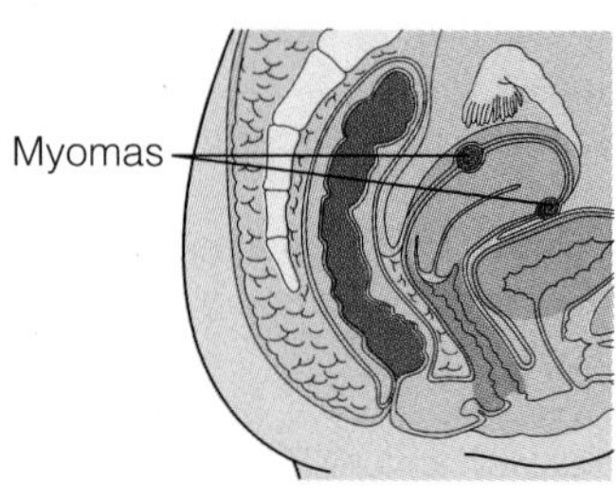 Myomas/ fibroids	◆ May be influenced by estrogen.	◆ May be asymptomatic. ◆ May cause excessive bleeding during menses. ◆ Uterus may become enlarged. ◆ May cause abdominal distention, pain, intestinal obstruction, frequent urination, and constipation.	◆ Depends upon symptoms, and whether the woman is currently pregnant or wishes to become pregnant. ◆ Surgery.
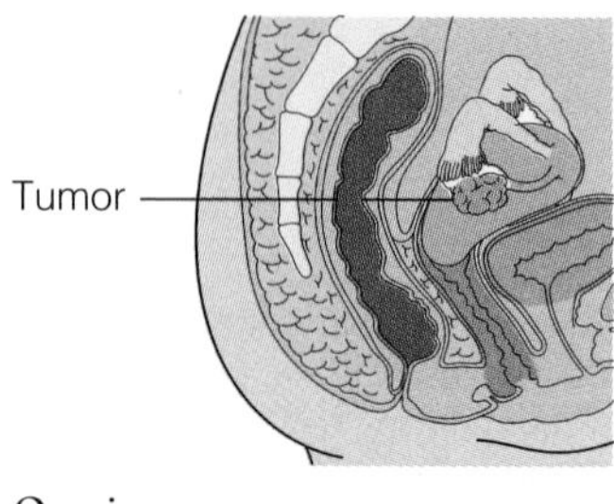 Ovarian cancer	◆ Incidence higher in women of upper socioeconomic status, history of infertility, history of breast or uterine cancer.	◆ In early stages, may be asymptomatic. Some individuals experience gastrointestinal disturbances. ◆ Progression of tumor may lead to urinary frequency, constipation, pain.	◆ Depends upon the stage, but may include surgery, chemotherapy, radiation therapy.
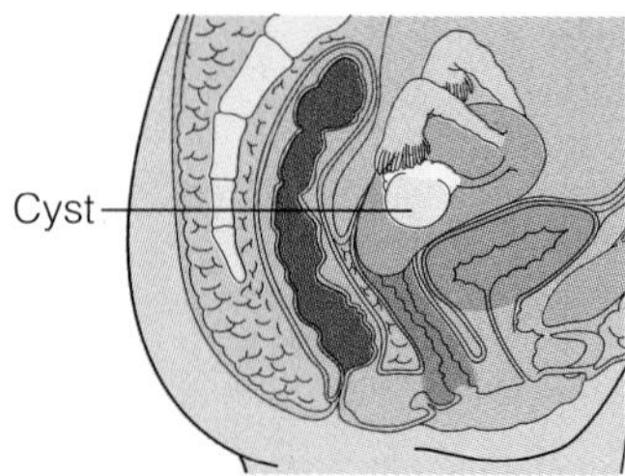 Ovarian cysts	◆ Nonmalignant cysts that may develop during puberty through menopause.	◆ Can be asymptomatic. ◆ Some individuals experience pelvic pain, abdominal distention, lower back pain.	◆ May be spontaneously resorbed within several months. ◆ Medications may include clomiphene citrate, progesterone, or hydrocortisone. ◆ Surgery may be indicated.

Table 15.5 Abnormal Cell Growth in Reproductive Organs (continued)

Disease	Characteristics	Signs and Symptoms	Treatment
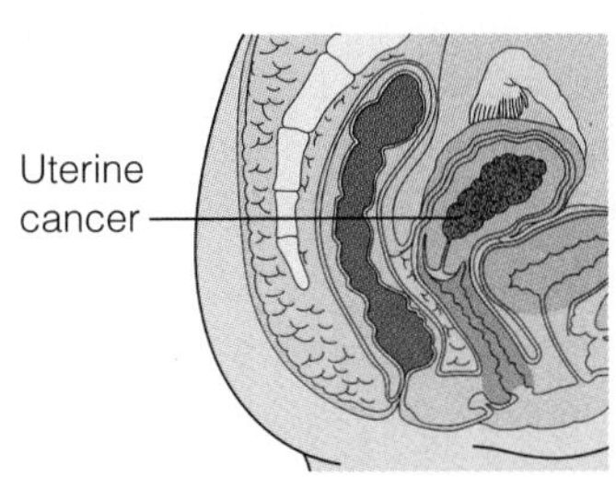 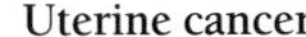 Uterine cancer	◆ May have a genetic predisposition. ◆ Most common type of female reproductive cancer. ◆ May be associated with hypertension, uterine polyps, estrogen therapy, infertility.	◆ Abnormal menstrual bleeding, bleeding recurring during menopause. ◆ Uterine enlargement.	◆ Surgery, radiation therapy, and/or hormonal therapy.
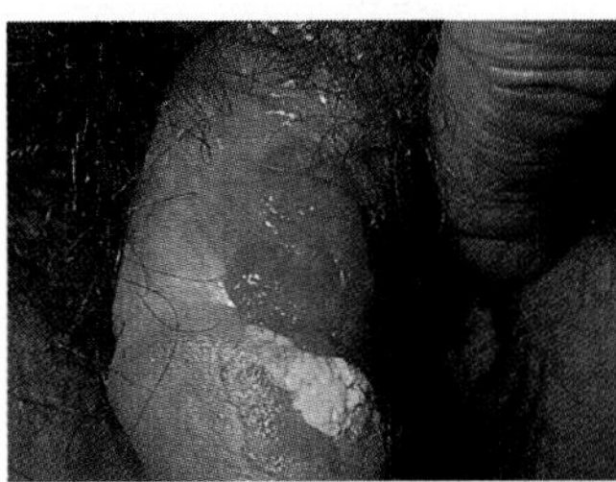 Penile carcinoma	◆ Higher incidence in uncircumcised males.	◆ Appears as a sore or lesion on the penis. ◆ Initially painless. ◆ Can progress to painful condition. ◆ Discharge may be watery, purulent, or possibly bloody.	◆ Depends on stage, but may include surgery, radiation, chemotherapy.
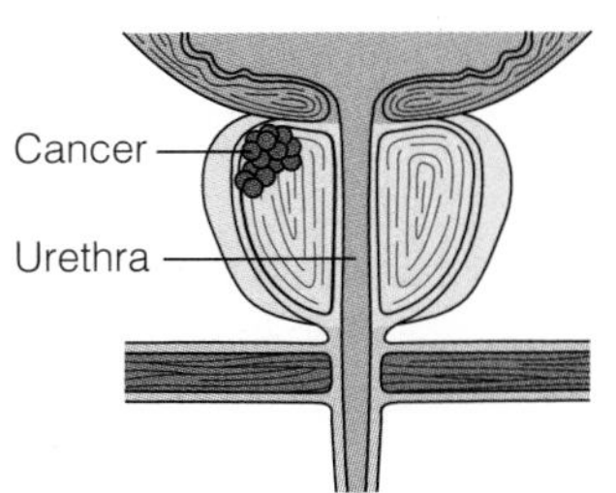 Prostate cancer	◆ Second leading cause of cancer-related death in men.	◆ Asymptomatic in early stages. ◆ Urinary retention, dribbling, difficulty in initiating flow.	◆ Variety of therapies, including surgery, radiation, hormone therapy.
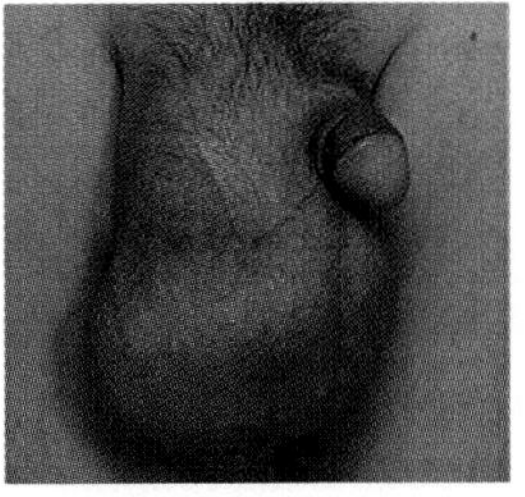 Testicular cancer	◆ Higher incidence in men with cryptorchidism, and in men whose mothers took DES during pregnancy.	◆ Initial stage is asymptomatic. ◆ A painless mass is often found on palpation. ◆ Later stages: pain, uretheral obstruction, weight loss.	◆ Surgery, radiation, chemotherapy.

Table 15.6 Inguinal Hernias

Type of Hernia	Characteristics	Signs and Symptoms
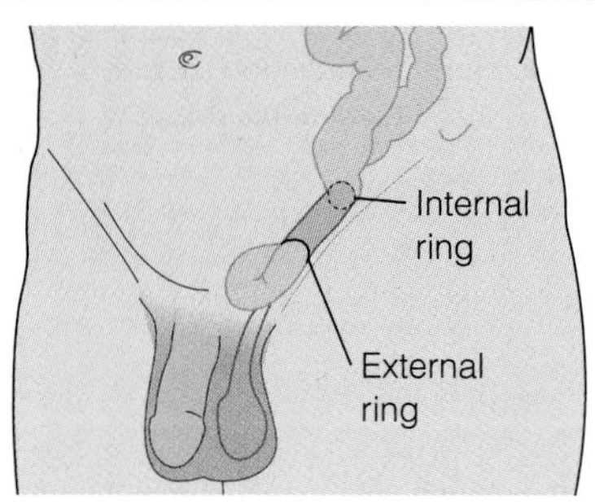 Direct hernia	◆ Extrusion of abdominal intestine into inguinal ring. ◆ Bulging occurs in the area around the pubis. ◆ Occurs much more commonly in men.	◆ Most often is painless. ◆ Appears as a swelling. ◆ During palpation, have the client cough. You will feel pressure against the side of your finger.
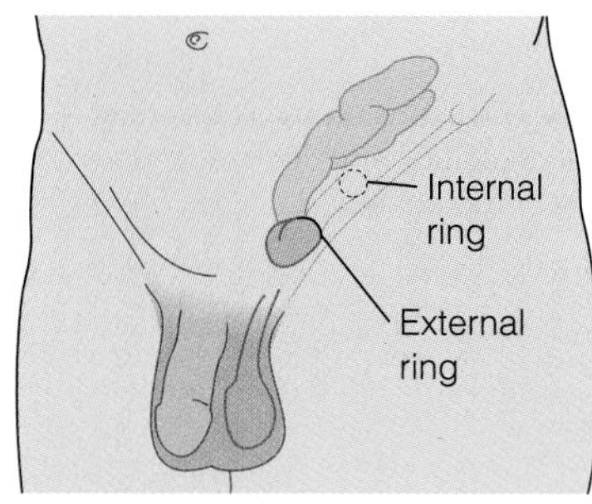 Indirect hernia	◆ Abdominal intestine may remain within the inguinal canal or extrude past the external ring. ◆ Most common type of hernia.	◆ Appears as a swelling. ◆ During palpation, have the client cough. You will feel pressure against your finger-tip.
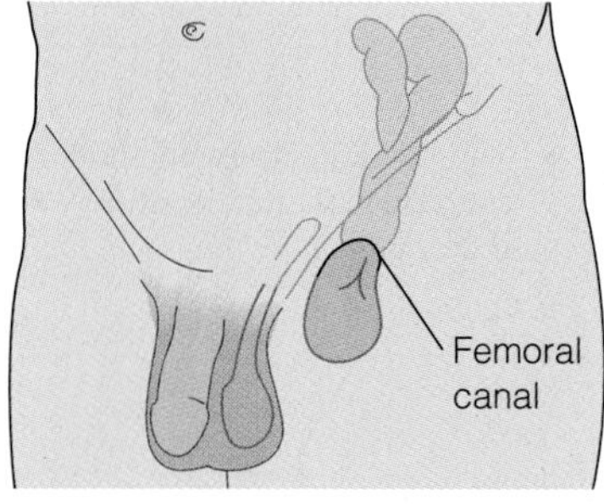 Femoral hernia	◆ Located within the femoral canal. ◆ Bulge occurs over the area of the femoral artery. The right femoral artery is affected more frequently than the left. ◆ Lowest incidence of all three hernias.	◆ Palpable soft mass. ◆ May not be painful; however, once strangulation occurs, pain is severe.

Health Promotion and Client Education

Promoting the General Health of the Reproductive System

To promote the general health of the female and male reproductive system, advise clients to

- Maintain cleanliness and prevent infections by daily washing, keeping the genitals dry, and changing underclothing daily.
- Seek counseling and support on issues of sexual function, bleeding problems in women, sexual satisfaction, and sexual orientation.
- Seek health care for:

  Abnormal colored discharge from genitals

  Foul smelling discharge from genitals

  Intense itching of genitals

  Genital rashes, warts, lesions, swelling, or discoloration

  Any masses, lesions, or lumps in the genitals or abdominal area

  Any pain or tenderness in the genital or abdominal area

Changes in libido, ability to achieve or maintain an erection, painful erection, inability to ejaculate, painful intercourse, and persistent inability to achieve orgasm

Promoting Healthy Menstruation

Advise the client to observe the pattern and characteristics of the menstrual cycle and report any significant changes such as increased pain, bleeding, clotting, skipped periods, and breakthrough bleeding.

Menstrual cramps are often caused by the release of prostaglandins. Treatment options include aspirin, ibuprofen, naproxen (Naprosyn), application of heat such as warm baths or showers, heating pads, and warm drinks such as herbal teas. Some medications and the use of heat may increase the flow of blood.

Tampons and pads should be changed frequently to ensure cleanliness, prevent leakage, and reduce the chances of developing infections. Some of the chemicals used in tampons and pads to prevent odor can cause contact dermatitis or harm the vaginal mucosal lining. Superabsorbent tampons may absorb not only the menstrual flow but also other fluid, thus contributing to vaginal dryness. Also, because the use of superabsorbent tampons has been associated with toxic shock syndrome, a potentially fatal infection, they should be used only during heaviest flow. The symptoms of toxic shock syndrome include temperature of 101F or greater, diarrhea, vomiting, muscle aches, and a rash that looks like a sunburn. The client should understand that these are serious findings and warrant *immediate* attention.

Although the cause of premenstrual syndrome (PMS) is still unknown, self-help treatment options include regular exercise, vitamin supplementation, and reduction of salt in the diet. Medical treatments include diuretics, prostaglandin inhibitors, and administration of alprazolam (Xanax). These should be prescribed and monitored under a physician's care.

Vaginal sprays and douches may be harmful. They have been known to contribute to vaginal irritation, itching, and rashes as well as infections. Daily bathing and cleaning of genital areas, changing underclothing daily, and keeping the genital area dry are sufficient to maintain cleanliness.

Preventing Sexually Transmitted Diseases

To prevent sexually transmitted diseases (STDs), advise the client that the risk of contracting an STD increases with the number of sexual partners. Intercourse exposes the client to all of the other people with whom the partner has had sex for the past 5 years or more. Other than abstinence, the condom is the best contraceptive method currently available for protection from STDs. However, other methods, such as the diaphragm, cervical cap, sponge, and spermicides alone offer some protection. Absence of symptoms does not mean absence of infection. If infection is suspected, the client should be evaluated. Table 15.4 on page 450 describes various sexually transmitted diseases.

Preventing Cancers of the Reproductive System

Factors related to prevention and detection of cancers of the reproductive tract should be discussed with the client. Uterine, cervical, and ovarian cancers threaten the lives of many women, and although testicular cancer is rare, it is the most common cancer in men between the ages of 20 and 35. Prostatic cancer is the second leading cause of cancer-related death in men. The risk factors for developing these cancers are

Cervical cancer

- Multiple sex partners
- Early and frequent sexual activity
- Sexually transmitted diseases
- Smoking

Uterine cancer

- Menstruation before age 12
- No children or infertility
- Hypertension
- Diabetes mellitus
- Obesity
- Menopause that begins after age 50
- Long-term estrogen replacement therapy without progestin

Ovarian cancer

- Family history of ovarian, breast, or uterine cancer
- No children, infertility, or first pregnancy after 30 years of age
- Repeated problems with failure to ovulate regularly

Testicular cancer

The risk profile is not clear but may include

- Cryptorchidism
- Peak age 20–40

Prostatic cancer

- Possibly smoking
- Family history of prostatic cancer

DIAGNOSTIC REASONING IN ACTION

Charlie Drake is a 16-year-old male who excels scholastically, is popular with his peers, and is a star athlete in his high school's varsity baseball and football programs. He comes into the school's health clinic and asks the nurse, Tammy Hassemi, RN, if he can ask her some questions privately. He initally seems embarrassed and somewhat reluctant to talk, but gathers his courage. "My girlfriend and I have decided to have sex, but she insists that I wear a condom. I don't want to use condoms. I've heard that they aren't foolproof and that the sex isn't as good." He continues, "I don't think we have to worry about my girlfriend getting pregnant anyway because we wouldn't be having sex all the time—probably just on Saturday nights when we can stay out late. My parents tried for 2 years before my mom got pregnant with me!"

Ms Hassemi asks Charlie some questions about his reproductive health; sexual function, satisfaction, and practices; and his self-care. She explores with Charlie his knowledge of sexually transmitted diseases, contraceptives, and his understanding of reproductive physiology.

After the focused interview, Ms Hassemi identifies the nursing diagnosis *Knowledge deficit* as appropriate for Charlie. She then collects some additional information. She examines why Charlie and his partner have decided to start to have sex at this time in their relationship. Are they experiencing any social pressure from their peers? She asks Charlie to describe what he has heard about condoms decreasing sexual pleasure. She also examines what Charlie knows about the use of condoms: how to acquire them, what types are available, how and when to apply them, and how often a new one should be used. She explores with Charlie whether abstinence is a feasible option for his relationship with his partner. She also explains to Charlie that alcohol and drugs may lead to impaired decisions and increase his likelihood of engaging in unprotected sex. Finally, she discusses with Charlie the importance of protecting himself and his partner from sexually transmitted diseases. She gives Charlie brochures describing contraceptive options and methods for preventing sexually transmitted diseases, and suggests Charlie and his girlfriend visit the local Planned Parenthood clinic.

All women should know the warning signals of uterine and cervical cancer. Instruct the client to see her physician if she exhibits any of these symptoms:

- Unusual vaginal discharge
- Bleeding outside of the normal menstrual period
- Bleeding after menopause

Annual pelvic exams with a general physical examination are recommended as a screening tool for sexually active women (now or in the past) who have reached 18 years of age. The Pap smear is very effective in detecting cervical cancer, and partially effective as a screening tool for endometrial cancer. To date, no effective screening tool has been discovered for ovarian cancer, which is sometimes called a "silent disease" because it frequently progresses to an advanced stage before it is diagnosed.

Testicular cancer has no early warning signs. Thus, males should perform a testicular self-exam monthly, beginning in adolescence. Describe to the client how to perform the exam:

- The best time to perform the exam is in the shower or bath, since the heat and steam will warm your hands and the water will help your hands to glide over the skin surface. If your hands are cold, a reflex response will occur, causing your testicles to move up against your body. They will then be more difficult for you to feel.
- Feel each testicle by applying gentle pressure with your thumb, index, and middle fingers. If your testicle hurts while you feel it, you are pressing too hard.
- The contour of the testicle should be smooth, rounded, and firm.
- You will feel the epididymis on top of and behind each testicle.
- You should not feel any distinct lumps or areas of hardness, nor should your testicle be enlarged. If any of these signs are present, make an appointment with your physician immediately.

Table 15.5 on page 452 describes various types of abnormal cell growths in the reproductive system.

Summary

Assessment of the reproductive system requires an understanding of normal anatomy and physiology for various age groups, good interviewing and communication skills, skill in inspecting and palpating, and the use of special equipment such as the vaginal speculum. You must keep thorough and accurate documentation to facilitate communication with other caregivers and to follow trends in relation to the client's state of health. The physical assessment of the reproductive system requires you to use tremendous sensitivity in responding to the client's need for privacy and respect of personal boundaries. As with the assessment of other body systems, you use diagnostic reasoning to develop nursing diagnoses and to identify collaborative problems based on your assessment data. Teaching is a primary tool in promoting reproductive health.

Key Points

- ✓ Assessing the male reproductive system requires a sound knowledge of the anatomy and physiology of the male reproductive organs, including the scrotum, testes, spermatic cord, the duct system, accessory glands, and penis.
- ✓ Assessing the female reproductive system requires a sound knowledge of the anatomy and physiology of the female reproductive organs, including the mons pubis, labia majora and minora, Skene's glands, Bartholin's glands, clitoris, ovaries, vagina, uterus, and uterine tubes.
- ✓ During the focused interview, perform a general survey of reproductive health, sexual function, pregnancy, fertility, sexual satisfaction, sexual practices, and self-care.
- ✓ During the physical assessment, inspect the genitals of both males and females for variations such as discoloration, inflammation, lesions, vesicles, warts, signs of trauma, rashes, swelling, masses, asymmetry, and discharge.
- ✓ Palpate the male and female genitals to assess for nodules, areas of hardness, lumps, masses, asymmetry, and irregularities.
- ✓ Take cultures and smears as appropriate.
- ✓ Refer any significant findings to the physician.
- ✓ Nursing diagnoses commonly associated with the reproductive system include *Rape-trauma syndrome, Sexual dysfunction, Altered sexuality patterns, High risk for infection, Altered growth and development, Knowledge deficit,* and others.
- ✓ Encourage clients to know their risk factors for developing reproductive system cancers and sexually transmitted diseases. Provide information on strategies for modifying those factors and for incorporating changes into their lifestyle.
- ✓ Encourage clients to report any unsual symptoms to their physicians. These include unusual discharge, masses, swelling, itching, inflammation, and rashes. Women should report significant changes in their menstrual pattern, and breakthrough bleeding postmenopause. Men should perform monthly testicular exams and report lumps or enlarged testicles.
- ✓ Clients must be referred if there is any suspicion of sexual abuse.

Chapter 16

Assessing the Peripheral Vascular and Lymphatic Systems

The peripheral vascular system is made up of the blood vessels of the body. Together with the heart and the lymphatic vessels, they make up the body's circulatory system, which transports blood and lymph throughout the body. This chapter discusses assessment of the 60,000-mile network of veins and arteries that make up the peripheral vascular system, as well as the peripheral lymphatic vessels. The cervical lymphatics are discussed in Chapter 9, and the lymph nodes of the breasts and axillae are discussed in Chapter 12.

The vascular system plays a key role in the development of heart disease, one of the leading causes of death. People with high blood pressure have three to four times the risk of developing coronary heart disease and as much as seven times the risk of a stroke as do those with normal blood pressure (U.S. Department of Health and Human Services 1990). Unfortunately, hypertension does virtually all of its damage before any symptoms are experienced and that characteristic has tended to undermine efforts at treatment.

Therefore, your efforts as a nurse must be directed at prevention of problems of the circulatory system and promotion of a healthful way of life. A client's psychosocial health, self-care practices, and factors related to the client's family, culture, and environment all influence vascular health. Figure 16.1 gives an overview of some important factors to consider when you assess the vascular system.

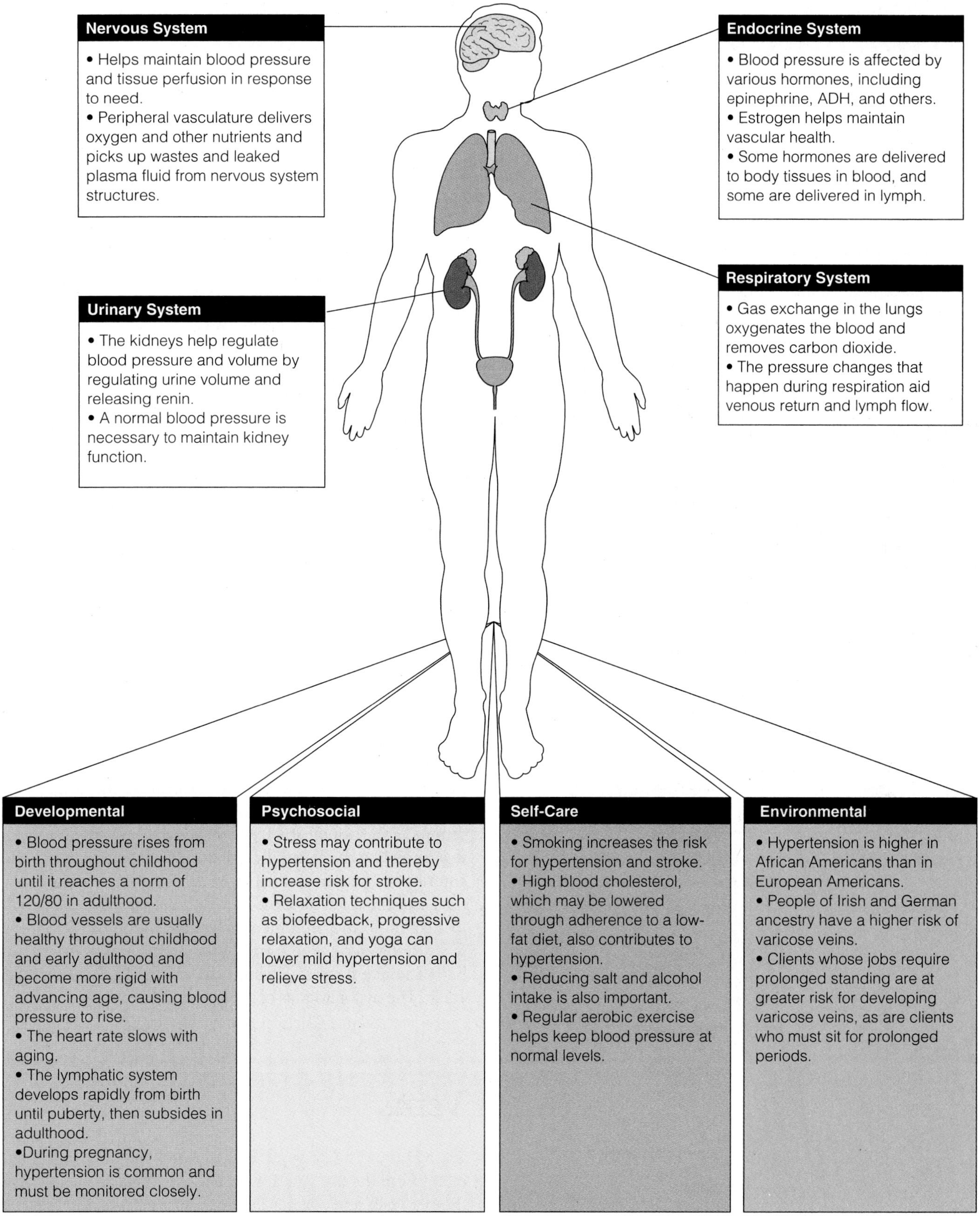

Nervous System

- Helps maintain blood pressure and tissue perfusion in response to need.
- Peripheral vasculature delivers oxygen and other nutrients and picks up wastes and leaked plasma fluid from nervous system structures.

Endocrine System

- Blood pressure is affected by various hormones, including epinephrine, ADH, and others.
- Estrogen helps maintain vascular health.
- Some hormones are delivered to body tissues in blood, and some are delivered in lymph.

Urinary System

- The kidneys help regulate blood pressure and volume by regulating urine volume and releasing renin.
- A normal blood pressure is necessary to maintain kidney function.

Respiratory System

- Gas exchange in the lungs oxygenates the blood and removes carbon dioxide.
- The pressure changes that happen during respiration aid venous return and lymph flow.

Developmental

- Blood pressure rises from birth throughout childhood until it reaches a norm of 120/80 in adulthood.
- Blood vessels are usually healthy throughout childhood and early adulthood and become more rigid with advancing age, causing blood pressure to rise.
- The heart rate slows with aging.
- The lymphatic system develops rapidly from birth until puberty, then subsides in adulthood.
- During pregnancy, hypertension is common and must be monitored closely.

Psychosocial

- Stress may contribute to hypertension and thereby increase risk for stroke.
- Relaxation techniques such as biofeedback, progressive relaxation, and yoga can lower mild hypertension and relieve stress.

Self-Care

- Smoking increases the risk for hypertension and stroke.
- High blood cholesterol, which may be lowered through adherence to a low-fat diet, also contributes to hypertension.
- Reducing salt and alcohol intake is also important.
- Regular aerobic exercise helps keep blood pressure at normal levels.

Environmental

- Hypertension is higher in African Americans than in European Americans.
- People of Irish and German ancestry have a higher risk of varicose veins.
- Clients whose jobs require prolonged standing are at greater risk for developing varicose veins, as are clients who must sit for prolonged periods.

Figure 16.1 Important factors to consider when assessing the peripheral vascular system.

Anatomy and Physiology Review

Arteries

The **arteries** of the peripheral vascular system receive oxygen-rich blood from the heart and carry it to the organs and tissues of the body. The pumping heart creates a high pressure wave or *pulse* that causes the arteries to expand and contract. This pulse propels the blood through the vessels and is palpable in arteries near the skin or over a bony surface. The thickness and elasticity of arterial walls help them to withstand these constant waves of pressure and to propel the blood to the body periphery.

Arterial pulses are palpable over areas where an artery lies over a bone and just deep to the skin. In the arm, the pulsations of the *brachial artery* can be palpated in the antecubital region. The divisions of the brachial artery, the *radial* and *ulnar arteries*, can be palpated for pulsations over the anterior wrist. The major arteries of the arm are shown in Figure 16.2.

In the leg, the pulsations of the femoral artery can be palpated inferior to the inguinal ligament, about halfway between the anterior superior iliac spine and the symphysis pubis. The *femoral artery* continues down the thigh, and becomes the *popliteal artery* as it passes behind the knee. Pulsations of the popliteal artery are palpable over the popliteal region. Below the knee, the popliteal artery divides into the anterior and posterior tibial arteries. The *anterior tibial artery* travels to the dorsum of the foot, and its pulsation can be felt just lateral to the prominent extensor tendon of the big toe close to the ankle. Pulsations of the *posterior tibial artery* can be felt where it passes behind the medial malleolus of the ankle. The major arteries of the leg are shown in Figure 16.3.

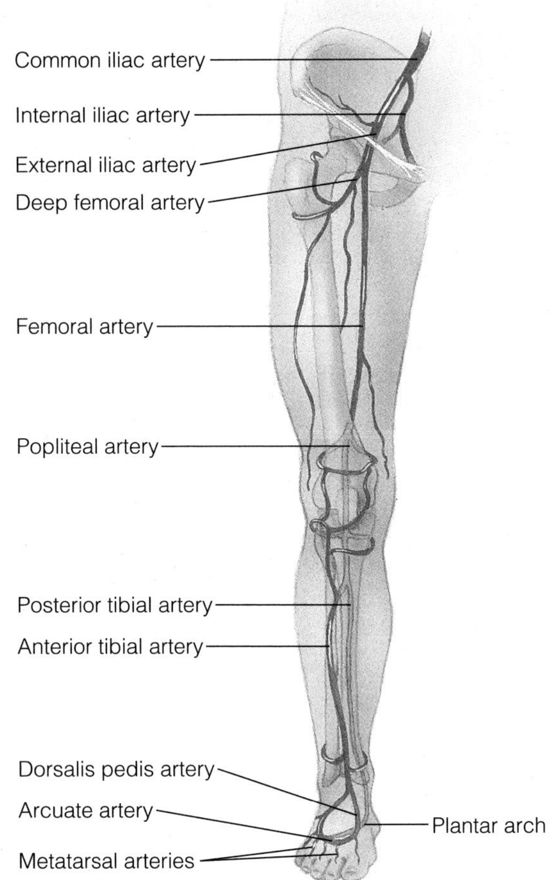

Figure 16.3 The main arteries of the leg.

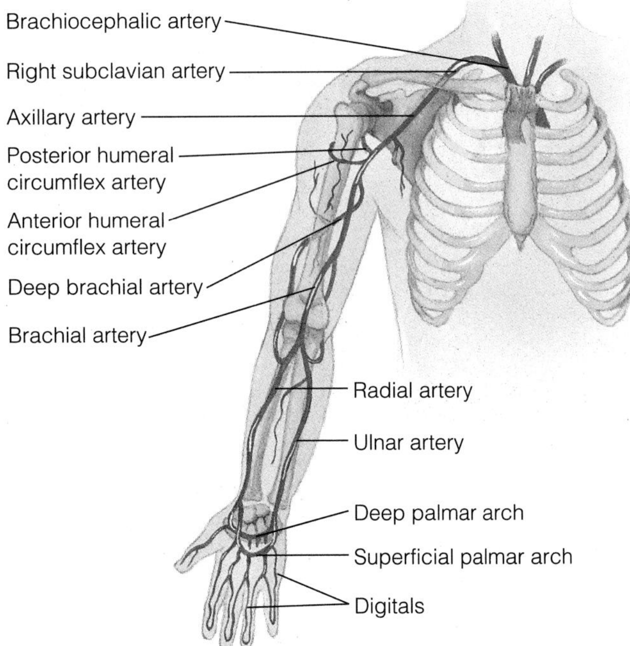

Figure 16.2 The main arteries of the arm.

Veins

The **veins** of the systemic circulation deliver deoxygenated blood from the body periphery back to the heart. Veins have thinner walls and a larger diameter than arteries and are able to stretch and dilate to facilitate venous return. Venous return is assisted by contraction of skeletal muscles during activities such as walking, and by pressure changes related to inspiration and expiration. In addition, veins have one-way intraluminal valves that close tightly when filled to prevent backflow. Thus, venous blood flows only toward the heart. Problems with the lumen or valves of the leg veins can lead to *stasis,* or pooling of blood in the veins of the lower extremities.

The femoral and the popliteal veins are deep veins of the legs and carry about 90% of the venous return from the legs. The great and small saphenous veins are superficial veins that are not as well supported as the deep veins by surrounding tissues and therefore are more susceptible to venous stasis. The major veins of the leg are shown in Figure 16.4.

Capillaries

Exchanges of gases and nutrients between the arterial and venous systems are conducted within beds of **capillaries**, the smallest vessels of the circulatory system. Blood pressure in the arterial end of the capillary bed forces fluid out across the capillary membrane and into the body tissues.

Lymphatic Vessels

Lymphatic vessels form their own circulatory system and provide a network of defense against invading microorganisms. During circulation, as blood continues through the capillary bed toward the smallest veins, called *venules*, more fluid leaves the capillaries than can be absorbed by the veins. The lymphatic system retrieves this excess fluid, called *lymph*, from the tissue spaces and carries it to the lymph nodes throughout the body. Lymph nodes are clumps of tissue located along the lymphatic vessels either deep or superficially in the body. The lymph nodes usually are covered and protected by connective tissue, and are therefore not palpable. Some of the more superficial nodes are located in the neck, the axillary region, and the inguinal region. Deeper clusters

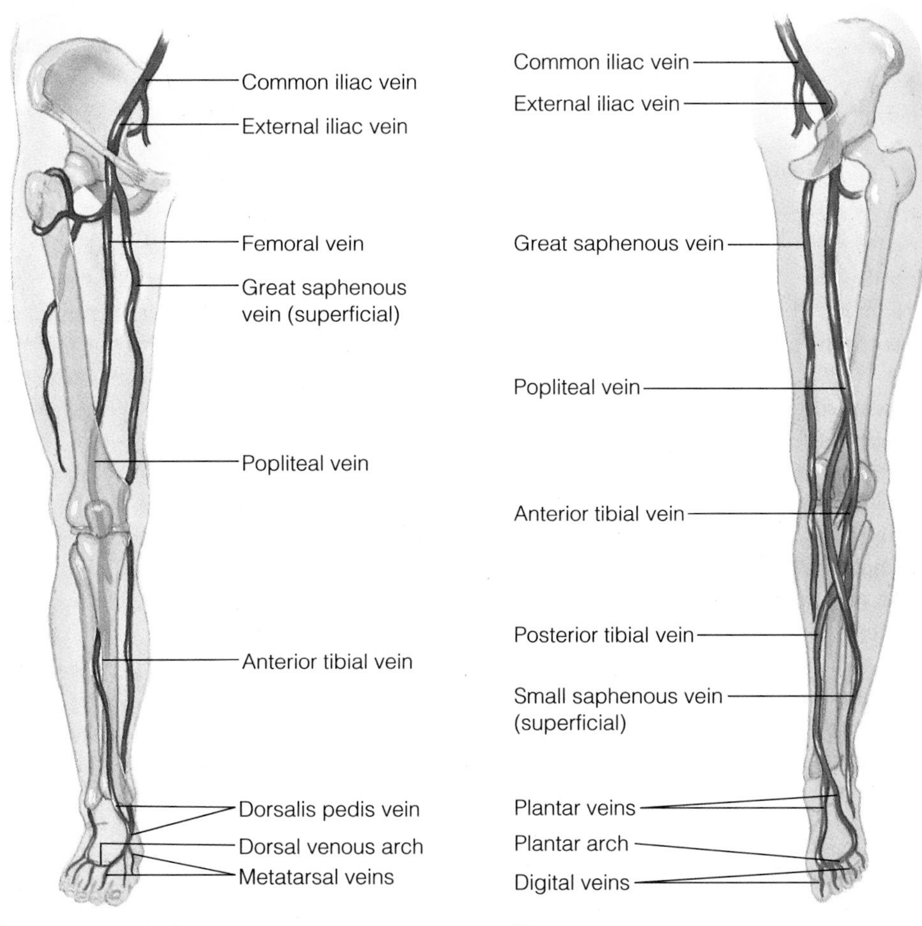

Figure 16.4 The main veins of the leg. *A*, anterior view; *B*, posterior view.

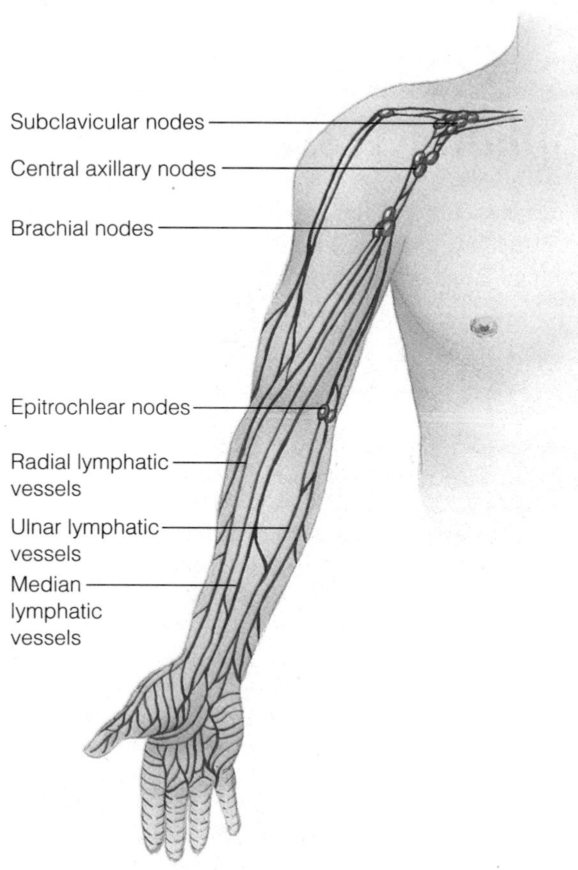

Figure 16.5 The main lymph nodes of the arm.

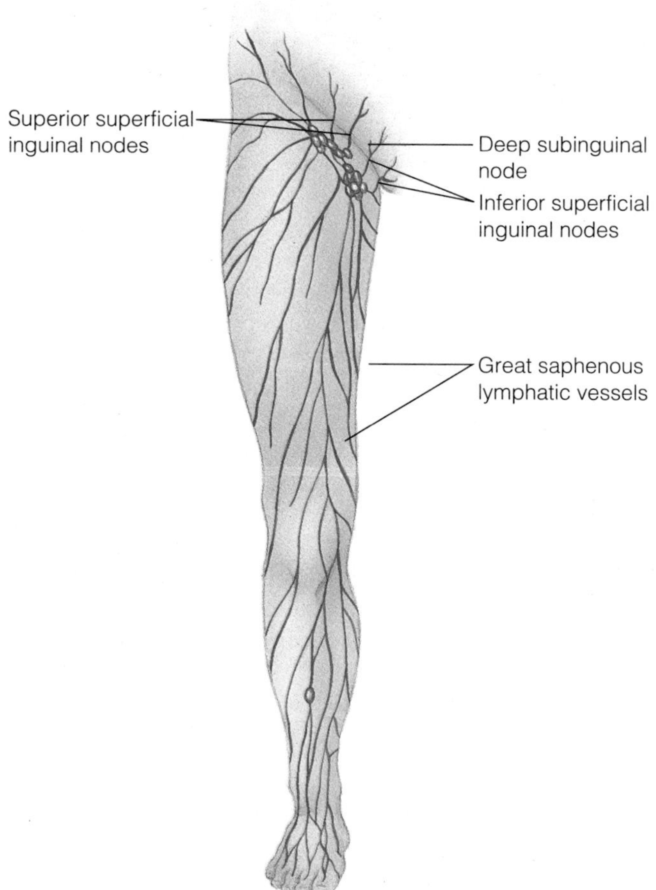

Figure 16.6 The main lymph nodes of the leg.

are located in the abdomen and thoracic cavity. The lymph nodes filter lymph fluid, removing any pathogens before the fluid is returned to the bloodstream.

The *epitrochlear node* located on the medial surface of the arm above the elbow drains the ulnar surface of the forearm, the ring and little finger, and the middle finger. The nodes in the axilla of the arm drain the rest of the arm. The major lymph nodes of the arm are shown in Figure 16.5.

The legs have two sets of superficial inguinal nodes—a vertical group and a horizonal group. The vertical group is located close to the saphenous vein and drains that area of the leg. The horizontal group of nodes is found below the inguinal ligament; it drains the skin of the abdominal wall, the external genitals, the anal canal, and the gluteal area. The major lymph nodes of the leg are shown in Figure 16.6.

The functions of the peripheral vascular and lymphatic systems are

- Delivering oxygen and nutrients to tissues of the body
- Transporting carbon dioxide and other waste products from the tissues for excretion
- Removing pathogens from the body fluid by filtering lymph

Gathering the Data

Focused Interview

Clients who have peripheral vascular changes may or may not be aware of any alteration in health. Therefore, the focused interview is essential to obtain data reflecting the current health status of the client's peripheral vascular system. It should build on information gathered during the health history and cardiovascular assessment described in Chapters 2 and 11. The data obtained should reflect the client's level of wellness, existing peripheral vascular problems, and interventions being implemented. Identifying pain and skin changes in the extremities is particularly important when you assess the peripheral vascular system.

1. Do you know of any problems you are having or have had with your circulation? If so, please describe the problem, including any treatment and resolution.
2. Have you or any member of your family ever had heart problems, respiratory disease, or diabetes? *These problems can damage the peripheral circulation, and they tend to be hereditary.*
3. Have you noticed any skin changes on your arms or legs? If so, describe the changes. Have you noticed any swelling or shiny skin, particularly on your legs? *Shiny skin and swelling is sometimes caused by fluid leaking into tissue spaces because of incompetent valves in the veins.*
4. *If the client reports swelling:* Is the swelling in one leg or both legs? When did this swelling start? Is the swelling worse in the morning or at the end of the day, or is the swelling constant? What relieves the swelling? *Answers to these questions may help you to determine the reason for the swelling.*
5. Have you noticed any changes in temperature in your arms or legs, such as extreme coolness or heat? *Extreme coolness may indicate arterial insufficiency.*
6. Have you noticed any skin changes such as sores or ulcers on your legs? If so, Is there any pain associated with the sores? *Leg ulcers can be an indication of chronic arterial or venous problems.*
7. Have you noticed any changes in the feeling in your legs, such as numbness or tingling? *Decreased circulation in the lower extremities can cause a loss of sensation, particularly in persons with diabetes.*
8. Do you ever have pains in your legs, or leg cramps? If so, please describe the pain or cramp, the location, and the time it most often occurs. *Pain associated with arterial insufficiency is usually described as gnawing, sharp, or stabbing and increases with exercise. Pain is relieved with the cessation of movement and when legs are dangling. The pain is most commonly in the calf of the leg but it may also be in the lower leg or top of the foot. Venous insufficiency pain is described as aching or a feeling of fullness and intensifies with prolonged standing or sitting in one position. Swelling and varicosities in the legs may also be present. The condition is relieved by elevating the legs or by walking.*
9. Do you smoke? If so, how long have you smoked? How many cigarettes, cigars, or pipes of tobacco do you smoke per day? *Nicotine is a vasoconstrictor and aggravates peripheral vascular disease.*
10. *For male clients:* Have you experienced any difficulty in achieving an erection? *Impotence may occur as a result of a diminished arterial flow to the pelvic arteries. This condition is a common finding in peripheral vascular disease and is not always reported because of client embarrassment.*
11. What medications are you taking, either over-the-counter or prescription? *Oral contraceptives have been associated with blood clots in the peripheral vascular system. Aspirin is an anticoagulant.*
12. Do you have any swollen glands? If so, where are they in your body? How long have they been enlarged? Is there any pain or redness associated with these enlarged glands? Have you had any other symptoms such as fever, fatigue, or bleeding? *Enlarged lymph glands usually are associated with an infectious process in the body.*
13. Do you exercise regularly? If so, describe your exercise routine. How often do you exercise? For how long? *Exercise not only helps to prevent vascular disease but also improves the survival rate of people who have already suffered a heart attack and reduces the likelihood of their suffering a second attack. Even modest levels of physical activity are beneficial, according to the American Heart Association.*

Note: No additional questions are required for children, adolescents, childbearing clients, or older clients.

Physical Assessment

Preparation

☑ **Review the guidelines below for palpating peripheral pulses. Review Chapter 7 for technique for auscultating blood pressure.**

Assessing Peripheral Pulses

Assess peripheral pulses by palpating with gentle pressure over the artery. Use the pads of your first three fingers.

Note the following characteristics:

- Rate—the number of beats per minute
- Rhythm—the regularity of the beats
- Symmetry—pulses on both sides of body should be similar
- Amplitude—the strength of the beat, assessed on a scale of 0 to 4:
  - 4 = Bounding
  - 3 = Increased
  - 2 = Normal
  - 1 = Weak
  - 0 = Absent or nonpalpable

☑ **Gather the equipment:**

examination gown	stethoscope
examination gloves	sphygmomanometer

☑ **Wash your hands.**

☑ **Ask the client to don the examination gown.** The client need not remove underwear, but should remove socks. Have the client remove watches and tight bracelets, which may interfere with the physical assessment.

☑ **Adjust the room lighting if necessary.**

Remember

- Provide a warm, comfortable environment.
- Explain the procedure to the client to allay any fear or apprehension.
- Ensure the client's privacy.
- If you notice breaks in the skin, put on gloves before proceeding with the assessment.
- Lymph nodes are small and normally not palpable. During the assessment, you palpate body regions where superficial nodes are located. Palpable nodes are usually enlarged and painful to touch.

ASSESSMENT TECHNIQUE/NORMAL FINDINGS | SPECIAL CONSIDERATIONS

Blood Pressure

Step 1 *Position the client.*

- Place the client in a sitting position on the examination table with the examination gown closed (Figure 16.7).

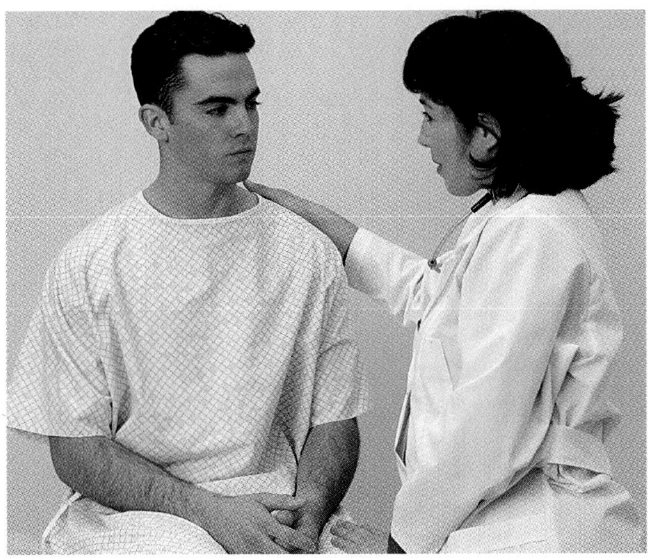

Figure 16.7 Positioning the client.

Step 2 *Take the blood pressure in both arms.*

Step 3 *Assist the client to a supine position.*

Step 4 *Take the blood pressure in both arms.*

Step 5 *Take the blood pressure in both legs.*

Blood pressure normally can be affected by factors such as exercise, anxiety, pain, eating, drinking, or smoking.

A systolic reading over 140 or a diastolic reading over 90 is considered elevated. If you obtain such a reading, wait 30 minutes and repeat the procedure. If the second reading is still abnormal, you should refer the client to a physician.

The blood pressure normally does not vary more than 5 to 10 mm Hg in each arm. The blood pressure in the popliteal artery is usually 10 to 40 mm Hg higher than that in the brachial artery.

A difference of 10 mm Hg or more between the arms may indicate an obstruction of arterial flow to one arm.

Referral

A systolic reading below 90 or a diastolic reading under 60 may be an early indication of shock, which requires immediate medical attention.

ASSESSMENT TECHNIQUE/NORMAL FINDINGS | SPECIAL CONSIDERATIONS

Carotid Arteries

Step 1 *Palpate the carotid pulses.*

- Place the flat surface of your first three fingers on the client's neck between the trachea and the sternocleidomastoid muscle, just below the angle of the jaw (Figure 16.8).

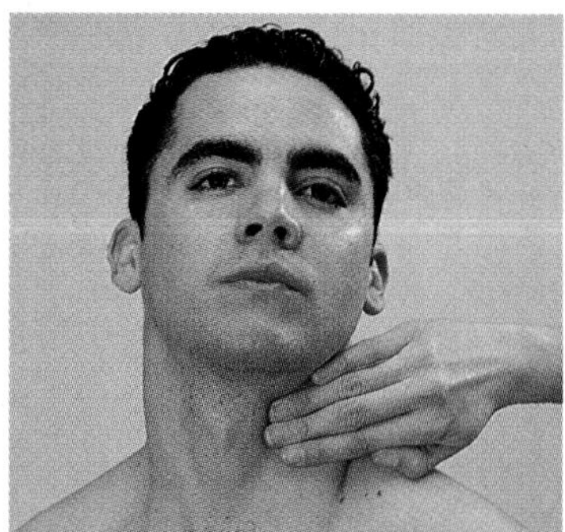

Figure 16.8 Palpating the carotid pulse.

- Ask the client to turn the head slightly toward your hand to relax the sternocleidomastoid muscle.
- Palpate firmly, but not so hard that you occlude the artery.
- Palpate one side of the neck at a time.
- If you are having difficulty finding the pulse, try varying the pressure of your fingers, feeling carefully below the angle.

If both carotid arteries are palpated at the same time, the result can be a drop in blood pressure or a reduction in the pulse rate.

- Note the rate, rhythm, amplitude, and symmetry of the carotid pulses.

A rate over 90 beats per minute is considered abnormal unless the client has recently been exercising, smoking, or is anxious. A rate below 60 is also considered abnormal. However, some athletes have a resting pulse as low as 50 beats per minute. An irregular rhythm, or a pulse with extra beats or period pauses is considered abnormal. An exaggerated pulse or a weak, thready pulse is abnormal. A discrepancy between the two carotid pulses is abnormal.

Step 2 *Auscultate the carotid arteries.*

- Using the diaphragm of the stethoscope, auscultate each carotid artery high in the neck and medial to the sternocleidomastoid muscle.
- Auscultate each carotid artery over the lateral end of the clavicle and the posterior margin of the sternocleidomastoid muscle. Ask the

ASSESSMENT TECHNIQUE/NORMAL FINDINGS | SPECIAL CONSIDERATIONS

client to hold the breath for several seconds to decrease trachial sounds. You may need to have the client turn the head slightly to the side not being examined.

- Repeat the procedure using the bell of the stethoscope.

ALERT!

Be careful not to put pressure on the bell of the stethoscope or you may occlude the sounds in the blood vessel.

While auscultating, you should hear a very quiet sound. Normal heart sounds could be transmitted to the neck, but there should be no swishing sounds..

A swishing sound indicates the presence of a bruit, an obstruction causing turbulence, such as a narrowing of the vessel due to the build up of cholesterol.

An increased cardiac output such as seen in hyperthyroidism or anemia also will produce a bruit.

Arms

Step 1 ***Assess the hands.***

- Take the client's hands in your hands.
- Note the color of skin and nailbeds, the temperature and texture of the skin, and the presence of any lesions or swelling.
- Look at the fingers and nails from the side and observe the angle of the nail base. The angle should be about 160 degrees.

Flattening of the angle of the nail and enlargement of the tips of the fingers (clubbing) is a sign of oxygen deprivation in the extremities. In clients with chronic hypoxia (oxygen deprivation), there may be a rounding of the tip of the finger described as "turkey drumsticks." The nail may feel spongy instead of firm, and there may be a blue discoloration of the nail.

Step 2 ***Observe for capillary refill in both hands.***

- Holding one of the client's hands in your hand, apply pressure to one of the client's fingernails for 5 seconds.

The area under pressure should turn pale.

- Release the pressure and note how rapidly the normal color returns.

In a healthy client, the color should return in less than 1 to 2 seconds.

- Repeat the procedure for the other hand.

A delayed capillary refill could indicate decreased cardiac output or constriction of the peripheral vessels. However, cigarette smoking, anemia, or cold temperatures can also cause delayed capillary refill.

Step 3 ***Place both arms together and compare their size.***

They should be nearly equal in size.

Edema (increased accumulation of fluid) in the arms could indicate an obstruction of the lymphatic system.

ASSESSMENT TECHNIQUE/NORMAL FINDINGS

Step 4 ***Palpate both radial pulses.***

The radial pulses are found on the ventral side of each wrist.

- Ask the client to extend one hand, palm up.

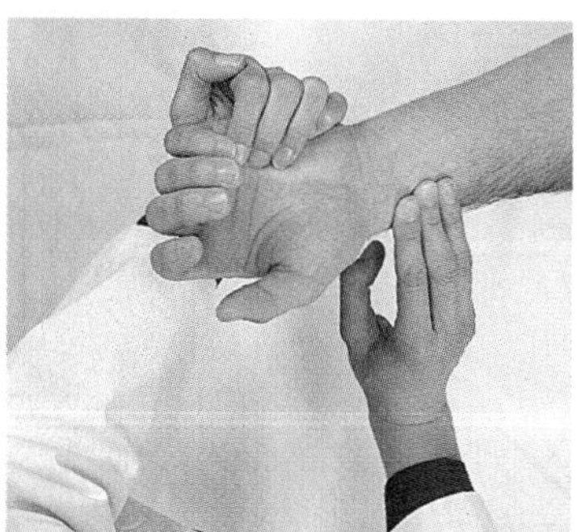

Figure 16.9 Palpating the radial pulse.

- Palpate with two fingers over the lateral wrist (Figure 16.9).
- Repeat the procedure for the other arm.
- Note the rate, rhythm, amplitude, and symmetry of the pulses.
- Grade the amplitude on the four-point scale as described in the chart on page 464.

SPECIAL CONSIDERATIONS

You do not need to palpate the ulnar pulses, located medial to the ulna on the flexor surface of the wrist. They are deeper than the radial pulses and are difficult to palpate.

Step 5 ***Palpate both brachial pulses.***

The brachial pulses are found just medial to the biceps tendon.

- Ask the client to extend the arm.
- Palpate over the brachial artery just superior to the antecubital region (Figure 16.10).

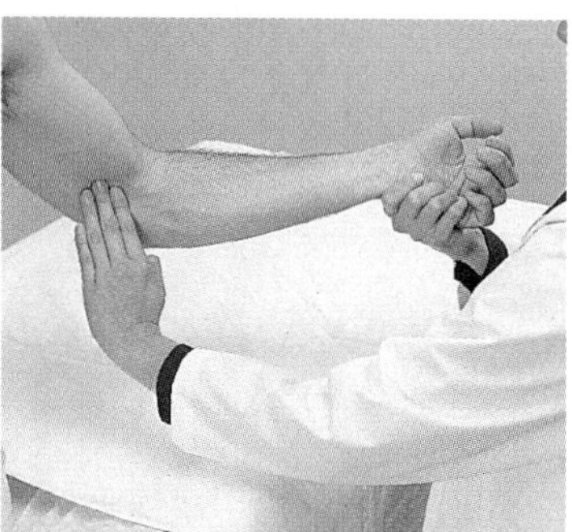

Figure 16.10 Palpating the brachial pulse.

- Repeat the procedure for the other arm.
- Note the rate, rhythm, amplitude, and symmetry of the pulses.
- Grade the amplitude on the four-point scale as before.

If you have difficulty palpating any pulses, use a Doppler flowmeter. When positioned over a patent artery, this device emits sound waves as the blood moves through the artery. (See Chapter 7.)

ASSESSMENT TECHNIQUE/NORMAL FINDINGS	SPECIAL CONSIDERATIONS

Step 6 ***Perform the Allen test.***

If you suspect an obstruction or insufficiency of an artery in the arm, the Allen test may determine the patency of the radial and ulnar arteries.

- Ask the client to place the hands on the knees with palms up.
- Compress the radial arteries of both wrists with your thumbs.
- Now ask the client to open and close the fist several times.
- While you are still compressing the radial arteries, ask the client to open the hands.

The palms should become pink immediately, indicating patent ulnar arteries.

If normal color does not return, the ulnar arteries may be occluded.

- Next occlude the ulnar arteries and repeat the same procedure to test the patency of the radial arteries.

If normal color does not return, the radial arteries may be occluded.

Step 7 ***Palpate the epitrochlear lymph node in each arm.***

The epitrochlear node drains the forearm and the third, fourth, and fifth finger.

- Hold the client's right hand in your right hand.
- With your left hand reach behind the elbow to the groove between the biceps and triceps muscles (Figure 16.11).

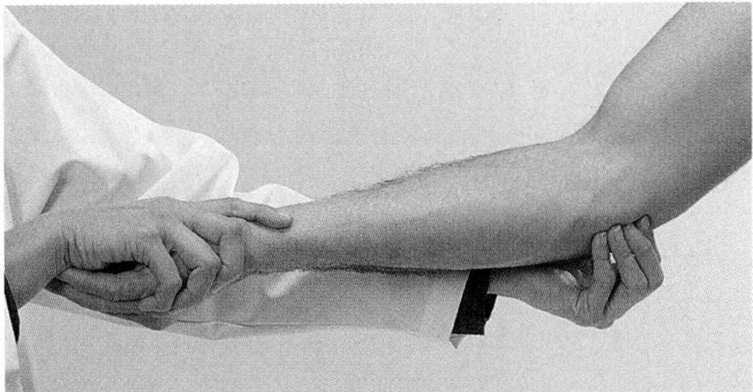

Figure 16.11 Palpating the epitrochlear lymph node.

- Note the size and consistency of the node. Normally it is not palpable or is barely palpable.

An enlarged node may indicate an infection in the hand or forearm.

- Repeat the procedure for the left arm.

Legs

Step 1 ***Inspect both legs.***

- Observe skin color, hair distribution, and any skin lesions.

Skin color should match the skin tone of the rest of the body. Hair is normally present on the legs. If the hair has been removed, there is still

If the peripheral vessels are constricted, the skin will be a paler than the rest of the body. If the vessels are dilated, the skin will have a reddish tone.

ASSESSMENT TECHNIQUE/NORMAL FINDINGS	SPECIAL CONSIDERATIONS

usually hair on the dorsal surface of the great toes. Hair growth should be symmetric. The skin should be intact with no lesions.

A rusty discoloration over the anterior tibial surface with the skin intact is associated with decreased arterial circulation. The characteristic color stems from blood leaking out of a vessel with decreased capacity for it to be reabsorbed.

If skin lesions or ulcerations are present, note the size and location. Ulcers occurring as a result of arterial deficit tend to occur on pressure points, such as tips of toes and lateral malleoli. Venous ulcers occur at medial malleoli because of fragile tissue with poor drainage.

> ***Referral***
>
> **If you discover any tissue which has become blackened, refer the client immediately. The presence of blackened tissue can indicate tissue death (necrosis).**

Step 2 ***Compare the size of both legs.***

They should be symmetric in size. If the legs are unequal in size, measure the circumference of each leg at the widest point. It is important to measure each leg at the same point.

A discrepancy in the size of the legs could indicate an accumulation of fluid (edema) resulting from increased pressure in the capillaries or an obstruction of a lymph vessel. Unequal size of the legs could also indicate a blood clot in the deep vessels of the leg.

Step 3 ***Palpate the legs for temperature.***

- Palpate from the feet up the legs, using the dorsal surface of your hands.
- Note any discrepancies.

The skin should be the same temperature on both legs.

If the peripheral vessels are constricted, the skin will feel cool. If the peripheral vessels are dilated, the skin will feel warm. A difference in the temperature of the feet may be a sign of arterial insufficiency.

Step 4 ***Assess the legs for the presence of superficial veins.***

- With the client in a sitting position, legs dangling from the examination table, inspect the legs.
- Now ask the client to elevate the legs.

The veins may appear as nodular bulges when the legs are in the dependent position, but any bulges should disappear when the legs are elevated.

- Palpate the veins for tenderness or inflammation (phlebitis).

Varicosities (distended veins) frequently occur in the anterolateral aspect of the thigh and lower leg or on the posterolateral aspect of the calf. These bulging veins do not disappear when legs are elevated. Varicose veins are dilated but have a diminished blood flow and an increased intravenous pressure. Varicosities are caused by an incompetent valve, a weakness in the vein wall, or an obstruction in a proximal vein.

ASSESSMENT TECHNIQUE/NORMAL FINDINGS	SPECIAL CONSIDERATIONS

Step 5 ***Perform the manual compression test.***

If varicose veins are present, you can determine the length of the varicose vein and the competency of its valves with the manual compression test.

- Ask the client to stand.
- With the fingers of one hand, palpate the lower part of the varicose vein.
- Keeping that hand on the vein, compress the vein firmly at least 15 to 20 cm higher with the fingers of your other hand (Figure 16.12).

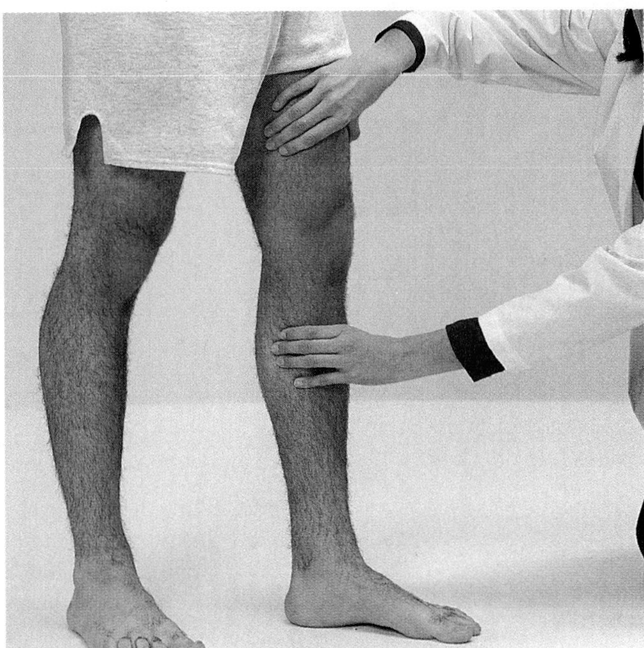

Figure 16.12 Performing the manual compression test.

You will not feel any pulsation beneath your lower fingers if the valves of the varicose vein are still competent.

If the valves are incompetent, you will feel an impulse in the vein between your two hands.

Step 6 ***Perform the Trendelenburg test.***

A second test to evaluate valve competence in the presence of varicosities is the Trendelenburg test.

- Assist the client to a supine position.
- Elevate the leg to 90 degrees until the venous blood has drained from the leg.
- Place a tourniquet around the upper thigh (Figure 16.13, *A*).
- Help the client to stand.
- Watch for filling of the venous system (Figure 16.13, *B*).

A rapid filling of the superficial veins from above indicates incompetent valves.

ASSESSMENT TECHNIQUE/NORMAL FINDINGS | SPECIAL CONSIDERATIONS

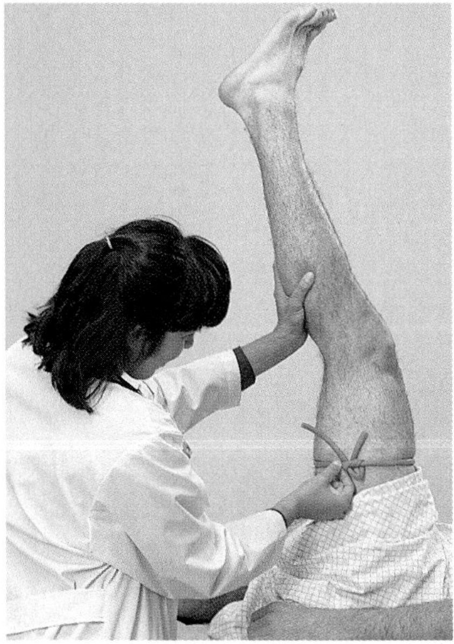

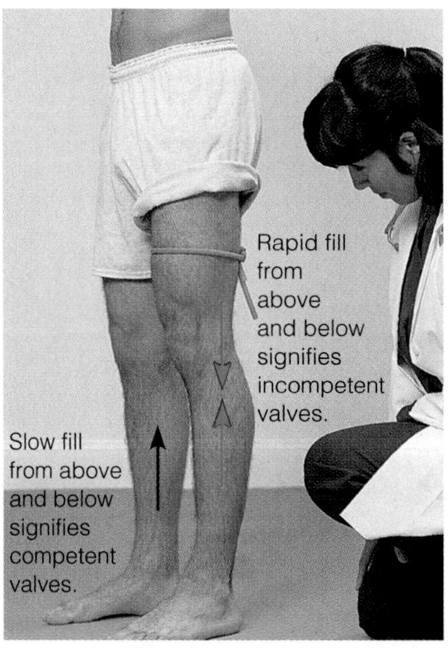

Figure 16.13 Performing the Trendelenburg test. *A,* Applying tourniquet. *B,* Watching for filling.

The saphenous vein should fill from below in about 30 to 35 seconds.

- After the client has been standing for 20 to 30 seconds, remove the tourniquet and note whether the varicose veins fill from above.

Competent valves prevent sudden retrograde filling.

A sudden filling of superficial veins after removing the tourniquet indicates backward filling past incompetent valves.

Step 7 ***Test for Homan's sign.***

- Assist the client to a supine position.
- Flex the client's knee about 5°.
- Now sharply dorsiflex the client's foot (Figure 16.14).

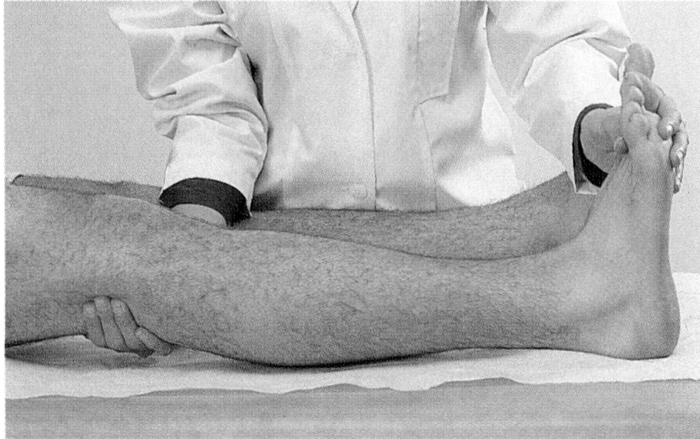

Figure 16.14 Testing for Homan's sign.

A positive Homan's sign could indicate a blood clot in one of the deep veins of the leg. However, a positive Homan's sign could also indicate an inflammation of one of the superficial leg veins or an inflammation of one of the tendons of the leg. The reliability of Homan's sign in indicating disease has been shown to be inconsistent.

ASSESSMENT TECHNIQUE/NORMAL FINDINGS | SPECIAL CONSIDERATIONS

- Ask whether the client feels calf pain.

This maneuver exerts pressure on the posterior tibial vein and should not cause pain.

Step 8 ***Palpate the inguinal lymph nodes.***

- Move the client's gown aside over the inguinal region.
- Palpate over the top of the medial thigh (Figure 16.15).

Lymph nodes that are larger than 1 cm or tender may be an indication of an infection in the legs.

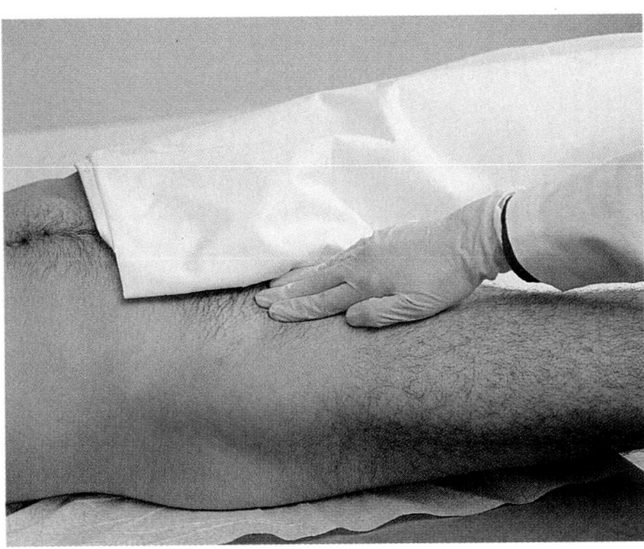

Figure 16.15 Palpating the inguinal lymph nodes.

If the nodes can be palpated, they should be movable and not tender.

- Repeat the procedure for the other leg.

Step 9 ***Palpate both femoral pulses.***

The femoral pulses are inferior and medial to the inguinal ligament.

- Ask the client to bend the knee out to the side.
- Palpate over the femoral artery (Figure 16.16).

If you are unable to palpate the femoral pulse, an artery may be occluded.

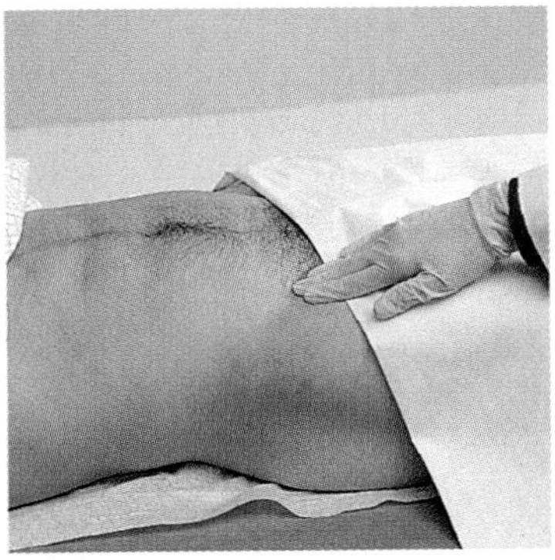

Figure 16.16 Palpating the femoral pulse.

ASSESSMENT TECHNIQUE/NORMAL FINDINGS	SPECIAL CONSIDERATIONS

The femoral artery is deep, and you may need to place one hand on top of the other to locate the pulse.

- Repeat the procedure for the other leg.
- Note the rate, rhythm, amplitude, and symmetry of the pulses.
- Grade the amplitude on the four-point scale.

Step 10 *Palpate both popliteal pulses.*

The pulsations of the popliteal artery can be palpated deep in the popliteal fossa lateral to the midline.

- Ask the client to flex the knee and relax the leg.
- Palpate the popliteal pulse.
- If you cannot locate the pulse, ask the client to roll onto the abdomen and flex the knee (Figure 16.17).

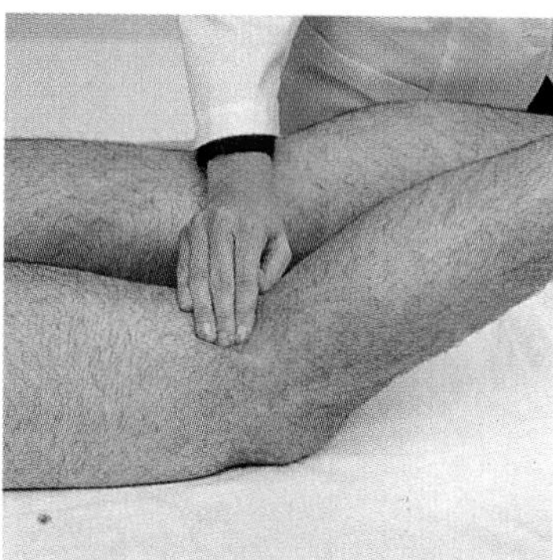

Figure 16.17 Palpating the popliteal pulse.

- Palpate deeply for the pulse.
- Repeat the procedure for the other leg.
- Note the rate, rhythm, amplitude, and symmetry of the pulses.
- Grade the amplitude on the four-point scale.

If you are unable to palpate the popliteal pulse, an artery may be occluded.

Step 11 *Palpate both dorsalis pedis pulses.*

The dorsalis pedis pulses may be felt on the medial side of the dorsum of the foot.

- Palpate the pulse lateral to the extensor tendon of the great toe (Figure 16.18).

The absence of a dorsalis pedis pulse may not be indicative of occlusion because another artery may be supplying blood to this area of the foot. Edema in the foot will make palpation difficult.

ASSESSMENT TECHNIQUE/NORMAL FINDINGS

SPECIAL CONSIDERATIONS

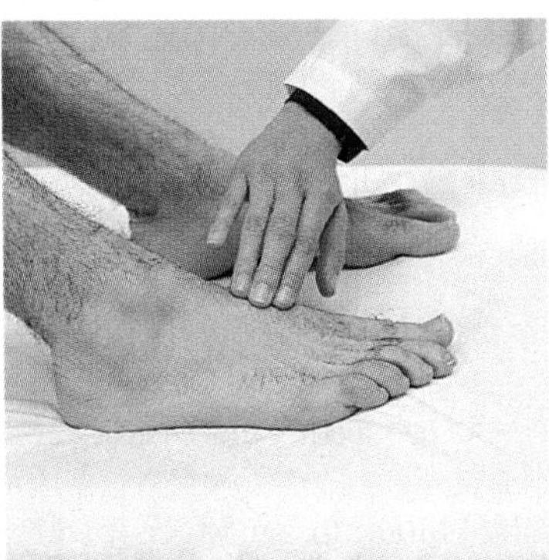

Figure 16.18 Palpating the dorsalis pedis pulse.

- Use light pressure.
- Repeat the procedure for the other foot.
- Note the rate, rhythm, amplitude, and symmetry of the pulses.
- Grade the amplitude on the four-point scale.

Step 12 *Palpate both posterior tibial pulses.*

The posterior tibial pulses may be palpated behind and slightly inferior to the medial malleolus of the ankle, in the groove between the malleolus and the Achilles tendon.

- Palpate the pulse by curving your fingers around the medial malleolus (Figure 16.19).

If you are unable to palpate the posterior tibial pulse, an artery may be occluded.

If the client has edematous ankles, this pulse may be difficult to palpate.

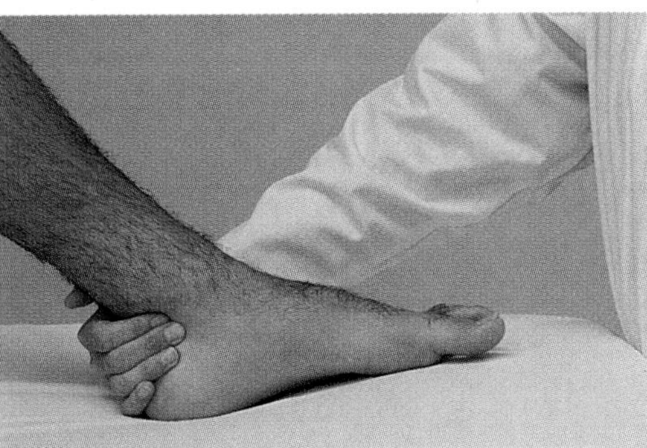

Figure 16.19 Palpating the posterior tibial pulse.

- Repeat the procedure for the other foot.
- Note the rate, rhythm, amplitude, and symmetry of the pulses.
- Grade the amplitude on the four-point scale.

ASSESSMENT TECHNIQUE/NORMAL FINDINGS

Step 13 *Assess for arterial supply to the lower legs and feet.*

- If you suspect an arterial deficiency, test for arterial supply to the lower extremities.
- Ask the client to remain supine.
- Elevate the client's legs 12 inches above the heart.
- Ask the client to move the feet up and down at the ankles for 60 seconds to drain the venous blood (Figure 16.20).

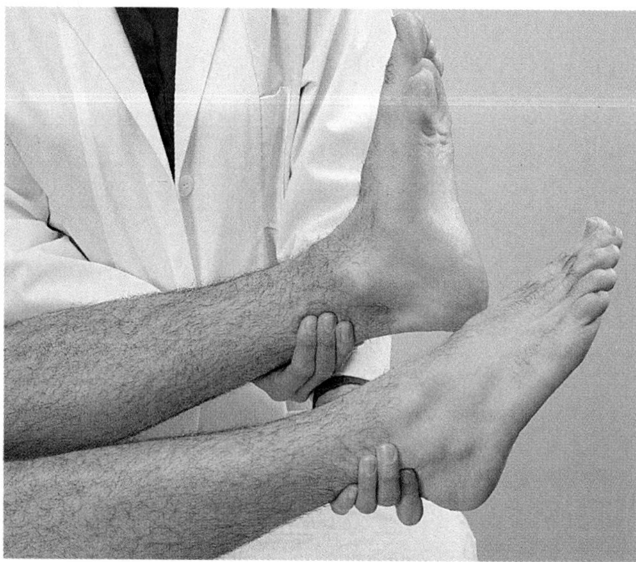

Figure 16.20 Testing arterial supply to the lower extremities.

The skin now will be lighter in color because only arterial blood is present.

- Now ask the client to sit up and dangle the feet.
- Compare the color of both feet.

The original color should return in about 10 seconds.

The superficial veins in the feet should fill in about 15 seconds.

The feet of a dark-skinned person may be difficult to evaluate, but the soles of the feet should reflect a change in color.

Step 14 *Test the lower legs for muscle strength.*

See Chapter 17, "Assessing the Musculoskeletal System."

Step 15 *Test the lower legs for sensation.*

See Chapter 18, "Assessing the Neurologic System."

Step 16 *Check for edema of the legs.*

SPECIAL CONSIDERATIONS

Marked pallor of the elevated extremities may indicate arterial insufficiency.

A marked bluish red color of the dependent feet occurs with severe arterial insufficiency. This color is due to a lack of oxygenated blood to the area, which leads to a loss of vasomotor tone and venous stasis. Delayed filling of the superficial veins of the feet also could indicate arterial insufficiency.

Motor loss may occur with arterial insufficiency.

Sensory loss may occur with arterial insufficiency.

Pitting edema can be related to a failure of the right side of the heart or an obstruction of the lymphatic system. Edema in only one leg may indicate an occlusion of a large vein in the leg.

Diminished arterial flow thickens toenails, which often become yellow and loosely attached to the nail bed. Clients with diabetes often acquire fungal and bacterial infections of the nail because of increased glucose collecting in the skin under the nail.

ASSESSMENT TECHNIQUE/NORMAL FINDINGS | SPECIAL CONSIDERATIONS

- Press the skin for at least 5 seconds over the tibia, behind the medial malleolus, and over the dorsum of each foot (Figure 16.21).

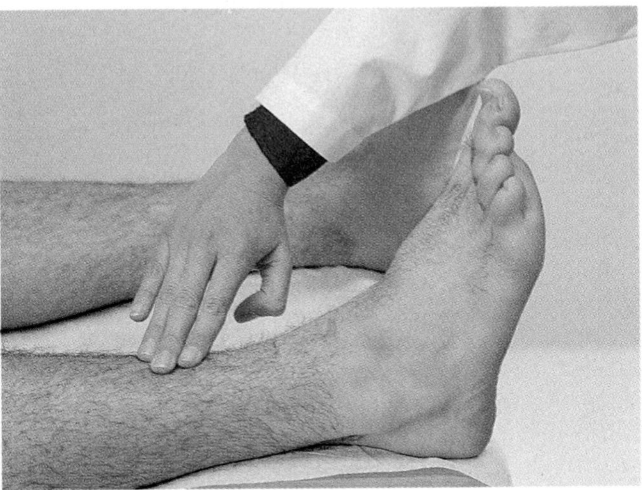

Figure 16.21 Palpating for edema over the tibia.

- Look for a depression in the skin (called pitting edema) caused by the pressure of your fingers.
- If edema is present, you should grade it on scale of 1+ (mild) to 4+ (severe) (see Figure 8.13 on page 136).

Step 17 *Inspect the toenails for color and thickness.*

Nails should be pink and not thickened. Clubbing should not be present.

Reminders

- In addition to the above steps, consider the common variations in physical assessment findings for the different groups discussed below.
- After completing the physical assessment, answer any questions the client may have, and provide appropriate client teaching for health promotion and self-care (see page 481).
- Confirm that the client is comfortable and has no adverse effects from the procedure, then dim the lights and leave the client to rest or to get dressed.
- Document the assessment findings as described in Chapter 1. See pages 471–480 for information on identifying nursing diagnoses commonly associated with the peripheral vascular system.

Developmental Considerations

Infants, Children, and Adolescent Clients

Assessing the blood pressure of a baby under 1 year of age is difficult without special equipment. It is usually not necessary if the infant is moving well and the skin color is good. However, if the child is lethargic and tires easily during feeding or the skin becomes cyanotic when the infant cries, the blood pressure should be measured with a Doppler flowmeter (see Chapter 7).

A newborn's blood pressure is much lower than that of an adult and gradually increases with age. The systolic pressure of a newborn is 50–80 mm Hg; the diastolic pressure is 25–55 mm of Hg.

All children 18 months of age and older should have their blood pressure evaluated during their well-child examination. The cuff should be no larger than two-thirds or smaller than half of the length of the child's arm between the elbow and the shoulder. Pediatric blood pressure cuffs are available.

In young children, the blood pressure should be measured on the thigh to rule out a significant difference between upper and lower extremity pressure. Such a difference in pressure could indicate a narrowing (coarctation) of the aorta. In a baby less than 1 year old, the systolic pressure in the thigh should equal that of the arm. A child over 1 year will have a systolic pressure in the thigh that is 10 to 40 mm Hg higher than that in the arm. The diastolic pressure in the thigh equals that in the arm.

The pulse increases if the child has a fever. For every degree of fever, the pulse may increase 8 to 10 beats per minute. The lymphatic system develops rapidly from birth until puberty, then subsides in adulthood. The presence of enlarged lymph nodes in a child may not indicate illness. However, if an infection is present, the nodes may enlarge considerably. Chapter 19 describes a complete assessment of infants, children, and adolescents.

Childbearing Clients

Blood pressure should be monitored throughout the pregnancy to test for pregnancy-induced hypertension. A reading of 140/90 mm Hg is considered hypertensive during pregnancy. Blood volume during pregnancy almost doubles. In the second trimester, blood pressure may decrease because of the dilation of the peripheral vessels. However, blood pressure usually returns to the prepregnancy level by the third trimester. If the client has a history of hypertension prior to her pregnancy, the blood pressure may increase dramatically during the third trimester, posing the threat of cerebral hemorrhage. Pressure from the uterus on the lower extremities can obstruct venous return and lead to hypotension when the client is lying on her back, or it can cause edema, varicosities of the leg, and hemorrhoids. Chapter 20 describes a complete assessment of the childbearing client.

Older Clients

The aging process causes arteriosclerosis or calcification of the walls of the blood vessels. The arterial walls lose elasticity and become more rigid. This increase in peripheral vascular resistance results in increased blood pressure. The enlargement of calf veins can pose the risk of blood clots in leg veins. However, the amount of circulatory inadequacy at any given age is not predictable. The aging process may not cause any symptoms in some persons.

The normal blood pressure reading for an adult over 50 years of age should be no higher than 140 mm Hg systolic and 90 mm diastolic. Most hypertension is asymptomatic, but a severe elevation may produce a headache, epistaxis (nosebleed), shortness of breath, or chest pain.

When evaluating the various arterial pulses, keep in mind that the heart rate slows with aging. Some persons may normally have a rate of 50 beats per minute; however, the client should be evaluated if the pulse is below 60 beats per minute. Likewise, it is common for older patients to manifest irregular pulses often with occasional pauses or extra beats. Again, any client with an irregular pulse should be referred for further examination. Chapter 21 describes a complete assessment of the older client.

Psychosocial Considerations

Most experts believe that, although stress does not cause hypertension and cerebrovascular accidents (or CVAs, commonly called strokes), stress may contribute to the overall risk and merits some attention. A CVA is an interruption in blood supply to the brain. Oxygen deprivation rapidly kills brain cells, which cannot regenerate. The primary means of preventing a stroke is to control hypertension. A growing body of evidence shows that job strain by itself may contribute to hypertension. In general, blood pressure levels for most individuals tend to be higher at work than at home. In addition, people who hold high-stress jobs, such as air-traffic controllers, have been shown to have higher blood pressure than individuals in other professions. Jobs that demand careful attention to detail but give the worker little latitude for decision-making and offer little person satisfaction are most commonly associated with hypertension. A sense of control is apparently an important characteristic in controlling stress.

Studies have shown that relaxation techniques such as biofeedback, progressive relaxation, and yoga can lower mild hypertension by up to 5 mm Hg and may also relieve stress.

Self-Care Considerations

The most effective means of preventing a CVA is the control of hypertension. Reducing risk factors, such as cigarette smoking and high serum cholesterol levels, help to prevent CVAs.

Varicose veins occur in at least 10% of men and 40% of women, and the incidence increases dramatically after age 60 (*Johns Hopkins Medical Letter* 1993a). The condition occurs as veins begin to stretch and lose their elasticity. Eventually the valves no longer close properly, and blood flows backward and pools in the affected vein, which swells into twisted, bulging masses just beneath the skin. Clients who spend a significant part of the day standing or sitting in one position are at risk. Other factors include crossing the legs and wearing garters or other constricting garments on the legs. Elevating the legs above the level of the heart promotes circulation.

Any client who has poor circulation, including persons who have diabetes mellitus, must be vigilant in caring for the legs and feet. The risk of infection is high, especially as the client ages. All people should always wear properly fitting shoes and socks, and older adults should inspect their feet daily for blisters or abrasions. Any type of foot care, such as removing corns or calluses, should be performed by a podiatrist. Toenails should be trimmed straight across to avoid ingrown toenails.

Family, Cultural, and Environmental Considerations

There is a greater incidence of hypertension in persons of African descent. Thirty-eight percent of African-Americans have high blood pressure (readings equal to or above 140/90) versus 29% of European-Americans. In 1987, the death rate from strokes was 51.2 per 100,000 African-Americans (U.S. Department of Health and Human Services 1990).

Risk factors for varicose veins include Irish and German descents, family history of varicosities, and a sedentary lifestyle.

Clients whose jobs require them to stand for most of the day, such as hairdressers and cashiers, are at greater risk for developing varicose veins. Desk jobs that require sitting for prolonged periods also contribute to venous stasis and varicose veins.

Organizing the Data

After carrying out the focused interview and conducting the physical assessment of the peripheral vascular system, begin to group the related data into clusters leading to nursing diagnoses, which require nursing interventions such as client teaching (discussed on pages 481–485), or alterations in health, which require consultation with other members of the health care team.

Identifying Nursing Diagnoses

Nursing assessment of the peripheral vascular system may lead to the diagnosis of *Altered tissue perfusion* if the client has impaired circulation related to diabetes mellitus, or an obstruction of blood flow related to a blood clot or vascular disease (Table 16.1 on page 480). *Activity intolerance* may apply if the client is unable to perform activities of daily living because of pain or weakness in a lower limb (Table 16.1). *Body image disturbance* might be an appropriate diagnosis for a client who has severe varicosities in the legs. For a client who has suffered a stroke and is unable to eat, bathe, dress, or perform other self-care activites, the nursing diagnosis *Self-care deficit* is appropriate.

Other nursing diagnoses which may apply are *Disuse syndrome, Fear, Impaired mobility, High risk for injury,* and *Impaired skin integrity.*

Table 16.1 Nursing Diagnoses Commonly Associated with the Peripheral Vascular System

ALTERED TISSUE PERFUSION: PERIPHERAL

Definition: The state in which an individual experiences a decrease in nutrition and oxygenation at the cellular level due to a deficit in capillary blood supply (NANDA).

RELATED FACTORS

Interruption of arterial flow, Interruption of venous flow, Exchange problems, Hypovolemia, Hypervolemia.

DEFINING CHARACTERISTICS

Skin temperature
Cold extremities
Blue or purple skin on dependent extremity
Skin pale when extremity is lifted
Color does not return when leg is lowered
Diminished arterial pulsations
Shiny skin
Lack of lanugo
Round scars covered with atrophied skin
Gangrene
Slow-growing, dry, brittle nails
Claudication
Blood pressure changes in extremities
Bruits
Slow healing of lesions

ACTIVITY INTOLERANCE

Definition: A state in which an individual has insufficient physiologic or psychologic energy to endure or complete required or desired daily activities (NANDA).

RELATED FACTORS

Anxiety, Arrhythmias, Imbalance between oxygen supply and demand, Acute Pain, Chronic Pain, Weakness/fatigue, Sedentary lifestyle, Others specific to client (specify).

DEFINING CHARACTERISTICS

Complaints of fatigue and weakness
Abnormal heart rate or blood pressure in response to activity
Exertional discomfort or dyspnea
EKG changes during activity reflecting arrhythmias or ischemia

DIAGNOSTIC REASONING IN ACTION

Mitchell Terry is a 56-year-old stockbroker who comes to his firm's employee wellness clinic to have his blood pressure measured. He tells nurse Wendy Shimmon that during his last physical his physician told him that he had "mild hypertension." However, he says he has no symptoms and does not understand what this diagnosis means. Mrs. Shimmon measures Mr. Terry's blood pressure at 144/92. She explains that anyone who has a blood pressure reading above 140/90 has a very real risk of heart disease or stroke. Sixty percent of the deaths attributed to hypertension-induced coronary artery disease in the US occur in people with so-called mild hypertension (*Johns Hopkins Medical Letter* 1993b).

Mr. Terry is 6' tall and weighs 240 pounds. He states, "I used to be able to eat whatever I wanted without gaining an ounce, but since my fiftieth birthday, I seem to have gained a few pounds every year." When asked about his diet, he says that he eats meat twice a day and usually has a chocolate bar in the mid-afternoon "to keep me going." Mr. Terry does not exercise regularly. He smokes two packs of cigarettes a day and consumes 2 to 3 cocktails before dinner.

Mrs. Shimmon clusters this information and arrives at the following nursing diagnoses:

- *Knowledge deficit* related to lack of information about hypertension
- *Altered nutrition: more than body requirements* related to excessive intake, decreased metabolic requirements, and lack of physical exercise.

Mrs. Shimmon tells Mr. Terry that with just a few changes in his lifestyle he may be able to reduce his blood pressure without the use of medication. Mrs. Shimmon then gives Mr. Terry some suggestions for eliminating or reducing his alcohol intake, provides him with a low-fat diet emphasizing complex carbohydrates, and offers him a referral to a smoking-cessation clinic. Although a regular exercise program would be most beneficial, she suggests that Mr.Terry do some additional walking each day.

Mrs. Shimmon suggests that Mr. Terry return to the clinic in 1 month for a follow-up evaluation of his blood pressure.

Common Alterations in the Health of the Peripheral Vascular and Lymphatic Systems

Common alterations in the health of the peripheral vascular and lymphatic systems include insufficiency of the venous and arterial systems as well as the complications arising from these insufficiencies. Table 16.2 on page 482 provides a list of normal and abnormal pulses, their characteristics, arterial waveform pattern, and the conditions that might contribute to these pulses. Table 16.3 on page 483 describes some of the most common alterations in peripheral vascular health.

Health Promotion and Client Education

At the conclusion of the assessment, answer any questions the client may have. All clients need information on promoting and maintaining the health of the peripheral vascular system. Clients with current alterations in peripheral vascular health need counseling on how to prevent their current health problem from worsening.

Promoting the Health of the Peripheral Vascular System

Diseases of the heart and blood vessels are among the leading causes of death and disability in the United States. Current research demonstrates that a reduction in high blood pressure can significantly reduce the chances of both stroke and heart attack. Recent evidence indicates that cigarette smoking is also a risk factor for stroke and that smoking cessation will reduce the risk of a stroke. Progressive kidney failure is a serious complication of high blood pressure; 26% of all cases of kidney failure are due to high blood pressure (U.S. Department of Health and Human Services 1990). The principal damage done by high blood pressure is to the wall of the smaller arteries, which both thicken and lose their strength from prolonged exposure to high pressure. As a result, blood flow to tissues is reduced, and arteries become prone to rupture. The consequences can include strokes, kidney damage, and loss of vision due to injured blood vessels in the eye.

Losing excess weight is an important measure to lower blood pressure. The best strategy for weight control combines regular aerobic exercise with a low-fat diet. Aerobic exercise,

Text continues on page 485

Table 16.2 Normal and Abnormal Pulses

Name of Pulse	Characteristics	Arterial Waveform Pattern	Contributing Conditions
Normal	◆ Regular, even in intensity		◆ Normal
Absent	◆ No palpable pulse, no waveform		◆ Cardiac arrest ◆ Arterial line disconnected
Weak/thready	◆ Intensity of pulse is +1 ◆ May wax and wane ◆ May be difficult to find		◆ Shock ◆ Severe peripheral vascular disease
Bounding	◆ Intensity of pulse is +4 ◆ Very easy to observe in arterial locations near surface of skin ◆ Very easy to palpate and difficult to obliterate with pressure from fingertips		◆ Hyperdynamic states such as seen with hyperthyroidism, exercise, anxiety, vasodilation seen in high cardiac output syndromes ◆ May be due to normal aging secondary to arterial wall stiffening ◆ Aortic regurgitation ◆ Anemia
Biferiens	◆ Has two systolic peaks with a dip in between ◆ Easier to detect in the carotid location ◆ In the case of hypertrophic obstructive cardiomyopathy, only one systolic peak palpated, but waveform demonstrates double systolic peak		◆ Aortic regurgitation ◆ Combination of aortic regurgitation and stenosis ◆ Hypertrophic obstructive cardiomyopathy
Pulsus alternans	◆ Alternating strong and weak pulses ◆ Equal interval between each pulse		◆ Aortic regurgitation ◆ Terminal left ventricular heart failure ◆ Systemic hypertension
Pulsus bigeminus	◆ Alternating strong and weak pulses, but the weak pulse comes in *early* after the strong pulse		◆ Regular bigeminal dysrhythmias such as PVCs and PACs
Pulsus paradoxus	◆ Reduced intensity of pulse during inspiration versus expiration	Inspiration Expiration	◆ Cardiac tamponade ◆ Acute pulmonary embolus ◆ Pericarditis ◆ May be present in clients with chronic lung disease ◆ Hypovolemic shock ◆ Pregnancy
Water-Hammer, Corrigan's pulse	◆ Rapid systolic upstroke and no dicrotic notch secondary to rapid		◆ Aortic regurgitation
Unequal	◆ Difference in intensity or amplitude between right and left pulses	Right femoral Left femoral	◆ Dissecting aneurysm (location of aneurysm determines where the difference in amplitude is felt)

Table 16.3 Common Alterations in the Health of the Peripheral Vascular and Lymphatic Systems

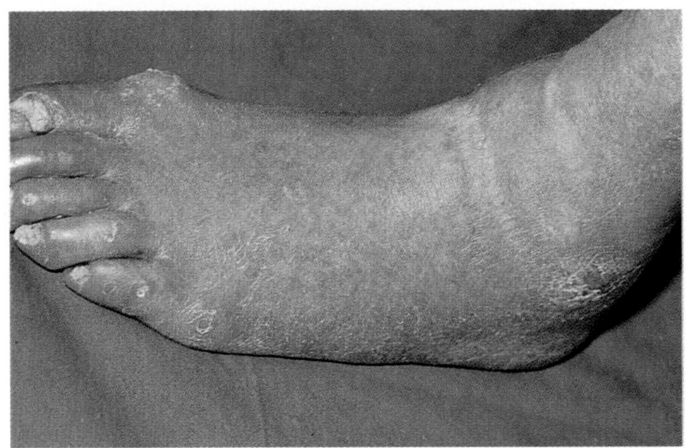 Arterial Insufficiency	Inadequate circulation in the arterial system usually due to the build-up of fatty plaque and/or calcification of the arterial wall resulting in diminished pulses; cool, shiny skin; absence of hair on toes; pallor on elevation, red color when dependent; and deep muscle pain, usually in the calf or lower leg aggravated by activity and elevation of the limb. Pain is quickly relieved by rest. Ulcers due to arterial insufficiency are usually seen on the toes or areas of trauma of the feet or lateral malleolus. The ulcer is pale in color with well-defined edges and no bleeding.
Arterial Aneurysm	A bulging or dilation caused by a weakness in the wall of an artery. It can occur in the aorta and abdominal, renal, or femoral arteries. Aneurysms can sometimes be detected by a characteristic bruit over the artery; however, if they are located deep in the abdomen, they can be difficult to discover.
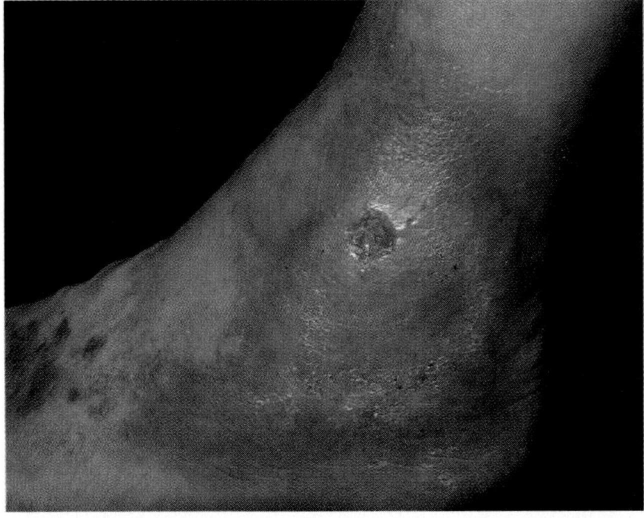 Venous Insufficiency	Inadequate circulation in the venous system usually due to incompetent valves in deep veins or a blood clot in the veins. Temperature of skin is normal, but edema is usually present accompanied by a feeling of fullness in the legs. Skin around the ankles may be thickened and have a brown discoloration. Discomfort is aggravated by prolonged standing or sitting and is relieved by rest but only after several hours. Ulcers related to venous insufficiency are often found on the medial malleolus and are characterized by bleeding, uneven edges. There is minimal pain associated with the ulcer, and the skin surrounding the ulcer is coarse.

Table 16.3 Alterations in the Health of the Peripheral Vascular and Lymphatic Systems (continued)

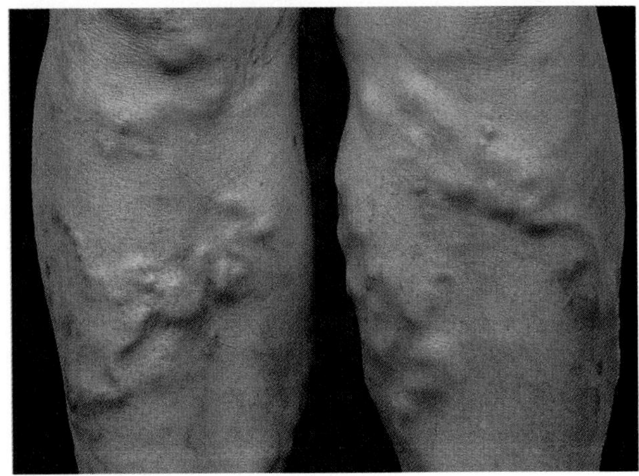

Varicose Veins

Veins that have become dilated and have a diminished rate of blood flow and increased intravenous pressure. The condition may be the result of incompetent valves that permit the reflux of blood or an obstruction of a proximal vein.

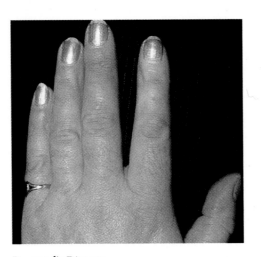

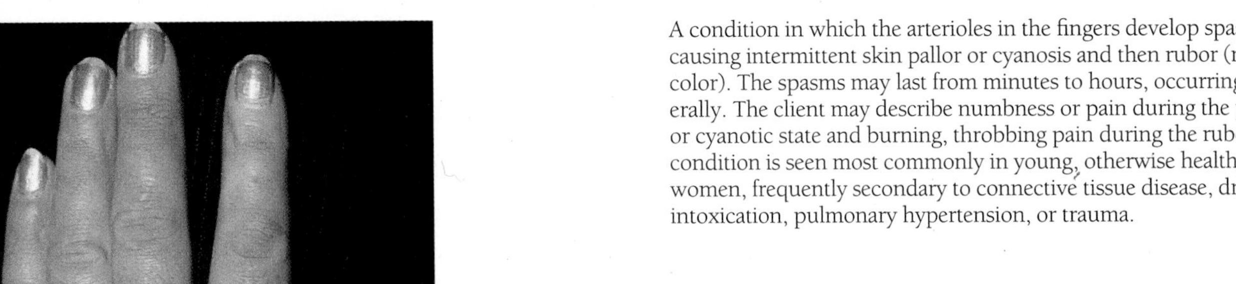

Raynaud's Disease

A condition in which the arterioles in the fingers develop spasms, causing intermittent skin pallor or cyanosis and then rubor (red color). The spasms may last from minutes to hours, occurring bilaterally. The client may describe numbness or pain during the pallor or cyanotic state and burning, throbbing pain during the rubor. This condition is seen most commonly in young, otherwise healthy women, frequently secondary to connective tissue disease, drug intoxication, pulmonary hypertension, or trauma.

Deep Vein Thrombosis

The occlusion of a deep vein, such as in the femoral or pelvic circulation, by a blood clot. There may be no symptoms, or the client may describe intense, sharp pain along the iliac vessels, in the popliteal space, or in the calf muscles. Pain may increase with sharp dorsiflexion of the foot (Homan's sign), but this maneuver is not absolutely reliable for diagnosis. There may also be slight swelling of the leg, some edema, low-grade fever, and tachycardia (rapid heartbeat). This condition requires immediate referral because of the danger of the clot migrating to the lung, resulting in a pulmonary embolism.

when regularly performed, helps keep blood pressure at normal levels, reduces the risk of heart disease, and aids in weight control. In hypertensive individuals who exercise regularly, studies have found a decrease in blood pressure about 10 mm Hg systolic and 8 mm Hg diastolic (*Harvard Medical School Health Letter* 1989).

Although research findings are controversial, high salt intake seems to play a relatively minor role in *causing* high blood pressure. However, once hypertension is established, salt restriction can help with control (*Harvard Medical School Health Letter* 1988). Reduction of salt intake by itself is rarely sufficient to normalize high blood pressure. Most authorities seem to agree that it makes sense to keep the daily intake of salt to less than 3000 mg, slightly more than a teaspoon of salt.

There is convincing evidence that alcohol contributes to raising blood pressure, independently of any other factors. Currently, estimates are that alcohol intake accounts for 5–25% of all cases of primary essential hypertension—the type that occurs without a detectable basis in some other disease (*Harvard Medical School Health Letter* 1987). Consuming one drink a day has very little influence on blood pressure, but more than three drinks can measurably raise it. Fortunately, the effect appears to be reversible, and heavy drinkers who eliminate alcohol can lower both their systolic and diastolic pressures by more than 10 points.

Medications to control hypertension are associated with certain unpleasant side effects. Some individuals complain of dizziness, nausea, headache, and lack of energy. Men frequently complain of an onset of impotence with this therapy. Therefore, noncompliance with treatment is a major limiting factor in reducing hypertension. Client education is crucial in these circumstances. Adequate control of high blood pressure with a minimum of side effects requires close cooperation between client and physician. You can play an important role in interpreting these facts to the client.

Clients who have venous or arterial insufficiency in the lower limbs must take special care to avoid infections of the feet and legs. Some helpful self-care measures include:

- Apply lotion to feet daily (but not between the toes) to keep skin moist.
- Test water temperature before putting feet in the tub to avoid burning the skin.
- Inspect the legs and feet daily for abrasions, blisters, or any sign of trauma that might lead to infection.
- Wear support hose or stockings to promote venous return.
- Clients who have diabetes should control blood glucose to prevent vascular complications and avoid wearing garments that might inhibit circulation in the legs.

Summary

The peripheral vascular and lymphatic system provides the circulation for the body by means of arteries, veins, and lymphatic vessels. Knowledge of the anatomy and physiology of the circulatory system helps you perform the assessment and understand normal variations that occur in certain client groups. The interview concerning the circulatory system allows you to identify any significant factors in the client's history that you should pursue in depth during the physical assessment. During the physical assessment, you identify any variations from the norms that may indicate the need for referral to a physician. After performing the health assessment and identifying any appropriate nursing diagnoses, provide the client with the information needed to promote the health of the peripheral vascular system.

Key Points

- ✓ The peripheral vascular system consists of arteries, veins, capillaries, and the lymphatic vessels. The major function of the vascular system is to deliver oxygen to the tissues, release carbon dioxide from the tissues into the lungs, transport waste products for excretion, and produce lymphocytes to prevent the invasion of foreign substances.
- ✓ A focused interview is conducted to gather specific information about the structures of the vascular system, including the client's health history; self-care practices; and family, cultural, and environmental factors.
- ✓ During the physical assessment of the peripheral vascular system, you use the techniques of inspection, palpation, and auscultation.
- ✓ Nursing diagnoses commonly associated with the head and neck include *Altered peripheral tissue perfusion, Activity intolerance, Body image disturbance, Impaired skin integrity,* and *Self-care deficit.*
- ✓ Provide the client with information needed to promote health of the peripheral vascular system.

Chapter 17

Assessing the Musculoskeletal System

The primary function of the musculoskeletal system is to provide structure and movement for the human body. Its 206 bones and accompanying skeletal muscles allow the body to stand erect and move, support and protect body organs, produce red blood cells, store fat and minerals, and generate heat.

A thorough assessment of the musculoskeletal system provides data relevant to activity, exercise, nutrition, and metabolism. Because the musculoskeletal system extends throughout the body, the physical assessment is extensive, requiring a head-to-toe approach. Also, because every other body system is affected by or affects this system, the musculoskeletal assessment is usually combined with assessments of other body systems to obtain data reflecting the client's total health status. Figure 17.1 shows the relationship between the musculoskeletal system and some other body systems. Included in this figure are selected developmental, psychosocial, self-care, and environmental considerations that you should keep in mind while assessing the musculoskeletal system for each individual client.

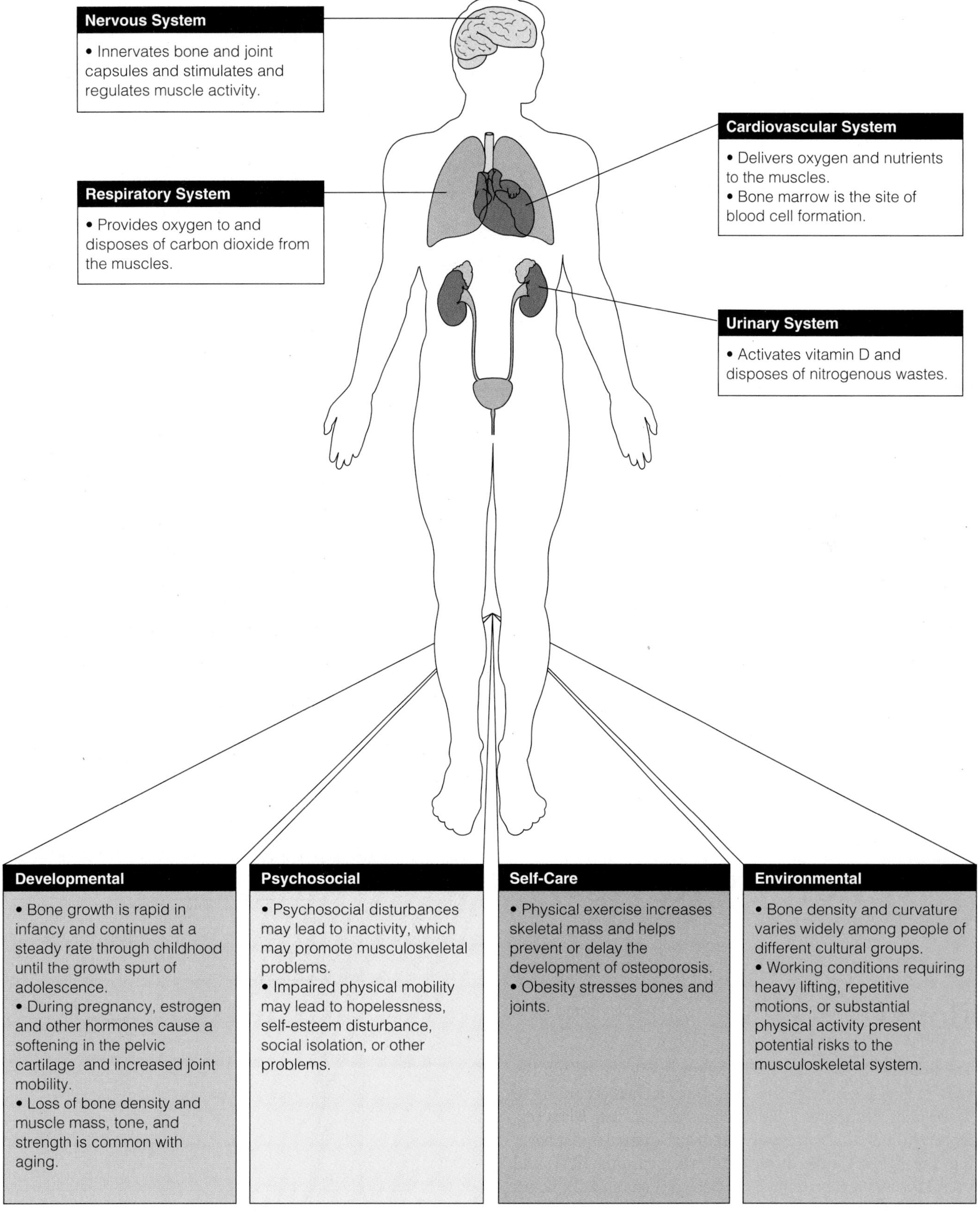

Nervous System
• Innervates bone and joint capsules and stimulates and regulates muscle activity.
Respiratory System
• Provides oxygen to and disposes of carbon dioxide from the muscles.
Cardiovascular System
• Delivers oxygen and nutrients to the muscles.
• Bone marrow is the site of blood cell formation.
Urinary System
• Activates vitamin D and disposes of nitrogenous wastes.
Developmental
• Bone growth is rapid in infancy and continues at a steady rate through childhood until the growth spurt of adolescence.
• During pregnancy, estrogen and other hormones cause a softening in the pelvic cartilage and increased joint mobility.
• Loss of bone density and muscle mass, tone, and strength is common with aging.
Psychosocial
• Psychosocial disturbances may lead to inactivity, which may promote musculoskeletal problems.
• Impaired physical mobility may lead to hopelessness, self-esteem disturbance, social isolation, or other problems.
Self-Care
• Physical exercise increases skeletal mass and helps prevent or delay the development of osteoporosis.
• Obesity stresses bones and joints.
Environmental
• Bone density and curvature varies widely among people of different cultural groups.
• Working conditions requiring heavy lifting, repetitive motions, or substantial physical activity present potential risks to the musculoskeletal system.

Figure 17.1 An overview of important factors to consider when assessing the musculoskeletal system.

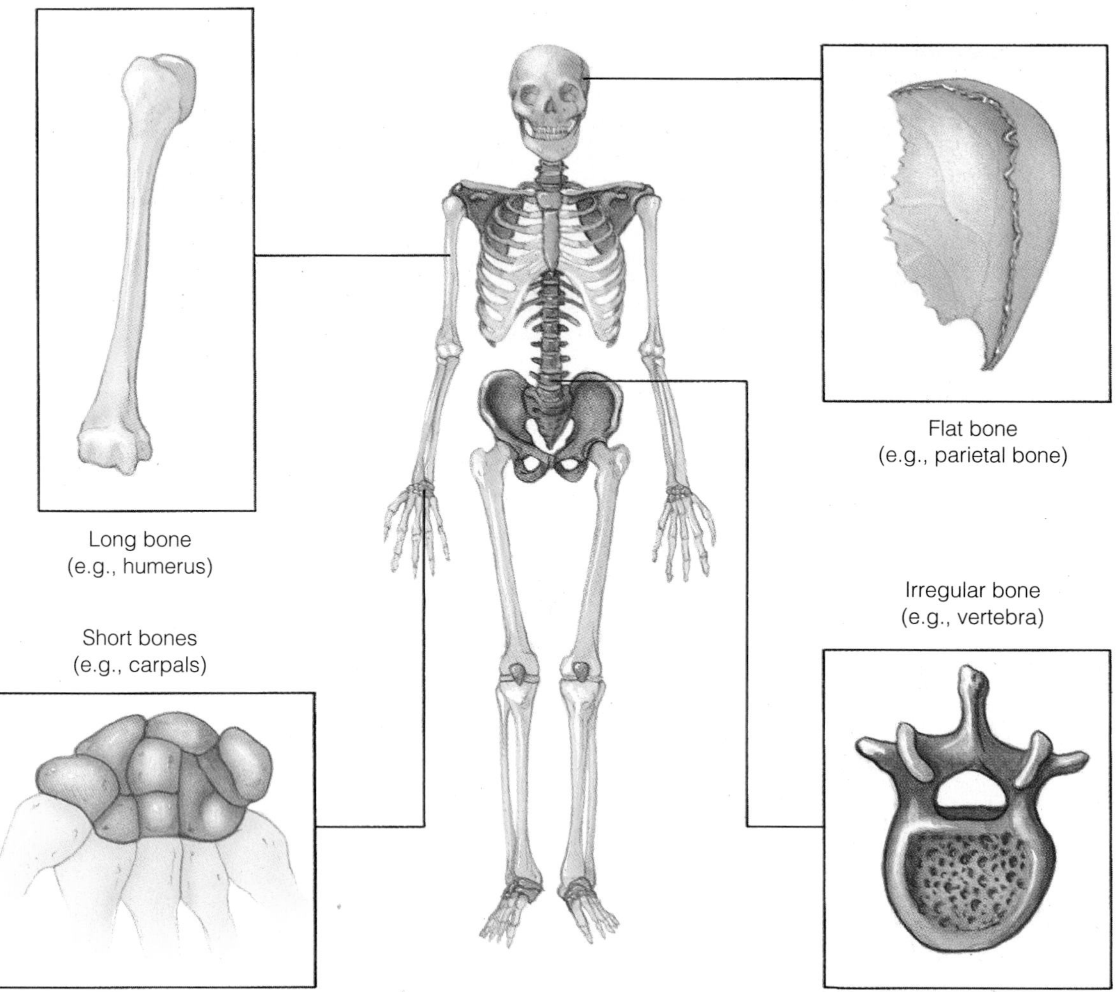

Figure 17.2 Classification of bones according to shape.

Anatomy and Physiology Review

Bones

The **bones** support and provide a framework for the soft tissues and organs of the body. They are classified according to shape and composition. Bone shapes include *long bones* (eg, femur, humerus), *short bones* (eg, carpals, tarpals), *flat bones* (eg, the parietal bone of the skull, the sternum, ribs), and *irregular bones* (eg, vertebrae, hip bones) (Figure 17.2). Bones are composed of osseous tissue that is arranged in either a dense, smooth, compact structure, or a cancellous, spongy structure with many small open spaces (Figure 17.3). The bones of the human skeleton are illustrated in Figure 17.4.

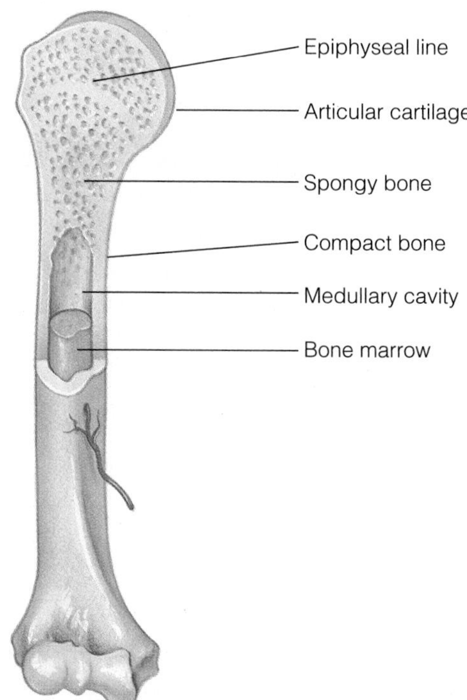

Figure 17.3 Composition of a long bone.

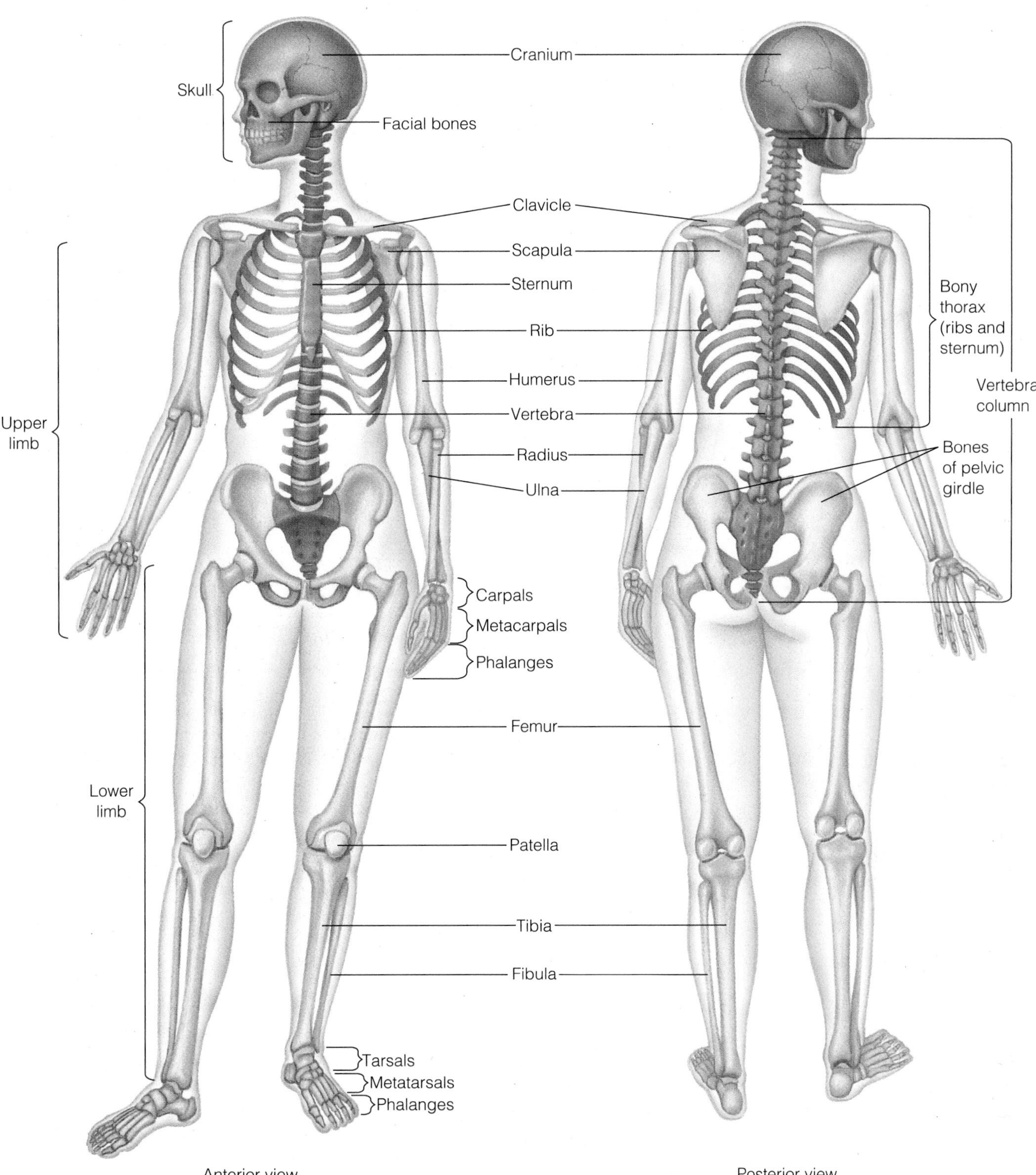

Figure 17.4 Bones of the human skeleton.

The major functions of the bones are

- Providing a framework for the body
- Anchoring inner organs
- Protecting body structures
- Acting as levers for movement
- Storing fat and minerals
- Producing blood cells

Skeletal Muscles

A **skeletal muscle** is composed of hundreds of thousands of elongated muscle cells or *fibers* arranged in striated bands that attach to skeletal bones (Figure 17.5). Although some skeletal muscles react by reflex, most skeletal muscles are voluntary and are under an individual's conscious control. Figures 17.6, *A* and *B* show the muscles of the human body.

The major functions of the skeletal muscles are

- Providing for movement
- Maintaining posture
- Generating heat

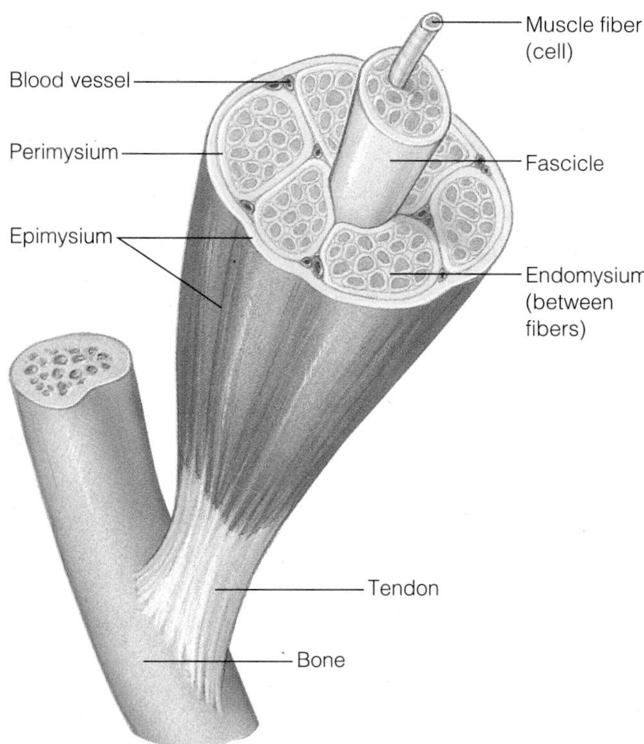

Figure 17.5 Composition of a skeletal muscle.

Joints

A **joint** (or *articulation*) is the point where two or more bones of the body meet. Joints may be classified structurally as fibrous, cartilaginous, or synovial. Bones joined by fibrous tissue, such as the sutures joining the bones of the skull, are called *fibrous joints*. Bones joined by cartilage, such as the vertebrae, are called *cartilaginous joints*. Bones separated by a fluid-filled joint cavity are called *synovial joints*. The structure of synovial joints allows tremendous freedom of movement, and all joints of the limbs are synovial joints. Most synovial joints are reinforced and strengthened by a system of *ligaments*, bands of flexible tissue that attach bone to bone. Some are protected from friction by small, synovial-fluid-filled sacs called *bursae*. *Tendons* are tough fibrous bands that attach muscle to bone, or muscle to muscle. In tendons subjected to continuous friction, an elongated fluid-filled bursa called a *tendon sheath* wraps itself around the tendon to protect it from damage.

During the assessment of the musculoskeletal system, you should assess the joint, its range of motion, and its surrounding structures of muscles, ligaments, tendons, and bursae (see Table 17.1 on page 493 for a description of joint types and movements). A description of selected joints to be examined during an assessment of the musculoskeletal system follows.

Temporomandibular Joint

The **temporomandibular joint** permits articulation between the mandible and the temporal bone of the skull (Figure 17.7 on page 496). Lying just anterior to the external auditory meatus, the temporomandibular joint allows an individual to speak and chew. Temporomandibular movements include

- Opening and closing of the jaw
- Protraction and retraction
- Side-to-side movement of lower jaw

Shoulder

The **shoulder joint** is a ball-and-socket joint in which the head of the humerus articulates in the shallow glenoid cavity of the scapula (see Table 17.1). It is supported by the rotator cuff, a sturdy network of tendons and muscles, as well as a series of ligaments (Figure 17.8 on page 497). The major landmarks include the scapula, acromion process, greater tubercle of the humerus, and the coracoid process. The subacromial bursa, which allows the arm to abduct smoothly and with ease, lies just below the acromion process. Movements of the shoulder include:

- Abduction (180°)
- Adduction (50°)

Text continues on page 497

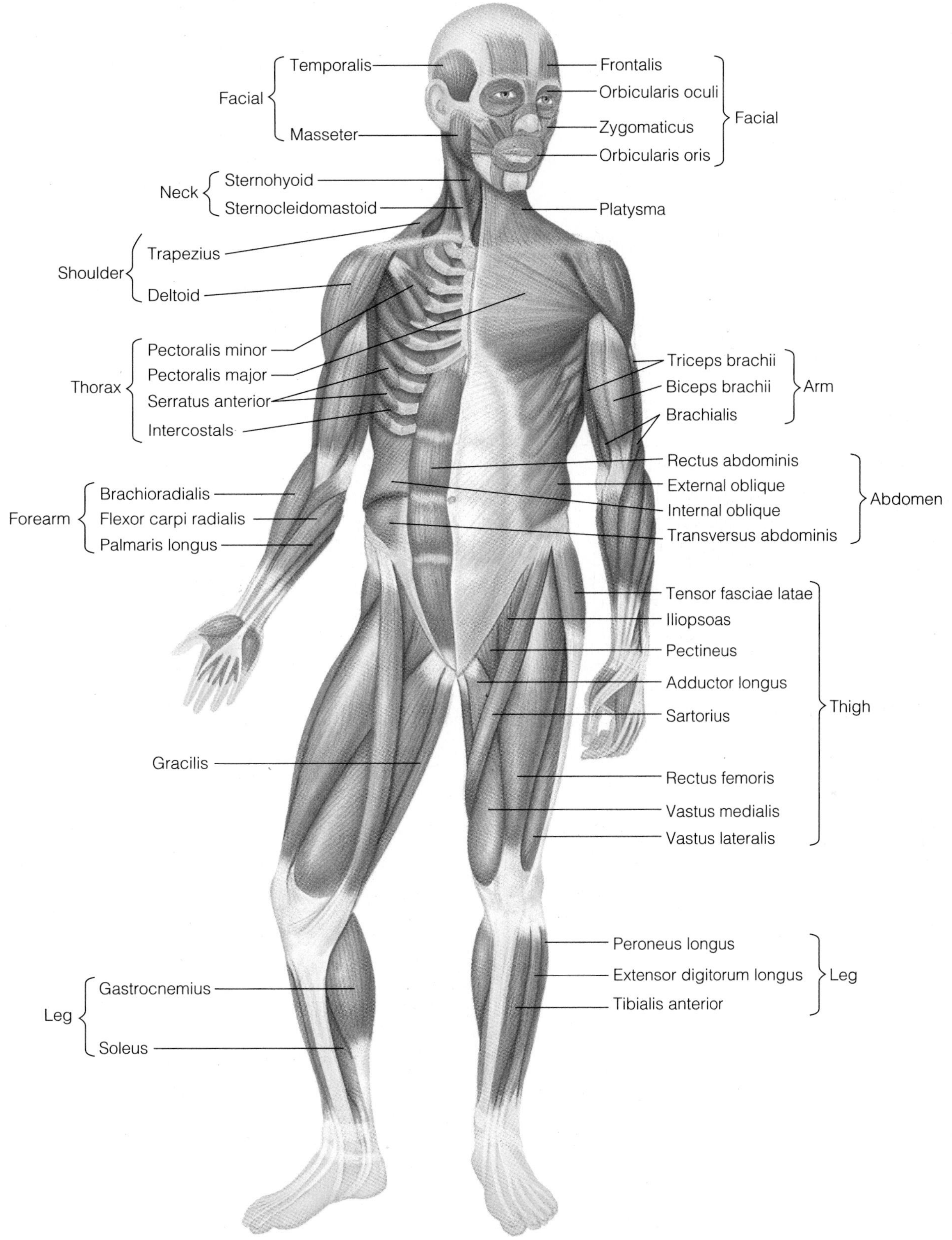

Figure 17.6 Muscles of the human body.

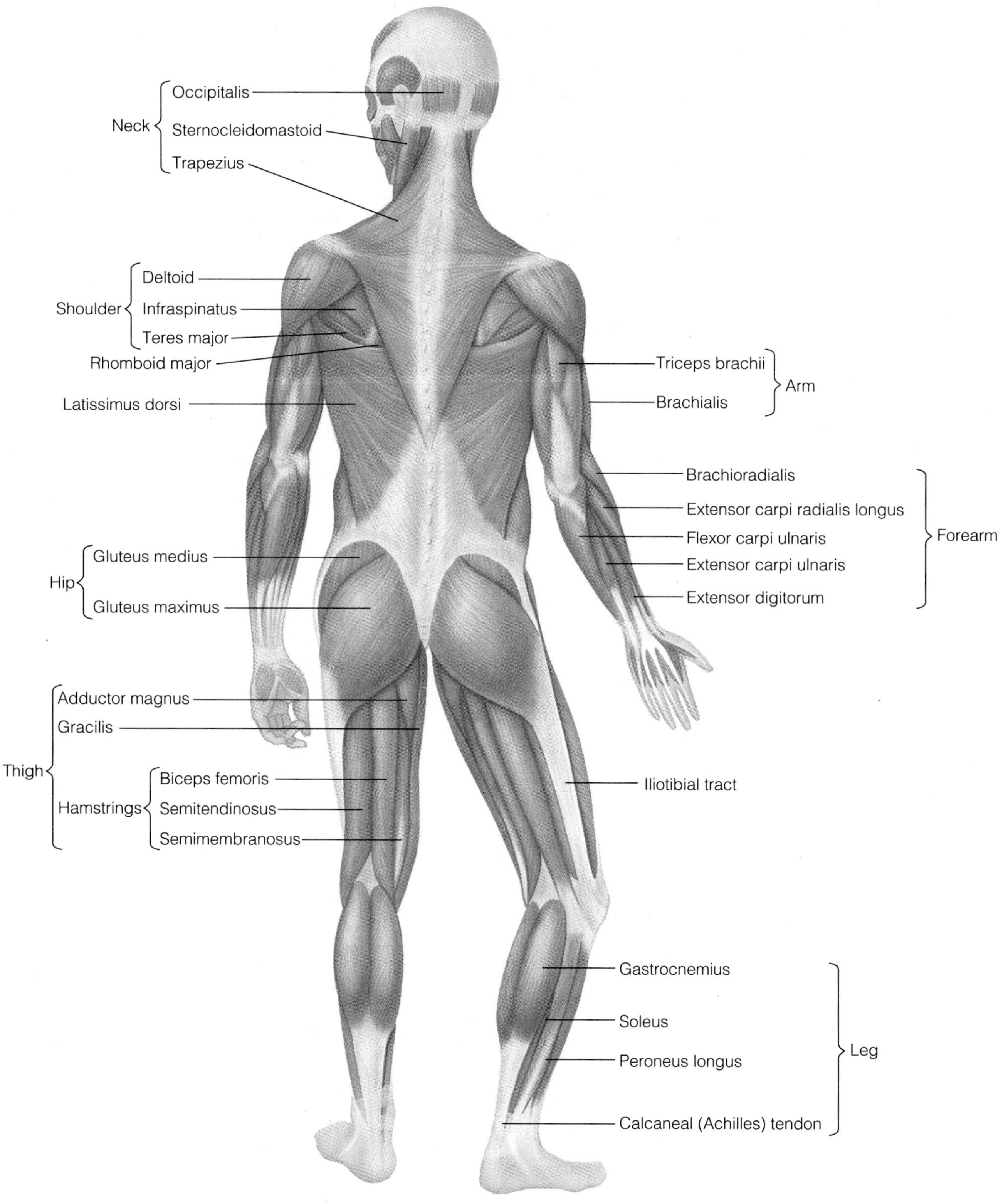
Neck
Occipitalis
Sternocleidomastoid
Trapezius
Shoulder
Deltoid
Infraspinatus
Teres major
Rhomboid major
Latissimus dorsi
Triceps brachii
Brachialis
Arm
Brachioradialis
Extensor carpi radialis longus
Flexor carpi ulnaris
Extensor carpi ulnaris
Extensor digitorum
Forearm
Hip
Gluteus medius
Gluteus maximus
Thigh
Adductor magnus
Gracilis
Hamstrings
Biceps femoris
Semitendinosus
Semimembranosus
Iliotibial tract
Gastrocnemius
Soleus
Peroneus longus
Calcaneal (Achilles) tendon
Leg
B

Figure 17.6 Muscles of the human body.

Table 17.1 Synovial Joints: Classification and Movements

Type of Joint

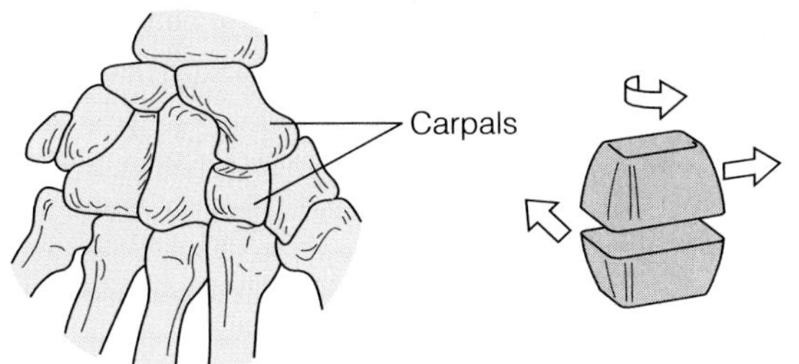

A Plane joint

In *plane joints*, the articular surfaces are flat, allowing only slipping or gliding movements. Examples include the intercarpal and intertarsal joints, and the joints between the articular processes of the ribs.

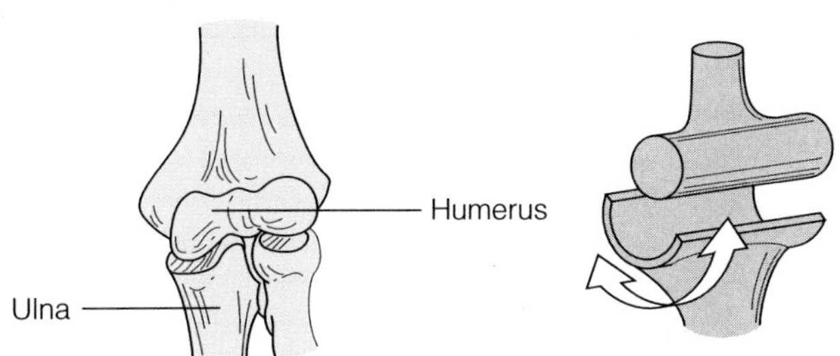

B Hinge joint

In *hinge joints*, a convex projection of one bone fits into a concave depression in another. Motion is similar to that of a mechanical hinge. These joints permit flexion and extension only. Examples include the elbow and knee joints.

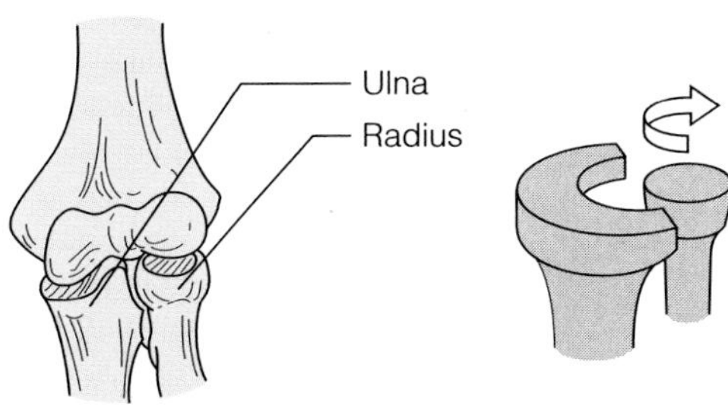

C Pivot joint

In *pivot joints*, the rounded end of one bone protrudes into a ring of bone (and possibly ligaments). The only movement allowed is rotation of the bone around its own long axis or against the other bone. An example is the joint between the atlas and axis of the neck.

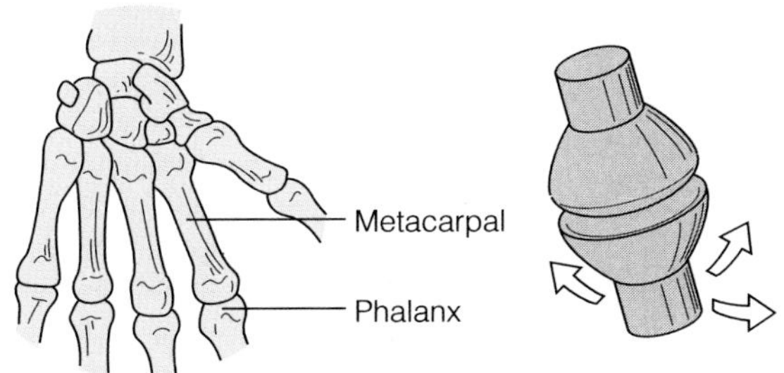

D Condyloid joint

In *condyloid joints*, the oval surfaces of two bones fit together. Movements allowed are flexion and extension, abduction, adduction, and circumduction. An example is the radiocarpal (wrist) joints.

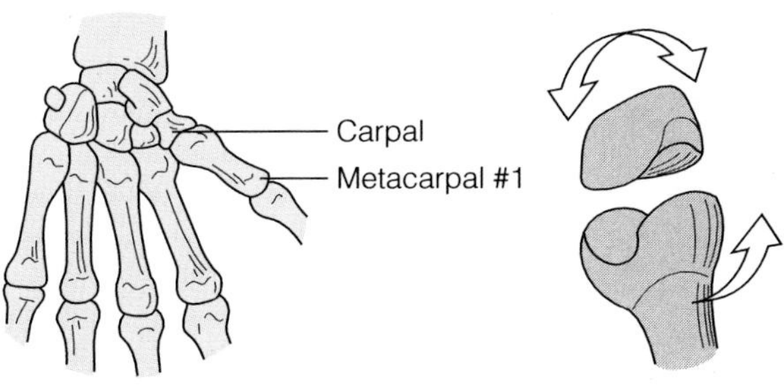

E Saddle joint

In *saddle joints*, each articulating bone has both concave and convex areas (resembling a saddle). The opposing surfaces fit together. The movements allowed are the same as for condyloid joints, but the freedom of motion is greater. The carpometacarpal joints of the thumbs are an example.

Table 17.1 Synovial Joints: Classification and Movements (continued)

Type of Joint (continued)

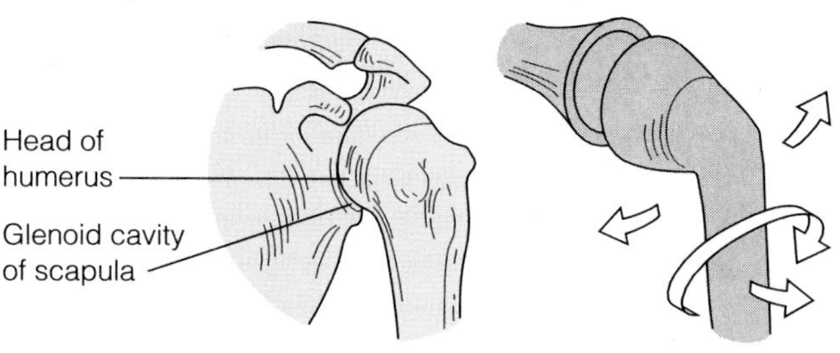

F Ball-and-socket joint

In *ball-and-scoket joints*, the ball-shaped head of one bone fits into the concave socket of another. These joints allow movement in all axes and planes, including rotation. The shoulder and hip joints are the only examples in the body.

Type of Movement

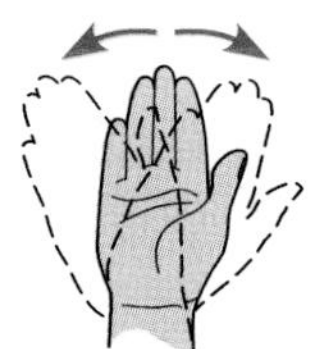

Gliding movements are the simplest type of joint movements. One flat bone surface glides or slips over another similar surface. The bones are merely displaced in relation to one another.

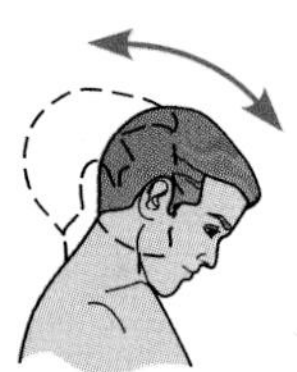

Flexion is a bending movement that decreases the angle of the joint and brings the articulating bones closer together. *Extension* increases the angle between the articulating bones. (*Hyperextension* is a bending of a joint beyond 180°.)

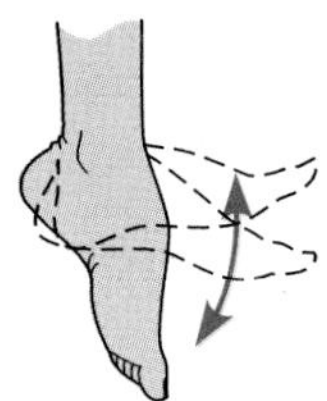

Flexion of the ankle so that the superior aspect of the foot approaches the shin is called *dorsiflexion*. Extension of the ankle (pointing the toes) is called *plantar flexion*.

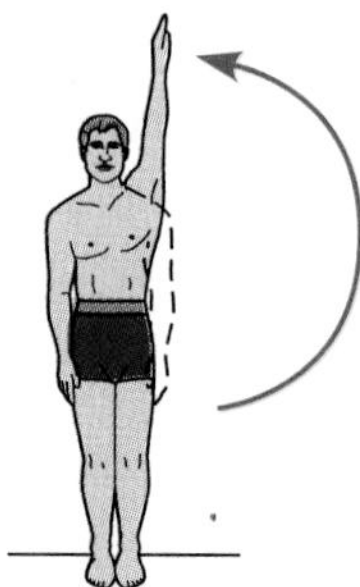

Abduction is movement of a limb away from the midline or median plane of the body, along the frontal plane. When the term is used to describe movement of the fingers or toes, it means spreading them apart. *Adduction* is the movement of a limb toward the body midline. Bringing the fingers close together is adduction.

Table 17.1 Synovial Joints: Classification and Movements (continued)

Type of Movement (continued)

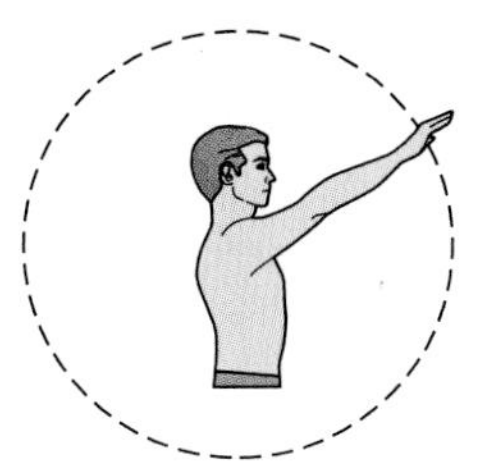

Circumduction is the movement in which the limb describes a cone in space: while the distal end of the limb moves in a circle, the joint itself moves only slightly in the joint cavity.

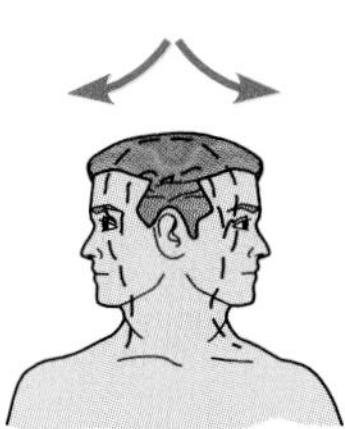

Rotation is the turning movement of a bone around its own long axis. Rotation may occur toward the body midline or away from it.

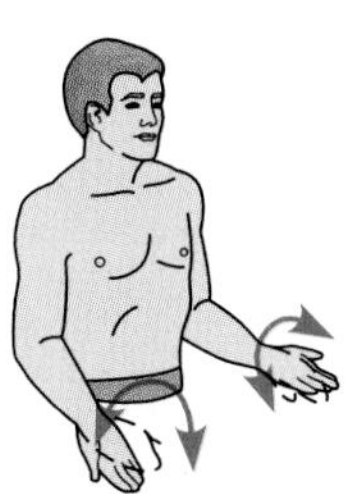

The terms *supination* and *pronation* refer only to the movements of the radius around the ulna. Movement of the forearm so that the palm faces anteriorly or superiorly is called *supination*. In *pronation*, the palm moves to face posteriorly or inferiorly.

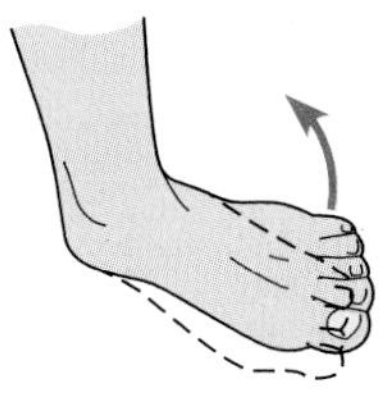

The terms *inversion* and *eversion* refer to movements of the foot. In *inversion*, the sole of the foot is turned medially. In *eversion*, the sole faces laterally.

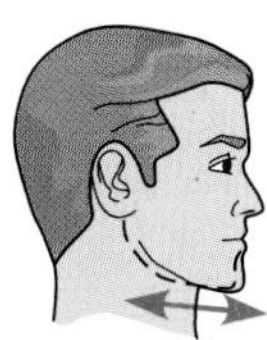

Protraction is a nonangular anterior movement in a transverse plane. *Retraction* is a nonangular posterior movement in a transverse plane.

Table 17.1 Synovial Joints: Classification and Movements (continued)

Type of Movement (continued)

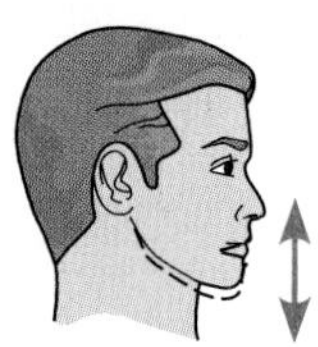

Elevation is a lifting or moving superiorly along a frontal plane. When the elevated part is moved downward to its original position, the movement is called *depression*. Shrugging the shoulders and chewing are examples of alternating elevation and depression.

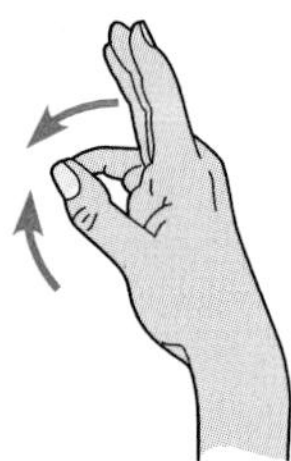

Opposition of the thumb is only allowed at the saddle joint between metacarpal 1 and the carpals. It is the movement of touching the thumb to the tips of the other fingers of the same hand.

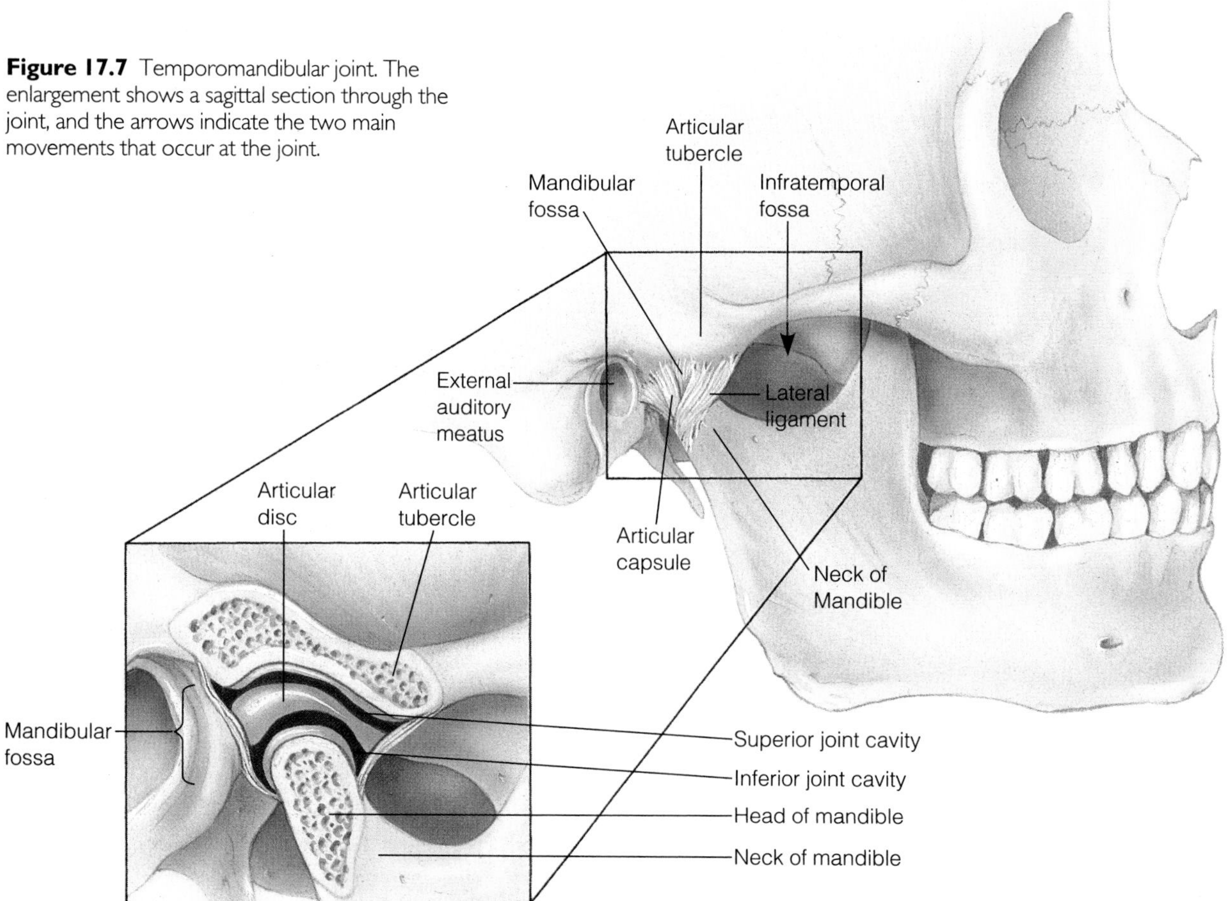

Figure 17.7 Temporomandibular joint. The enlargement shows a sagittal section through the joint, and the arrows indicate the two main movements that occur at the joint.

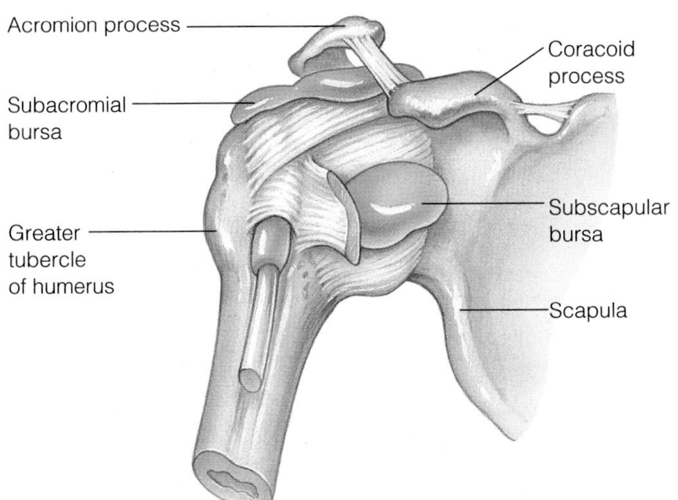

Figure 17.8 Shoulder joint. Anterior view.

- Horizontal forward flexion (180°)
- Horizontal backward extension (50°)
- Circumduction (360°)
- External rotation (90°)
- Internal rotation (90°)

Elbow

The **elbow** is a hinge joint that allows articulation between the humerus of the upper arm, and the radius and ulna of the forearm (Figure 17.9). Landmarks include the lateral and medial epicondyles on either side of the distal end of the humerus, and the olecranon process of the ulna. The olecranon bursa sits between the olecranon process and the skin. The ulnar nerve travels between the medial epicondyle and the olecranon process. When inflamed, the synovial membrane is palpable between the epicondyles and the olecranon process. Elbow movements include

- Flexion of the forearm (160°)
- Extension of the forearm (160°)
- Supination of the forearm and hand (90°)
- Pronation of the forearm and hand (90°)

Wrist and Hand

The **wrist** (or *carpus*) consists of two rows of eight short carpal bones connected by ligaments (Figure 17.10 on page 498). The distal row articulates with the metacarpals of the hand. The proximal row includes the scaphoid and lunate bones, which articulate with the distal end of the radius to form the wrist joint. Wrist movements include

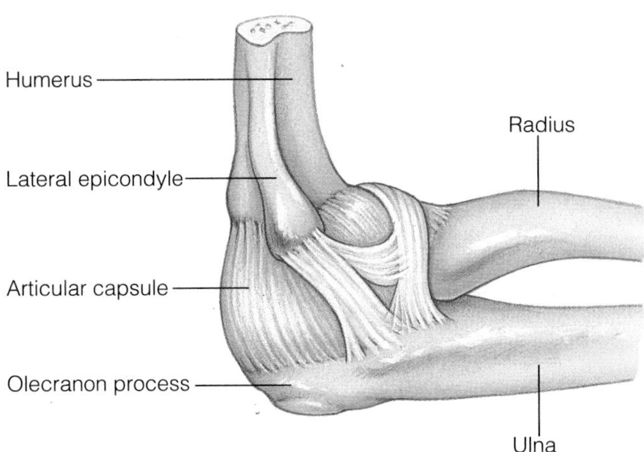

Figure 17.9 Elbow joint. Lateral view of the right elbow.

- Extension (70°)
- Flexion (90°)
- Hyperextension (30°)
- Radial deviation (20°)
- Ulnar deviation (55°)

Each hand has **metacarpophalangeal joints**, and each finger has **interphalangeal joints**. Finger movements include

- Abduction (20°)
- Extension
- Hyperextension (30°)
- Flexion (90°)
- Circumduction

Thumb movements include

- Extension
- Flexion (80°)
- Opposition

Hip

The **hip joint** is a ball-and-socket joint composed of the rounded head of the femur as it fits deep into the *acetabulum*, a rounded cavity on the right and left lateral sides of the pelvic bone (Figure 17.11 on page 498). Although not as mobile as the shoulder, the hip is surrounded by a system of cartilage, ligaments, tendons, and muscles that contribute to its strength and stability. Landmarks include the iliac crest (not shown), the greater trochanter of the femur, and the anterior inferior iliac spine. Hip movements include

- Extension (90°)
- Hyperextension (15°)

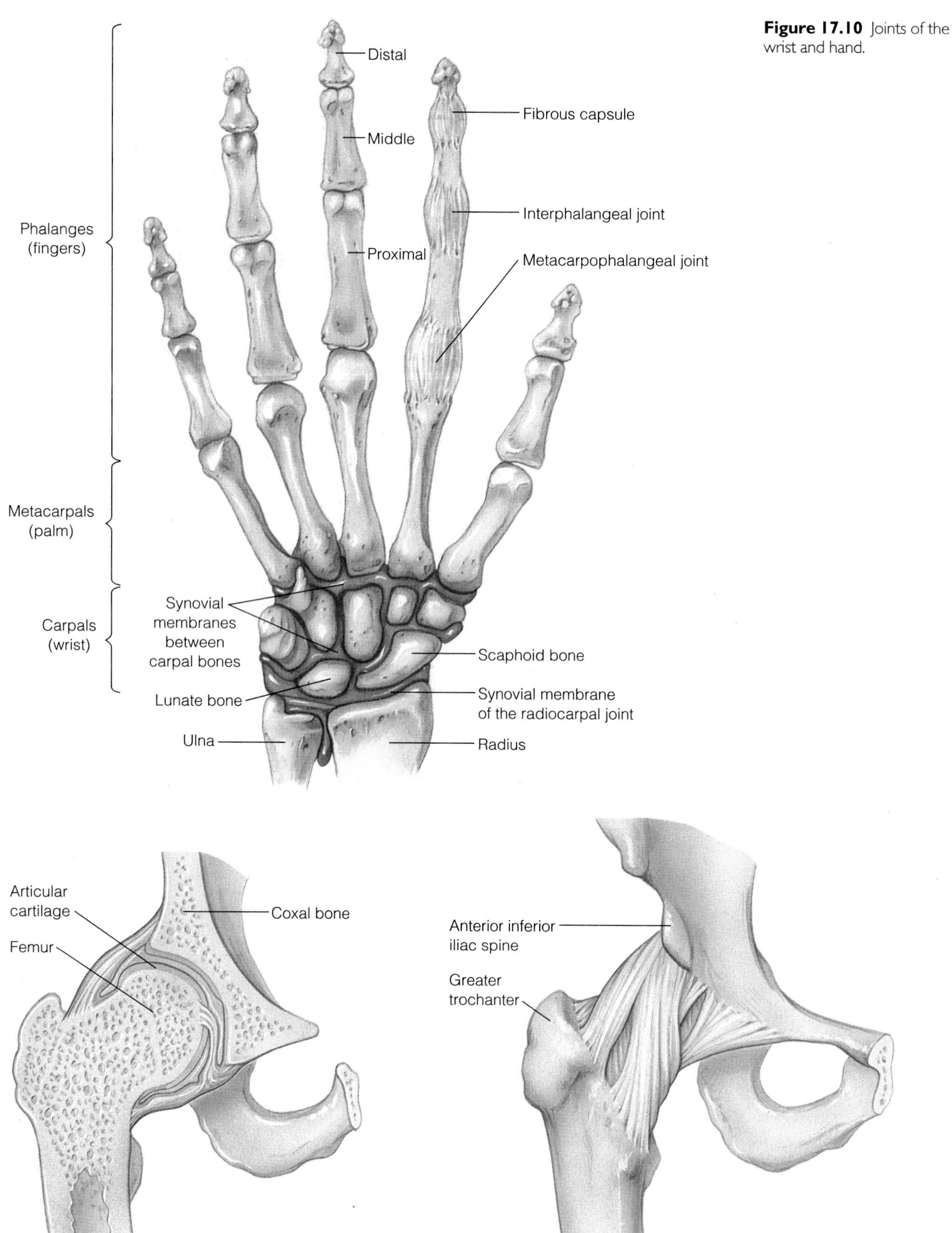

Figure 17.10 Joints of the wrist and hand.

Figure 17.11 Hip joint. *A*, Frontal section. *B*, Anterior view.

- Flexion with knee flexed (120°)
- Flexion with knee extended (90°)
- Internal rotation (40°)
- External rotation (45°)
- Abduction (45°)
- Adduction (30°)

Knee

The **knee** is a complex joint consisting of the patella (kneecap), femur, and tibia (Figure 17.12). It is supported and stabilized by the cruciate and collateral ligaments, which have a stabilizing effect on the knee and prevent dislocation. The landmarks of the knee include the tibial tuberosity and the medial and lateral condyles of the tibia. Knee movements include

- Extension
- Flexion (130°)

Ankle and Foot

The **ankle** is a hinge joint that accommodates articulation between the tibia, fibula, and *talus*, a large, posterior tarsal of the foot (Figure 17.13 on page 500). The *calcaneus* (or "heel-bone") is just inferior to the talus. It is stabilized by a set of taut ligaments that are anchored from bony prominences at the distal ends of the tibia and fibula (the lateral and medial malleoli), then extend and attach to the foot. Movements of the ankle and foot include

- Dorsiflexion of ankle (20°)
- Plantar flexion of ankle (45°)
- Inversion of foot (30°)
- Eversion of foot (20°)

Movements of the toes include

- Extension
- Flexion
- Abduction (10°)
- Adduction (20°)

Spine

The **spine** is composed of 26 irregular bones called **vertebrae** (Figure 17.14 on page 501). There are 7 *cervical vertebrae*, which support the base of the skull and the neck. All 12 of the *thoracic vertebrae* articulate with the ribs. The 5 *lumbar vertebrae* support the lower back. They are heavier and denser than the other vertebrae, reflecting their weight-bearing function. The *sacrum* shapes the posterior wall of the pelvis, offering strength and stability. The *coccyx* is a small, triangular "tailbone" at the base of the spine.

Viewed laterally, the spine has cervical and lumbar concavities and a thoracic convexity. As a person bends forward, the

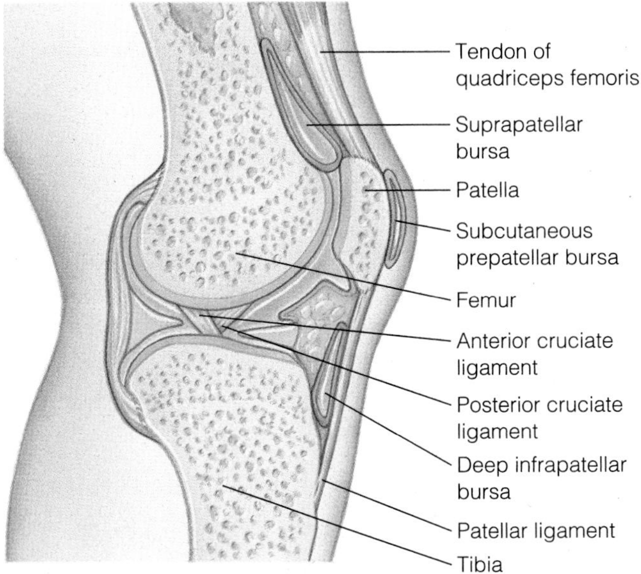

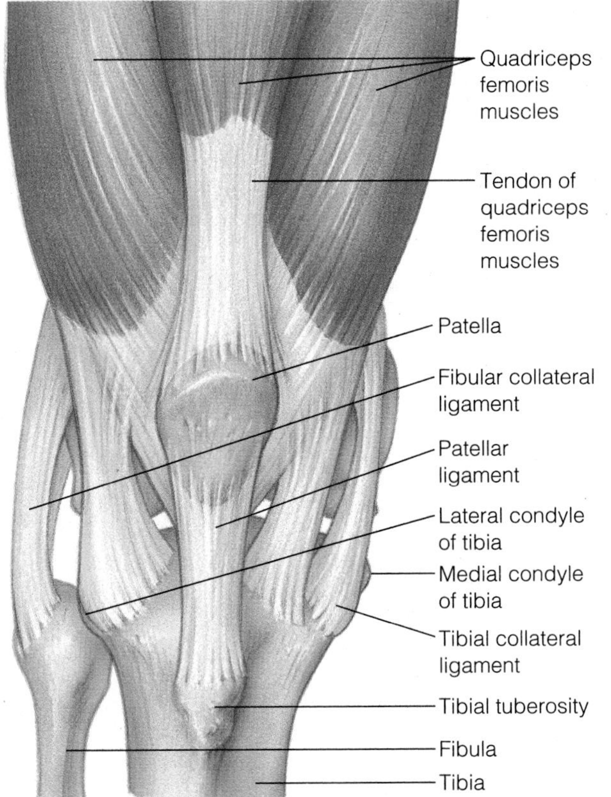

Figure 17.12 Knee joint. *A*, Sagittal section through the right knee. *B*, Anterior view.

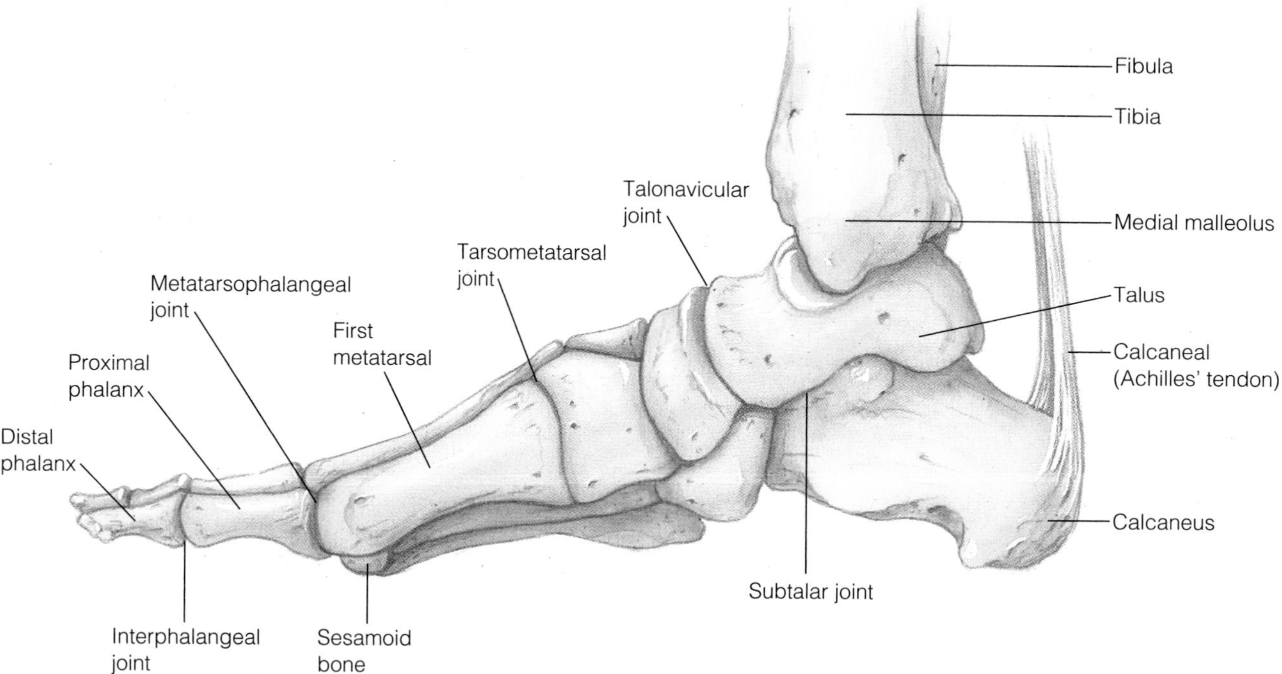

Figure 17.13 Joints of the ankle and foot.

normal concavity should flatten, and there should be a single convex C-shaped curve.

Figure 17.6, *B* on page 492 shows the main muscles of the neck and spine.

Movements of the neck include

- Flexion (45°)
- Extension (55°)
- Lateral flexion (bending) (40°)
- Rotation (70°)

Movements of the spine include

- Lateral flexion (35°)
- Extension (30°)
- Flexion (90°)
- Rotation (30°)

Gathering the Data

Focused Interview

If you are conducting the musculoskeletal assessment as part of a total physical assessment, you should review your findings from the rest of the assessment to determine if there are relationships between the client's musculoskeletal health status and the health of other body systems. For example, a client who works on a computer eight hours a day and complains of pain in the wrists and hands may have problems with innervation or circulation. When gathering additional information during the focused interview, be guided by any problems the client may have discussed during the initial interview.

See Chapter 2 for a discussion of the general health history. The following questions are suggested as part of the focused assessment of the musculoskeletal system.

General Survey of the Musculoskeletal System

1. Describe your mobility today, 2 months ago, and 2 years ago. Tell me about any changes you have experienced in your ability to walk, sit, stand, eat, dress, or perform other simple activities free of pain. *Musculoskeletal problems affect daily activities because of factors such as pain and decreased mobility.*
2. Please describe any musculoskeletal problems of any family member. *Some conditions such as rheumatoid arthritis are familial and recur in a family.*
3. Tell me about any swelling, heat, redness, or stiffness you have had in your muscles or joints, or any infections in your bones, muscles, or joints. *Osteomyelitis, an infection of the bone, frequently recurs in clients with a history of previous infections. Infections in the bones, muscles,*

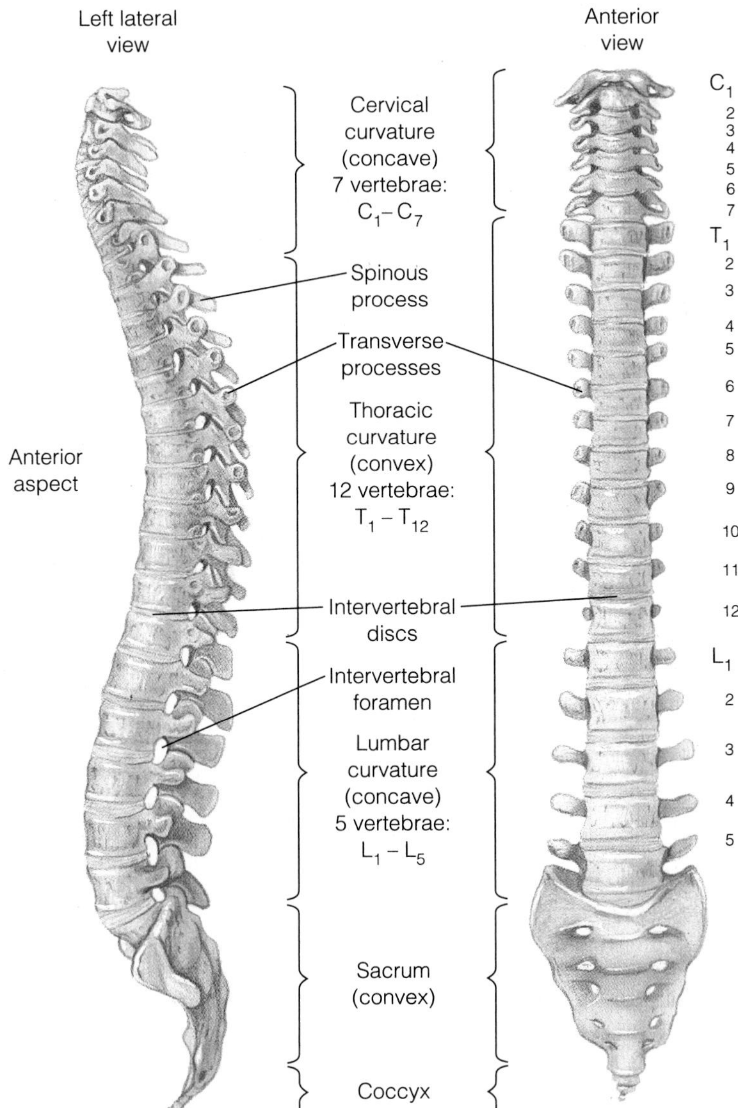

Figure 17.14 The spine.

or joints can lead to musculoskeletal complications that may require surgical intervention.

4. Do you have any chronic diseases such as diabetes mellitus, sickle cell anemia, lupus, or rheumatoid arthritis? If so, describe the disease and its progression, treatment, and effects on daily activities. *These conditions can predispose the client to musculoskeletal problems such as osteomyelitis.*
5. *Ask the premenopausal woman:* Describe your menstrual periods. *Women who have decreased amounts of estrogen production are more prone to the development of osteoporosis, a degeneration of bone tissue.*
6. Have you had any fractures? If so, tell me about the frequency, cause, injuries, treatment, and present problems with daily activities. *Older adults who have osteoporosis and osteomalacia (adult vitamin D deficiency) are prone to develop multiple fractures of the bone. Physical abuse should always be considered when an individual has a history of frequent fractures.*
7. Have you ever experienced any penetrating wounds? If so, please describe them. *Penetrating wounds may be a causative factor for osteomyelitis.*
8. Describe your typical daily diet. Do you have problems eating or drinking dairy products? If so, describe the problems you experience. *Protein deficiency interferes with bone growth and muscle tone; calcium deficiency predisposes an individual to low bone density resulting in osteo-*

porosis; vitamin C deficiency inhibits bone and tissue healing. Clients with intolerance to milk products frequently ingest low amounts of calcium, leading to musculoskeletal problems such as osteoporosis.

9. Tell me about your exercise program. *A sedentary lifestyle leads to muscle weakness and incoordination and predisposes postmenopausal women to osteoporosis.*
10. Have you had any recent weight gain? If so, how much weight? *Increased weight puts added stress on the musculoskeletal system.*
11. How much sunlight do you get each day? *Twenty minutes of sunshine each day helps the body manufacture vitamin D. Vitamin D deficiency can lead to osteomalacia.*
12. Do you smoke? If so, how much? How much caffeine do you consume each day? How many cups of coffee, tea, cola? How much alcohol do you drink? *Smoking, caffeine consumption, and alcohol consumption increase the client's risk for osteoporosis.*
13. What kind of work do you do? *Frequent repetitive movements may lead to misuse syndromes such as carpal tunnel syndrome, an inflammation of the tissues of the wrist that causes pressure on the median nerve. Work that requires heavy lifting or twisting may lead to lower back problems.*
14. Are you currently taking any medications such as steroids, estrogen, muscle relaxants, or any other drugs? *These drugs may cause a variety of symptoms that could affect the musculoskeletal system.*

Pain and Discomfort

1. Please describe any pain you experience in your bones, muscles, or joints. When did the pain begin? What were you doing at the time that the pain began? What activities increase the pain? What activities seem to decrease or eliminate the pain? Does this pain radiate from one place to another? Do you experience any unusual sensations such as a tingling feeling along with the pain? *These questions help determine if the pain had a sudden or gradual onset. Also, certain activities such as lifting heavy objects can strain ligaments and vertebrae in the back, causing acute pain. Weight-bearing activities might increase the pain if the client has degenerative disease of hip, knee, and vertebrae. The pain from hiatal hernia and from cardiac, gallbladder, and pleural conditions may be referred to the shoulder. Lumbosacral nerve root irritation might cause pain to be felt in the leg. Sensations of burning, tingling or prickling (paresthesia) may accompany compression of nerves or blood vessels in that body region.*
2. Do you experience constipation and/or abdominal distention? *These diagnostic cues commonly occur in clients who have decreased mobility, atrophy of the abdominal muscles, or spinal deformity.*
3. Do you have difficulty breathing? If so, describe. *Spinal deformities, osteoporosis, and any other condition that restricts trunk movement may interfere with normal breathing movements.*

Additional Questions with Infant, Children, and Adolescent Clients

1. Were you told about any trauma to your infant during labor and birth? If so, describe the trauma. *Traumatic births increase the risk for fractures, eg, of the clavicle.*
2. Did your baby require resuscitation after delivery? *Periods of anoxia can result in decreased muscle tone.*
3. Have you noticed any deformity of your child's spine or limbs, or any unusual shape of the feet and toes? If yes, please describe these deformities and any treatment your child has had. *Some deformities correct themselves as the child grows. Others may require physical therapy or surgery.*
4. Please describe any dislocations or broken bones your child has had, including any treatment. *Dislocations or broken bones are more common in children with certain developmental disabilities or sensory or motor disorders, or they may signal physical abuse.*
5. Ask the school-age child: Do you play any sports at school or after school? If so, describe the sports activities. *Some sports activities such as football can cause musculoskeletal injuries, especially if played without adequate adult supervision.*

Additional Questions with Childbearing Clients

- Please describe any back pain you are experiencing. Tell me about the effects of the pain on your daily activities. *Lordosis may occur in the last months of pregnancy along with complaints of back pain.*

Additional Questions with Older Clients

1. Has your height changed in recent years? *There is a decrease in height as part of the normal aging process because of the bone wasting of osteoporosis. This wasting may be heightened by lack of physical activity, dietary factors, and lack of exposure to sunlight.*
2. Have you noticed any muscle weakness over the past few months? If so, explain what effect this muscle weakness has on your daily activities. *Muscle weakness is common as a person ages, especially in people with sedentary lifestyles.*

3. Have you fallen in the past 6 months? If so, how many times? What prompted the fall(s)? Describe your injuries. What treatment did you receive? What effect did your injuries have on your daily activities? *Older adults have an increased rate of falls because of a change in posture that can affect their balance. Loss of balance may also be caused by sensory or motor disorders, inner-ear infections, the side effects of certain medications, and other factors.*
4. Do you use any aids such as a cane or walker to help you get around? If so, please describe the aid or show it to me. *These aids help the older adult ambulate, but they can also cause falls, especially if the client does not use the device properly.*
5. *Ask postmenopausal women:* Do you take estrogen? Do you take calcium supplements? *Estrogen replacement threrapy and calcium supplementation may slow the development of some of the musculoskeletal changes associated with age, such as osteoporosis.*

Physical Assessment

Preparation

☑ **Gather the equipment:**

examination gown
drape
examination gloves
examination light
goniometer and tape measure

☑ **Wash your hands.**

☑ **Ask the client to put on the examination gown.**

Remember

- Provide a warm, comfortable environment.
- Explain the procedure to the client to allay any fear or apprehension.
- Ensure the client's privacy.
- Drape for full visualization of the body part you are examining, without unnecessary exposure of your client.
- To increase your client's comprehension and compliance, demonstrate the range-of-motion movement to the client while giving verbal instructions in language appropriate to the client's developmental and cognitive level.
- When assessing range of motion, do not push the joint beyond its normal range. If the client complains of discomfort, stop!
- Whenever range of motion appears limited, measure the joint angle with a goniometer.
- Always compare the two sides of the body for symmetry.
- Examine the client in an orderly manner: head to toe, proximal to distal. The order of the examination of each joint is: inspection, palpation, assessment of range of motion, and assessment of muscle strength.
- A complete musculoskeletal assessment may exhaust some clients with compromised health status. Provide adequate rest periods, or schedule two or more sessions to complete the assessment.

ASSESSMENT TECHNIQUE/NORMAL FINDINGS | SPECIAL CONSIDERATIONS

Temporomandibular Joint

Step 1 ***Position the client.***

- Place the client in a sitting position with the examination gown on.

Step 2 ***Inspect the temporomandibular joint on both sides.***

The joints should be symmetric and not swollen or painful.

An enlarged or swollen joint shows as a rounded protuberance.

Step 3 ***Palpate the temporomandibular joints.***

- As the client opens and closes the mouth, palpate the temporomandibular joints with your index and middle fingers (Figure 17.15).

Discomfort, swelling, crackling sounds, and limited movement of the jaw are unexpected findings that require further evaluation.

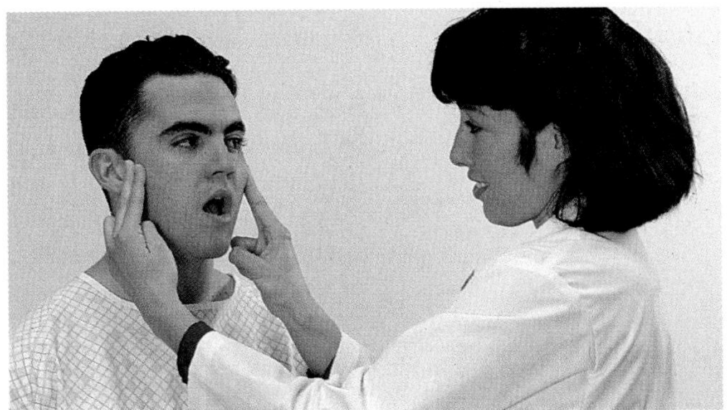

Figure 17.15 Palpating the temporomandibular joints.

- As the client's mouth opens, your fingers should glide into a shallow depression. Confirm the smooth motion of the mandible.

The joint may audibly and palpably click as the mouth opens. This is normal.

Step 4 ***Palpate the muscles of the jaw.***

- Instruct the client to clench the teeth as you palpate the masseter and temporalis muscles.

Confirm that the muscles are symmetric, firm, and nontender.

Swelling and tenderness suggest arthritis and myofascial pain syndrome.

Step 5 ***Test for range of motion of the temporomandibular joints.***

- Ask the client to open the mouth as wide as possible. Confirm that the mouth opens with ease to as much as 3 to 6 cm between the upper and lower incisors.
- With the mouth slightly open, push out the lower jaw. Return lower jaw to neutral position. The jaw should protrude and retract with ease.
- Move the lower jaw from side to side.

Confirm that the jaw moves laterally from 1 to 2 cm without deviation or dislocation.

Suspect temporomandibular joint dysfunction if facial pain and limited jaw movement accompany clicking sounds as the jaw opens and closes.

ASSESSMENT TECHNIQUE/NORMAL FINDINGS

SPECIAL CONSIDERATIONS

- Close the mouth. The mouth should close completely without pain or discomfort.

Step 6 ***Test for muscle strength and cranial nerve V function.***

- Instruct the client to repeat the movements in step 5 as you provide opposing force.

The client should be able to perform the movements against your resistance. The strength of the muscles on both sides of the jaw should be equal.

For more detailed testing of cranial nerve V, see Chapter 18.

Shoulders

Step 1 ***With the client facing you, inspect both shoulders.***

- Compare the shape and size of the shoulders, clavicles, and scapula. Confirm that they are symmetric and similar in size both anteriorly and posteriorly.

Swelling, deformity, atrophy, and malalignment, combined with limited motion, pain, and crepitus (a grating sound caused by bone fragments in joints), suggest degenerative joint disease, traumatized joints (strains, sprains), and inflammatory conditions (rheumatoid arthritis, bursitis, or tendinitis).

Step 2 ***Palpate the shoulders and surrounding structures.***

- Begin palpating at the sternoclavicular joint, then move laterally along the clavicle to the acromioclavicular joint.
- Palpate downward into the subacromial area and the greater tubercle of the humerus. Confirm that these areas are firm and nontender, the shoulders symmetric, and the scapula level and symmetric.

Referral

Shoulder pain without palpation or movement may result from insufficient circulation to the myocardium. This cue can be a precursor to a myocardial infarction (heart attack). If the client exhibits other symptoms such as chest pain, indigestion, and cardiovascular changes, obtain medical assistance immediately.

Step 3 ***Test the range of motion of the shoulders.***

Instruct the client to use both arms for the following maneuvers:

- Shrug the shoulders by flexing them forward and upward.
- With the elbows extended, raise the arms forward and upward in an arc. The client should demonstrate a forward flexion of 180°.
- Return the arms to the sides. Keeping the elbows extended, move the arms backward as far as possible (Figure 17.16). Client should demonstrate an extension of as much as 50°.

If the client expresses discomfort, determine if the pain is referred. Conditions that increase intra-abdominal pressure, such as hiatal hernia, may cause pain in the shoulder area.

ASSESSMENT TECHNIQUE/NORMAL FINDINGS

SPECIAL CONSIDERATIONS

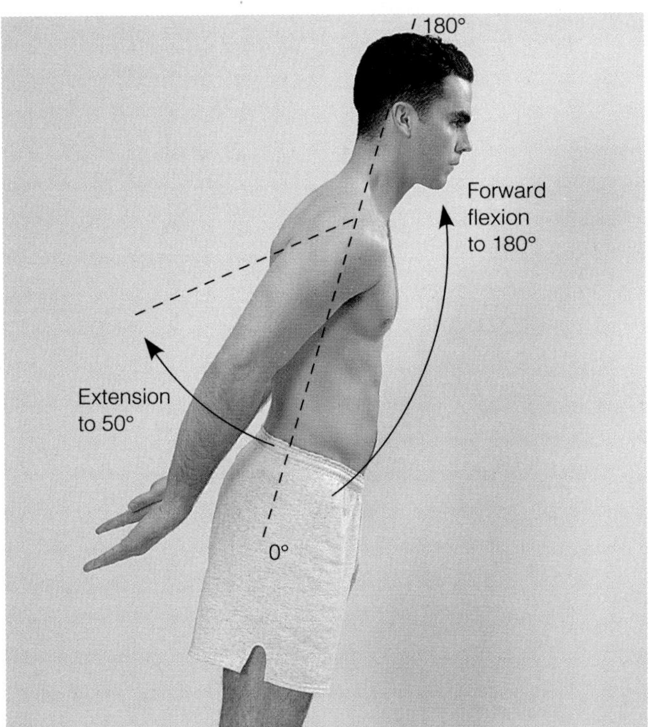

Figure 17.16 Flexion and extension of the shoulders.

- Place back of hands against back as close as possible to scapulae (internal rotation) (Figure 17.17).

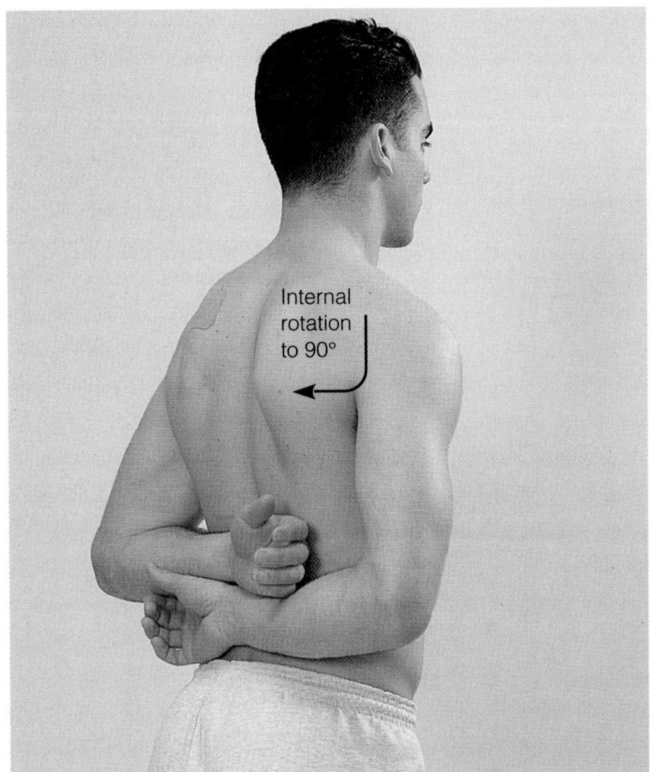

Figure 17.17 Internal rotation of the shoulders.

ASSESSMENT TECHNIQUE/NORMAL FINDINGS	SPECIAL CONSIDERATIONS

- Clasp hands behind head (external rotation) (Figure 17.18).

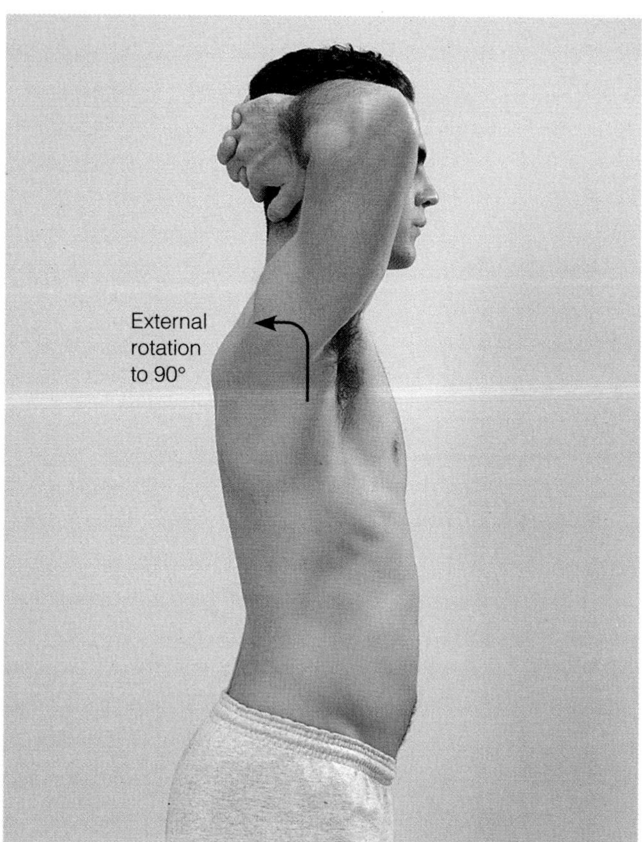

Figure 17.18 External rotation of the shoulders.

- With the elbows extended, swing arms out to the sides in arcs, touching palms together above the head. The client should demonstrate abduction of 180°.
- With the elbows extended, swing each arm toward midline of body (Figure 17.19). The client should demonstrate adduction of as much as 50°.

In rotator cuff tears, the client is unable to perform abduction without lifting or shrugging the shoulder. This sign is accompanied by pain, tenderness, and muscle atrophy.

ASSESSMENT TECHNIQUE/NORMAL FINDINGS | SPECIAL CONSIDERATIONS

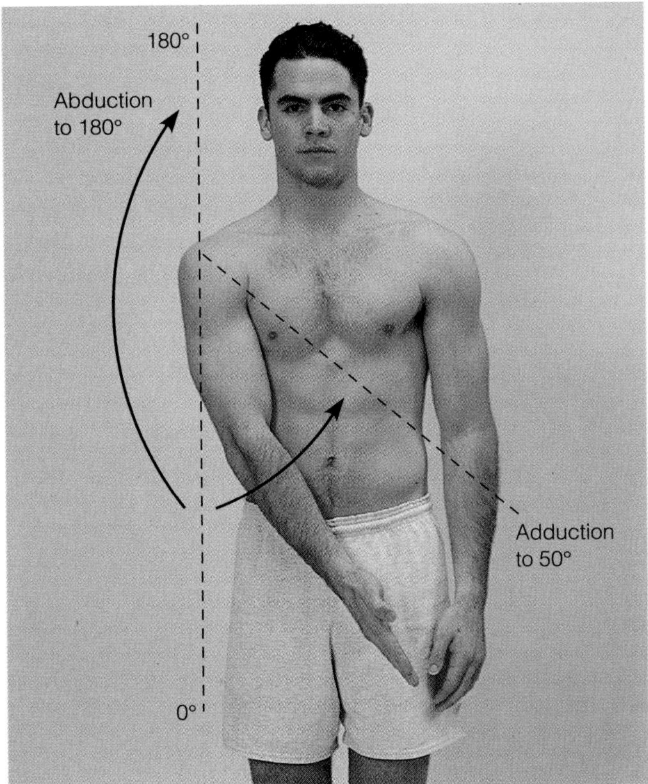

Figure 17.19 Abduction and adduction of the shoulder.

Step 4 *Test for strength of the shoulder muscles.*

- Instruct the client to repeat the movements in step 3 as you provide opposing force.

The client should be able to perform the movements against your resistance. The strength of the shoulder muscles on both sides should be equal.

Full resistance during the shoulder shrug indicates adequate cranial nerve XI (spinal accessory) function. See Chapter 18 for more detail.

Elbows

Step 1 *Support the client's arm and inspect the lateral and medial aspects of each elbow.*

The elbows should be symmetric.

Swelling, deformity, or malalignment requires further evaluation. If there is a subluxation (partial dislocation), the elbow looks deformed, and the forearm is misaligned.

Step 2 *Palpate the lateral and medial aspects of the olecranon process.*

- Use your thumb and middle fingers to palpate the grooves on either side of the olecranon process.

In the presence of inflammation, the grooves feel soft and spongy, and the surrounding tissue may be red, hot, and painful. Inflammatory conditions of the elbow include arthritis, bursitis, and epi-

ASSESSMENT TECHNIQUE/NORMAL FINDINGS

The joint should be free of pain, thickening, swelling, or tenderness.

Step 3 *Test the range of motion of each elbow.*

Instruct the client to perform the following movements:

- Bend the elbow by bringing the forearm forward and touching the fingers to the shoulder (Figure 17.20).

The elbow should flex to 160°.

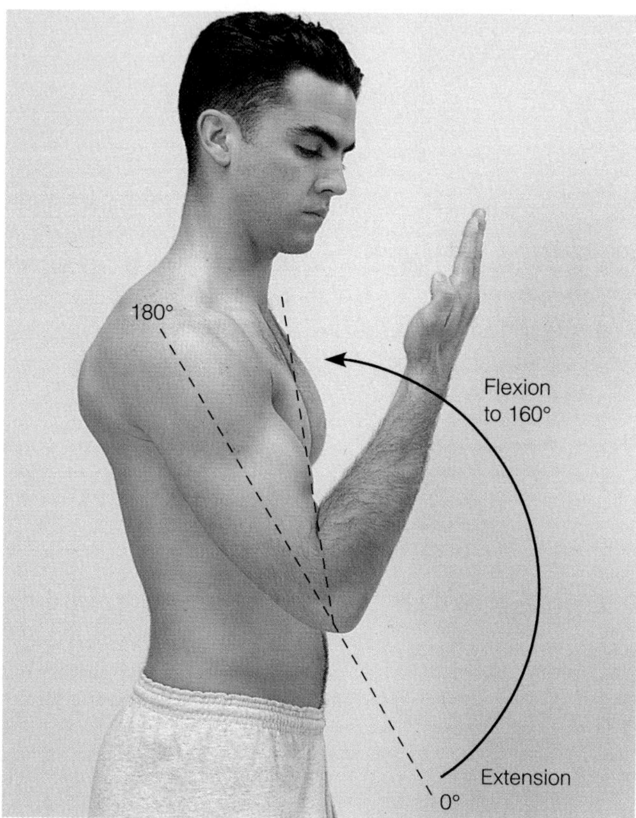

Figure 17.20 Flexion and extension of the elbow.

SPECIAL CONSIDERATIONS

condylitis (see Table 17.3 on page 535). *Rheumatoid arthritis* may result in nodules in the olecranon bursa or along the extensor surface of the ulna. Nodules are firm, nontender, and not attached to the overlying skin. *Lateral epicondylitis* (tennis elbow) results from constant repetitive movements of the wrist and/or forearm. Pain occurs when the client attempts to extend the wrist against resistance. *Medial epicondylitis* (pitcher's elbow) results from constant repetitive flexion of the wrist. Pain occurs when the client attempts to flex the wrist against resistance.

ASSESSMENT TECHNIQUE/NORMAL FINDINGS | SPECIAL CONSIDERATIONS

- Straighten the elbow.

The lower arm should form a straight line with the upper arm. The elbow in a neutral position is at 0° extension. The elbow should extend to 0°.

- Holding the arm straight out, turn the palm upward facing the ceiling, then downward facing the floor (Figure 17.21).

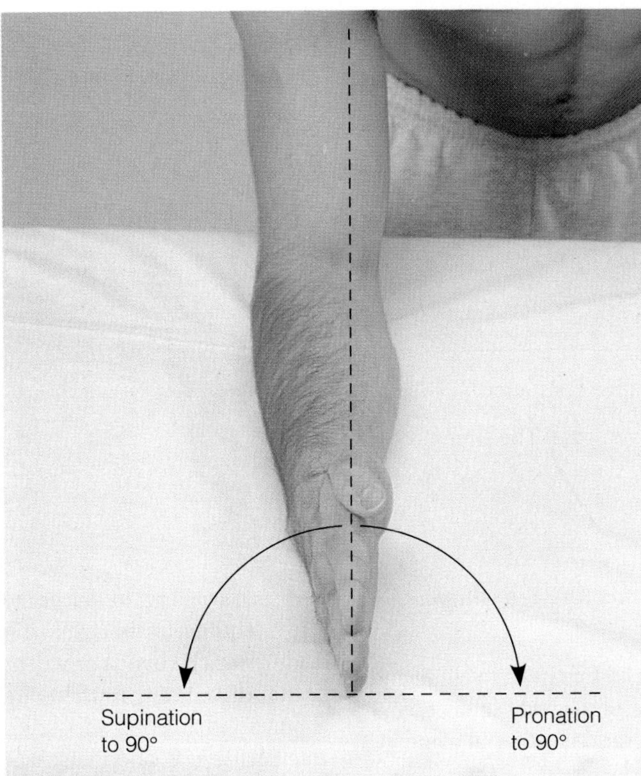

Figure 17.21 Supination and pronation of the elbow.

The elbow should supinate and pronate to 90°.

The client should be able to put each elbow through the normal range of motion without difficulty or discomfort.

Step 4 *Test for muscle strength.*

- Stabilize the client's elbow with your nondominant hand while holding the wrist with your dominant hand.
- Instruct the client to flex the elbow while you apply opposing resistance (Figure 17.22 on page 512).

ASSESSMENT TECHNIQUE/NORMAL FINDINGS | SPECIAL CONSIDERATIONS

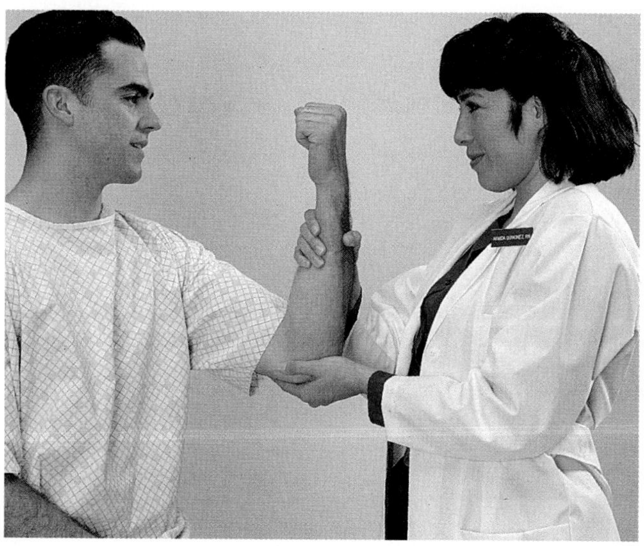

Figure 17.22 Testing muscle strength of the elbow.

- Instruct the client to extend the elbow against resistance.

The client should be able to perform the movements. The strength of the muscles in each elbow should be equal.

Wrists and Hands

Step 1 ***Inspect the wrists and dorsum of the hands for size, shape, symmetry, and color.***

The wrists and hands should be symmetric and free from swelling and deformity. The color should be similar to that of the rest of the body. The ends of either the ulna or radius may protrude further in some individuals.

Redness, swelling, or deformity in the joints requires further evaluation. Note any nodules on the hands or wrists, or atrophy of the surrounding muscles. In acute rheumatoid arthritis, the wrist, proximal interphalangeal, and metacarpophalangeal joints are likely to be swollen, tender, and stiff. As the disease progresses, the proximal interphalangeal joints deviate toward the ulnar side of the hand, the interosseous muscles atrophy, and rheumatoid nodules form, giving the rheumatic hand its characteristic appearance (see Table 17.3 on page 535).

Step 2 ***Inspect the palms of the hands.***

There is a rounded protuberance over the thenar eminence (the area proximal to the thumb).

Carpal tunnel syndrome is a nerve disorder in which an inflammation of tissues in the wrist causes pressure on the median nerve (which innervates the hand). Thenar atrophy is a common finding associated with carpal tunnel syndrome; however, some atrophy of the thenar eminence occurs with aging.

ASSESSMENT TECHNIQUE/NORMAL FINDINGS

SPECIAL CONSIDERATIONS

Step 3 *Palpate the wrists and hands for temperature and texture.*

The temperature of the wrists and hands should be warm and similar to the rest of the body. The skin should be smooth and free of cuts. The skin around the knuckles may have a rougher texture.

Step 4 *Palpate each joint of the wrists and hands.*

- Move your thumbs from side to side gently but firmly over the dorsum, with your fingers resting beneath the area you are palpating (Figure 17.23, *A* and *B*). As you palpate, make sure you keep the client's wrist straight.

A ganglion is a typically painless, round, fluid-filled mass that arises from the tendon sheaths on the dorsum of the wrist and hand. It may require surgery. Ganglions that are more prevalent when the wrist is flexed do not interfere with range of motion or function.

- To palpate the sides of the interphalangeal joints, pinch them gently between your thumb and index finger (Figure 17.23, *C*). All joints are firm and nontender, with no swelling.

A cool temperature in the extremities may indicate compromised vascular function, which may in turn influence muscle strength.

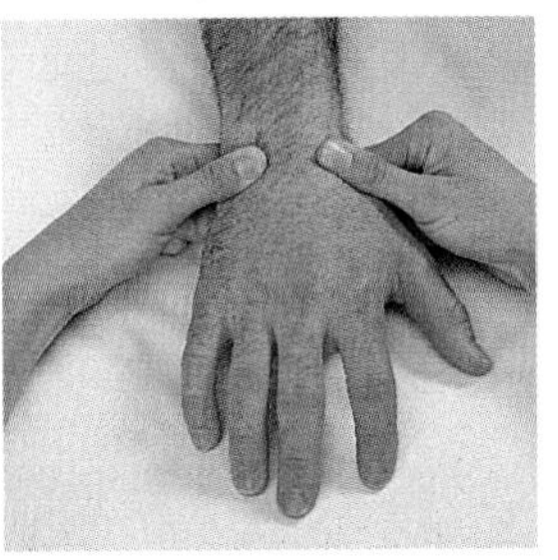
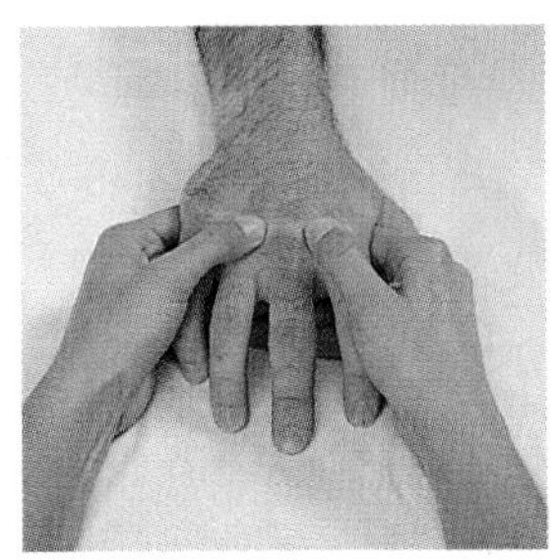
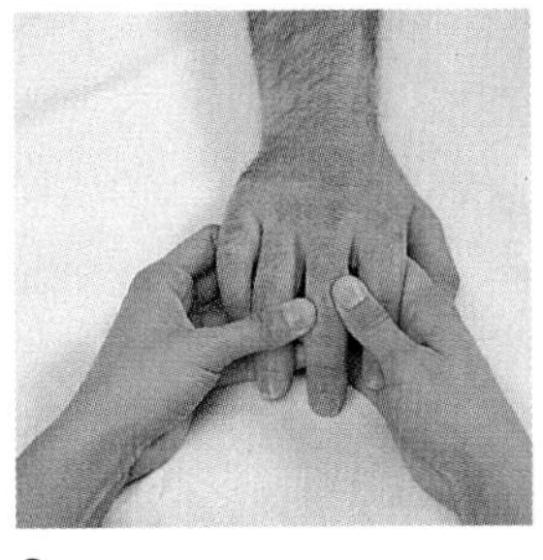

A **B** **C**

Figure 17.23 Palpating the wrist (*A*), hand (*B*), and fingers (*C*).

- As you palpate, note the temperature of the client's hand.

Step 5 *Test the range of motion of the wrist.*

Instruct the client to perform the following movements:

- Straighten the hand (extension).
- Using the wrist as a pivot point, bring the fingers backward as far as possible, then bend the wrist downward (Figure 17.24 on page 514). The wrist should hyperextend to 70° and flex to 90°.

ASSESSMENT TECHNIQUE/NORMAL FINDINGS

SPECIAL CONSIDERATIONS

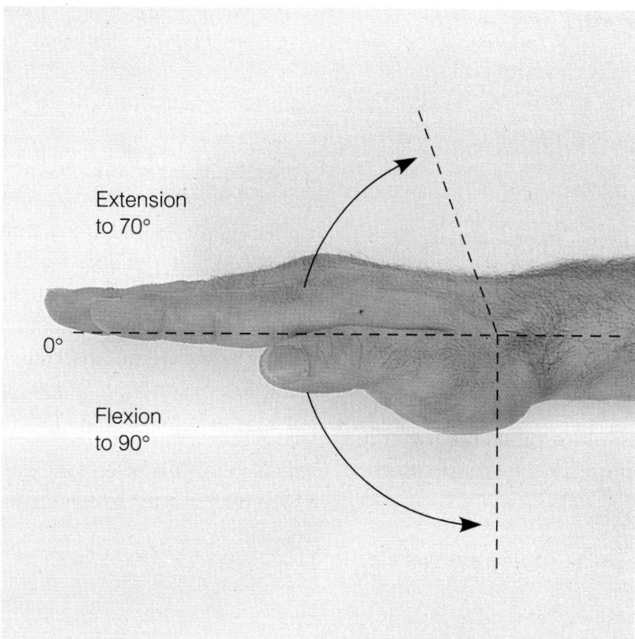

Figure 17.24 Hyperextension and flexion of the wrist.

- Turn the palms down, then move the hand laterally toward the fifth finger, then medially toward the thumb (Figure 17.25). Be sure the movement is from the wrist and not the elbow. Ulnar deviation should reach as much as 55°; radial deviation should reach as much as 20°.

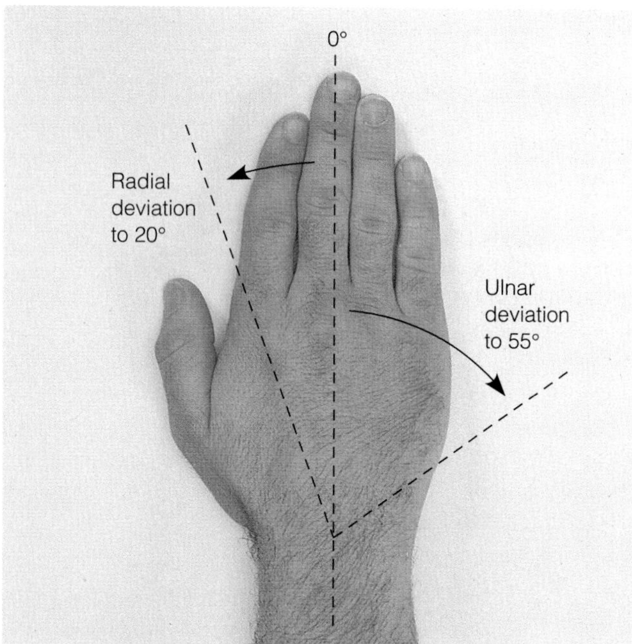

Figure 17.25 Ulnar and radial deviation of the wrist.

ASSESSMENT TECHNIQUE/NORMAL FINDINGS

- Bend the wrists downward and press the backs of both hands together (*Phalen's test*) (Figure 17.26). This causes flexion of the wrists to 90°. Normally clients experience no symptoms with this maneuver.

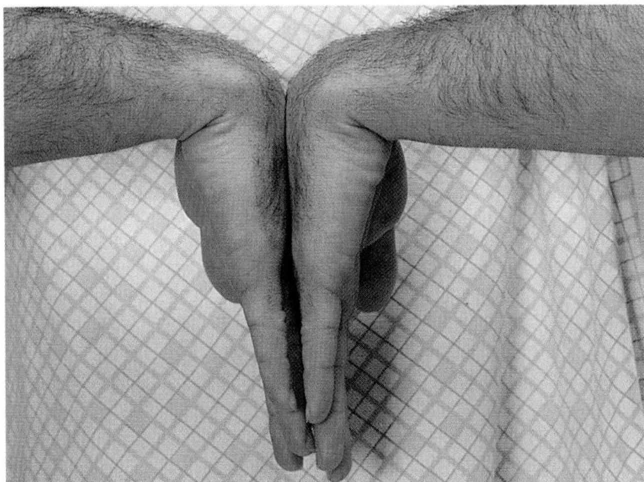

Figure 17.26 Phalen's test.

Step 6 *Test the range of motion of the hands and fingers.*

Instruct the client to perform the following movements:

- Make a tight fist with each hand with the fingers folded into the palm and the thumb across the knuckles (thumb flexion).
- Open the fist and stretch the fingers (extension).
- Point the fingers downward toward the forearm, then back as far as possible (Figure 17.27). Fingers should flex to 90° and hyperextend to as much as 30°.

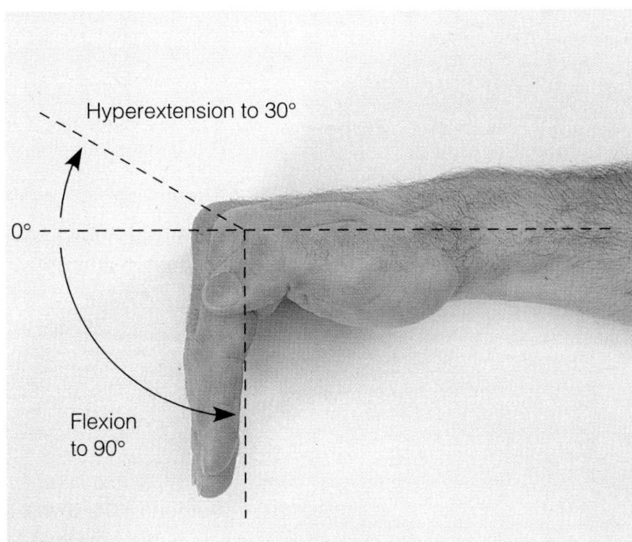

Figure 17.27 Flexion and extension of the fingers.

SPECIAL CONSIDERATIONS

When Phalen's test is used on individuals with carpal tunnel syndrome, 80% experience pain, tingling, and numbness that radiates to the arm, shoulder, neck, or chest within 60 seconds. If you suspect carpal tunnel syndrome, check for Tinel's sign by percussing lightly over the median nerve in each wrist. If carpel tunnel syndrome is present, the client feels numbness, tingling, and pain along the median nerve.

ASSESSMENT TECHNIQUE/NORMAL FINDINGS

- Spread the fingers far apart, then back together. Fingers should abduct to 20° and should adduct fully (to touch).
- Move the thumb toward the ulnar side of the hand and then away from the hand as far as possible.
- Touch the thumb to the tip of each of the fingers and to the base of the little finger.

SPECIAL CONSIDERATIONS

In *Dupuytren's contracture,* the client is unable to extend the fourth and fifth fingers. This is a progressive, painless, inherited disorder that causes severe flexion in the affected fingers, is usually bilateral, and is more common in middle-aged and older males.

Step 7 *Test for muscle strength of the wrist.*

- Place the client's arm on a table with the palm facing up.
- Stabilize the client's forearm with one hand while holding the hand with your other hand.
- Instruct the client to flex the wrist while you apply opposing resistance (Figure 17.28).

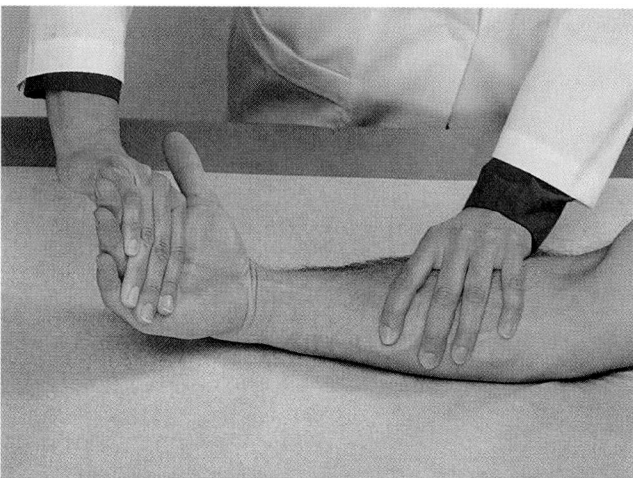

Figure 17.28 Testing the muscle strength of the wrist.

The client should be able to provide full resistance.

Step 8 *Test for muscle strength of the fingers.*

- Ask the client to spread the fingers, then try to force the fingers together.
- Ask the client to touch the little finger with the thumb while you place resistance on the thumb in order to prevent the movement.

Clients with carpal tunnel syndrome manifest weakness when attempting opposition of the thumb.

Hips

Step 1 *Assist the client to a supine position.*

Step 2 *Inspect the position of each hip and leg.*

The legs should be slightly apart and the toes should point toward the ceiling.

External rotation of the lower leg and foot is a classic sign of a fractured femur.

ASSESSMENT TECHNIQUE/NORMAL FINDINGS	SPECIAL CONSIDERATIONS

Step 3 ***Palpate each hip joint and the upper thighs.***

The hip joints are firm, stable, and nontender.

Pain, tenderness, swelling, deformity, limited motion (especially limited internal rotation), and crepitus are diagnostic cues that signal inflammatory or degenerative joint diseases in the hip. Suspect a fractured femur if the joint is unstable and deformed.

Step 4 ***Test the range of motion of the hips.***

ALERT!

Do not ask clients who have undergone hip replacement to perform these movements without the permission of the physician, because these motions can dislocate the prosthesis.

Instruct the client to

- Raise each leg straight off the bed or table (Figure 17.29). The other leg should remain flat on the bed. Hip flexion with straight knee should reach 90°. Return the leg to its original position.

This maneuver produces back and leg pain along the course of the sciatic nerve in the client with a herniated disc.

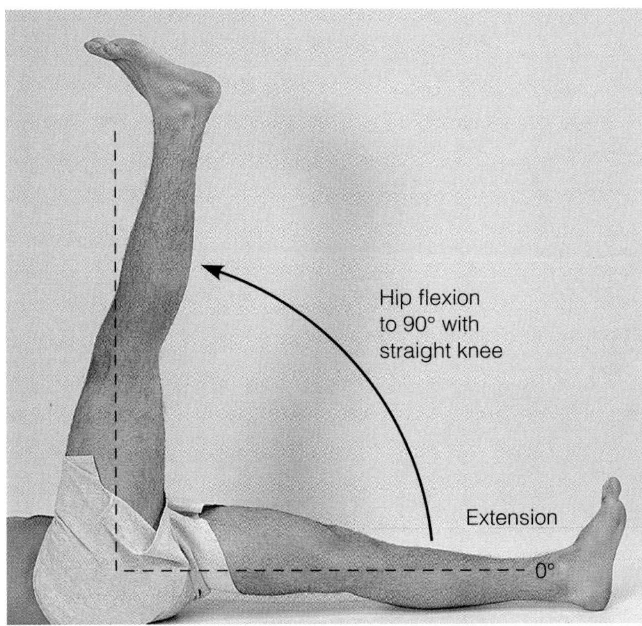

Figure 17.29 Flexion of the hip with straight knee.

- Raise the leg with the knee flexed toward the chest as far as it will go (Figure 17.30 on page 518). Hip flexion with flexed knee should reach 120°. Return the leg to its original position.

ASSESSMENT TECHNIQUE/NORMAL FINDINGS

SPECIAL CONSIDERATIONS

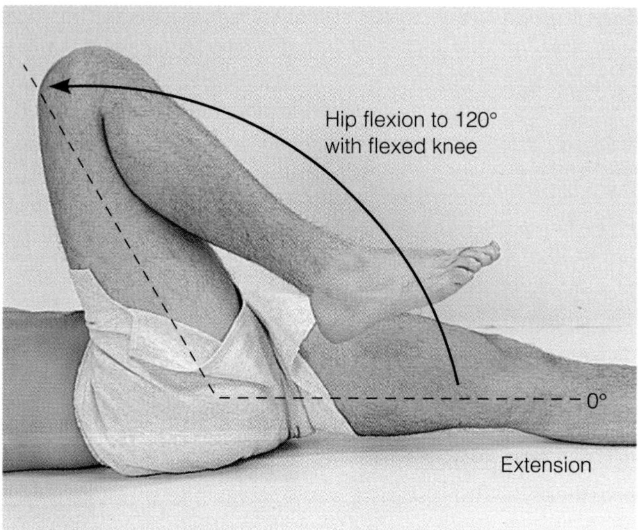

Figure 17.30 Flexion of the hip with flexed knee.

- Move the foot away from the midline as the knee moves toward the midline (Figure 17.31). Internal hip rotation should reach 40°.
- Move the foot toward the midline as the knee moves away from the midline. External hip rotation should reach 45°.

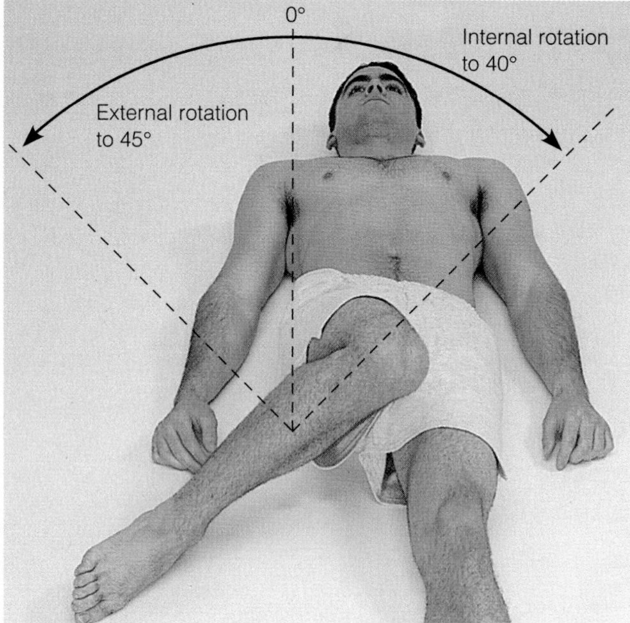

Figure 17.31 Internal and external hip rotation.

ASSESSMENT TECHNIQUE/NORMAL FINDINGS

SPECIAL CONSIDERATIONS

- Move the leg away from the midline (Figure 17.32), then as far as possible toward the midline. Abduction should reach 45°. Adduction should reach 30°.

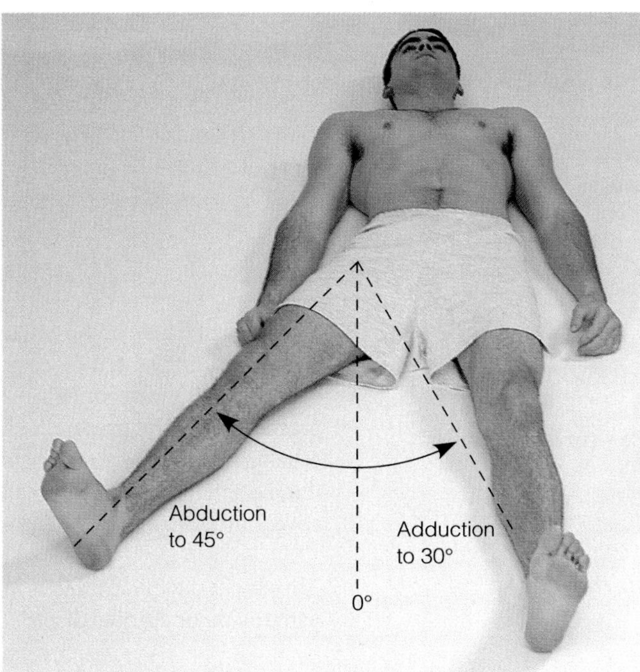

Figure 17.32 Abduction and adduction of the hip.

- Assist the client to turn onto the abdomen. With knee extended, raise each leg backward and up as far as possible (Figure 17.33). Hips should hyperextend to 15°. (You may also perform this test later, during assessment of the spine, with the client standing.)

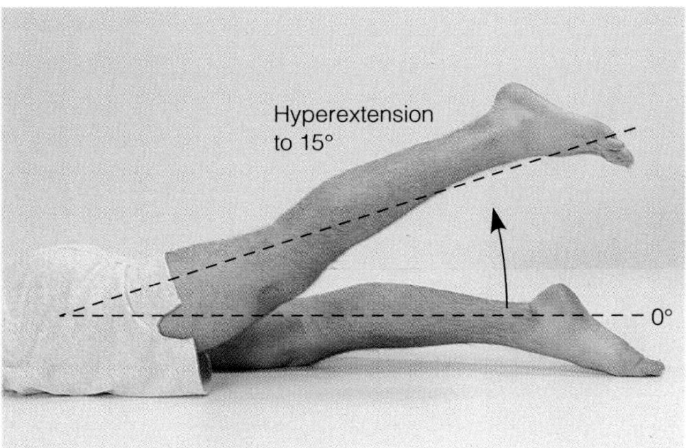

Figure 17.33 Hyperextension of the hip.

ASSESSMENT TECHNIQUE/NORMAL FINDINGS	SPECIAL CONSIDERATIONS

Step 5 ***Test for muscle strength of the hips.***

- Assist the client in returning to the supine position.
- Press your hands on the client's thighs and ask the client to raise the hip.
- Place your hands outside the client's knees and ask the client to spread both legs against your resistance.
- Place your hands between the client's knees, and ask the client to bring the legs together against your resistance.

Knees

Step 1 ***Inspect the knees.***

The patella should be centrally located in each knee. The normal depressions along each side of the patella should be sharp and distinct. The skin color should be similar to that of the surrounding areas.

Swelling and signs of fluid in the knee and its surrounding structures require further evaluation. Fluid accumulates in the suprapatellar bursa, the prepatellar bursa, and other areas adjacent to the patella when there is inflammation, trauma, or degenerative joint disease.

Step 2 ***Inspect the quadriceps muscle in the anterior thigh.***

Atrophy in the quadriceps muscles occurs with disuse or chronic disorders.

Step 3 ***Palpate the knee.***

- Using your thumb, index, and middle fingers, begin palpating approximately 10 cm above the patella with the thumb, index, and middle fingers (Figure 17.34). Palpate downward, evaluating each area.

Note any pain, swelling, thickening, or heat as you palpate. These diagnostic cues occur when the synovium is inflamed. Painless swelling frequently occurs in degenerative joint disease. A painful localized area of swelling, heat, and redness in the knee is caused by the inflammation of the bursa (bursitis), for example, *prepatellar bursitis* (housemaid's knee).

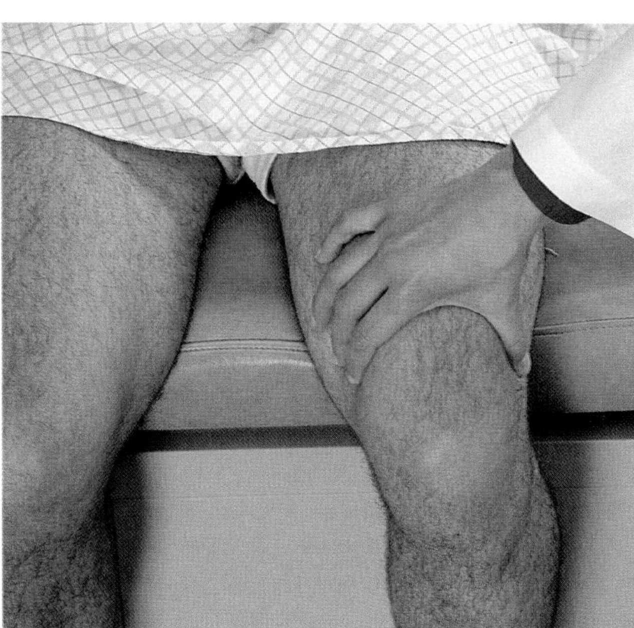

Figure 17.34 Palpating the knee.

ASSESSMENT TECHNIQUE/NORMAL FINDINGS | SPECIAL CONSIDERATIONS

The quadripceps muscle and surrounding soft tissue should be firm and nontender. The suprapatellar bursa is usually not palpable.

Step 4 ***Palpate the tibiofemoral joint.***

- With the knee still in the flexed position, use your thumbs to palpate deeply along each side of the tibia toward the outer aspects of the knee.
- Then palpate along the lateral collateral ligament.

The joint should be firm and nontender.

Signs of inflammation, including pain and tenderness, occur when the joint is inflamed or damaged and may indicate degenerative joint disease, synovitis, or a torn meniscus. Bony ridges or prominences in the outer aspects of the joint occur with osteoarthritis.

Step 5 ***Test for the bulge sign.***

This procedure detects the presence of small amounts of fluid (4 to 8 ml) in the suprapatellar bursa.

- With the client in the supine position, use firm pressure to stroke the medial aspect of the knee upward several times, displacing any fluid (Figure 17.35, *A*).
- Apply pressure to the lateral side of the knee while observing the medial side (Figure 17.35, *B*).

The medial side of the knee bulges if fluid is in the joint.

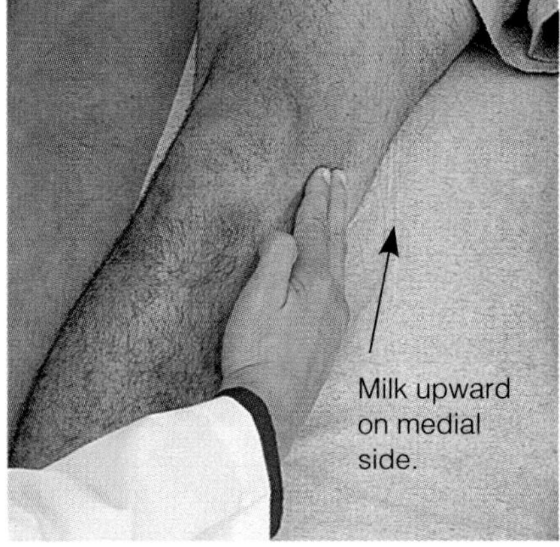

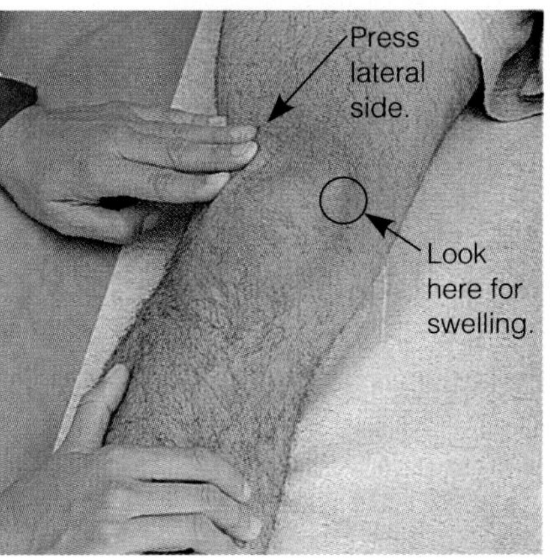

Figure 17.35 Testing for the bulge sign. *A*, Stroking the knee. *B*, Observing the medial side.

Normally no fluid is present.

Step 6 ***Perform ballottement.***

Ballottement is a technique used to detect fluid, or to examine or detect floating body structures: the examiner displaces body fluid and then palpates the return impact of the body structure.

- To detect large amounts of fluid in the suprapatellar bursa: With your thumb and fingers, firmly grasp the thigh just above the knee. This action causes any fluid in the suprapatellar bursa to move between the patella and the femur.

When there are abnormal fluid levels, fluid forced between the patella and femur causes the patella to "float" over the femur. A palpable click is felt when the patella is snapped back against the femur when fluid is present.

ASSESSMENT TECHNIQUE/NORMAL FINDINGS | SPECIAL CONSIDERATIONS

- With the fingers of your left hand, quickly push the patella downward upon the femur (Figure 17.36).

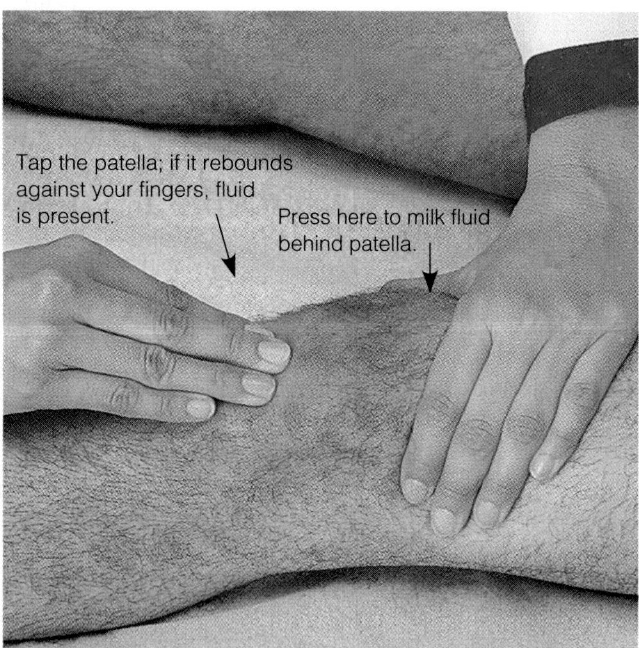
Tap the patella; if it rebounds against your fingers, fluid is present.
Press here to milk fluid behind patella.

Figure 17.36 Testing for ballottement.

Normally the patella sits firmly over the femur, allowing little or no movement when pressure is exerted over the patella.

Step 7 ***Test the range of motion of each knee.***

Instruct the client to:

- Bend each knee against the chest as far as possible (flexion) (Figure 17.37), then return the knee to its extended position.

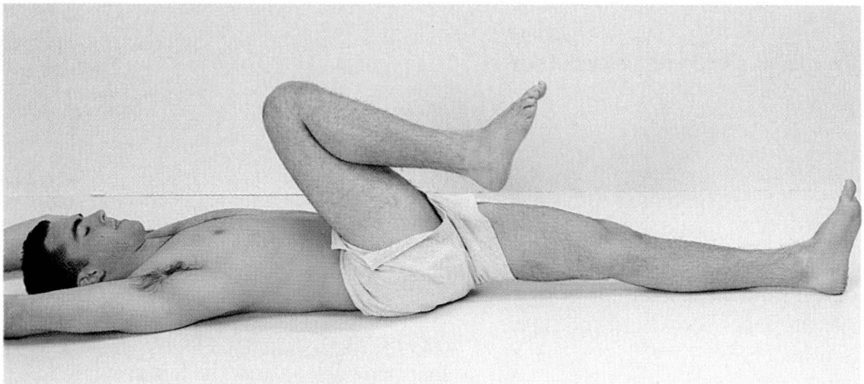

Figure 17.37 Flexion of the knee.

ASSESSMENT TECHNIQUE/NORMAL FINDINGS	SPECIAL CONSIDERATIONS

- Walk at a comfortable pace and with a relaxed gait.

Step 8 ***Test for muscle strength.***

- Instruct the client to flex each knee while you apply opposing force. Now instruct the client to extend the knee again.

The client should be able to perform the movement against resistance. The strength of the muscles in both knees is equal.

Step 9 ***Inspect the knee while the client is standing.***

- Ask the client to stand erect. If the client is unsteady, allow the client to hold onto the back of a chair.

The knees should be in alignment with the thighs and ankles.

Look for genu varum (bowlegs), genu valgum (knock-knees), or genu recurvatum, (excessive hyperextension of the knee with weight bearing due to weakness of quadriceps muscles).

Ankles and Feet

Step 1 ***Inspect the ankle and foot with the client sitting, standing, and walking.***

The color of the ankles and feet should be similar to that of the rest of the body. They should be symmetric, and the skin should be unbroken. The feet and toes should be in alignment with the long axis of the lower leg. No swelling should be present, and the client's weight should fall on the middle of the foot.

The following abnormalities require further evaluation (see Table 17.3 on page 535):

Gouty arthritis: The metatarsophalangeal joint of the great toe is swollen, hot, red, and extremely painful.

Hallux valgus (bunion): The great toe deviates laterally from the midline, crowding the other toes. The metatarsophalangeal joint and bursa become enlarged and inflamed, causing a bunion.

Hammertoe: Flexion of the proximal interphalangeal joint of a toe, while the distal metatarsophalangeal joint hyperextends. A callus or corn frequently occurs on the surface of the flexed joint from external pressure.

Pes planus (flat foot): The arch of the foot is flattened, sometimes coming in contact with the floor. The deformity may be noticeable only when an individual is standing and bearing weight on the foot.

Step 2 ***Palpate the ankles.***

- Grasp the heel of the foot with the fingers of both hands while palpating the anterior and lateral aspects of the ankle with your thumbs (Figure 17.38 on page 524).

Pain or discomfort on palpation and movement frequently indicates degenerative joint disease.

ASSESSMENT TECHNIQUE/NORMAL FINDINGS	SPECIAL CONSIDERATIONS

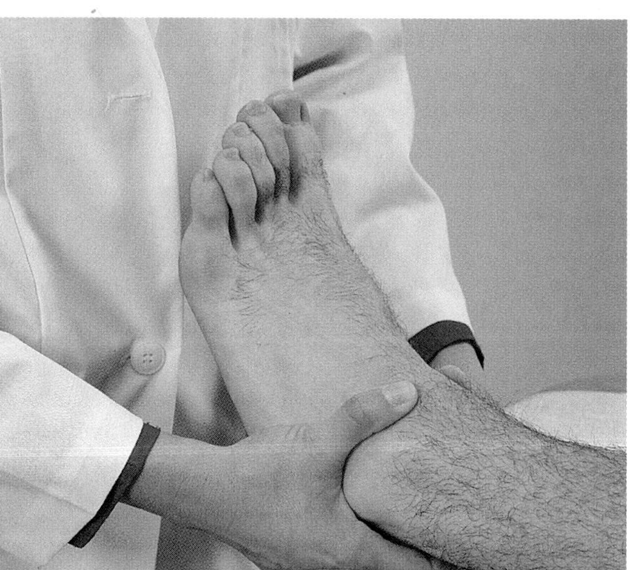

Figure 17.38 Palpating the ankle.

The ankle joints should be firm, stable, and nontender.

Step 3 ***Palpate the length of the calcaneal (Achilles) tendon at the posterior ankle.***

The calcaneal tendon should be free of pain, tenderness, and nodules.

Look for pain and tenderness along the tendon, which may indicate tendinitis or bursitis. Small nodules sometimes occur in clients with rheumatoid arthritis.

Step 4 ***Palpate the metatarsophalangeal joints just below the ball of the foot.***

The metatarsophalangeal joints should be nontender.

Pain and discomfort with this maneuver suggest early involvement of rheumatoid arthritis. Acute inflammation of the first metatarsophalangeal joint suggests gout.

Step 5 ***Deeply palpate each metatarsophalangeal joint.***

The joints should be firm and nontender.

Pain, swelling, or tenderness may be associated with inflammation or degenerative joint disease.

Step 6 ***Palpate each interphalangeal joint.***

Pain, swelling, or tenderness may be associated with inflammation or degenerative joint disease.

- As you did for the hand, note the temperature of the extremity. Confirm that it is similar to the temperature of the rest of the client's body.

A temperature in the lower extremities that is significantly cooler than the rest of the body may indicate vascular insufficiency, which in turn may lead to musculoskeletal abnormalities.

Step 7 ***Test the range of motion of the ankles and feet.***

Instruct the client to:

- Point the foot toward the nose. Dorsiflexion should reach 20°.

Limited range of motion and painful movement of the foot and ankle without signs of inflammation suggest degenerative joint disease.

ASSESSMENT TECHNIQUE/NORMAL FINDINGS	SPECIAL CONSIDERATIONS

- Point the foot toward the floor. Plantar flexion should reach 45°.
- Point the sole of the foot outward, then inward. The client is able to evert the ankle to 20° and invert the ankle to 30° (Figure 17.39.).

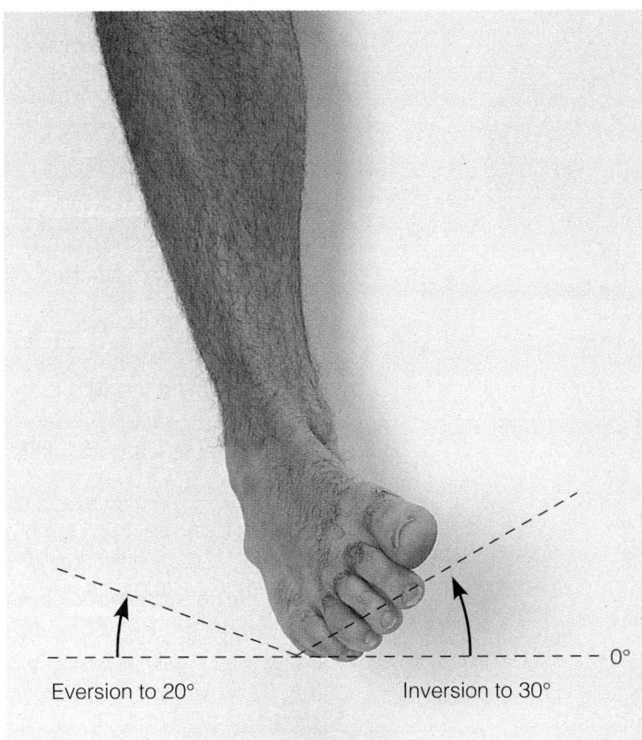

Figure 17.39 Eversion and inversion of the ankles.

- Curl the toes downward (flexion).
- Spread the toes as far as possible (abduction), then bring the toes together (adduction).

Step 8 *Test muscle strength of the ankle.*

- Ask the client to perform dorsiflexion and plantar flexion against your resistance.

Step 9 *Test muscle strength of the foot.*

- Ask the client to flex and extend the toes against your resistance.

Spine

Step 1 *Inspect the spine.*

- With the client in a standing position, move around the client's body to check the position and alignment of the spine from all sides:

Lack of symmetry of the scapulae may indicate thoracic surgery. A scapula may appear higher if a lung has been removed on that side. In addition, the following

ASSESSMENT TECHNIQUE/NORMAL FINDINGS

- Confirm that the cervical and lumbar curves are concave, and that the thoracic curve is convex (Figure 17.40, *A*).

- Imagine a vertical line falling from the level of T1 to the gluteal cleft. Confirm that the spine is straight (Figure 17.40, *B*).

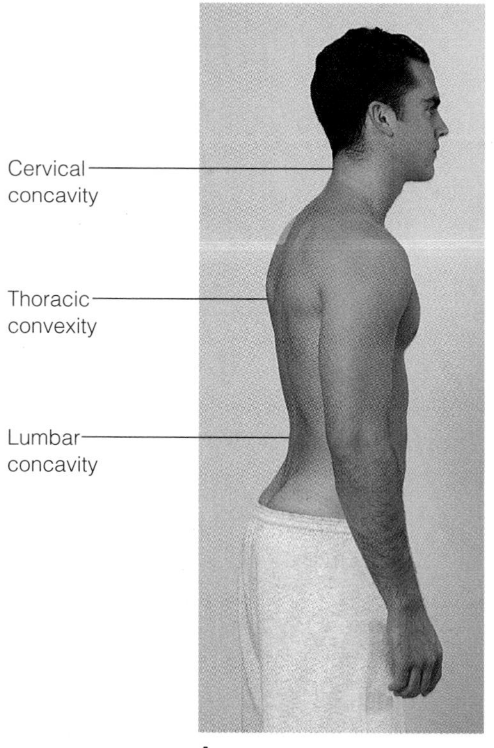

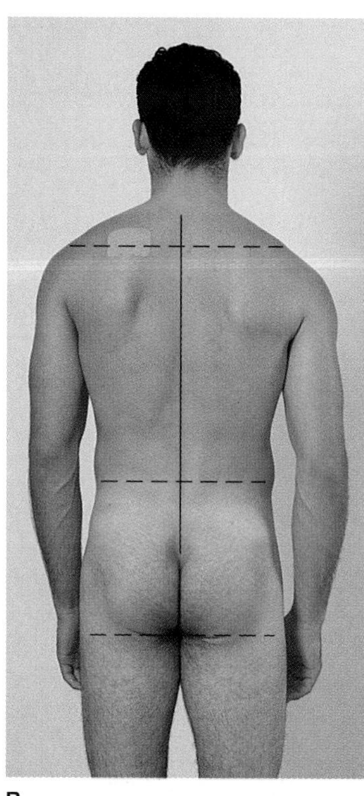

Figure 17.40 Lateral view (*A*) and posterior view (*B*) of the normal spine.

- Imagine a horizontal line across the top of the scapulae. Confirm that the scapulae are level and symmetric (Figure 17.40, *B*).

- Similarly, check that the heights of the iliac crests and the gluteal folds are level (Figure 17.40, *B*).

SPECIAL CONSIDERATIONS

abnormalities require further evaluation (see Table 17.3 on page 537 for more information):

Kyphosis: An exaggerated thoracic dorsal curve that causes asymmetry between the sides of the posterior thorax.

Lordosis: An exaggerated lumbar curve that compensates for pregnancy, obesity, or other skeletal changes.

Flattened lumbar curve: A concave lumbar curve. This change frequently occurs when spasms affect the lumbar muscles.

List: The spine leans to the left or right: a plumb line drawn from T1 does not fall between the gluteal cleft. This condition may occur with spasms in the paravertebral muscles or a herniated disc.

Scoliosis: The spine curves to the right or left, causing an exaggerated thoracic convexity on that side. The body compensates, and a plumb line dropped from T1 falls between the gluteal cleft. Unequal leg length may contribute to scoliosis; therefore, if you suspect scoliosis, measure the client's leg length. With the client supine, measure the distance from the anterior superior iliac spine to the medial malleolus, crossing the tape measure at the medial side of the knee (Figure 17.41).

ASSESSMENT TECHNIQUE/NORMAL FINDINGS	SPECIAL CONSIDERATIONS

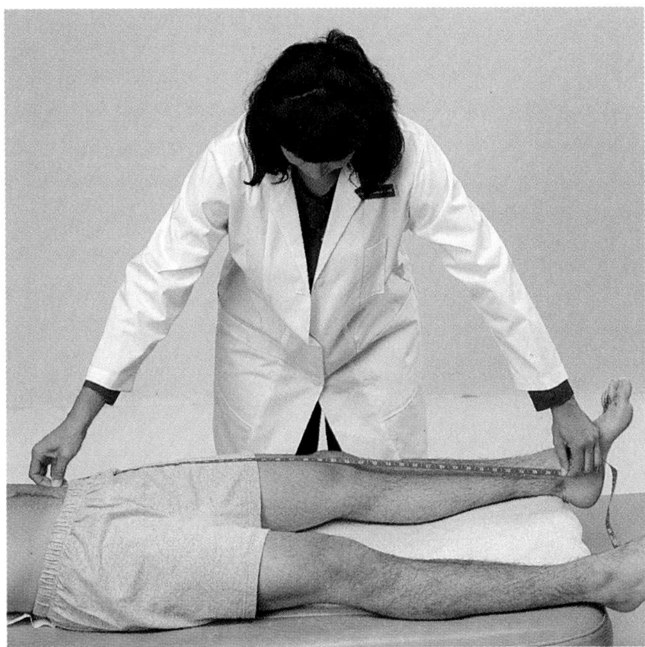

Figure 17.41 Measuring leg length.

Step 2 *Palpate each vertebral process with your thumb.*

The vertebral processes should be aligned, uniform in size, firm, stable, and nontender.

Consider a *compression fracture* if the client is elderly, complains of pain and tenderness in the back, and has restricted back movement. T8 and L3 are the most common sites for compression fractures.

Step 3 *Palpate the muscles on both sides of the neck and back.*

The neck muscles should be fully developed and symmetric, firm, smooth, and nontender.

Muscle spasms feel like hardened or knotlike formations. When they occur, the client may complain of pain and restricted movement. Muscle spasms may be associated with temporomandibular joint dysfunction or with *spasmodic torticollis,* a disorder in which the spasms cause the head to be pulled to one side.

Step 4 *Test the range of motion of the cervical spine.*

Instruct the client to:

- Touch the chest with the chin (flexion).
- Look up toward the ceiling (hyperextension).
- Attempt to touch each shoulder with the ear on that side, keeping the shoulder level (lateral bending or flexion).
- Turn the head to face each shoulder as far as possible (rotation).

Step 5 *Test the range of motion of the thoracic and lumbar spine.*

- Sit or stand behind the standing client.

Stabilize the pelvis with your hands and ask the client to

- Bend sideways to the right and to the left. Right and left lateral flexion should reach 35° (Figure 17.42 on page 528).

Limited range of motion, crepitation, or pain on movement in the joint require further evaluation. If the client complains of sharp pain that begins in the lower back and radiates down the leg, perform the straight-leg-raising test: Keeping the knee extended, raise the client's leg until pain

ASSESSMENT TECHNIQUE/NORMAL FINDINGS

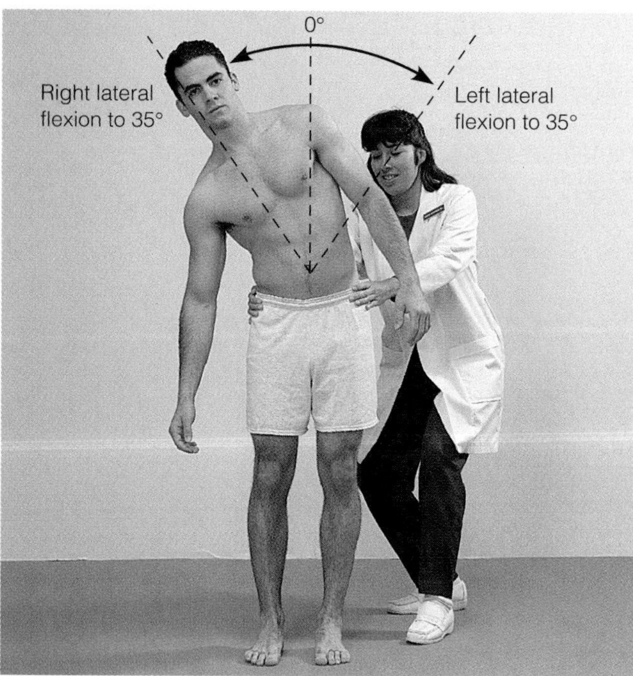

Figure 17.42 Lateral flexion of the spine.

- Bend forward and touch the toes (flexion). Confirm that the lumbar concavity disappears with this movement, and the back assumes a single **C**-shaped convexity (Figure 17.43).

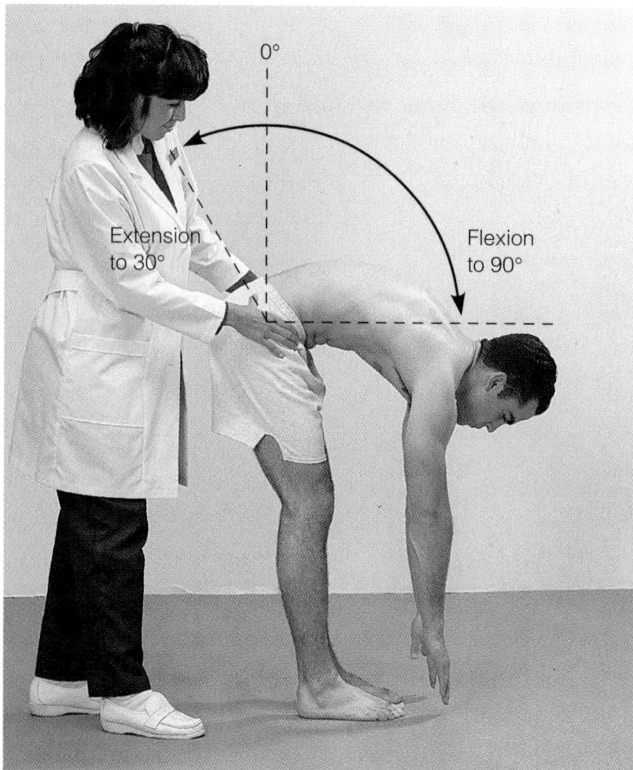

Figure 17.43 Forward flexion of the spine.

SPECIAL CONSIDERATIONS

occurs, then dorsiflex the client's foot. Record the distribution and severity of the pain and the degree of leg elevation at the time the pain occurs. Also record whether dorsiflexion increases the pain. Pain with straight-leg raising may indicate a herniated disc.

ASSESSMENT TECHNIQUE/NORMAL FINDINGS | SPECIAL CONSIDERATIONS

- Bend backward as far as is comfortable. Hyperextension should reach 30°.
- Twist the shoulders to the left and to the right. Rotation should reach 30° (Figure 17.44).

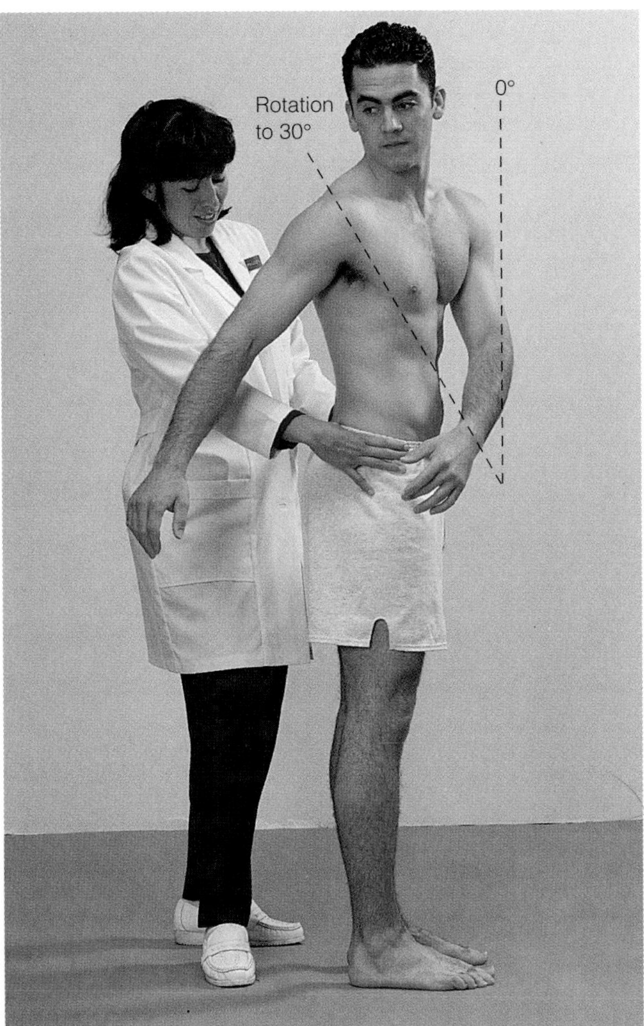

Figure 17.44 Rotation of the spine.

Reminders

- In addition to the above steps, consider the common variations in physical assessment findings for the different groups discussed in the following sections.
- After completing the physical assessment, answer any questions the client may have, and provide appropriate client teaching for health promotion and self-care (see page 538).
- Confirm that the client is comfortable and has no adverse effects from the procedure, then dim the lights and leave the client to rest or to get dressed.
- Document the assessment findings as described in Chapter 1. See pages 533–534 for information on identifying nursing diagnoses commonly associated with the musculoskeletal system.

Developmental Considerations

Infant, Children, and Adolescent Clients

Infants Examine the infant without clothing. When examining newborns, make sure to use a warming table to prevent hypothermia. Observe spontaneous movement and posture in the supine, prone, and sitting positions. As you observe the infant, check for achievement of developmental milestones such as the following:

- From about the age of 2 months, forearm strength is usually sufficient to enable the infant to lift the head and trunk from the prone position.
- From about 4 months, the infant normally is able to roll from the prone to supine position.
- At about 8 months, the infant should be able to sit alone without support, and the earlier kyphosis of the spine has disappeared.
- At about 9 months, most infants begin crawling.
- At about 15 months, most infants are able to walk without support.

(For more information, use the Denver Developmental Screening Test II, and refer to Chapter 19 of this text.)

Fetal positioning and the birth experience may cause musculoskeletal anomalies in the infant. These include *tibial torsion*, a curving apart of the tibias, and *metatarsus adductus*, a tendency of the forefoot to turn inward. Many such anomalies correct themselves spontaneously as the child grows and walks.

Newborns normally have flat feet; arches develop gradually during the preschool years. Before learning to walk, infants tend to exhibit genu varum (bowlegs). Then, as the child begins to walk, this tendency gradually reverses until, by the age of 4, most children tend to exhibit genu valgum (knock-knees). This condition also resolves spontaneously, usually by late childhood or early adolescence.

Inspect the newborn's spine. Any tuft of hair, cyst, or mass may indicate spina bifida and requires further evaluation. Palpate the length of the clavicles at each office visit, noting any lumps or irregularities and observing the range of motion of the arms. The clavicle is frequently fractured during birth, and the fracture often goes unnoticed until a callus forms at the fracture site.

Assess the infant for congenital hip dislocation at every office visit until 1 year of age. (For the procedure, see Chapter 19.) Additionally, use the *Allis sign* to detect unequal leg length: Position yourself at the child's feet. With the infant supine, flex the knees, keeping the femurs aligned. Compare the height of the knees. An uneven height indicates unequal leg length (Figure 17.45).

Hold the infant with your hands beneath the axillae. Shoulder muscle strength is adequate if the infant remains upright between your hands. Muscle weakness is indicated if the infant begins to slip through your hands (Figure 17.46).

Children and Adolescents Bone growth is rapid during infancy and continues at a steady rate during childhood until

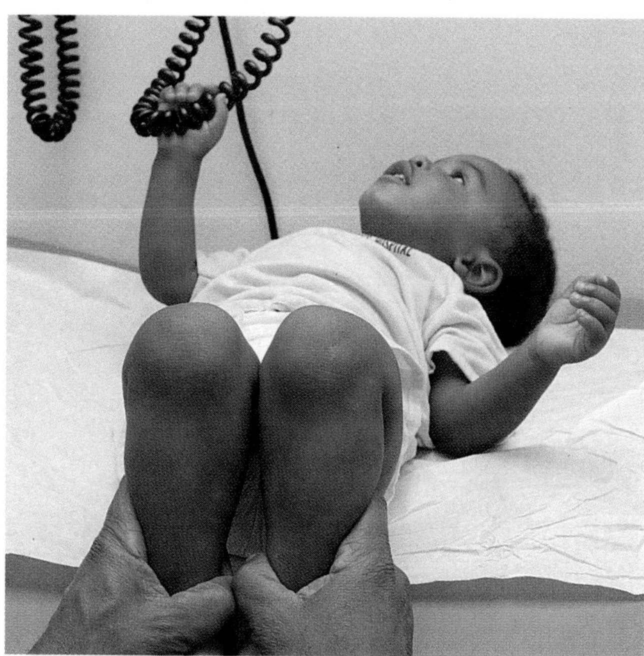

Figure 17.45 Checking for the Allis sign.

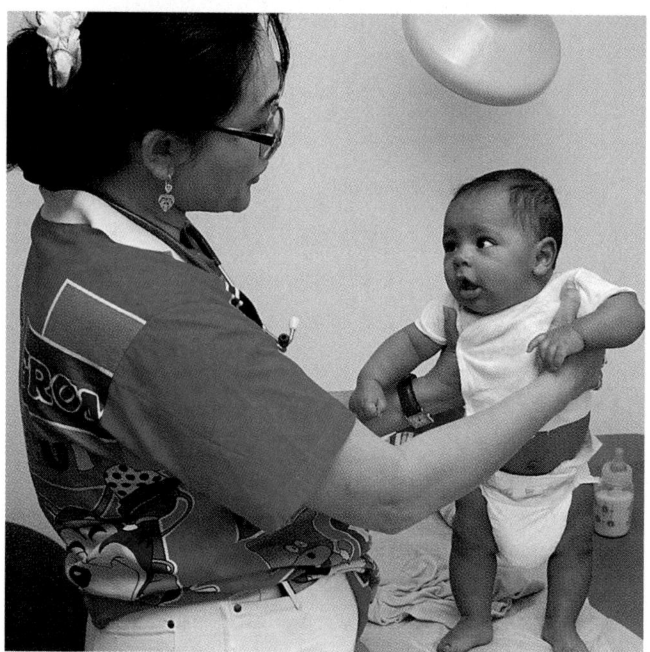

Figure 17.46 Assessing shoulder muscle strength in an infant.

adolescence, at which time both girls and boys experience a growth spurt. Long bones increase in width because of the deposition of new bony tissue around the diaphysis (shaft). They increase in length because of a proliferation of cartilage at the growth plates at the epiphyses (ends) of the long bones. Longitudinal growth ends at about 21 years of age, when the epiphyses fuse with the diaphysis. Throughout childhood, ligaments are stronger than bones. Therefore, childhood injuries to the long bones and joints tend to result in fractures instead of sprains. Individual muscle fibers grow throughout childhood, but growth is especially increased during the adolescent growth spurt. Muscles vary in size and strength due to genetics, exercise, and diet.

Much of the exam of the child and adolescent includes the same techniques of inspection, palpation, and assessment of range of motion and muscle strength used in the examination of the adult. But children also have unique assessment needs. Take advantage of the wonderful opportunities children present for assessing range of motion and muscle strength as they play with toys in the waiting area or examination room. Encourage children to jump, hop, skip, and climb for you. You'll find that most children are eager to "show off" their abilities.

At each office visit, ask children to show you their favorite sitting position. If a child assumes the *reverse tailor position* (Figure 17.47), common when watching television, encourage the child to try other sitting positions. Explain to the parent that the reverse tailor position stresses the hip, knee, and ankle joints of the growing child.

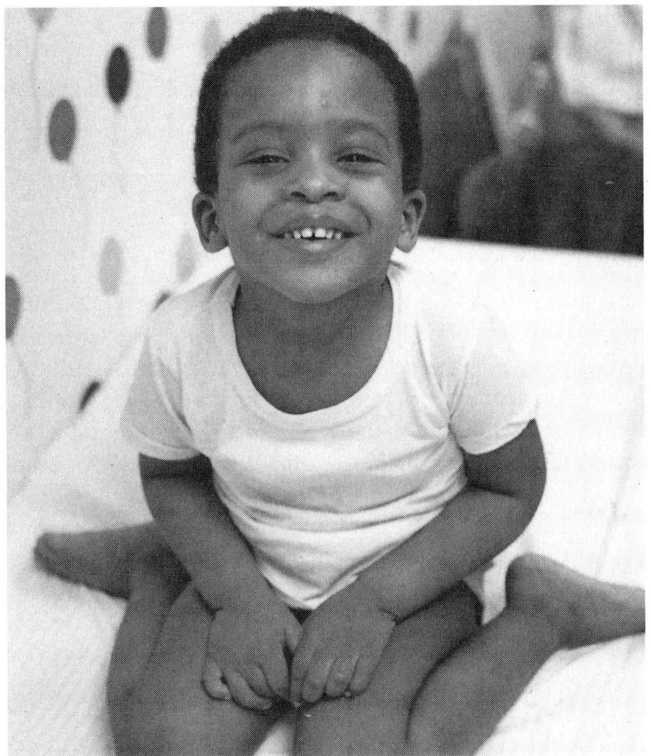

Figure 17.47 Reverse tailor position.

Ask the child to lie supine, then to rise to a standing position. Normally, the child rises without using the arms for support. Generalized muscle weakness may be indicated if the child places the hands on the knees and pushes the trunk up (*Gower sign*).

Assess the child's spine for scoliosis at each office visit. Inspect the child's shoes for signs of abnormal wear, and assess the child's gait. Before age 3, the gait of the child is normally broad-based. After age 3, the child's gait narrows. At each visit, assess the range of motion of each arm. Subluxation of the head of the radius occurs commonly when adults dangle children from their hands or remove their clothing forcibly.

Make sure you have complete information on any sports activity the child or adolescent engages in, because participation in these can indicate the need for special assessments or preventive teaching. For a comprehensive health assessment of infants, children, and adolescents, see Chapter 19.

Childbearing Clients

Estrogen and other hormones soften the cartilage in the pelvis and increase the mobility of the joints, especially the sacroiliac, sacrococcygeal, and symphysis pubis joints. As the pregnancy progresses, *lordosis* compensates for the enlarging fetus: as the woman's center of gravity shifts forward, she shifts her weight farther back on the lower extremities. This shift strains the lower spine, causing the lower back pain so common during late pregnancy.

As the woman's pregnancy progresses, she may develop a waddling gait because of her enlarged abdomen and the relaxed mobility in her joints. Typically, a woman resumes her normal posture and gait shortly after the pregnancy. For a comprehensive health assessment of the childbearing client, see Chapter 20.

Older Clients

As an individual ages, physiologic changes take place in the bones, muscles and connective tissue, and joints. These changes may affect the older client's mobility and endurance.

Bone changes include decreased calcium absorption and reduced osteoblast production. If the individual has a chronic illness, such as chronic obstructive lung disease or hyperthyroidism, or takes medications containing glucocorticoids or anticonvulsants, bone strength may be greatly compromised. Elderly persons who are housebound and immobile or whose dietary intake of calcium and vitamin D is low may also experience reduced bone mass and strength. With aging, bone resorption occurs more rapidly than new bone growth, resulting in the loss of bone density typical of osteoporosis. The entire skeleton is affected, but the vertebrae and long bones are especially vulnerable. Most older adults develop some degree of osteoporosis, but it is more marked in Caucasian females, especially those of Scandinavian ancestry.

The decreased height of the aging adult occurs because of a shortening of the vertebral column, which results from two factors: a thinning of the intervertebral disks during middle age, and an erosion of individual vertebrae due to osteoporosis. There is an average decrease in height of 1 to 2 inches from the twenties through the seventies, and a further decrease in the eighties and nineties because of further collapse of the vertebrae. *Kyphosis* (exaggerated convexity of the thoracic region of the spine) is common. When the older adult is standing, you may notice a slight flexion of the hips and knees. These changes in the vertebral column may cause a shift in the individual's center of gravity, which in turn may put the older adult at an increased risk for falls.

The size and quantity of muscle fibers tend to decrease by as much as 30% by the eightieth year. The amount of connective tissue in the muscles increases, and they become fibrous or stringy. Tendons become less elastic. As a result, the older client experiences a progressive decrease in reaction time, speed of movements, agility, and endurance.

Degeneration of the joints causes thickening and decreased viscosity of the synovial fluid, fragmentation of connective tissue, and scarring and calcification in the joint capsules. In addition, the cartilage becomes frayed, thin, and cracked, allowing the underlying bone to become eroded. Because of these changes, the joints of older people are less shock absorbent and have decreased range of motion and flexibility. These normal degenerative joint changes that occur from aging and wear and tear are referred to as *osteoarthrosis*. In some individuals, *Heberden's nodes*—hard, typically painless, bony enlargements associated with osteoarthritis—may occur in the distal interphalangeal joints.

The gait of an older client alters as the bones, muscles, and joints change with advancing age. Both men and women tend to walk slower, supporting themselves as they move. Elderly men tend to walk with the head and trunk in a flexed position, using short, high steps, a wide gait, and a smaller arm swing. The bowlegged stance that older women assume is due to reduced muscular control. It alters the normal angle of the hip, leading to increased susceptibility to falls and subsequent fractures.

As one ages, there is a general decrease in reaction time and speed of performance of tasks. This can affect mobility and safety, especially with unexpected environmental stimuli (eg, objects on the floor, loose carpeting, wet surfaces). In addition, any health problem that contributes to decreased physical activity tends to increase the chance of alterations in the health of the musculoskeletal system. A well-balanced diet and regular exercise help to slow the progression of these musculoskeletal changes.

The physical assessment of the musculoskeletal system of the elderly person is similar to that of any other adult. When testing range of motion, be careful not to cause pain, discomfort, or damage to the joint. Because elderly clients often have health problems that affect endurance, conduct the musculoskeletal exam at a slower pace when necessary. For a comprehensive health assessment of older adults, see Chapter 21.

Psychosocial Considerations

Psychosocial disturbances such as anxiety, depression, fear, body-image disturbance, or a disturbance in self-esteem may promote inactivity and/or isolation, which in turn may lead to musculoskeletal degeneration. By the same token, any health problem that contributes to inactivity may trigger or contribute to psychosocial disturbances. Impaired physical mobility may lead to stress, hopelessness, ineffective coping, social isolation, or other problems.

Physical abuse should be considered if a client has a history of frequent fractures, sprains, or other musculoskeletal trauma. Follow your state's guidelines for referring the client to social or protective services.

Self-Care Considerations

Lifestyle affects musculoskeletal changes. A sedentary lifestyle hastens musculoskeletal degeneration, and excessive weight puts additional stress on the bones. By contrast, physical exercise increases skeletal mass and helps prevent or delay the development of osteoporosis.

Sudden musculoskeletal changes such as fractures and degenerative changes such as arthritis affect one's ability to perform activities of daily living. Any client with changes in the musculoskeletal system should be evaluated for the presence or risk for activity intolerance, injury, self-care deficit, and other alterations in health.

Dietary factors influence musculoskeletal health. Deficiencies of protein, calcium, or vitamin D can inhibit bone growth and muscle strength. Excessive intake of caffeine or alcohol can predispose a client to osteoporosis.

Family, Cultural, and Environmental Considerations

The bone density of people of African ancestry is significantly higher than that of people of European heritage, whereas the bone density of Asians typically is lower than that of Europeans. The curvature of long bones varies widely among cultural groups and seems to be related to genetics and body weight. Thin people have less curvature than people of average weight; obese people display an increased curvature.

The number and distribution of vertebrae vary with different populations. While 24 vertebrae is the average (present in about 85–90% of all people), 23 or 25 verterbrae is not uncommon.

Certain working conditions present potential risks to the musculoskeletal system. Workers required to lift heavy objects may strain and injure the back. Jobs requiring substantial physical activity, such as those of construction workers, firefighters, or athletes, increase the likelihood of musculoskeletal injuries such as sprains, strains, and fractures.

Frequent repetitive movements may lead to misuse disorders such as carpal tunnel syndrome, pitcher's elbow, or vertebral degeneration.

Organizing the Data

After carrying out the focused interview and conducting the physical assessment of the musculoskeletal system, group the related data into clusters leading to either nursing diagnoses, which require interventions such as client teaching (discussed on pages 538–539), or alterations in health, which require consultation with other members of the health care team.

Identifying Nursing Diagnoses

Impaired physical mobility (see Table 17.2) is the NANDA diagnosis that most often reflects a client's response to musculoskeletal problems. The diagnosis may be appropriate, for example, when the client has a fracture, a degenerative bone disorder, or decreased muscle strength and is unable or reluctant to move about. In most cases, clients who are diagnosed with impaired physical mobility must also be assessed for potential problems such as *High risk for disuse syndrome, High risk for injury,* and *High risk for trauma.*

High risk for disuse syndrome is the state in which an individual is at risk for deterioration of body systems as the result of prescribed or unavoidable inactivity (NANDA). When an individual is unable to move a body part, the muscle and soft tissue in the affected part atrophy, and contractures develop in the affected muscles. Some of the related factors that contribute to disuse syndrome include neurologic disorders such as multiple sclerosis and Parkinson's disease; musculoskeletal disorders such as fractures, sprains, and arthritis; and surgical/orthopedic procedures such as amputation, traction, casts, and splints.

Individuals with impaired mobility are always at high risk for trauma or injury because their disorder does not allow them to protect themselves from various hazards. *High risk for injury* is the state in which an individual is at risk for injury as a result of environmental conditions interacting with the individual's adaptive and defensive resources (NANDA).

The nursing diagnosis *High risk for trauma* is more specific, and is defined as an accentuated risk of accidental tissue injury (eg, wound, burn, fracture) (NANDA). The risk factors for both diagnoses are similar: impaired mobility, sensory

Table 17.2 The Nursing Diagnosis Most Commonly Associated with the Musculoskeletal System

IMPAIRED PHYSICAL MOBILITY	
Definition: A state in which the individual experiences a limitation of ability for independent physical movement (NANDA). Level I: Independently uses equipment or device Level II: Requires help from another person for assistance, supervision, or teaching Level III: Requires help from another person and equipment/device Level IV: Is dependent and does not participate in activity Specify level _______	
DEFINING CHARACTERISTICS	
Reluctance to attempt movement Impaired motor coordination, muscle strength Limited range of motion	Inability to move purposefully within the physical environment Imposed restrictions of movement, including mechanical and/or medical protocol
RELATED FACTORS	
Pain/discomfort; Perceptual/cognitive impairment; Medically prescribed limitations; Musculoskeletal impairment; Neuromuscular impairment; Decreased strength and endurance secondary to (specify); Depression/severe anxiety; Others specific to client (specify).	

DIAGNOSTIC REASONING IN ACTION

Luisa Suarez is an 89-year-old female who moved to the Northeastern United States from her native Puerto Rico. She is unmarried and has no immediate family. Five years ago, she suffered a spinal injury that left her lower extremities weak. Although frail, Ms Suarez is fiercely independent and cares for herself whenever possible.

One morning, while trying to go to the bathroom without assistance, Ms Suarez fell and fractured her pelvis. While in the hospital, Ms Suarez experienced severe pain and did not recover as quickly as was expected. Because of her deteriorating condition, Ms Suarez was admitted to a nursing care center.

After 2 weeks in the center, Diane DeVito, RN, Ms Suarez's primary nurse, called a care planning conference for her client. She stated, "Ms Suarez is becoming weaker each day. Because of her pain, she moves only when she has to and resists being turned or moved by the nurses and aides. Even though several weeks have passed since the injury, she still refuses to attempt ambulation. Range of motion in her arms and legs is being compromised by lack of activity, and she is unable even to stand at the bedside without assistance."

The nursing assessment of Ms Suarez provided the following subjective and objective data:

- 89-year-old frail female
- Lower extremity weakness (from prior spinal cord injury)
- Reluctant to move after fracturing her pelvis
- Complains of severe pain at fracture site
- Reluctant to move by herself and resists being moved by nurses and aides
- Refuses to attempt ambulation
- Some limitation of range of motion in arms and legs

To cluster the information, Ms DeVito

- Notes that reluctance to attempt movement, impaired muscle strength, limited range of motion, and inability to move purposefully within the physical environment are defining characteristics of *Impaired physical mobility.*
- Notes that musculoskeletal impairment, pain/discomfort, injury, age (elderly), decreased muscle strength, and decreased joint flexibility are related factors for the diagnosis *Impaired physical mobility.*

The nurse arrives at the following nursing diagnoses:

1. *Impaired physical mobility* related to physiologic impairment, pain at fracture site
2. *High risk for disuse syndrome* related to reluctance to move in bed and refusal to ambulate secondary to fracture of pelvis
3. *High risk for injury* related to age, impaired mobility
4. *Pain* related to fractured pelvis
5. *Activity intolerance* related to pain
6. *Self-care deficit* related to pain and musculoskeletal impairment

Ms DeVito consults with Ms Suarez's physician and physical therapist, then develops a care plan to minimize Ms Suarez's pain and increase her activity.

deficits, presence of environmental hazards, and lack of knowledge of safety concerning environmental hazards.

Several other nursing diagnoses also are commonly associated with the musculoskeletal system. These include *Pain* related to degeneration of soft tissue in the joints; *Activity intolerance* related to immobility; *Social isolation* and *Body image disturbance* related to musculoskeletal changes; and *Knowledge deficit* related to inadequate information concerning self-care. The entire group of self-care deficits relating to feeding, bathing/hygiene, dressing/grooming, toileting, and instrumental self-care activities are also possible nursing diagnoses for the client with a musculoskeletal disorder.

Common Alterations in Health Associated with the Musculoskeletal System

Common alterations in health associated with the musculoskeletal system include degenerative disorders, misuse syndromes, trauma-induced disorders, and others. (See Table 17.3.) A comparison of position, precipitating factors, quality, and other descriptors of pain related to three common musculoskeletal disorders is provided in Table 17.4 on page 538.

Table 17.3 Common Alterations in the Health of the Musculoskeletal System

Joint Disorders

Carpal tunnel syndrome	Numbness, pain, and paresthesia caused by compression of the median nerve of the hand(s). The pain may radiate from the fingers down the hand. Common in persons who engage in repetitive motion, such as switchboard operators and data-entry clerks.
Lateral epicondylitis (tennis elbow)	Chronic disabling disease causing pain and tenderness occurring at the lateral epicondyles of the humerus. Persons who are involved in activities that combine pronation and supination of the forearm with an extended wrist (eg, tennis, racquet ball) are most prone to developing this problem.
Medial epicondylitis (pitcher's elbow)	Pain and tenderness at the medial epicondyles of the humerus following repetitive wrist flexion, such as in throwing a baseball. Wrist flexion increases the pain at the medial epicondyle site.
TMJ (temporomandibular joint) syndrome	Unilateral or bilateral facial pain that worsens with movement of the jaw. May be caused by congenital anomalies, trauma, stress, malocclusion, or arthritis. The pain may be referred to other parts of the face, neck, shoulder, and arm.
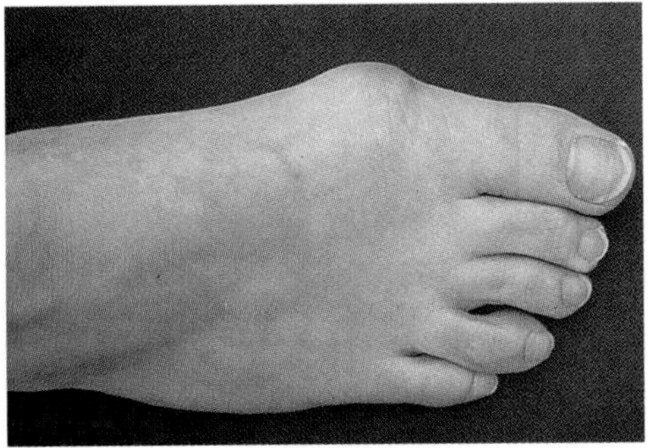 Bunion	A thickening and inflammation of the bursa of the joint of the great toe. There is a lateral displacement of the toe along with marked enlargement of the joint.
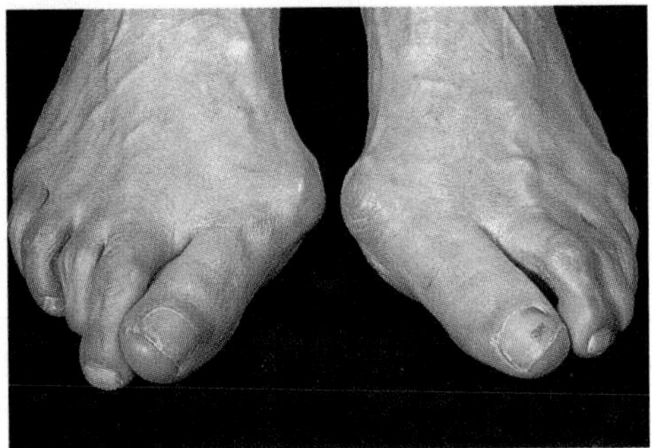 Hallux valgus	An abnormal adduction of the great toe at the metatarsophalangeal joint.
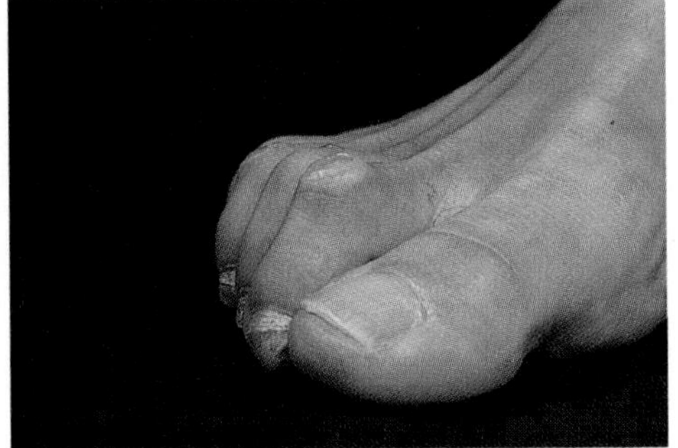 Hammertoe	A hyperextension at the metatarsophalangeal joint along with flexion of the interphalangeal joint of the toe. Corns sometimes develop at pressure points on the toe, such as at the proximal interphalangeal joints.

Table 17.3 Common Alterations in the Health of the Musculoskeletal System (continued)

Bone Disorders

Osteitis deformans (Paget's disease)	A chronic, inflammatory thickening and swelling of the bones with bowing of the long bones.
Osteoarthritis	A chronic, noninflammatory, nonsystemic disorder causing a deterioration of articular cartilage and formation of new bone at joint surfaces. The incidence increases with age.
Osteomyelitis	An infection in the bone caused by a pathogenic organism resulting from an open wound or fracture.
Osteoporosis	A decrease in bone mass and density of the skeleton involving mainly the long bones and vertebral column. This disease occurs because bone resorption is more rapid than bone deposition. Bones tend to be fragile and susceptible to spontaneous fractures. Approximately 29% of older women and 18% of older men are affected.
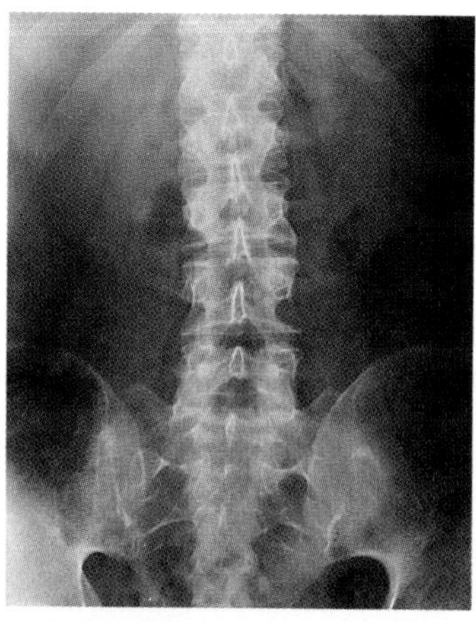 Ankylosing spondylitis (Marie-Strumpell disease)	A hereditary, chronic, inflammatory disease that begins with an inflammation around the sacroiliac joint. The disease is progressive, leading to eventual deformity and fusion of the spine. Sometimes considered a variation of rheumatoid arthritis. Men are affected more frequently than women (10:1 ratio) usually beginning in the twenties or thirties.
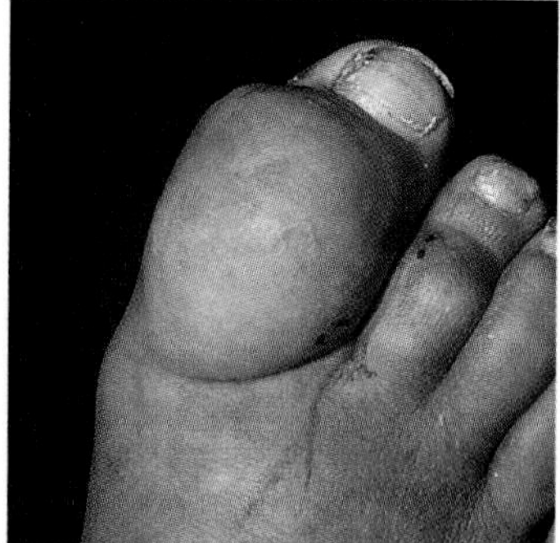 Gout (gouty arthritis)	An inflammatory metabolic disorder of purine metabolism. There is usually an elevation of serum uric acid with uric acid deposits in the joint spaces. The phalanx of the great toe is most commonly affected. Primarily affects men over age 40.
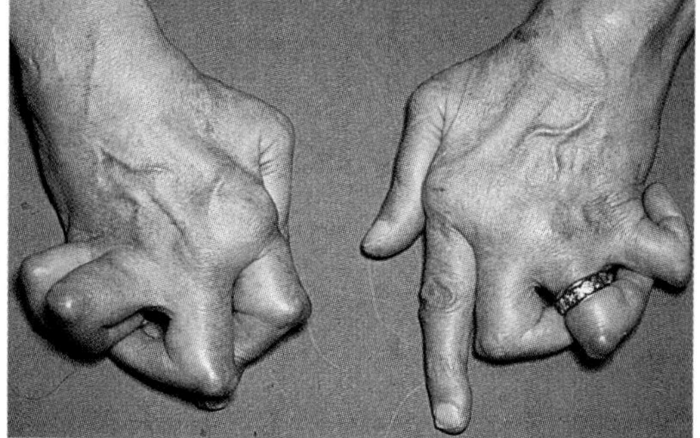 Rheumatoid arthritis	A chronic, inflammatory, systemic disease of the joints and connective tissue. Inflammation of the synovial membranes leads to thickening and fibrosis, causing moderate to severe joint enlargement and limitation in motion. Onset may occur at any age. More females are affected than males. The joint changes associated with rheumatoid arthritis tend to be symmetric, whereas the changes attributed to osteoarthritis are not.

Table 17.3 Common Alterations in the Health of the Musculoskeletal System (continued)

Spinal Disorders

List

The spine leans to the left or right: a plumb line drawn from T1 does not fall between the gluteal cleft. This condition may occur with spasms in the paravertebral muscles or a herniated disc.

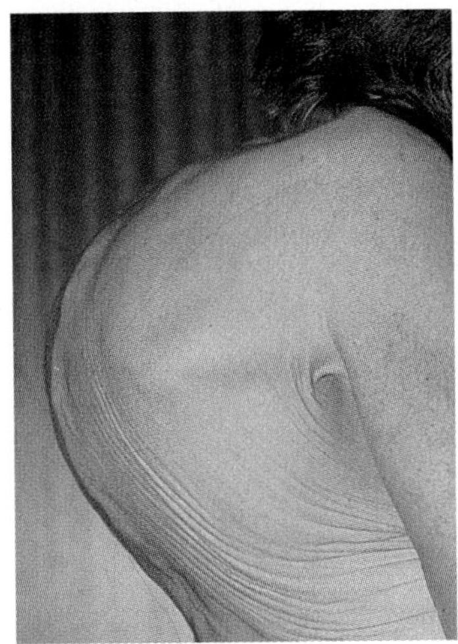

Kyphosis (hunchback)

A rounded convexity of the thoracic spine commonly seen in older adults, especially women.

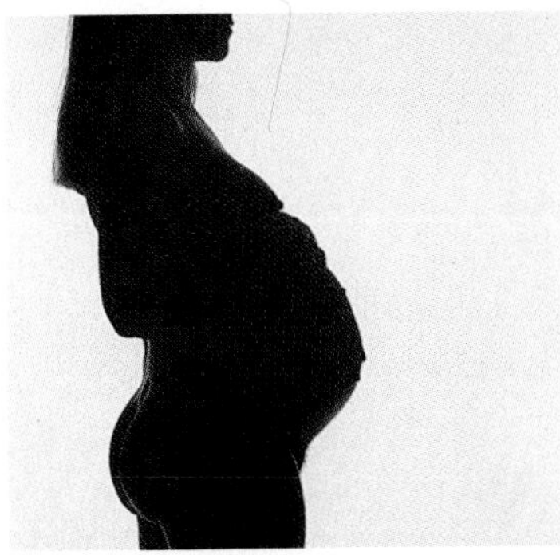

Lordosis (swayback)

An exaggeration of the normal lumbar curve that develops to compensate for the protuberant abdomen accompanying marked obesity or pregnancy.

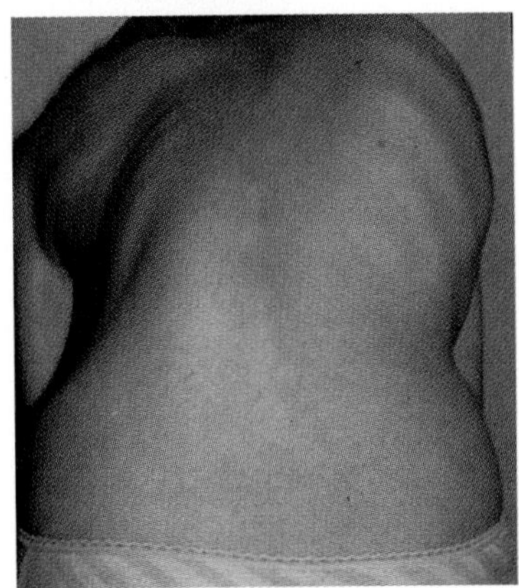

Scoliosis

A lateral curvature of the spine. *Structural scoliosis* may arise from a spinal deformity. It is accentuated with forward flexion: the thorax appears higher on the affected side because of the protrusion and spreading of the ribs, and the hip on the affected side is more prominent. *Functional scoliosis* may be caused by other irregularities of the body, such as unequal leg length. Functional scoliosis disappears with forward flexion. When scoliosis is severe, pulmonary ventilation may be compromised, leading to respiratory failure as an individual grows older.

Table 17.3 Common Alterations in the Health of the Musculoskeletal System (continued)

Trauma-Induced Disorders	
Dislocation	A displacement of the bone from its usual anatomic location in the joint.
Muscle sprain	A stretching or tearing of the capsule or ligament of a joint due to forced movement beyond the joint's normal range.
Fracture	A partial or complete break in the continuity of the bone from trauma.
Muscle strain	A partial muscle tear resulting from overstretching or overuse of the muscle.

Table 17.4 Descriptors of Pain Related to Common Musculosketal Disorders

	Costochronditis	Cervical Disc Syndrome or Cervical Radiculitis	Thoracic Outlet Syndrome
Definition	An inflammatory process of the cartilage that joins the ribs to the sternum. Pain, tenderness, and edema are present over more than one junction, most commonly the junction at the second rib.	Compression of a cervical root nerve from degenerative changes of the vertebrae, repeated trauma, or aging causes a persistent pain in neck and upper extremity.	Compression of subclavian artery, subclavian vein, and brachial nerve plexus by the first rib, muscles of the upper thorax or clavicle. Symptoms of pain, numbness, or tingling are directly related to the structures being compressed.
Position	Pain in upper costrochrondral cartilages, usually anterior chest	No specific position	Raising arm, have patient abduct and externally rotate arm
Precipitating Factors	Movement of the chest wall, coughing, deep breathing, usually associated with trauma	Worsens with neck movement, coughing, sneezing	Cause of claudication
Quality	Imitates the pain of an MI, may also feel tender	May be sharp, boring in nature depending upon the site of origin	Anterior chest pain
Radiation	Usually none, more localized	Usually none	To arm, shoulder, scapula
Relief	Usually by stopping movement of the chest wall, mild analgesia	Stop movement of neck, stop coughing, sneezing	Stop precipitator of claudication
Severity	Variable on a 1–10 scale	Variable on a 1–10 scale	Variable on a 1–10 scale
Timing	With thoracic movement	With precipitators	With cause of claudication
Duration	May last for days	Hours, days	Variable

Health Promotion and Client Education

At the conclusion of the assessment, answer any questions the client may have and stress any of the following guidelines for maintaining the health of the musculoskeletal system that may be appropriate for the individual client.

Promoting Healthy Bones and Muscles

To promote the general health of the musculoskeletal system

- Maintain a healthy weight. Obesity strains the muscles, bones, and joints.
- Do weight-bearing exercises and muscle-toning such as walking or low-impact aerobics at least three times a week (Figure 17.48).
- Eat a well-balanced diet, including approximately 800 mg of calcium daily to reduce the incidence of osteoporosis in later life. Foods rich in calcium include dairy products, dark green, leafy vegetables, and sardines. Additionally, consume an adequate amount of protein and vitamin C and D daily to maintain bone health and muscle tone, and to promote tissue healing.
- Avoid smoking. Research suggests a relationship between smoking and osteoporosis.
- Avoid alcohol and caffeine. Research suggests a relationship between osteoporosis and ingestion of alcohol and caffeine.

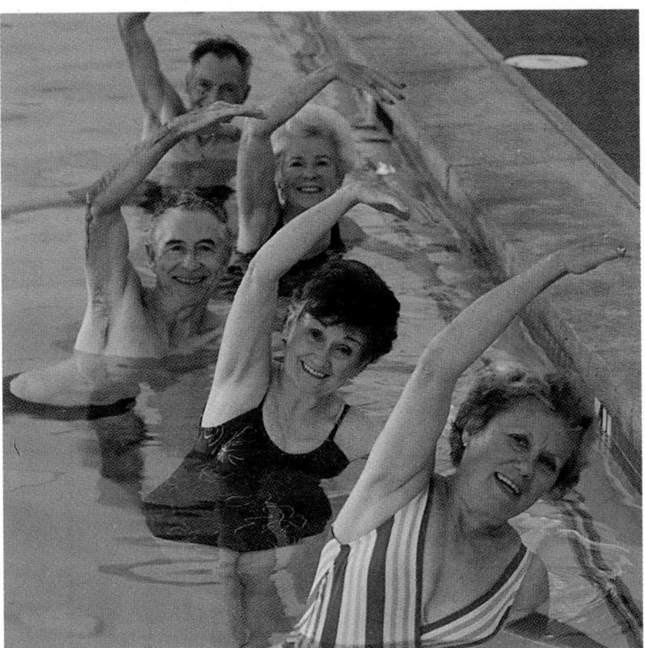

Figure 17.48 Weight-bearing exercise reduces the risk of osteoporosis.

Preventing Injuries to the Musculoskeletal System

To prevent injuries to the musculoskeletal system

- Use proper body mechanics. When lifting an object, bend the knees, not the back, letting the strong thigh muscles do the work. Position yourself as closely as possible to the object to help you maintain your center of gravity.
- Use the longest and strongest muscles of arms and legs when doing strenuous exercise.
- Maintain an erect posture.
- Maintain a safe environment to prevent slips and falls. Use night lights and remove loose rugs (throw rugs) from the floors. In the bathtub, use handrails and non-slip mats.
- Use the handrails for support and balance when walking up and down stairs.
- Wear properly fitting shoes with low, broad heels to prevent back strain and loss of balance.
- Use seat belts and observe speed limits for motor vehicles.
- Wear glasses if needed to enhance perception and prevent falls.
- Use assistive devices such as walkers and canes when needed to maintain balance when walking.

Summary

The musculoskeletal system provides the basic framework for the human body. To perform a comprehensive assessment of the system, you use a systematic head-to-toe approach to assess the major muscles, bones, and joints. During the focused interview, gather data about the client's family history, physical history, self-care, environment, pain and discomfort, and psychosocial factors that may have contributed to the onset of musculoskeletal problems. The nursing diagnosis most commonly identified with the musculoskeletal system is *Impaired physical mobility.* Other nursing diagnoses that may be appropriate include *High risk for disuse syndrome, High risk for injury, Pain,* and *Activity intolerance.* After performing the health assessment and identifying any appropriate nursing diagnoses, provide the client with the information needed to promote the health of the musculoskeletal system.

Key Points

- ✓ The primary function of the musculoskeletal system is to provide a framework for the human body. The skeletal system contains 206 bones and is responsible for posture, support of body organs, production of red blood cells, and the storage of fat and minerals. The major functions of the skeletal muscles are to provide movement, maintain posture, and generate heat. A joint is the articulation point where two or more bones of the body meet. Joints are classified as fibrous, cartilaginous, or synovial.
- ✓ During the focused interview, gather information about the client's musculoskeletal system, including mobility, family and physical history, self-care, environment, pain and discomfort, and psychosocial factors that may have contributed to musculoskeletal problems.
- ✓ During the physical examination, use the techniques of inspection and palpation to assess the health status, range of motion, and muscle strength of the major muscles, bones, and joints of the body.
- ✓ Assess all of the following joints of the body during the musculoskeletal exam: temporomandibular joint, shoulders, elbows, wrists, hands and fingers, hips, knees, ankles, feet and toes, and spine.
- ✓ Examine the client in an orderly, systematic manner—head to toe, proximal to distal, on both sides of the body.
- ✓ The nursing diagnosis most commonly associated with the musculoskeletal system is impaired physical mobility.
- ✓ Encourage the client to maintain a healthy weight, get plenty of weight-bearing exercise such as walking, eat a well-balanced diet with plenty of protein and calcium, use proper body mechanics, and use safety measures to prevent musculoskeletal injury or trauma.

Chapter 18

Assessing the Neurologic System

The complex integration, coordination, and regulation of body systems and ultimately all body functions are achieved through the mechanics of the nervous system. The intricate nature of the nervous system permits the individual to (a) perform all physiologic functions, (b) perform all activities of daily living, (c) function in society, and (d) maintain a degree of independence. A threat to any aspect of neurologic function is a threat to the total person. A neurologic deficit could alter self-concept, produce anxiety related to decreased function and loss of self-control, and restrict the client's mobility. Thus, it is essential to assess the psychosocial health status of a client experiencing a neurologic deficit. Because factors such as diet, alcohol intake, smoking, and other health-care practices can influence neurologic health, you must consider the client's self-care practices when assessing the client's neurologic system. Factors relating to the client's job, environment, and genetic background also contribute to the total database. These factors, as well as the relationship between the neurologic system and other body systems, are depicted in Figure 18.1.

A thorough neurologic assessment gives you detailed data regarding the client's health status and self-care practices. It is imperative for you to develop and refine your assessment skills regarding the wellness and normal parameters of the neurologic functions in the body. You need to foster a keen discriminatory skill concerning the subtle changes that could be occurring in the client. Neurologic assessment is an integral aspect of the total database used by the professional nurse.

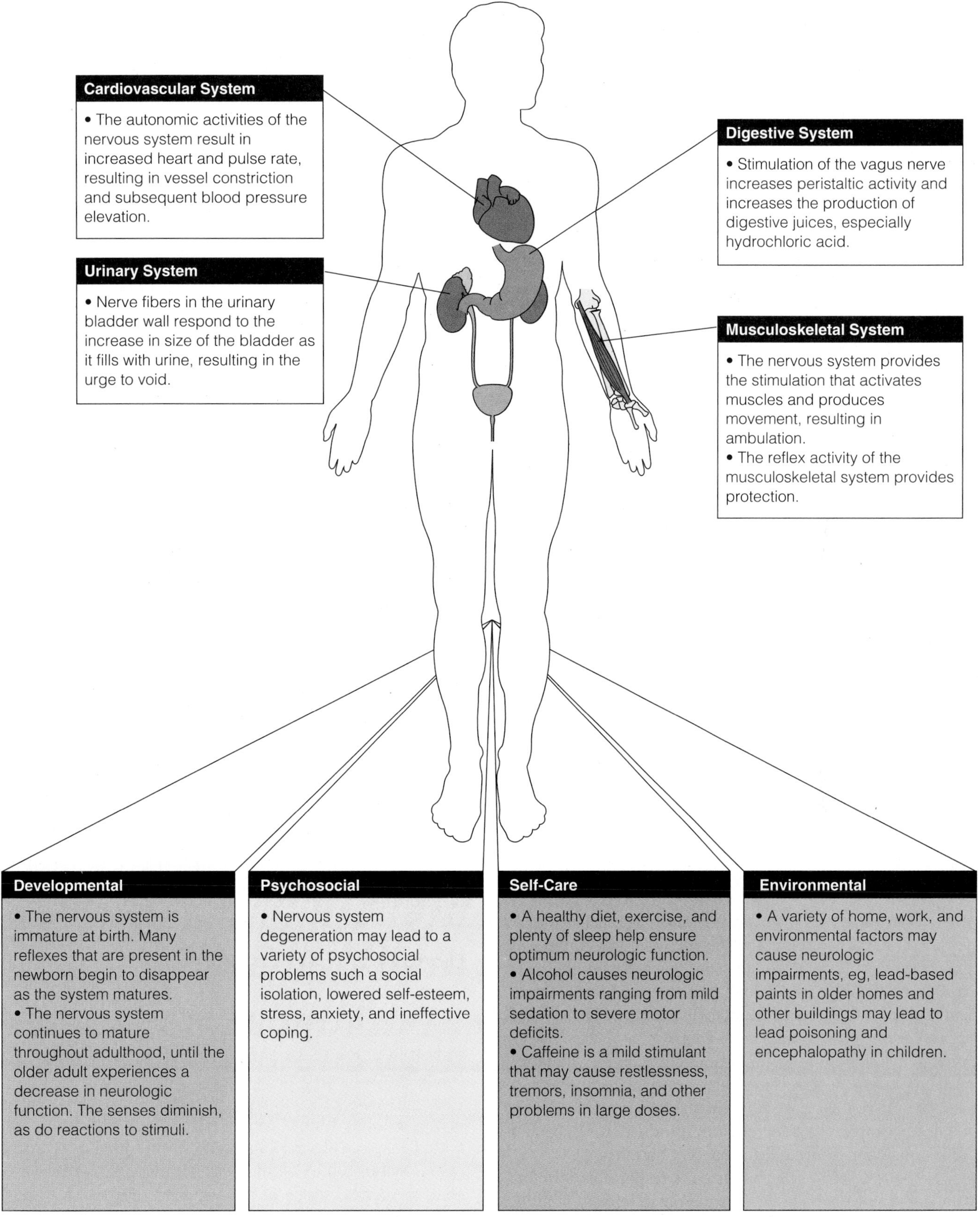

Cardiovascular System
• The autonomic activities of the nervous system result in increased heart and pulse rate, resulting in vessel constriction and subsequent blood pressure elevation.
Urinary System
• Nerve fibers in the urinary bladder wall respond to the increase in size of the bladder as it fills with urine, resulting in the urge to void.
Digestive System
• Stimulation of the vagus nerve increases peristaltic activity and increases the production of digestive juices, especially hydrochloric acid.
Musculoskeletal System
• The nervous system provides the stimulation that activates muscles and produces movement, resulting in ambulation.
• The reflex activity of the musculoskeletal system provides protection.
Developmental
• The nervous system is immature at birth. Many reflexes that are present in the newborn begin to disappear as the system matures.
• The nervous system continues to mature throughout adulthood, until the older adult experiences a decrease in neurologic function. The senses diminish, as do reactions to stimuli.
Psychosocial
• Nervous system degeneration may lead to a variety of psychosocial problems such a social isolation, lowered self-esteem, stress, anxiety, and ineffective coping.
Self-Care
• A healthy diet, exercise, and plenty of sleep help ensure optimum neurologic function.
• Alcohol causes neurologic impairments ranging from mild sedation to severe motor deficits.
• Caffeine is a mild stimulant that may cause restlessness, tremors, insomnia, and other problems in large doses.
Environmental
• A variety of home, work, and environmental factors may cause neurologic impairments, eg, lead-based paints in older homes and other buildings may lead to lead poisoning and encephalopathy in children.

Figure 18.1 Important factors to consider when assessing the neurologic system.

Anatomy and Physiology Review

The neurologic system, a highly integrated and complex system, is divided into two principal parts, the central nervous system (CNS) and the peripheral nervous system (PNS). The central nervous system consists of the brain and the spinal cord, whereas the cranial nerves and the spinal nerves make up the peripheral nervous system. The two systems work together to receive an impulse, interpret it, and initiate a response, enabling the individual to maintain a high level of adaptation and homeostasis. The nervous system is responsible for control of cognitive function and both voluntary and involuntary activities.

Central Nervous System

Brain

The **brain** is the largest portion of the central nervous system. It is covered and protected by the meninges, the cerebrospinal fluid, and the bony structure of the skull. The **meninges** are three connective tissue membranes that cover, protect, and nourish the central nervous system. The **cerebrospinal fluid** also helps to nourish the central nervous system; however, its primary function is to cushion the brain and prevent injury to the brain tissue. The brain is made up of the cerebrum, diencephalon, cerebellum, and brainstem (Figure 18.2).

Cerebrum

The **cerebrum** is the largest portion of the brain. The outermost layer of the cerebrum, the *cerebral cortex,* is composed of gray matter. Responsible for all conscious behavior, the cerebral cortex enables the individual to perceive, remember, communicate, and initiate voluntary movements. The lobes of the cerebrum are shown in Figure 18.3.

The *frontal lobe* of the cerebrum helps control voluntary skeletal movement, speech, emotions, and intellectual activities. The prefrontal cortex of the frontal lobe is involved with intellect, complex learning abilities, production of abstract ideas, judgment, reasoning, and concern for others.

The *parietal lobe* of the cerebrum is responsible for conscious awareness of sensation, and somatosensory stimuli, including temperature, pain, shapes, and two-point discrimination.

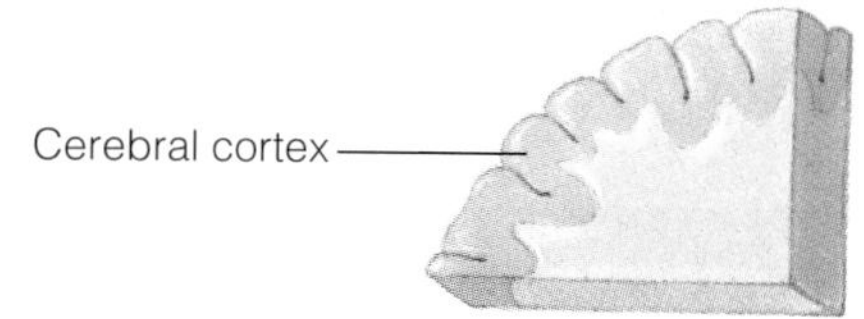

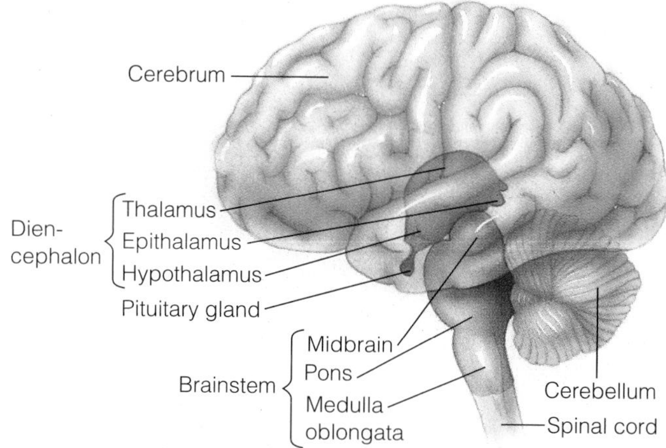

Figure 18.2 Regions of the brain.

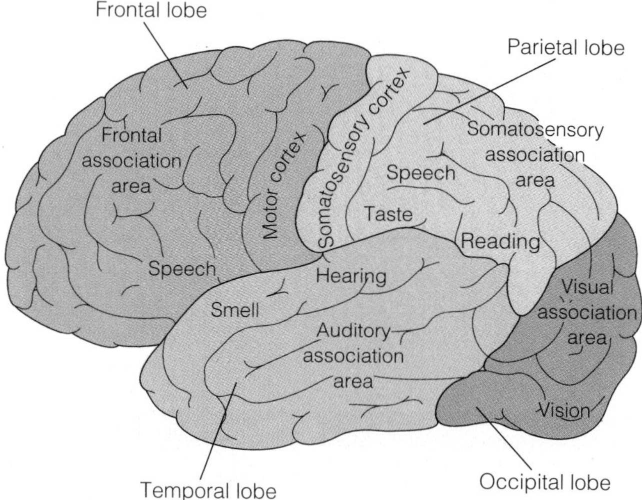

Figure 18.3 Lobes of the cerebrum.

The visual cortex, located in the *occipital lobe,* receives stimuli from the retina and interprets the visual stimuli in relation to past experiences.

The *temporal lobe* of the cerebrum is responsible for interpreting auditory stimuli. Impulses from the cochlea are transmitted to the temporal lobe and are interpreted regarding pitch, rhythm, loudness, and perception of what we hear. The olfactory cortex is also in the temporal lobe and transmits impulses related to smell.

Diencephalon

The **diencephalon** is composed of the thalamus, hypothalamus, and epithalamus.

The *thalamus* is the gateway to the cerebral cortex. All inputs channeled to the cerebral cortex are processed by the thalamus.

The *hypothalamus*, an autonomic control center, influences activities such as blood pressure, heart rate, force of heart contraction, digestive motility, respiratory rate and depth, and perception of pain, pleasure, and fear. Regulation of body temperature, food intake, water balance, and sleep cycles are regulated by the hypothalamus.

The *epithalamus* helps control moods and sleep cycles. It contains the choroid plexus, where the cerebrospinal fluid is formed.

Cerebellum

The **cerebellum** is located below the cerebrum and behind the brainstem. It coordinates stimuli from the cerebral cortex to provide precise timing for skeletal muscle coordination and smooth movements. The cerebellum also assists with maintaining equilibrium and muscle tone.

Brainstem

The **brainstem** contains the midbrain, pons, and medulla oblongata. Located between the cerebrum and spinal cord, it connects pathways between the higher and lower structures. Ten of the twelve pairs of cranial nerves originate in the brainstem. As an autonomic control center, it influences blood pressure by controlling vasoconstriction. It also regulates respiratory rate, depth, and rhythm as well as vomiting, hiccuping, swallowing, coughing, and sneezing.

Spinal Cord

The **spinal cord** is a continuation of the medulla oblongata. About 42 cm (17 inches) in length, it passes through the skull at the foramen magnum and continues through the vertebral column to the first lumbar vertebra (see Figure 18.6). The spinal cord is protected by the meninges, cerebrospinal fluid, and the bony vertebrae. The spinal cord has the ability to transmit impulses to and from the brain via the ascending and descending pathways. Some reflex activity takes place within the spinal cord; however, this activity must be interpreted by the brain to be useful.

Reflexes

Reflexes are stimulus-response activities of the body. They are fast, predictable, unlearned, inborn, and involuntary reactions to stimuli. The individual is aware of the results of the reflex activity and not the activity itself. The reflex activity may be simple and take place at the level of the spinal cord, with interpretation at the cerebral level. For example, if the tendon of the knee is sharply stimulated with a reflex hammer, the impulse follows the afferent nerve fibers, a synapse occurs in the spinal cord, the impulse is transmitted to the efferent nerve fibers, leading to an additional synapse and stimulation of muscle fibers. As the muscle fibers contract, the lower leg moves, causing the knee-jerk reaction. The individual is aware of the reflex after the lower leg moves and the brain has interpreted the activity. Figure 18.4 illustrates two simple reflex arcs.

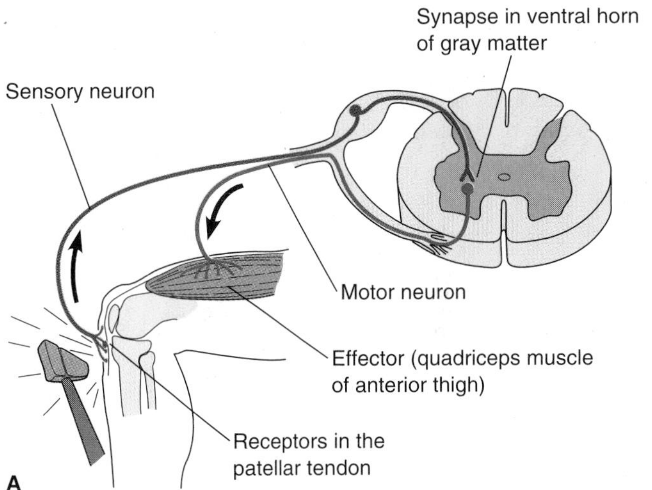

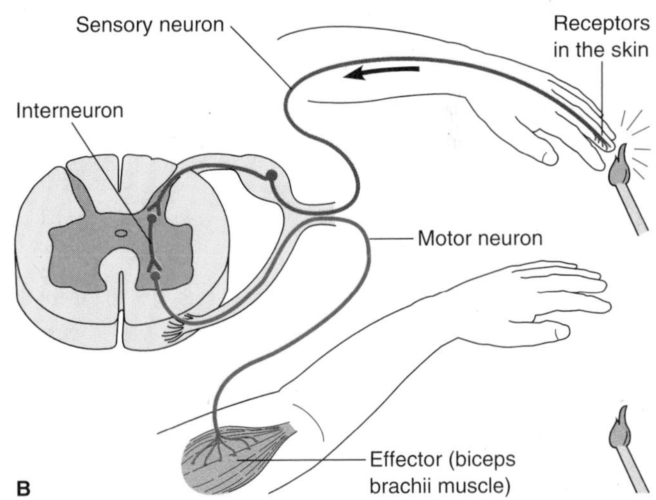

Figure 18.4 Two simple reflex arcs: *A*, In the two-neuron reflex arc, the stimulus is transferred from the sensory neuron directly to the motor neuron at the point of synapse in the spinal cord. *B*, In the three-neuron reflex arc, the stimulus travels from the sensory neuron to an interneuron in the spinal cord, and then to the motor neuron. (Sensory nerves are shown in blue; motor nerves, in red.)

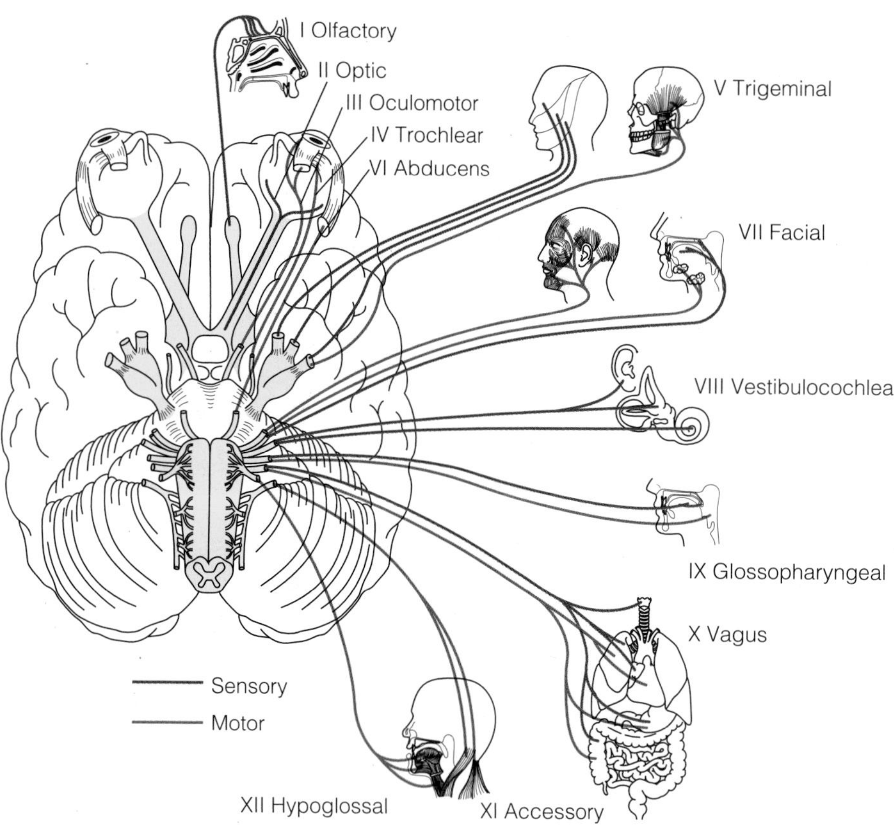

Figure 18.5 Cranial nerves and their target regions. (Sensory nerves are shown in blue; motor nerves, in red.)

Table 18.1 Cranial Nerves

Name	Number	Function	Activity
Olfactory	I	Sensory	Sense of smell.
Optic	II	Sensory	Vision.
Oculomotor	III	Motor	Pupillary reflex, extrinsic muscle movement of eye.
Trochlear	IV	Motor	Eye-muscle movement.
Trigeminal	V	Mixed	*Ophthalmic branch*: Sensory impulses from scalp, upper eyelid, nose, cornea, and lacrimal gland. *Maxillary branch*: Sensory impulses from lower eyelid, nasal cavity, upper teeth, upper lip, and palate. *Mandibular branch*: Sensory impulses from tongue, lower teeth, skin of chin, and lower lip. Motor action includes teeth clenching, movement of mandible.
Abducens	VI	Mixed	Extrinsic muscle movement of eye.
Facial	VII	Mixed	Taste (anterior two-thirds of tongue). Facial movements such as smiling, closing of eyes, frowning. Production of tears and salivary stimulation.
Vestibulocochlear	VIII	Sensory	*Vestibular branch*: Sense of balance or equilibrium. *Cochlear branch*: Sense of hearing.
Glossopharyngeal	IX	Mixed	Produces the gag and swallowing reflexes. Taste (posterior third of the tongue).
Vagus	X	Mixed	Innervates muscles of throat and mouth for swallowing and talking. Other branches responsible for pressoreceptors and chemoreceptor activity.
Accessory	XI	Motor	Movement of the trapezius and sternocleidomastoid muscles. Some movement of larynx, pharynx, and soft palate.
Hypoglossal	XII	Motor	Movement of tongue for swallowing, movement of food during chewing, and speech.

Peripheral Nervous System

Cranial Nerves

The 12 pairs of **cranial nerves** originate in the brain and serve various parts of the head and neck (Figure 18.5). Pairs I and II originate in the anterior brain, and the remaining 10 pairs originate in the brainstem. The vagus nerve is the only cranial nerve to serve a body region below the neck. The cranial nerves are numbered using roman numerals and many times are discussed by number rather than name. Composition of the cranial nerve fibers varies, producing sensory nerves, motor nerves, and mixed nerves. A summary of the name, number, function, and activity of the cranial nerves is presented in Table 18.1.

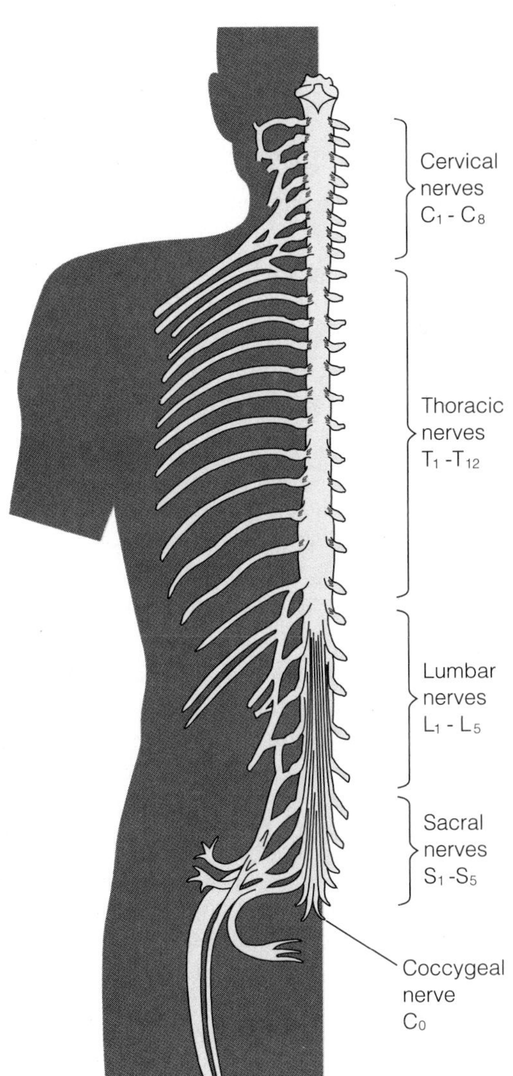

Figure 18.6 Spinal nerves.

Spinal Nerves

The spinal cord supplies the body with 31 pairs of **spinal nerves** that are named according to the vertebral level of origin (Figure 18.6).

There are 8 pairs of cervical nerves, 12 pairs of thoracic nerves, 5 pairs of lumbar nerves, 5 pairs of sacral nerves, and 1 pair of coccygeal nerves. At the cervical level, the nerves exit superior to the vertebra except for the eighth cervical nerve. This nerve exits inferior to the seventh cervical vertebra. All remaining descending nerves exit the spinal cord and vertebral column inferior to the same-numbered vertebrae. Spinal nerves are all classified as mixed nerves because they contain motor and sensory pathways that produce motor and sensory activities. Each pair of nerves is responsible for a particular area of the body. The nerves provide some overlap of body segments they serve. This overlap is more complete on the trunk than on the extremities.

A *dermatome* is an area of skin innervated by the cutaneous branch of one spinal nerve. An anterior view of the dermatomes of the body is shown in Figure 18.7.

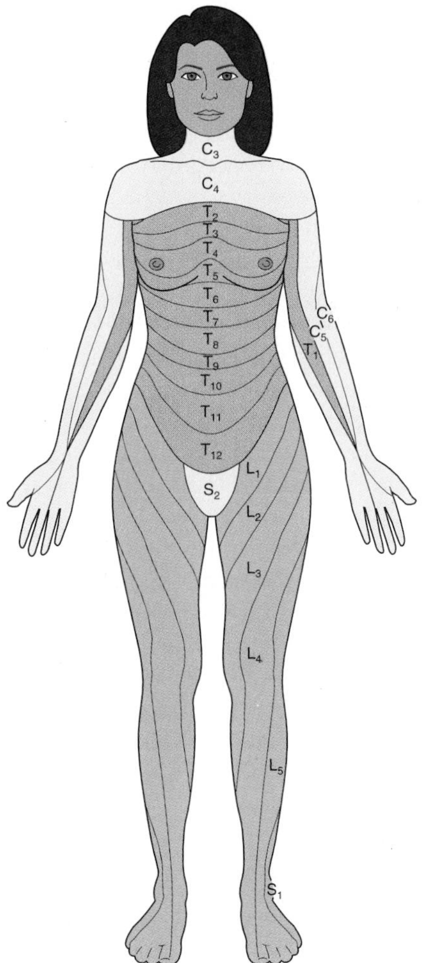

Figure 18.7 Anterior dermatomes.

Gathering the Data

The neurologic assessment provides you with detailed data regarding the health status of the client. Because of the natural complexity of the neurologic system, you may at first feel uncomfortable when performing this aspect of the total assessment.

As a professional nurse you will perform selected aspects of the neurologic assessment on a daily basis with all clients. The data-gathering process begins with the initial nurse-client interaction. As you meet clients, you make observations regarding their general appearance, personal hygiene, ability to walk to the chair, and ability to sit down. The ability to perform these activities is directly related to cerebral function.

The data-gathering process is twofold. The first step, the focused interview, builds on the data obtained in the health history. You must be sensitive to the needs and concerns of the client when asking questions related to neurologic function. Clients fear loss of control of bodily functions and loss of independence. Clients may attempt at times to mask or conceal data. Time is an additional variable to take into consideration. Many clients need extra time to comprehend and respond to questions. It may also be necessary to have a family member present.

The physical assessment is the second source for data gathering. Organize your assessment strategies by working in a cephalocaudal and distal-to-proximal pattern, always comparing corresponding body parts. Most likely, you will begin by assessing the 12 cranial nerves as discussed shortly. If an in-depth assessment of the head and neck has been completed, then the cranial nerves may have been tested. If so, you need to vary the organizational pattern you use. The organizational pattern will also vary according to the physical condition of the client.

Because of the complexity of the neurologic system, several tests are available to assess a function, and several functions may be assessed simultaneously. For example, asking the client to smile tests cranial nerve VII (facial), which is responsible for facial movement. This test also assesses cranial nerve VIII for hearing and cerebral cortex functioning, indicated by the client's ability to follow directions and initiate voluntary movements.

Focused Interview

While taking the health history, you most likely ascertained information regarding a history of hypertension, stroke, meningitis, encephalitis, the use of alcohol and drugs, and prescribed medications. The data you obtain now provides additional information regarding client strengths, weaknesses, and health-care practices related to the neurologic system. You use this data to formulate a nursing diagnosis and develop a plan for care.

Questions Related to the Neurologic System

Before beginning the interview, review the available data. This database could include assessment of other systems, X-ray studies, MRI and tomographic scans, blood studies, EEG reports, and any other diagnostic work that has been completed.

1. Ask the client to complete the sentence: "After I get out of bed in the morning, a typical day in my life includes—" *You are asking for the activities of daily living. If this data has been obtained in another area of the assessment, then alter the lead statement accordingly. The client usually perceives this opening as nonthreatening. It places a focus on activities, self-care practices, and the client's level of wellness. Employ therapeutic communication skills to seek clarification, and encourage the client to relate all of the activities of the day.*
2. Explain to me what brings you here today. *This open-ended statement allows the client to state what is important. It increases the client's control in what may be a stressful situation, thereby producing a less threatening environment. Based on the client's response, adjust the sequence of questions to explore the client's concern.*
3. Have you ever had a work or sports injury to your head or back? If so, please explain what happened. When did this happen? What treatments did you receive? As a result of this injury, what problems do you have today? *The database being developed relates to past incidents and residual deficits.*
4. Describe your memory. Do you need to make a list or write things down so you won't forget? Do you lose things easily? What did you do today before you came here? *Memory loss is indicative of the aging process and neurologic or psychiatric disease. You are developing a baseline regarding the client's memory and the ability to recall recent and distant events.*
5. Do you get headaches? If so, describe them. Where are they located? Are they always in the same area? How often do they occur? Are you able to function with these headaches? What do you think causes your headaches? What do you do to help relieve the pain? Does this remedy work? On a scale of 1 to 10, rate the severity of your headaches. *You are developing the database to determine if headaches are migraines, tension, cluster, unilateral, bilateral, or associated with other disease.*

Another possibility is the side effect to a prescribed medication. See Chapter 9 for a description of types of headaches.

6. Do you have fainting spells? Do you have a history of seizures or convulsions? If so, when did you have your first seizure? What happens to you immediately before the seizure? What have you been told about what your body does during the seizure? How do you feel after the seizure? What medications do you take? Do you take your medications regularly? When was the last time you had a seizure? *Encourage the client to identify the type of seizure—petite mal or grand mal. The questions focus on an aura, muscular activity, postictal period, and use of medications. Lifestyle changes are important, because these individuals need to be cautioned regarding driving and the use of dangerous equipment. (Epilepsy is described later in this chapter.)*
7. Has your vision changed in any way? Do you ever see two objects when you know there is just one? Are you able to see off to the sides without turning your head? When you go from a bright room to a darker room, do your eyes adjust to the change rapidly? *While near and far vision and other ocular diseases are assessed with the head and neck, these changes may indicate problems with the cranial nerves, a brain tumor, or increased intracranial pressure.*
8. What changes, if any, have you noticed in your hearing? Have you noticed any ringing in the ears? *Hearing is assessed with the head and neck. Changes in hearing and ringing in the ears may indicate a problem with cranial nerve function.*
9. Have you noticed any change with your ability to smell or taste? *Smell and taste are assessed with the head and neck. A change in the ability to smell or taste may also indicate a problem with cranial nerve function.*
10. Describe your balance. Are you steady on your feet? Are you able to function without difficulty? Is one leg stronger than the other? Do you notice any tremors? Could you bend down to pick up a straight pin and stand up again? Do you drop things easily? Do you find yourself being very clumsy—tripping, spilling things, knocking things over? If so, how long have the symptoms been present? Are the symptoms continuous? Are they getting worse? What do you do to control or limit the symptoms? *All of these questions relate to activities of the cerebellum.*
11. Are you having any pain? If so, where is it? When did the pain begin? Is the pain constant or intermittent? What relieves or decreases the pain? What increases the pain? Does the pain interfere with your daily activities? How would you describe the pain—sharp, dull, acute, burning, stabbing, or stinging? On a scale of 1 to 10 with 10 being highest, how would you rate the pain? *Pain, a completely subjective experience, can be acute or chronic. This database provides information regarding cultural variations, self-care practices, and placement on the health-illness continuum.*
12. Are you now or have you ever been exposed to environmental hazards such as insecticides, organic solvents, lead, toxic wastes, or other pollutants? If so, which one, when, and for what period of time were you exposed? What treatment did you seek? Are you left with any problems because of the exposure? *Such exposure could contribute to neurologic deficits and neoplastic activity in the body.*

Additional Questions with Infants, Children, and Adolescents

1. Ask the mother or other caretaker: Describe if you can the pregnancy with this child, including any health problems, medications taken, or alcohol or drugs used. Was the child premature, at term, or late? Describé the birth of the child, including any complications during or shortly after the birth. *Problems during the antepartal period, including the use of medications, alcohol, or drugs, may affect the neurologic health of the child. Similarly, complications during or shortly after birth may have residual effects. For example, research indicates that some cases of epilepsy, a seizure disorder, may be due to prenatal or birth trauma.*
2. Has the child had any seizures? If so, how often has this happened? Describe what happens when your child has a seizure. Has the child had a high fever when the seizures occurred? *Seizures in feverish infants and toddlers are not uncommon. Seizures without accompanying fever may indicate a seizure disorder such as epilepsy.*
3. For toddlers and older children: Have you noticed any clumsiness in your child's activities? For example, does your child frequently drop things, have difficulty manipulating toys, bump into things, have problems walking or climbing stairs, or fall frequently? *These signs may indicate neurologic disease.*
4. Are you aware of any surfaces in your home that are painted with lead-based paint? Have you ever seen your child eating paint chips? *Lead poisoning may lead to developmental delays, peripheral nerve damage, or brain damage.*
5. For school-aged children: How is your child doing in school? Does your child seem to be able to concentrate on homework assignments and complete them on time? Have you ever been told that your child has a learning disability? That your child is hyperactive? Do you agree with this assessment? Why or why not?

Additional Questions with Childbearing Clients

1. Have you had a past history of seizures or any seizures during this pregnancy or previous pregnancies? If so, how often? Please describe the seizures.
2. Are you taking any vitamins or other nutritional supplements? Please describe these. *Prenatal supplements are important to provide for the neurologic health of the growing fetus. For example, vitamin A is required for nerve myelinization, and folic acid has been shown to reduce the incidence of neural-tube defects.*

Additional Questions with Older Adults

1. Do you require more time to perform tasks today than perhaps 2 years ago? Five years ago? Explain.
2. When you stand up, do you have trouble starting to walk? *Trouble initiating movement may indicate Parkinson's disease, which is more common in older adults.*
3. Do you notice any tremors? *Tremors may indicate motor nerve disease, or they may be attributable to certain medications or excessive consumption of caffeine.*
4. What safety features have you added to your home? *Safety precautions are essential to prevent neurologic trauma from falls and other accidents.*

Physical Assessment

Preparation

☑ **Gather the equipment:**

- percussion hammer
- tuning fork
- sterile cotton balls
- penlight
- ophthalmoscope
- stethoscope
- sterile needle
- tongue blade
- applicator
- hot and cold water in test tubes
- objects to touch, such as paper clip, safety pin, penny, dime, and quarter
- substances to smell, such as coffee, vanilla, and perfume
- substances to taste, such as salt, lemon, and sugar
- drape for client
- examination gown
- examination gloves

☑ **Wash your hands.**

☑ **Ask the client to remove all clothing except underwear and put on an examination gown.**

☑ **Ensure that the room is warm and free of drafts, with full lighting.**

Remember

- Ensure client privacy.
- Ensure client safety.
- Vary your approach according to the physical condition of the client.
- When possible, perform the nonthreatening, easily performed tasks first.
- Use universal precautions throughout the neurologic assessment.
- Explain all procedures to the client. A client with a neurologic deficit may require a more detailed explanation and more time to respond to a question or direction.
- The neurologic assessment begins with the first contact you have with the client. Before beginning the physical assessment, make a rapid survey to determine the client's ability to participate. Also determine whether any aspects have been tested with other body systems.
- Work in an organized manner, taking a head-to-toe and distal-to-proximal approach. Assess mental status, cranial nerves, motor function, sensory function, and reflexes.

ASSESSMENT TECHNIQUE/NORMAL FINDINGS | SPECIAL CONSIDERATIONS

Mental Status

You assess the mental status of the client when you meet the client for the first time. This process begins with the taking of the health history and continues with each client contact. The assessment of the client's mental status is discussed fully in Chapter 7. If necessary, review this material before proceeding.

Step 1 *Position the client.*

The client should be sitting on the examination table wearing the examination gown (Figure 18.8).

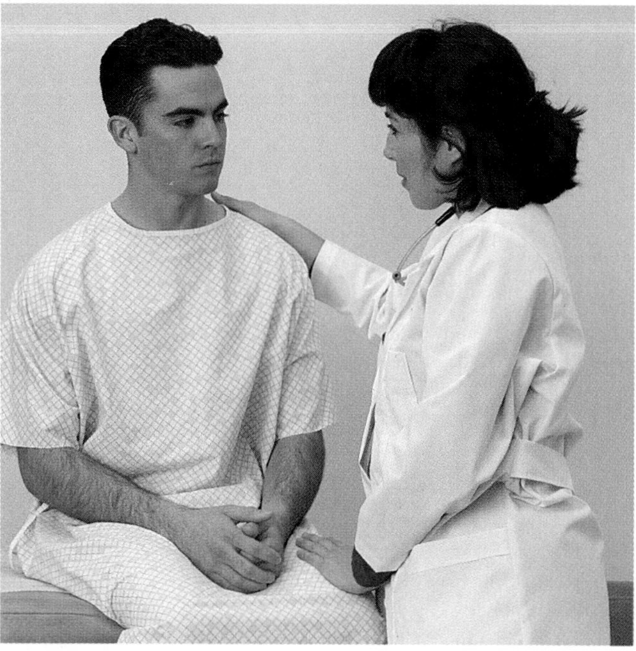

Figure 18.8 Positioning the client.

Step 2 ***Observe the client's hygiene, grooming, posture, body language, gait, facial expressions, speech, and ability to follow directions.***

Changes could be indicative of depression, schizophrenia, organic brain syndrome, or obsessive-compulsive disorder.

Step 3 ***Note the client's speech and language abilities.***

- Throughout the assessment, note the client's rate of speech, ability to pronounce words, loudness or softness, and ability to talk smoothly and clearly.
- Assess the client's choice of words, ability to respond to questions, and ease with which a response is made.

Changes in speech could reflect anxiety, Parkinson's disease, depression, or various forms of aphasia.

Step 4 ***Assess the client's sensorium.***

- Determine the client's orientation to date, time, place, and reason for being here.

Neurologic disease can produce a sliding or changing degree of alertness. Change in the level of consciousness may be related to cortical or brainstem disease. A stroke,

ASSESSMENT TECHNIQUE/NORMAL FINDINGS	SPECIAL CONSIDERATIONS

- Grade the level of alertness on a scale from full alertness to coma.

seizure, or hypoglycemia could also contribute to a change in the level of consciousness.

Step 5 *Assess the client's memory.*

- Ask the client for date of birth, Social Security number, name and ages of any children or grandchildren, educational history with dates and events, work history with dates, and job descriptions.

Loss of long-term memory may indicate cerebral cortex damage, such as occurs in Alzheimer's disease.

Step 6 *Assess the client's ability to calculate problems.*

- Start with a simple problem, such as 4 + 3, 8 + 7, and 15 – 4.
- Progress to more difficult problems, such as (10 × 4) – 8, or ask the client to start with 100 and subtract 7 (100 – 7 = 93, 93 – 7 = 86, 86 – 7 = 79, and so on).
- Remember to use problems that are appropriate for the developmental, educational, and intellectual level of the client.

Inability to calculate simple problems may indicate the presence of organic brain disease, or it may simply indicate lack of exposure to mathematical concepts, nervousness, or an incomplete understanding of the examiner's language. In an otherwise unremarkable assessment, a poor response to calculations should not be considered an abnormal finding.

Step 7 *Assess the client's ability to think abstractly.*

- Ask the client to identify similarities and differences between two objects or topics, such as wood and coal, king and president, orange and apple, and pear and celery.
- Quote a proverb and ask the client to explain its meaning. For example

  "A stitch in time saves nine."

  "The empty barrel makes the most noise."

  "Don't put all your eggs in one basket."

The client's responses should reflect an ability to think abstractly.

Responses made by the client may reflect lack of education, mental retardation, or dementia. Bizarre responses may be made by clients with personality disorders.

Cranial Nerves

Step 1 *Test the olfactory nerve (CN I).*

- If you suspect the client's nares are obstructed with mucus, ask the client to blow the nose.
- Ask the client to close both eyes and to close one naris. Place a familiar odor under the open naris (Figure 18.9 on page 554).

Anosmia, the absence of the sense of smell, may be due to cranial nerve dysfunction, colds, rhinitis, or zinc deficiency, or it may be genetic. A unilateral change in this sense may be indicative of a brain tumor.

ASSESSMENT TECHNIQUE/NORMAL FINDINGS

SPECIAL CONSIDERATIONS

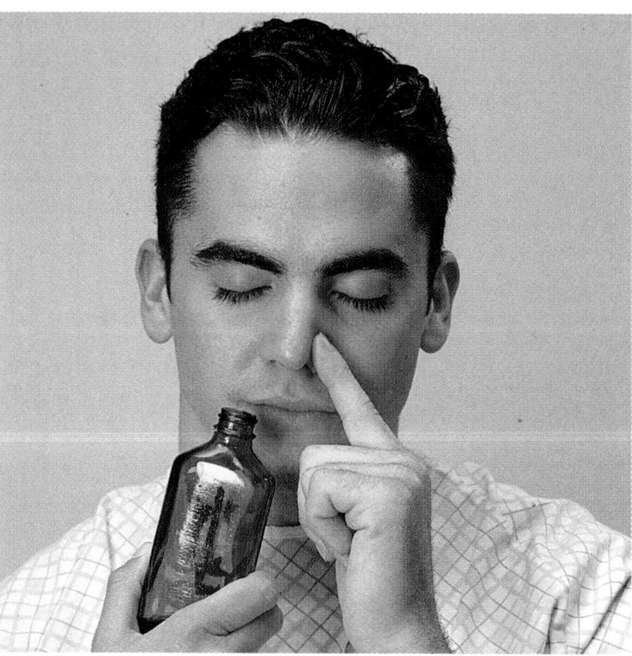

Figure 18.9 Olfactory nerve assessment.

- Ask the client to sniff and identify the odor. Use coffee, vanilla, perfume, cloves, and so on.
- Repeat with the other naris.

Step 2 *Test the optic nerve (CN II).*

- Test near vision by asking the client to read from a magazine, newspaper, or prepared card. Observe closeness or distance of page to face. Also note the position of the head.
- Use the Snellen chart to test distant vision and color.
- Use the ophthalmoscope to inspect the fundus of the eye. Locate the optic disc and describe the color and shape.

See Chapter 9 for a detailed description of the technique for all of these activities.

Pathologic conditions of the optic nerve include retrobulbar neuritis, papilledema, and optic atrophy. *Retrobulbar neuritis* is an inflammatory process of the optic nerve behind the eyeball. Multiple sclerosis is the most common cause.

Papilledema (or *choked disc*) is a swelling of the optic nerve as it enters the retina. A symptom of increased intracranial pressure, papilledema can be indicative of brain tumors or intracranial hemorrhage.

Referral

Immediate medical attention is required if intracranial hemorrhage is suspected.

Optic atrophy produces a change in the color of the optic disc and decreased visual acuity. It can be a symptom of multiple sclerosis or brain tumor.

ASSESSMENT TECHNIQUE/NORMAL FINDINGS	SPECIAL CONSIDERATIONS

Step 3 ***Test the oculomotor, trochlear, and abducens nerves (CN III, IV, and VI).***

- Test the six cardinal points of gaze.
- Test direct and consensual pupillary reaction to light.
- Test convergence and accommodation of the eyes.

These three tests are described in detail in Chapter 9.

Pathologic conditions include nystagmus, strabismus, diplopia, or ptosis of the upper lid. *Nystagmus* is the constant involuntary movement of the eyeball. A lack of muscular coordination, *strabismus*, causes deviation of one or both eyes. *Diplopia* is double vision. A dropped lid, or *ptosis* of the lid, is usually related to weakness of the muscles.

Step 4 ***Test the trigeminal nerve (CN V).***

Test the sensory function.

- Ask the client to close both eyes.
- Touch the face with a wisp of cotton (Figure 18.10).

Document any loss of sensation, pain, or noted fasciculations.

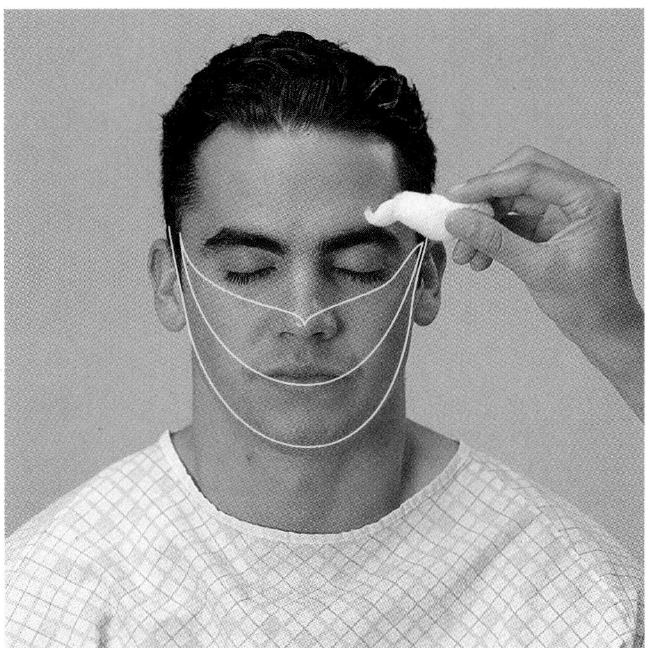

Figure 18.10 Testing sensory function of the trigeminal nerve.

- Direct the client to say "now" every time the cotton is felt.
- Repeat the test using sharp and dull stimuli.

Be random with the stimulation. *Do not* establish a pattern when testing. Be sure all three branches of the nerve are assessed.

Test the corneal reflex.

- Ask the client to look straight ahead.
- Use a wisp of cotton to touch the cornea from the side.
- Anticipate a blink.

Clients using contact lenses need to remove them before testing. Most likely these clients will have a decreased or absent reflex.

Details for this procedure are presented in Chapter 9.

ASSESSMENT TECHNIQUE/NORMAL FINDINGS	SPECIAL CONSIDERATIONS

Test the motor function of the nerve.

- Ask the client to clench the teeth tightly.
- Bilaterally palpate the masseter and temporalis muscles, noting muscle strength (Figure 18.11).
- Ask the client to open and close the mouth several times. Observe for symmetry of movement of the mandible without deviation from midline.

Muscle pain, spasms, and deviation of the mandible with movement can indicate myofascial pain dysfunction.

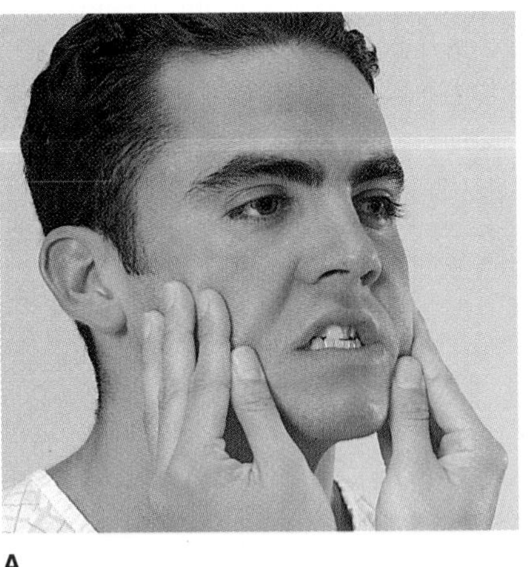
A

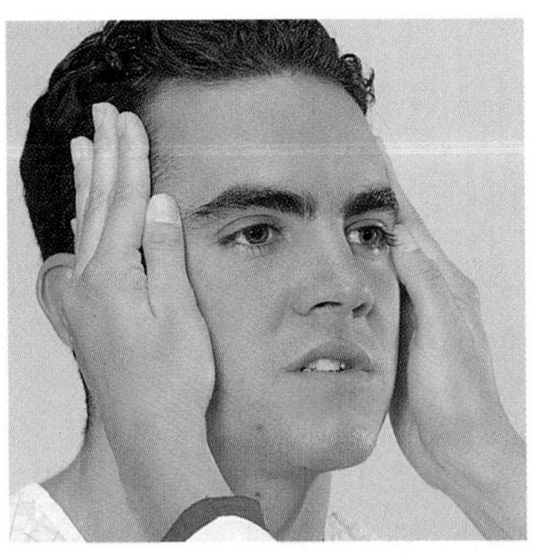
B

Figure 18.11 Testing the strength of the *(A)* masseter and *(B)* temporalis muscles.

Step 5 *Test the facial nerve (CN VII).*

Test the motor activity of the nerve.

- Ask the client to perform several functions such as: smile, show your teeth, close both eyes, puff your cheeks, frown, and raise your eyebrows. (Figure 18.12).
- Look for symmetry of facial movements.

Asymmetry or muscle weakness may indicate nerve damage. Muscle weakness includes drooping of the eyelid and changes in the nasolabial folds.

Inability to perform motor tasks could be the results of a lower or upper motor neuron disease.

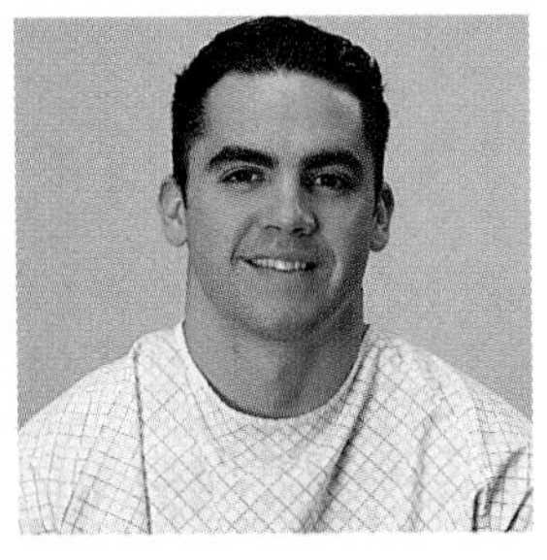
A

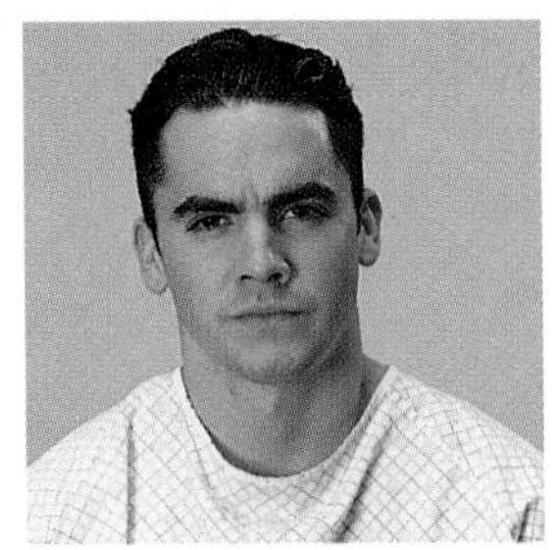
B

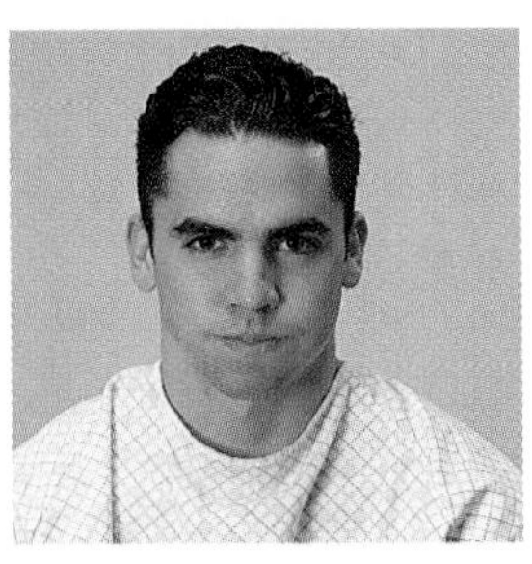
C

Figure 18.12 Testing the facial nerve with *(A)* smile, *(B)* frown, and (C) puffing cheeks.

ASSESSMENT TECHNIQUE/NORMAL FINDINGS | SPECIAL CONSIDERATIONS

Test the muscle strength of the upper face.

- Ask the client to close both eyes tightly and keep them closed.
- Try to open the eyes by retracting the upper and lower lids simultaneously and bilaterally (Figure 18.13).

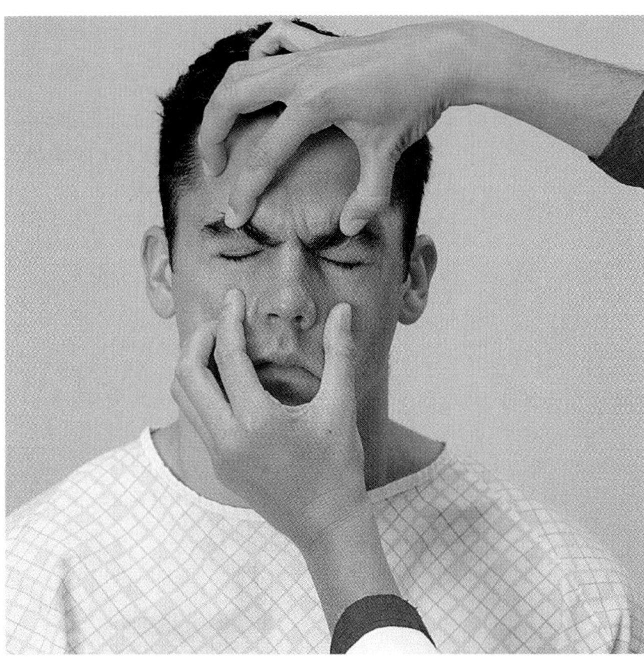

Figure 18.13 Testing the strength of the facial muscles.

Test the muscle strength of the lower face.

- Ask the client to puff cheeks.
- Apply pressure to the cheeks, attempting to force the air out of the lips.

Test the sense of taste.

- Moisten three applicators and dab one in each of the samples of sugar, salt, and lemon.
- Touch the client's tongue with one applicator at a time and ask the client to identify the taste. Water may be needed to rinse the mouth between tests.

Test the corneal reflex.

- This may have been tested with the trigeminal nerve assessment. The motor response of this reflex is regulated by the cranial nerve VII.

Step 6 ***Test the vestibulocochlear nerve (CN VIII).***

- Test the auditory branch of the nerve by performing the Weber test. This test uses the tuning fork and provides lateralization of the sound.

Tinnitus and deafness are deficits associated with the cochlear or auditory branch of the nerve, while vertigo is associated with the vestibular portion.

ASSESSMENT TECHNIQUE/NORMAL FINDINGS

- Perform the Rinne test. This compares bone conduction of sound with air conduction.

Both the Weber and Rinne tests are described in detail in Chapter 9.

The vestibular portion of the nerve is not usually tested at this time. The caloric test, or ice water test as it is sometimes called, tests the vestibular portion of the nerve. Consult a neurology text for description of this technique.

Step 7 ***Test the glossopharyngeal and vagus nerves (CN IX and X).***

Test the motor activity.

- Ask the client to open the mouth.
- Depress tongue with tongue blade.
- Ask client to say "Ah."
- Observe the movement of the soft palate and uvula (Figure 18.14).
- Normally, the soft palate rises and the uvula remains in the midline.

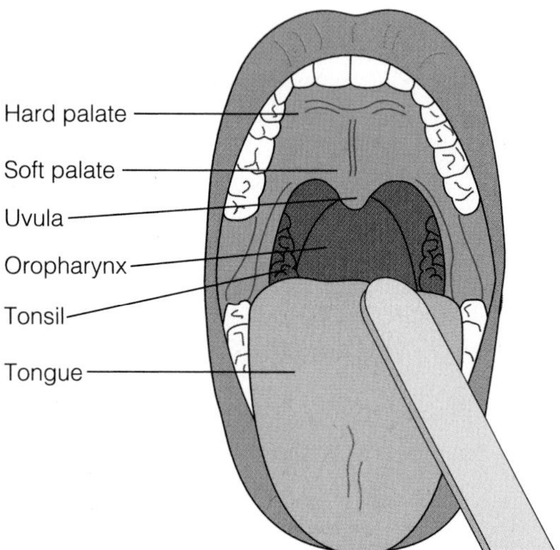

Figure 18.14 Testing cranial nerves IX and X.

Test the gag reflex. This tests the sensory aspect of CN IX and the motor activity of CN X.

- Inform the client that you are going to place an applicator in the mouth and lightly touch the throat.
- Touch the posterior wall of the pharynx with the applicator.
- Observe pharyngeal movement.

SPECIAL CONSIDERATIONS

Unilateral palate and uvula movement indicate disease of the nerve on the opposite side.

Referral

Clients having a diminished or absent gag reflex have an increased potential for aspiration and need medical evaluation.

ASSESSMENT TECHNIQUE/NORMAL FINDINGS	SPECIAL CONSIDERATIONS

Test the motor activity of the pharynx.

- Ask the client to drink a small amount of water and note the ease or difficulty of swallowing.

Dysphagia, difficulty with swallowing, could be related to cranial nerve disease.

- Note the quality of the voice or hoarseness when speaking.

Vocal changes could be indicative of lesions, paralysis, or other conditions.

Step 8 ***Test the accessory nerve (CN XI).***

Abnormal findings include muscle weakness, muscle atrophy, fasciculations, uneven shoulders, and inability to raise chin following flexion.

Test the trapezius muscle.

- Ask the client to shrug the shoulders. Observe the equality of the shoulders, symmetry of action, and lack of fasciculations.

Test the sternocleidomastoid muscle.

- Ask the client to turn the head to the right.
- Ask the client to turn the head to the left.
- Ask the client to try to touch the right ear to the right shoulder without raising the shoulder.
- Ask the client to try to touch the left ear to the left shoulder without raising the shoulder.
- Observe ease of movement and degree of range of motion.

Test trapezius muscle strength.

- Have the client shrug the shoulders while you provide resistance with your hands (Figure 18.15).

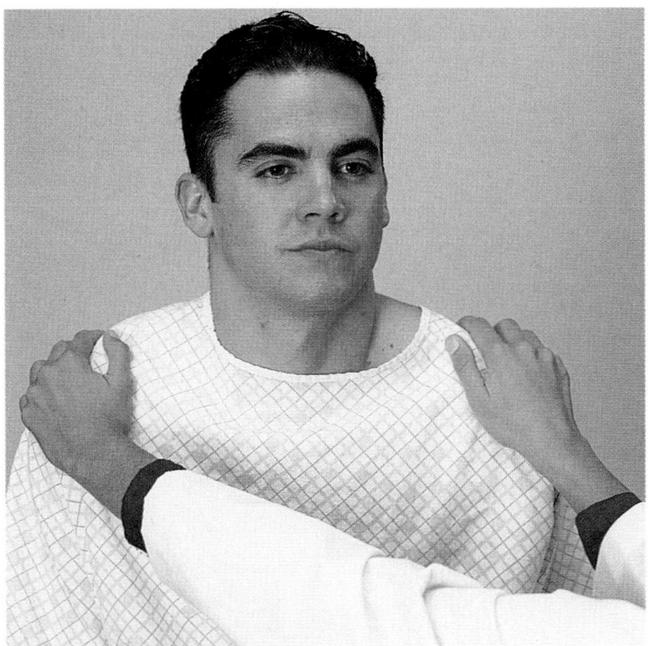

Figure 18.15 Testing the strength of the trapezius muscle against resistance.

ASSESSMENT TECHNIQUE/NORMAL FINDINGS

Test sternocleidomastoid muscle strength.

- Ask the client to turn the head to the left to meet your hand.
- Attempt to return the client's head to midline position (Figure 18.16).
- Repeat the preceding steps with the client turning to the right side.

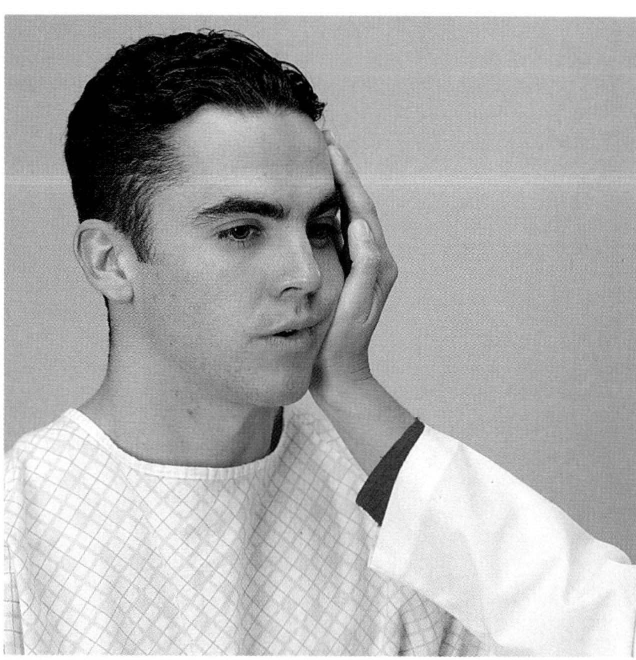

Figure 18.16 Testing the strength of the sternocleidomastoid muscle against resistance.

Step 9 ***Test the hypoglossal nerve (CN XII).***

Test the movement of the tongue.

- Ask the client to protrude the tongue.
- Ask the client to retract the tongue.
- Ask the client to protrude the tongue and move it to the right and then to the left.
- Note ease of movement and equality of movement.

Test the strength of the tongue.

- Ask the client to push against the inside of the cheek with the tip of the tongue.
- Provide resistance by pressing your two fingers against the client's outer cheek (Figure 18.17).
- Repeat on the other side.

SPECIAL CONSIDERATIONS

Note atrophy, tremors and paralysis. An ipsilateral paralysis will demonstrate deviation and atrophy of the involved side.

ASSESSMENT TECHNIQUE/NORMAL FINDINGS | SPECIAL CONSIDERATIONS

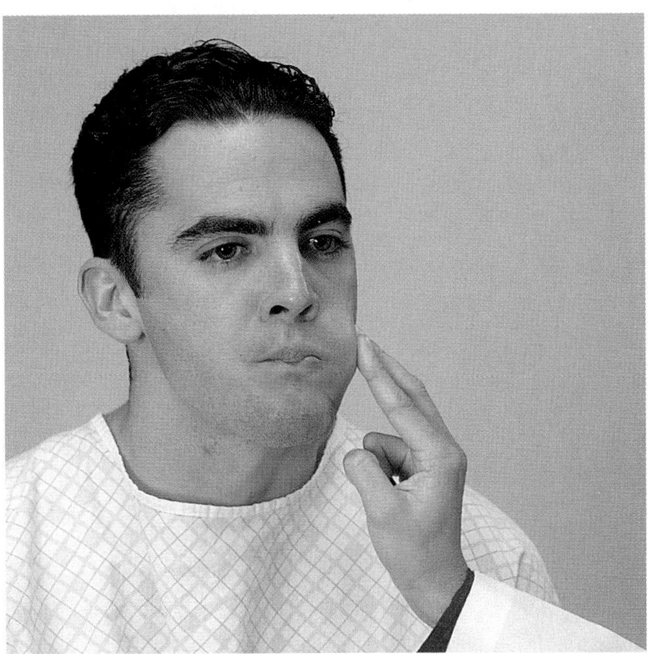

Figure 18.17 Testing the strength of the tongue.

Motor Function

Motor function requires the integrated efforts of the musculoskeletal and the neurologic systems. Assessment of the musculoskeletal system is discussed in detail in Chapter 17. The neurologic aspect of motor function is directly related to activities of the cerebellum, which is responsible for coordination and smoothness of movement, and equilibrium. All tests to be discussed focus on activities of the cerebellum.

ALERT!

Be ready to support and protect the client to prevent an accident, injury, or fall.

Step 1 *Assess the client's gait and balance.*

- Ask the client to walk across the room and return.
- Ask the client to walk heel-to-toe (or tandem), by placing the heel of the left foot in front of the toes of the right foot, then the heel of the right foot in front of the toes of the left foot. Continue this pattern for several yards (Figure 18.18 on page 562).

A change in gait could be indicative of drug or alcohol intoxication, motor neuron weakness, or muscle weakness.

ASSESSMENT TECHNIQUE/NORMAL FINDINGS	SPECIAL CONSIDERATIONS

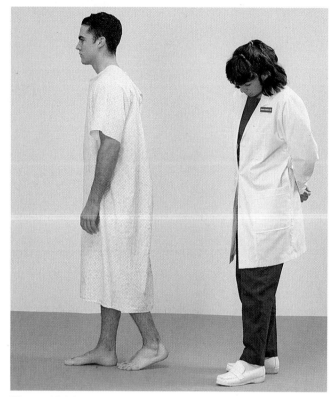

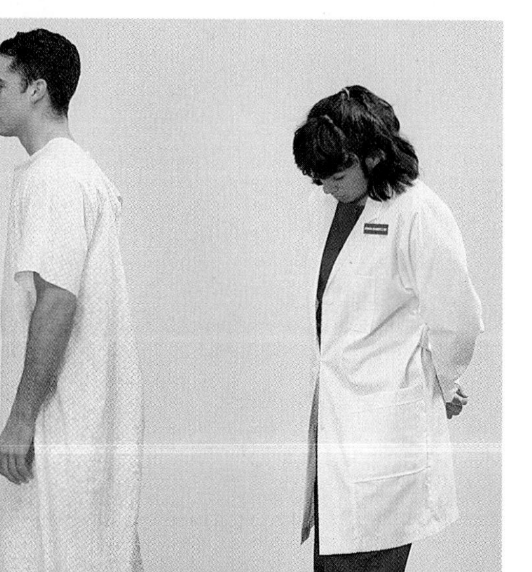

Figure 18.18 Heel-to-toe walk.

- Ask the client to walk on toes.
- Ask the client to walk on heels.
- Observe the client's posture. Does the posture demonstrate stiffness or relaxation?
- Note the equality of steps taken, the pace of walking, the position and coordination of arms when walking, and the ability to maintain balance during all activities.

Step 2 ***Perform the Romberg test.***

The Romberg test assesses coordination and equilibrium. See Figure 9.38 on page 194.

- Ask the client to stand with feet together, arms at side. The client's eyes are open.
- Stand next to the client to prevent falls.
- Observe for swaying.
- Ask the client to close both eyes without changing position.
- Observe for swaying with the eyes closed. Swaying normally increases slightly when the eyes are closed.

If swaying greatly increases and/or the client falls, suspect disease of the posterior columns of the spinal cord. When the eyes are open, the same client maintains the position.

ASSESSMENT TECHNIQUE/NORMAL FINDINGS	SPECIAL CONSIDERATIONS

Step 3 *Perform the finger-to-nose test.*

The finger-to-nose test also assesses coordination and equilibrium. It is sometimes called the pass-point test.

- Ask the client to resume a sitting position.
- Ask the client to extend both arms from the sides of the body.
- Ask the client to keep both eyes open.
- Ask the client to touch the tip of the nose with the right index finger, then return the right arm to an extended position.
- Ask the client to touch the tip of the nose with the left index finger, then return the left arm to an extended position.
- Repeat the procedure several times.
- Ask the client to close the eyes and repeat the alternating movements (Figure 18.19).
- Observe the movement of the arms, the smoothness of the movement, and the point of contact of finger. Does the finger touch the nose, or is another part of the face touched?

With the eyes closed, the client with cerebellar disease will reach beyond the nosetip, because the sense of position is affected.

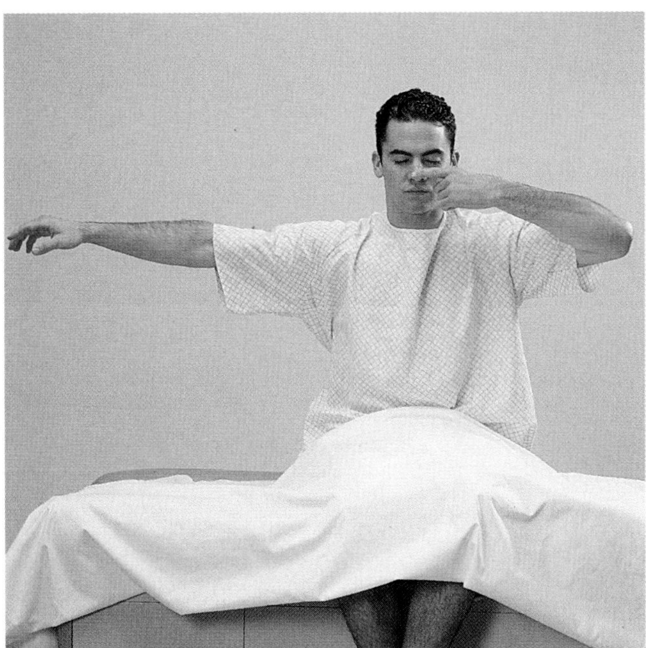

Figure 18.19 Finger-to-nose test.

Step 4 *Assess the client's ability to perform a rapid alternating action.*

- Ask the client to place the hands palms-down on the thighs (Figure 18.20, *A*).
- Ask the client to turn the hands palms-up (Figure 18.20, *B*).
- Ask the client to return the hands to a palms-down position.

Inability to perform this task could indicate upper motor neuron weakness.

ASSESSMENT TECHNIQUE/NORMAL FINDINGS	SPECIAL CONSIDERATIONS

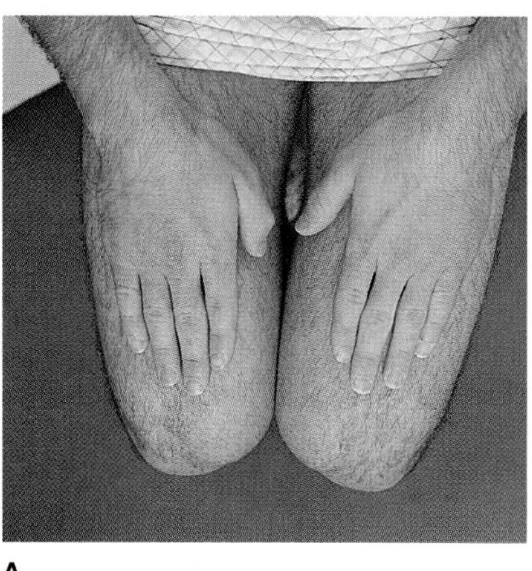
A

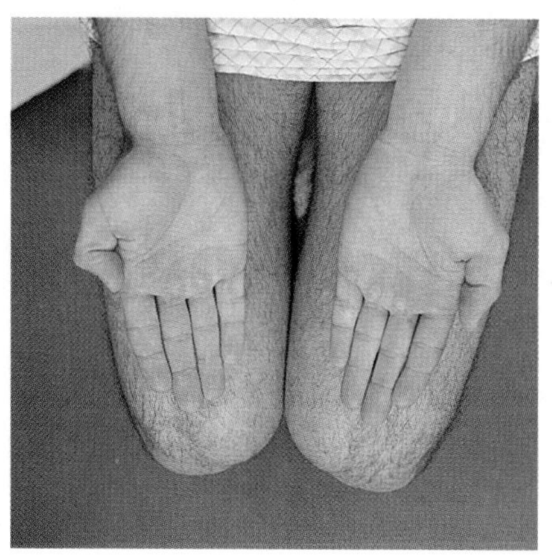
B

Figure 18.20 Testing rapid alternating movement, *(A)* to *(B)*.

- Ask the client to alternate the movements at a faster pace.
- If you suspect any deficit, test one side at a time.
- Observe the rhythm, rate, and smoothness of the movements.

Step 5 ***Ask the client to perform the heel-to-shin test.***

- Assist the client to a supine position.
- Ask the client to place the heel of the right foot below the left knee.
- Ask the client to slide the right heel along the "shin bone" to the ankle (Figure 18.21).

Inability to perform this test could indicate disease of the posterior spinal tract.

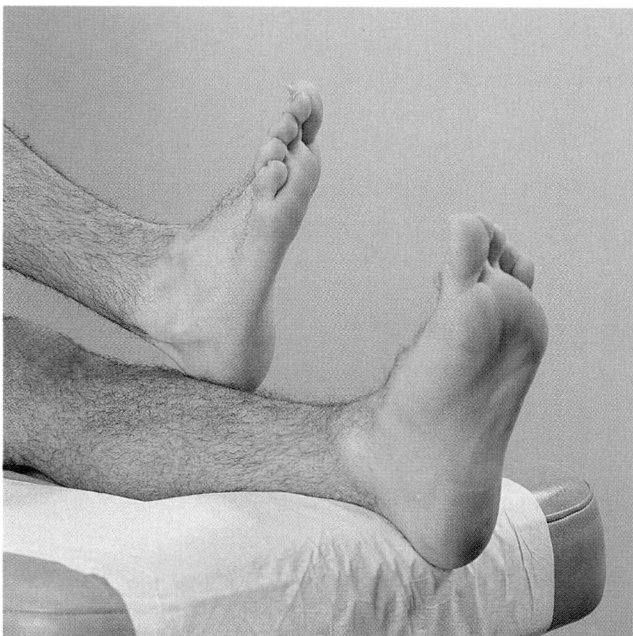

Figure 18.21 Heel-to-shin test.

ASSESSMENT TECHNIQUE/NORMAL FINDINGS

- Ask the client to repeat the procedure, reversing legs.
- Observe the smoothness of the action. The client should be able to move the heel in a straight line so that it doesn't fall off the lower leg.

Sensory Function

This part of the physical assessment evaluates the client's response to a variety of stimuli. This assessment tests the peripheral nerves, the sensory tracts, and the cortical level of discrimination. A variety of stimuli are used, including light touch, hot/cold, sharp/dull, and vibration. Stereognosis, graphesthesia, and two-point discrimination are also assessed.

ALERT!

The client may tire during these procedures. If this happens, stop the assessment and continue at a later time. Be sure to test corresponding body parts. Take a distal-to-proximal approach along the extremities. When the client describes sensations accurately at a distal point, you usually do not need to proceed to a more proximal point. If you detect a deficit at a distal point, then it becomes imperative to proceed to proximal points while attempting to map the specific area of the deficit. Repeat testing to determine accuracy in areas of deficits.

Remember, always ask the client to describe the stimulus and the location. Do not suggest the type of stimulus or location. Tell the client to keep the eyes closed during testing. To promote full client understanding, you might have to demonstrate what you will do.

Step 1 ***Assess the client's ability to identify light touch.***

- Using a wisp of cotton, touch various parts of the body, including feet, hands, arms, legs, abdomen, and face (Figure 18.22).

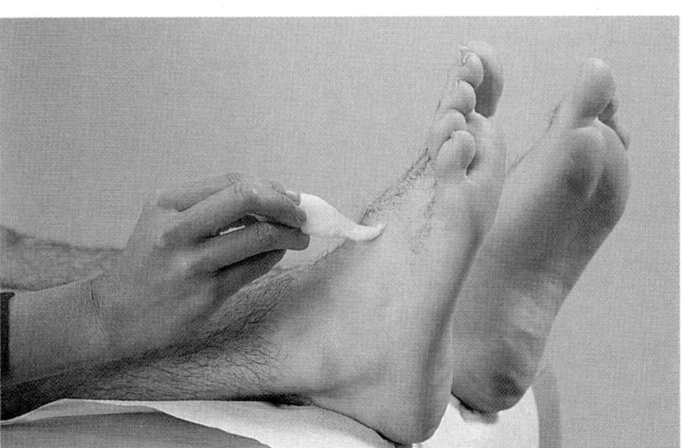

Figure 18.22 Evaluation of light touch.

SPECIAL CONSIDERATIONS

Anesthesia is the inability to perceive the sense of touch. *Hyperesthesia* is an increased sensation, whereas *hypoesthesia* is a decreased but not absent sensation.

ASSESSMENT TECHNIQUE/NORMAL FINDINGS	SPECIAL CONSIDERATIONS

- Touch at random locations and random time intervals.
- Ask the client to say "yes" or "now" when the stimulus is perceived.
- Be sure to test corresponding dermatomes.

Step 2 ***Assess the client's ability to distinguish the difference between sharp and dull.***

- Ask the client to say "sharp" or "dull" when something sharp or dull is felt on the skin.
- Touch the client with the tip of a sterile safety pin (Figure 18.23, *A*).
- Now touch the client with the blunt end of the pin (Figure 18.23, *B*).

The absence of pain sensation is called *analgesia*. Decreased pain sensation is called *hypalgesia*.

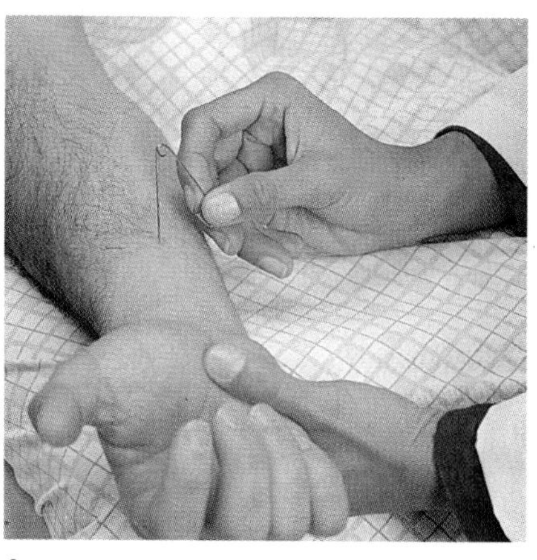

A

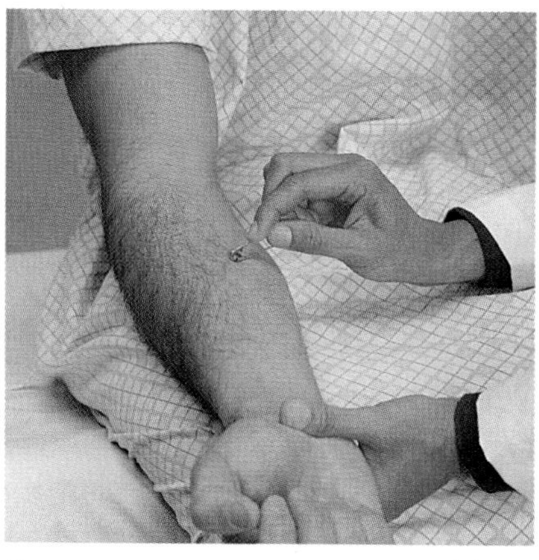

B

Figure 18.23 Testing client's ability to distinguish between *(A)* sharp and *(B)* dull sensations.

- Alternate between sharp and dull stimulation.
- Touch at random times and with random and alternating patterns.
- Be sure to test corresponding body parts.
- Discard the pin.

Step 3 ***Assess the client's ability to distinguish temperature.***

- Perform this test only if the client demonstrates an absence or decrease in pain sensation.
- Randomly touch the client with test tubes containing warm and cold water.
- Ask the client to describe the temperature perceived.
- Be sure to test corresponding body parts.

Step 4 ***Assess the client's ability to feel vibrations.***

- Set a tuning fork in motion and place it on bony parts of the body, such as the toes, ankle, knee, iliac crest, spinal process, fingers, sternum, wrists, or elbows (Figure 18.24).

Loss of vibration sense many times indicates a neuropathy. This may be associated with aging, diabetes, intoxication, or posterior column disease.

ASSESSMENT TECHNIQUE/NORMAL FINDINGS

SPECIAL CONSIDERATIONS

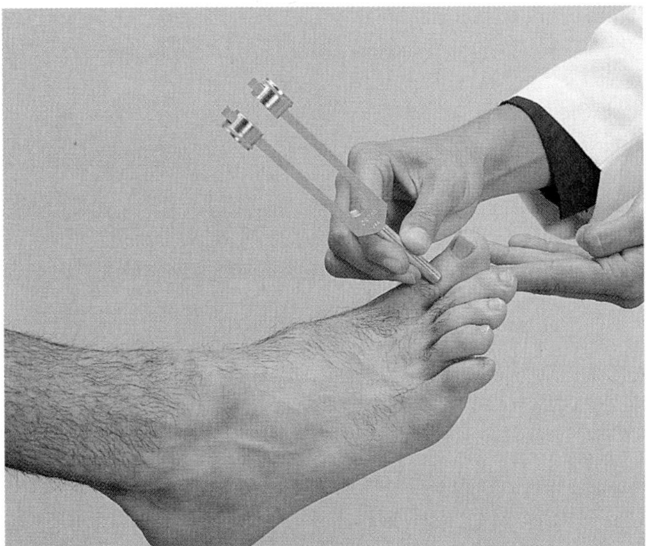

Figure 18.24 Testing the client's ability to feel vibrations.

- Ask the client to say "now" when the vibration is perceived and "stop" when it is no longer felt.
- If the client's perception is accurate when you test the most distal aspects (toes, ankles, fingers, and wrist), end the test at this time.
- Proceed to proximal points if distal perception is diminished.

Step 5 ***Test stereognosis, the ability to identify an object without seeing it.***

Inability to identify a familiar object could indicate cortical disease.

- Direct the client to close both eyes.
- Place a safety pin in the right hand and ask the client to identify it (Figure 18.25).

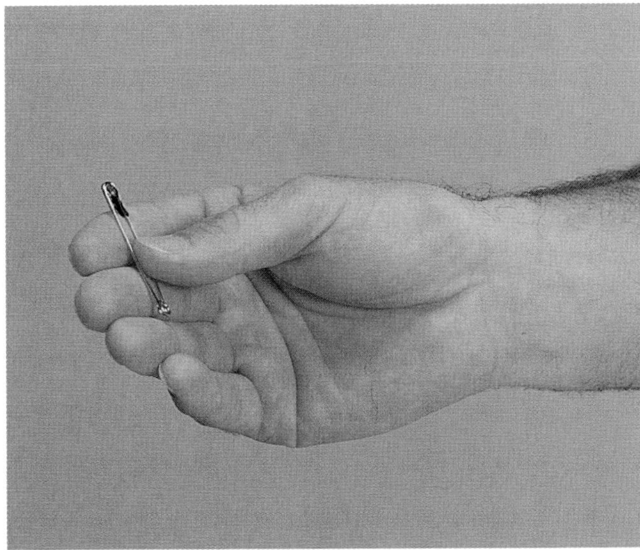

Figure 18.25 Testing stereognosis.

ASSESSMENT TECHNIQUE/NORMAL FINDINGS	SPECIAL CONSIDERATIONS

- Place a paper clip in the left hand and ask the client to identify it.
- Place a coin in the right hand and ask the client to identify it.
- Place a different coin in the left hand and ask the client to identify it.

The objects you use must be familiar and safe to hold (no sharp objects). Test each object independently.

Step 6 ***Test graphesthesia, the ability to perceive writing on the skin.***

Inability to perceive the character on the skin may indicate cortical disease.

- Direct the client to keep eyes closed.
- Using the non-cotton end of an applicator or the base of a pen, scribe a number such as 3 into the palm of the right hand (Figure 18.26).

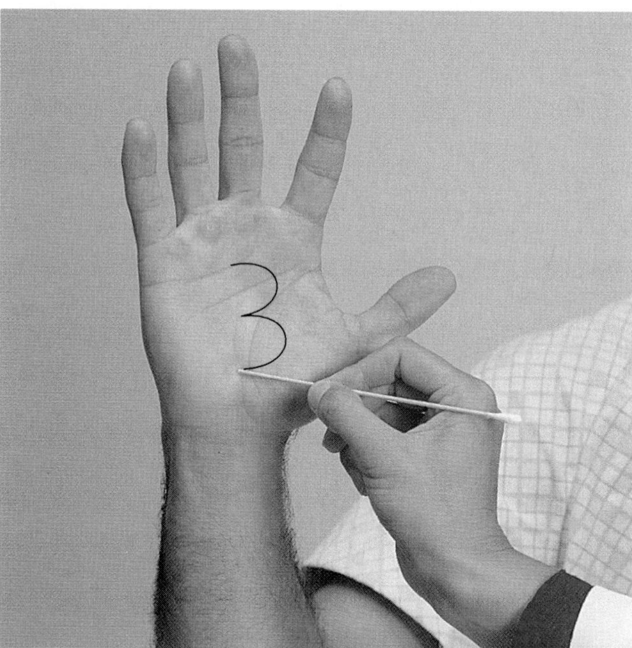

Figure 18.26 Testing graphesthesia.

- Ask the client to identify the number.
- Repeat in the left hand using a different number such as 5 or 2.
- Ask the client to identify the number.

Step 7 ***Assess the client's ability to discriminate between two points.***

An inability to perceive two separate points within normal distances may indicate cortical disease.

- Simultaneously touch the client with two stimuli over a given area (Figure 18.27).

ASSESSMENT TECHNIQUE/NORMAL FINDINGS | SPECIAL CONSIDERATIONS

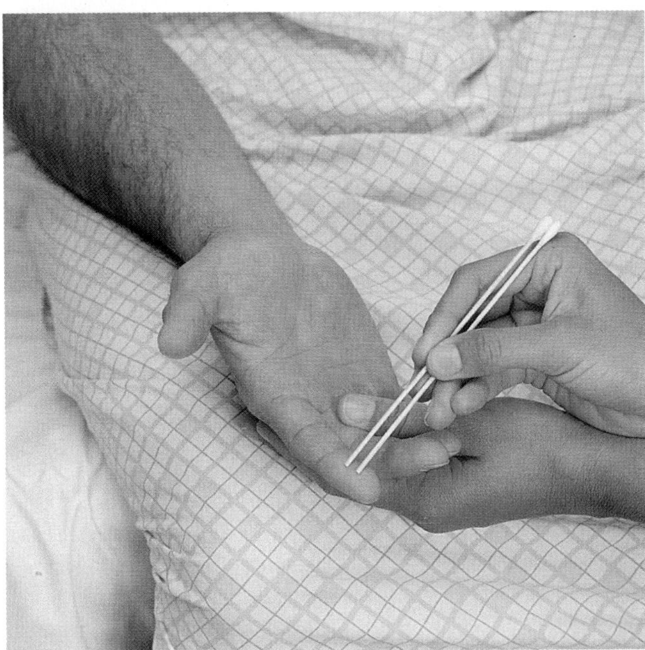

Figure 18.27 Two-point discrimination.

Use the unpadded end of two applicators or two 25-gauge sterile needles. Vary the distance between the two points according to the body region being stimulated. The more distal the location, the more sensitive the discrimination. Normally, the client is able to perceive two discrete points at the following distances and locations:

Finger tips	0.3–0.6 cm
Hands and feet	1.5–2 cm
Lower leg	4 cm

- Ask the client to say "now" when the two discrete points of stimulus are first perceived.
- Note the smallest distance between which the client can perceive two distinct stimuli.
- Discard the needles or applicators.

Step 8 ***Assess topognosis, the ability of the client to identify an area of the body that has been touched.***

This need not be a separate test. You can include it in any of the previous steps by asking the client to identify what part of the body was involved. You can also ask the client to point to the area you touched.

Inability of the client to identify a touched area demonstrates sensory and/or cortical disease.

Reflexes

Reflex testing is usually the last part of the neurologic assessment. The client is usually in a sitting position; however, you can use a supine

ASSESSMENT TECHNIQUE/NORMAL FINDINGS

SPECIAL CONSIDERATIONS

position if the client's physical condition so requires. Position the client's limbs properly to stretch the muscle partially.

Hold the handle of the reflex hammer in your dominant hand between your thumb and index finger. Proper wrist action provides a brisk, direct, smooth arc for stimulation. After striking the tendon, remove the hammer immediately.

Proper use of the reflex hammer requires practice. Hold the handle of the reflex handle in your dominant hand between your thumb and index finger. Use your wrist, not your hand or arm, to generate the striking motion. Proper wrist action will provide a brisk, direct, smooth arc for stimulation. Stimulate the reflex arc with a brisk tap to the tendon, not the muscle. Through continued practice and experience, you will learn the amount of force to use. Strong force will cause pain, and too little force will not stimulate the arc. After striking the tendon, remove the hammer immediately.

Evaluate the response on a scale from 0 to 4+:

0 = no response

1+ = diminished

2+ = normal

3+ = brisk, above normal

4+ = hyperactive

Neuromuscular disease, spinal cord injury, or lower motor neuron disease may cause absent or diminished reflexes. Hyperactive reflexes may indicate upper motor neuron disease. *Clonus*, rhythmically alternating flexion and extension, confirms upper motor neuron disease.

Before concluding that a reflex is absent or diminished, repeat the test. Encourage the client to relax. It may be necessary to distract the client to achieve relaxation of the muscle before striking the tendon.

Step 1 ***Assess the biceps reflex (C5, C6).***

- Support the client's lower arm with your nondominant hand and arm. The arm needs to be slightly flexed at the elbow with palm up.
- Place the thumb of your nondominant hand over the biceps tendon.
- Using the reflex hammer, briskly tap your thumb (Figure 18.28).
- Look for contraction of the biceps muscle and slight flexion of the forearm.

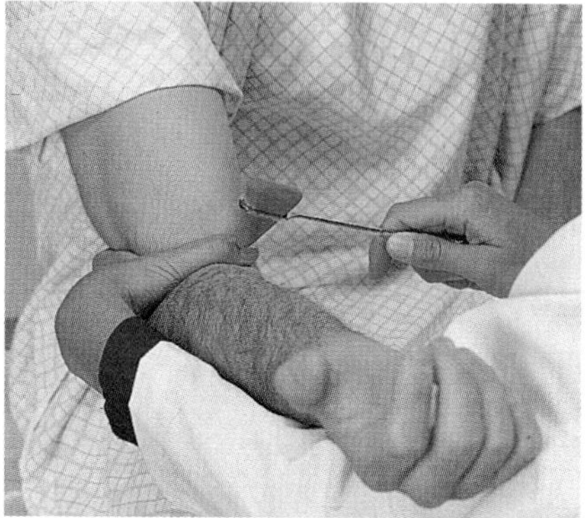

Figure 18.28 Testing the biceps reflex.

ASSESSMENT TECHNIQUE/NORMAL FINDINGS	SPECIAL CONSIDERATIONS

Step 2 *Assess the triceps reflex (C6, C7).*

- Support the client's elbow with your nondominant hand.
- Sharply percuss the tendon just above the olecranon process with the reflex hammer (Figure 18.29).
- Observe contraction of the triceps muscle with extension of the lower arm.

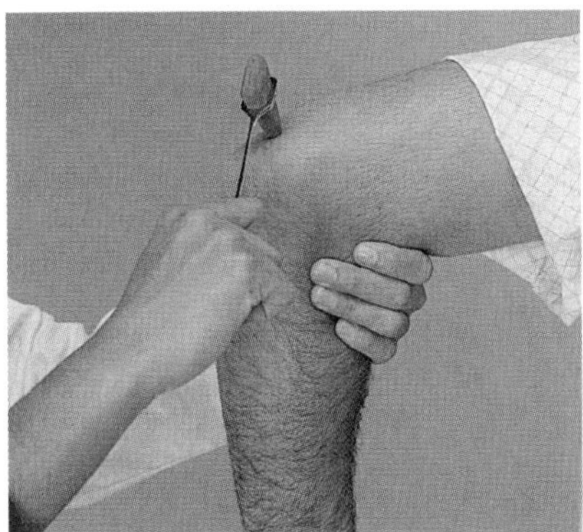

Figure 18.29 Testing the triceps reflex.

Step 3 *Assess the brachioradialis reflex (C5, C6).*

- Position the client's arm so the elbow is flexed and the hand is resting on the lap with palm down (pronation).
- Using the reflex hammer, briskly strike the tendon toward the radius about 2 or 3 inches above the wrist (Figure 18.30).
- Observe flexion of the lower arm and supination of the hand.

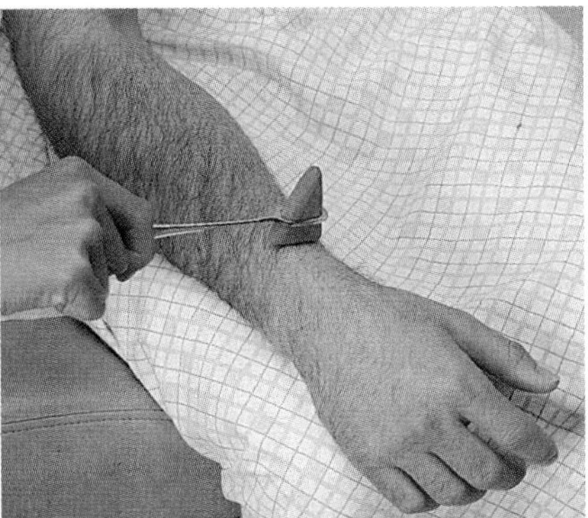

Figure 18.30 Testing the brachioradialis reflex.

Step 4 *Assess the patellar (knee) reflex (L2, L3, L4).*

- Flex the leg at the knee.
- Palpate the patella to locate the patellar tendon inferior to the patella.
- Briskly strike the tendon with the reflex hammer (Figure 18.31 on page 570).

ASSESSMENT TECHNIQUE/NORMAL FINDINGS | SPECIAL CONSIDERATIONS

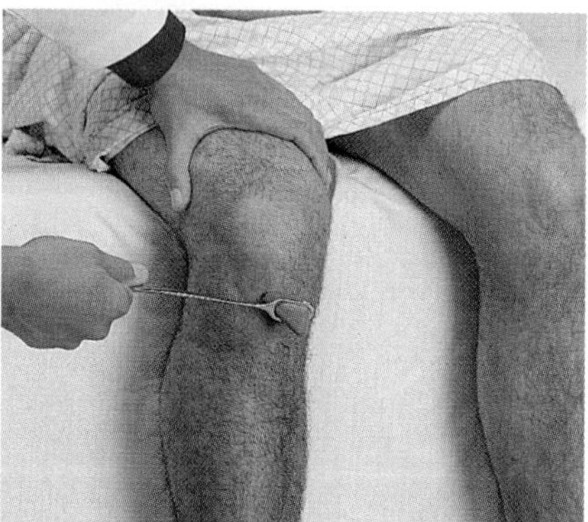

Figure 18.31 Testing the patellar reflex.

- Note extension of lower leg and contraction of the quadriceps muscle.

Step 5 *Assess the Achilles tendon (ankle) reflex (S1).*

- Flex the leg at the knee.
- Dorsiflex the foot of the leg being examined.
- Hold the foot lightly in the nondominant hand.
- Strike the Achilles tendon with the reflex hammer (Figure 18.32).
- Observe plantar flexion of the foot: the heel will "jump" from your hand.

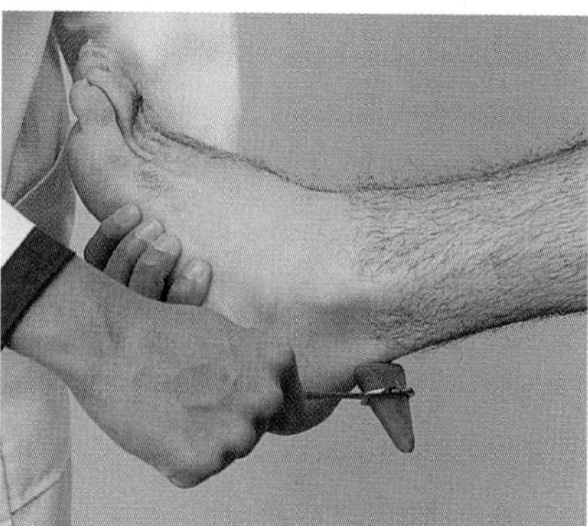

Figure 18.32 Testing the Achilles tendon reflex.

Step 6 *Assess the plantar reflex (L5, S1).*

- Position the leg with a slight degree of external rotation at the hip.
- Stimulate the sole of the foot from the heel to the ball of the foot on the lateral aspect.
- Continue the stimulation across the ball of the foot to the great toe.
- Observe for plantar flexion, in which the toes curl toward the sole of the foot (Figure 18.33). It may be necessary to hold the ankle to prevent movement.

A *Babinski response* is the fanning of the toes with the great toe pointing toward the dorsum of the foot (Figure 18.34). This is called dorsiflexion of the toe and is considered an abnormal response in the adult. It may indicate upper motor neuron disease.

ASSESSMENT TECHNIQUE/NORMAL FINDINGS	SPECIAL CONSIDERATIONS

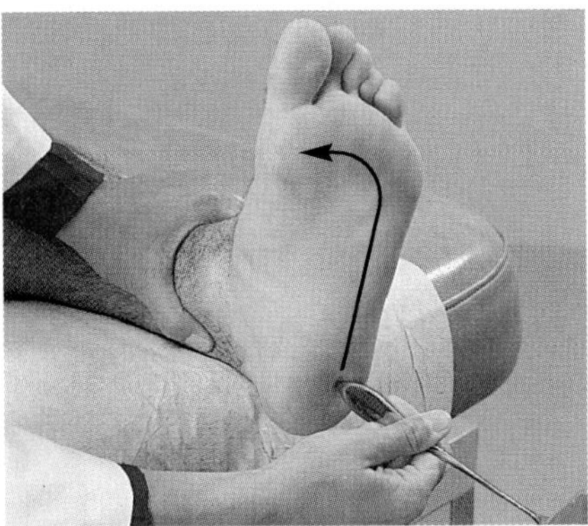

Figure 18.33 Testing the plantar reflex.

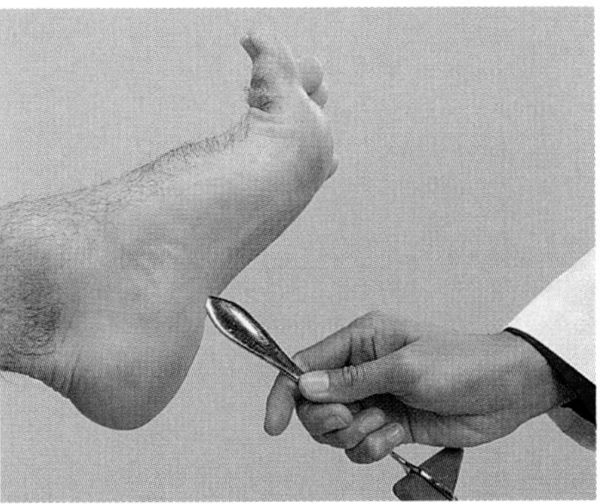

Figure 18.34 Babinski response.

Step 7 *Assess the abdominal reflexes (T8, T9, T10 for upper and T10, T11, T12 for lower).*

- Using an applicator or tongue blade, briskly stroke the abdomen from the lateral aspect toward the umbilicus (Figure 18.35).

Obesity and upper and lower motor neuron pathology can decrease or diminish the response.

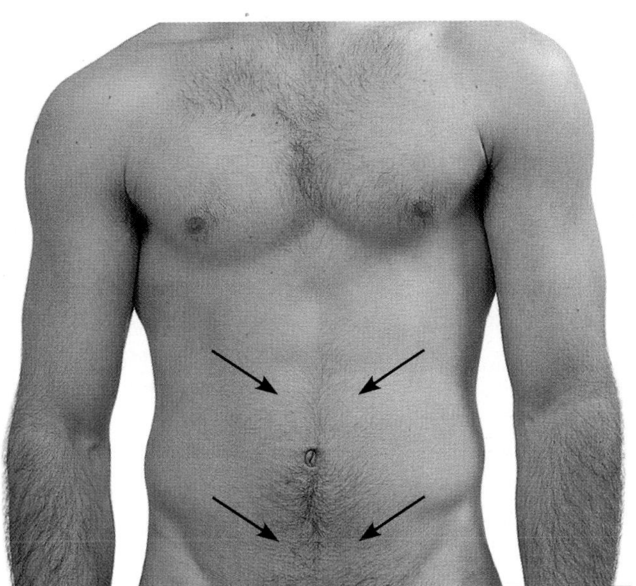

Figure 18.35 Abdominal reflex testing pattern.

- Observe muscular contraction and movement of the umbilicus toward the stimulus.
- Repeat this procedure in the other three quadrants of the abdomen.

Additional Assessment Techniques

Carotid Auscultation

Auscultation of the carotid arteries may be performed with the assessment of the head and neck or as part of the peripheral vascular assess-

ASSESSMENT TECHNIQUE/NORMAL FINDINGS | SPECIAL CONSIDERATIONS

ment. You may need to review your assessment notes for findings of carotid artery auscultation.

A bruit may be indicative of an obstructive disease process such as atherosclerosis. The amount of blood flow to the brain may be diminished. This decrease in oxygen could be responsible for subtle changes in client responses.

Meningeal Assessment

ALERT!

Be sure to use universal precautions if meningitis is suspected.

Ask the client to flex the neck by bringing the chin down to touch the chest. Observe the degree of range of motion and the absence or presence of pain. The client should be able to flex the neck about 45 degrees without pain.

When the client complains of pain and has a decrease in the flexion motion, you will observe for the *Brudzinski sign*. With the client in a supine position, assist the client with neck flexion. Observe the legs. The sign is positive when neck flexion causes flexion of the legs and thighs.

When the meningeal membranes are irritated or inflamed, as in meningitis, the client will experience *nuchal rigidity* or stiffness of the neck.

Use of Glasgow Coma Scale

The *Glasgow coma scale* assesses the level of consciousness of the individual on a continuum from alertness to coma (Figure 18.36). The scale tests three body functions: verbal response, motor response, and eye response. A maximum total score of 15 indicates the person is alert, responsive, and oriented. A total score of 3, the lowest achievable score, indicates a nonresponsive comatose individual. For more information on use of the Glasgow coma scale, consult a neurologic nursing text.

Syncope is a brief loss of consciousness and is usually sudden. *Coma* is a more prolonged state with pronounced and persistent changes.

Referral

A client experiencing any loss of consciousness needs immediate medical interventions.

GLASCOW COMA SCALE
BEST EYE-OPENING RESPONSE 4 = Spontaneously 3 = To speech 2 = To pain 1 = No response **(Record "C" if eyes closed by swelling)**
BEST MOTOR RESPONSE to painful stimuli 6 = Obeys verbal command 5 = Localizes pain 4 = Flexion—withdrawal 3 = Flexion—abnormal 2 = Extension—abnormal 1 = No response **(Record best upper limb response)**
BEST VERBAL RESPONSE 5 = Oriented X 3 4 = Conversation—confused 3 = Speech—inappropriate 2 = Sounds—incomprehensible 1 = No response **(Record "E" if endotracheal tube in place, "T" if tracheostomy tube in place)**

Figure 18.36 Glasgow coma scale.

Reminders

- After completing the neurologic assessment of your client, be sure the client is comfortable and has no adverse effects from the procedures. Assist the client with dressing or returning to a more comfortable position.
- Answer any questions the client has, discuss the findings, and provide client teaching to decrease risk factors and promote health and self-care. It may be necessary to have a family member present at this time.
- In addition to the previous steps of physical assessment, consider the variations for different client groups discussed in the following section.
- Document the assessment findings as described in Chapter 1. See pages 574–575 for data regarding nursing diagnoses commonly associated with the neurologic system.

Developmental Considerations

Infants, Children, and Adolescent Clients

The growth of the nervous system during the fetal period is very rapid. This rate of growth does not continue during infancy.

Some research indicates that no neurons are formed after the third trimester of fetal life. It is believed that during infancy the neurons mature, allowing for more complex actions to take place. The cerebral cortex thickens, brain size increases, and myelinization occurs. The maturational advances in the nervous system are responsible for the cephalocaudal and proximal-to-distal refinement of development, control, and movement. Primitive reflexes begin to disappear, and the child takes on more controlled and complex activity.

The cry of the newborn helps you place the infant on the health-illness continuum. *Strong* and *lusty* are terms used to describe the cry of a healthy newborn. An absent, weak, or a "cat-like" or shrill cry usually indicates cerebral disease.

Throughout infancy and the early childhood years, it is important to assess the fine and gross motor skills, language, and personal-social skills of the child. You need to identify "bench marks" or "mileposts" related to age and level of functioning of the child and compare the child's actual functioning to an anticipated level of functioning. Developmental delays or learning disabilities may be related to neurologic conditions. See Chapter 19 for a full discussion of the assessment of infants, children, and adolescents.

Childbearing Clients

As the uterus grows to accommodate the fetus, pressure may be placed on nerves in the pelvic cavity, thus producing neurologic changes in the legs. As the pressure is relieved in the pelvis, the changes in the lower extremities are resolved. As the fetus grows, the center of gravity of the female shifts, and the lumbar curvature of the spine is accentuated. This change in posture can place pressure on roots of nerves, causing sensory changes in the lower extremities. These sensory changes are reversible following relief of pressure and postural changes. Hyperactive reflexes may indicate pregnancy-induced hypertension (PIH). See Chapter 20 for a full assessment of the childbearing client.

Older Clients

As the individual ages, many neurologic changes occur. Some of these changes are readily visible, whereas others are internal and are not easily detected. The internal changes could be primary in nature, or secondary to other changes and contribute to the aging process.

In general, the aging process causes a subtle, slow, but steady decrease in neurologic function. These changes can be more pronounced and more troublesome for the individual when they are accompanied by a chronic illness. Impulse transmission decreases, as does reaction to stimuli. Reflexes are diminished or disappear, and coordination is not as strong as it once was. Deep tendon reflexes are not as brisk. Coordination and movement may be slower and not as smooth as it was at one time.

The senses—hearing, vision, smell, taste, and touch—are not as acute as they once were. Taste is not as strong; therefore, the older adult tends to use more seasonings on food. Visual acuity and hearing begin to diminish.

As muscle mass decreases, the individual moves and reacts more slowly than during youth. The client's gait may now include short, shuffling, uncertain, and perhaps unsteady steps. The posture of the older adult demonstrates more flexion than in earlier years.

Assessment techniques used with the older adult are the same as those used for the younger or middle-aged adult. However, because the older adult tires more easily, you may need to do the total assessment in more than one visit. Remember to allow more time than usual when you perform the neurologic assessment of the older adult. It is also imperative that you obtain a detailed history, because chronic health problems can influence the findings. See Chapter 21 for a complete assessment of older adults.

Psychosocial Considerations

Changes in nervous system functioning may alter an individual's ability to control body movements, speech, or elimination patterns, and to engage in activities of daily living. Inevitably, these changes will affect the individual's psychosocial health. Clients' self-esteem may suffer as they suddenly or progressively become unable to carry out the roles they previously assumed in their family and society. Another common psychosocial problem associated with neurologic disorders is social isolation, as for example when an individual in the first stage of Alzheimer's disease declines invitations to social functions because the person feels anxious and confused in unfamiliar surroundings. Such problems indicate a need for improved or increased support systems and coping strategies.

As stresses accumulate, an individual becomes increasingly susceptible to neurologic problems, such as forgetfulness, confusion, inability to concentrate, sleeplessness, and tremors. For example, a college senior who is studying for examinations, writing applications for graduate school, and has just broken up with her boyfriend might experience one or all of these symptoms. Chronic stress may also contribute to clinical depression in some clients.

Self-Care Considerations

Accidents are responsible for many neurologic problems, including head trauma, spinal cord injury, infections, and toxicity. Safety precautions must be practiced at home, at work, and during recreation. Some safety practices related to the neurologic system are discussed later in this chapter.

The nervous system is in constant need of glucose for optimum functioning. Proper nutrition and timing of meals throughout the day may prevent hyper- or hypoglycemia.

Regular aerobic exercise increases tissue oxygenation throughout the body, including the brain. Studies indicate that regular exercise can improve alertness and alleviate depression in some clients.

Caffeine stimulates the central nervous system. Very large daily doses of caffeine (eg, the amount in 7 or more cups of brewed coffee) can lead to restlessness, insomnia, trembling, palpitations, and diarrhea.

When consumed in small amounts (eg, one glass of wine with dinner), alcohol has a mild tranquilizing effect. In higher doses, it may cause significant neurologic impairments, such as memory loss, inability to concentrate, and severe motor deficits. Chronic heavy drinking can cause the brain to shrink in size and the ventricles (the fluid-filled cavities within the brain) to enlarge.

In recent years, researchers have noted increasing cases of sleep deprivation among people with busy schedules and multiple roles, eg, men and women who hold full-time jobs, raise children, and care for aging parents. Lack of sleep may contribute to neurologic impairments such as forgetfulness, inability to concentrate, and impaired memory. Remember that some medications also may cause sleeplessness in some clients.

Family, Cultural, and Environmental Considerations

Huntington's disease is a genetically transferred neurologic disorder. However, the genetic link to most other degenerative neurologic disorders, such as Alzheimer's disease, multiple sclerosis, myasthenia gravis, and others, is unclear.

Research is also inconclusive on the effects of environmental toxins on the development of degenerative neurologic disorders; however, some studies suggest that Alzheimer's disease in some clients may be due to aluminum intoxication. Other research indicates that some cases of Parkinson's disease may be caused by toxins such as carbon monoxide, manganese, and mercury. Peripheral neuropathy, damage to the peripheral nerves, occurs more often among farm workers exposed to the organophosphates in many insecticides.

Lead poisoning also causes peripheral neuropathy and encephalopathy. Although not as common as in the past, the risk for lead poisoning still remains high among preschool children who live in old apartments or houses in which walls are painted with lead-based paints. Note that lead poisoning is not limited to those who live in low-cost, inner-city dwellings, but may also occur in wealthy families living in restored older homes.

Organizing the Data

After completing the focused interview and the neurologic assessment of the client, you will review and organize the data collected. You integrate the recently obtained neurologic data with all other data and form clusters. These newly conceptualized clusters become the basis for nursing diagnoses. Nursing interventions help maintain or promote wellness, reduce risk factors, foster self-care, or help limit the deficit while providing safety and rehabilitation. When collaborative problems are identified, confer with other members of the health care team to identify interventions that promote continuity and consistency of care.

Identifying Nursing Diagnoses

Because the neurologic system integrates all body systems and contributes to many functions of the body, the nursing diagnoses reflect this integration. A problem or deficit within the nervous system influences the total person. Besides having an effect on the nervous system, the deficit alters other physiologic systems. It influences self-esteem, roles the client occupies, and relationships with other people. This influence is especially profound if the client is unable to perform activities independently.

Nursing diagnoses commonly used with clients experiencing a neurologic deficit include *Altered thought processes* (Table 18.2); *Sensory/perceptual alterations* (see Chapter 9); *Impaired verbal communication* (Table 18.2); and *Impaired physical mobility* (see Chapter 17). Each diagnostic statement has a unique definition and characteristics and a distinct interrelationship. For example, the client who has recently experienced a cerebrovascular accident (CVA) may have a right-sided paralysis and not be able to communicate. Although each problem has a definite set of interventions, they influence each other, and both problems influence the self-esteem of the client.

Table 18.2 Nursing Diagnoses Commonly Associated with the Neurologic System

ALTERED THOUGHT PROCESSES	
Definition: A state in which an individual experiences an impairment in cognitive operations, such as conscious thought, reality orientation, problem solving, and judgment. These impairments are a result of mental/personality or chronic organic disorders that may be exacerbated by situational crises.	
RELATED FACTORS	
Mental disorder (specify), Personality disorder (specify), Organic mental disorder (specify), Substance abuse, Others specific to patient (specify).	
DEFINING CHARACTERISTICS	
Fearful thoughts	Memory deficit/problems
Hallucinations	Inaccurate interpretation of environment
Irritability	Distractibility
IMPAIRED VERBAL COMMUNICATION	
Definition: The state in which an individual experiences a decreased or absent ability to use or understand language in human interaction (NANDA).	
RELATED FACTORS	
Acute confusion, Aphasia, Developmental disability, Psychologic impairment (specify), Inability to speak or speak clearly, Intubation, Primary language other than English, Tracheostomy, Others specific to patient (specify).	
DEFINING CHARACTERISTICS	
Major	**Minor**
Speaks or verbalizes with difficulty	Absence of audible speech
Unable to speak dominant language	Medical regimen/disease process interfering with ability to make audible sounds (eg, CVA, ET tube, trach)
Difficulty expressing thoughts verbally	Sign language as primary mode of communication
Does not or cannot speak	Anatomic defect
Difficulty forming words or sentences	Hearing deficit

DIAGNOSTIC REASONING IN ACTION

Mr. John Phelps, age 65, is an African-American male who comes to the community health clinic. He and his wife Helen recently celebrated their 40th wedding anniversary. He has a daughter 35 years old, a son 32 years old, and three grandchildren. Mr. Phelps retired 4 months ago from a busy accounting firm where he worked as a CPA for 25 years. He and his wife planned the retirement and traveling across the country to visit family.

Mr. Phelps's chief complaint is tremors that seem to be getting worse over the past few months. He noticed the tremors about 6 months ago and thought they were related to fatigue, since the office was very busy and he was working late hours. He anticipated that the tremors would stop after he retired and became rested. Mrs. Phelps indicates her husband's handwriting has become small and almost illegible and that she had to write several checks for him last week. His wife also comments that her husband seems depressed about his recent retirement, since he has a "blank look" to his face and his speech is slow. Lynette Chung, RN, conducts a focused interview and then proceeds with the physical assessment. She gathers the following objective and subjective data:

Mood swings

Tremors, movement of thumb and index finger in a circular fashion

Shuffling gait, falls easily

Constipation

Fatigue

Loss of 10 lbs

Drooling

Speaks in a monotone, voice slow, weak and soft

Rigidity during passive ROM

Jerky movements

Muscle pain and soreness

Decrease in corneal response

Posture not erect, forward flexion

Unable to perform finger-to-nose test and rapid alternating movement

Difficulty standing from sitting position without assistance

To cluster the data, Ms Chung:

Considers the data regarding tremors, posture, gait, falls, rigidity, and muscle pain and soreness.

Considers data regarding drooling, weight loss, fatigue, and constipation.

Considers data regarding jerky movements, inability to touch finger to nose, facial mask, and slow, weak, monotone voice.

Ms Chung arrives at the following nursing diagnoses:

1. *Impaired physical mobility* related to neuromuscular impairment
2. *Impaired verbal communication* related to inability to speak clearly as evidenced by soft, weak voice and slow, monotonous speech pattern
3. *High risk for injury* related to frequent falls, forward flexion, jerky movements

Ms Chung consults with the clinic physician. After further evaluation, Mr. Phelps is admitted to the neurologic unit of the community hospital with a diagnosis of Parkinson's disease (described in the next section).

Common Alterations in the Health of the Neurologic System

Problems commonly associated with the neurologic system include changes in motor function, including gait and movement, seizures, spinal cord injury, infections, degenerative disorders, and cranial nerve dysfunction. These conditions are described below and in Tables 18.3 and 18.4 on page 578.

Seizures

Seizures are sudden, rapid, and excessive discharges of electrical energy in the brain. They are usually centered in the cerebral cortex. Some seizure disorders stem from neurologic problems that occur before or during birth, or they can develop secondary to childhood fevers. In children and adults, seizures can result from a variety of factors including trauma, infections, cerebrovascular disease, environmental toxins, and withdrawal from alcohol, sedatives, or antidepressants. *Epilepsy* is a chronic seizure disorder.

Spinal Cord Injury

Recall that the spinal cord extends from the medulla oblongata of the brainstem. As it continues down the back, it is protected by the cervical, thoracic, and lumbar vertebrae. Spinal cord injuries result from trauma to the vertebrae, which causes dislocation fractures that in turn compress or transect the spinal cord. The most common causes of this type of trauma are automobile and motorcycle accidents, sports accidents such as football and diving accidents, and penetrating injuries such as stab wounds. In general, the higher the level of the injury, the greater the loss of neurologic function. Injuries to the cervical region are the most common and the most devastating.

Infections of the Neurologic System

Meningitis is caused by a virus or bacteria that infects the coverings, or meninges, of the brain or spinal cord. Meningitis may result from a penetrating wound, fractured skull, or upper respiratory infection, or it may occur secondary to facial or cranial surgery.

In some cases, meningitis may spread to the underlying brain tissues, causing encephalitis. *Encephalitis* is defined as an inflammation of the tissue of the brain. It usually results from a virus, which may be transmitted by ticks or mosquitos, or it may result from a childhood illness such as chickenpox or the measles.

Myelitis is an inflammation of the spinal cord. Poliomyelitis and herpes zoster infection are two common causes. It may develop after an infection such as measles or gonorrhea, or it may follow vaccination for cowpox or rabies.

A *brain abscess* is usually the result of a systemic infection. It is marked by an accumulation of pus in the brain cells. Most brain abscesses develop secondary to a primary infection. Others result from skull fractures or penetrating injuries, as from gunshot wounds.

Lyme disease is an infection caused by a spirochete transmitted by a bite from an infected tick that lives on deer. Its major symptoms are arthritis, a flulike syndrome, and a rash. If untreated, lyme disease may cause neurologic disorders.

Degenerative Neurologic Disorders

Alzheimer's disease is a progressive degenerative disease of the brain that leads to dementia. Although it is more common in people over age 65, its onset may occur as early as middle adulthood. Symptoms include a loss of memory, particularly of recent events, shortened attention span, confusion, and disorientation. Eventually, the client with Alzheimer's disease may experience paranoid fantasies and hallucinations.

Amyotrophic lateral sclerosis is a chronic degenerative disease involving the cerbral cortex and the motor neurons in the spinal cord. The result is a progressive wasting of skeletal muscles that eventually leads to death. Although the cause is unknown, research has implicated viral infection.

Huntington's disease is an inherited disorder characterized by uncontrollable jerking movements, called *chorea*, which literally means *dance*. It typically progresses to mental deterioration and ultimately death. Symptoms usually first appear in early middle age; thus, those with Huntington's disease often have had children before they know they have the disorder.

Multiple sclerosis is the deterioration of the protective sheaths, composed of *myelin,* of the nerve tracts in the brain and spinal cord. The first attack usually occurs between the ages of 20 and 40. Early symptoms include temporary tingling, numbness, or weakness that may affect only one limb or one side of the body. Other symptoms include unsteadiness, blurred vision, slurred speech, and difficulty in urinating. Some individuals experience repeated attacks that progress in severity. In these individuals, permanent disability with progressive neuromuscular deficits develops.

Myasthenia gravis is a chronic neuromuscular disorder involving increasing weakness of voluntary muscles with activity, and some abatement of symptoms with rest. Onset is gradual and usually occurs in adolescence or young adulthood. The precise etiology is unknown, but it is believed that myasthenia gravis is an *autoimmune* disorder: that is, the individual's immune system attacks the individual's own normal cells rather than foreign pathogens. Some of the most common symptoms include ptosis (drooping eyelids), diplopia (double vision), a flat affect, and a weak, monotonous voice.

Parkinson's disease is a degeneration of the basal nuclei of the brain, which are collections of nerve cell bodies deep within the white matter of the cerebrum. These nuclei are responsible for initiating and stopping voluntary movement. Parkinson's is characterized by slow movements, a continuous "pill-rolling" tremor of the forefinger and thumb, a rhythmic shaking of the hands, a bobbing of the head, and difficulty in initiating movement. The individual may have a masklike facial expression, difficulty in speaking clearly, and difficulty maintaining balance while walking. Although the precise etiology is unknown, research indicates that some cases of Parkinson's may be caused by environmental toxins such as carbon monoxide or certain metals. It may also result from previous encephalitis.

Table 18.3 Problems with Motor Function

Gait

Ataxic Gait
A walk characterized by a wide base, uneven steps, feet slapping, and a tendency to sway. This type of walk is associated with posterior column disease or decreased proprioception regarding extremities. Seen in multiple sclerosis and drug or alcohol intoxication.

Scissors Gait
A walk characterized by spastic lower limbs and movement in a stiff, jerky manner. The knees come together; the legs cross in front of one another; and the legs are abducted as the individual takes short, progressive, slow steps. This is seen in individuals with multiple sclerosis.

Steppage Gait
Sometimes called the "foot drop" walk. The individual flexes and raises the knee to a higher than usual level yielding a flopping of the foot when walking. This usually is indicative of lower motor neuron disease. Seen in individuals with alcoholic neuritis and progressive muscular atrophy.

Festination Gait
Referred to as the "Parkinson's walk." The individual has stooped posture, takes short steps, and turns stiffly. There is a slow start to the walk and frequent, accelerated steps. This gait is associated with basal ganglia disease.

Movement

Fasciculation
Commonly called a twitch, this is an involuntary, local, visible muscular contraction. It is not significant when it occurs in tired muscles. It can be associated with motor neuron disease.

Tic
Commonly called a *habit,* a tic is usually psychogenic in nature. The involuntary spasmodic movement of the muscle is seen in a muscle under voluntary control, usually in the face, neck, or shoulders.

Tremor
A rhythmic or alternating involuntary movement from the contraction of opposing muscle groups. Tremors vary in degree and are seen in Parkinson's disease, multiple sclerosis, uremia (a form of kidney failure), and alcohol intoxication.

Athetoid Movement
A continuous, involuntary, repetitive, slow, "wormlike," arrhythmic muscular movement. The muscles are in a state of hypotoxicity, producing a distortion to the limb. This movement is seen in cerebral palsy.

Dystonia
Similar to athetoid movements, dystonia involves larger muscle groups. The twisting movements yield a grotesque change to the individual's posture. Torticollis, or wry neck, is an example of dystonia.

Myoclonus
A continual, rapid, short spasm involving a muscle, part of a muscle, or even a group of muscles. Frequently occurs in an extremity as the individual is falling asleep. Myoclonus is also seen in seizure disorders.

Table 18.4 Problems Associated with Dysfunction of Cranial Nerves

Cranial Nerve		Dysfunction
I	Olfactory	Unilateral or bilateral anosmia.
II	Optic	Optic atrophy, papilledema, amblyopia, field defects.
III	Oculomotor	Diplopia, ptosis of lid, dilated pupil, inability to focus on close objects.
IV	Trochlear	Convergent strabismus, diplopia.
V	Trigeminal	Tic douloureux, loss of facial sensation, decreased ability to chew, loss of corneal reflex, decreased blinking.
VI	Abducens	Diplopia, strabismus.
VII	Facial	Bell's palsy, decreased ability to distinguish tastes.
VIII	Vestibulocochlear	Tinnitus, vertigo, deafness.
IX.	Glossopharyngeal	Loss of "gag" reflex, loss of taste, difficulty swallowing.
X	Vagus	Loss of voice, impaired voice, difficulty swallowing.
XI	Accessory	Difficulty with shrugging of shoulders, inability to turn head to left and right.
XII	Hypoglossal	Difficulty with speech and swallowing, inability to protrude tongue.

Health Promotion and Client Education

At the conclusion of the neurologic assessment, answer the client's questions. If a family member was present during the assessment, answer their questions. Stress the importance of a healthy nervous system. Topics to cover include safety, prevention of limitations, limiting an existing problem, and rehabilitation to restore function to as high a level as possible.

Prevention is especially important in regard to the neurologic system. Many neurologic problems or pathologic processes cause permanent, nonreversible deficit. Therefore, the focus is on prevention rather than cure.

Safety Measures for Promoting the Health of the Neurologic System

Safety is a primary concern, and all aspects need to be encouraged. Safety measures must be observed at work, during recreation, and in the home.

DIAGNOSTIC REASONING IN ACTION

Anita Espitia comes to the wellness center of a large financial services corporation for a wellness assessment. She is 33 years old and is the mother of a 7-year-old daughter. She and her husband divorced 7 months ago. She has been an accounting manager for the corporation for 4 years but has never before visited its wellness center because she is "just too busy. I'm up at five to go for my run, then I have to get myself and my daughter ready for the day. I'm at the office by seven-thirty and don't leave until six. Then I pick up my daughter at day care, make us dinner, put her to bed, call my mother to see if she's OK, do some paperwork, watch the eleven o'clock news, then go to bed myself. Who has time for a wellness check-up? I shouldn't even be here now, but my boss insisted that I come."

The wellness center nurse, Claire Stevenson, RN, asks Ms Espitia why she feels her boss insisted that she come that day. Ms Espitia sighs, "Well, it probably has something to do with the fact that I forgot about two meetings last week, and I made some pretty serious errors in my calculations in a report I handed in yesterday. This morning, a client called me, and I couldn't even remember who he was or who I'd assigned his file to. I had to ask my boss if she'd ever heard of him! I was so embarrassed. This isn't like me!"

Ms Stevenson begins a focused interview, eliciting further information about Ms Espitia's neurologic health history, daily routine, diet, memory, and sleep patterns. Ms Espitia says she has no trouble falling asleep at night. "Are you kidding? I'm always so exhausted I'm asleep almost before my head hits the pillow."

Ms Stevenson performs a neurologic assessment, which reveals normal sensory and motor function, normal long-term memory, and full alertness. She then asks Ms Espitia to calculate $7 - 3 + 12 \times 3$. In response, Ms Espitia sighs, "You know, I just feel too tired to hold all those numbers in my head." Her eyes fill with tears. "Is there something wrong with me?" she asks.

Ms Stevenson clusters the subjective and objective data. She notes that an inability to maintain usual routines and verbalization of unremitting and overwhelming lack of energy are major defining characteristics for the nursing diagnosis *Fatigue*, and that minor defining characteristics include an inability to concentrate and decreased performance. She notes that one of the related factors for the diagnosis is excessive role demands. She therefore identifies the following nursing diagnoses:

1. *Fatigue* related to excessive role demands
2. *Knowledge deficit* related to lack of information about time management, role strain, and physiologic requirements for sleep and rest

Ms Stevenson explains to Ms Espitia the physiologic benefits of sleep and rest, and the harmful effects of inadequate sleep. She explores with Ms Espitia some ways in which she can increase the amount of sleep she gets each night, such as waiting until her lunch break to go for her run, arriving at work no earlier than eight, leaving no later than five-thirty, and watching the ten o'clock news instead of the later program. She suggests that Ms Espitia discuss frankly with her boss her need to maintain a manageable workload so that she will not have to bring paperwork home with her at night and instead can spend that time with her daughter. Finally, she schedules Ms Espitia for the company's next class on time management.

- Use safety gear at work, eg, hard hats, filtering masks, protective eye gear.
- Use safety gear during recreation, eg, helmets for skateboarding, bicycle riding, motorcycle riding, and contact sports.
- Use seat belts for all passengers in automobiles, school buses, or other vehicles, and use carseats for babies and young children.
- Safe driving and good road habits are important. Observe speed limits, do not pass stopped school buses, and do not drive when intoxicated.
- Firearms, drugs, and alcohol are responsible for many accidents that cause neurologic deficits. It is imperative to control the use and misuse of these objects. A complete discussion of safety and legislation regarding these three areas is beyond the scope of this text.
- Use prescription medications correctly. Follow directions for use, and become familiar with side effects. Cardiac medications indirectly increase perfusion to the cerebral tissue and may produce neurologic symptoms. Insulin in excess causes convulsive seizures.

General Measures to Promote Neurologic Health

- Take measures to prevent repeated systemic viral and bacterial infections. Meningitis and encephalitis can be a complication of a systemic infection. A healthy diet, vitamin supplements, nutritional supplements, rest, and regular exercise all promote a healthy immune system and may help to ward off infections.
- Keep stress at a minimum. Stress increases blood pressure, and sustained elevation of blood pressure leads to hypertension. A cerebrovascular accident (CVA), or *stroke*, is a common complication of hypertension. The client should adopt a healthful lifestyle, including plenty of rest, regular exercise, and stress-reduction techniques such as meditation and coping strategies.
- Use proper body mechanics in all daily activities. This topic is considered in the discussion of the musculoskeletal system; however, it applies to the neurologic system as well. For example, lifting a heavy object improperly may sprain the lumbosacral muscles. Muscle spasms place pressure on spinal nerve roots, causing pain and altered function. Repeated sprains can lead to a rupture of the vertebral disc, requiring the individual to undergo surgery.

Summary

You obtain valuable data regarding the overall health status from the neurologic assessment. You need knowledge of the anatomy, physiology, and complex integration of the nervous system with other body systems. This detailed knowledge base enhances your ability to perform the assessment techniques and observe the overt and covert changes demonstrated by the client. The data from the health history and focused interview serves as a foundation for the physical assessment. From this extensive data you formulate a plan to proceed with the assessment. Because many of the neurologic functions are integrated, it may not be necessary to perform numerous tests. Then organize the data obtained during the neurologic assessment, formulate nursing diagnoses, and develop a plan of care. Share this information with the client, and encourage the client to take an active role in the planning process. Client participation is most important, because neurologic deficits threaten self-esteem, and participation in the plan of care fosters self-esteem and gives the client a feeling of control. All interventions should foster wellness, limit the disability, and be appropriate for the individual.

Key Points

- ✓ The neurologic system has two main divisions, the central nervous system and the peripheral nervous system. The brain and the spinal cord make up the central nervous system, and the 12 pairs of cranial nerves and 31 pairs of spinal nerves make up the peripheral nervous system. The primary function of the nervous system is to receive an impulse, interpret the impulse, and provide a response to protect and maintain the integrity of the individual.
- ✓ Conduct a focused interview to obtain specific data regarding the health of the client's neurologic system. Together with data from the health history, the data from the focused interview gives you a comprehensive database. This data includes strengths, weaknesses, habits, risk factors, health practices, and cultural and environmental factors.
- ✓ Assess mental status, cranial nerves, motor function, sensory function, and reflexes. Because of the complexity and integrated function of the system, one test assesses several functions. You may need to capitalize on this concept.
- ✓ Organize your assessment techniques to conserve the client's energy. Take a head-to-toe and distal-to-proximal approach to assessment. Remember to integrate as many activities as possible.

- ✓ Nursing diagnoses commonly associated with the neurologic system include *Altered thought processes, Sensory/perceptual alterations, Impaired verbal communication, Impaired physical mobility,* and others.
- ✓ Common alterations in the health of the neurologic system include seizures, spinal cord injury, infections, degenerative disorders, cranial nerve dysfunction, and others.
- ✓ Provide the client with information needed to promote the health of the neurologic system, including information on safety measures, stress reduction, diet, exercise, and sleep and rest.

Unit Three

Integrated Health Assessments

Chapter 19

Assessing Infants, Children, and Adolescents

Much of the information in earlier chapters applies to the infant, child, or adolescent as well as to the adult client. However, children are not simply smaller versions of adults. For this reason, with each region or system assessment in Unit Two, specific variations for infants, children, and adolescents were discussed. Additionally, because the pediatric client is developmentally unique, this chapter presents an overview of the anatomy and physiology of the healthy child, focused interview questions, one possible exam sequence, some common nursing diagnoses and alterations in health, and some client teaching tips that may be appropriate for this group. Before continuing, you might find it helpful to review the developmental tasks of the various stages of childhood, discussed in Chapter 3. For more information, consult a pediatric nursing textbook.

Anatomy and Physiology Review

Children are constantly growing and developing; thus, their anatomy and physiology are changing and different from those of an adult. The challenge to the caregiver is to determine whether the variations are normal for the child's developmental stage, or whether they represent unexpected findings. The following sections list some normal variations in the anatomy and physiology of infants, children, and adolescents.

General Appearance and Vital Signs

The height, weight, head circumference, temperature, pulse, respirations, and blood pressure vary depending on the age of the child.

Integumentary System

Because of the trauma of birth, newborns may evidence bruising or localized edema in the presenting part. The bruising and edema usually resolve during the newborn period. Areas of hyperpigmentation over the buttocks, known as mongolian spots, are a normal finding in infants with darker skin tones. Because newborn skin is thin, smooth, and elastic, the infant is at greater risk for fluid and heat loss. Temperature regulation is not effective.

In children, the epidermis is thicker, tougher, darker, and better lubricated than in the infant. Bluish pigmentation in the gums, nail beds, and buccal mucosa of dark-skinned children is normal. The amount of hair and rate of hair growth varies from one child to another. In adolescents, subcutaneous fat deposits increase, and the apocrine sweat glands and sebaceous glands are more active. Coarse pubic hair and axillary hair develops, and males develop coarse facial hair. Females develop breast tissue, and the areolae enlarge and darken.

Head and Neck

The heads of most newborns are misshapen because of the molding of the head that occurs during vaginal deliveries. Molding of the head is made possible by the fontanelles and by overriding of the **sutures**, or junction lines that connect the eight bones of the cranium. Within a week, the newborn's head usually regains its symmetry.

The newborn's skull contains six **fontanelles**, unossified membranous gaps between the bones that allow for growth of the brain during the first year (see Figure 9.48). The five smaller fontanelles gradually close during the first 8 weeks after birth. The largest fontanelle, the *anterior fontanelle*, is about 4 to 6 cm in diameter. The anterior fontanelle can increase in size for several months after birth. After about 6 months, the size gradually decreases until closure occurs between 9 and 16 months. Head size is greater than chest circumference at birth. By the time the child is about 6 years, approximately 90% of the adult head size is reached.

Visual abilities are present in the newborn. Focusing, tracking movements, and neural development leading to recognition, such as recognition of facial features, begin at birth. Recent studies using sophisticated measuring devices show that by 6 months the infant's visual acuity may be 20/20 to 20/40—nearly that of an adult.

The infant's auditory tube is shorter and wider and its postion is more horizonal than the adult's, making it easier for pathogens from the nasopharynx to migrate through to the middle ear. The auditory canals of infants and children under the age of 2 or 3 curve upward, and so you pull the ear lobe gently down and out before examining with an otoscope (Figure 19.1). The auditory canals of older children and adults are longer and curve downward; therefore, you pull the top of the pinna up and back.

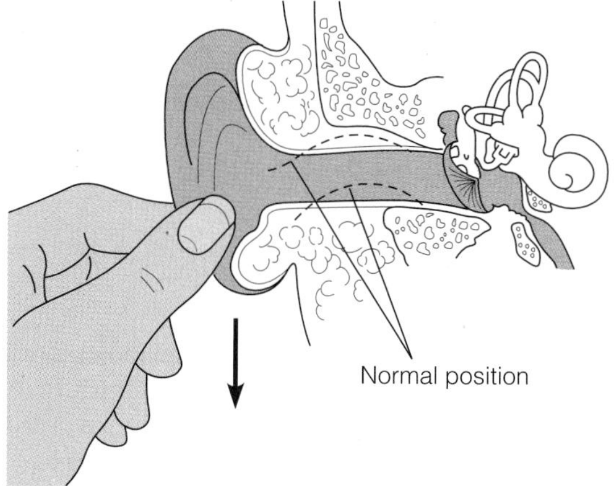

Figure 19.1 Straightening the auditory canal of a young child by pulling the pinna down and out.

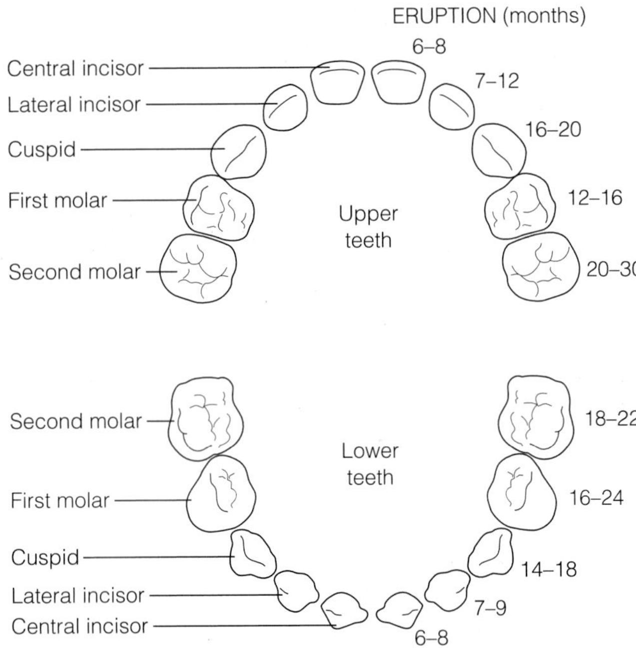

Figure 19.2 Temporary teeth and their times of eruption (stated in months).

Maxillary and ethmoid sinuses are developed at birth. The frontal sinuses develop by age 7 or 8, and the sphenoid sinus develops after puberty.

Teeth begin to erupt at about 6 months of age. By 30 months of age, all 20 deciduous teeth usually have erupted (Figure 19.2). Between ages 5 and 6, they often begin to shed. Permanent teeth begin to erupt at approximately 6 years of age and continue erupting until all 32 teeth are present.

The white nodules often seen in the palate of the newborn are a normal finding. Tonsils are generally small in infancy, appear large in preschool years, and become smaller as the child nears puberty.

The neck is short in infancy and lengthens at 2 to 3 years of age. Head control is related to control of neck muscles. The thyroid gland is not easily palpable until adolescence.

Respiratory System

The lung assessment of an infant or child on percussion normally reveals hyperresonance (a booming sound) because of the thinness of the chest wall. Breath sounds are usually harsher or louder in children for the same reason. Infants are obligatory nose breathers. In children under 6 or 7 years of age, respirations are abdominal. Older children are commonly thoracic breathers. Respiratory development continues throughout childhood, with increases in diameter and length of airways and increases in size and number of alveoli until adolescence, when maturation is complete.

Cardiovascular System

In the fetus, about two-thirds of the blood is shunted through an opening in the atrial septum, the *foramen ovale*, into the left side of the heart, where it is pumped out through the aorta. A small amount of blood goes to the lungs. The rest of the oxygenated blood is pumped by the right side of the heart out the pulmonary artery and is detoured through the ductus arteriosus into the aorta, bypassing the lungs. Inflation and aeration of the lungs at birth produce circulatory changes and closure of the foramen ovale and ductus arteriosus, usually within the first day of birth.

In children under the age of 8, the heart lies more horizontally, with the apex left of the nipple line. The point of maximal impulse (PMI) may therefore be located higher than the fifth intercostal space and more medially than the midclavicular line. In children, a pleural friction rub will stop if the breath is held, whereas a precordial friction rub will persist. An S3 gallop rhythm is often normal in children because of vibrations during ventricular filling.

Breasts

Newborns may display breast enlargement with a white discharge from the nipples as a normal result of maternal estrogen. This effect should disappear within 1 to 2 weeks. By late childhood, during the preadolescent period, estrogen hormones stimulate breast changes in females. The breasts enlarge, mostly because of extensive fat deposition. Although the age of onset of breast development varies widely, the five stages of breast development follow Tanner's sexual maturity rating (Figure 19.3).

Abdomen

Present in the newborn is the umbilical cord, which contains two arteries and one vein. The liver takes up proportionately more space in the abdomen at birth. Its lower edge may be

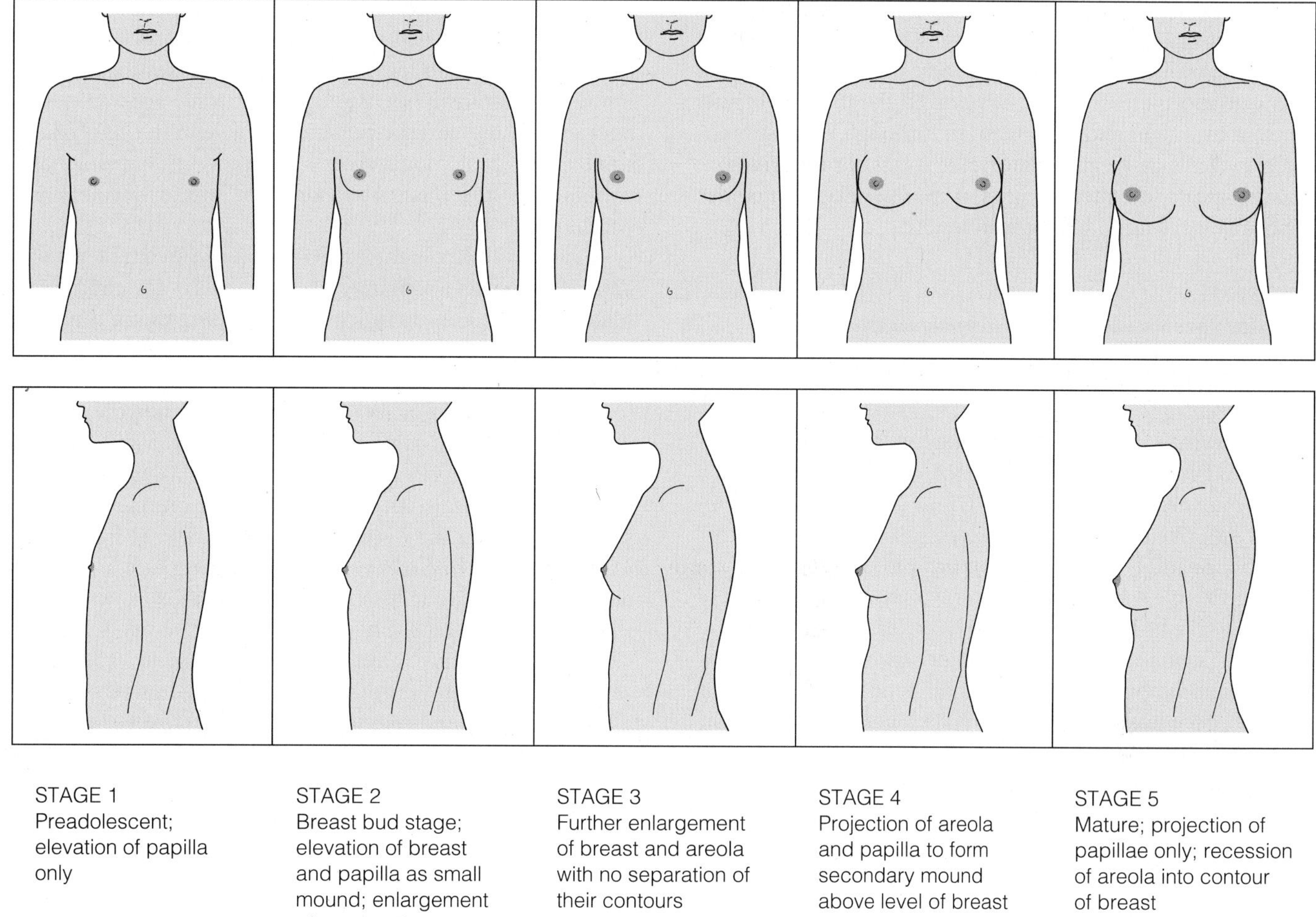
STAGE 1
Preadolescent; elevation of papilla only
STAGE 2
Breast bud stage; elevation of breast and papilla as small mound; enlargement of areolar diameter.
STAGE 3
Further enlargement of breast and areola with no separation of their contours
STAGE 4
Projection of areola and papilla to form secondary mound above level of breast
STAGE 5
Mature; projection of papillae only; recession of areola into contour of breast

Figure 19.3 Maturational stages of female breast development.

palpated 0.5 to 2.5 cm below the right costal margin, and the spleen may extend 1 to 2 cm below the left costal margin. Umbilical hernias less than 5 cm in size are common up to 1 to 2 years of life, and some may not close until 6 years of age, particularly in infants of African ancestry. Infants and young children normally exhibit a "potbelly" contour that often disappears by age 3 to 5.

Lymphatic System

The lymphatic system is well developed at birth and grows rapidly until about age 10. At approximately age 6, the lymphoid tissue reaches adult size. It surpasses adult size by puberty, and then it slowly atrophies. The excessive antigen stimulation in children may cause the early rapid growth of lymphoid tissue.

Genitourinary and Reproductive System

Bladder capacity increases with age from approximately 15–20 ml at birth to 700 ml in adulthood. When the bladder reaches a certain volume, stretch receptors stimulate bladder contraction and relaxation of the urethral sphincter. The urinary bladder is located higher in the abdomen in children than in adults.

Undescended testes should descend spontaneously in most males by 1 year of age. The first visible sign of sexual maturation in the male is testicular enlargement, which begins between 10 and 13 years of age and is completed between 14 and 18 years of age. Penile growth occurs later than testicular and scrotal growth. Male pubic hair is initially distributed at the base of the scrotum, then at the base of the penis; eventually it spreads over the pubic area. (See Chapter 15.)

The clitoris normally may be large in the female newborn because of maternal hormones. During puberty, the external female reproductive organs, especially the clitoris, become enlarged and increase in sensitivity, and the internal organs increase in weight and musculature. Although the first menstrual cycles may be anovulatory, the onset of menstruation, which appears just after the peak of growth velocity, provides confirmation of reproductive maturation.

Musculoskeletal System

Bone growth is rapid during infancy, steady during childhood, and rapid during adolescence. Young children often have *genu varum* (bowlegs) until 1 to 2 years of age (Figure 19.4a). *Genu valgum* (knock-knees) is normal from 2 to 7 years of age and is due to overcompensation for genu varum (Figure 19.4b). A broad-based gait is normal until 3 years of age. Feet may be flat until the child has been walking for 1 to 2 years. A spinal curve that is evident when the child stands upright but disappears when the child bends forward usually indicates poor posture, not congenital scoliotic curvature. The skeleton contributes to linear growth, and muscles and fat are significant for weight increase.

Neurologic System

At birth the neurologic system is not completely developed. There is little cortical control, and the neurons are not yet myelinated. Movements are directed primarily by primitive reflexes, such as the *tonic neck reflex* that is elicited when the head is forcibly turned to one side. In response, the infant extends the arm and leg on that side and flexes the opposite limbs. An infant will not crawl until the tonic neck reflex disappears. With gradual acquisition of myelin in the cephalocaudal and proximodistal order (head, neck, trunk, and extremities), the infant's sensory and motor development continues.

You need to know the expected developmental level of a child at any given age to interpret the status of the child's neurologic system. For example, when assessing motor function, consider that fine motor coordination is not fully developed until 4 to 6 years of age. Younger children are not able to perform sophisticated fine motor function tests; however, a pincer grasp should be present at 9 months, and a child should be able to stack blocks at 12 months. When assessing proprioception, expect a young child to balance on one foot for 5 seconds. A child over 4 years of age may be able to balance for 15 seconds and hop on one foot, staying in place and maintaining balance. Younger children have difficulty with hopping. When assessing memory, you can expect a 4-year-old child to repeat three numbers, a 5-year-old to repeat four numbers, and a 6-year-old to repeat five numbers. When assessing cortical motor integration, you can expect a 3-year-old child to draw a circle, a 4-year-old to draw a square, and a 5-year-old to draw a triangle. Older children usually can draw diamonds and more complicated figures. The Denver II is a helpful tool for assessing neurodevelopmental status in an infant or young child. The test assesses gross and fine motor skills, language skills, and social skills and compares the findings with other children the same age (Figure 19.5).

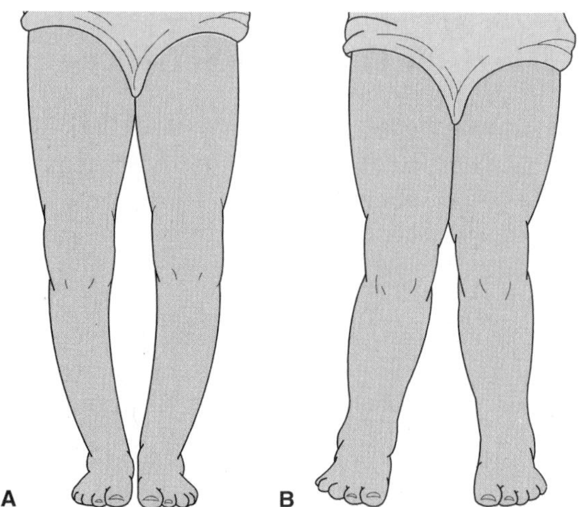

Figure 19.4 *A*, Genu varum. *B*, Genu valgum.

Gathering the Data

Focused Interview

Guidelines for Interviewing the Parent or Caregiver

When taking the history of an infant or young child, gather most of the data from the parent or other caregiver. Here are some guidelines for talking with the parent or other caregiver of an infant or young child:

- Always clarify the relationship to the child. For convenience through the remainder of this chapter, we use the

Text continues on page 591

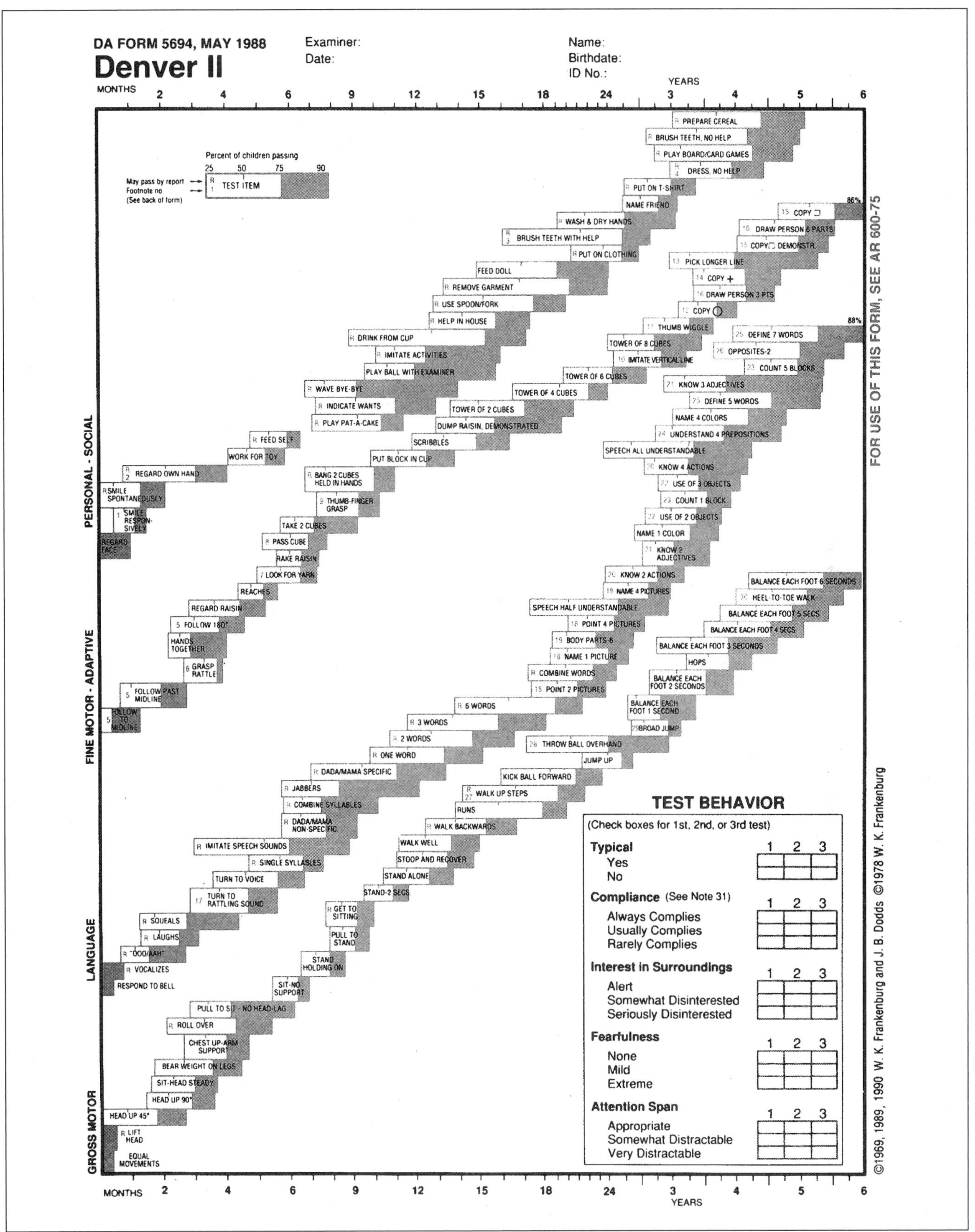

DA FORM 5694, MAY 1988

Denver II

Examiner:
Date:

Name:
Birthdate:
ID No.:

MONTHS 2 4 6 9 12 15 18 24 | YEARS 3 4 5 6

Percent of children passing 25 50 75 90
May pass by report → R
Footnote no → 1
(See back of form)
TEST ITEM

PERSONAL - SOCIAL

PREPARE CEREAL
BRUSH TEETH, NO HELP
PLAY BOARD/CARD GAMES
DRESS, NO HELP
PUT ON T-SHIRT
NAME FRIEND
WASH & DRY HANDS
BRUSH TEETH WITH HELP
PUT ON CLOTHING
FEED DOLL
REMOVE GARMENT
USE SPOON/FORK
HELP IN HOUSE
DRINK FROM CUP
IMITATE ACTIVITIES
PLAY BALL WITH EXAMINER
WAVE BYE-BYE
INDICATE WANTS
PLAY PAT-A-CAKE
FEED SELF
WORK FOR TOY
REGARD OWN HAND
SMILE SPONTANEOUSLY
SMILE RESPONSIVELY
REGARD FACE

FINE MOTOR - ADAPTIVE

COPY □ 86%
DRAW PERSON 6 PARTS
COPY □ DEMONSTR.
PICK LONGER LINE
COPY +
DRAW PERSON 3 PTS
COPY ○
THUMB WIGGLE
TOWER OF 8 CUBES
IMITATE VERTICAL LINE
TOWER OF 6 CUBES
TOWER OF 4 CUBES
TOWER OF 2 CUBES
DUMP RAISIN, DEMONSTRATED
SCRIBBLES
PUT BLOCK IN CUP
BANG 2 CUBES HELD IN HANDS
THUMB-FINGER GRASP
TAKE 2 CUBES
PASS CUBE
RAKE RAISIN
LOOK FOR YARN
REACHES
REGARD RAISIN
FOLLOW 180°
HANDS TOGETHER
GRASP RATTLE
FOLLOW PAST MIDLINE
FOLLOW TO MIDLINE

LANGUAGE

DEFINE 7 WORDS 88%
OPPOSITES-2
COUNT 5 BLOCKS
KNOW 3 ADJECTIVES
DEFINE 5 WORDS
NAME 4 COLORS
UNDERSTAND 4 PREPOSITIONS
SPEECH ALL UNDERSTANDABLE
KNOW 4 ACTIONS
USE OF 3 OBJECTS
COUNT 1 BLOCK
USE OF 2 OBJECTS
NAME 1 COLOR
KNOW 2 ADJECTIVES
KNOW 2 ACTIONS
NAME 4 PICTURES
SPEECH HALF UNDERSTANDABLE
POINT 4 PICTURES
BODY PARTS-6
NAME 1 PICTURE
COMBINE WORDS
POINT 2 PICTURES
6 WORDS
3 WORDS
2 WORDS
ONE WORD
DADA/MAMA SPECIFIC
JABBERS
COMBINE SYLLABLES
DADA/MAMA NON-SPECIFIC
IMITATE SPEECH SOUNDS
SINGLE SYLLABLES
TURN TO VOICE
TURN TO RATTLING SOUND
SQUEALS
LAUGHS
"OOO/AAH"
VOCALIZES
RESPOND TO BELL

GROSS MOTOR

BALANCE EACH FOOT 6 SECONDS
HEEL-TO-TOE WALK
BALANCE EACH FOOT 5 SECS
BALANCE EACH FOOT 4 SECS
BALANCE EACH FOOT 3 SECONDS
HOPS
BALANCE EACH FOOT 2 SECONDS
BALANCE EACH FOOT 1 SECOND
BROAD JUMP
THROW BALL OVERHAND
JUMP UP
KICK BALL FORWARD
WALK UP STEPS
RUNS
WALK BACKWARDS
WALK WELL
STOOP AND RECOVER
STAND ALONE
STAND-2 SECS
GET TO SITTING
PULL TO STAND
STAND HOLDING ON
SIT-NO SUPPORT
PULL TO SIT - NO HEAD-LAG
ROLL OVER
CHEST UP-ARM SUPPORT
BEAR WEIGHT ON LEGS
SIT-HEAD STEADY
HEAD UP 90°
HEAD UP 45°
LIFT HEAD
EQUAL MOVEMENTS

TEST BEHAVIOR

(Check boxes for 1st, 2nd, or 3rd test)

	1	2	3
Typical			
Yes			
No			
Compliance (See Note 31)			
Always Complies			
Usually Complies			
Rarely Complies			
Interest in Surroundings			
Alert			
Somewhat Disinterested			
Seriously Disinterested			
Fearfulness			
None			
Mild			
Extreme			
Attention Span			
Appropriate			
Somewhat Distractable			
Very Distractable			

MONTHS 2 4 6 9 12 15 18 24 | 3 4 5 6 YEARS

FOR USE OF THIS FORM, SEE AR 600-75

Figure 19.5 The Denver II is used to assess neurodevelopmental status in an infant or young child.

DIRECTIONS FOR ADMINISTRATION

1. Try to get child to smile by smiling, talking or waving. Do not touch him/her.
2. Child must stare at hand several seconds.
3. Parent may help guide toothbrush and put toothpaste on brush.
4. Child does not have to be able to tie shoes or button/zip in the back.
5. Move yarn slowly in an arc from one side to the other, about 8" above child's face.
6. Pass if child grasps rattle when it is touched to the backs or tips of fingers.
7. Pass if child tries to see where yarn went. Yarn should be dropped quickly from sight from tester's hand without arm movement.
8. Child must transfer cube from hand to hand without help of body, mouth, or table.
9. Pass if child picks up raisin with any part of thumb and finger.
10. Line can vary only 30 degrees or less from tester's line.
11. Make a fist with thumb pointing upward and wiggle only the thumb. Pass if child imitates and does not move any fingers other than the thumb.

12. Pass any enclosed form. Fail continuous round motions.

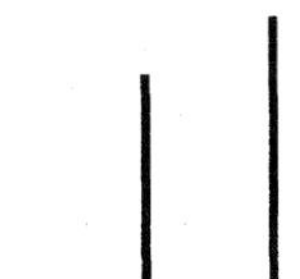

13. Which line is longer? (Not bigger.) Turn paper upside down and repeat. (pass 3 of 3 or 5 of 6)

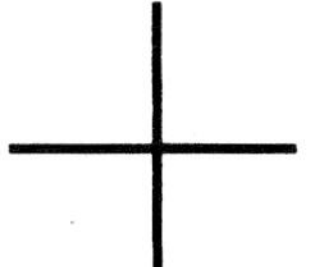

14. Pass any lines crossing near midpoint.

15. Have child copy first. If failed, demonstrate.

When giving items 12, 14, and 15, do not name the forms. Do not demonstrate 12 and 14.

16. When scoring, each pair (2 arms, 2 legs, etc.) counts as one part.
17. Place one cube in cup and shake gently near child's ear, but out of sight. Repeat for other ear.
18. Point to picture and have child name it. (No credit is given for sounds only.) If less than 4 pictures are named correctly, have child point to picture as each is named by tester.

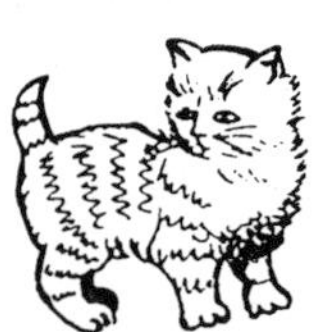
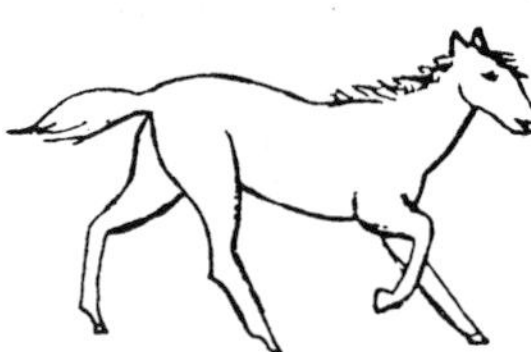
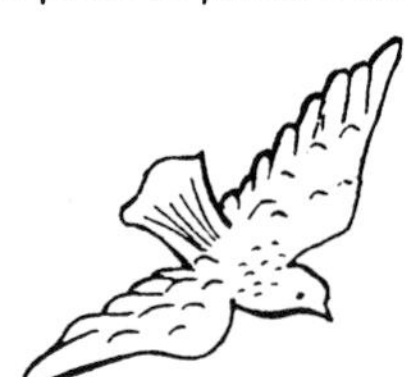
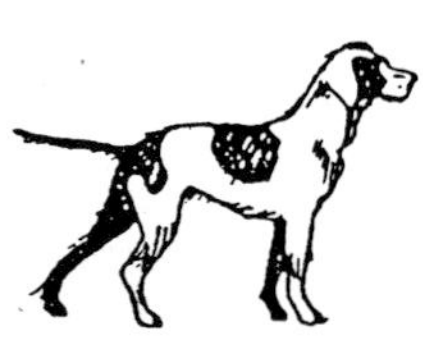
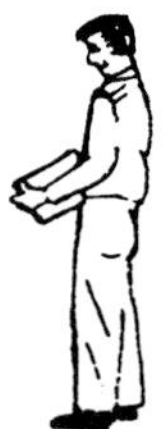

19. Using doll, tell child: Show me the nose, eyes, ears, mouth, hands, feet, tummy, hair. Pass 6 of 8.
20. Using pictures, ask child: Which one flies?... says meow?... talks?... barks?... gallops? Pass 2 of 5, 4 of 5.
21. Ask child: What do you do when you are cold?... tired?... hungry? Pass 2 of 3, 3 of 3.
22. Ask child: What do you do with a cup? What is a chair used for? What is a pencil used for? Action words must be included in answers.
23. Pass if child correctly places and says how many blocks are on paper. (1, 5).
24. Tell child: Put block **on** table; **under** table; **in front of** me, **behind** me. Pass 4 of 4. (Do not help child by pointing, moving head or eyes.)
25. Ask child: What is a ball?... lake?... desk?... house?... banana?... curtain?... fence?... ceiling? Pass if defined in terms of use, shape, what it is made of, or general category (such as banana is fruit, not just yellow). Pass 5 of 8, 7 of 8.
26. Ask child: If a horse is big, a mouse is __? If fire is hot, ice is __? If the sun shines during the day, the moon shines during the __? Pass 2 of 3.
27. Child may use wall or rail only, not person. May not crawl.
28. Child must throw ball overhand 3 feet to within arm's reach of tester.
29. Child must perform standing broad jump over width of test sheet (8 1/2 inches).
30. Tell child to walk forward, ⊂⊃⊂⊃⊂⊃⊂⊃→ heel within 1 inch of toe. Tester may demonstrate. Child must walk 4 consecutive steps.
31. In the second year, half of normal children are non-compliant.

OBSERVATIONS:

Figure 19.5 The Denver II, continued.

word *parent* to denote the person accompanying the child to the health care facility. Do not assume, however, that an adult accompanying a child is the child's parent. Often a child is brought to a clinic or hospital by a step-parent, a grandparent, an aunt or uncle, a nanny, a babysitter, or another caretaker. You need a complete understanding of the relationship between the adult and the child to conduct an accurate health assessment.

- Additionally, do not assume that the child's parents are married to each other. For example, when taking the family health history, you might ask the child's mother, "How old is Jennifer's father?" rather than, "How old is your husband?"
- Make the parents feel good about both themselves and the child by commenting favorably on aspects of the child's growth and abilities.
- Refer to the child by name rather than as "him," "her," or "the baby."
- Parents may interpret their child's illness as a failure on their part. Try to be supportive rather than judgmental. For instance, rather than asking a child's father, "Why didn't you bring Derek in sooner?" you might ask, "What treatments have you tried for Derek since he began vomiting last night?"
- If a child is crying or excessively fussy, you might try to distract the child with toys or encourage the parent to rock the child until he or she quiets down and you can continue the interview. When interviewing the parent of a child who is seriously ill, you might need to begin interventions before you are able to complete the entire health history.
- Finally, always use open-ended questions that encourage the parent to bring up other reasons for the visit and reveal all concerns. A parent who brings a child in for a "routine checkup" may not voice worries about the child's growth rate, appetite, bed-wetting, bad dreams, or a variety of other concerns. You may help the parent to open up by simply asking, "Is there anything else you'd like to talk about today?"

Guidelines for Interviewing a Child or Adolescent

From about the age of 5 years, a child will be able to respond meaningfully to questions about his or her health or illness independently of an adult. You may want to interview the older child alone, especially in cases when the child seems embarrassed, sullen, or confused, eg, because of bed-wetting, poor grades in school, eating disorders, substance abuse, sexually transmitted infections, or possible physical or sexual abuse.

Again, begin with open-ended questions, and be patient, especially with adolescent clients who may have difficulty confiding in adults. You may find that beginning the interview by chatting about the client's school, social life, hobbies, sports activities, or job might help to establish a trusting relationship.

When adolescents seek health care on their own, it is important (and in some states mandated by law) to respect their confidentiality. If the findings from the examination indicate that the parents should be notified of the adolescent's health status, follow state laws and institutional guidelines for parental notification, always including the adolescent in the notification process.

Respecting the Child's Individuality

Modify the focused interview for the pediatric client according to the age of the child, the reason for the visit, and whether or not the child has been seen previously in this setting. For instance, the 3-year-old child who comes to the clinic for a routine checkup and has been followed by the same health care team since birth has very different needs from the 16-year-old who has had no routine health care and comes alone to the emergency room because of difficulty breathing.

Base the interview of the child upon the same clusters of questions you use to take the health history of the adult. These include, for example, questions regarding the child's present problem or illness, if any; the child's past medical history, immunizations, and allergies; the family's health history; and a review of the child's body systems. For a discussion of these interview questions, see Chapter 2. In addition, the interview of the pediatric client might include some or all of the following questions.

Questions Related to the Birth History

1. Describe this pregnancy. *Make sure the mother reveals parity, problems, length of the pregnancy, diet, weight gain, and use of medications, street drugs, tobacco, and alcohol during pregnancy. Events during pregnancy can have long-term physical and psychosocial effects on the child.*
2. Describe your labor. *Encourage the mother to discuss the course and duration of labor, use of analgesia and anesthesia, any obstetric procedures, type of birth, birth weight, Apgar scores, and any medical problems. Events of the perinatal period can have long-term physical and psychosocial effects on the child.*
3. How was the postnatal period for you and your baby? *Encourage the mother to talk about problems in the nursery or after the baby was discharged, including feeding problems, colic, diarrhea, sleeping problems, postnatal depres-*

sion, and problems within the family. Events of the perinatal period can have long-term physical and psychosocial effects on the child.

4. *If the mother does not accompany the child, ask the father or other caretaker:* Describe the pregnancy and perinatal period as thoroughly as possible. *Try to gather data as indicated in the above questions.*

Questions Related to the Child's Growth and Development

1. At what age did the child first (a) hold the head erect? (b) roll over? (c) sit up independently? (d) walk alone? (e) say words with meaning? (f) speak in sentences? (g) tie shoes? (h) dress without help? At what age did the child's first tooth come in? At what age was the child toilet-trained? *The age at which children reach developmental milestones may be an indication of their overall health status.*
2. Do you believe that the child's development has been normal? If so, why? If not, why not? How do you think the child's development compares with that of siblings or other children of the same age? *The parent's or caretaker's response to this question may reveal concerns about the child's growth and development. It may also provide information about familial patterns of development.*

Questions Related to the Child's Psychosocial Health

1. Describe the child's typical day. *Responses to this question may provide significant information about the routine and structure, the environment, and the amount of stimulation or deprivation.*
2. *Ask the older child or adolescent:* Describe a typical school day. *Responses to this question may provide significant information about the child's sleep patterns, stress level, extracurricular activities, employment, self-care, personal goals, and family coping.*
3. *Ask the older child or adolescent:* How much alcohol do you consume each day? How many cigarettes do you smoke each day? Describe your typical daily diet. How much water do you drink each day? *Responses to these questions may reveal a self-care deficit, knowledge deficit, or other problem.*
4. *Ask the adolescent:* Describe your present level of sexual activity. *If the adolescent is sexually active, encourage the adolescent to discuss the number of sexual partners, the steadiness of the relationship, the type of contraception used, if any, and the protection taken again sexually transmitted infections. Whether or not the adolescent is sexually active or has been in the past, encourage the adolescent to discuss feelings and concerns about sexuality. Responses to these questions may reveal a self-care deficit, knowledge deficit, self-esteem disturbance, impaired social interaction, body-image disturbance, or other problem.*

Physical Assessment

Preparation

☑ **Gather the equipment:**

- examination gloves
- examination gown
- drape
- centimeter measuring tape
- ophthalmoscope
- otoscope with pneumatic bulb and ear pieces of various sizes
- stethoscope with diaphragm and bell
- sphygmomanometer and blood pressure cuff of appropriate size

☑ **Wash your hands.**

☑ **Before beginning the assessment, encourage the toilet-trained child to void. When examining infants, leave the diaper on except when weighing or examining the perineum.**

Remember

- You will use the techniques of inspection, palpation, percussion, and auscultation. In addition, you use the sense of smell to identify odors.
- Provide a warm, quiet environment with good lighting.
- Ensure the child's privacy.
- The presence of parents may provide comfort and reduce fear and anxiety, especially in infants and young children. Permit the child to remain on the parent's lap for as much of the examination as possible. Allow the preschool child to manipulate assessment equipment or to perform a simultaneous assessment on a stuffed animal or doll to decrease the child's fears and increase cooperation.
- Maintain eye contact. Smile and speak in a calm, friendly voice.
- Explain what you will do before each assessment step and discuss how the child or parent can help. Provide simple reasons why the child needs to lie down or assume a particular position. Reassure the child and parent that examinations are not painful and that you will respect the child's modesty.
- The most accurate assessment is obtained from a quiet child. Anxiety and crying alter vital signs, diminish the accuracy of lung and heart auscultation, and make abdominal palpation more difficult. If a child is crying, encourage the child to play with a doll or toy, or suggest that the parent rock or walk the child. Remember that an infant or toddler may cry because of hunger or a wet diaper.
- Approach the assessment systematically, varying the sequence of the examination according to the child's age and degree of cooperation. Begin the examination of infants and young children with the least threatening procedures. Postpone parts of the assessment that the child may perceive as threatening—such as laying the child down and examining the child's ears, mouth, and throat—until the end. You can examine older children and adolescents in a head-to-toe sequence.
- Integrate cultural knowledge and sensitivity into the examination. Before beginning the examination, determine any concerns the family may have and proceed in a manner that they will perceive as least offensive.
- Use gloves to examine mucous membranes and to assess skin lesions, wounds, or any areas with blood, drainage, or body fluids.

ASSESSMENT TECHNIQUE/NORMAL FINDINGS | SPECIAL CONSIDERATIONS

General Appearance and Mental Status

Step 1 *Observe physical appearance, body structure, mobility, and behavior.*

Obvious abnormalities, limitations of movement, inappropriate behavior for age, or poor hygiene may indicate the need for further investigation or parent and child education.

Step 2 *Observe the interaction between the child and parents.*

- Note how a parent is holding an infant. Does the parent seem to be reading the infant's cues? Are the parent's expectations appropriate for the age of the child?

A parent who holds an infant facing away, avoids eye contact with an infant, or is unable to read an infant's cues may lack attachment. Early intervention is imperative.

- Note whether the child looks to the parent for comfort and whether the parent provides support. Listen to how the parent and child relate to each other.

Expecting a young child to sit quietly indicates a knowledge deficit of normal child development.

An extremely negative or hostile interaction may indicate a disturbed parent-child relationship. Intervention and referral are required.

Step 3 *Listen to the child's speech.*

- Note articulation, quantity, and organization of the child's speech, as well as the child's thought processes. Does the older infant or toddler label objects and have names for significant others? Is the preschool child able to ask and answer questions? Are older children and adolescents able to contribute to the health history and answer age-appropriate questions?

Speech should be understandable by about 3 years of age. Speech delay or articulation problems may indicate a hearing deficit, a lack of environmental stimulation, a bilingual environment, or a generalized developmental delay.

An older child who is not able to express thoughts in an expected manner may have a hearing deficit, learning disability, or language problem related to a bilingual environment.

Growth and Development

Step 1 *Obtain accurate height and weight measurements (see Chapter 7 for technique).*

- Plot the measurements on an age- and gender-appropriate growth chart.

Figure 19.7 on page 596 provides growth charts for boys. Figure 19.8 on page 597 provides growth charts for girls. Measurements are evaluated in relation to each other and the child's age. Table 19.1 on page 598 provides average height and weight gain per year of life through puberty.

Both height and weight measurements should fall in approximately the same percentile. A single measurement is of limited value; serial measurements provide a more accurate assessment of rate of growth.

Great discrepancies between height and weight percentile require further evaluation. Low weight for height may indicate inadequate nutrition, cardiac problems, renal problems, or chronic systemic disease. High weight for height may indicate overnutrition or a metabolic problem.

ASSESSMENT TECHNIQUE/NORMAL FINDINGS

Step 2 ***Measure the head circumference of the child under 2 years of age.***

- Measure the head by placing the tape measure around the head just above the eyebrows and the ear pinna and around the most prominent area of the occiput (Figure 19.6).

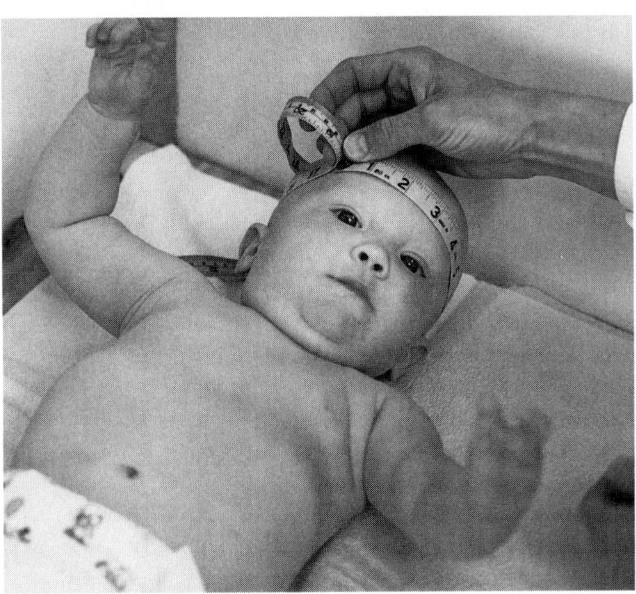

Figure 19.6 Measuring an infant's head circumference around the skull, above the eyebrows.

- Plot the measurement on an appropriate growth chart (see Figures 19.7 and 19.8 on pages 596 and 597).

Rapid growth of the skull and the structures it encases makes the head vulnerable to developmental abnormalities.

SPECIAL CONSIDERATIONS

A single head circumference measurement that falls above the 95th percentile or below the 5th percentile for the child's age requires further evaluation.

Infants born to mothers who used cocaine or alcohol during pregnancy may have smaller heads than expected for age. *Microcephaly*, a small head, may result in severe developmental delay because the brain is unable to grow normally. *Macrocephaly*, a large head, may be the result of rapid head growth due to a tumor or *hydrocephalus*, excessive cerebrospinal fluid within the skull.

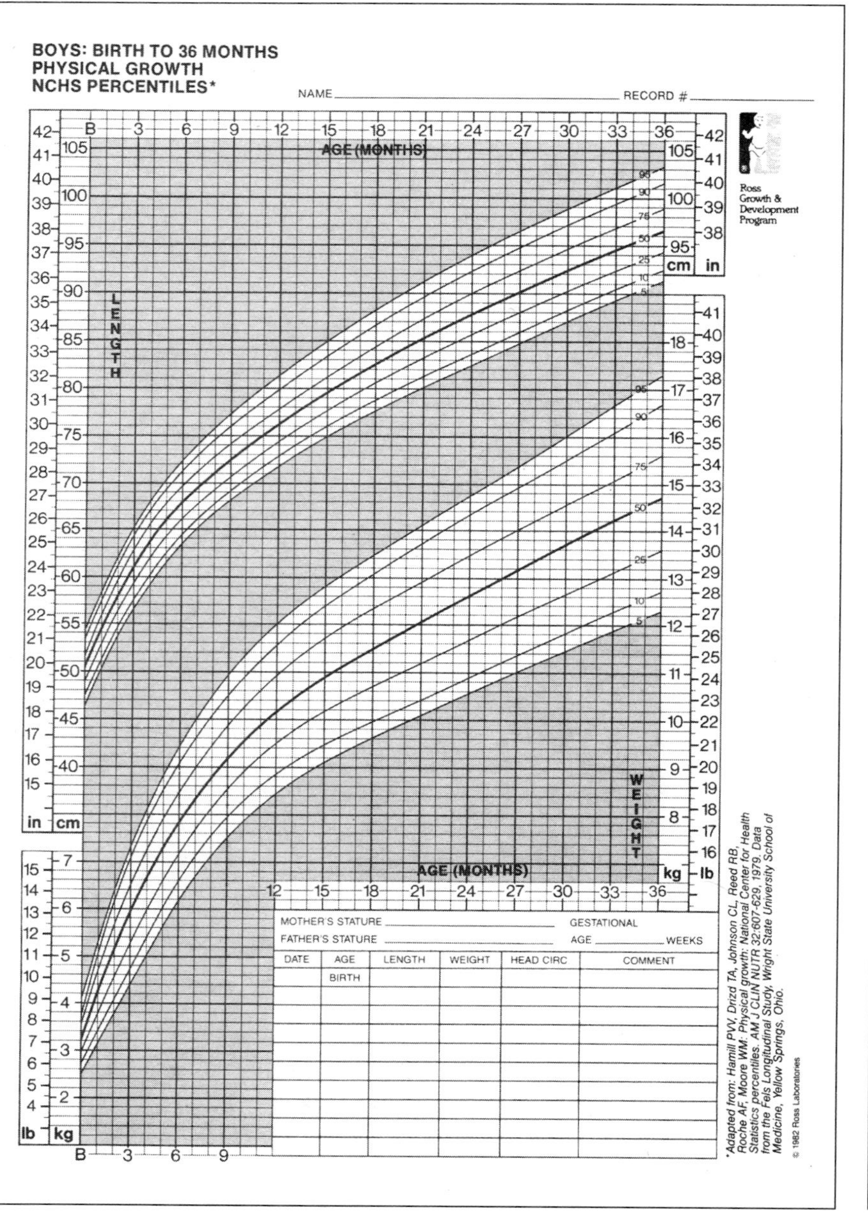

A

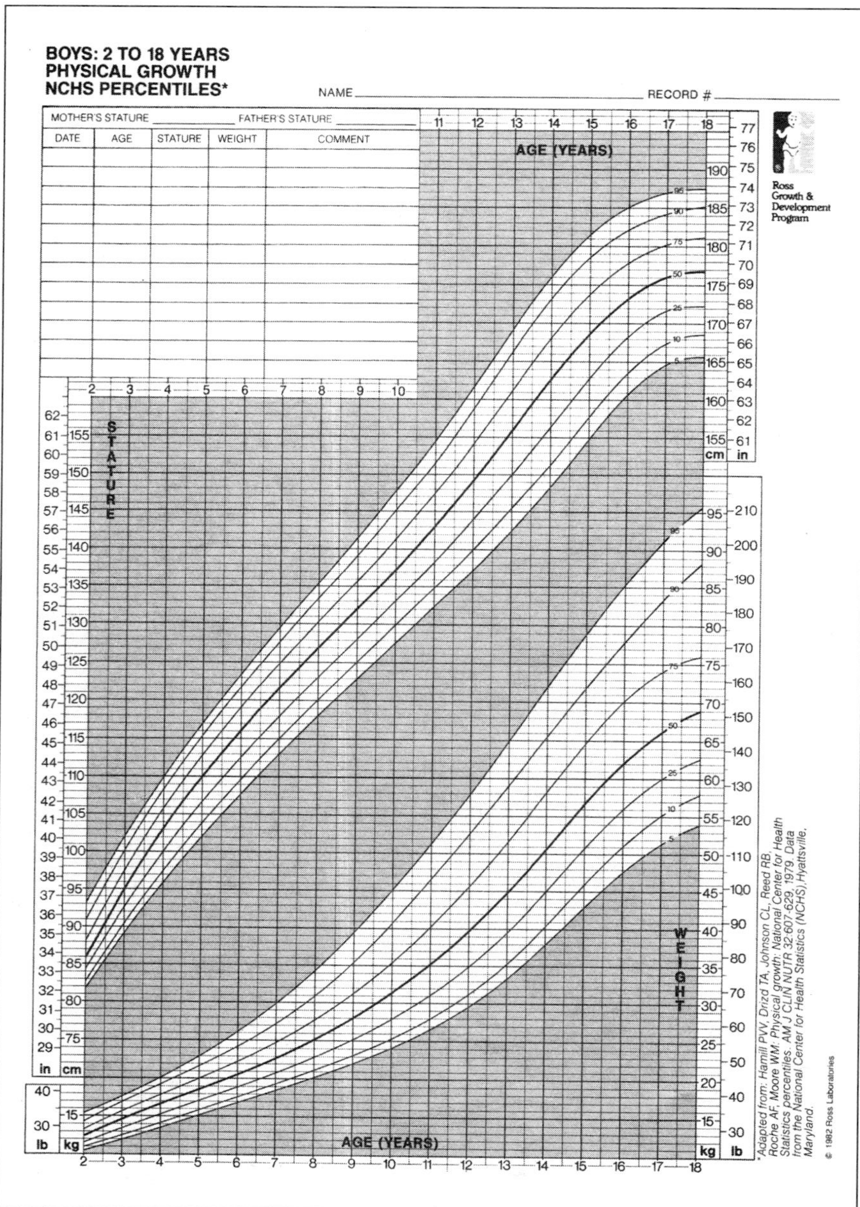

B

Figure 19.7 Growth charts for boys. *A,* National Center for Health Statistics (NCHS) percentiles for boys birth to 36 months, weight, length, and head circumference. *B,* NCHS percentiles for boys 2–18 years.

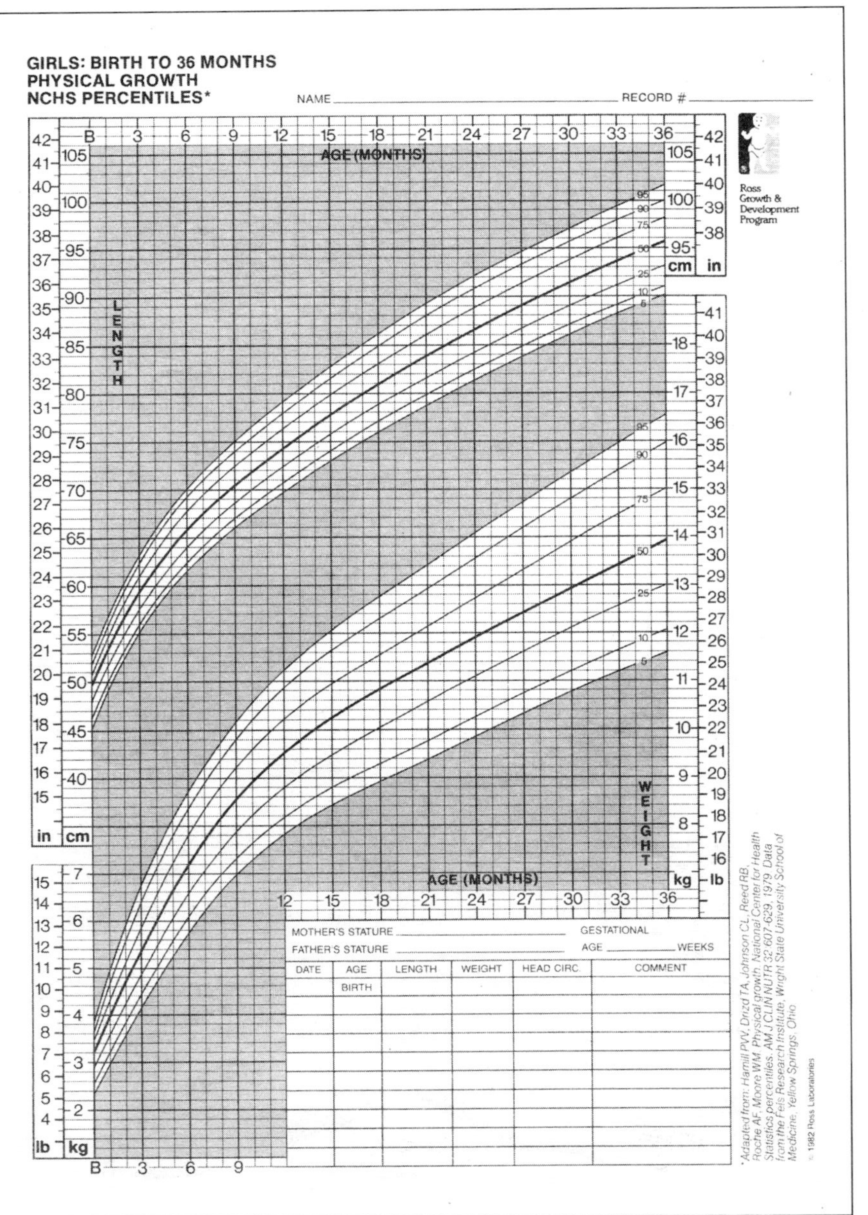

A

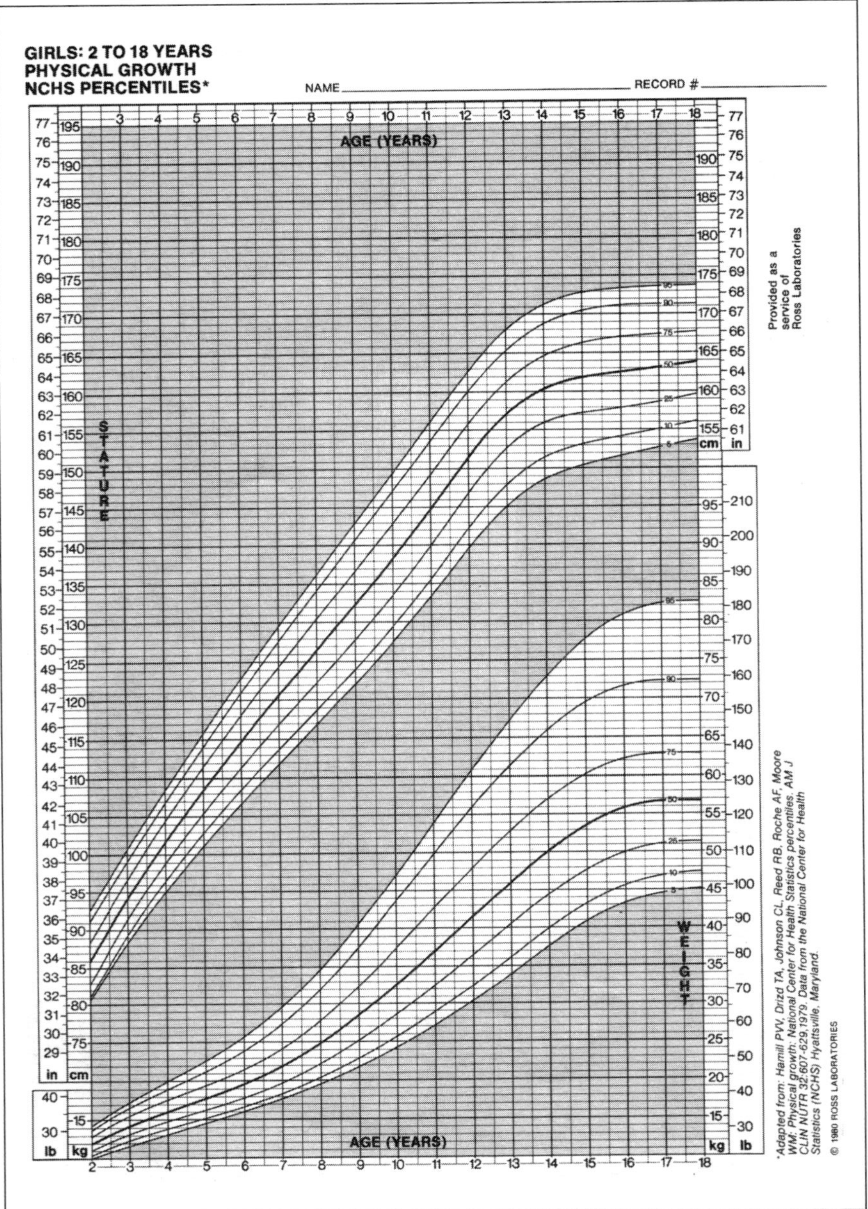

B

Figure 19.8 Growth charts for girls. *A*, NCHS percentiles for girls birth to 36 months; weight, length, and head circumference. *B*, NCHS percentiles for girls 2–18 years.

ASSESSMENT TECHNIQUE/NORMAL FINDINGS | SPECIAL CONSIDERATIONS

Table 19.1 Average Height and Weight Gain per Year of Life

Age	Linear growth per year	Weight gain per year
0–12 months	10 in (25 cm)	13–18 lb (6–8 kg)
13–24 months	5 in (12.5 cm)	5–8 lb (2.5 kg)
25–36 months	4 in (10 cm)	4–6 lb (2 kg)
37–48 months	3 in (8 cm)	3–5 lb (1–2 kg)
4 years to puberty	2.0–2.5 in (5.0–6.5 cm)	4–6 lb (2–3 kg)

Step 3 *Assess the child's developmental status.*

- For children under 6 years of age, use a standardized tool such as the Denver II (see Figure 19.5, earlier).
- For older children, assess development by discussing school progress, including specific questions about any grades repeated, report cards, achievement on standardized tests, and any special help the child receives in school.

Infants and children with suspected developmental delays or learning problems require referral for additional testing. Early identification and intervention promote a better outcome.

Skin, Hair, and Nails

Step 1 *Position the client.*

- Help the child into a comfortable sitting position on the examination table (Figure 19.9).

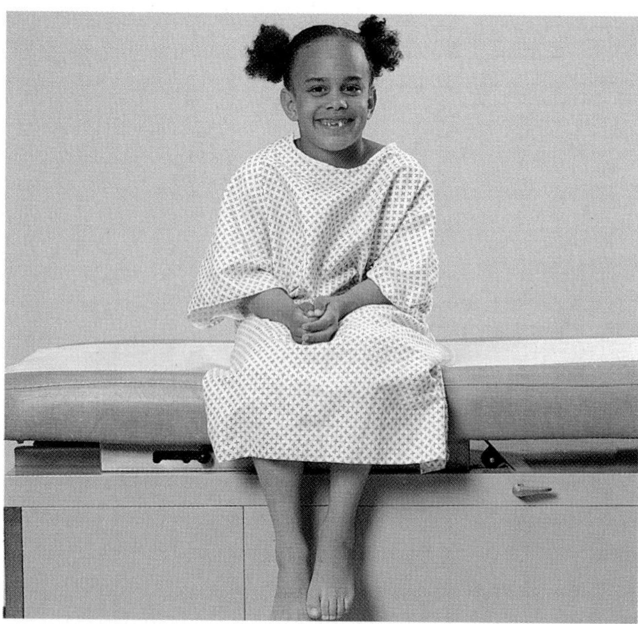

Figure 19.9 Positioning the child at the beginning of the assessment.

ASSESSMENT TECHNIQUE/NORMAL FINDINGS	SPECIAL CONSIDERATIONS

For infants and toddlers, you may ask the parent to hold the child while you perform many of the following techniques.

Step 2 ***Inspect and palpate the skin for general condition.***

- Note the texture, consistency, and temperature of the skin.
- Gently spread all creases to adequately assess the skin, especially in infants and obese children.

Peeling hands may be seen after scarlet fever or with *Kawasaki's disease*, a lymphatic disorder of unknown etiology.

Intertrigo, a bright pink, moist excoriation, is sometimes found in deep skin folds like those of the infant's neck and groin.

- Palpate the skin for dryness, firmness, turgor, and temperature.

The skin should be smooth, warm, and even.

Excessive dryness may be seen in children with eczema, after overexposure to the sun, or in nutritional deficiency.

Excessive moisture may be indicative of perspiration or shock. Poor skin turgor is indicative of dehydration.

Generalized hyperthermia may be seen in children with fever or sunburn. Localized hyperthermia may indicate local infection or a burn. Generalized hypothermia may indicate exposure to cold in an infant or shock in an older child. Localized hypothermia is sometimes a result of exposure to cold.

Step 3 ***Inspect the skin for color and pigmentation.***

- Confirm uniformity of color.

Generalized erythema may be seen in febrile children. Localized erythema may be seen with infection or sunburn.

Generalized pallor may be indicative of shock, circulatory failure, or chronic disease and requires evaluation.

- Inspect for cyanosis.

Circumoral cyanosis or slight peripheral cyanosis may normally be seen in infants during the first few weeks of life, especially if they are chilled. Striking cyanosis of the lower extremities may be seen in children with coarctation of the aorta. Cyanosis in older infants and children is indicative of inadequate oxygenation and requires immediate referral.

- Inspect for jaundice.

Natural daylight provides the best light for assessing jaundice. When jaundice is present or suspected, press gently on the tip of the nose and abdomen, blanching the skin. Observe for degree of jaundice, comparing the nose to the abdomen. Because jaundice progresses from the head down, in severe jaundice the abdomen will appear the same degree of yellow as the nose.

Yellowing of the skin and sclera is indicative of *jaundice*. Jaundice appearing in infants during the first 12 hours of life requires medical treatment. Physiologic jaundice appears about 24 hours after birth, disappears by the second week of life, and usually requires no treatment. Jaundice sometimes occurs in breast-fed infants after the third day of life, may continue for several weeks, and usually requires no treatment. Because jaundice

ASSESSMENT TECHNIQUE/NORMAL FINDINGS	SPECIAL CONSIDERATIONS

may indicate ABO incompatibility, sepsis, hepatitis, or bile duct obstruction, a medical evaluation is always warranted.

Yellow skin with clear sclera is indicative of *carotenemia*, a yellowing of the skin caused primarily by excessive intake of yellow vegetables, especially in older infants. Skin color returns to normal when intake of yellow vegetables is reduced.

Step 4 ***Inspect and palpate the skin for lesions.***

- Note the distribution, size, shape, color, and consistency of birthmarks and lesions.

Café-au-lait spots are flat, light brown patches on the skin. They may be an early indication of neurofibromatosis.

Mongolian spots are flat, blue patches found on infants or young children with dark skin pigmentation. Usually found on the buttocks or sacral area, these spots gradually fade. You need to learn to distinguish them from bruises.

Capillary hemangiomas appear as flat, pink lesions soon after birth, become raised and red during the first year, then gradually fade. They may be anywhere on the body.

Bruises may be seen on the anterior lower legs and are usually round or oval. Bruising on the face or trunk should be questioned as should any bruises that are linear or of an unusual shape or pattern, eg, suggestive of the use of a belt or stick. Bite marks, burns, and any other unusual skin lesions suggestive of assault should be thoroughly investigated.

Referral

With any of the above diagnostic cues, suspect child abuse. Obtain medical assistance and follow your state's legal requirements to notify the police or local protective agency.

Impetigo, a common skin infection, may be crusted or bullous; topical or systemic antibiotic treatment is required.

Vesicular lesions are seen with varicella (chicken pox), herpes simplex or poison ivy.

Petechiae are seen in severe systemic disease such as meningococcemia.

ASSESSMENT TECHNIQUE/NORMAL FINDINGS	SPECIAL CONSIDERATIONS

Step 5 *Inspect the scalp, hair, and nails.*

- Separate the hair to inspect the scalp.

Oily flakes on the scalp are indicative of seborrheic dermatitis (cradle cap).

- Note the distribution and texture of the hair on the head and body.

The hair should be clean and shiny, be generally the same color all over, and should cover the head. Infants may normally have areas of baldness on the back and sides of the head.

Most children do not have pubic or axillary hair before puberty, but they may have fine body hair.

Areas of baldness in older infants and children may be the result of local infection, tinea capitis (ringworm), traction from pulling hair into braids, or hair pulling (self-inflicted or child abuse).

Small white spots adhering to the hair shaft are indicative of pediculosis (head lice). Unlike dandruff, pediculosis nits adhere to the hair.

Pubic hair in a young child is an indication for referral.

Tufts of hair along the spinal column may be indicative of a spinal abnormality.

- Inspect the nails for color, shape, and condition. Nails should be convex with the ends covering the edges of the fingers.

Paronychia, an infection around the nail, sometimes occurs in children who bite their nails. An ingrown toenail may precipitate sepsis in an infant.

Head, Face, and Neck

Step 1 *Inspect and palpate the head.*

- Observe the head shape from all directions.

Premature infants often have long, narrow heads throughout infancy. A flat area of the head may result from an infant lying in one position or from *craniosynostosis*, premature closure of a cranial suture. Referral is indicated.

- Palpate the head, noting any irregularities such as masses or prominent ridges (Figure 19.10).

In the first few days of life some infants have *caput succedaneum*, a large, edematous mass of the scalp resulting from birth trauma. The mass generally crosses the suture line and lasts only a few days.

Cephalhematoma, also the result of birth trauma, appears similar to caput succedaneum but is the result of subperiosteal hemorrhage. It is normally restricted to one bone and takes several weeks or longer to resorb.

ASSESSMENT TECHNIQUE/NORMAL FINDINGS	SPECIAL CONSIDERATIONS

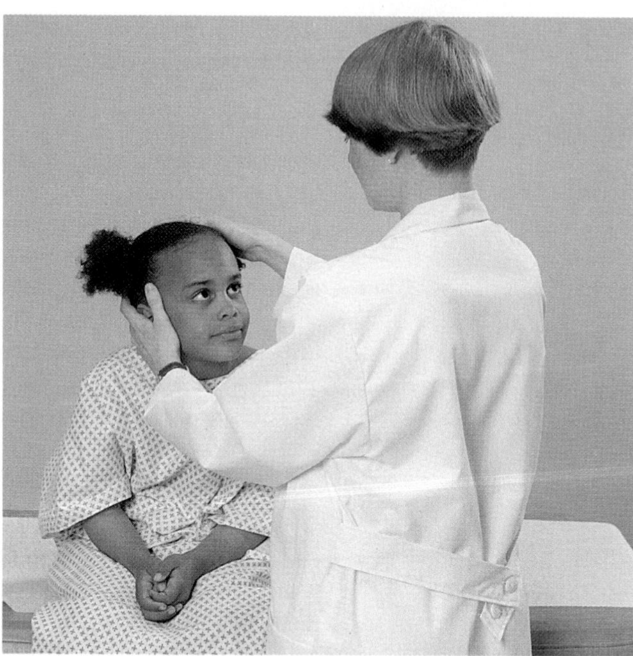

Figure 19.10 Palpating the child's head.

- Attempt to palpate the lymph nodes in the occipital region.

Palpable occipital lymph nodes indicate an inflammation or lesion of the scalp. The scalp should be reexamined to investigate the source of the problem.

- In infants, palpate the anterior and posterior fontanelles with the infant quiet and in a sitting position.

Bulging of the anterior fontanelle is indicative of increased intracranial pressure and requires further evaluation. A depressed fontanelle is indicative of dehydration.

- Note the size of the fontanelles.

A fontanelle may normally feel full in a crying infant or when the infant is lying down.

Large fontanelles with separated suture lines may be indicative of hydrocephalus. A small fontanelle may indicate abnormal head growth.

Step 2 ***Assess head control and position.***

- Observe head control for strength, steadiness, and position.

The head should be held straight and have full range of motion.

Poor head control after the age of 3–4 months may indicate developmental delay, neurologic problems, or muscle weakness.

Tremor may indicate a neurologic problem. Head tilt may indicate a hearing or vision deficit, or a muscle contracture.

- Carefully move the head in all directions to determine range of motion.

Resistance to flexion may indicate meningeal irritation.

ASSESSMENT TECHNIQUE/NORMAL FINDINGS	SPECIAL CONSIDERATIONS

Step 3 *Assess facial features.*

- Look at the facial features as a whole, individually, and in relation to each other.

Lowset ears may be associated with mental retardation or renal abnormalities.

- Compare one side to the other for symmetry.

An asymmetric smile or frown may indicate muscle weakness or nerve damage. Facial palsy may give the appearance of a flattened face.

Eyes should be level and the same size, nostrils should be the same size, the lips symmetric, and the ears set at the same level on both sides. Slight asymmetry may be normal.

Normally you can describe an imaginary line across the top of the pinna of the ears from the lateral corner of the eye to the most prominent protuberance of the occiput.

Step 4 *Assess the neck.*

- To inspect the neck of an infant, place the infant first in a supine position and then in a prone position. The toddler or older child remains sitting upright.

Retracting in the suprasternal area at the upper edge of the sternum may indicate respiratory distress.

- Observe for symmetry, size, shape, and pulsations.
- Palpate the neck to locate the trachea and thyroid.

Lung problems may cause the trachea to shift from the midline.

The thyroid may not be palpable in infants, but in older children the gland is normally a firm, smooth mass that moves up with swallowing. The thyroid often enlarges with the onset of puberty. However, an enlarged or nodular thyroid may indicate disease and requires evaluation.

- Palpate the lymph nodes using both hands and compare the findings.
- Note the location, size, mobility, consistency, and tenderness of palpable cervical lymph nodes.

Enlarged or tender nodes require further examination of the area drained by the nodes.

Cervical lymph nodes up to 1 cm in diameter that are discrete, movable, and nontender are normal in children up to 12 years of age.

Eyes and Vision

Step 1 *Inspect the external eyes.*

- Observe the eyes together, in relation to each other, and separately.
- Note size and placement.

Wide-set or closely set eyes may be a clue to a congenital disorder. Eyes slanting upward are seen in children with Down syndrome.

- Inspect the lids for movement, shape, and condition.

Ptosis, drooping of the lid, may be congenital or indicative of nerve damage. It may obstruct vision. Red, crusted, scaly lid edges may be seen in children with seborrhea. Eyes may become irritated.

ASSESSMENT TECHNIQUE/NORMAL FINDINGS	SPECIAL CONSIDERATIONS
◆ Note the color and character of any discharge. ◆ Inspect the eyebrows and lashes for distribution and condition.	Unilateral clear tearing in a young infant is indicative of a blocked lacrimal duct. Continuous tearing or a discharge may indicate infection, allergy, or a blocked lacrimal duct.
Step 2 ***Inspect the sclera for color, hemorrhage, or lesions.***	The sclera of newborns may appear slightly blue. Jaundice causes yellow-tinged sclera. Scleral hemorrhages may occur with birth trauma, severe vomiting, or severe coughing. They resolve spontaneously.
Step 3 ***Assess extraocular movements.***	
• Have the child watch a toy as you move it through the six cardinal directions of gaze (see Chapter 9).	Inability to move the eye fully through all fields of gaze indicates paralysis of an extraocular muscle. Referral is indicated. A few beats of nystagmus, a tremorlike movement, may normally occur when the child gazes at the outer limits of visual fields. Continuous nystagmus is abnormal.
◆ Shine a light into the eyes and observe for the reflection in exactly the same spot on each pupil.	Strabismus is present if the light reflection on the pupil is not in exactly the same spot on each pupil. Transient strabismus, an imbalance of the extraocular muscles, may be normal in infants under 6 months of age. Consistent strabismus or strabismus that persists after 6 months of age is abnormal and requires referral. *Amblyopia*, loss of vision in one eye, occurs when strabismus is not corrected during the first few years of life.
◆ Perform the cover-uncover test (see Chapter 9).	Any movement of the eye when it is uncovered indicates strabismus.
Step 4 ***Assess the internal eye structures.***	
◆ Inspect the iris for irregularities.	
◆ Observe the pupils for size, equality, and direct and consensual reaction to light.	Unequal pupils or failure of the pupils to react to light may be indicative of a central nervous system abnormality.
◆ Hold the ophthalmoscope, set at +8 to +10, about 12 inches from the child and look for the red reflex and any opacities.	Absence of a red reflex is abnormal. Opacities are indicative of cataracts or other serious conditions.
Step 5 ***Assess vision.***	Unidentified visual problems can interfere with an infant's or child's ability to respond, leading to developmental delay.

ASSESSMENT TECHNIQUE/NORMAL FINDINGS	SPECIAL CONSIDERATIONS
◆ Evaluate the vision of an infant by having the infant fixate on and follow a bright toy or face.	An infant who does not follow the toy or face should be referred for a full ophthalmologic examination.
◆ In children over 3 or 4 years of age, you can use a standard vision test such as Snellen E to evaluate vision.	A difference in visual acuity between eyes requires referral. Visual acuity of 20/40 or less in children 4 years and older requires referral.

Ears and Hearing

Step 1 ***Inspect the outer ear for structure, placement, and position.***

- Note any difference in structure of the ears.

Normally the ears are vertically placed, with the top of the auricle falling on an imaginary line drawn from the lateral eye to the occipital prominence.

Low-set ears may be associated with congenital anomalies.

Protruding ears may indicate swelling behind the ear or congenital lop-ears.

- Palpate the outer ear for consistency (Figure 19.11).

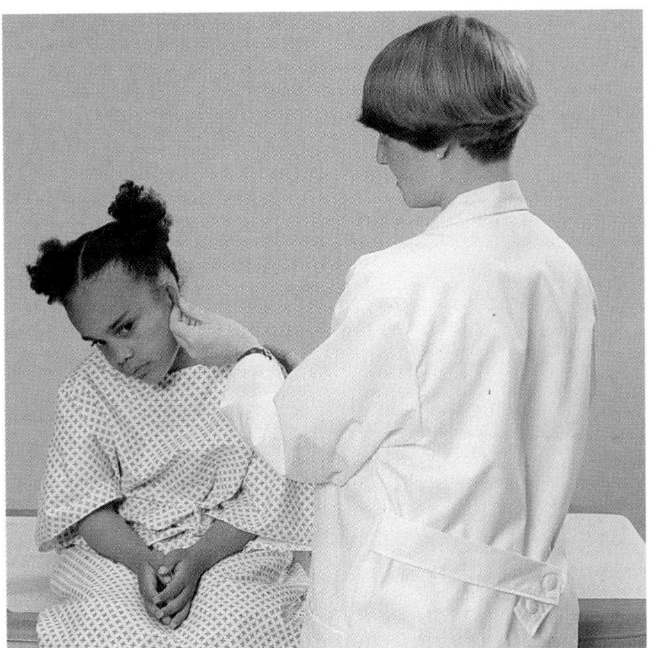

Figure 19.11 Palpating the outer ear.

Ears should feel like firm cartilage. Newborns' ears may be flat against the head and feel like thin tissue.

- Inspect the opening to the ear canal for wax or discharge; note the color, consistency, and amount.

A brownish wax discharge is normal.

A purulent, foul-smelling discharge is indicative of ear infection with perforation of the tympanic membrane or infection of the ear canal.

ASSESSMENT TECHNIQUE/NORMAL FINDINGS	SPECIAL CONSIDERATIONS

Step 2 ***Inspect the ear canal and tympanic membrane using an otoscope.***

- Hold the otoscope underhand, or as a pencil.
- Keep the lateral hand and little finger in constant contact with the child's head. If the child's head moves, the otoscope moves with it, avoiding injury to the ear canal.
- Attach a pneumatic bulb (insufflator) to the otoscope.
- Use a speculum of the appropriate size. Select one that will easily enter the canal but form a seal when inserted ¼ to ½ inch.
- Straighten the ear canal by pulling the pinna gently down and out for children younger than 3 years (see Figure 19.1), and up and back in older children.
- Place the hand holding the otoscope in contact with the child's head before beginning to insert the speculum.
- Slowly insert the speculum into the canal and inspect the canal for foreign bodies, lesions, edema, discharge, and cerumen.

Erythema and edema of the ear canal are seen in otitis externa or swimmer's ear.

- Inspect the tympanic membrane.

The tympanic membrane is normally pearly gray but may be erythematous in a crying or febrile child.

A red, bulging tympanic membrane with diffuse light reflex usually signals acute otitis media. Lesions or bubbles on the surface of the tympanic membrane indicate possible trauma or myringitis. A visible fluid level or bubbles behind the tympanic membrane are indicative of serous otitis media. See Chapter 9.

- Assess mobility of the tympanic membrane by depressing the pneumatic bulb.

Normally the tympanic membrane "flaps" or moves well.

Decreased or absent movement of the tympanic membrane indicates fluid or pus behind the membrane.

Step 3 ***Assess hearing.***

- Observe if infant or toddler turns toward the direction of a bell or clapping hands that are out of the visual field.
- Test children 4 years and older with an audiometer.

Hearing disorders may cause delays in language, speech, and social development. Parental concern or suspicion about an infant's hearing is sufficient reason for a full hearing evaluation.

ASSESSMENT TECHNIQUE/NORMAL FINDINGS | SPECIAL CONSIDERATIONS

Nose and Sinuses

Step 1 *Inspect the nose for shape, placement, symmetry, and proportion to other facial features.*

The nose should be straight and placed in the midline.

- Note any unusual shape, deformity, asymmetry of the nose and nares, and inflammation or lesions.
- Note any nasal flaring in infants.

Nasal flaring is an indication of increased respiratory effort and distress in infants. Because infants are obligatory nose breathers up to the age of about 3 months, they are predisposed to compromise of the upper airway.

- Note the amount, color, smell, and consistency of any discharge.

Unilateral discharge, often with a foul smell and sometimes with unilateral swelling, is indicative of a foreign body in the nose. A thin, watery discharge may indicate an upper respiratory infection or allergic rhinitis. A thick, yellow-green or green discharge is associated with infection. A clear nasal discharge following a head injury may be cerebrospinal fluid.

Step 2 *Palpate the nose for irregularities and tenderness.*

- In infants, press each naris closed to evaluate patency.

Smell is not usually evaluated during a routine examination.

Step 3 *Inspect the inner nose.*

Use an otoscope with a short, broad speculum.

- Lift the nose slightly by placing mild pressure on the tip.
- Gently insert the speculum into the rim of the naris.
- Note the color and condition of the mucous membrane and turbinates as well as any foreign body.
- Observe the septum for deviation to one side, perforation, lesions, or areas of bleeding.

Bright red, edematous turbinates are seen in infection. Pale, boggy, gray turbinates are indicative of allergy.

The nasal turbinates are normally pink and moist.

Step 4 *Assess the sinuses.*

- Because the sinuses are poorly developed in infancy, evaluate nasal discharge as a possible indication of infection.

Purulent nasal discharge is indicative of sinus infection.

- In older children, inspect the areas over the frontal and maxillary sinuses for swelling.

Swelling or pain over a sinus area is indicative of sinus infection.

ASSESSMENT TECHNIQUE/NORMAL FINDINGS	SPECIAL CONSIDERATIONS

- Evaluate the frontal sinuses by pressing with thumbs below the eyebrows.
- Evaluate the maxillary sinuses by pressing below the cheekbones.

Mouth and Throat

Step 1 ***Inspect the mouth.***

- Proceed from outside to inside observing color, symmetry, moisture, and condition of the lips.
- Note any dryness, swelling, sores, fissures, or cyanosis.
- Using a tongue depressor, gently retract the lips and cheeks away from the gums and observe every surface of the mucous membrane.

Normally the mucous membrane is pink, firm, smooth, moist, and free of lesions.

The mucous membranes are dry and tacky in dehydration. White, ulcerated sores may be the result of trauma (eg, from a toothbrush hitting the side of the mouth, or from forced feeding) or viral infection. White, curdy patches that are not easily scraped off are indicative of thrush, a monilial yeast infection of the mouth, common in young infants. It may also be seen in older children with immune deficiency.

- Observe the tongue for color, surface characteristics, movement, and size.
- Look under the tongue to inspect the frenulum and note any lesions.

A protruding tongue is seen in children with Down syndrome or cerebral palsy. A red tongue with prominent papilla (strawberry tongue) is sometimes seen in children with scarlet fever.

- Have older children stick their tongues out to note any deviation or tremor (Figure 19.12).

Deviation or tremor of the tongue is indicative of nerve damage.

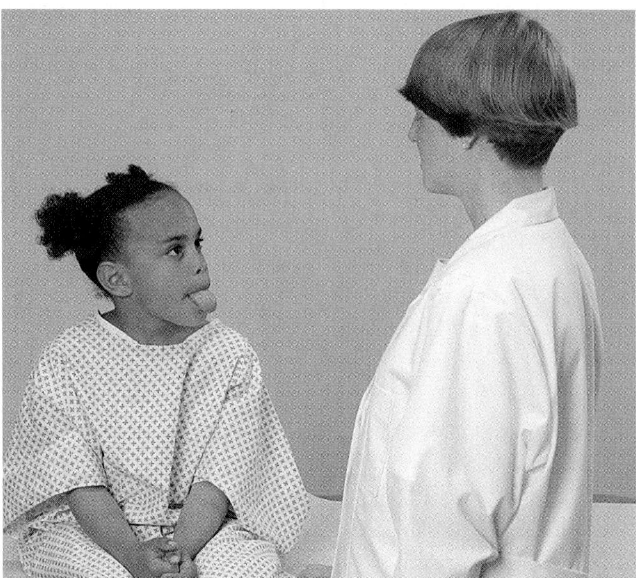

Figure 19.12 Inspecting the tongue.

ASSESSMENT TECHNIQUE/NORMAL FINDINGS	SPECIAL CONSIDERATIONS
◆ Observe the gums and teeth for color, condition, and hygiene.	Red, swollen, bleeding gums may indicate poor oral hygiene, poor nutrition, or infection. Caries of the central and lateral incisors usually indicate prolonged bottle feeding. A temporary gray discoloration of the teeth may be seen in children taking liquid iron.

Step 2 *Inspect the hard and soft palates and uvula.*

The hard palate should appear intact with a mild arch.

The soft palate and uvula should rise with crying or when the child says "ahh."

A high, arched palate may interfere with sucking.

A thin membrane in the midline of the palate may indicate an underlying cleft.

Deviation or lack of movement of the soft palate or uvula is indicative of nerve damage.

Petechiae may be seen on the soft palate of a child with strep throat.

A bifid or split uvula may indicate a submucosal cleft of the palate and requires further evaluation.

Step 3 *Inspect the tonsils and posterior pharynx.*

Do not use a tongue depressor in cooperative children, because many children become upset and uncooperative at the sight of a tongue depressor. In uncooperative children, you may try demonstrating the technique on the parent or a doll, or postponing the assessment until a later time.

Never use a tongue depressor on a child suspected of having epiglottitis, because the depressor may cause total laryngeal obstruction.

- Gently depress the tongue and inspect the tonsils and posterior pharynx.
- Assess the tonsils for size, position, and condition.

Tonsils are usually not visible in newborns, but they are quite large in preschool and school-aged children. They recede at about the age of 12 years.

Normal tonsils may have crypts that look like linear pits. The crypts may trap white debris.

Do not confuse this debris with the exudate associated with infection and found on the tonsillar surface.

- Observe the posterior pharyngeal wall for postnasal discharge.

Postnasal discharge from the sinuses may be seen along the posterior pharyngeal wall in children with sinus infections.

Chest and Lungs

Step 1 *Inspect the entire chest.*

- Proceed from neck to abdomen, front to back, including the sides and under the arms.
- Note the shape, movement, symmetry, and abnormalities.

Protuberance of the sternum indicates *pectus carinatum* (pigeon chest). When severe, it may compromise lung expansion.

Depression of the sternum indicates *pectus excavatum* (funnel chest), which may compromise lung expansion if severe.

ASSESSMENT TECHNIQUE/NORMAL FINDINGS	SPECIAL CONSIDERATIONS

The thoracic cage of a newborn is nearly round. It gradually grows in transverse diameter to achieve the elliptic adult shape at about 6 years of age. The infant's thoracic cage is relatively soft, allowing it to pull in during labored breathing.

Asymmetry of the chest may indicate a pneumothorax.

- Note the shape, color, and placement of nipples.

Supernumerary nipples occasionally occur along the milk line and are considered normal.

- Note the respiratory depth, rate, and effort.

In infants and children younger than 6 or 7 years, respirations are primarily diaphragmatic or abdominal. Breathing is less regular during infancy than in later childhood.

Rapid respirations are seen in infants and children with fever and respiratory or general illness.

Retracting, a "pulling in" during inspiration, may be supraclavicular, suprasternal, substernal, or intercostal; it is seen in children with increased respiratory effort. A prolonged expiratory phase is seen in obstructive respiratory problems such as asthma.

Step 2 ***Palpate the chest to evaluate chest expansion, swelling, pain, and respiratory vibration.***

- To evaluate expansion, place a palm with fingers spread on each side of the chest.

Asymmetric expansion indicates unilateral lung abnormality.

Chest expansion is normally symmetric.

- Palpate the nipple area for breast tissue, noting the size in relation to the age of the child.
- Evaluate breasts in girls by Tanner staging (see Figure 19.3), and perform a full breast examination.

Both male and female infants often have some breast tissue because of maternal hormonal influences.

Normal breast development may begin as early as 8 or 9 years of age and is most often unilateral.

Breast tissue in young children may indicate precocious puberty. *Gynecomastia*, breast tissue in a pubertal boy, is usually unilateral and temporary, although you need to consider evaluation for hormonal imbalance.

- Palpate fremitus by having the child repeat "ninety-nine" while palpating all areas of the chest.

In palpating fremitus, you feel vibrations of equal intensity on corresponding areas of each side of the chest.

The intensity of the fremitus diminishes over areas of lung collapse or pleural effusion. The fremitus intensifies over areas of consolidation.

Step 3 ***Percuss the chest.***

- Move symmetrically and systematically, comparing one side with the other.
- Assess the front, sides, and back of the chest using indirect percussion over the intercostal spaces.

Resonance is normally heard over the lung surfaces. Dullness is heard normally over the heart and liver.

Dullness heard over the lungs is abnormal and may indicate fluid or a mass.

ASSESSMENT TECHNIQUE/NORMAL FINDINGS

SPECIAL CONSIDERATIONS

Step 4 *Auscultate the lungs.*

- Listen first with the unaided ear for any sounds associated with breathing.
- Next listen with the diaphragm of the stethoscope (Figure 19.13).

Grunting respirations in an infant indicate respiratory distress.

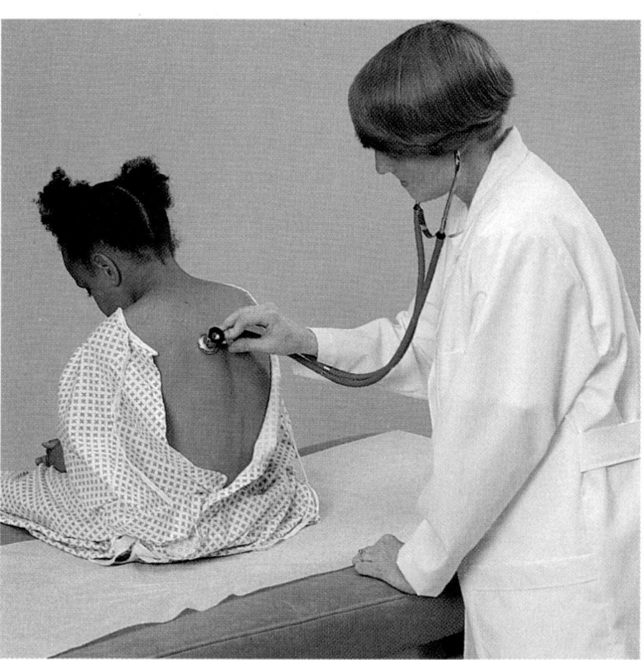

Figure 19.13 Auscultating the lungs.

Auscultation with the stethoscope should be systematic, symmetric, and proceed from apex to base (top to bottom). Listen in a specific spot on one side then in the same spot on the other side.

Transmitted upper airway sounds from mucus in the nose or throat may be confused with adventitious sounds. You can differentiate upper airway sounds by holding the stethoscope near the nose and mouth and listening for the sounds.

- Compare air exchange, character of breath sounds, and adventitious sounds, and evaluate the character of any coughing.

Because infants and children have thin chest walls, their breath sounds are louder and harsher than those of adults. Breath sounds are generally vesicular throughout the lung field.

Rales are heard in children with pneumonia or congestive heart failure. Rhonchi and wheezes that clear with coughing are indicative of bronchiolitis.

Scattered expiratory wheezing is heard in children with asthma, although the absence of wheezing in an asthmatic child may indicate that the child has considerably diminished air exchange and is in distress. Unilateral wheezing, usually on the right side, is indicative of foreign body aspiration. The right bronchus is shorter, wider, and angled less sharply than the left, allowing easier entry of foreign bodies.

ASSESSMENT TECHNIQUE/NORMAL FINDINGS | SPECIAL CONSIDERATIONS

Cardiovascular System

Step 1 *Measure blood pressure.*

Generally, you measure blood pressure on all children 3 years of age and older (see Chapter 7). A blood pressure may be required on a younger child who is ill.

- Ensure that the cuff covers ½ to ⅔ of the upper arm for an accurate reading. The thigh may be used if trauma or the presence of an IV line prevents the use of the arms.

Table 19.2 lists normal blood pressures for various ages.

Step 2 *Inspect the chest for visible pulsation.*

- Note the location of any pulsations.
- Note any obvious bulge or heave.

The apical impulse is often visible in children with thin chest walls.

A precordial bulge to the left of the sternum signals cardiac enlargement.

Step 3 *Palpate the pulses in all extremities for rate, rhythm, and strength.*

Normal heart rates vary with the age of the child (Table 19.3). Pulses should be strong and equal throughout the child's body.

Absent or diminished femoral pulses suggest coarctation of the aorta.

- Palpate the chest gently with the fingers to locate the apical impulse or point of maximal impulse (PMI).

With cardiac enlargement, the PMI moves laterally.

The PMI in children younger than 4 years is normally felt in the fourth intercostal space just to the left of the midclavicular line.

Table 19.2 Normal Blood Pressure for Various Ages (mm Hg)

Age	Systolic	2 SD	Diastolic	2 SD
1 day	78	14	42	14
1 mo	86	20	54	18
6 mo	90	26	60	20
1 yr	96	30	65	25
2 yr	99	25	65	25
4 yr	99	20	65	20
6 yr	100	15	60	10
8 yr	105	15	60	10
10 yr	110	17	60	10
12 yr	115	19	60	10
14 yr	118	20	60	10
16 yr	120	16	65	10

NOTE: The figures under 1 year were obtained by the Doppler method. From 1 year on, the figures were obtained by auscultation, using the first change in sound to indicate diastolic pressure.

SOURCE: Lowrey GH: *Growth and Development of Children*. 7th ed. Year Book, 1978, p. 450.

ASSESSMENT TECHNIQUE/NORMAL FINDINGS | SPECIAL CONSIDERATIONS

Table 19.3 Average Heart Rate for Children at Rest

Age	Average rate	2 SD
Birth	140	50
1st mo	130	45
1–6 mo	130	45
6–12 mo	115	40
1–2 yr	110	40
2–4 yr	105	35
5–10 yr	95	30
10–14 yr	85	30
14–18 yr	82	25

Source: Lowrey GH: *Growth and Development of Children.* 7th ed. Year Book, 1978, p. 228.

The PMI gradually changes location with growth. It is found in the fourth intercostal space at the midclavicular line between 4 and 6 years, and in the fifth intercostal space at the midclavicular line by about 7 years.

- Palpate the chest with the ulnar surface of the hand feeling for thrills, and note the location and timing.

A thrill indicates organic heart disease.

Step 4 *Percuss or use the "scratch" method to determine cardiac borders.*

Enlargement of the heart indicates cardiac disease.

- For the scratch method, place the stethoscope over the heart and scratch longitudinally with a finger beginning in the axillary line and moving toward the heart in 1 cm increments. When you scratch over the heart, you will hear a change in the intensity of the scratch sound through the stethoscope.

Step 5 *Auscultate the heart.*

- Begin with the diaphragm of the stethoscope, then use the bell.
- Begin with the child sitting upright, then lying supine.
- Proceed systematically: inch the stethoscope along from one listening area to the next (Figure 19.14).

ASSESSMENT TECHNIQUE/NORMAL FINDINGS | SPECIAL CONSIDERATIONS

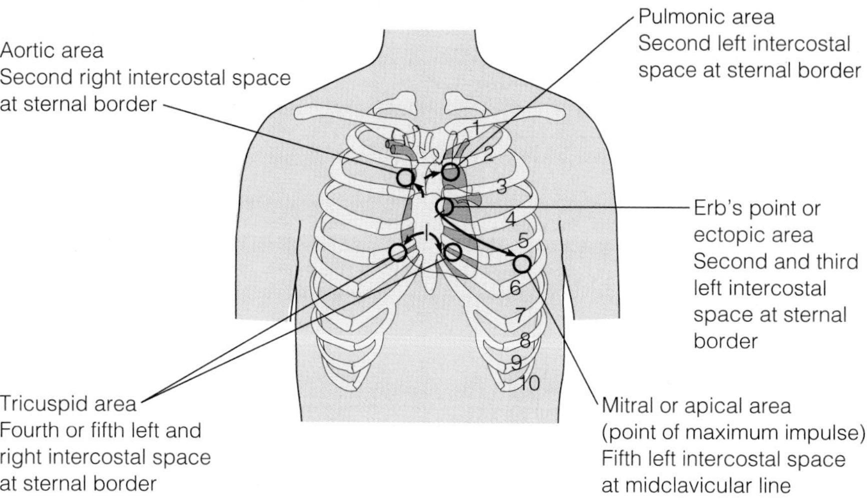

Figure 19.14 Heart auscultation sites in the child.

- Note the heart rate and rhythm. At each stop, listen for S1 and S2, noting the strength, character, and any split of each sound.

Children's heart sounds are higher-pitched and of shorter duration than those heard in adults. Heart sounds are also louder in children because their chest walls are thinner.

Sinus arrhythmia is normally heard in children of all ages, especially in adolescents. S1 is loudest at the apex, and S2 is loudest at the base of the heart. Splitting of S2 can be heard in most young children at the second left intercostal space.

- Then listen to the systole and diastole for any murmurs, clicks, or snaps. Listen in diastole for S3 or S4.

Some children have a physiologic S3, which is heard best at the apex.

- Listen to the back for any radiating murmurs.

A venous hum is commonly heard in children and is not pathologically significant. It is a continuous, low-pitched sound that is loudest in diastole and heard above or below the clavicles. It disappears when the child lies down.

A murmur is the sound of turbulent blood flow. It is described by its timing, pitch, location, radiation, quality, and grade of intensity. (See Chapter 11.) Many children have innocent or functional murmurs that are characteristically systolic, vibratory, short, and medium-pitched. They are of grade 1 to 2 in intensity, do not radiate, and are usually heard along the left sternal border. Murmurs of grade 3 or louder, those associated with a thrill, and those heard during diastole almost always indicate heart disease.

ASSESSMENT TECHNIQUE/NORMAL FINDINGS | SPECIAL CONSIDERATIONS

Abdomen

Step 1 *Inspect the contour and movement of the abdomen.*

- The child is in a supine position.
- Note any localized fullness.

Young children normally have a potbelly that appears flat when they lie down.

A protuberant abdomen in infants or a concave appearance in older children may indicate malnutrition. A midline protrusion is seen in *diastasis recti abdominis* when the two halves of the rectus abdominis muscle are separated. It can be a normal variant. Distention may indicate pregnancy in menstruating girls. Distention also may indicate organomegaly, feces in the bowel, or a tumor. Peristaltic waves indicate obstruction or, in young infants, possible pyloric stenosis.

- Inspect the umbilicus, noting any irritation, discharge, or odor. The umbilicus should be clean and dry.

An umbilical hernia may cause umbilical protrusion in children up to the age of 6 years. It requires no intervention.

Umbilical discharge in a young infant may indicate a granuloma or infection. Infection is often accompanied by a foul odor.

Step 2 *Auscultate the abdomen.*

- Firmly place the diaphragm of the stethoscope on the abdomen.
- Listen for peristalsis in all four quadrants.

High-pitched, tinkling sounds are heard in children with diarrhea or obstruction.

Auscultation precedes palpation and percussion because palpation and percussion may disturb normal abdominal sounds.

Gurgling bowel sounds are usually heard every 10 to 30 seconds.

Before determining that bowel sounds are absent, listen for a full 5 minutes.

Absence of bowel sounds is indicative of paralytic ileus.

Step 3 *Percuss all areas of the abdomen in a systematic manner.*

- Use indirect percussion.
- You may use the scratch method to further define organ borders.

Tympany is heard over most of the abdomen. Dullness is heard over the liver margin, 2–3 cm below the right costal margin. Dullness may be heard over a full bladder or large masses of feces.

Step 4 *Palpate the abdomen twice, first superficially, then deeply.*

In a crying child, palpation is best accomplished during inspiration. In an older child, flexion of the knees helps to relax the abdominal muscles (Figure 19.15 on page 616).

The spleen is not usually felt except in very young infants. When enlarged, the spleen feels like the tip of a nose or a thumb below the left costal margin.

The liver may normally be palpated as a superficial mass a few centimeters below the right costal margin. Feces may occasionally be palpated as a firm mass in the left lower quadrant. All masses other than those identified as feces require further evaluation.

ASSESSMENT TECHNIQUE/NORMAL FINDINGS | SPECIAL CONSIDERATIONS

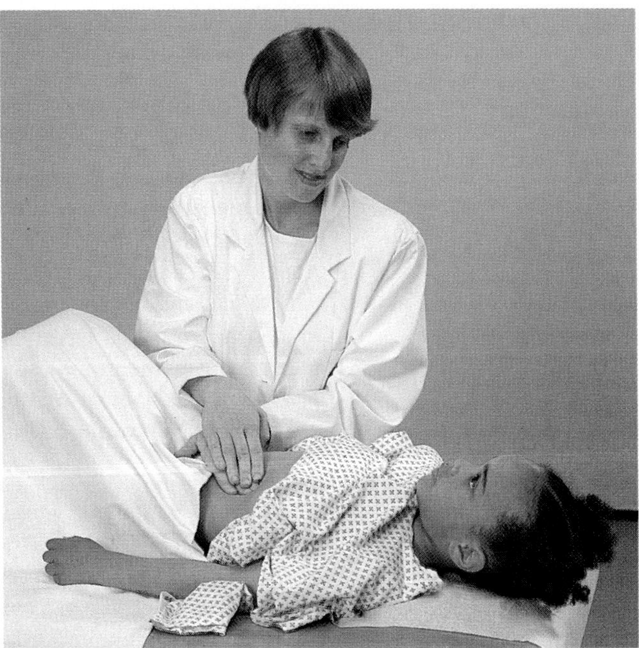

Figure 19.15 Palpating the abdomen.

- Palpate any painful area last.
- Begin at the lower left abdomen, inching up to the left costal margin.
- Repeat the procedure in the midline and then on the right.
- Note tenderness, lesions, and muscle tone.

Genitals

Inspection of the vagina and cervix with the speculum is not usually part of the examination of preadolescent girls. For a description of this assessment for adolescents and adults, see Chapter 15.

Step 1 ***Inspect the external genitals.***

The child should still be supine.

- Uncover only the area to be examined, and be sensitive to the child's modesty.
- Note the presence and distribution of hair.
- In girls, gently spread the labia majora to inspect the mucous membrane, clitoris, and urethral and vaginal openings. Note any edema, erythema, discharge, or lesions.

Labial adhesions in girls may obscure the vaginal and urethral openings. Treatment is recommended. A foul-smelling vaginal discharge may indicate a foreign body, infection, or poor hygiene.

ASSESSMENT TECHNIQUE/NORMAL FINDINGS	SPECIAL CONSIDERATIONS

- In boys, note the penis size and the presence of testes in the scrotum. Note whether or not the boy has been circumcised. Inspect the urinary meatus and note any discharge.

In boys, the urinary meatus is normally a slitlike opening at the tip of the penis.

Step 2 ***Palpate the external genitals and inguinal areas.***

- In girls, palpate the mons pubis and labia majora for masses.

Any mass of the mons pubis or labia majora is abnormal and requires evaluation.

- In boys, gently attempt to retract the foreskin.

You may find that having the boy sit crosslegged on the examining table will help during this assessment.

- Note any adhesions on circumcised boys.

The foreskin of an uncircumcised boy is not expected to retract fully until about 3 years of age. It is never appropriate to retract the foreskin forcibly.

- Palpate the testes for size, consistency, shape, and mobility.

Testes not in the scrotum usually can be milked down into the scrotum from the inguinal canal, where they often ascend. Again, having the child sit crosslegged often helps.

A testis that cannot easily be brought down into the scrotum of a child over 3 years of age may indicate *cryptorchidism*, or undescended testicle. In this condition, the testicle remains in the abdomen or inguinal canal. Surgery may be required.

- Palpate the inguinal areas of both boys and girls, noting any masses or lymph nodes.

Small, moveable lymph nodes in the inguinal area are normal in a young child.

The continuous presence of fluid in the scrotum of an infant is likely a hydrocele, which will resorb over time. Intermittent scrotal fluid, usually unilateral, is indicative of an inguinal hernia. A single bulge or mass in the inguinal area is indicative of an inguinal hernia.

Anus

A digital rectal examination is not usually part of a routine examination.

Step 1 ***Inspect the anal area.***

- Help the child to a prone position. Alternatively, the child may lie on one side.
- Spread the buttocks to view the anal area.
- Note hygiene, the presence of stool, marks, fissures, tears, scars, hemorrhoids, polyps, or skin tags.

The presence of stool may indicate *encopresis*, fecal incontinence without an organic cause. Evidence of scratching is suggestive of pinworms. Fissures are commonly seen in children with hard stools. Irregular tears or scars may indicate sexual abuse.

Step 2 ***Assess the anal reflex.***

- Stroke the anal area lightly with a tongue depressor to elicit the anal reflex.

Absence of the anal reflex may indicate sexual abuse.

ASSESSMENT TECHNIQUE/NORMAL FINDINGS | SPECIAL CONSIDERATIONS

Musculoskeletal System

Step 1 ***Observe the child move, walk, crawl, and play prior to the examination.***

Limping indicates an abnormality that requires evaluation.

- Note any asymmetry, lack of limb use, or favoring one side.

Toddlers tend to walk bowlegged with a wide-based gait.

Step 2 ***Inspect and palpate the upper body.***

- Have the child sit upright.
- Inspect and palpate the clavicles, noting any irregularities.
- Inspect and palpate the surrounding muscles, noting symmetry and strength.
- Palpate the muscles down both arms, feeling for muscle consistency and irregularities.

A fracture of the clavicle resulting from birth trauma may be recognized by a hard, fixed mass on the clavicle.

- Inspect the palms.

Simian creases (transverse palmar creases) may be seen in some normal children but may be an indication of Down syndrome.

- Assess the range of motion of all joints (see Chapter 17).

Step 3 ***Inspect and palpate the back.***

- Infants may be examined lying prone. Inspect the back of a school-aged child or adolescent with the child standing straight.
- Inspect and palpate the scapulae, vertebrae, and muscles, noting any asymmetry.

Asymmetry may indicate scoliosis, a lateral curvature of the spine.

When the child is standing, the shoulders, scapulae, and hips should be level and the spine straight.

- Have the child bend at the waist and note any unilateral fullness.
- Palpate the spine while the child is bending.

When bending, a unilateral fullness or obvious curvature of the spine is indicative of scoliosis.

Step 4 ***Inspect and palpate the hips.***

- Note any pain, limitation of movement, or asymmetry.
- In infants, note symmetry of gluteal skin folds.

Unequal gluteal skin folds may indicate congenital dislocation of the hips.

- Test infants for *Ortolani's sign* of hip dislocation (Figure 19.16). With the infant supine on a firm surface, place thumbs on the inside of both thighs with fingertips resting over the trochanter muscles. Flex both hips and knees and fully abduct each knee. Normally, nothing is heard or felt.

Early identification and treatment of congenital dislocated hips eliminate the need for surgical intervention and prevent disability. Unequal or limited abduction may indicate hip dislocation.

Ortolani's sign is positive for hip dislocation when a click is heard or felt. Ortolani's sign is most reliable in infants less than 4 months old.

ASSESSMENT TECHNIQUE/NORMAL FINDINGS | SPECIAL CONSIDERATIONS

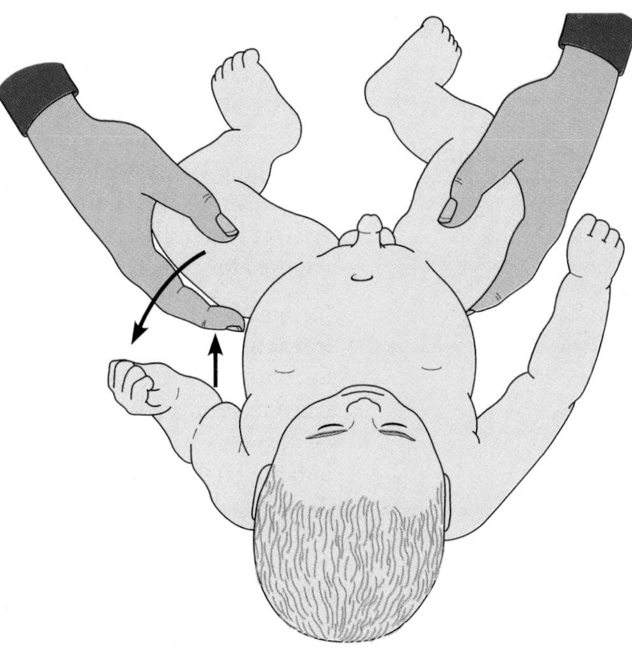

Figure 19.16 Ortolani's test to assess congenital dislocation of the hip.

- Perform *Barlow's maneuver* to test infants for dislocated hip (Figure 19.17). With the infant supine on a firm surface, flex and slightly adduct both hips while lifting the femur and applying pressure to the trochanter. Normally, no movement is felt.

Barlow's maneuver is positive when movement of the femoral head is felt as it slips out onto the posterior lip of the acetabulum, then as it returns. Although not diagnostic, a positive maneuver indicates that the infant requires close observation for congenital dislocated hip.

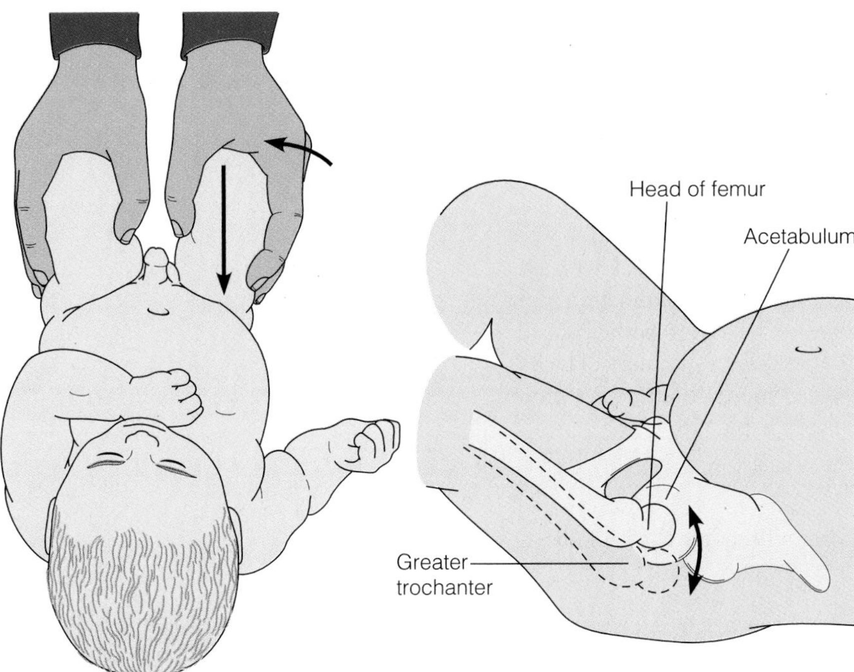

Figure 19.17 Barlow's test to assess congenital dislocation of the hip.

ASSESSMENT TECHNIQUE/NORMAL FINDINGS	SPECIAL CONSIDERATIONS

Step 5 ***Inspect and palpate the lower extremities.***

- In children who can walk, inspect the leg and foot position while the child is standing.

The feet of infants and toddlers are flat. The arch develops gradually in early childhood.

The legs appear bowed until walking is firmly established. Severe bowing, called genu varum, requires evaluation for rickets (see Figure 19.5, *A*). Knock-knees (genu valgum) are normal until 7 or 8 years of age (see Figure 19.5, *B*). Referral is required for persistent knock-knees.

- Manipulate the ankles and feet to assure that they move easily to a neutral position.

Infants often have turned-in ankles and feet as a result of fetal positioning. If the feet and ankles are easily straightened when manipulated, frequent massage may be the only treatment required. Referral is indicated if the feet or ankles cannot be easily straightened.

- Assess the range of motion of all joints (see Chapter 17).

Neurologic System

Step 1 ***Assess mental status.***

Assess the mental status of infants and young children as they respond to their parents and the examination.

- Note the child's ability to understand and follow directions. Is the behavior appropriate for the child's age?
- Note evidence of short attention span, impulsivity, or hyperactivity.
- Assess the child's speech.

It is important to differentiate normal, busy activity of a young child from impulsivity and hyperactivity. Impulsive, hyperactive children with short attention spans require evaluation and early intervention to improve their ability to function and avoid developing a poor self concept.

Step 2 ***Assess the child's development as described on pages 594–598.***

Step 3 ***Assess cranial nerve function.***

Cranial nerves II (optic), III (oculomotor), IV (trochlear), and VI (abducens) are tested during assessment of the eye. Cranial nerves X (vagus) and XII (hypoglossal) are evaluated during examination of the mouth. Infants and young children may not be able to participate adequately in some of the tests. Table 19.4 provides a summary of techniques for testing cranial nerve function in young children. For more information on testing cranial nerves, see Chapter 18.

Step 4 ***Assess infant reflexes.***

During the first few months of life, infant reflexes are a good indication of neurologic function.

- Test for Babinski sign.

The toes fan and the big toes dorsiflex in response to stroking the sole of the foot along the outer edge from heel to toe. This reflex is present during the first 2 years.

A positive Babinski test in a child older than 2 years suggests a lesion in the extrapyramidal tract.

ASSESSMENT TECHNIQUE/NORMAL FINDINGS | SPECIAL CONSIDERATIONS

Table 19.4 Testing Cranial Nerve Function in Young Children

Cranial nerves	Procedures and observations
CN I	Use familiar non-noxious smells such as orange or soap. *Not* routinely tested.
CN II	Use the Snellen E or Picture Chart to test vision. Test visual fields while immobilizing the head as needed.
CN III, IV, and VI	Move an object through the cardinal points of gaze and have the child follow it with the eyes.
CN V	Observe bilateral jaw strength while the child chews a cookie or cracker.
	Touch the child's forehead and cheeks with cotton and watch the child bat it away.
CN VII	Observe the child's face when smiling, frowning, and crying.
	Ask the child to show the teeth.
	Demonstrate puffed cheeks and ask the child to imitate.
CN VIII	Observe the child turn to sounds such as a bell or whisper.
	Whisper a commonly used word, such as "doggie," behind the child's back and have the child repeat the word.
CN IX and X	Elicit the gag reflex
CN XI and XII	Ask an older child to stick out the tongue and shrug the shoulders or raise the arms.

- Test the blinking reflex.

The eyes close in response to bright light. This reflex is present during the first year.

Absence of the reflex suggests blindness.

- Test the extrusion reflex.

The tongue extends outward when touched with the tip of a tongue depressor. This reflex disappears at 4 months.

Persistence of the reflex after 4 months may indicate Down syndrome.

- Test the Moro reflex.

In response to an abrupt change of position or jarring, the infant's arms extend, the fingers fan, the head is thrown back, the legs may flex weakly, the arms return to center with hands clasped, and the spine and lower extremities extend. The reflex disappears by 3–4 months.

Asymmetry is indicative of hemiparesis, clavicle fracture, or injury to the brachial plexus. Persistence beyond 4 months suggests brain damage.

- Test the palmar grasp reflex.

The infant's fingers curve around a finger placed in the infant's palm from the ulnar side. The reflex disappears by 3–4 months.

Asymmetric grasp is indicative of paralysis; persistence is indicative of cerebral disorder.

- Test the plantar grasp reflex.

The infant's toes flex in response to a finger pressed against the sole of the infant's foot. The reflex disappears at 8–10 months.

Persistence is abnormal.

- Test the rooting reflex.

The infant turns the head in the direction of the cheek that is stroked. The reflex disappears at 3–4 months but may persist for up to 12 months, especially during sleep.

Absence is indicative of severe neurologic disorder.

- Test the stepping reflex.

When the feet lightly touch a firm surface, the infant moves the feet up and down as if walking. The reflex disappears by 1–2 months.

Persistence is abnormal.

ASSESSMENT TECHNIQUE/NORMAL FINDINGS	SPECIAL CONSIDERATIONS
◆ Test the sucking reflex. With a gloved finger, assess the strength and character of the suck.	Suck should be strong and even. Weak suck may indicate neurologic abnormality.
◆ Test the tonic neck reflex. The infant assumes a fencing position when the head is turned to one side; the arm and leg extend on the side to which the head is turned and flex on the opposite side. This response does not occur each time head is turned. The reflex appears at about 2 months and disappears at 6 months.	This reflex is abnormal if a response occurs each time the head is turned. Persistence indicates major cerebral damage.
Step 5 ***Assess deep tendon reflexes.*** Assess these reflexes only in school-aged children and adolescents (see Chapter 18). ◆ Compare the symmetry and strength of reflexes.	Hyperactivity of the reflexes may indicate upper motor neuron lesion, hypocalcemia, or hyperthyroidism. Decreased or absent reflexes may indicate a lower motor neuron lesion, muscular dystrophy, or paralysis.
Step 6 ***Assess motor function during the musculoskeletal examination and developmental assessment.***	

Reminders

- Developing expertise in pediatric assessment requires you to use a system that is comfortable, systematic, thorough, and adaptable for children of various ages. Experience will sharpen your observational skills and provide the opportunity to integrate the various components of the examination with ease.
- Integrate age-appropriate anticipatory guidance throughout the pediatric assessment. After completing the exam, answer any questions that the child or parent may have, and provide appropriate teaching for health promotion and self-care (see pages 627–633).
- Confirm that the child is comfortable and has no adverse effects from the procedure, then dim the lights before leaving the room.
- Document the assessment findings as described in Chapter 1. Nursing diagnoses applicable to infants, children, and adolescents are discussed in the next section.

Organizing the Data

After conducting the interview and physical assessment, group related data into clusters leading to either nursing diagnoses, which require independent nursing actions, or alterations in health, which require you to work with other members of the health care team.

Identifying Nursing Diagnoses

The physical assessment of the infant, child, or adolescent is likely to reveal one of three general findings: (1) The child's physical development is within normal limits. (2) The child exhibits the potential for physical problems caused by rapid growth, factors in the child's environment, family conflict, or other factors. (3) The child's physical condition deviates from the norm in some way. In most instances, the diagnosis of an alteration in one or more physiologic processes usually indicates referral to a physician.

Table 19.5 Nursing Diagnoses Commonly Associated with Infants, Children, and Adolescents

FEAR

Definition: Feeling of dread related to an identifiable source which the person validates (NANDA).

RELATED FACTORS

Environmental stressor/hospitalization, Powerlessness, Real or imagined threat to own well-being, Implications for future pregnancies, Real or imagined threat to child, Others specific to client (specify).

DEFINING CHARACTERISTICS

Ability to identify object of fear

ALTERED GROWTH AND DEVELOPMENT

Definition: The state in which an individual demonstrates deviations in norms from his/her age group (NANDA).

RELATED FACTORS

Inadequate prenatal care, Congenital anomaly, Fetal distress during or after birth/delivery, Prematurity, Neonatal disease, Unhealthy maternal lifestyle during pregnancy, Maternal acute/chronic disease, Maternal age, Inadequate caretaking, Poverty, Changes in family system, Inadequate bonding, Lack of stimulation in environment, Abuse, Traumatic separation, Loss, Rapid growth, Serious illness/injury, Prescribed dependence/limitations, Indifference, Inconsistent responsiveness, Multiple caretaking, Separation from significant others, Enrivonment and stimulation deficiencies, Effects of physical disability, Prescribed dependence, Others specific to client (specify).

DEFINING CHARACTERISTICS

Major	Minor
Delay or difficulty in performing skills (motor, social, or expressive) typical of age group	Flat affect
Altered physical growth	Listlessness
Inability to perform self-care or self-control activities appropriate for age	Decreased responses
	Infant irritability

DIAGNOSTIC REASONING IN ACTION

Nicky is a 6-year-old boy whose father brings him to the clinic for evaluation of bed-wetting for the past 2 months. Nicky appears alert and happy and plays with the blocks in the examining room while the nurse, Cordelia Jordan, RN, interviews his father. Mr. Kasvin reports that Nicky is doing well in first grade and seems to get along well with the other children. He believes that his son is generally healthy. Although Nicky had three colds during the past year, he recovered from all of them within a few days. Ms Jordan asks Mr. Kasvin about any changes in Nicky's environment other than his entering first grade. Mr. Kasvin reports that his wife returned to work a few weeks after Nicky started school after having been at home with Nicky throughout his preschool years. Nicky is an only child, and Mr. Kasvin states that there are no other children his age in the neighborhood. Ms Jordan then asks Mr. Kasvin to describe the frequency and time of the enuresis. Mr. Kasvin states that Nicky wets his bed two or three times a week, between midnight, when he checks his son before retiring, and 6:00 AM, when Nicky gets up for school. He doesn't believe his son has ever had an episode of enuresis during the day. Ms. Jordan then asks Mr. Kasvin about the following factors:

- Perinatal complications
- Developmental or physical problems
- Management of the home routine
- Hours he and Mrs. Kasvin work, and amount of time they spend with Nicky
- Nicky's toilet-training history
- Nicky's daily voiding pattern (number of daily voids, duration, description of urine stream)
- Any history of urinary tract infections
- Any food sensitivities
- Type and amount of fluids consumed
- Problems relayed by Nicky's teacher

Ms Jordan performs a thorough physical assessment of Nicky and obtains urine for a routine urinalysis and culture and sensitivity. The exam reveals that Nicky's growth and development are normal for his age, and he has no signs or symptoms of infection or of any current alteration in his physiologic health.

Ms Jordan asks Mr. Kasvin to step into the waiting room and talks to Nicky alone. She asks Nicky about school, and Nicky says that it's "OK, but I don't like Christopher very much." She asks Nicky who Christopher is, and Nicky reveals that he is a boy in second grade who has been teasing him and some of the other first-graders. Nicky also reveals that he is afraid he might wet his pants at school and everyone will laugh at him. Finally, she asks Nicky how he feels about his bed-wetting. Nicky answers, "I don't mean to do it. Mom started crying yesterday when she woke me up and my bed was wet. I know I'm bad."

The nursing assessment of Nicky Kasvin provides the following subjective and objective data:

- Normal growth and development
- Nocturnal incontinence
- Verbalization of negative feelings about self
- Expression of guilt

To cluster the information, Ms Jordan

- Notes that incontinence is a defining characteristic for the nursing diagnosis *Altered urinary elimination* and that the psychosocial stressors of beginning school, conflict with schoolmates, and the return of a parent to work might be related factors.
- Notes that Nicky's verbalization of negative feelings about himself and his expression of guilt are defining characteristics of the nursing diagnosis *Self-esteem disturbance* and that Nicky's new role in beginning school and his guilt at being unable to control his nocturnal enuresis might be related factors.

Based on this analysis and the normal findings from the urinalysis and urine culture, Ms Jordan arrives at the following nursing diagnoses:

1. *Altered urinary elimination* related to psychogenic factors such as beginning school, conflict with schoolmates, and return of a parent to work
2. *Self-esteem disturbance,* related to assumption of a new role and guilt at being unable to control his enuresis

Ms Jordan assures Nicky and Mr. Kasvin that in the absence of physical causes and with passage of time, nocturnal enuresis, a common problem, will resolve without treatment. She also teaches Nicky and Mr. Kasvin some methods for preventing and coping with enuresis (see page 632). Finally, she suggests that Mr. and Mrs. Kasvin make an appointment with Nicky's teacher or school counselor to discuss Nicky's adjustment to first grade and his relationships with his schoolmates.

Nursing diagnoses for pediatric clients may be as varied as those for adults. Some of the most common include:

- *Fear:* Feeling of dread related to an identifiable source that the child validates. This diagnosis may be related to the child's illness, unfamiliar surroundings, forced contact with strangers, treatments and procedures, and hospitalization. Defining characteristics include uncooperativeness, regressive behavior, restlessness, constant crying, tachypnea, tachycardia, and diaphoresis (Table 19.5 on page 623).
- *Altered growth and development:* The state in which an individual demonstrates deviations in norms from his or her age group (NANDA). Defining characteristics include altered physical growth and delay or difficulty in performing skills typical of age group. (See Table 19.5.)
- *Knowledge deficit Child/Family:* A state in which the child or family does not comprehend, learn, or demonstrate knowledge of health care measures necessary to maintain or improve the health of the child (NANDA). This diagnosis may be related to cognitive or cultural language limitations, sensory overload, misinterpretation of information, lack of motivation, or inability to recognize signs and symptoms, or it may be related to the disease state itself.
- *High risk for injury:* A state in which the child is at risk for injury as a result of environmental conditions interacting with the individual's adaptive and defensive resources (NANDA). This diagnosis may be related to a wide variety of internal and external factors, including physical, developmental, chemical, and psychologic factors.

Common Alterations in the Health of Infants, Children, and Adolescents

Problems commonly associated with infants, children, and adolescents may involve maternal or congenital factors, birth-related stressors, developmental problems, childhood infections, psychosocial stressors, and a variety of altered functioning patterns that also might be seen in an adult. The following brief discussion outlines some of the more common conditions of infants, children, and adolescents. Consult a pediatric nursing textbook for more information.

Fetal Alcohol Syndrome

Fetal alcohol syndrome (FAS) is a cluster of malformations that occurs in about 1–3 live births per 1000 as a result of maternal chronic alcohol consumption. Signs of FAS include prenatal or postnatal retardation, central nervous system dysfunction, and facial dysmorphology, which may include microcephaly, microphthalmia, short palpebral fissures, a poorly developed philtrum, thin lips, or a flattened maxillary area (See figure in Table 9.2 on page 210). Reports of the amount of alcohol consumption necessary to produce FAS vary, and "safe" amounts of alcohol consumption during pregnancy have not been determined.

Otitis Media

Otitis media is infection or inflammation of the middle ear. It is caused by microorganisms or allergies that cause closure of the auditory tube (See figure in Table 9.4 on page 215). Infants and children under the age of 5 are more commonly affected because their auditory tubes are shorter and straighter than those of older children and adults. Organisms from the nasopharynx therefore have a shorter, easier route to the middle ear. Otitis media frequently follows an upper respiratory infection. The affected child may experience pain in the ear, a fever which may run as high as 104F (40C), cervical lymph node enlargement, irritability, dizziness, anorexia, and nausea. Antibiotics are the common treatment. See page 629 for teaching tips for the child prone to otitis media.

Chronic Allergic Rhinitis

Allergic rhinitis is a hypersensitivity disorder that results from the release of chemical mediators in response to allergens in the nasal passages. These mediators cause nasal congestion, sneezing, increased secretion of mucus, and itching. Allergic rhinitis is one of the most common allergic conditions affecting children; in the United States, it affects approximately 6 million children. Children suffering from this condition may not be able to breathe through their noses at all; thus, their mouths may be open continuously. Additionally, the child may have edema and discoloration of the skin beneath the eyes (called "allergic shiners"). The child may also have a horizontal groove on the nose from constantly rubbing it upward with the palm of the hand. Treatment includes removal of the allergen and antihistamine therapy.

Asthma

Asthma, the most common chronic illness in childhood, occurs in approximately 3 to 5% of the population. *Asthma* is a reversible obstructive respiratory disease characterized by an increased responsiveness of the trachea and bronchi to a variety of stimuli. These stimuli cause episodic bronchospasm. The child's airways narrow from the edema and increased thick, tenacious mucus, and the child has dyspnea, wheezing, and excessive coughing. The obstructive process is the body's response to triggers such as pollen, animal dander, and feathers. Treatment of asthmatic children varies with the severity of the disease. First-line treatment is environmental modification and bronchodilators by nebulizer, inhaler, or mouth. Additional medications are used as needed.

Cystic Fibrosis

Cystic fibrosis is an autosomal recessive disorder characterized by widespread dysfunction of the exocrine glands, which causes oversecretion of a viscous mucus that clogs the respiratory passages and impairs digestion. It accounts for about 5% of childhood deaths. In newborns, the most common sign is small-bowel obstruction from inspissated meconium. The infant or young child may exhibit growth failure, steatorrhea, voracious appetite, constipation/bowel obstruction, and respiratory disease, characterized by a dry and hacking or loose and productive cough with excessive secretion. Medical treatment includes inhalation therapy, clapping/percussion and postural drainage, and breathing exercises to maintain airway patency. Gastrointestinal involvement is treated with dietary therapy, vitamin and iron supplementation, and replacement of pancreatic enzymes.

Acne Vulgaris

Acne vulgaris, which affects 80 to 90% of all adolescents, may be due to rising levels of androgens that stimulate the sebaceous glands to increase production of sebum and promote changes in keratinization in the wall of the hair follicles. These physiologic changes in turn lead to a sequence of pathologic changes that result in the formation of comedones, pustules,

Table 19.6 Signs and Symptoms of Physical Abuse

Indication of abuse	Assessment findings
Bruises or welts on ears, eyes, mouth, lips, torso, buttocks, genital areas, calves	Injuries may be in the shape of the object used to produce them (eg, sticks, belts, hairbrushes, buckles)
	Injuries located on parts of body not usually injured, such as bruising behind the ear, pinch marks on genitals (normal bruises commonly appear on forehead, shins, knees, elbows)
	Injuries often in various stages of healing
Burns	Shape suggests type of burn
Immersion burns	Immersion burns on feet have "socklike," on hands "glovelike," on buttocks or genitals "donutlike" appearance
Pattern burns	Pattern suggests object used (eg, iron, stove grate, electric burner, heater); small, circular burns on feet, face, hands, chest, or buttocks suggest cigar or cigarette
Friction burns	Friction burns on legs, arms, neck, or torso may be cause by child having been tied up with rope
Scald burns	Caused by hot liquid poured over trunk or extremities; multiple splash marks may appear on body; depth of burn varies with temperature of liquid, length of contact, and presence of clothing
Fractures of skull, face, nose, orbit, long bones, ribs	Multiple or spiral fractures caused by twisting motion
	Evidence of epiphyseal separations and periosteal shearing
	Shaft fractures from direct blows
	Fractures may be in various stages of healing if earlier fractures went untreated
Lacerations or abrasions on mouth, lips, gums, eyes, genitals	Human bite marks, especially those of adult size, may be evident
	Torn frenulum in infant from forcing object into mouth
	Puncture wounds or deep scratch marks from fingernails around face or genital area
Head trauma	Evidence of increased intracranial pressure in infant (eg, bulging fontanelle)
	Subdural hematomas from being dropped on the head or from receiving blows to the head; if abuse is repetitive, separation of cranial sutures may be evident due to chronic subdural hematoma
	Areas of baldness and swelling from hair being pulled out when dragging the child by the hair
Neck trauma	Limited range of motion from whiplash injury due to being shaken
	Dislocation or subluxation of neck
Somatic	Persistent vomiting or abdominal pain
	Rigid abdomen due to internal bleeding
	Shock
Child's behaviors	Extreme aggressiveness or withdrawal; wariness of adults; fear of going home; apprehension when other children cry
	Appears disinterested or frightened of parents, shows no emotion when parents leave or return
	Indiscriminate friendliness and immediate affection shown toward anyone providing attention
	Vacant stare; no eye contact
	Surveys environment but remains motionless
	Stiffens when approached as if expecting punishment of a physical nature
	Inappropriate response to painful procedures

Table 19.7 Signs of Sexual Abuse

Physical signs	Behavioral signs
Laceration of labia, vagina, or perineum	Advanced knowledge of adult sexual behavior
Irritation, pain, or injury to genital area	Discussion of or implied involvement in sexual activity
Hematomas in genital area	Expression of severe emotional conflict at home with fear of intervention
Vaginal or penile discharge	Reluctance to participate in sports, showers, changing of clothes
Dysuria or urinary frequency	Excessive bathing
Sexually transmitted disease in young child (on eyes, mouth, anus, or genitals)	Sitting carefully because of injuries
Pregnancy	Unusual interest in genital area (eg, "French kissing" or fondling of genitals, excessive masturbation)
Itching, bruises, or bleeding in genital area	Sexual acting out with peers
Unexplained vaginal or rectal bleeding	Sleep disturbances (eg, nightmares, fear of sleeping alone)
Enlarged vaginal or rectal orifice	Reluctance to participate in activities with a particular person or at a particular place
Foreign objects in vagina or rectum	Increased number of new fears
Increased rectal pigmentation	Fear of being alone
Gait disturbance	Poor peer relations
	Depression
	Change in performance at school
	Eating disorders
	Vague somatic complaints
	Extreme shyness
	Increased aggressive or hostile behavior
	Encopresis
	Enuresis
	Self-destructive or suicidal behaviors
	Substance abuse
	Runaway behaviors

and cysts (see Figure 8.23 on page 149). The lesions are usually located on the face and chest but may occur on the back, neck, and arms. Topical therapy, systemic medications, and phototherapy are treatments commonly used.

Physical and Sexual Abuse of Children

Physical abuse of children involves nonaccidental physical injury or injuries that result from acts or omissions on the part of the child's parents or caregivers. These physical injuries may include both old and new bruises, X-ray evidence of fractures, and skin lesions whose shape suggests the implements used to inflict trauma, such as a belt buckle, rope, coat hanger, or cigarette lighter. The child may seem sad and noncommunicative or may seem concerned with pleasing the abusing parent. Table 19.6 lists other signs and symptoms of physical abuse.

Sexual abuse is the exploitation of a child for the sexual gratification of an adult. The physical and behavioral signs of sexual abuse are listed in Table 19.7.

Health Promotion and Client Education

At the conclusion of the assessment of the infant, child, or adolescent, answer any questions the parent or child may have and provide teaching targeted to address the individual client's health-care needs. General tips for teaching children of different ages about health are listed in Table 19.8 on page 628. The following section provides teaching tips for promoting a healthy childhood.

Preventing Infection

Prevention of infection begins with immunization. The goal of immunization is to prevent infectious disease by introducing an antigen or antibody to the child. Immunization guidelines are provided in the box on page 629, and a recommended

text continues on page 629

Table 19.8 Developmental Approach to Health Education

Age	Developmental characteristic	Learning style	Teaching strategy
Infancy (birth to 18 months)	Depends on others to meet health care needs; beginning cognitive development requires stimulation; expression of needs by crying, moving, and so forth; developing trust versus mistrust; beginning development of coping mechanisms	Sensorimotor (Piaget); stimulation for adequate growth; preverbal	Help parents clarify roles; encourage attachment; assist parents to meet universal self-care demands and foster a nurturing environment; teach parents health care measures—importance of regular well-child checkups, immunizations, and environmental modification
Early childhood (18 months to 4½ years)	Tendency to demand; aggressive and protest behavior; fantasy and fears; focus on control of elimination; positive or negative attitudes learned from environment; self-protection decreased due to increased curiosity; seeks autonomy	Preconceptual; trial and error; use of fantasy and drama; short attention span requires varied presentation; needs repetition to learn	Teach parents importance of continuing immunization and well-child visits; continue environmental protection; teach cleanliness and safety by role modeling; encourage beginning responsibility for self-care—bathing, dressing, dental care; teach parents appropriate criteria for choosing a preschool; encourage positive self-image; coordinate teaching with periods of optimal wakefulness and attention; encourage regular rest periods
Middle childhood (5–8 years)	High activity level; increased emphasis on physical prowess; increasing intellectual development; increasing spiritual and moral development; emphasis on following rules; awareness of socially acceptable behavior; increasing identification with peers	Beginning to be a concrete thinker and problem solver; language skills improving; learns best by manipulating objects	Continue to emphasize well-child care; encourage participatory care and control over own health; teach rules of safety; encourage self-esteem by positive reinforcement; give clear, concise answers to questions regarding death and moral issues; explore values and how they relate to peers' values; encourage independence in meeting self-care demands; encourage parents to provide a wide variety of experiences and opportunities to solve problems; begin education in areas of sex, substance abuse, and child abuse; allow for questions; use humor as a teaching tool to gain and keep affection
Late childhood (8–12 years)	Increasing awareness of causes of disease may lead to psychosomatic complaints; peer group important; need to achieve competence in school and sports; beginning exposure to abusable substances; increased self-direction (eg, will initiate visits to school nurse)	Concrete, with beginning development of abstract conceptual thought; problem-solving capability; well-developed language skills	Focus on safety principles; use influence of peer group to alter health behaviors; encourage parental support and continued role modeling; use the media to encourage positive health habits; teach health education in the schools to foster positive health habits and prevent substance abuse; use problem situations and discussion groups to teach health concepts and grapple with moral issues
Adolescence	Physical maturation; peer pressure most influential; accidents increase, particularly automobile; substance abuse; sexual activity can lead to pregnancy or sexually transmitted disease; focus on social rather than healthful aspects of living	Abstract; problem solving; future oriented	Emphasize enhancing self-esteem; identify and reinforce positive behaviors; use peer counseling and alter group rather than individual behaviors; minimize the negative; discuss choices, goals, and moral and ethical dilemmas of behavior

schedule for active immunization of normal infants and children is provided in Table 19.9.

Teach the family members some simple precautions for minimizing droplet-spread diseases such as the common cold:

- Cover the mouth while coughing or sneezing.
- Discard tissues immediately after use.
- Avoid sharing towels, napkins, and eating utensils.
- Wash the hands frequently, particularly when family members are ill.

Immunization Guidelines

- Live viruses should be given 1 month apart if not administered on the same day.
- There should be intervals of 2 weeks to a month between the administration of inactivated viruses (see recommended schedule).
- Live viruses and inactivated viruses may be given simultaneously at different sites or together orally.
- Live viruses may be given in licensed combinations, such as MR and MMR.
- Killed viruses may be given simultaneously at different sites.
- Live virus vaccination should not be administered sooner than 3 months following passive immunization with immune serum globulin.
- Immune serum globulin should not be given, except in emergency circumstances, for 2 weeks after a vaccine is administered.
- Persons known to experience side effects from vaccines should receive vaccines on separate occasions; avoid simultaneous administration.

Finally, share the following tips for deterring contact diseases such as impetigo, pediculosis, fungal infections, and parasitic infections:

- Wash the hands thoroughly after elimination.
- Do not share articles of clothing, particularly hats and underwear, with other children.
- Do not share cosmetics, hair clips or barrettes, or brushes or combs with other children.
- Do not share towels or pillows with other children.

Preventing Accidents

Injuries are the leading cause of childhood disease, disability, and death; thus, the importance of client teaching in this area cannot be overemphasized. Safety education is directed to parents initially and then to children according to their cognitive and developmental stage. Table 19.10 on page 630 lists the most common potential hazards of different developmental stages, along with their preventive strategies.

Preventing Poisoning

Review the principles of poison safety with the parents before the infant is crawling. Most poison control centers provide educational materials such as "Mr. Yuk" stickers, pamphlets, and posters upon request. In addition, stress the tips in the box on page 633 at well-child visits.

Precautions for Children Prone to Otitis Media

Give parents of children prone to otitis media the following suggestions for reducing the risk for recurrence:

- Feed the infant or young child in an upright position and keep the child upright for 15 to 30 minutes following feedings to prevent passage of fluids into the middle ear.

text continues on page 632

Table 19.9 Recommended Schedule for Normal Active Immuniation

Birth	HBV	
2 mo	DTP1, OPV1, HbCV1	OPV and DTP can be given earlier in areas of high endemicity or during epidemics
4 mo	DTP2, OPV2, HbCV2	Interval of 6 weeks to 2 months between OPV doses
6 mo	DTP3, HbOC3, HBV	An additional dose of OPV is optional in high risk areas
15 mo	MMR, DTP4, OPV3, HbCV3, or HbCV4	Completion of primary series of DTP and OPV
4–6 yr	DTP5, OPV4, measles	At or before school entry
11–12 yr	MMR	At entry to middle school unless second dose was given at age 4–6 years at time of school entry
14–16 yr	Td	Repeat every 10 years throughout life

Table 19.10 Developmental Approach to Accident Prevention

Age	Potential hazard	Preventive strategy
Infancy		
0–3 months	Can catch arms or fingers between loose-fitting mattress and frame of crib	Use crib sides and bumpers; stuff towels between mattress and crib side; cribs should have slats no more than 2⅜" apart
	Suffocation in crib	Do not use pillows or excess blankets
	Automobile accidents	Infant car seats should be used from birth
	Sudden movement leading to falls	Do not leave infant alone on high places, particularly on an adult bed or infant seat; keep crib sides raised; keep a hand on infant at all times, especially during bathing when infant is slippery with soap; on stairs, hold infant with two hands
	Burns and punctures from bathing and changing; poisoning from spoiled or incorrectly mixed formula	Test bath water for lukewarm temperature; be careful of sharp points of diaper pins near infant's skin; store formula in cool, dry place; protect infant from sunburn
3–6 months	Harmful objects within infant's immediate reach	Keep potential hazards such as hot coffee while infant is sitting on parent's lap; protect infant from hot faucet while bathing in sink; toys should have no removable parts or sharp edges that could be put in infant's mouth or eyes; do not allow access to plastic bags
	Sharp fingernails	Parents can cut infant's fingernails while infant sleeps
	Falls	Crib mattress in lowest position; change infant on the floor; remove large stuffed animals from crib
6–9 months	Glass breakage if dropped	Use plastic bottles
	Range of grasp increases with mobility	Cover electrical outlets and wind cords on appliances to keep them out of reach; lock lower cabinets or remove any dangerous objects (eg, glass jars, soap powders); eliminate lead paint hazards, assess environment for lead
	Increased access to hazardous fixtures and furniture	Use gates to protect from stairways; fence off woodburning stoves and space heaters; supervise constantly when infant is in walker, swing, jumper, or high chair; wastebaskets, plants, and household cleaners contain potential poisons and should be placed out of infant's reach; remove hazardous machinery such as fans and humidifiers from floor level; have syrup of ipecac in the home; have poison control number readily available; have smoke detectors and check them regularly
	As teeth develop, infants enjoy teething biscuits	Supervise for choking; do not leave infant unattended while eating
9–12 months	Falls	Bicycle passenger safety
	Mobility and range of grasp increase further	Turn pot handles in on stove; remove stove burner knobs if within reach; remove dangerous objects from counters and tables; teach about "hot"
	Hazardous fixtures become increasingly accessible	Screen windows and use gates on stairways if not already done; use playpens with sides up and corrals with net siding if infant is out of visual range; teach descending stairs backward
	Choking on small objects	Cut food into small pieces; no peanuts or popcorn; child should eat while sitting; easy-to-handle eating utensils; check toys for small pieces; keep money out of reach
12–18 months	Body control not highly developed, resulting in an unsteady walk; would rather run than walk	Keep furniture with sharp edges, glass coffee tables, and the like out of child's way; keep house clutter-free; lock up poisonous substances if not previously done; pull-toy strings should not be greater that 12" in length
	Bath—temperature of water and slippery tub	Lukewarm water at low level in tub; teach child not to stand in tub; never leave child unattended during bath time; run cold water first before mixing with hot

Table 19.10 (continued)

Age	Potential hazard	Preventive strategy
Early childhood		
18–24 months	Accidents are more frequent when parents are preoccupied such as at mealtimes and in the morning	Parents can share responsibility for preparing meals and watching children; children's television programs can hold attention during meal preparation; parents should be alert to children's whereabouts
	Fire begins to be a hazard, especially charcoal fires in the summer	Parents should begin to educate children about danger of fire; place matches out of reach; teach fire safety
	Curiosity makes household and yard plants more interesting	Teach child not to put any plants, leaves, or berries in mouth
	Climbing accidents become more frequent, especially climbing out of crib	Child can sleep with crib sides lowered temporarily until a bed is obtained or on a mattress on the floor
2–3 years	Injury from riding toys	Parents should teach child not to ride tricycles in streets or behind cars; plastic tricycles are lower to the street and slower than metal ones, but are harder for passing motorists to see
	Children are attracted to brightly colored objects such as pills	Child should be taught never to take pills unless given by parent; medicine should not be made to "taste good"
	Drowning—children who have been taught to swim might get careless in the water	Pools should be fenced and children carefully supervised at beaches; even children who swim should be observed
	Wandering, streets	Needs safe, enclosed area when outside
3–5 years	Injury from playground equipment	Safety teaching should include not walking in front of swings and no pushing and shoving off equipment
	Foreign objects in Halloween candy	Parents should check Halloween treats before allowing child to eat them; throw away any loose or open candy
	Choking	Teach children not to run with candy or other objects in their mouths
	Increasing freedom out of doors; contact with unleashed animals	Encourage cooperative play; teach street safety—looking both ways, crossing at corners, watching lights; teach children to avoid strangers and keep parents informed of their whereabouts; teach children not to allow anyone to touch them inappropriately; teach children to walk quietly near animals and to avoid approaching them if parents are not present
	Craft toys	Provide safety scissors and age-appropriate activities
Middle and late childhood		
5–12 years	Imitates action seen on television	Teach critical television viewing and talk to children about their favorite shows
	Dogs and cats	Teach child to avoid all strange animals, not to break up an animal fight even when own pet is involved, not to tease animals, and to behave appropriately when encountering a strange animal (stand still, move slowly, keep an eye on the animal)
	Skateboard misuse, particularly in populated areas	Caution children to remember street safety on skates or skateboards; extra control is needed for downhill runs; discourage jumps; encourage protective gear and helmet
	Bicycle accidents are common	Teach bicycle safety; provide bicycle helmet
	Drowning—ice or water	Teach children water safety; do not allow skating unless ice thickness is proven safe; never swim or skate alone

Table 19.10 Developmental Approach to Accident Prevention (continued)

Age	Potential Hazard	Preventive strategy
Middle and late childhood (continued)	Sports injuries	Teach parents and children sports safety
	Automobiles	Require seatbelts at all times; teach child not to hide or play near cars
	Nighttime accidents increase as child is allowed more freedom	Parents should encourage children to be home before dark; wear light-colored clothing and reflective material when walking at night
	Vacant buildings, excavations, quarries, sand pits, house foundations	Teach children to avoid these areas and not to play around heavy machinery, and not to hide in refrigerators or piles of leaves
	Fire	Review home fire drills
	Tools	Teach proper use of home workshop tools, including use of protective equipment
	Flying objects—balls, darts, arrows, stones	Any target sport should be carefully supervised; targets should be in isolated areas or against walls; teach children not to throw objects at people or moving vehicles
	Abusable substances—effect of drugs and alcohol on coordination and judgment lead to accidental injury	Keep inaccessible in locked cabinet
	Firearms	Teach rules for hunting and proper care of firearms; keep firearm unloaded and locked up and hidden away
Adolescence		
Older than 12 years	Abusable substances	
	Vehicle hazards—cars, motorcycles	Driver safety; parents need to set firm limits on car use, particularly regarding drinking and driving; use seatbelts and motorcycle helmet
	Outdoor activities such as swimming, jogging, or boating are no longer under direct parental supervision	Encourage adolescents to do activities in a group so others can obtain help in case of injuries; review safety rules
		Parental role modeling regarding safety and hazards leading to injury can affect their children's safety practices; open communication between parents and children is a powerful preventive measure

Note: These ages are not exact. Parents should be taught to anticipate their children's development and to take preventive action according to individual developmental patterns.

- Breastfeed the infant. Breast milk appears to protect against invasion of the middle ear by pathogens and also prevents allergic reactions to bovine milk proteins.
- Since cigarette smoke may play a role in persistent otitis media, advise parents to provide a smoke-free environment.
- Note any food that the child may be sensitive to and avoid those foods, because they may play a role in persistent otitis media.

Coping with Nocturnal Enuresis

Reassure the parents and the child that enuresis that is not due to physical causes eventually will resolve without treatment. In the meantime, encourage the parents to

- Praise or reward the child for periods of bladder control.
- Avoid scolding or punishing the child when enuresis occurs.
- Allow the child to assume responsibility for changing clothes and stripping the bed.
- Restrict certain irritating beverages, such as sodas and caffeine drinks.
- Schedule bathroom trips just before retiring for the night (usually 2 or more hours after the child's bedtime).
- Consider using a urine-sensing device. These commercially available units use a buzzer or bell to awaken the child when a pad attached to the child's bedding or clothing senses moisture. The child learns to delay urination to avoid being awakened by the alarm.

Family Teaching — Poison Prevention

1. Keep all household products out of the reach of young children when not in use. When these products are in use, they should never be out of sight of adults—even if it means taking them along when answering the telephone or the doorbell.
2. Chose cleaning supplies with childproof or hard-to-open containers. Containers should be rinsed before discarding.
3. Keep household products in their original containers. They should never be stored in food containers or soft-drink bottles.
4. Label all products properly and read the label before using.
5. Don't save medicine. Discard leftover medications by flushing them down the toilet or putting them in a hazardous waste garbage collection. Current medications should be stored separately from other household products, preferably locked up. Metal boxes with locks commonly used to store checks are difficult for a child to open and can be used to store medications.
6. Return medication to safe storage immediately after using. Never leave any medication, including vitamins, aspirin, or acetaminophen by the sink or on the dining table.
7. Always turn the light on when giving or taking medications.
8. Do not take medications in front of children because youngsters tend to imitate adults.
9. Refer to medications as "medicine" and never as "candy."
10. Use safety packaging properly and close securely after use.
11. Ask the nursery for the botanic name of any new plant purchased and record it. Do not place poisonous plants in areas easily accessible to young children. Alert family members where potentially poisonous plants are already planted and supervise children carefully in those areas.
12. Always keep syrup of ipecac in the house—at least one ounce for each child—and call poison control before administering it.

- Demonstrate love and acceptance, emphasizing the child's strengths and successes.

Summary

The physical assessment of the infant, child, or adolescent incorporates many elements of the adult history and assessment. In assessing this population, however, you must also consider the influence of the child's developmental stage on the findings, including normal developmental variations in anatomy and physiology, and developmental tasks. Finally, be aware of the common health alterations in childhood, and provide health teaching to the child and family as appropriate.

Key Points

- ✓ Infants, children, and adolescents exhibit a variety of normal variations in anatomy and physiology according to their developmental stage.
- ✓ The interview of the pediatric client and parent/caregiver focuses on collection of baseline data about the child's birth history, growth and development, and psychosocial health status.
- ✓ The physical assessment of the infant, child, or adolescent consists of an assessment of general appearance and mental status, an assessment of growth and development, and a complete systems assessment.
- ✓ Nursing diagnoses associated with infants, children, and adolescents are as varied as for adults. Some of the most common include *Fear, Altered growth and development, Knowledge deficit,* and *High risk for injury.*
- ✓ Some common alterations in the health of infants, children, and adolescents include fetal alcohol syndrome, otitis media, chronic allergic rhinitis, asthma, cystic fibrosis, acne vulgaris, and physical and sexual abuse. Injuries are the leading cause of childhood disease, disability, and death.
- ✓ Client teaching is provided to the pediatric client and family as appropriate to the child's developmental stage. Some important areas for pediatric client teaching include information on preventing injuries, infections, accidents, and poisoning.

Chapter 20

Assessing the Childbearing Client

In the 1980s, the health care community increasingly began to view pregnancy as a healthy condition requiring support and monitoring rather than an alteration in health requiring medical intervention. Thus, the nurse's role in caring for the childbearing client has expanded, particularly in the area of assessment. In fact, the nurse often has the first contact with the client in the prenatal clinic or obstetrician's office, and certified nurse-midwives and nurse practitioners typically share assessment responsibilities with the physician.

Assessment of the childbearing client is directed primarily at the maintenance and promotion of health for the client and her fetus. Because pregnancy produces physical and psychosocial changes that affect all body systems, you need a knowledge of the anatomic and physiologic variations of pregnancy to care for the childbearing client. In addition, this chapter provides interview questions, one possible exam sequence, and a brief overview of some common alterations in the health of the childbearing client. Finally, some tips for promoting a healthy pregnancy also are provided. For more information, consult a maternity nursing textbook.

Anatomy and Physiology Review

Pregnancy initiates physiologic and anatomic changes in each body system that promote fetal growth and prepare the woman's body for childbirth. These changes may be quite subtle, or they may be striking alterations that would be considered abnormal, or even life-threatening, in a nonpregnant client.

Integumentary System Changes

Integumentary system changes are caused primarily by hormonal factors and the growth of the abdomen and breasts. Many of these are illustrated in Chapter 8.

Striae gravidarum, also called stretch marks, are pinkish-red streaks (in light-skinned women) with slight depressions appearing over the abdomen, breasts, and sometimes the buttocks and thighs. In dark-skinned women, the striae appear lighter than the surrounding skin. One may note silver lines in multiparous women or dark purple lines in dark-skinned women. The weight gain experienced during pregnancy, along with the expanding uterus, stretch the skin's underlying connective tissue. Striae are most noticeable in the second and third trimesters.

Changes in skin pigmentation begin early in pregnancy under the influence of estrogen, progesterone, ACTH, and melanocyte-stimulating hormone. These changes include the *linea nigra,* a dark line extending from the umbilicus to the mons pubis, and *chloasma,* a darkening of the skin on the face also referred to as the "mask of pregnancy." Other areas in which pigmentation may be altered include the breasts, the axillae, the anal area, the vulva, and the inner thighs.

Estrogen secretion also contributes to the development of pregnancy-specific vascular markings. These include *spider nevi,* tiny, bright red angiomas that appear mostly on the face, neck, chest, arms, and legs. *Palmar erythema,* a well-delineated pink area on the palmar surface of the hands, may appear in 60% of Caucasian and 35% of black women. A dusky appearance or pallor in the palms or nail beds of black women may indicate anemia. Increases in hair growth, called *hirsutism,* and increased nail growth are sometimes associated with pregnancy. Some women find a softening or thinning of the nails by the sixth week. Acne may become more pronounced or clear up completely.

Many of these integumentary changes fade or disappear completely after pregnancy. Striae become silvery white, and facial chloasma, the linea nigra, and the various vascular markings fade. Heightened breast pigmentation may remain.

Respiratory System Changes

Nasal stuffiness and a tendency toward epistaxis is common in pregnancy. During mid to late pregnancy, the diaphragm is displaced upward by approximately 4 cm. Progesterone causes relaxation of the ligaments that join the rib cage, allowing the rib cage to flare and expand.

Increased cellular growth in the client and her fetus increases oxygen requirements during pregnancy. Simultaneously, certain functional changes improve gas exchange in the alveoli. These changes include

- 30% to 40% increase in tidal volume (volume of gas moved in and out of the respiratory tract with each breath)
- 50% increase in minute volume (volume of air breathed in a minute) by term
- Increase in respiratory rate by approximately two breaths per minute
- Decreased Pa_{CO_2}, facilitating diffusion of carbon dioxide from the fetus
- Decreased functional residual capacity causing slight hyperventilation

Breasts and Axillae

Anatomic and physiologic changes in the breasts are due to the effects of estrogen and progesterone. As pregnancy progresses

- The woman may experience tingling and tenderness (in the first trimester).
- The breasts increase in size and become more nodular.
- The nipples enlarge, and the areolae darken.
- The tubercles of Montgomery enlarge.
- Superficial veins become more prominent.
- Striae may develop.
- Colostrum may be present (in the third trimester).

Cardiovascular System Changes

During pregnancy, the heart enlarges slightly because of increased blood volume and cardiac output. Additionally, the heart is displaced upward and rotated toward the left, occasionally producing systolic murmurs. Dependent edema is common as pregnancy advances. Other alterations include:

- Increase in heart rate of 10 to 15 beats per minute above prepregnant baselines
- 50% increase in cardiac output by week 32 due to increased oxygen demands
- Increased venous pressures due to uterine pressure on the inferior vena cava, called *vena caval syndrome* (Figure 20.1), sometimes accompanied by supine hypotension
- Decreased arterial blood pressure in the second trimester due to the vasodilatory effects of progesterone
- An increased risk of clot formation due to decreased venous return and increased clotting factors
- 40% increase in blood volume with a disproportionate increase in blood plasma compared to red blood cells, producing a physiologic anemia
- Elevated white blood cell counts, producing a physiologic leukocytosis
- Decreased hematocrit and hemoglobin (Blood tests should be performed to obtain a baseline. Rh factor and blood type are also important.)

Gastrointestinal System Changes

Nausea and vomiting are common in the first trimester, perhaps because of higher levels of human chorionic gonadotropin (hCG), but this relation is not proven. Emotional factors may also play a part.

Changes in the gastrointestinal system during the second and third trimesters include the following: The gums bleed more easily because of hypertrophy and increased vascularity, which are effects of estrogen. *Ptyalism,* an increase in saliva production, may occur. Mechanical pressure from the growing uterus contributes to displacement of the small intestine and reduces motility. The increased secretion of progesterone further reduces motility because of decreased gastric tone and increased smooth muscle relaxation; thus, the emptying time of the stomach and bowel is prolonged, and constipation is common. Progesterone's relaxing effect on smooth muscle also accounts for the prolonged emptying time of the gallbladder, and gallstone formation may result. Heartburn (regurgitation of the acidic contents of the stomach into the esophagus) may be related to the enlarging uterus displacing the stomach upward and to a decrease in gastrointestinal motility. Hemorrhoids are another common factor in the third trimester. They may result from the increasing size of the uterus creating pressure on the veins. If the mother is constipated, the pressure on the venous structures from straining to move the bowels can lead to hemorrhoids.

Urinary System Changes

The growing uterus causes displacement of the ureters and kidneys, especially on the right side. A slower flow of urine through the ureters causes physiologic hydronephrosis and hydroureter. Estrogen causes increased bladder vascularity, predisposing the mucosa to bleed more easily. Urinary frequency occurs in the first trimester as the uterus grows and puts pressure on the bladder. Relief from frequency occurs after the uterus moves out of the pelvis, only to return in the third trimester when the enlarged uterus again presses on the bladder.

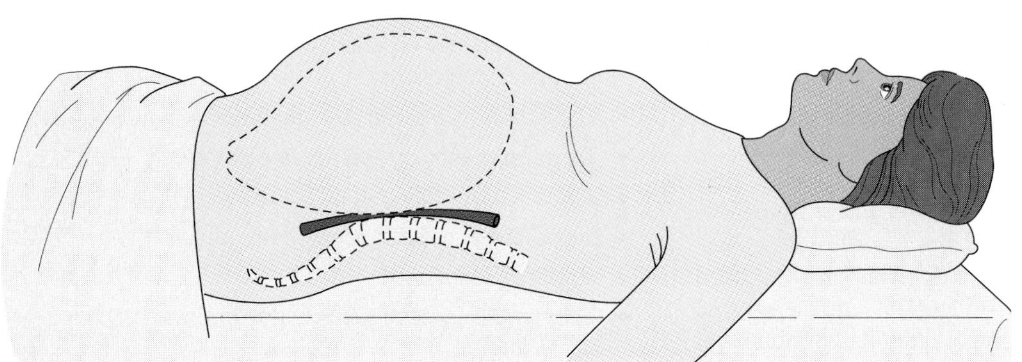

Figure 20.1 Vena caval syndrome. When the pregnant woman is supine, the uterus compresses the vena cava, reducing venous return to the heart. This in turn increases venous pressure, and may cause hypotension, faintness, and dizziness.

The functional changes in the urinary system include

- Increased renal blood flow by as much as 50% by the third trimester
- Increased glomerular filtration rate by as much as 50% above prepregnancy levels
- Decreased resorption of filtered glucose in the renal tubules, contributing to glycosuria

Reproductive System Changes

Externally, the labia majora, labia minora, clitoris, and vaginal introitus enlarge because of hypertrophy and increased vascularity, which also gives the vagina a bluish tinge. During pregnancy, the isthmus of the uterus softens (Hegar's sign), as does the cervix (Goodell's sign). Because of increased vascularity, the cervix takes on a bluish tinge (Chadwick's sign). Cervical mucus is thick and tenacious, forming a mucous plug that protects the uterus.

Internal reproductive changes result from hormonal influences and the growth of the fetus. The formation of ovarian follicles and ovulation cease once conception occurs. The uterine endometrium thickens, and uterine blood vessels increase in number and size.

Uterine size increases to approximately 28 × 24 × 21 cm, and uterine weight increases to about 1000 g (Figure 20.2). The growing uterus can be palpated abdominally by about 10–12 weeks, at which time the uterine fundus is slightly above the symphysis pubis. At 16 weeks, the fundus is halfway between the symphysis and umbilicus. Between 20 and 22 weeks, the fundus reaches the umbilicus. Fundal height after midpregnancy is variable, but you should observe a consistent increase in fundal height until 36 weeks. Between 38 and 40 weeks, fetal descent occurs, and the fundal height drops gradually. (See Figure 20.7 on page 646.)

Musculoskeletal System Changes

Anatomic changes in the musculoskeletal system result from the influence of hormones, growth of the fetus, and maternal weight gain. As pregnancy advances, the growing uterus tilts the pelvis forward, increasing the lumbosacral curve and creating a gradual lordosis. The enlarging breasts pull the shoulders forward, and the client may assume a stoop-shouldered stance. The pelvic joints and ligaments are relaxed by progesterone and relaxin. The rectus abdominis muscles may separate during the third trimester, allowing the abdominal contents to protrude. The weight of the uterus and breasts, along with the relaxation of the pelvic joints, changes the client's center of gravity, stance, and gait. Backaches are a common

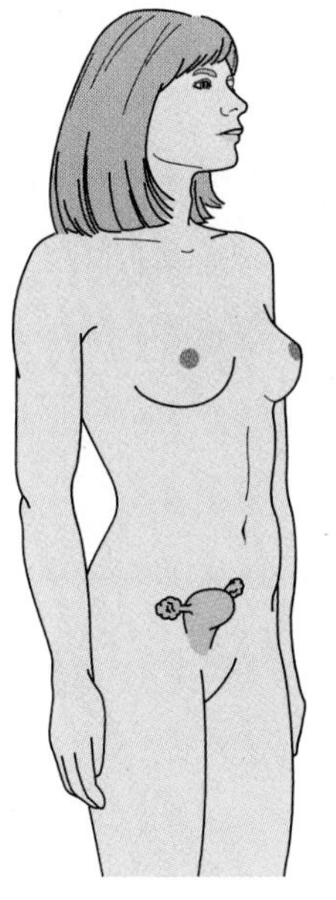

A before conception

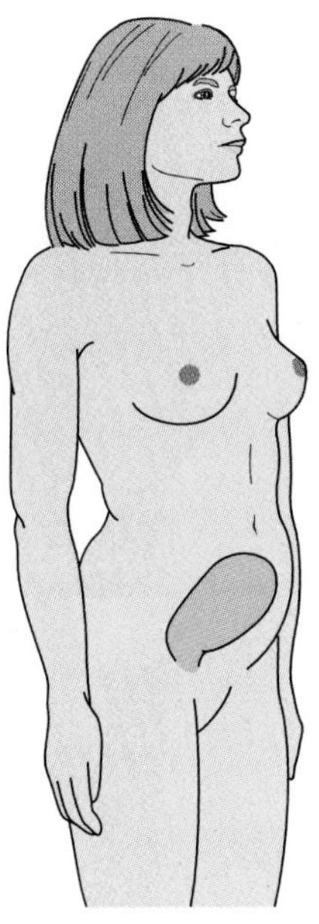

B 4 months

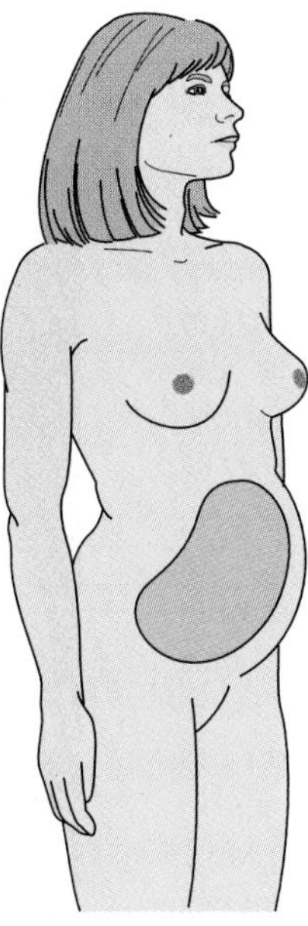

C 7 months

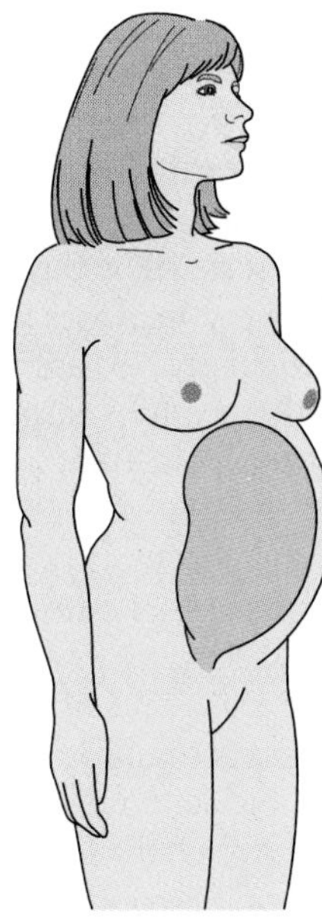

D 9 months

Figure 20.2 Relative size of the uterus before conception and at different stages of pregnancy.

complaint. Shoe size, especially width, may increase permanently.

Neurologic System Changes

Neurologic changes frequently associated with pregnancy include

- Entrapment neuropathies due to mechanical pressures in the peripheral nervous system
- *Meralgia paresthetica* (pain, numbness, and a prickly or tingling feeling in the thigh) caused by pressure on the lateral femoral cutaneous nerve
- Carpal tunnel syndrome (pressure on the median nerve beneath the carpal ligament of the wrist) causing burning, tingling, and pain in the hand
- Leg cramps, which may be caused by inadequate intake of calcium
- Dizziness and light-headedness, which may be associated with vena caval syndrome.

Endocrine System Changes

Changes in the endocrine system facilitate the metabolic functions that maintain maternal and fetal health throughout the pregnancy. The pituitary, thyroid, parathyroid, and adrenal glands enlarge because of estrogen stimulation and increased vascularity. Oxytocin, secreted by the posterior pituitary, stimulates uterine contractions and causes milk ejection in the mammary glands. Prolactin, secreted by the anterior pituitary, facilitates lactation after delivery. Increases in the production of thyroid hormones, particularly T3 and T4, increase the basal metabolic rate (BMR), cardiac output, vasodilation, heart rate, and heat intolerance. The BMR may increase by as much as 30% by term.

In early pregnancy, insulin production increases in response to the rise in serum levels of estrogen, progesterone, and other hormones. In addition, the mother's body tissues develop an increased sensitivity to insulin, thus decreasing the mother's need. The result is a build-up of insulin during the first half of pregnancy. This build-up of insulin ensures an adequate supply of glucose, which the fetus requires in large amounts. In the second half of pregnancy, maternal hormones cause an increased resistance to insulin, resulting in a breakdown of insulin stores during fasting periods. A disruption in this delicate homeostatic balance results in gestational diabetes mellitus.

Gathering the Data

Focused Interview

The first prenatal visit focuses on collection of baseline data about the client and her partner, identification of risk factors, and establishment of a trusting nurse-client relationship (Figure 20.3). The format and questions vary with the stage of pregnancy. Most of the following questions are appropriate for an initial visit in the first trimester. Note that the following questions amplify the information gathered during the complete health history as described in Chapter 2. If the complete health history is not available prior to the first prenatal visit, be sure to collect this information during the first prenatal visit.

1. What is your age? *Women under the age of 15 and over the age of 35 have increased age-related risks during pregnancy. The adolescent client is at increased risk for inadequate dietary intake, leading to iron-deficiency anemia, pregnancy-induced hypertension, sexually transmitted dis-*

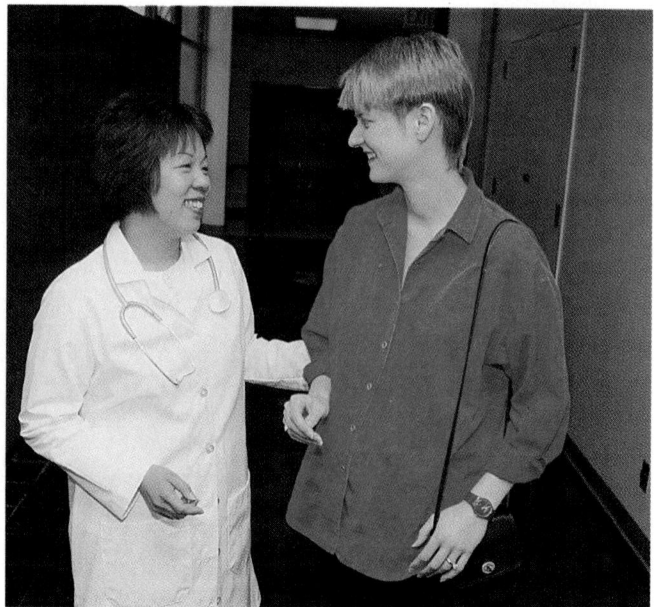

Figure 20.3 Greeting the pregnant client.

eases, preterm delivery, and a low-birth-weight infant. The client over 35 years is at increased risk for pregnancy-induced hypertension, cesarean delivery, and neonatal morbidity and mortality related to chromosomal abnormalities.

2. Who lives at home with you? *This question explores marital status in an indirect manner, thus decreasing the anxiety that unwed pregnant women may feel. In addition, identifying significant persons with whom the client resides gives you insight into the family structure and possible support systems.*

Present Pregnancy

1. What leads you to believe you are pregnant? *The client will most likely report subjective signs of pregnancy, such as absence of menstrual periods, nausea, vomiting, breast tenderness, fatigue, abdominal enlargement, or urinary frequency.*
2. When was the date of your last menstrual period (LMP)? *The estimated date of delivery (EDD) is usually calculated by using the first day of the LMP, which may also be useful in estimating gestational age.*
3. Describe your usual menstrual cycle. *The typical menstrual cycle is 28 days in length. Prolonged, shortened, or irregular menstrual cycles affect the EDD.*
4. Have you had any cramping, bleeding, or spotting since your LMP? *Cramping, bleeding, or spotting may indicate a problem with hormonal support of the endometrium and may lead to a spontaneous abortion.*
5. Was this pregnancy planned? *Confirmation of pregnancy usually causes ambivalent feelings whether or not the pregnancy was planned. If the pregnancy was unplanned, you need to assess the couple's desire to maintain the pregnancy and explain available options. If the pregnancy was planned, the couple usually develops more positive thoughts as it progresses.*
6. Have you experienced any discomfort or unusual occurrences since your LMP? *The client's response allows you to evaluate whether the symptoms reported are expected or if they suggest development of a complication. Client teaching and other nursing interventions can also be identified.*
7. Do you perform a monthly breast self-examination? If so, describe the procedure you follow. *This information gives insight into the client's self-care practices.*
8. What is your typical food intake in a 24-hour period? What are your food likes and dislikes? *The increased growth of the mother and fetus requires an increased intake of nutrients, especially carbohydrates and proteins. Assessment of present nutritional status provides a diet history that serves as a basis for future teaching and intervention.*
9. What is your regular exercise pattern? *Assessment of exercise or physical activity provides information regarding the client's self-care practices. See the tips for exercise later in this chapter.*
10. What type of health care do you typically receive? *Assessment of the client's pre-pregnant health care provides information regarding the client's self-care practices. Although many young women may not be frequent users of the health care system, activities such as regular dental and vision exams and annual Papanicolaou smears indicate good self-care.*
11. Do you have a cat? If so, how do you change its litter? *Toxoplasmosis from infected cat litter may have teratogenic effects on the developing fetus.*
12. How much alcohol, tobacco, and caffeine do you consume each day? *Alcohol exposure may harm the fetus. Women who smoke give birth to smaller infants than those who do not smoke. Caffeine intake has been associated with newborn withdrawal behaviors.*
13. Do you use any drugs such as marijuana, cocaine, or heroin? If so, which ones and how much do you use each day? *These drugs are addicting to both the client and the fetus, and increase the risk of complications during pregnancy and birth. Additionally, use of addicting drugs increases the risk of poor nutrition, and IV drug use increases the risk of infections such as hepatitis B and HIV.*

Previous Pregnancies and Outcomes

1. Have you been pregnant before? How many times? *Multiparity, especially if there have been more than three previous pregnancies, increases the maternal risks of antepartal and postpartal hemorrhage and fetal/neonatal anemia.*
2. Have you had any spontaneous or induced abortions? *Previous history of spontaneous abortion (miscarriage or stillbirth) places the client at higher risk for subsequent spontaneous abortions. Induced abortions may cause trauma to the cervix and may interfere with cervical dilation and effacement during labor.*
3. Describe any previous pregnancies, including the length of the pregnancy, the length of labor, problems during pregnancy, medications taken during pregnancy, prenatal care received, type of birth; and your perception of the experience. *Discussion of the client's previous pregnancies helps you anticipate needs and complications of the current pregnancy.*
4. Describe your birth experience, including labor or delivery complications, the infant's condition at birth, the infant's weight, and whether the infant required additional treatment or special care after birth. *Reviewing the client's previous birth experience(s) helps you to anticipate needs and complications of the current pregnancy and to assess the client's current knowledge base and the success with which the client integrated the previous birth experience into her life experiences.*

5. Do you attend or plan to attend prenatal education classes? *Assessment of prenatal education provides information on the client's current knowledge base and attitude toward education for self-care.*
6. What are your expectations for this pregnancy? *Identification of the client's desires helps you provide guidance in formulating the birth plan in the present pregnancy.*

Gynecologic History

1. Do you experience any discomfort during menstruation? If so, describe the discomfort. *Secondary dysmenorrhea involving pain in various pelvic locations may indicate anatomic anomalies or endometriosis, which may cause complications during pregnancy or birth.*
2. Have you ever had a vaginal infection or sexually transmitted infection? *Reproductive system infections may be transmitted to the fetus transplacentally or through contact with the birth canal.*
3. Have you had any reproductive tract surgery? *Previous uterine surgery increases the client's risk for spontaneous preterm labor and birth.*
4. What birth-control method did you use prior to this pregnancy? *If the woman became pregnant while using birth control pills, the fetus is at risk for birth defects. If the woman became pregnant while using an intrauterine device (IUD), the risk of spontaneous abortion increases.*
5. When was your last Pap smear, and what was the result? *Papanicolaou smears identify normal and abnormal cervical cells to detect the presence of cancer.*

Family Health History

1. Is there a history of genetic or congenital birth defects in your family or your partner's family? If so, please describe these. *Genetic or congenital birth defects may be familial. You may need to explain to the client what genetic and congenital defects are.*
2. Have any members of your family or your partner's family had any of the following conditions: diabetes mellitus, heart disease, hypertension, kidney problems, multiple gestations, bleeding disorders, or allergies? *You need to assess the family medical history to identify and investigate risk factors thoroughly.*

Psychosocial Health History

1. Describe your feelings about your pregnancy. *Confirmation of pregnancy frequently produces ambivalent feelings in the client. Further assessment may be required.*
2. Describe how you usually cope with stress. *Pregnancy is both physically and psychologically stressful. Early assessment of the client's abilities helps you identify nursing diagnoses related to the client's problem-solving abilities.*
3. Have you ever had any emotional problems? If so, describe them. *Pregnancy can be a time of crisis for the client with a history of emotional disturbances. Frequent psychosocial assessments help you detect any problems early. The client may require referral for psychologic care.*
4. How do you think your religious beliefs will affect your pregnancy? *Religious beliefs may influence health practices during pregnancy. For example, some religions prohibit blood transfusions.*
5. How does your partner feel about the pregnancy? *The attitude of the client's partner may influence the psychologic health of the client. A nonsupportive attitude may adversely affect the client's health, and a positive attitude may help the client cope with the stress of pregnancy.*
6. Who are your most important support persons? *You need to encourage active involvement of the support persons during the client's pregnancy.*
7. What is your highest educational level? *The client's educational level may influence her attitude about the pregnancy, her understanding about the changes of pregnancy, and her decisions regarding her prenatal care and birthing plans.*
8. What is your occupation? *Identifying the client's occupation helps you identify environmental teratogens, physically exhausting work, level of job stress, and in some cases, the client's economic status.*

Partner's Health History

1. Does your partner have any of the following conditions: congenital or genetic diseases, bleeding disorders, cancer, cardiac disease, diabetes, epilepsy, hepatitis, hypertension, renal disease, or psychiatric problems? *Assessment of the partner's health history provides information on potential inherited disorders and the psychologic stability of the partner.*
2. How much alcohol and tobacco does your partner consume each day? *Alcohol abuse in the partner may affect the client's health. Exposure to second-hand smoke poses risks similar to those of smoking.*
3. Does your partner use any drugs such as marijuana, cocaine, or heroin? If so, which ones and how much does he use? *Substance abuse in the partner may affect the client's health. If the partner uses IV drugs, the client is at risk for HIV transmission.*
4. What is your partner's educational level and occupation? *Knowledge of the partner's educational level and occupation provides information about socioeconomic status and the partner's ability to offer support to the client.*
5. What is your partner's blood type and Rh factor? *The partner's blood type and Rh factor is significant to the Rh-negative client. If the client is Rh negative and her partner is Rh positive, then she will receive RhoGAM at 28–32 weeks as a preventive measure.*

Physical Assessment

Preparation

- ☑ **Gather the equipment:**

sterile specimen container	stethoscope
dipsticks	Doppler stethoscope or fetoscope
examination light	pelvimeter
examination gloves	water-soluble lubricant
examination gown	vaginal speculum
drape	cotton applicators
centimeter measuring tape	cervical spatula
sphygmomanometer	glass slides

- ☑ **Wash your hands.**
- ☑ **Ask the client to void before beginning the exam to decrease discomfort with the pelvic exam. Instruct the client in providing a clean-catch, midstream urine specimen, and give the client a sterile container. Perform a dipstick check for glucose, protein, ketones, and albumin. Send the remaining urine to the laboratory for a urinalysis if this is the client's first prenatal visit.**
- ☑ **The following blood tests are common at the first prenatal visit: CBC, blood type, Rh status, rubella titer, serologic test for syphilis, and sickle-cell anemia screen for clients of African ancestry. Clients with a history of IV drug use, sexual intercourse with an IV drug user, or multiple sexual partners should be tested also for hepatitis B and HIV. In most clinical settings, these tests are performed by a laboratory technician, but you should be comfortable explaining the rationale for these tests to the client.**

Remember

- Provide a warm, comfortable environment.
- Explain the procedure to the client to allay any fear or apprehension.
- Ensure the client's privacy.
- Before assessing the pelvic region, put on gloves. As always, if you notice any skin drainage, blood, or other body fluids, put on gloves before proceeding with the exam.

ASSESSMENT TECHNIQUE/NORMAL FINDINGS | SPECIAL CONSIDERATIONS

General Survey

Step 1 ***Measure the client's height and weight.***

At the initial exam, you take these measurements to establish a baseline (Figure 20.4). In the first trimester, the client should gain 2–4 pounds. The client should gain an additional 11–12 pounds in both the second and the third trimesters, for a total weight gain of about 24–28 pounds, an average of 2.7–3.1 pounds per month.

A gain of 6 pounds or more per month may be associated with pregnancy-induced hypertension and fluid retention, and a gain of less than 2.5 pounds per month may indicate insufficient nourishment or insufficient utilization of nutrients.

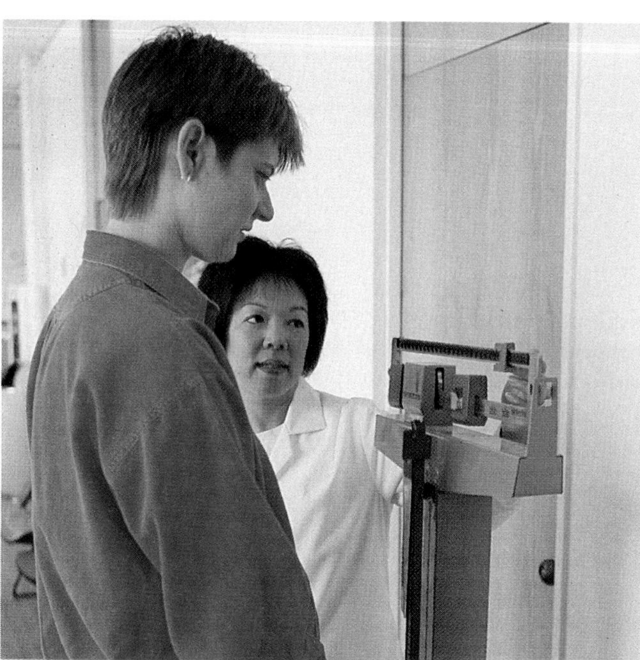

Figure 20.4 Weighing the client.

Step 2 ***Assess the client's general appearance and mental status.***

Marked anxiety or apathy may indicate unresolved issues related to acceptance or rejection of the pregnancy.

Step 3 ***Take the client's vital signs.***

- Assess the client's temperature, pulse, respirations, and blood pressure.

An elevated temperature may be related to a vaginal or urinary tract infection. Slight hyperventilation may accompany pregnancy because the uterus applies pressure to the diaphragm. After 20 weeks increased blood pressure readings may be associated with pregnancy-induced hypertension (PIH), and decreases may indicate supine hypotensive syndrome.

Step 4 ***Observe the client in sitting and standing positions.***

In pregnancy, there is usually an accentuated lumbar spinal curve, and the shoulders may be slumped forward, causing backaches (Figure 20.5).

ASSESSMENT TECHNIQUE/NORMAL FINDINGS	SPECIAL CONSIDERATIONS

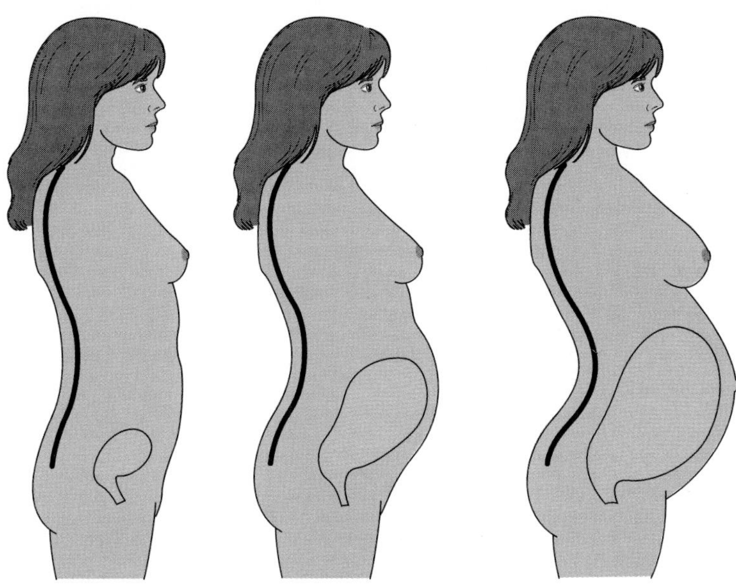

Figure 20.5 Postural changes during pregnancy.

Step 5 *Help the client into a sitting position* (Figure 20.6).

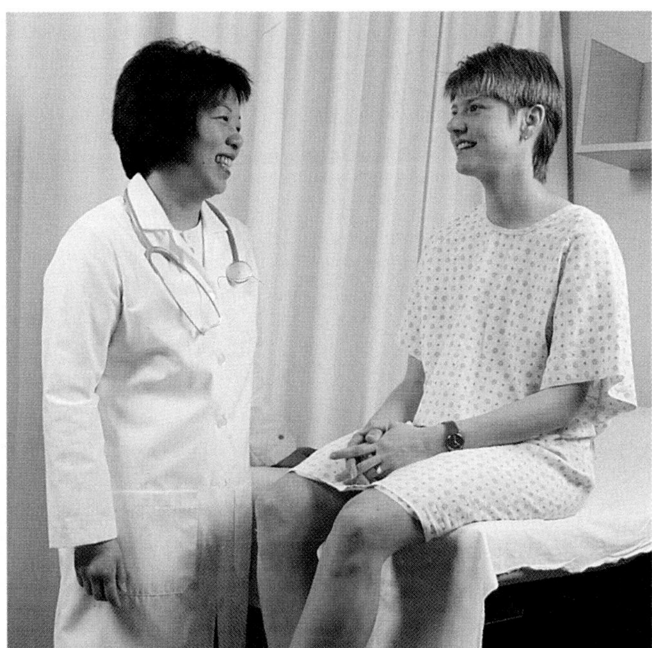

Figure 20.6 Positioning the client.

ASSESSMENT TECHNIQUE/NORMAL FINDINGS	SPECIAL CONSIDERATIONS

Skin

Step 1 ***Observe the skin for pigmentary changes associated with pregnancy.***

These include spider nevi, striae gravidarum, and chloasma. Remember the differences in skin changes in dark-skinned women.

Step 2 ***Observe the skin for the vascular markings associated with pregnancy.***

These include angiomas, palmar erythema, and palmar pallor.

Head and Neck

Step 1 ***Inspect the nasal mucosa.***

- Look for changes related to pregnancy, such as edema and redness. Nasal stuffiness or nosebleeds may occur in response to increased estrogen.

Step 2 ***Inspect the mouth.***

- Look for hypertrophy of the gingival tissue.

Inflammation of gingival tissue may indicate infection. Paleness of the gums may indicate anemia. Bleeding may occur with toothbrushing or dental exams.

Step 3 ***Palpate the neck for nontender, small, mobile nodes.***

Hard, tender, fixed, or prominent nodes could indicate infection or carcinoma.

Step 4 ***Palpate the thyroid.***

- Assess for slight hyperplasia after the third month of pregnancy.

Enlargement of the thyroid indicates hyperthyroidism.

The Lungs

Step 1 ***Inspect, palpate, and percuss the chest.***

- Note diaphragmatic expansion and character of respirations. Later in pregnancy, pressure from the growing uterus produces a change from abdominal to thoracic breathing.

Intercostal space retractions with inspiration, bulging with expiration, or unequal expansion are signs of respiratory distress.

- Observe for symmetric expansion with no retraction or bulging of the intercostal spaces.

Step 2 ***Auscultate breath sounds.***

- Confirm that the lungs are clear in all fields.

Rales, rhonchi, wheezes, rubs, absence of sounds, and unequal breath sounds are signs of respiratory distress.

ASSESSMENT TECHNIQUE/NORMAL FINDINGS | SPECIAL CONSIDERATIONS

The Heart

Step 1 *Assist the client to a supine position.*

Step 2 *Auscultate heart sounds.*

Confirm that the rhythm is regular and that the rate is from 70–90 beats per minute. The heart rate in pregnancy increases 10–15 beats per minute above the baseline. Short systolic murmurs are due to increased blood volume and displacement of the heart.

Thrills, thrusts, skipped beats, gross irregularity, and gallop rhythm may signal cardiac disease.

Breasts and Axillae

Step 1 *Inspect the breasts.*

Pregnancy-associated changes include enlargement, increased pigmentation of the areolae, presence of prominent superficial veins, presence of striae, enlargement of tubercles of Montgomery, and presence of colostrum after the twelfth week.

Flat or inverted nipples will interfere with breast-feeding. Nipple rolling and stimulation with a towel are controversial. The client may be able to use a syringe to evert nipples after delivery for breast feeding (Kesaree et al 1993).

Step 2 *Palpate the breasts for tenderness and nodules.*

Breasts become nodular and tingling sensations may be felt during pregnancy.

Abdomen

Step 1 *Auscultate bowel sounds.*

Step 2 *Inspect and palpate the abdomen.*

- Note the appearance of the skin, linea nigra, and the size and the contour of the abdomen. Confirm the absence of masses.

Palpable masses or nodules may indicate cancer or ectopic pregnancy. A distended bladder and inability to void may indicate urinary retention.

Step 3 *Assess fundal height.*

- Measure the distance in centimeters from the top of the symphysis pubis to the top of the fundus (Figure 20.7).

Increased fundal height is associated with multiple pregnancies, polyhydramnios, and hydatidiform moles. Decreased fundal height is associated with fetal growth retardation, fetal death, and fetal abnormalities. Variations may also indicate an error in the calculation of the gestational week.

ASSESSMENT TECHNIQUE/NORMAL FINDINGS | SPECIAL CONSIDERATIONS

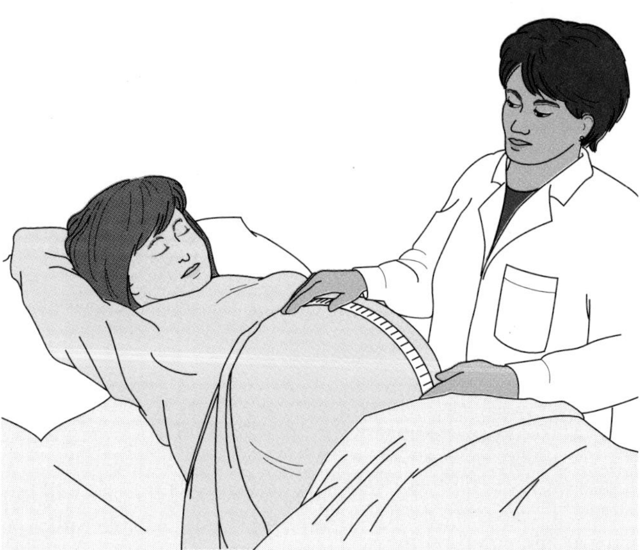

Figure 20.7 Measuring fundal height.

At 12 weeks, the fundus is at the symphysis pubis. At 20 weeks, the fundus is at the level of the umbilicus. After 20 weeks, the fundus approximates the weeks of gestation; for example, fundal height of 28 cm indicates 28 weeks gestation (Figure 20.8).

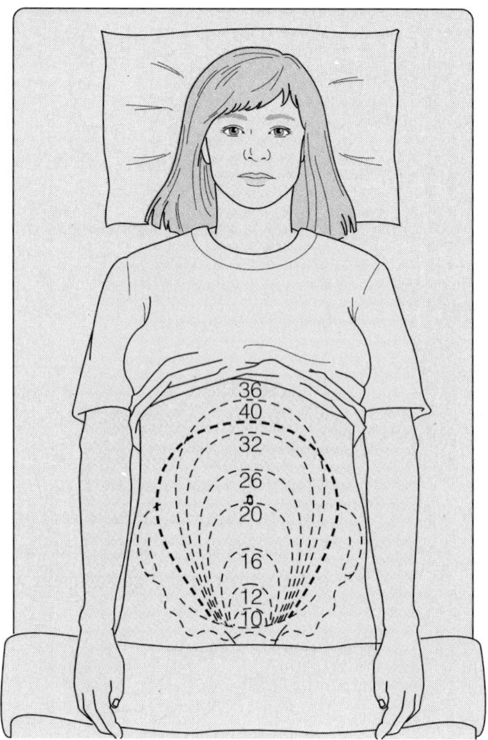

Figure 20.8 Fundal height measurements during specific gestational weeks.

ASSESSMENT TECHNIQUE/NORMAL FINDINGS | SPECIAL CONSIDERATIONS

Extremities

Step 1 *Inspect the lower extremities for varicose veins.*

Mild varicose veins in later pregnancy are normal.

Step 2 *Inspect and palpate the extremities for edema.*

In the late second and third trimester, edema in the hands and ankles is normal.

Marked edema requires physician referral. Redness, heat, and pain in the legs may indicate thrombophlebitis.

Step 3 *Assess the patellar reflexes*

Normal response is +2; reflexes should be equal in both extremities.

Hyperreflexia (+3) and clonus are signs of preeclampsia, a type of pregnancy-induced hypertension (PIH). Refer to a physician.

Pelvic Region

See Chapter 15 for a complete discussion of assessment of the pelvic region, including specific instructions for using a speculum and taking a Papanicolaou smear.

Step 1 *Assist the client into the lithotomy position with the thighs flexed.*

- Ask the client to move her buttocks slightly beyond the end of the examination table and position her legs in the stirrups (Figure 20.9).

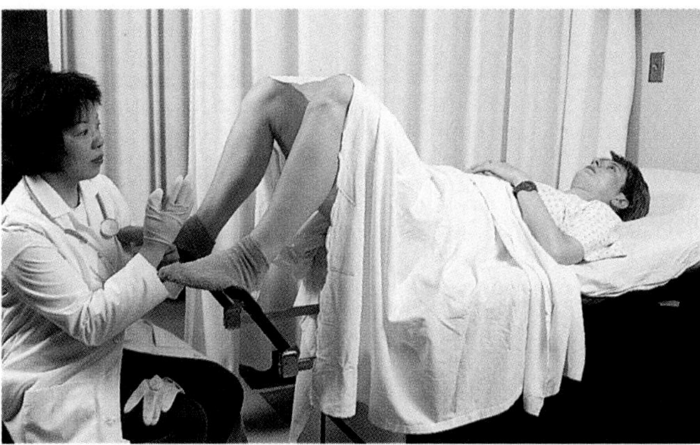

Figure 20.9 Assisting the client into the lithotomy position.

- Drape the client's legs so that a flap is over the perineum, allowing easy exposure.
- Wash your hands and put on gloves.

Step 2 *Inspect the external genitals.*

- Note appearance, pubic hair distribution, and vaginal discharge.

The labia should be pink or purplish in color, and there may be a slight increase in white discharge.

Redness or irritation of the external genitals may indicate irritation or infection. Bloody, pink, mucousy, or watery discharge may signal preterm labor. Bloody discharge may also signal placental separation. A yellowish-white discharge may indicate infection.

ASSESSMENT TECHNIQUE/NORMAL FINDINGS	SPECIAL CONSIDERATIONS

Step 3 *Visualize the cervix.*

- Gently insert a prewarmed vaginal speculum until the cervix can be visualized. (See Chapter 15.)

Step 4 *Inspect the cervix.*

- Note position and color.

There should be no lesions or ulcerations. A clear or white odorless discharge is normal. The cervix of the pregnant client at 8–11 weeks is a bluish color (Chadwick's sign). In the mulitpara, the cervix has a slit-like appearance.

An infection of the cervix may present with a thick, purulent discharge of mucus, as with gonorrhea; pinpoint vesicles in a reddened base as with herpes simplex II; profuse whitish bubbly discharge and petechial spots on the vaginal wall as in trichomoniasis; or a thick white "cheesy" discharge with monilial infection.

Step 5 *Obtain a Papanicolaou smear if indicated.*

- Remember to swab the endocervix, cervical os, and vaginal pool. (See Chapter 15.)

Step 6 *Unlock and remove the speculum.*

If the speculum is not unlocked and partially collapsed, it will cause excessive stretching and pain.

- Observe the walls of the vagina as you withdraw the speculum.

Early in pregnancy, the vagina assumes a bluish color. As the pregnancy progresses, the vagina distends, becomes smooth, and there is a localized dryness of the mucosa.

Step 7 *Palpate the uterus bimanually.*

- Insert the lubricated index and middle fingers of one gloved hand into the vagina.
- Palpate the woman's abdomen with the other, pressing down toward the hand in the vagina until the uterus is palpated between the two hands (Figure 20.10).

An extremely retroverted uterus will not be palpable abdominally.

ASSESSMENT TECHNIQUE/NORMAL FINDINGS	SPECIAL CONSIDERATIONS

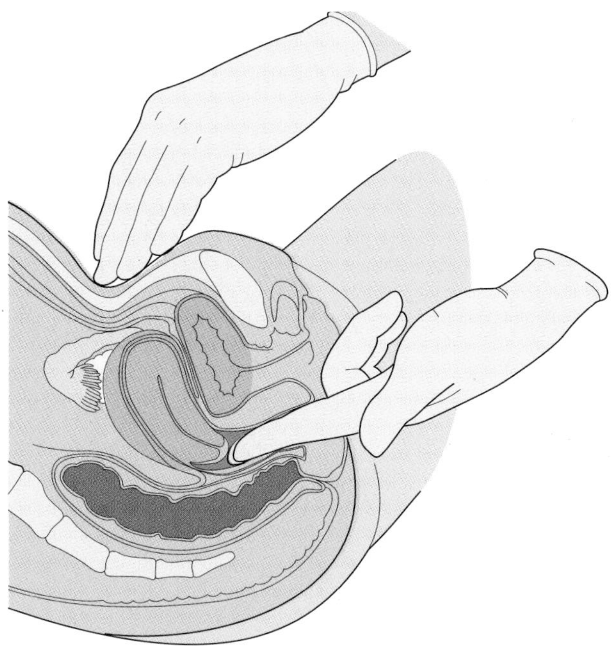

Figure 20.10 Bimanual palpation of the uterus.

Step 8 *Palpate the ovaries bimanually.*

Palpable ovarian cysts require physician referral.

Pelvic Adequacy

The pelvis is assessed to determine whether its size is adequate for a vaginal birth. Physicians and nurses with special preparation may perform this assessment and interpret pelvimetry findings. Clinical pelvimetry is performed in a systematic manner, beginning with the anterior pelvis, proceeding to the lateral walls, and concluding with the posterior and inferior portions.

Step 1 *Estimate the angle of the subpubic angle.*

- Confirm that the angle is slightly more than 90 degrees (Figure 20.11).

Vaginal birth may be difficult if the subpubic angle is less than 90 degrees.

ASSESSMENT TECHNIQUE/NORMAL FINDINGS	SPECIAL CONSIDERATIONS

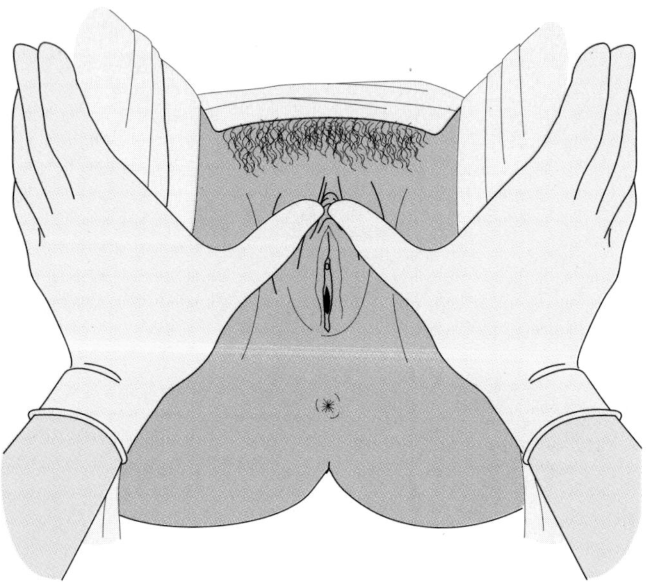

Figure 20.11 Estimating the angle of the subpubic angle.

Step 2 *Estimate the height and inclination of the symphysis pubis.*

The height should be short and the inclination gradual, not steep (Figure 20.12).

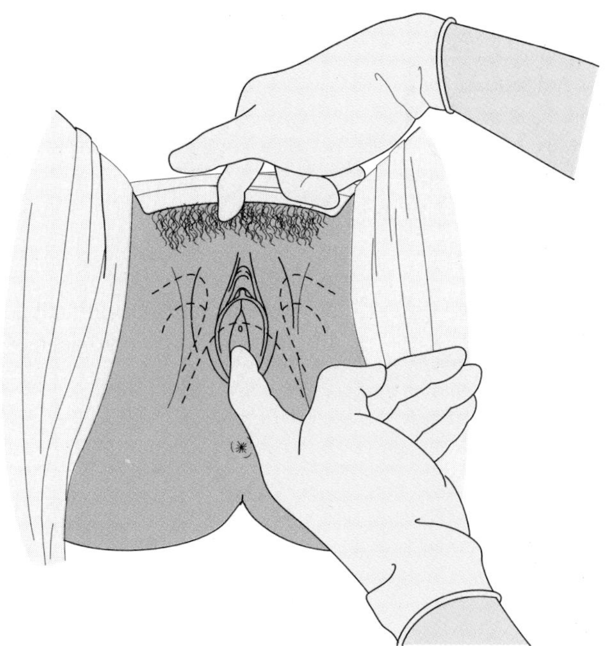

Figure 20.12 Measuring height and inclination of symphysis pubis.

ASSESSMENT TECHNIQUE/NORMAL FINDINGS	SPECIAL CONSIDERATIONS

Step 3 *Palpate the lateral walls of the pelvis.*

- Determine if they are straight, convergent, or divergent.

Convergent side walls make the internal pelvis more narrow as it approaches the vagina and may interfere with a vaginal birth.

Step 4 *Palpate the ischial spines.*

- Move the examining fingers in a straight line from one spine to the other.

Ischial spines are normally small and not prominent, and the interspinous diameter is at least 10.5 cm (Figure 20.13).

Prominent ischial spines and/or large spines decrease the interspinous diameter, impeding fetal passage through the pelvic cavity.

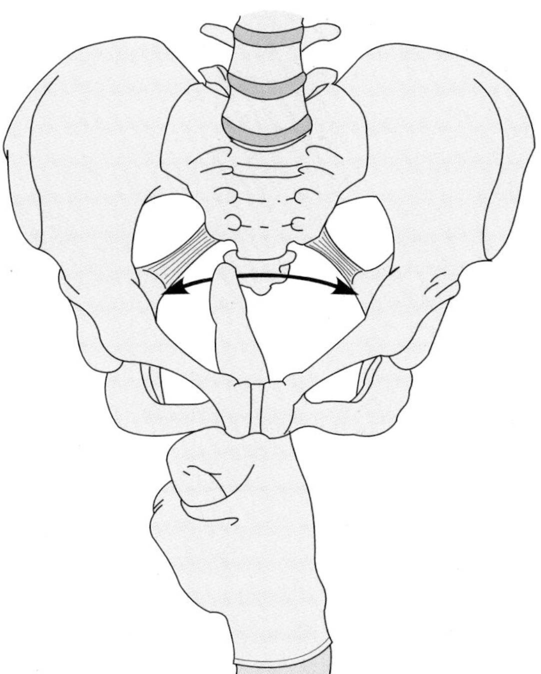

Figure 20.13 Palpating the ischial spines to measure interspinous diameter.

Step 5 *Examine the sacrum and the coccyx.*

- Sweep the fingers down the sacrum, noting whether it is concave, straight, or convex.
- Gently press the coccyx back to determine its mobility.

A pelvis with a deeply curved or flat sacrum and an immobile coccyx may inhibit vaginal birth.

Step 6 *Measure the diagonal conjugate.*

The diagonal conjugate suggests the anteroposterior diameter of the pelvic inlet, the first opening through which the fetal head must pass.

- Gently press inward and upward until your middle finger touches the sacral prominence (Figure 20.14, *A*).

Because the diameter of the fetal head at term is approximately 9 cm, a diagonal conjugate of less than 12.5 cm may prevent a vaginal birth.

ASSESSMENT TECHNIQUE/NORMAL FINDINGS

SPECIAL CONSIDERATIONS

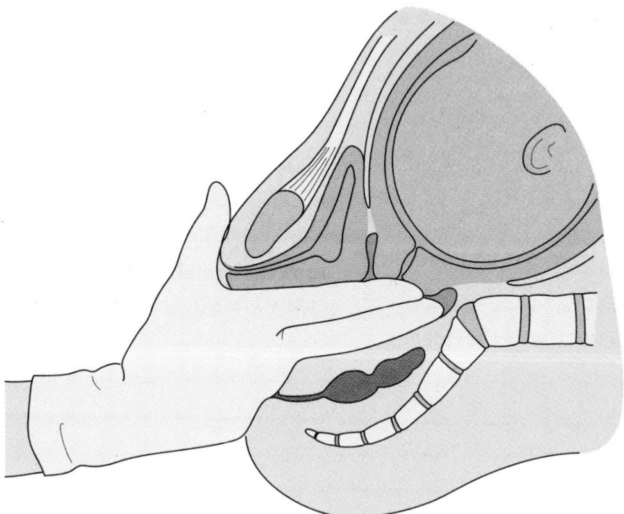

A

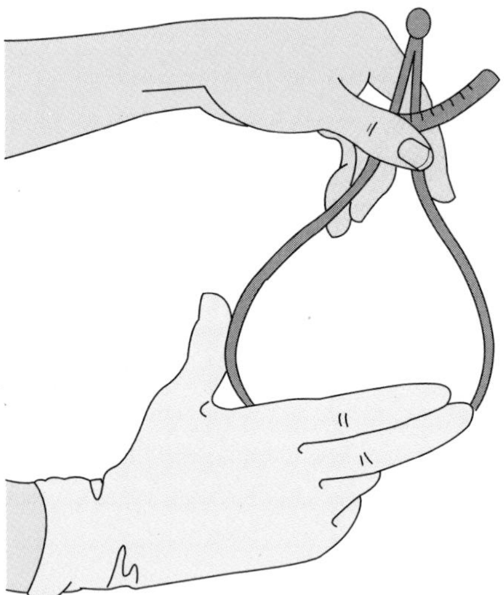

B

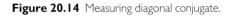

Figure 20.14 Measuring diagonal conjugate.

- Using your other hand, mark the part of the examining hand that is directly below the symphysis pubis.
- With the pelvimeter, measure the distance from the tip of your middle finger to the spot marked. (Figure 20.14, *B*). Pelvic adequacy is expected if this measurement is 12.5 cm or more.

ASSESSMENT TECHNIQUE/NORMAL FINDINGS | SPECIAL CONSIDERATIONS

Step 7 *Calculate the obstetric conjugate.*

The obstetric conjugate, also called the true conjugate (or conjugate vera), is the smallest anteroposterior diameter through which the fetal head must pass.

- Subtract 1.5 to 2 cm from the diagonal conjugate. The obstetric conjugate should measure 10.5 to 11 cm.

If the measurement is less than 10.0 cm, the fetal head may not be able to pass through the pelvis.

Step 8 *Measure the transverse diameter of the pelvic outlet.*

- Make a fist and place it between the ischial tuberosities (Figure 20.15). The diameter is usually 10 to 11 cm.

You must know the measurement of your own fist to use this technique.

Diameters of less than 10 cm may inhibit fetal descent toward the vagina.

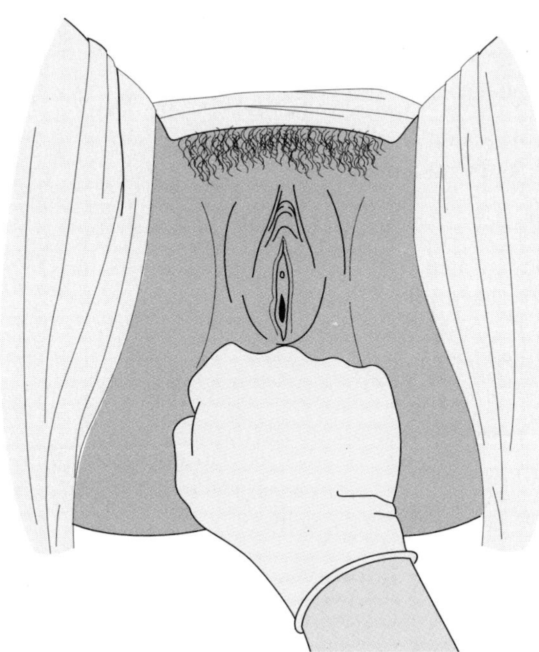

Figure 20.15 Measuring the transverse diameter of the pelvic outlet with a closed fist.

Anus and Rectum

Step 1 *Assist the client to a lateral position.*

Step 2 *Inspect the anus and rectum.*

- Lift the buttocks and inspect.

The mucosa should be pink, intact, and free from lumps, lesions, tears, or discharge.

Hemorrhoids or varicosities of the veins around the anus and rectum may be present. These are caused by pressure from the gravid uterus and constipation. Masses or nodules may indicate cancer.

ASSESSMENT TECHNIQUE/NORMAL FINDINGS

SPECIAL CONSIDERATIONS

Assessing the Fetus

Assessment of fetal activity, heart rate, and position provides you with data regarding fetal well-being.

Step 1 *Assist the client to a supine position.*

Step 2 *Ask the client about her fetus' activity patterns.*

The first movement should be felt at 18 weeks in multiparous clients and 20 weeks in primiparous clients. After 27 to 28 weeks, the client should report more than 10 fetal movements in a 12-hour period.

> ### Referral
> Marked decrease in fetal activity, or cessation of movement, may indicate fetal compromise, requiring immediate physician referral.

Step 3 *Auscultate the fetal heart rate.*

After 10–12 weeks' gestation, the fetal heart rate is audible with a Doppler stethoscope and should be assessed at each prenatal visit.

- Place the Doppler (with conductive gel) on the client's abdomen midway between the umbilicus and the symphysis, in the midline.
- Move the Doppler until you hear the fetal heartbeat.

Note that after 19–20 weeks, an ordinary fetoscope may be used. The fetoscope is placed over the area where the fetal back has been palpated.

The normal fetal heart rate is between 120–160 beats per minute, and the rhythm is regular.

If the fetal heart rate is above 160 or below 120 beats per minute, refer the client to a physician.

Step 4 *Assess fetal lie.*

- Inspect the client's abdomen to determine whether the uterus is longest longitudinally or transversely.

At term, most clients will demonstrate a longitudinal lie.

The fetus in a persistent transverse lie or breech will most likely require a cesarean delivery.

Step 5 *Assess the position and presentation of the fetus.*

After 32–34 weeks, the position, presentation, and attitude of the fetus can be assessed through four abdominal palpations referred to as Leopold's maneuvers (Table 20.1).

Table 20.1 Leopold's Maneuvers to Determine Fetal Position and Presentation

Leopold's maneuvers are a systematic way of palpating the maternal abdomen. These maneuvers require frequent practice and skill and may be difficult to perform on an obese person or a person who has excessive amniotic fluid. Note that the woman's bladder should be empty. The woman should be supine with the knees bent.

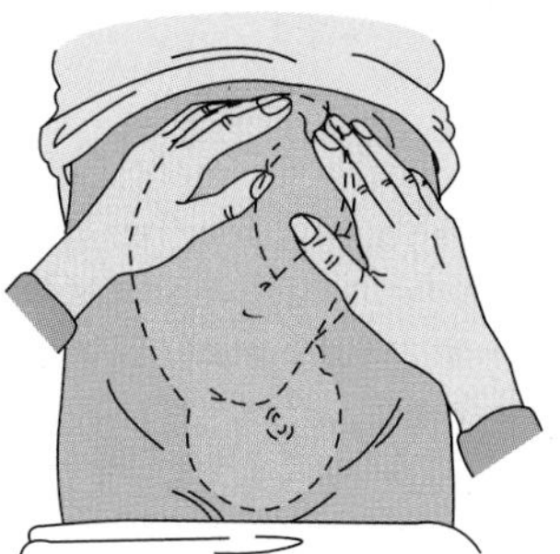

First Maneuver

Determine the part of the fetus in the fundus by facing the woman and palpating the upper abdomen with both hands. Note the shape, consistency, and mobility of the palpated part. A fetal head feels firm, hard, and round, and moves independently of the trunk. The buttocks feel irregular, softer, and are more difficult to move because they move with the trunk.

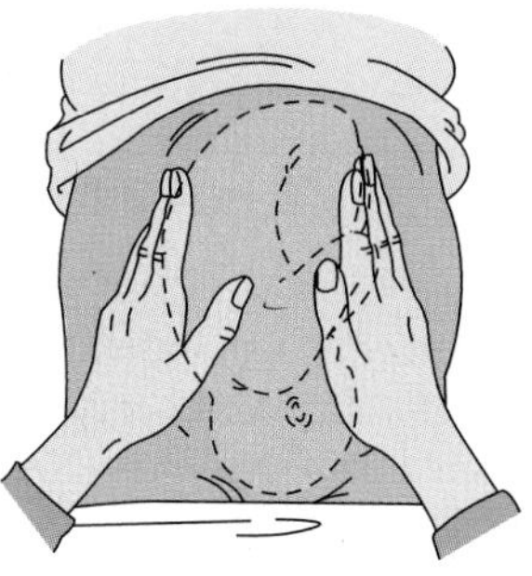

Second Maneuver

After ascertaining whether the head or the buttocks occupies the fundus, determine the location of the fetal back and note whether it is on the right or left side of the mother's abdomen. Still facing the woman, continue to palpate with the palms of the hands. Keep the right hand steady while the left hand explores the right side of the uterus, and then reverse the maneuver. Locate the back, arms, and legs by moving the hands down toward the pelvis. The fetal back feels smooth and offers resistance as you palpate. The arms, legs, and feet feel knobby and lumpy.

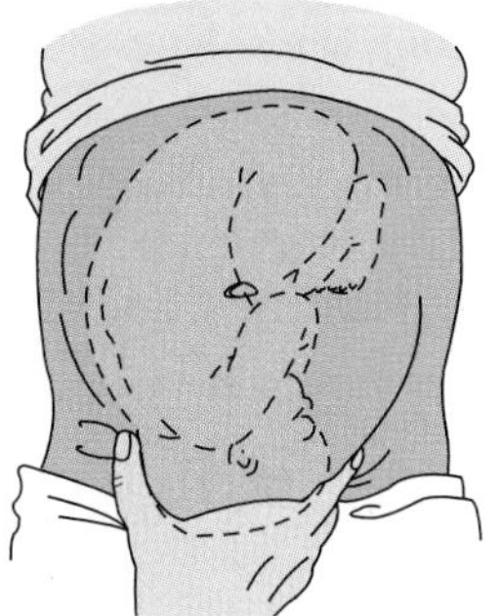

Third Maneuver

Determine what part is lying above the pelvic inlet by cupping the abdomen just above the symphysis pubis with the thumb and fingers of one hand. Note whether the palpated part feels like the head or the buttocks. This maneuver is performed to confirm the fetal position determined in the first maneuver.

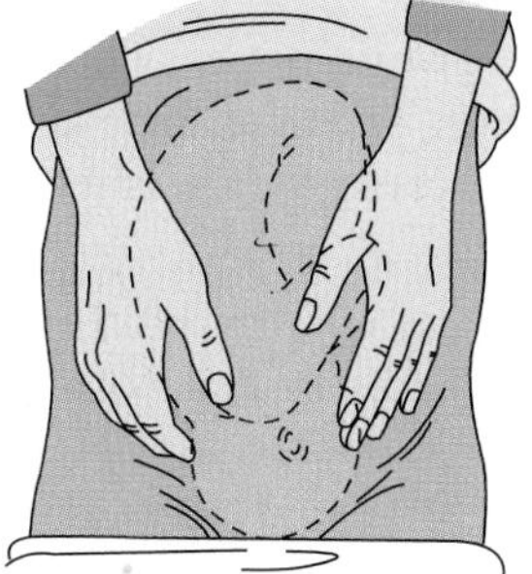

Fourth Maneuver

In later stages of pregnancy, determine the degree of cephalic flexion and engagement by facing the woman's feet and attempting to locate the cephalic prominence (or brow). Palpate the lower abdomen with both hands, moving the hands down the sides of the uterus toward the pubis. The cephalic prominence is located on the side that presents the greatest resistance to the descent of the fingers toward the pubis.

Reminders

- At the conclusion of each prenatal assessment, assist the client to an upright position. Answer any questions the client may have, and provide the client with anticipatory guidance for health promotion (see pages 661–664). Then leave the client to dress in privacy.
- Document assessment findings as described in Chapter 1. Nursing diagnoses commonly related to antepartal assessment are discussed in the next section.
- Perform a psychosocial assessment at each prenatal visit to assess the client's emotional responses to the pregnancy. You collect the psychosocial assessment data during the focused interview.
- Continue to collect data regarding the client's health throughout the pregnancy, performing nursing assessments at each prenatal visit. Most prenatal visits are scheduled at regular intervals throughout the pregnancy. It is usual to schedule nine visits for nulliparous and seven for multiparous women. For the first 28 weeks of pregnancy, assess the client every 4 weeks. From weeks 28–36, schedule client visits every 2 weeks. From 36 weeks until the birth, assess the client weekly. High-risk mothers will, of course, be seen more often. During subsequent prenatal assessments, focus on documentation of normal physiologic adaptations; early identification of high-risk symptoms; client teaching and other interventions related to comfort, self-care, and recognition of the danger signs of pregnancy; and evaluations to determine future care.

Organizing the Data

After conducting the focused interview of the childbearing client and performing the physical assessment, begin to group the related data into clusters leading to either nursing diagnoses, which require interventions such as client teaching, or collaborative problems, which require you to work with other members of the health care team.

Identifying Nursing Diagnoses

Many nursing diagnoses apply to the childbearing client because of the tremendous physiologic and psychosocial changes accompanying pregnancy. Some of the most common are

- *Activity intolerance:* A state in which an individual has insufficient physiologic or psychologic energy to endure or complete required or desired daily activities (NANDA) (see Table 20.2)
- *Impaired adjustment:* The state in which an individual is unable to modify her lifestyle/behavior in a manner consistent with a change in health status (NANDA)
- *Anxiety:* A vague, uneasy feeling whose source is often nonspecific or unknown to the individual (NANDA)
- *Constipation:* A state in which an individual experiences a change in normal bowel habits characterized by a decrease in frequency and/or passage of hard, dry stools (NANDA)
- *Ineffective family coping:* A state in which a family is unable to provide support that the client may need to manage tasks related to her health challenge (NANDA) (see Table 20.2)
- *Fatigue:* An overwhelming sustained sense of exhaustion and decreased capacity for physical and mental work (NANDA)
- *Knowledge deficit:* A state in which the individual/family does not comprehend, learn, or demonstrate knowledge of health care measures necessary to maintain or improve health (NANDA)
- *Altered nutrition: less than body requirements:* The state in which an individual experiences an intake of nutrients insufficient to meet metabolic needs (NANDA) (see Table 20.2)

Table 20.2 NANDA Nursing Diagnoses Related to Pregnancy

HIGH RISK FOR ACTIVITY INTOLERANCE	
Definition: State in which an individual is at risk of experiencing insufficient physiologic or psychologic energy to endure or complete required or desired daily activities (NANDA).	
RISK FACTORS	
History of previous intolerance, Deconditioned status, Presence of circulatory/respiratory problems, Inexperience with the activity, Others specific to client (specify).	
COMPROMISED INEFFECTIVE FAMILY COPING	
Definition: A state in which a usually supportive family member/close friend provides ineffective comfort/support that may be needed by the client to manage or master adaptive tasks related to his/her health challenge (adapted from NANDA).	
RELATED FACTORS	
Inadequate or incorrect information or understanding by family member/close friend, Temporary preoccupation of family member/close friend with own emotional conflicts and personal suffering, Temporary family disorganization and role changes, Situational crisis (specify), Developmental crisis (specify), Client's diminished support of family member/close friend, Chronic illness or disability, Economic problems, Unrealistic expectations/demands, Lack of mutual decision-making skills, Shift in family's normal power structure, Others specific to client (specify).	
DEFINING CHARACTERISTICS	
Client expresses concern/complaint regarding family members' response	Family verbal interaction with client is absent or decreased
Family member overassists client	Family expresses a lack of knowledge
Family member underreacts—eg, withdraws, ignores, minimizes, refuses to assist	Family attempts to assist with client care but is unsuccessful
Family member interferes with necessary medical/nursing interventions	Family is preoccupied with own stressors/conflicts/crises
Family members are divisive and form unsupportive coalitions	Family displays emotional lability
	Family displays rigid role boundaries

- *Altered sexuality patterns:* The state in which an individual expresses concern regarding her sexuality patterns (adapted from NANDA)
- *Sleep pattern disturbance:* A state in which the individual experiences a disruption in the amount of and/or quality of sleep that interferes with desired lifestyle (adapted from NANDA)

Common Alterations in the Health of the Childbearing Client

Alterations in health commonly associated with the childbearing client typically involve preexisting health problems or altered functioning patterns that develop as a result of preg-

Table 20.2 NANDA Nursing Diagnoses Related to Pregnancy (continued)

ALTERED NUTRITION: LESS THAN BODY REQUIREMENTS	
Defintion: The state in which an individual experiences an intake of nutrients insufficient to meet metabolic needs (NANDA).	
RELATED FACTORS	
Chemical dependence (specify), Difficulty in chewing, Difficulty in swallowing, Psychologic impairment (specify), Food intolerance, High metabolic needs, Lack of basic nutritional knowledge, Limited access to food, Loss of appetite, Nausea/vomiting, Inadequate sucking reflex in the infant, Parental neglect, Chronic illness, Economic factors, Others specific to client (specify).	
DEFINING CHARACTERISTICS	
Abdominal pain	Satiety immediately after ingesting food
Difficulty in swallowing/chewing	Perceived inability to ingest food
Indigestion/stomach cramps	Inadequate food intake of less than recommended daily allowance
Aversion to eating	Pale conjunctival and mucous membranes
Alteration in taste sensation	Poor muscle tone
Body weight 20% or more under ideal for height and frame	Excessive loss of hair
Refusal to eat	Weakness of muscles required for swallowing or masticiation
Weight loss with adequate food intake	Capillary fargility
Ulcerated oral mucosa	Lack of interest in food
Diarrhea and/or steatorrhea	Lack of information, misinformation
Hyperactive/hypoactive bowel sounds	Misconceptions
Reported or evidence of lack of food	

nancy. High-risk conditions existing prior to pregnancy include anemia, diabetes, infection, and cardiac disease. Socioeconomic and self-care factors, such as substance abuse, smoking, diet, and poverty, also have an effect on the pregnancy. Additionally, age-related concerns involving the adolescent client or the client over the age of 35 affect maternal and fetal health.

Some of the most common complications of the childbearing client are discussed briefly in the following sections. See a maternity nursing textbook for more information.

Gestational Diabetes Mellitus

Diabetes can have a severe effect on pregnancy. If the mother is diagnosed as having type III diabetes, called gestational diabetes mellitus, she can often be managed by dietary controls during pregnancy. If she has insulin-dependent diabetes mellitus (Type I IDDM), control of the diabetes is a delicate balancing act taking into account the needs of both the mother and the developing fetus and the effects of gestational hormones on insulin and glucose uptake. The woman with IDDM and her fetus are at risk for perinatal mortality and congenital anomalies. Control of blood glucose levels, use of insulin, and fetal monitoring have improved the outcomes for both the pregnant woman and the fetus.

Hyperemesis Gravidarum

Hyperemesis gravidarum is pernicious vomiting during the first trimester of pregnancy, progressing to a point at which the woman vomits everything she swallows. In severe cases, the condition may lead to fluid-electrolyte imbalances. Severe potassium loss may disrupt cardiac functioning, and starvation may cause severe protein and vitamin deficiencies. Embryonic, fetal, or maternal death may result. The nurse monitors a client with hyperemesis gravidarum carefully for episodes of vomiting, intake and output, fetal heart rate, and evidence of jaundice or bleeding. Because emotional factors may play a role in this condition, the nurse monitors the woman's emotional state and refers her for psychotherapy as indicated.

DIAGNOSTIC REASONING IN ACTION

Sara Wolkovich, a 17-year-old high school student, comes into the student nurse's office complaining of nausea, vomiting, and fatigue. She states that for the last few weeks, she has had an aversion to food and that when she does eat, she often "throws up." She also says that she is so tired she can barely stay awake in her classes. While taking her health history, Lucy Retta, RN, asks Sara the date of her last menstrual period. Sara responds that she can't remember but that she doesn't think she has had her period "for a while." She states that she has been sexually active "for about 2 years" but has never been pregnant. Ms Retta asks Sara about her method of contraception, and Sara states, "I leave it up to the guy to stop in time." When Ms Retta asks Sara if she thinks she could be pregnant, Sara shrugs her shoulders and mumbles, "I hope not."

Ms Retta also questions Sara about her self-care habits. Sara states that she smokes cigarettes when she is at school or out with her friends. She states that she doesn't drink much alcohol. She exercises daily. She does not eat breakfast, and her typical lunch is a salad from the school cafeteria. She works five nights a week at a fast-food restaurant and usually eats a fish sandwich, french fries, and a diet cola. She states that she thinks her diet is "okay, because I eat a salad every day."

Ms Retta asks Sara about her family and home environment. Sara's parents are divorced, and she and her brother live with her mother.

Ms Retta's physical assessment reveals that Sara is 5'6" tall and weighs 105 lb. Her temperature, pulse rate, respirations, blood pressure, and heart and lung sounds are normal.

When Ms Retta tells Sara that the information provided suggests that Sara may be pregnant, Sara begins to cry. She states: "I can't be pregnant. I can't handle it. I don't know how to take care of a baby. I don't even know who the father is!"

The nursing assessment of Sara Wolkovich provides the following subjective and objective data:

- Nausea and vomiting
- Fatigue
- Aversion to food
- Absence of menstruation
- Sexually active
- Ineffective method of contraception
- Smoking (approximately three packs per week)
- Inadequate food intake of less than the recommended daily allowance
- Lack of basic nutritional knowledge
- Client is underweight for her height
- Verbalization of inability to cope

To cluster the information, Ms Retta:

- Notes that Sara's aversion to food and inadequate food intake of less than the recommended daily allowance are defining characteristics for the nursing diagnosis *Altered nutrition: less than body requirements*. Her nausea, vomiting, and lack of basic nutritional knowledge are related factors for this diagnosis.
- Notes that Sara's verbalization of her lack of understanding about contraception, nutrition, self-care, and the signs of pregnancy is a defining characteristic of the nursing diagnosis *Knowledge deficit*. Sara's limited exposure to information about contraception, nutrition, and the signs of pregnancy is a related factor for this diagnosis.
- Notes that Sara's verbalization of inability to cope with the pregnancy is a defining characteristic of the nursing diagnosis *Ineffective individual coping*.

Based on the above analysis, Ms Retta arrives at the following nursing diagnoses:

1. *Altered nutrition: less than body requirements,* related to nausea, vomiting, and lack of basic nutritional knowledge
2. *Knowledge deficit,* related to lack of information about contraception, nutrition, and the signs of pregnancy
3. *Ineffective individual coping,* related to personal vulnerability in the crisis of an unplanned pregnancy

Ms Retta notes that the following nursing diagnoses may also apply: *Altered health maintenance, Impaired adjustment,* and *Ineffective denial.*

Ms Retta discusses with Sara the need for her to have a complete physical examination and laboratory tests to confirm the pregnancy. They decide together that Sara will go to the local family planning clinic, and Ms Retta makes an appointment for Sara for the next day. Since Sara states that she does not wish to carry the pregnancy to term, Ms Retta discusses with Sara the surgical methods for terminating pregnancy. She teaches Sara about various contraceptive methods and she also teaches her about the harmful effects of smoking. Finally, she makes an appointment for Sara with the school's dietitian for nutritional counseling.

Iron-Deficiency Anemia

Iron-deficiency anemia is a form of anemia that results from an inadequate supply of iron for optimal formation of red blood cells. The deficiency leads to depleted red blood cell mass, decreased concentration of hemoglobin, and a resultant inability to transport oxygen efficiently throughout the body. During pregnancy, iron-deficiency anemia is diagnosed when the hemoglobin level is below 11 g/dL and the hematocrit is below 32%. The nurse monitors the childbearing client for adverse effects of the anemia and monitors the fetus for evidence of fetal distress related to insufficient delivery of oxygen.

Placenta Previa

Placenta previa is implantation of the placenta in the lower portion of the uterus. In some cases, the placenta may partially or completely cover the cervical os (Figure 20.16). Thus, as the uterus contracts and the cervix begins to dilate in the later weeks of pregnancy, the placental villi are torn, and bleeding begins. Typically the woman reports painless, bright red vaginal bleeding occurring after 20 weeks' gestation. At first, the bleeding may be scanty, but heavier bleeding episodes generally occur. In some instances, hemorrhage and shock may occur. Nursing assessments include monitoring maternal vital signs, blood loss, pain, and uterine contractility as well as fetal heart rate.

Pregnancy-Induced Hypertension

Pregnancy-induced hypertension (PIH) is the most common hypertensive disorder in pregnancy. It is characterized by hypertension and proteinuria. Edema may or may not occur. PIH is defined as a blood pressure of 140/90 mm Hg or higher during the second half of pregnancy in a previously normotensive woman, or an increase of 30 mm Hg systolic and/or 15 mm Hg diastolic above the baseline confirmed in two readings taken 6 hours apart. Thus a reading of 120/76 would indicate PIH in a woman whose baseline is 90/60. If unchecked, PIH may progress from mild preeclampsia, which may be asymptomatic, to severe preeclampsia, with edema, weight gain, blood pressure readings of 160/100 or higher, frontal headaches, blurred vision, nausea, vomiting, irritability, and other symptoms. If the woman is not treated, the disease may progress to eclampsia, which is characterized by a grand mal seizure of both tonic and clonic type. The woman with mild preeclampsia usually is placed on bed rest and is prescribed a diet high in protein. The woman with severe preeclampsia is hospitalized.

Preterm Labor

Preterm labor (labor between weeks 20 and 37) is the primary cause of perinatal and neonatal problems. The etiology is often unknown. Maternal factors may include infection, renal disease, cardiovascular disease, PIH, diabetes, or cervical incompetence. Fetal factors may include infections, hydramnios (an excess of amniotic fluid), or multiple gestations. Placenta previa and abruptio placentae can also cause preterm labor. Interventions depend on the gestational age, etiology, and maternal and fetal condition. The gestational age at which preterm labor occurs determines the extent of the interventions that will be required for the mother and fetus/infant.

Rh Incompatibility

Mothers who are Rh negative run the risk of having an infant with Rh incompatability if the infant is Rh positive. The first pregnancy is rarely affected because the maternal Rh antibodies usually are not stimulated until the fetus' Rh-positive blood cells enter the mother's circulation at birth. However, once the mother is sensitized, each succeeding pregnancy carries a high risk for an incompatibility reaction, marked by destruction of red blood cells and severe anemia in the fetus. Modern techniques of giving RhoGAM (Rh immune globulin) both before and immediately after birth have dramatically decreased the frequency of this condition in the past few years. Mothers must be counseled to obtain RhoGAM with each pregnancy and/or abortion.

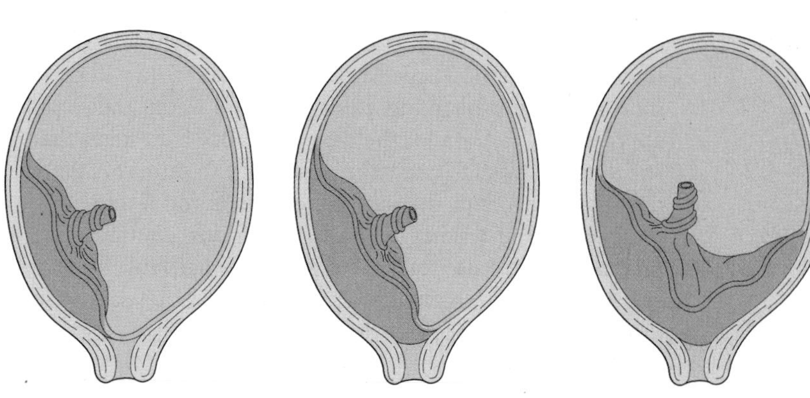

Figure 20.16 Placenta previa. *A*, Low placental implantation. *B*, Partial placenta previa. *C*, Complete placenta previa.

Spontaneous Abortion

Sources differ regarding the incidence of spontaneous abortions (miscarriages and stillbirths), but they may occur in as many as 20 to 60% of all pregnancies. It is believed that many women abort within the first few days after conception without knowing they are pregnant. Those who are aware of the spontaneous abortion often seek a reason for it so that they can change the causative factor for the future. This may not be possible, because the precise reason for a spontaneous abortion is almost always unclear.

Substance Abuse

Alcohol abuse in pregnancy may lead to a cluster of mental and physical health problems, called *fetal alcohol syndrome,* in the developing fetus. A safe level of alcohol intake has not been established; therefore, the childbearing client should be cautioned against consuming any alcohol during pregnancy. Smoking may cause a small-for-gestational-age (SGA) infant. Drugs such as cocaine may cause not only premature labor but also withdrawal symptoms in the infant.

Health Promotion and Client Education

At the conclusion of the assessment, answer any questions the client may have and provide the client with information on potential risk factors during pregnancy, measures to promote a healthy pregnancy, and measures to eliminate or alleviate the discomforts of pregnancy.

Risk Factors During Pregnancy

To reduce the potential health risks in pregnancy, provide the client with anticipatory guidance regarding the danger signs during pregnancy. Advise all antepartal clients to report immediately any of the following signs and symptoms:

- Sudden gush of or leaking fluid from the vagina
- Vaginal bleeding
- Temperature above 101F (38.3C) and chills
- Abdominal pain or cramps
- Epigastric pain
- Persistent vomiting
- Severe headache
- Dizziness, blurred or double vision, or spots before eyes
- Edema of the hands, face, legs, and feet
- Muscular irritability or convulsions
- Painful urination or decreased urine output
- Absence of or marked decrease in fetal movement

Measures for Promoting a Healthy Pregnancy

Health promotion begins with a review of the client's current health practices and resources. Pregnancy produces marked physiologic and psychologic adaptations, and the client's usual health practices may require modifications, such as those described here, to accommodate these changes.

Breast Care

1. Wear a well-fitting support bra with wide nonelastic straps, at least three back hooks, and a cup that covers the entire breast.
2. Keep the nipples dry with nonplastic, lined breast pads.
3. Avoid using soap on the nipples.
4. The client who plans to breast-feed should practice gently rolling and pulling the nipple. Oral stimulation from the client's sexual partner is also effective. However, the client with a history of preterm labor should avoid nipple stimulation.
5. Teach the client with inverted nipples how to perform Hoffman's exercises (Figure 20.17) or advise the client to wear breast shields (Figure 20.18 on page 662). Be aware, however, that neither of these methods is universally accepted as beneficial.

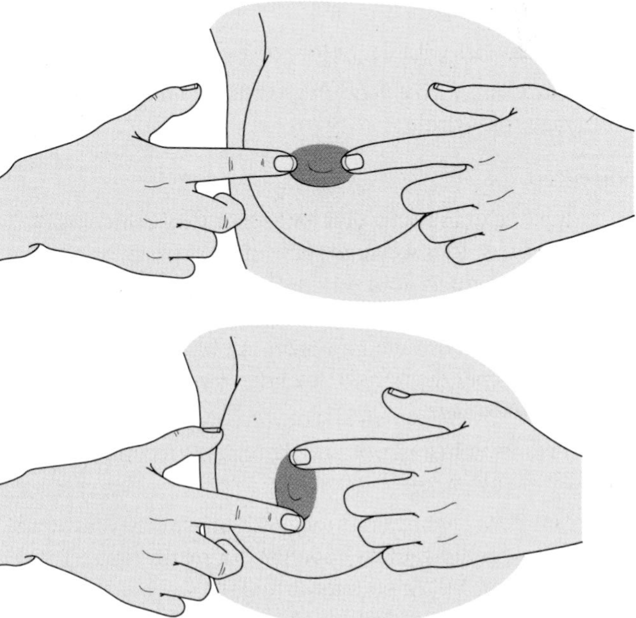

Figure 20.17 Hoffman's exercises are designed to increase nipple protactility. The client is instructed to place her thumbs or index fingers opposite each other near the edge of the areola. She then presses into the breast and stretches outward to break any adhesions. This is done both horizontally and vertically.

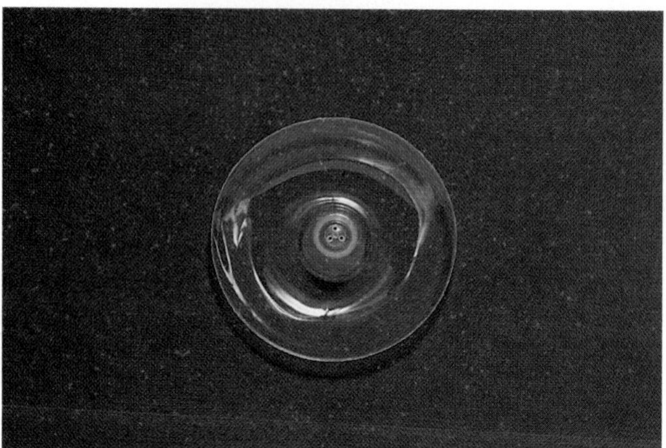

Figure 20.18 Breast shield.

Rest

1. Increase the number of hours of sleep to at least 8–10 hours each night.
2. Rest in the left lateral position (Figure 20.19).
3. Use relaxation techniques such as meditation and focused breathing to promote rest.
4. If possible, plan rest periods during waking hours.
5. Teach the client about positioning the body for comfort and safety, especially in the third trimester.

Clothing

1. Wear loose-fitting clothing.
2. Wear cotton underwear.
3. Wear shoes with flat or low wedge heels.
4. The client with a pendulous abdomen may wear a maternity girdle.

Nutrition

1. Include in the daily diet four servings of milk or milk products; four servings of bread, rice, pasta, or other grain products; four servings of fruits and vegetables; and three servings of eggs, meat, fish, beans, soy foods, or other foods high in protein. An increase of 300–500 calories per day is recommended for pregnant and lactating women.
2. Take vitamin and iron supplements as recommended by the physician.
3. Monitor weight gain throughout pregnancy. Ideally, the client should gain 2–4 pounds during the first trimester, 11–12 pounds during the second trimester, and 11–12 pounds during the third trimester.
4. Folic acid is necessary for fetal growth and helps prevent anemia in pregnancy. Most women in the U.S. receive an adequate supply of folic acid in a well-balanced diet (leafy green vegetables, yeast, organ meats, peanuts, and small amounts in dairy products), but some women may need supplemental folic acid.

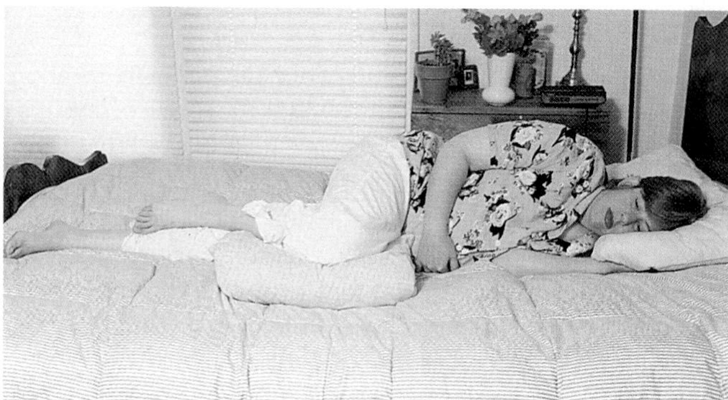

Figure 20.19 Pregnant client resting in the left lateral position.

Exercise

1. Warm up and stretch before exercising.
2. Stop exercises if heart rate increases above 140.
3. Decrease the intensity of exercise as the pregnancy progresses.
4. Avoid overheating and fatigue.
5. Avoid exercises that require balance.
6. Cool down after exercise with mild activity.
7. Wear loose clothing, supportive shoes, and a supportive bra.
8. Rest in the left lateral position after exercise.
9. Stop exercising if you experience excessive fatigue, dizziness, shortness of breath, abdominal pain, vaginal bleeding, or tingling or numbness to extremities.
10. Walking is one of best exercises for pregnant women.

Travel

1. Wear shoulder and lap belts in the car. The lap belt should rest below the uterus.
2. Get out of the car and stroll for 10 minutes for every 2 hours of driving.
3. Avoid flying in the final weeks of pregnancy.

Substance Use

1. Stop smoking.
2. Avoid alcohol.
3. Avoid illicit drugs (eg, cocaine, heroin, marijuana).
4. Consult with the physician or nurse before taking any over-the-counter medications.

Occupation

1. Plan rest periods during work hours.

2. Do not engage in strenuous physical activity.
3. Avoid sitting or standing for long periods of time.
4. Elevate the legs whenever possible.
5. Avoid environmental toxins and other hazards.

Sexual Activity

1. Continue sexual activity throughout the pregnancy as desired except in the presence of vaginal bleeding, ruptured membranes, or signs of preterm labor.
2. Recognize that desire may change at different stages of the pregnancy because of the effects of changing levels of hormones, fatigue, and physical discomfort. (Desire often decreases in the first and third trimesters and increases in the second.)

Childbirth Exercises

1. Practice the pelvic tilt to decrease back discomfort.
2. When walking, squeeze the buttocks together to help maintain erect posture and support the lower back.
3. Practice Kegel exercises (squeeze perineal muscles as if to stop urination) to increase the strength of the muscles of the pelvic floor.

Childbirth Education

1. Attend childbirth education and parenting classes throughout the pregnancy.
2. Discuss pregnancy, childbirth, and parenting frequently with other parents.

Measures for Promoting a Comfortable Pregnancy

Help the client identify the discomforts associated with her advancing pregnancy and teach self-care measures to eliminate or reduce them.

Vomiting

1. Avoid odors that initiate symptoms.
2. Eat dry carbohydrates such as crackers or toast before rising in the morning.
3. Drink liquids between meals.
4. Eat small, frequent meals every 2 to 3 hours.
5. Avoid spicy or greasy foods.
6. Contact a physician if vomiting occurs more than once a day.

Urinary Frequency and Urgency

1. Drink at least eight 8-oz glasses of fluid per day.
2. Decrease fluid intake in the evening to prevent nocturia.
3. Urinate at least every 2 to 3 hours to prevent stasis.
4. Report to the physician immediately any signs of urinary tract infection such as burning on urination, painful urination, or fever.

Breast Tenderness

1. Wear a well-fitting support bra.
2. Avoid the use of soap on the nipples.

Leukorrhea

1. Cleanse the perineal area daily with a mild soap and water.
2. Wear cotton underwear.
3. Avoid restrictive, tight-fitting clothes.
4. Avoid pantyhose.
5. Report foul-smelling, purulent vaginal discharge to the physician immediately.

Nasal Stuffiness or Nosebleeds

1. Use a cool mist vaporizer when sleeping.
2. Gently pinch the nose during acute bleeding episodes.
3. Avoid the use of decongestants.

Excessive Salivation

1. Use an astringent mouthwash regularly.
2. Chew gum or suck on hard candy.

Heartburn

1. Eat small meals every 2 to 3 hours.
2. Avoid eating highly seasoned or fried foods.
3. Avoid lying down after eating.
4. Avoid the use of sodium bicarbonate. Use an antacid recommended by a physician.

Ankle Edema and Varicose Veins

1. Elevate the legs above the hips when sitting.
2. Avoid prolonged sitting or standing.
3. Practice dorsiflexion of the foot frequently.
4. Avoid restrictive bands such as knee-high or thigh-high stockings on the legs.
5. Wear supportive hose.
6. Avoid crossing the legs.

Hemorrhoids

1. Consume foods high in fiber.
2. Drink 8 to 10 glasses of fluid per day.
3. Avoid straining when having a bowel movement.
4. Apply ice packs, warm packs, and ointments as prescribed by physician.
5. Gently reinsert hemorrhoids as necessary.

Constipation

1. Consume foods high in fiber.
2. Drink 8 to 10 glasses of fluid per day.
3. Exercise regularly.
4. Establish regular bowel elimination times.
5. Use stool softeners as recommended by the physician.

Backache

1. Practice the pelvic tilt.
2. Avoid lifting heavy objects. When lifting, use leg muscles instead of back muscles, squatting rather than bending (Figure 20.20).
3. Use proper body mechanics and good posture.
4. Avoid high-heeled shoes.

Leg Cramps

1. Dorsiflex the affected leg to relieve the cramp.
2. Apply a warm towel to relieve the cramp.
3. Assess the diet for calcium/phosphorus imbalance.

Faintness or Dizziness

1. Avoid lying on the back. Use the left lateral position.
2. Change body position slowly, eg, when moving from lying down to sitting or standing.
3. Avoid standing for prolonged periods.
4. When feeling lightheaded, sit down and place the head between the legs.

Dyspnea

1. Use proper posture when sitting or standing.
2. Use pillows for support of the back.
3. Place the hands over the head and perform deep breathing.

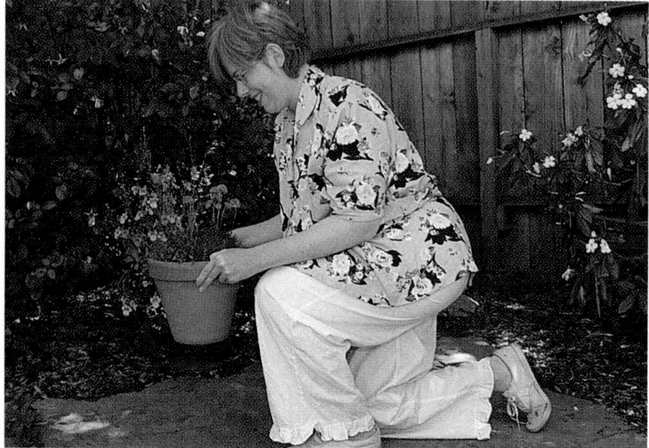

Figure 20.20 The pregnant client should practice proper body mechanics, such as squatting rather than bending to pick up objects

DIAGNOSTIC REASONING IN ACTION

Amelia Cipriano is a 36-year-old attorney who is at the clinic for her second prenatal visit. She is 9 weeks pregnant, and this is her first pregnancy. Doris Duke, RN, performs a health assessment, which reveals no unexpected findings except that Mrs. Cipriano has lost 2 pounds in the 4 weeks since her last visit and is currently 4 pounds below the minimum for her height and age. When Ms Duke tells Mrs. Cipriano about the weight loss, she responds, "I'm not surprised. I haven't had much of an appetite. I feel nauseated all the time, and I vomited three times last week." As they talk further, Mrs. Cipriano reveals that she has had almost no sexual desire for the past month. "I'm so tired all the time," she says. "I guess that's the reason. But I think my husband is beginning to worry that now that I'm about to become a mother, I'll never want sex again."

Ms Duke clusters the information gathered during the assessment and arrives at the following nursing diagnoses:

1. *Altered nutrition: less than body requirements* related to nausea and vomiting
2. *Knowledge deficit* related to lack of information about the expected changes of pregnancy

Ms Duke explains to Mrs. Cipriano the importance of consuming enough calories each day to meet the needs of her heightened metabolism and her growing fetus. She also advises Mrs. Cipriano to avoid any odors that precipitate nausea; to eat dry carbohydrates such as crackers before rising in the morning; to eat small, frequent meals every 2 to 3 hours rather than larger meals three times a day; to avoid spicy or greasy foods, and to contact the clinic if she vomits more than once a day. She also asks Mrs. Cipriano to monitor her own weight. Ms Duke informs Mrs. Cipriano that when she is beyond the early stages of her pregnancy, she will probably gain weight appropriately.

Additionally, Ms Duke reassures Mrs. Cipriano that her decreased sexual desire is a common change in early pregnancy and is due to both hormonal changes and simple fatigue. She encourages Mrs. Cipriano to discuss her feelings openly with her husband and to try having sexual intercourse in the mornings or early evenings when she might be less tired. Finally Ms. Duke assures Mrs. Cipriano that this change is not permanent and that most women experience an increase in sexual desire in the second trimester.

Summary

Pregnancy initiates physiologic and anatomic changes in all body systems, making early and continued assessment of the childbearing client essential. Assessment data is derived from the client's health history, a focused interview, and a thorough physical assessment. In addition to assessing the client, the nurse identifies appropriate nursing diagnoses and plans interventions such as client teaching to assist the client in maintaining optimum health throughout pregnancy.

Key Points

- ✓ Pregnancy produces a wide variety of anatomic and physiologic changes. The skin may exhibit striae gravidarum, heightened vascularity, or changes in pigmentation. Respiration may become labored. Gastric motility decreases, and urine flows more slowly through the ureters. The reproductive organs change markedly in response to hormonal changes and the growth of the fetus. The breasts enlarge and become more nodular, and the areolae darken. Body posture and alignment change as the uterus enlarges. The childbearing woman may experience dizziness and light-headedness associated with vena caval syndrome. Marked changes in the endocrine system facilitate the metabolic functions that maintain maternal and fetal health throughout the pregnancy. For example, hormonal changes increase cardiac output, vasodilation, heart rate, and heat intolerance, and the BMR may increase by as much as 30% by term.
- ✓ The initial prenatal interview of the childbearing client focuses on collection of baseline data about the client and her partner, identification of risk factors, and establishment of a trusting nurse-client relationship. If the complete health history is not available, it is gathered during the initial prenatal visit.
- ✓ The physical assessment of the childbearing client consists of laboratory tests, a complete systems assessment, assessment of pelvic adequacy, and assessment of the health and position of the fetus.
- ✓ Nursing diagnoses commonly associated with the childbearing client include *Impaired adjustment, Anxiety, Constipation, Ineffective individual coping, Knowledge deficit, Altered nutrition: less than body requirements, Altered sexuality patterns, Sleep pattern disturbance,* and others.
- ✓ Common alterations in the health of the childbearing client include gestational diabetes, hyperemesis gravidarum, iron-deficiency anemia, placenta previa, pregnancy-induced hypertension, preterm labor, Rh incompatibility, spontaneous abortion, and substance abuse.
- ✓ The nurse provides information to assist the client in identifying the health risks of pregnancy, to promote a healthy pregnancy, and to eliminate or alleviate the discomforts of pregnancy.

Chapter 21

Assessing the Older Adult

According to the Bureau of the Census, 30.3 million men and women, more than 12% of the United States population, were 65 years of age or older in the United States in 1990. Americans are living longer: 2.9 million were over the age of 85 in 1990, which is an increase of 0.6 million from 1980. Because the range of 65 to 100 years of age is so great, it is difficult to generalize about older adults and the changes that occur with aging. However, if you keep in mind that aging is a process that occurs over time, then you can distinguish the physiologic and psychologic changes of normal aging from the pathologic and pathophysiologic changes of disease.

In general, older adults of the 1990s are better educated, hold more advanced degrees, and are better off financially than in previous decades (Eliopoulos 1993). Many live in their own homes, have access to significant others, and participate in meaningful work or volunteer activities. Many older people, including the very old, enjoy vigorous good health and minimal disease.

Even those with a healthy lifestyle, however, experience a decline in functioning that affects all body systems over time. Studies have identified five common characteristics of aging:

1. The changes are gradual.
2. The more complex a function, the more apparent the decline.
3. Individual differences are significant.
4. Vulnerability to disease increases with age.
5. Vulnerability to stress increases with age.

Eliopoulos (1993) notes that although elderly people have fewer acute illnesses than younger adults, these illnesses are more serious when they strike older adults. Recovery takes longer, and they are more likely to lead to a chronic disorder.

Anatomy and Physiology Review

Numerous, often overlapping, theories have been put forth to explain the changes of aging. The **genetic mutation theory** proposes that as one ages, the DNA controlling the reproduction and activities of somatic cells becomes altered. The DNA no longer provides an accurate blueprint for cellular replication, and the result is synthesis of defective proteins. These changes lead to the death of cells, autoimmune disorders, decreased production of enzymes and antibodies, and decreased resistance to disease. The **cross-linking theory** suggests that, over time, the double strands of the DNA molecules become glued together, damaging the chromosomes and altering cellular reproduction. This alteration especially affects collagen and elastic tissues, leading to wrinkling. The **lipofusin theory** proposes that the end products, or debris, of cell metabolism accumulate and replace cells, especially nerve cells and myocardial cells. A related theory is the **free radical theory**, which proposes that free radicals generated from oxygen metabolism damage proteins and enzymes, creating genetic disorder. It is believed that vitamin E and selenium may help eliminate the accumulated end products. Finally, recent genetic research points to a genetically programmed life expectancy of each person's cells, suggesting that the longevity of one's relatives is significant (Eliopoulos 1993, Kimmel 1980, Schuster and Ashburn 1986).

Another relevant factor is the presence of chronic illnesses. The health status of older individuals varies greatly according to genetic predisposition and lifestyle. Statistics show that increasing age is correlated with increasing physician and hospital visits, many as the result of chronic illnesses that have festered over time, coming to a head in the period known as "old age." The effect of chronic illness is thus an important consideration in the assessment of the older adult.

Integumentary System Changes

Because of a decrease in collagen, subcutaneous fat, glutamic acid, and lysine needed for elastin formation, the skin loses strength and elasticity with age, giving the physical appearance of wrinkling and sagging. The dehydration of the outer layer of the skin due to loss of sebaceous and sweat glands leads to the common problem of dry skin, called **xerosis**, and associated scaliness, itching, and scratching. Thinning of the skin begins with decreases in gonadal hormones in both men and women and progresses with advancing age until the skin looks transparent. Pruritus and thinness may lead to abrasions and excoriations from trauma or scratching.

Melanocytes diminish with age and become deposited irregularly. This leads to overall pallor in the very old or a lightening of dark skins as well as "white freckles" or small, patchy areas of pigment loss. Do not confuse these with vitiligo (see Chapter 8). The irregular deposition of melanocytes can result in patchy areas of increased pigmentation as well, especially when circulation to the area is impaired. A common complaint, liver spots, also known as **lentigo senilis**, occurs as the melanocytes increase at the dermal-epidermal junction. Loss of melanocytes is responsible for the graying of hair seen with aging. Skin of all colors is at risk for sun-generated cancer, but fair skins have an increased risk for basal-cell carcinoma.

The aging skin is subject to a variety of lesions (Figure 21.1 on page 668). The cause is unknown but may be related to altered DNA causing a change in cell types. **Xanthelasma** is a tiny, tumorlike fatty deposit on the eyelid that may be related to hyperlipidemia. **Acrochordons**, or skin tags, are pedunculated, flesh-colored lesions of collagen and subcutaneous tissue that occur on the neck, axillary area, and eyelids. **Actinic keratoses** are normal aging growths, especially in fair skins, but are considered precancerous. They appear as calluslike red, yellow, or flesh-colored plaques appearing on exposed areas such as ears, cheeks, lips, nose, upper extremities, or balding scalp. **Seborrhea keratoses** are benign, greasy, wartlike lesions that are yellow-brown in color. They can appear anywhere on the body but are seen more frequently on the neck, chest, and back. Vascular lesions can include **cherry angiomas**, which are nonsignificant tiny red spots, either macules or papules, rarely larger than 3–4 mm, seen usually on the trunk. Another more serious vascular lesion is **senile purpura**, which can occur spontaneously or in response to minimal trauma in the very old client with fragile blood vessels. It is a coalescion of petechiae that begins as tiny individual red-to-purple spots caused by rupture of small capillaries. The petechiae converge to form large purple-to-brown patches.

The number of hair follicles declines by about one third by age 50 and continues to decrease with age. The amount of eventual loss is genetically determined: baldness is an X-linked recessive genetic trait. Hair distribution is controlled by testosterone in both sexes. As testosterone production decreases with age, body hair, especially axillary and pubic hair, diminishes. Estrogen levels also decrease with age, causing increased facial hair in women and increased hair growth inside the nose and ears in both sexes.

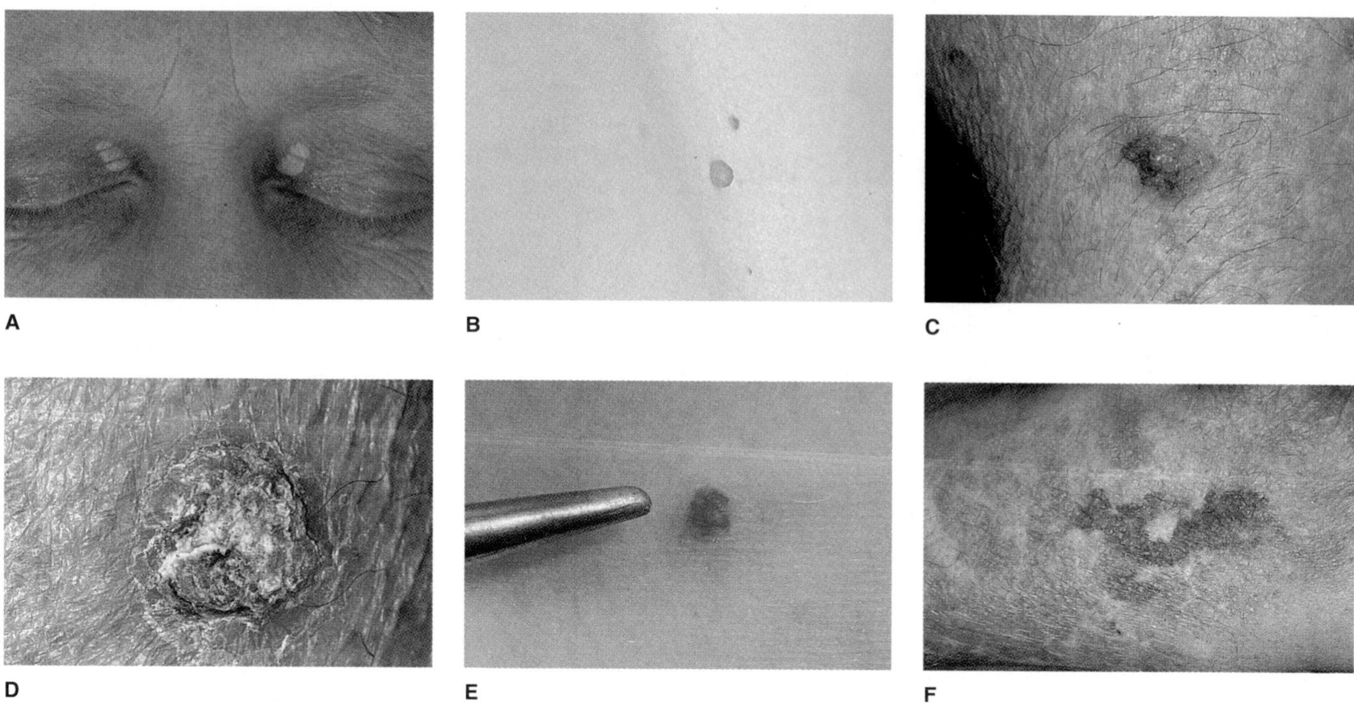

Figure 21.1 Lesions of the skin common in older clients. *A*, Xanthelasma. *B*, Acrochordon. *C*, Actinic keratosis. *D*, Seborrhea keratosis. *E*, Cherry angioma. *F*, Senile purpura.

Head and Neck Changes

Skull, Face, and Neck

The major age-related changes that occur in the head, face, and neck are related to loss of the supporting network of collagen and subcutaneous fat. The bones appear more prominent and the hollows more deep. The larynx becomes more visible, especially in men, and tendons and muscles are noticeable in the neck. A shortening of the platysma muscle gives a wattled appearance to the throat.

The eyes appear sunken, and the eyelids droop, sometimes covering the upper portion of the iris, resulting in a perpetually sleepy look. Tissue under the eyes thins, giving the appearance of bluish circles from underlying veins. Fluid may collect in this delicate tissue, resulting in puffiness under the eyes. In some older people, loss of muscle tone of the lower lid causes it to fall open, revealing a reddened palpebral conjunctiva; this condition is called **ectropion.** Alternatively, for an unknown reason, the lid may turn in. This condition, called **entropion,** causes the eyelashes to irritate the cornea.

The nose may enlarge, becoming bulbous and red if the person has had excessive exposure to the elements. The lips may thin and be subject to dryness. Also, with excessive salivation, which can occur with aging, cracking and soreness may be present in the corners of the mouth.

Eyes

Several changes may be noted upon inspection of the eyes: The pupils are normally from 2 to 3 mm. There may be a gray, white, or yellow ring around the **limbus** (the edge of the cornea where it joins the sclera) or just arcing over the top portion of the limbus. This ring is called **arcus senilis**. A stretch of fatty tissue extending from the limbus to either the medial or lateral canthus, called **pterygium,** may be present. The latter two conditions are sometimes related to altered fat metabolism or high cholesterol levels. The lens of aging eyes loses power, and the ability to accomodate to changes in distance and to decreased light levels. Called **presbyopia**, or the short-arm syndrome, this usually starts as early as age 40 and progresses slowly. The older person needs larger print and more light to read effectively. Glare intolerance and loss of depth perception are also normal findings. Visual acuity and peripherial vision may diminish with macular degeneration and the development of cataracts. All of these changes can have implications for the elderly driver.

Ears

Presbycusis is the term used to designate the decrease in hearing acuity associated with aging; hearing loss is first evidenced by diminished perception of high-frequency sounds. The hearing loss that normally accompanies aging is usually due to a loss of hair cells in the organ of Corti of the inner ear, but conductive losses can also occur because of thickening of the tympanic membrane or because of simple problems, such as accumulated wax. As hearing gradually diminishes, the older adult may have difficulty discriminating consonant sounds such as S, Z, T, F, and G. Competing sounds, such as a loud television or others talking nearby, can be distracting. Remember, however, that elderly people process language more slowly than before; therefore, do not interpret requests for something to be repeated as a definitive indication of hearing loss.

Mouth, Nose, and Throat

The senses of both smell and taste diminish with age because of a decrease in olfactory fibers, taste buds, and saliva production. (Some elderly people, however, experience increased salivation.) Many older people lose all or most of their teeth. Dentures may cease to fit well when the bones and tissues of the mouth shrink with age. All of these factors may have a profoundly negative influence on the nutritional status of older adults. With better dental care and personal oral hygiene, more older adults are keeping their own teeth throughout their lives.

Cardiovascular Changes

A variety of cardiovascular changes occur over time. Probably the most damaging is the development of atherosclerosis, a narrowing of the arteries and thickening of the heart valves. Researchers now believe that fatty streaks, precursors of plaque, begin in the teens and early twenties and ultimately lead to atherosclerosis. Development of these fatty streaks may be associated with genetic factors, gender, and lifestyle. Although many elderly people live to their 70s and beyond without significant heart disease, most have changes that gradually affect their functioning.

The size of the heart does not increase, but the heart muscle loses efficiency and contractile strength by about 1% per year. Stroke volume, isometric contraction, recovery, and cardiac output are all decreased. Older adults compensate by slowing down, but they are not always able to meet increased demand on the cardiovascular system. The heart rate can increase, but not as much as in younger adults, and the increase is sustained for a longer time. Though older adults tire more easily than younger adults, most non-ill elderly persons feel they have adequate energy to do what they need to do to maintain their daily lives.

The level of blood pressure that indicates hypertension in the elderly is still being debated because the older adult's thicker, more rigid, and less elastic vessels naturally increase systolic blood pressure and widen pulse pressure. Current conservative recommendations are to treat blood pressures of 140/90 or higher. Altered baroreceptor sensitivity results in problems with orthostatic hypotension, which can be made worse by diuretic and antihypertensive medications.

Pulmonary Changes

Structural changes, such as alterations in the shape and rigidity of the rib cage, kyphosis, and weakening of the intercostal muscles, affect respiratory function. Lungs enlarge, lose elasticity, and have less recoil, and lung alveoli decrease in number and elasticity. Most adults by 80 years of age have some degree of emphysema, both from these changes and from years of passively or actively inhaling noxious substances. As alveolar gas diffusion decreases and less oxygen becomes available to the tissues, older individuals may experience a decreased ability to respond to stress. The very old who function with relative ease in their home environment may thus become flustered and upset when rushed in a store or restaurant. This may be partially due to slower reflexes but can also be a manifestation of common physiologic changes, such as those noted previously.

Gastrointestinal Changes

As the basal metabolic rate decreases with age, fewer calories are required for maintenance. However, because of a variety of factors, including inadequate dental care, decreased salivation, limited money for food, and social isolation, older people may not have an adequate appetite or eat enough of a variety of foods to get the nutrients they need. The need to follow a special diet to manage a chronic illness exacerbates the problem. As one elderly client lamented, "You've taken away my cigarettes, alcohol, salt, and fat, and now you tell me I can't have sugar!" Thus, some older adults experience a decline in health because of malnutrition. Table 21.1 on page 670 lists the recommended dietary allowances for adults age 51 and older.

Water intake can also be a problem, because the thirst mechanism becomes less effective with age. In addition, because of a common problem with nocturia, older people may limit their fluid intake in the early afternoon and evening. Decreased gastrointestinal motility, often coupled with low fiber and water intake, results in the very common complaint of constipation, which the older person may make worse by the indiscriminate use of laxatives.

Heartburn, caused by reflux due to a relaxed gastroesophageal sphincter, and delayed gastric emptying are also

Table 21.1 Recommended Daily Dietary Allowances for Older Adults* as Revised in 1980 (Designed for the Maintenance of Good Nutrition of Practically All Healthy People in the United States)

Nutrient	Men 51+ yr	Women 51+ yr
Protein, g	56	44
Vitamin A, g RE†	1000	800
Vitamin D, g	5	5
Vitamin E, mg a-TE‡	10	8
Vitamin C, mg	60	60
Thiamine, mg	1.2	1
Riboflavin, mg	1.4	1.2
Niacin, mg NE§	16	13
Vitamin B_6, mg	2.2	2
Folacin, g	400	400
Vitamin B_{12}, mg	3	3
Calcium, mg	800	800
Phosphorus, mg	800	800
Magnesium, mg	350	300
Iron, mg	10	10
Zinc, mg	15	15
Iodine, g	150	150

* For men, the average height was 70 inches and the average weight 154 lb (70 kg). For women, the average height was 64 inches and the average weight 120 lb (55 kg).

† Retinol equivalents.

‡ Alphatocopherol equivalents.

§ Niacin equivalent = 1 mg niacin or 60 mg dietary tryptophan.

From *Recommended Daily Dietary Allowances,* 9th rev ed (1980). The National Academy of Sciences, Washington, D.C.

common complaints of aging. A decreased gag and cough reflex can put the older person at risk for aspiration.

Genitourinary Changes

By age 75 or 80, a 50% loss of nephrons has occurred; thus, glomerular filtering is decreased. This has major implications for drug toxicity in the elderly. Atherosclerosis of renal arteries can decrease renal blood flow and may lead to atrophy of the kidneys. Tubular function also diminishes, and urine is not as effectively concentrated as at a younger age: maximum specific gravity may be only 1.024.

Incontinence, the health problem older adults usually find most troubling, is related to diminished bladder elasticity, bladder capacity, and sphincter control. This results in the common complaints of frequency, urgency, and stress incontinence. New research shows a possible relationship with decreased estrogen levels in women. Prostatic enlargement, which occurs in 95% of all men by the age of 85, results in the additional problem of urinary retention.

Men do not lose the physical capacity for erection and ejaculation with age, but response time is slower. Women also do not lose the capacity for orgasm; in fact, some research indicates capacity may increase after menopause. However, the female genitals demonstrate many atrophic changes with aging due to hormonal changes: loss of subcutaneous fat and hair, flattening of the labia, loss of elastic tissue and vascularity in the vagina, decrease in vaginal secretions, and atrophy of the cervix, uterus, uterine tubes, and ovaries. Some of these, like the vaginal changes, can be averted or delayed with postmenopausal hormonal treatment, but atrophy eventually occurs.

Peripheral Vascular Changes

Circulation to the lower extremities decreases with aging, usually because of atherosclerosis, especially at the arteriole level, and because of a decrease in the competence of the valves of the veins. Diseases such as diabetes and a genetic or occupational proclivity to varicose veins increase the effects of aging on the circulation to the lower extremities. These circulatory changes may lead to thinning of the skin; decreased hair (also related to diminishing gonadal hormones); highly pigmented areas, especially in the inner aspects of the shin; and visible, tortuous veins if varicosities are present. Blue-hued vascular spiders frequently accompany visible veins. Pedal pulses may be diminished in strength. Because of long-standing pressure from shoes and circulatory changes, toenails are inclined to thicken, become yellow and grooved, and accumulate debris that is difficult to remove.

Musculoskeletal Changes

Bone and muscle mass decrease. The amount of loss appears to depend upon the bone density and muscle mass present in younger years, the amount of exercise, and the use of hormone therapy for postmenopausal women. Because men usually have more muscle mass and increased density, their loss is not as great; however, genetic factors and exercise patterns are also important for men. For light-boned persons, who are most at risk, pathologic fractures of the femur or vertebrae with minimal trauma (sometimes just stepping off a curb or sneezing vigorously) can result in permanent disability. Joint stiffness and enlargement from degenerative changes are not uncommon, especially in the weight-bearing joints of the obese. In all older adults, the intevertebral disks dry and flatten, providing less support and resulting in a shortening of the spine. This spinal compression accounts for the loss of several inches of height after age 65 (Figure 21.2).

Decreased baroreceptor sensitivity decreases the older adult's ability to compensate for gravitational effects on blood pressure. In addition, the older adult's sense of balance, which is mediated by several brain centers including the cerebellum, is altered. These factors make the older person more prone to falls. Interestingly, whereas younger people usually fall forward and may break their wrists, older people typically fall sideways and fracture their hips.

The loss of subcutaneous fat and muscle mass gives the older person a more gaunt appearance, with hollows and bony prominences. The loss of insulation, decreased sweating, and altered hypothalamic sensitivity to temperature tend to make the older person less tolerant to temperature extremes.

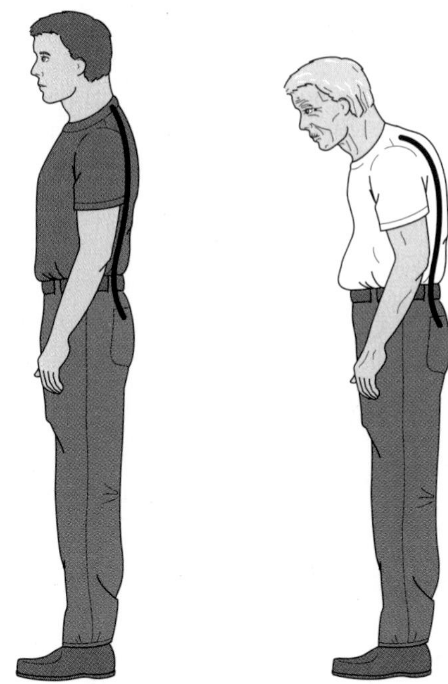

Figure 21.2 Loss of height from spinal compression in the older adult.

Neurologic Changes

Starting at age 25, an individual loses several thousand neurons a day. Fortunately there is much redundancy—billions of neurons. Blood flow to the brain of a 75-year-old under nondisease conditions is about 90% that of a 30-year-old. Thus, the main cause of mental deterioration associated with aging usually is related to disease, such as severe arteriosclerosis, or genetically dictated disorders, such as Alzheimer's disease.

The common changes of aging are usually due to decreased speed of impulse transmission, manifested as a decrease in reaction time, slowness in new learning, and possible loss of short-term memory. The word *possible* is used because some investigators propose that there is no loss but rather "computer overload with increased search time." In other words, normal older people do not lose memory, they just have more stored information and, because of slowed neural impulses, they need more time to search through that larger volume of information.

Although many of the changes that occur with aging are seen as negative, research has shown that intelligence, abstract thinking, problem solving, and especially creativity do not diminish with age but in fact are enhanced by experience. This fact, coupled with a mellow and relaxed outlook that can result from having conquered a number of life's problems, means that people should not dread aging but anticipate and enjoy it by adopting a healthy lifestyle.

Gathering the Data

Focused Interview

Guidelines for Interviewing Older Adults

When assessing older adults, keep the following points in mind:

- Grant older persons the dignity they have earned: call clients by their last names unless instructed otherwise. When greeting clients and introducing yourself, offer to shake hands, or touch their hands.
- Begin with clients' concerns and listen carefully to their explanations of their health status and problems, as well as their understanding of their current medical regimen. Elderly people in today's media-dominated culture are often very knowledgeable about health matters, and if not, you have excellent data to begin health teaching. Use open-ended questions to follow up on areas that need further investigation.
- Take into consideration changes in vision and hearing. Sit close enough to the person to be heard easily, speak clearly in a low-pitched voice, do not shout, and reduce noise levels in the environment. Adjust the lighting for adequate brightness, but avoid glare. Sit where the client can easily see you. Be sure that glasses, dentures, and hearing aids are available if needed.
- Make sure the client is in a comfortable and safe position. Ask if the room is warm enough. If possible, conduct the assessment in familiar surroundings: the client's hospital room or private bedroom at home.
- Remember that elderly individuals sometimes tire easily. Monitor their tolerance level and plan to complete the assessment in more than one meeting if necessary. Ask clients to tell you if they are getting too tired. If possible, try to determine ahead of time whether the client prefers a morning or afternoon meeting.
- Do not rush the interview or examination. Maintain a relaxed and patient attitude; allow for some life review to elicit long-term patterns of functioning and social support. You may need to refocus the interview if the life review tends to dominate the assessment.
- Assessments should focus on functional abilities rather than just deviations.
- Encourage the discussion of strategies used in the past to resolve health and other problems. Give positive feedback about the clients' strategies for managing their health.
- To decrease anxiety during mental status testing (eg, if you administer the Mini Mental Status Examination or the Geriatric Depression Scale), introduce these procedures with qualifiers about how the information helps you individualize care.
- It is often helpful to get collaborative information from significant others or reliable caretakers, but be sure to include clients in the discussion. Especially avoid talking about clients in their presence.
- Consider that some elderly clients may not report some of their symptoms, possibly because of fear of institutionalization, embarrassment, or not wanting to be considered old and sick. Others may overemphasize minor problems, seeking attention or sympathy. It helps to be objective in evaluating the data and to seek validation of problems from family members if necessary.
- Bear in mind that in some cultures illness is considered punishment for deviations from social/cultural norms or for real or imagined sins. Clients may withhold information about physical problems because of fear of being ostracized or extreme guilt.
- Keep an open mind about health practices that you consider questionable. In many cultures a variety of activities and folk medicines are believed to be important in preventing disease and treating illness. Medical research is just now beginning to prove the validity of many folk medicine practices. Unless the practice has been documented as harmful, support clients in their beliefs, although it might be useful to offer alternatives.

Questions for the Client

Many of the questions you use to collect data from younger adults are appropriate, but you need to focus on some special areas when assessing elderly individuals. In addition, if there is evidence of possible changes in mental status, direct some questions to caretakers or family members when not in the presence of the older person.

1. What would you like help with today? *Answers to this question will bring out the client's priority concerns, which you can then investigate with more specific questions.*
2. Describe what you do during a typical day. *Responses to this request may reveal sleep patterns, eating habits, social-*

ization, ability to manage the home environment, and ability to perform activities of daily living.

3. How often do you walk outside? Have you experienced any dizziness when you get up from bed or from a chair? *Answers to these questions may help identify those persons who are at risk for falls, especially for those older people who do not offer information about falls for fear of being removed from their homes. When people have experienced falls, they tend to self-limit outdoor walking activity. This can be an important cue, especially if they have been more active previously. Also, dizziness upon arising indicates orthostatic hypotension, which increases the risk of falls.*
4. Do you have any problem holding your urine? How many times do you get up at night to urinate? *Responses help to identify problems with incontinence due to diminished sphincter control or decreased bladder capacity. If you introduce the topic in this matter-of-fact manner, the older person is more likely to discuss the problem in more depth, whereas a question such as, "Do you have any problems with urinating or with your kidneys?" is apt to elicit a negative response.*
5. Do you have problems with your bowels? How frequently do you expect to have a bowel movement? What do you do to manage your bowel functioning? *Gastrointestinal motility decreases with age, and older people, recalling previous elimination patterns, may have unrealistic expectations regarding normal bowel functions (eg, daily bowel movements). Responses to these questions can help you determine whether the client needs health teaching regarding bowel functioning and whether a serious problem with constipation exists. The answers also may help you identify laxative abuse.*
6. Do you know what your medications are and why you are taking them? How long have you been taking each of these medications? *It is very important to ask elderly people these questions, because clients may have been taking some medications for many years without the knowledge of their current physician. Also, occasionally a person may be taking two identical medications with different names (eg, one generic name and one trade name). Information gained from these questions can point to a need for client teaching or medication management.*
7. Are you having pain or discomfort in any areas of your body? Tell me what this discomfort means to you. *These questions may encourage clients to report concerns that they are reluctant to mention because they do not want to be perceived as complainers or because they fear, and thus deny the possibility of, a serious health problem. In addition, differing cultural perceptions of and reactions to the pain experience may inhibit a direct response to questions about pain. Initiating a discussion may help to allay fears or facilitate a prompt referral to appropriate health care providers.*
8. Do you have enough energy to do the things you want to do each day? *Responses can pinpoint deterioration in function or gradual changes in physical or psychologic health.*
9. Do you feel you get enough sleep at night? Describe a typical night. What do you do to help yourself go to sleep? *Sleep problems are very common in elderly persons and can result in unnecessary fatigue and depression. Responses to these questions can help you identify sleep dysfunctions of which the client may be unaware, such as sleep apnea, restless leg syndrome, poor sleep habits, depression or anxiety, and possible misuse of sleeping medications.*
10. Do you have periods when you feel especially sad or lonely? Do you ever feel like you want to end your life? *Depression and suicide are major concerns with elderly people, especially those who have debilitating illnesses or who have recently lost a significant person. Older people seldom give warning that they are contemplating suicide; men are more at risk than women. The responses to these questions can help you identify those who may need psychologic intervention. You can use the Yesavage/Brink Geriatric Depression Scale (see the box on page 674) to explore any suspicious signs.*

Questions for Family Members or Caretakers

1. Have you noticed any forgetfulness or changes in the way (the client) normally does things? Has (the client) stopped doing any of his or her normal activities? Have you noticed any unusual behavior? *Responses can help you identify changes in mental status or deterioration of function, which might put the client at risk for injury. Even though the client may still be mentally competent, changes may be so subtle that the older person has gradually compensated for declining health*
2. Do you have any concerns about (the client) that you do not want to discuss with him or her? *This gives family members permission to share fears or ask questions that they are reluctant to mention for fear of worrying the older person.*

Geriatric Depression Scale

1. Are you basically satisfied with your life? (no)
2. Have you dropped many of your activities and interests? (yes)
3. Do you feel that your life is empty? (yes)
4. Do you often get bored? (yes)
5. Are you hopeful about the future? (no)
6. Are you bothered by thoughts that you just cannot get out of your head? (yes)
7. Are you in good spirits most of the time? (no)
8. Are you afraid that something bad is going to happen to you? (yes)
9. Do you feel happy most of the time? (no)
10. Do you often feel helpless? (yes)
11. Do you often get restless and fidgety? (yes)
12. Do you prefer to stay home at night, rather than go out and do new things? (yes)
13. Do you frequently worry about the future? (yes)
14. Do you feel that you have more problems with memory than most? (yes)
15. Do you think it is wonderful to be alive now? (no)
16. Do you often feel downhearted and blue? (yes)
17. Do you feel pretty worthless the way you are now? (yes)
18. Do you worry a lot about the past? (yes)
19. Do you find life very exciting? (no)
20. Is it hard for you to get started on new projects? (yes)
21. Do you feel full of energy? (no)
22. Do you feel that your situation is hopeless? (yes)
23. Do you think that most persons are better off than you are? (yes)
24. Do you frequently get upset over little things? (yes)
25. Do you frequently feel like crying? (yes)
26. Do you have trouble concentrating? (yes)
27. Do you enjoy getting up in the morning? (no)
28. Do you prefer to avoid social gatherings? (yes)
29. Is it easy for you to make decisions? (no)
30. Is your mind as clear as it used to be? (no)

Score one point for each response that matches the yes or no answer after the question.

Source: Adapted with permission from Yesavage JA, Brink TL. Development and Validation of a Geriatric Depression Screening Scale: A Preliminary Report. *J Psychiatr Res* 1983;17:41.

Physical Assessment

Preparation

☑ **Gather the equipment:**

examination gown	sphygmomanometerc
drape	centimeter measuring device
examination gloves	tongue blade
examination light	cotton
penlight	vision screener
stethoscope	tuning fork
ophthalmoscope	reflex hammer
otoscope	substances to taste and smell

☑ **Wash your hands in warm water.**

☑ **Warm your stethoscope.**

☑ **Ask whether the client needs to void before the examination.**

Remember

- To prevent discomfort due to temperature sensitivity, allow the elderly person to remain clothed, removing only what is necessary to examine a specific area.
- Lying or sitting on a hard examining table is difficult for many elderly people. Whenever possible conduct the exam in the client's home, with the client on the bed or in a chair.
- Conserve the client's energy by organizing the assessment so activities are grouped for a minimum of positional changes.
- Many older people are uncomfortable with a much younger examiner, especially if the examiner is of the opposite sex. Maintain a mature and professional attitude, but also be warm, caring, and sensitive to body image concerns.
- Explain each step as you proceed, but also ask questions about the findings. You can often put older clients at ease by allowing them to explain a scar or physical alteration. However, use care not to alarm them about a new and possibly frightening finding.
- You can conserve the energy of older adults and stimulate their memory by asking health history questions while examining the area under consideration. This pattern may seem more natural for you as well.
- Check whether the client would prefer to have a family member present during the examination or would rather have privacy. This preference varies considerably from culture to culture and from individual to individual.
- You can gain a great deal of information about the functional abilities of the person by observing movements, their ability to carry out requests (both physical ability and the ability to hear and understand the request), and communication and interaction with the examiner.
- Elderly people have good and bad days. They may not be as fully cooperative with the assessment on a bad day. Be flexible, and be open to rescheduling.

ASSESSMENT TECHNIQUE/NORMAL FINDINGS | SPECIAL CONSIDERATIONS

General Survey and Mental Status

Step 1 *Position the client.*

- Ensure that the client is seated comfortably at the beginning of the physical exam (Figure 21.3).

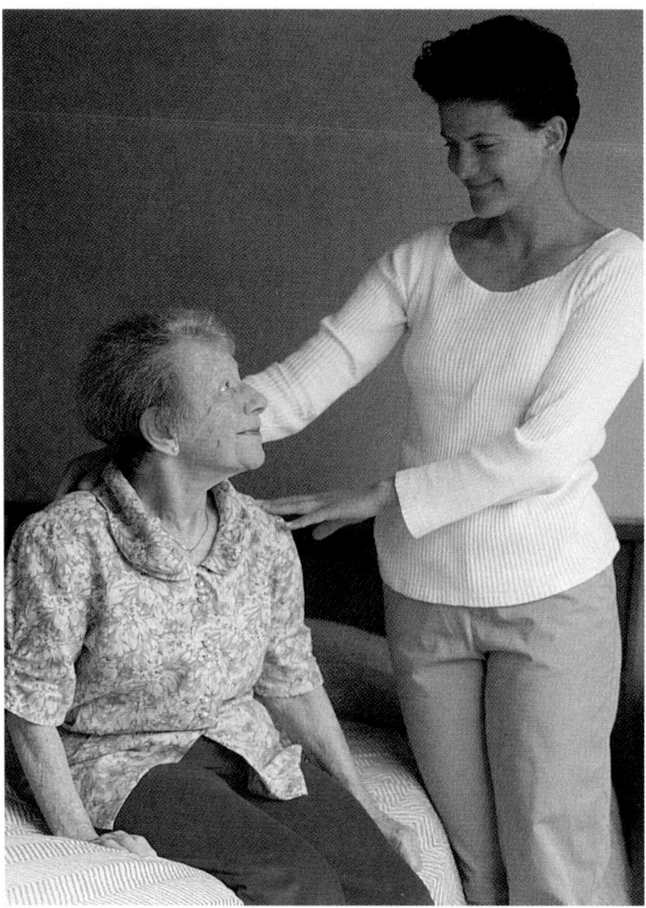

Figure 21.3 Seating the client in a comfortable position.

Step 2 *Observe the client.*

- Note signs of distress, quality of dress and hygiene, physical deformity, and so on.

Facial grimacing, pallor, or perspiration could indicate pain or anxiety; a perfectly groomed appearance might indicate someone who might not cope well with a disfiguring surgery; a deformity such as "dowager's hump" could indicate the need to probe for signs of pathologic fractures.

Step 3 *Observe the client's movements around the examining area.*

- Observe range of motion, gait, overall mobility, and posture (Figure 21.4).

Mobility is an indicator of safety, function, and self-care ability. Alterations can imply arthritis, neuromuscular disorders, stroke,

ASSESSMENT TECHNIQUE/NORMAL FINDINGS | SPECIAL CONSIDERATIONS

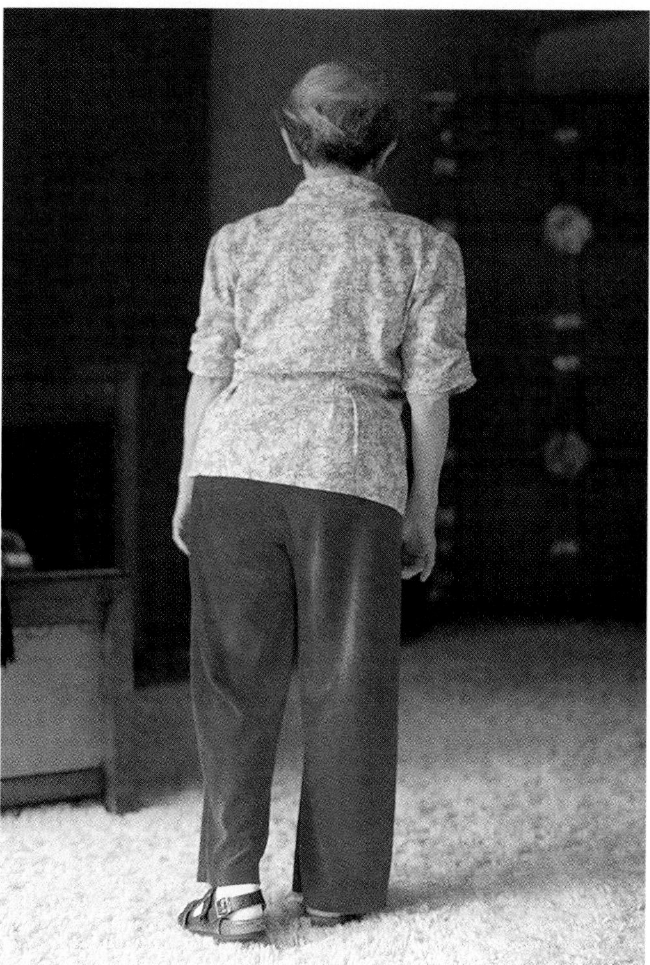

Figure 21.4 Checking the gait.

or degenerative disorders such as Parkinson's disease. Elderly people may slow down and become stooped. Men's gaits become more flexed with a wide base; women have a narrower base and tend to waddle, altering their balance. Both tend to take short steps, have decreased pick-up (shuffle), decreased velocity, and decreased arm swing.

Step 4 ***Evaluate the client's nutritional status.***

- Observe for a wasted or apathetic appearance.
- Measure height and weight and ask about usual values.
- Compare findings to height/weight scales especially designed for older adults (Table 21.2 on page 691).

Muscle and fat are normally lost with aging, but extreme loss might be due to inadequate nutrition or wasting diseases such as cancer.

Step 5. ***Observe the client's general hygiene, grooming, and dress.***

An unkempt appearance may be a sign of a physical inability to care for self, a sign of depression or other mental illness, or deteriorating mental functioning (eg, because of Alzheimer's disease or multi-infarct dementia). Also, abuse or neglect by caretakers must be considered.

ASSESSMENT TECHNIQUE/NORMAL FINDINGS	SPECIAL CONSIDERATIONS

Step 6 ***Note the client's interactions with family members or caretakers, and with you.***

- Observe for quality and quantity of interactions.

Excessive passivity or aggression can point to mental dysfunction, dysfunctional family system, or abuse. However, this interaction pattern might be typical for this family or culture.

Step 7 ***Observe the client's general attitude, behavior, communication, and ability to follow directions.***

- Specifically note speech defects, inattention, or failure to comply with spoken or written directions.

These observations can point out hearing or vision disruptions, alterations in mental status, depression, or neurologic disease. Speech problems include aphasia due to stroke of the dominant hemisphere, scanning due to cerebellar changes, or motor speech alterations such as slurring due to cranial nerve damage or brain tumors. Inability to follow directions could indicate hearing loss or receptive aphasia from stroke or dementias.

Step 8 ***Note any breath or body odors.***

The odor of urine/ammonia or feces is a sign of incontinence or neglect of personal hygiene; ammonia odor on breath and body may be due to renal failure. Fruity/acetone odor points to ketoacidosis in Type I diabetes but is rare in elderly Type II diabetes. It also can indicate starvation.

Step 9 ***Evaluate mental status.***

- Use a tool designed for older people such as the Mini Mental Status Examination (MMSE) or the Short Portable Mental Status Questionnaire (see page 692).

These tools can identify subtle changes in memory and judgment that the client could disguise in ordinary conversation by confabulation.

Step 10 ***Measure vital signs.***

- Take the blood pressure in both arms with the client reclining, sitting, and standing. Allow a minute or two between each measurement.
- Use a child-sized cuff for very thin, frail persons.
- Try Osler's maneuver: pump cuff above the systolic BP to see if the brachial artery is still palpable.
- Ask the client to resume a sitting position, assisting if necessary.

Orthostatic hypotension (drop of 20 mm Hg or more) is common with elderly people especially if the client is hypertensive or taking medications that affect blood pressure. Orthostatic hypotension increases risk of falls. Also, older people are more likely to have discrete differences of blood pressure in each arm. Loss of subcutaneous fat in small-boned persons makes the regular adult cuff too large, resulting in an erroneously low reading.

Osler's maneuver is used to evaluate hypertension. Because arteriosclerotic arteries do not compress as readily with the cuff, you may get a falsely high blood pressure reading (pseudohypertension). If the brachial artery is still palpable, pseudohypertension is likely, and the client should be referred to a physician for further evaluation. Hypertension is common

ASSESSMENT TECHNIQUE/NORMAL FINDINGS	SPECIAL CONSIDERATIONS
	in 35–50% of elderly people. A diastolic pressure of more than 90 should be watched, and the client should be referred if it persists.
◆ Take the pulse both apically and radially and compare, checking for pulse deficit. Note if pulse is irregular, either apically or radially, and check for extra or dropped beats.	Arrythmias are very common and affect the radial pulse, because weaker beats may be heard apically but not conduct radially. It is helpful to take radial and apical pulses simultaneously to check for pulse deficit, which is common in clients with atrial fibrillation and ventricular ectopic beats. If the apical beat is distant, verify with simultaneous radial palpation. Consider medications (eg, beta-blockers or digoxin) as a cause if the pulse is very slow, and adrenergic drugs or corticosteroids (taken orally or by inhaler) if the pulse too fast.
◆ Take a tympanic temperature if possible (see Chapter 7). Otherwise take an oral temperature using a glass or an electronic thermometer, holding it in place if client is unable to do so.	Temperature is commonly subnormal to low (95 to 97F) and may not become elevated with infection. Medications may also affect temperature.
◆ Observe respirations after listening to the apical beat while the stethoscope is still on the client's chest.	Older people may alter their respiratory rate when the examiner is listening with a stethoscope because of previous medical conditioning: "take a deep breath" or "hold your breath." By telling the client to breathe normally while you listen to the apical beat, you are able to assess respiratory rate more easily.
◆ Ensure that the client is not overly fatigued before proceeding with the exam.	

Integumentary System

ASSESSMENT TECHNIQUE/NORMAL FINDINGS	SPECIAL CONSIDERATIONS
Step 1 *Inspect the skin for color.* ◆ Note any overall redness, cyanosis, jaundice, or pallor. ◆ Check for erythema on bony prominences on the immobilized person and in moist areas such as the groin and under the breasts.	Elderly skin is paler and more transparent, but pallor could indicate anemia, malnutrition, or edema. Erythema could indicate an inflammation, irritation, or beginning decubitus ulcer. Differentiate visible veins, which cast a bluish color to lower extremities, from cyanosis.
Step 2 *Palpate the skin.* ◆ If any open sores or drainage is visible, put on gloves before proceeding with the assessment.	*Xerosis* (extreme dryness) is not uncommon, but moisturizers should be used to prevent cracking. Red and scaly skin may be *eczema*, and a silvery gray and scaly skin may indicate *psoriasis*. Skin temperature

ASSESSMENT TECHNIQUE/NORMAL FINDINGS	SPECIAL CONSIDERATIONS
◆ Note moisture or dryness, scaliness, temperature changes, and texture, especially wrinkling or thinness.	may be ambient or slightly cool, but specific areas of heat may indicate infection, and cold areas may signal impaired circulation due to, for instance, arterial insufficiency. Skin loses elasticity with age, so expect some wrinkling and decreased turgor. Extremely thin, fragile skin, especially in conjunction with underskin hemorrhages, excessive bruising, and *purpura*, may be seen in the very old; however, these signs more commonly signal long-term corticosteroid use. In this case, take special care to avoid tearing or other trauma.
Step 3 ***Measure and describe all skin lesions.*** ◆ Look for lesions that are common and nonsignificant in aging skin: *cherry angiomas, senile lentigos, seborrheic keratoses,* and *acrochordons*. (See Figure 21.1 on page 668.) Describe and measure these so that new lesions or changes in the old can be identified. ◆ Inspect precancerous *actinic keratoses* for cancerous lesions such as melanoma and basal- or squamous-cell carcinomas. ◆ Identify any areas of trauma and potential decubitus or vascular ulcers.	Altered pigmentation, especially in less vascular areas, is not unusual but may represent more easily traumatized tissue. Herpes zoster is more common in older adults: be suspicious of painful, red vesicular or pustular lesions that have a unilateral dermatome distribution. Ecchymoses, petechiae, or purpura may indicate a bleeding disorder. Excessive bruising, burns, or unexplained trauma could be a sign of abuse.
Step 4 ***Inspect the client's hair.*** ◆ Observe amount, distribution, and color of hair. ◆ Note excessive or total loss of hair; abnormal location of hair, especially gender related; and dry, brittle, or coarse hair.	Loss and growth of hair are variable with aging. Expect increased growth of facial hair in women, and more nasal and ear hair in both sexes. Altered distribution of hair, such as loss of chest and facial hair in men and excessive chest, arm, and facial hair in women could indicate hormonal disorders, use of gonadotropic hormones for cancer chemotherapy, or excessive use of corticosteroids. Gray or white hair is normal due to loss of melanocytes, but hair may be artificially colored, so check roots or ask about usual hair color. Dry, brittle hair may indicate malnutrition or overprocessing. Dull, dry, coarse hair could indicate hypothyroidism.
Step 5 ***Inspect the nails and nail beds.*** ◆ Note condition, hygiene, nail-bed angle, and blanching.	Nails can become thicker or more brittle, but extreme brittleness and tearing could indicate protein deficiency or diabetes. Very thick nails are seen in diabetes and vascular insufficiency. Long, dirty nails are a sign of caretaker neglect or inability to care for self. Increased nail-bed angle or absence of space when the nails are held

ASSESSMENT TECHNIQUE/NORMAL FINDINGS | SPECIAL CONSIDERATIONS

together indicates clubbing, which is related to chronic lung or cardiac diseases (see Chapter 8). Delayed blanching (longer than 6 seconds) is common with thickened, aging nails, especially toenails, and may not be an accurate reflection of circulatory status.

Head and Neck

Step 1 *Observe the face for sagging or drooping (Figure 21.5).*

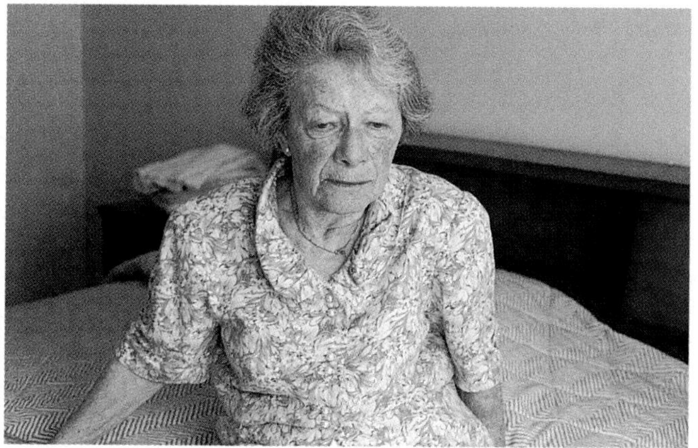

Figure 21.5 Observing for facial sagging.

Loss of muscle tone and collagen results in a sagging or jowly appearance, but drooping is usually a sign of a stroke or cranial nerve damage.

Step 2 *Inspect the eyelids, cornea, and iris.*

- Note the position of the lid on the iris, identifying any tumors or cloudiness of the cornea, rings over the limbus, irregularities of the iris, and inturning or drooping of lids.

The eyelids cover more of the iris in the aging eye because of decreased muscle tone, but frank *ptosis* in which the upper lid covers a considerable portion of the pupil, especially if unilateral, is a sign of dysfunction of cranial nerves III and IV, possibly due to stroke. Bilateral *ptosis* may be due to ocular myasthenia gravis. *Pterygium* is not significant, nor is *arcus senilis*. Cloudiness over the iris and pupil could be due to beginning cataracts. Irregularities of the iris may be genetic in origin but more likely due to previous surgery for glaucoma. *Entropion* and *ectropion* are the result of loss of muscle tone. (See Chapter 9.)

Step 3 *Check the pupils for size, equality, and reactivity.*

- Note both consensual and direct response to light.

For the best results, ensure that room is dimly lighted or that the client is facing away from sources of outside light.

Pupils decrease in size with age, and because of their smallness you may have difficulty eliciting pupillary constriction. Lack of consensual response or inequality of size may indicate damage to cranial nerve III. Unusually small pupils (smaller

ASSESSMENT TECHNIQUE/NORMAL FINDINGS	SPECIAL CONSIDERATIONS
	than 2 mm) may be due to ophthalmic miotic medications for glaucoma.
Step 4 *Measure visual acuity.* ◆ Be sure that the light is comfortably bright. ◆ Use a handheld Snellen vision screener, testing each eye separately while the client has glasses on. Then test both eyes together. ◆ Note if client holds screener more than the recommended 14 inches in order to read.	Loss of accommodation and power (holding the screener more than 14 inches away from eyes and requiring bright light to read by), called *presbyopia*, is a normal finding. Loss of central vision indicates macular degeneration. Blurring or cloudiness could be related to glaucoma, diabetic retinopathy, or cataracts.
Step 5 *Check peripheral fields of vision.* ◆ Especially note any losses of either left or right fields of vision.	A right or left hemispheric stroke can result in a loss in the contralateral visual field. Bilateral loss of peripheral vision may indicate cataracts or glaucoma.
Step 6 *Inspect the fundus of the eye with an ophthalmoscope.* ◆ Note any dark areas in the red reflex, changes in the optic disk, and appearance of the blood vessels.	Tiny pupils make fundoscopic inspection difficult. Changes of aging include narrower and straighter vessels. Black spots in the red reflex are signs of opacities as may be seen in cataracts. "Cupping" of the disk is a sign of glaucoma, and "fuzzy disk" indicates cerebral edema. Narrowing and tapering of the arterioles are seen in hypertensive disease, and small red spots or creamy round lesions are punctate hemorrhages and exudate seen in diabetic retinopathy.
Step 7 *Gently palpate the eyeball.* ◆ Ask the client to close the eyes. ◆ Note tension or firmness.	Very soft or boggy eyeballs indicate dehydration, whereas rock-hard orbits could mean glaucoma.
Step 8 *Evaluate the client's hearing.* ◆ Use the whisper, Rinne, and Weber tests (see Chapter 9). Use a 512 or 1024 tuning fork.	Hearing loss with aging begins with diminished perception of high-frequency sounds. You will find subtle changes when you use higher-frequency tuning forks. Sensorineural losses are more common than conductive losses in older adults because of loss of hair cells in the organ of Corti. This loss is called *presbycusis*. In sensorineural hearing loss, the Rinne test is normal (AC>BC), but the Weber test shows the sound lateralizing to the good ear or equal in both if hearing is diminished bilaterally.
Step 9. *Inspect the outer ear, ear canal, and tympanic membrane.* Use an otoscope to inspect the ear canal and ear drum. ◆ Note any excessive earwax or changes in tympanic membrane.	Excessive wax may cause a conductive hearing loss. Wax tends to be drier in older adults and may not be easy to remove. Improper ear-cleaning habits (eg, use of

ASSESSMENT TECHNIQUE/NORMAL FINDINGS	SPECIAL CONSIDERATIONS

cotton swabs) can pack wax tightly in the canal, interfering with hearing and obscuring visualization of the tympanic membrane. Scarring and sclerosis of the tympanic membrane from repeated inflammation or infection give a darkened appearance or dark lines.

Step 10 *Inspect the nose and nares.*

- Note color, size, and any excessive dryness.

Dryness is a sign of senile rhinitis, and redness in the nares may indicate chronic allergy. The nose tends to get larger with age, but a swollen, papular, red nose indicates **rhinophyma**, a severe rosacea of the lower half of nose. Usually seen in males, rhinophyma is characterized by lobulated overgrowth of sebaceous glands and epithelial connective tissue.

Step 11 *Evaluate the client's sense of smell.*

Use easily identifiable substances such as cloves or lemon.

Smell and taste diminish with age, but perceiving unusual odors may be a sign of temporal lobe epilepsy. An inability to distinguish pungent, common odors could be related to neurologic dysfunction such as stroke.

Step 12 *Inspect the oral mucous membranes, gums, throat, and tongue.*

- Note color, exudate, swelling, and lesions.
- Have the client say "ah" as you depress the tongue with a tongue blade. Check for symmetric elevation of soft palate.

Pale mucous membranes can indicate malnutrition or anemia; white patches could be precancerous *leukoplakia*. If the client's own teeth are present, redness and spongy swelling with recession of the gum from the neck of the tooth indicate periodontal disease. If the client is wearing dentures, redness and leukoplakia are signs of poorly fitting, irritating dentures. A bright red tongue could indicate thiamine (B_1) or vitamin C deficiency; a dark red, swollen tongue with white or yellow adherent patches is a sign of fungal infection, which older people on antibiotics commonly experience. A dry and red tongue with longitudinal furrows indicates dehydration, especially in people taking diuretics or having elevated blood sugar levels. Unequal elevation or loss of elevation of the soft palate occurs with impairment of cranial nerves IX and X, seen with stroke. In this case, the person is at risk for choking and aspiration.

Step 13 *Palpate and auscultate the carotid arteries.*

- Proceed gently, palpating one artery at a time.

Bruits are signs of carotid stenosis and impending stroke. If you hear bruits, check the aortic and pulmonic valve areas of the

ASSESSMENT TECHNIQUE/NORMAL FINDINGS	SPECIAL CONSIDERATIONS
◆ Auscultate with the bell of the stethoscope. ◆ Note any bruits.	chest for murmurs, which may be radiating into the neck.
Step 14 *Inspect and palpate the neck veins.* ◆ Assess the veins first with the client lying flat and then with the client elevated above 45 degrees. ◆ Note any firmness and distention.	All vessels enlarge with age and are more visible because of decreased subcutaneous tissue, but they are normally soft and compressible. If the veins are flat when the client is supine, suspect dehydration. If the neck veins are visible, firm to the touch, or tortuous when the client is elevated 45 degrees, suspect increased venous pressure and right heart failure.
Step 15 *Evaluate the range of motion of the neck.*	Limited range of motion in the neck is often related to cervical arthritis, degenerative disc disease, or muscle spasm. If *kyphosis* is present, hyperextension of the neck is difficult.

Heart and Lungs

ASSESSMENT TECHNIQUE/NORMAL FINDINGS	SPECIAL CONSIDERATIONS
Step 1 *Take the apical pulse.* ◆ Note rate, rhythm, and irregularities.	Arrythmias are quite common in healthy elders. Abnormally slow rates could indicate heart block or sinus arrest, especially if accompanied by syncope. Fast or grossly irregular rhythms point to potentially serious tachyarrythmias, especially if accompanied by chest pain or dizziness. After periods of immobilization, increased heart rate can indicate decompensation.
Step 2 *Auscultate the precordium.* ◆ Check for murmurs, clicks, and S3 or S4 gallops. ◆ Using the bell of the stethoscope, listen for low-pitched murmurs during S3 and S4. ◆ Using the diaphragm, listen for high-pitched murmurs, clicks, and snaps. ◆ If you hear a murmur, inch the stethoscope away from the site in several directions to check for radiation. ◆ Describe murmurs using specified criteria (see Chapter 11).	Murmurs, usually holosystolic and grade III without radiation, and S3 are common in older people because of decreased cardiac muscle tone. Loud murmurs grade IV or greater and with thrills and/or radiation suggest a failing heart, or valvular stenosis or incompetency. Murmurs that radiate from the apex to the anterior axillary area are usually of mitral origin. Murmurs that radiate from the base near the sternal border, right or left, up into the neck are usually related to aortic or pulmonic valve disease. Clicks and snaps are opening sounds and point to aortic or mitral calcifications. A fixed splitting of the second heart sound (not heard just on inspiration, but throughout the respiratory cycle) is noted in pulmonary hypertension or chronic obstructive pulmonary disease.

ASSESSMENT TECHNIQUE/NORMAL FINDINGS	SPECIAL CONSIDERATIONS

Step 3 *Inspect the shape of the thorax.*

- Look for increased anteroposterior diameter and spinal curvature abnormalities that may affect respiration.

Loss of bone density and weakened thoracic musculature result in an increased anteroposterior diameter. Severe barrel chest is a sign of chronic obstructive pulmonary disease. Also, kyphosis and scoliosis may decrease lung expansion (see Chapter 17).

Step 4 *Inspect and palpate the chest wall and ribs.*

- Assess pain or tenderness to touch, crepitus, or bruising.
- Palpate for tactile fremitus.

Pain upon palpation of the ribs is a sign of pathologic fractures of the ribs, which can occur without any major trauma in the client with osteoporosis. Also look for bruising in conjunction with rib pain, which could be due to falls or physical abuse.

Increased fremitus, especially in the periphery, indicates fluid accumulation or tissue consolidation.

Step 5 *Percuss the lung fields.*

- Check for hyperresonance or dullness.

Anticipate hyperresonance in the older adult with chronic obstructive pulmonary disease. Dullness indicates fluid accumulation from pulmonary edema or retained secretions. Dullness could also indicate tissue consolidation from a tumor or mass.

Step 6 *Auscultate the lung fields.*

- Note characteristics of sounds, decreased aeration or expansion, adventitious sounds such as rales or wheezes, and altered vocal resonance.

Scattered rales in the bases are quite common in healthy elderly persons. Rales that extend upward and do not clear with cough suggest pulmonary edema. Scattered or discrete rales can be due to alveolar or small airway exudate. Coarse, loud rales may be signs of pulmonary fibrosis seen in people with long-standing lung disease. Because lung expansion decreases with age, you will not hear breath sounds as far down as in younger adults; also, increased tactile fremitus and vocal resonance may be present because of decreased muscle and fat. If the person has increased trapped air from emphysema, which is present to some degree in the very old as a normal finding, breath sounds and vocal resonance will be diminished. Difficulty hearing any breath sounds, harsh ronchi, or bronchovesicular breath sounds in the periphery are indicative of advanced chronic lung disease.

ASSESSMENT TECHNIQUE/NORMAL FINDINGS | SPECIAL CONSIDERATIONS

Breasts

Step 1 ***Inspect and palpate the female and male breasts.***

- Note changes in symmetry, lumps or thickening of tissue, lesions or sores, inflammation, changes in the nipples, or drainage from open lesions or from the nipples.

Hormonal changes can increase breast tissue in males and put them at risk for breast cancer; however, the incidence is still very low for males. Females on postmenopausal hormone therapy are also at increased risk for breast cancer, especially if female relatives have had it. Decreased fat in the female breast may make masses easier to feel. Risk for all cancers increases with age, and early identification of tumors is vital.

Abdomen

Step 1 ***Inspect the abdomen.***

- Observe for shape, symmetry, pulsations, and visible tortuous veins, especially near the umbilicus.

Flaccid or "potbelly" abdomen is common because of loss of collagen and muscle, and deposition of fat. A scaphoid and flaccid abdomen is seen in the very old with additional fat loss but may also be a sign of rapid weight loss accompanying malnutrition or cancer. A distended abdomen is seen with fluid in the peritoneal cavity (ascites) or excessive gas. Asymmetry may indicate tumors, hernia, constipation, or bowel obstruction. Although the slight up-and-down pulsation from a normal aorta is more readily seen in clients with thin abdominal walls, lateral pulsations or soft, pulsatile masses indicate an aortic aneurysm. Visible tortuous veins on the abdominal wall near the umbilicus, in conjunction with a firm and distended abdomen, indicate portal hypertension with ascites.

Step 2 ***Auscultate the abdomen.***

- Note the number and quality of bowel sounds.
- Check for vascular bruits over the aorta, in flank areas for renal arteries, over the groin for femoral and iliac arteries.

Bowel sounds may be hypoactive. Borborygmi may be due to bleeding or inflammatory bowel disease. High-pitched hyperactive bowel sounds accompanied by colicky pain and distention are signs of small bowel obstruction, which occurs most often in elderly men. Bruits heard over any of the arteries are signs of stenosis or aneurysms.

Step 3 ***Percuss the abdomen.***

- Note tympany and dullness over most of the abdomen.
- Check for shifting dullness.
- Check for a distinct area of dullness in the lower abdomen above the symphysis pubis.

Because of the normally thinner abdominal wall, tympany may be more noticeable, but should still be within normal ranges. Areas of dullness in the lower left quadrant and sigmoid area are probably related to stool, but you must rule out tumors.

ASSESSMENT TECHNIQUE/NORMAL FINDINGS	SPECIAL CONSIDERATIONS

Shifting dullness, especially when accompanied by firm dullness, suggests ascites (Chapter 13).

Dullness above the symphysis pubis could indicate a full bladder.

Step 4 *Palpate the abdomen.*

- Note tenderness, firmness, rigidity, and masses.
- Palpate the costal margin at the right midclavicular line and midsternal line for liver enlargement.

Tenderness with moderate distention could be due to gas but could also indicate irritation of the stomach or bowel. The thinner abdominal wall of the older person makes it easier to feel the underlying bowel, and a soft mass or small firm masses felt in left lower quadrant may be stool, especially because constipation is common. Firmness is associated with fluid or excessive gas, but rigidity is a sign of peritoneal inflammation. Distention just above the symphysis pubis may be caused by bladder distention due to prostatic hypertrophy or incomplete emptying. If you can palpate the liver below the costal margins, the liver is probably enlarged. Enlargement may reflect passive congestion due to congestive heart failure or liver disease, especially if the liver feels nodular.

Genitourinary System

Female

Step 1 *Check the underclothing for staining.*

- If present, note color and odor.

Staining indicates incontinence or vaginal discharge.

Step 2 *Inspect the external genitals.*

- Note changes in the tissue, redness, swelling, or odor.

Atrophy of the labia is usual. Redness, swelling, or odor can indicate incontinence, yeast infections, inadequate self-care, or caretaker neglect. Fecal-like odor could signal a urinary tract infection.

Step 3 *Perform a pelvic examination.*

- Assist the client into the left lateral decubitus position.
- Perform the examination in the client's bed whenever possible, as this is much more comfortable for the elderly woman.

Bulging of tissue or muscle into the vagina or rectum indicates cystocele, rectocele, or uterine prolapse. Vaginal atrophy and dryness may make examination painful. Malodorous vaginal discharge could be a sign of cancer or infection.

Step 4 *Examine the rectum.*

- Note sphincter control.
- Check for hemorrhoids.
- Take a stool sample and check for occult blood.

Sphincter control decreases with age, resulting in incontinence. Rectal cancer is more common in older people; occult blood in the stool is a fairly early sign.

ASSESSMENT TECHNIQUE/NORMAL FINDINGS	SPECIAL CONSIDERATIONS

Male

Step 1 ***Check the underclothing for staining.***

- Note color and odor of any stains.

Staining indicates incontinence. Small amounts of dried blood could indicate intermittently bleeding hemmorrhoids.

Step 2 ***Examine the external genitals.***

- Observe for swelling, redness, or odor.

Testicular atrophy is normal, but swelling could be a sign of infection or prostatic hypertrophy. Swelling, redness, and odor can be a sign of infection, incontinence, poor self-care, or caretaker neglect.

Step 3 ***Perform a rectal exam.***

- Note sphincter control.
- Check for prostate enlargement and any rectal abnormalities such as hemorrhoids.
- Take a stool sample and check for occult blood.

Prostatic hypertrophy can be benign or malignant; encourage the client to get a PSA (prostate specific antigen) test. Elevated levels usually indicate carcinoma of the prostate.The occult blood test can detect colon cancer, which increases in incidence in men over 40. Hemorrhoids can cause bright red bleeding as well as a red stain on the stool. A mass in the rectum could be rectal cancer.

Musculoskeletal System

Step 1 ***Position the client.***

- Help the client to a comfortable sitting position.

Step 2 ***Inspect and palpate the spinal column.***

- Note abnormal curvatures, deformities, pain or tenderness with palpation of vertebrae, and bruising or other signs of trauma.

Shortening of the spine due to flattening of the discs is very common (see Figure 21.2). Loss of bone matrix and decreased muscle mass and tone can result in increased curvatures such as kyphosis, lordosis, or scoliosis. Arthritis and degenerative disc disease can cause spinal deformities. Pain upon palpation of the vertebrae and generalized back pain indicate pathologic fractures due to osteoporosis. Bruising or unusual lesions on the back could indicate falls or physical abuse.

Step 3 ***Inspect and palpate all joints.***

- Assess for pain, heat, redness, swelling, deformity, and range of motion.

Heat, redness, swelling, and pain on movement of joints indicate bursitis or gouty or septic arthritis. Rheumatoid arthritis also produces these symptoms but is more likely to be seen in younger adults. Osteoarthritis causes swelling and joint deformity with early morning stiffness and pain. Hands and weight-bearing joints, such as hips and knees, are most often affected. Chapter 17 describes different deformities of joints.

ASSESSMENT TECHNIQUE/NORMAL FINDINGS	SPECIAL CONSIDERATIONS

Step 4 *Inspect and palpate the feet.*

- Note color, skin integrity, any deformities, and signs of inflammation, infection, or ulcerations.
- Palpate pedal pulses.

Bunions and corns are common. If home remedies have been used to treat corns, inflammation and ulceration may result. Pedal pulses may diminish with aging, but the inability to palpate pulses, especially if the feet are red or dusky in color, indicates arterial insufficiency. Pitting edema of feet and legs due to venous incompetency or right-sided heart failure may be present. The box on page 693 outlines a lower extremity assessment for the older adult.

Neurologic System

Step 1 *Evaluate balance and coordination.*

- Assess the client's ability to walk heel-to-toe forward and backward.
- Ask the client to perform the *Romberg* test first with eyes opened, then with eyes closed.
- Look for swaying and loss of balance.
- Ask client to open the eyes. Stand next to client to prevent fall or injury.

The heel-to-toe walk is often impaired and is not indicative of any specific disease, but it can place the person at risk for falls. Older people have a tendency to fall sideways. Falling forward and a propulsive gait are indicative of Parkinson's disease. If the person can correct balance with the eyes open, the defect is probably proprioceptive rather than of basal ganglion or cerebellar origin.

Step 2 *Inspect for tremors of the head, face, and extremities.*

- Note the kind of tremor and whether it is present at rest or primarily with movement.

Gross tremor of the head (head bobbing), jaw, and tongue is called a *senile tremor* and is not treatable. A *resting tremor*, which diminishes with willed movement, and a pill-rolling tremor of the hands is seen in Parkinson's disease. People taking bronchodilator drugs have a fine tremor that increases with activity.

Step 3 *Evaluate motor strength.*

- Assess the client's arm drift. Have the client stand with the feet comfortably apart, and the arms held straight out at shoulder level. Check arm drift first with the client's eyes closed, then open (Figure 21.6 on page 690).

Subtle hemiparesis is indicated by slow downward drift and pronation of hand on affected side when the eyes are closed; if the client is able to correct drift when the eyes are opened, suspect proprioceptive dysfunction (sensory-position sense). Unilateral diminished grip and loss of strength against resistance can indicate a stroke. Loss of innervation to specific muscle groups or paralysis from stroke or other neurologic diseases results in atrophy and loss of or increased tone.

ASSESSMENT TECHNIQUE/NORMAL FINDINGS | SPECIAL CONSIDERATIONS

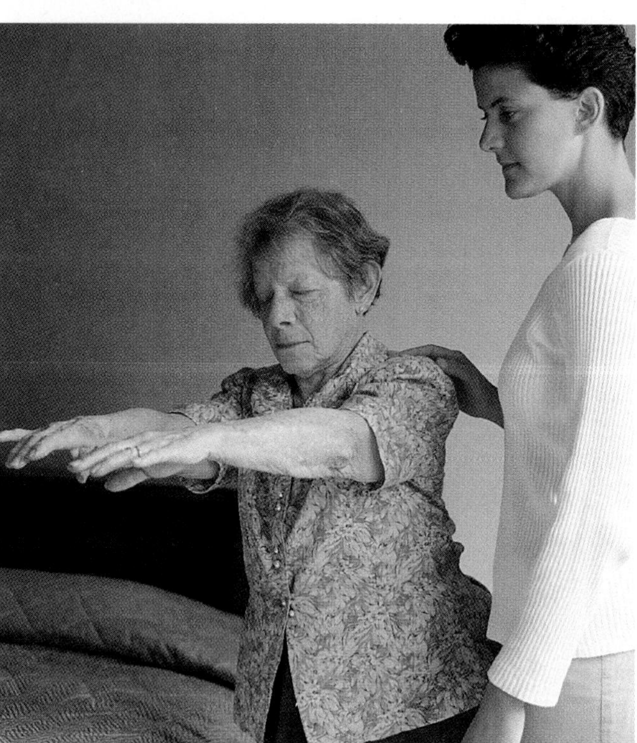

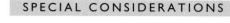

Figure 21.6 Assessing for hemiparesis.

- Assess the client's grip and extremity strength against resistance.
- Inspect the muscles for size, comparing one side with the other.
- Palpate muscles for tone.

Step 4 ***Evaluate sensation.***

- Assist the client to the sitting position.
- Ask the client to close the eyes for all sensory evaluation.
- Check various sites for sensitivity to touch (use sharp and dull objects) and vibration (use a tuning fork on joints). Ask the client to identify where sensation is felt by pointing or verbally identifying location.
- Assess stereognosis by asking the client to close the eyes and identify a key or other familiar object placed in the client's hand. Assess graphesthesia by asking the client to identify numbers you write with your finger on each of the client's hands.
- Evaluate proprioception by having the client identify the position to which you move a toe or finger. (See Chapter 18.)

Sensation and discrimination normally decrease in elderly people, as does vibratory sense in the toes. Suspect neurologic disease such as cerebrovascular accident if sensation is absent in any area, especially unilaterally. Diminished or absent sensation symmetrically in lower extremities is a sign of diabetic peripheral neuropathy.

Step 5 ***Evaluate the reflexes with a reflex hammer.***

- Note diminished or increased reflexes.

Reflexes normally diminish with aging. If they are absent, suspect upper motor neuron disease; if they are hyperactive, especially with clonus, suspect lower motor neuron disease.

Table 21.2 Height-Weight Scales for Older Adults

Average Weight in Pounds per Inch of Height in Women Aged 65–94

	Age (years)					
Height (inches)	65–68	69–74	75–79	80–84	85–89	90–94
58	133	125	123	–	–	–
59	134	127	124	116	110	–
60	135	129	126	118	113	–
61	137	131	128	121	116	–
62	139	134	131	124	120	119
63	141	137	134	128	124	119
64	144	140	137	132	133	120
65	147	144	140	136	138	124
66	151	147	143	140	142	129
67	155	151	146	144	–	–
68	159	155	–	–	–	–
69	164	160	–	–	–	–

Average Weight in Pounds per Inch of Height in Men Aged 65–94

	Age (years)					
Height (inches)	65–69	70–74	75–79	80–84	85–89	90–94
61	142	139	137	–	–	–
62	144	141	139	135	–	–
63	146	143	141	136	133	–
64	149	146	143	138	135	–
65	151	149	145	141	139	130
66	154	152	148	144	142	133
67	156	155	151	147	145	136
68	159	158	154	150	148	140
69	163	162	158	154	152	144
70	167	165	162	159	156	149
71	172	169	166	164	160	154
72	177	173	171	170	165	–
73	182	178	175	–	–	–

From O'Hanlon P, Kohrs M. Dietary studies of older Americans. *Am J Clin Nutr* 1978; 31:1257.

Short Portable Mental Status Questionnaire

Instructions: Ask questions 1 through 10 in this list and record all answers.
Ask question 4A only if client does not have a telephone. Record total number of errors based on 10 questions.

1. What is the date today? ______________________
   Month Day Year
2. What day of the week is it? ______________________
3. What is the name of this place? ______________________
4. What is your telephone number? ______________________

4A. What is your street address? ______________________
(Ask only if client does not have a telephone.)

5. How old are you? ______________________
6. When were you born? ______________________
7. Who is the president of the United States now? ______________________
8. Who was the president just before him? ______________________
9. What was your mother's maiden name? ______________________
10. Subtract 3 from 20 and keep subtracting 3 from each new number, all the way down.

Total Number of Errors

Scoring:

0–2 errors = intact mental function

3–4 errors = mild intellectual impairment

5–7 errors = moderate intellectual impairment

8–10 errors = severe intellectual impairment

Allow one more error if subject had only grade school education.

Allow one fewer error if subject has had education beyond high school.

Adapted from Pfeiffer E. A short portable mental status questionnaire for the assessment of organic brain deficit in elderly patients. *J Am Geriatr Soc* 1975; 23:433; used with permission.

Lower Extremity Assessment for the Older Adult

1. Mobility (check one):
   ❑ Walks without assistance ❑ Walks with help of equipment ❑ Does not walk—uses wheelchair ❑ Bedfast
2. Ask the client, "Does the condition of your feet or legs limit your activity in any way?" ❑ Yes ❑ No
   ❑ If *yes*, describe: ________________
3. Ask the client to walk approximately 10 feet. Is there any gait disturbance? ❑ Yes ❑ No

Remove the client's shoes and stockings

4. Cleanliness of feet: ❑ Acceptable ❑ Unacceptable
5. Are the stockings a good fit? ❑ Yes ❑ No
6. Does the client usually wear well-fitting, leather (synthetic) shoes that cover the feet completely?
   ❑ Yes ❑ No If *yes*, are they in good condition?
   ❑ Yes ❑ No
7. Does the client wear circular garters? ❑ Yes ❑ No

Dermatologic assessment

8. Skin lesions
   a. Fissure between the toes? ❑ Yes ❑ No
   b. Fissure on heel(s)? ❑ Yes ❑ No
   c. Ecoriation on legs or feet? ❑ Yes ❑ No
   d. Corn(s)? ❑ Yes ❑ No
      (Corn—painful, circular area of thickened skin, appearing on skin that is normally thin)
   e. Callus(es)? ❑ Yes ❑ No
      (Callus—thickened skin, occurring on skin that is normally thick, such as soles)
   f. Plantar wart? ❑ Yes ❑ No
   g. Other? ❑ Yes ❑ No
      Describe: ________________
9. Itching on legs or feet? ❑ Yes ❑ No
10. Rash on legs or feet? ❑ Yes ❑ No
11. Inspect pressure areas on the feet for localized areas of redness. Are any present? ❑ Yes ❑ No
    If *yes*, which foot? ❑ Right ❑ Left
12. Inspect legs, feet, and toes for localized swelling, warmth, tenderness, and redness. Is any present?
    ❑ Yes ❑ No If *yes*, specify location:
    ❑ R leg ❑ R foot ❑ L leg ❑ L foot
13. Toenails
    a. Ingrown? ❑ Yes ❑ No
       (Ingrown toenail—a sensitive and tender overhanging nail fold)
    b. Overgrown (long)? ❑ Yes ❑ No
    c. Thickened? ❑ Yes ❑ No
    d. Yellow discoloration? ❑ Yes ❑ No
    e. Black discoloration? ❑ Yes ❑ No

Circulatory status

Questions 14 to 18 relate to feet only.

14. Do the feet have any red, reddish blue, or bluish discoloration? ❑ Yes ❑ No
15. Is there any brownish discoloration around the ankles? ❑ Yes ❑ No
16. Is the dorsalis pedis pulse present?
    ❑ Yes ❑ No If *no*, in which foot is it absent?
    ❑ Right ❑ Left
17. Is the posterior tibial pulse present?
    ❑ Yes ❑ No If *no*, in which foot is it absent?
    ❑ Right ❑ Left
18. Is the skin dry? ❑ Yes ❑ No

Questions 19 to 23 relate to both feet and legs.

19. Is edema present? ❑ Yes ❑ No

Check the temperature of the legs and the feet with the backs of your fingers, comparing one extremity with the other

20. Are the feet the same temperature? ❑ Yes ❑ No
21. Are the legs the same temperature? ❑ Yes ❑ No
22. Does the client have any pain in legs or feet?
    ❑ Yes ❑ No If *yes*, describe:
    ____

Inspect the legs, sides of ankles, soles, and toes for ulceration

23. Is any ulceration present? ❑ Yes ❑ No
    If *yes* specify location: ❑ R leg ❑ R foot ❑ L leg ❑ L foot

Adapted from Eliopoulos C. *Health Assessment of the Older Adult,* 2d ed. (Redwood City, CA: Addison-Wesley Nursing, 1992).

Organizing the Data

After completing the focused interview and the physical examination, group the data into clusters to identify appropriate nursing diagnoses that require independent nursing actions, such as teaching, or to identify alterations in health that call for collaboration with other health care professionals.

Identifying Nursing Diagnoses

Problems for the older adult can fall into most of the diagnoses on NANDA's list. It is important that you review all diagnoses when analyzing clients over age 65, because multi-

DIAGNOSTIC REASONING IN ACTION

Lily Mae Kandsky is an 82-year-old female with insulin-dependent diabetes mellitus (IDDM) who lives alone. She has three adult children who take turns checking on her daily. The nurse is making a home visit on referral from Mrs. Kandsky's physician to evaluate her ability to manage at home and to monitor her compliance with the medical treatment plan. She was discharged home 2 days ago after being hospitalized for 10 days for diabetic ketoacidosis.

Although her children have wanted her to move in with one of them, Mrs. Kandsky adamantly refuses. Her daughter, Mary, who is present at the intake, reports that her mother has had a loss of her short-term memory gradually over the last 2 years but still functions very effectively, even though she occasionally forgets to take her medicines. She also indicates that her mother falls frequently and gets numerous bruises and abrasions but has not broken any bones or had an infection in any of the abrasions.

Mary tells the nurse, Kevin Greene, RN, that her mother will not let any of them come over and clean the house. Mary also states that her mother, who used to be energetic and loved to socialize, won't go anywhere with them anymore and won't even come over to her children's homes for dinner because she is embarrassed about how she looks.

She administers her own insulin: 45 units of NPH every morning and 15 units of NPH every evening. Her daughter draws up the insulin weekly. She also checks to make sure all injections were taken for the week but has noted that occasionally Mrs. Kandsky has forgotten the evening injection. They do not check her blood sugar, and neither mother nor daughter knows the signs and symptoms of hypoglycemia or hyperglycemia.

Mrs. Kandsky states, "I know all about what kind of diet I should be on—no cake or candy or sugar on anything. But lately I don't have much of an appetite—nothing tastes very good."

On assessment, Mr. Greene notes the following significant data:

- Height/weight: 64 inches, 98 pounds (with a loss of 15 pounds over the last year)
- Blood pressure: 138/60
- Apical pulse: 72 regular
- Respirations: 18
- Lungs clear
- Temperature: 97F
- Skin thin and dry with several 3 cm ecchymotic areas on left arm, 6 cm ecchymoses on left thigh, and several healed excorations on arms and legs
- Legs very thin with visible tortuous veins; dependent rubor noted 4 cm above ankles and feet with no palpable pulses
- Feet very dry and cracking, but skin intact; nails thickened, but trimmed neatly
- Unable to feel light touch or discriminate sharp from dull from the ankle down.
- Finger-stick blood sugar: 224 mg/%.

The nursing assessment of Lily Mae Kandsky reveals the following subjective and objective data:

- Insistence on living alone
- Refuses help with home maintenance
- Moderate loss of short-term memory
- Occasionally forgets to take medicines
- Frequent falls
- Bruises and healed excoriations on arms and legs
- Refuses to socialize with family
- Impaired circulation in legs: visible veins, dependent rubor, absent pedal pulses

system disorders are common and altered abilities not unusual. Some of the more common diagnoses include:

- *Activity intolerance:* A state in which an individual has insufficient physiologic or psychologic energy to endure or complete required or desired daily activities.
- *Body image disturbance:* Disruption in the way one perceives one's body image.
- *Caregiver role strain:* A caregiver's felt difficulty in performing the family caregiver role.
- *Perceived constipation:* A state in which an individual makes a self-diagnosis of constipation and ensures a daily bowel movement through use of laxatives, enemas, and suppositories.
- *Diversional activity deficit:* The state in which an individual experiences a decreased stimulation from or interest or engagement in recreational or leisure activities.
- *Ineffective family coping:* A usually supportive primary person is providing insufficient, ineffective, or compromised support, comfort, assistance, or encouragement that may

- Impaired sensation in ankles and feet
- Does not check blood sugar, takes insulin daily
- Current blood sugar elevated
- Lack of knowledge about complications of diabetes and its dietary management
- Diet inadequate in amount and basic nutrients
- Decreased appetite and altered taste sensation
- Below ideal body weight with 15% loss over one year

To cluster the data, Mr. Greene

- Notes that the reported frequent falls and verifying bruises and excoriations are defining characteristics for the diagnosis *High risk for injury.* Her impaired circulation, altered sensation in lower extremities, and loss of balance common at her age are related factors for this diagnosis.
- Notes that by forgetting to take her medication and failing to monitor her blood sugar while taking daily insulin, Mrs. Kandsky is demonstrating the defining characteristics of *Altered health maintenance.* Related factors are cognitive impairment and possibly lack of knowledge.
- Notes that Mrs. Kandsky's refusal to go out with her children or spend time at their homes are defining characteristics of the nursing diagnosis *Impaired social interaction.* Related factors appear to be self-concept disturbance and decreased energy.
- Notes that Mrs. Kandsky's low body weight, with a 15-pound loss over the last year, and inadequate food intake are defining characteristics for the diagnosis of *Altered nutrition: less than body requirements.* The related factors are loss of appetite and altered taste sensations secondary to diabetes and aging.
- Notes that Mrs. Kandsky and her daughter's lack of understanding about the complications of diabetes, appropriate diet for managing diabetes, and proper way to test blood sugar are defining characteristics of the nursing diagnosis *Knowledge deficit.* The related factors are unknown and need further exploration. Possible factors include lack of recall and incomplete information.

Based on the analysis of the assessment, Mr. Greene derives the following nursing diagnoses:

1. *Impaired home maintenance management* related to decreased energy and refusal of family help
2. *High risk for injury* related to impaired circulation, altered sensation and perception in lower extremeties, and loss of balance
3. *Altered health maintenance* related to memory loss and possibly lack of knowledge
4. *Impaired social interaction* related to self-concept disturbance and decreased energy
5. *Altered nutrition: less than body requirements* related to loss of appetite and impaired taste sensation
6. *Knowledge deficit* of diabetic management related to possible lack of recall or cognitive limitation

Mr. Greene sets up a contract with Mrs. Kandsky and her daughter for weekly home visits over a period of 2 months. During that time, Mr. Greene will teach both mother and daughter the various aspects of managing diabetes, including diet, proper technique for monitoring blood sugar by fingerstick, and the main complications that should be reported immediately to the nurse or doctor. Mr. Greene refers them to the Diabetic Society as a resource for obtaining a blood glucose monitor and for follow-up and support after the home visits are discontinued. Mr. Greene initiates a discussion with Mrs. Kandsky and Mary about ways that Mrs. Kandsky can conserve her energy, feel better about her appearance, and avoid falling and injuring herself. Mrs. Kandsky agrees to let her daughters clean her house once a week if she can supervise. Mr. Greene puts a note on Mrs. Kandsky's refrigerator, reminding her to take the evening insulin after dinner. Finally, Mr. Greene calls Mrs. Kandsky's physician and reports the client's status and the agreed-upon plan.

be needed by the client to manage or master adaptive tasks related to his or her health challenge.

- *Fatigue:* An overwhelming sustained sense of exhaustion and decreased capacity for physical and mental work.
- *Altered health maintenance:* Inability to identify, manage, or seek out help to maintain health.
- *Home maintenance management:* Inability to independently maintain a safe, growth-producing immediate environment.
- *Stress incontinence:* The state in which an individual experiences a loss of urine of less than 50 ml occuring with increased abdominal pressure.
- *High risk for injury:* A state in which the individual is at risk of injury as a result of environmental conditions interacting with the individual's adaptive and defensive resources.
- *Altered nutrition: less than body requirements:* The state in which an individual experiences an intake of nutrients insufficient to meet metabolic needs.
- *Chronic pain:* A state in which the individual experiences pain that continues for more than 6 months.
- *Self-care deficit:* Feeding, bathing/hygiene, dressing/grooming, toileting: The state in which an individual experiences an impaired ability to perform or complete activities of daily living.
- *Low self-esteem: situational:* Negative self-evaluation/feelings about self that develop in response to a loss or change in an individual who previously had a positive self-evaluation.
- *Impaired social interaction:* The state in which an individual participates in an insufficient or excessive quantity or ineffective quality of social exchange.

Common Alterations in the Health of the Older Adult

The previous case study illustrates the multisystem problems encountered by the elderly person. While many older adults, especially those in their 60s and 70s, are quite healthy, the older the person gets, the more likely that one or more chronic diseases will become evident. However, it is important to realize that many people with chronic diseases live full, satisfying lives. By following a prescribed medical regime, embracing healthful practices, and focusing on people and events other than their illnesses and discomforts, they ensure that their later years, unencumbered by the competitive drives of career and developing family, can be just as enjoyable (some say more enjoyable) as their youth and middle age. Although you are responsible for doing everything you can to empower the older client by encouraging active participation in managing health and disease, you will still encounter clients who feel unable to provide self-care. In these cases, help the client find reliable caretakers, either family members or hired professionals, and provide education and support to the caregivers. Finally, as an advocate for the client, supervise the quality of the care.

Arthritis

A common degenerative disorder of older people, osteoarthritis can result in pain and disability that impair mobility and interfere with carrying out ADLs. Although arthritis is not curable, most of the discomfort can be alleviated by use of nonsteroidal anti-inflammatory drugs, daily exercises prescribed by a physical therapist, and other specific interventions such as application of heat and cold, dietary changes, and weight loss, if appropriate.

The signs and symptoms of arthritis include enlarged or deformed, painful joints, commonly of the distal and proximal interphalanges, knees, hips, and vertebrae. Pain and stiffness are more common upon arising and during cold, damp weather.

Cancer

Because of the possiblity of age-related alterations in DNA, prolonged exposure to environmental carcinogens, and impaired immunity, elderly people are at risk for many cancers. The signs and symptoms relate to the areas of the body affected; no complaint of pain or altered body functioning should go uninvestigated. Fair-skinned people are commonly at risk for skin cancers because of a loss of melanocytes. Many skin cancers are easily treated. Older men are at a higher risk for prostate cancer and older women for breast cancer, especially if they are receiving postmenopausal hormone replacement therapy. Bowel cancer is also more common in the aging population. Clients need to be taught to recognize the seven signs of cancer (see the accompanying box) and to seek medical advice if they note any changes. Men should have a yearly PSA; women should have a yearly Papanicolaou smear and mammogram, especially if they are on hormone replacement therapy. Both men and women should have a test for occult blood in the stool and sigmoidoscopy.

Congestive Heart Failure

Whether the result of earlier myocardial damage, the ravages of long-term diabetes mellitus or undiagnosed hypertension, or just the gradual fatigue of a hard-working organ, heart failure can be recognized by several classic signs and symptoms: persistent dependent edema and ascites of right-sided heart failure; pulmonary edema (rales), dyspnea, and fatigue of left-sided failure. Often murmurs and gallops are heard. Conges-

The Seven Warning Signs of Cancer

C hange in bowel or bladder habits
A sore that does not heal
U nusual bleeding or discharge
T hickening or lump in breast or elsewhere
I ndigestion or difficulty in swallowing
O bvious change in wart or mole
N agging cough or hoarseness

If you have a warning sign, see your doctor!

tive heart failure can be managed by a variety of drugs that improve cardiac function, decrease fluid retention, decrease afterload, and improve circulation and oxygenation. To manage the disease, you need to monitor these clients closely and collaborate with the physician. Teach clients to conserve energy but stay active and involved within their limitations.

Constipation

Decreased gastrointestinal motility, often coupled with low fiber and water intake, results in the very common complaint of constipation, which the older person may aggravate by the indiscriminate use of laxatives. Many older people expect to have a bowel movement every day and fear becoming "toxic" if they do not. Experts feel that this erroneous idea comes from childhood conditioning. Whatever the cause, this is an excellent area for client teaching. See the teaching plan later in this chapter. One caution: small bowel obstruction is a real risk for older adults. The loss of fat and muscle tone in an older adult may result in the unsupported bowel twisting upon itself. This condition, called a *volvulus*, is the primary cause of bowel obstruction in elderly men. Adhesions from previous surgeries is another cause. Therefore, you need to do a thorough assessment before concluding that the constipation is due to dietary or other functional causes.

Diabetes

Non-insulin-dependent diabetes mellitus (NIDDM) is seen more often in older adults than younger people. Unfortunately, if NIDDM is poorly controlled, affected individuals can have the same devastating complications that accompany the insulin-dependent disease. One of the defining characteristics of NIDDM is that the individual has some circulating insulin but not enough, or that the receptor sites on the cell become resistant to insulin. The result is hyperglycemia, which often can be treated by diet management alone or a combination of diet and oral hypoglycemic agents that reduce resistance of the receptor sites to insulin. The reasons that this disease occurs in older individuals appear to be threefold. First, the beta cells "tire" with age and do not produce enough insulin. Second, obesity increases the amount of tissue needing insulin, putting more pressure on the beta cells to produce insulin, perhaps exacerbating insulin resistance. Finally, autoimmune processes may be a factor in insulin-resistant receptor sites, and the tendency toward autoimmunity increases with age. Include fingerstick blood glucose monitoring in the assessment of older adults, and pay careful attention to signs and symptoms of diabetes: polyuria, polydipsia, and polyphagia. In addition, you should explore signs and symptoms that point to any of the complications, such as peripheral neuropathy, retinopathy, nephropathy, or vascular changes, especially of the lower extremities. Refer clients with suspicious findings to appropriate medical practitioners.

Depression and Suicide

Although depression is not a normal response to aging, recent studies show that 10 to 25% of elderly people are clinically depressed. A substantial number of these depressed clients are successful in committing suicide because, unlike their younger counterparts, they do not signal their intent. The reasons for such devastating statistics are a pervasive sense of loss. Among the losses are occupation, income, prestige, spouse, children, friends, appearance, and social value. Physical disease and side effects of drugs worsen the situation. Although the elderly may not specifically verbalize suicidal intent, depression does have clinical manifestations that you can detect, and treatment can help. Appetite disturbances, loss of energy, loss of interest in previous activities, loss of pleasure, frequent complaints about multisystem problems, insomnia or sleeping too much, agitation or inactivity, expression of feelings of worthlessness, diminished ability to concentrate, crying without apparent reason, and recurrent thoughts of death or talking about death are all signs that you should note and investigate further. Because most people deny depression, suggesting a mental health referral may be difficult, but you should persist in getting help for a depressed client. The elderly client most at risk for suicide is a man 80 years or older who is recently widowed and drinks too much alcohol. (See the box on page 674 for the Geriatric Depression Scale.)

Drug and Alcohol Abuse

For some of the same reasons that cause depression, some elderly people use drugs, such as tranquilizers or alcohol, to cope with both physical and emotional pain. Because the afflicted client will minimize or deny use of substances, you need to collect adequate corroborative data before confronting the client with the problem. It is also helpful to consult the client's physician or a specialist in addiction to devise a team approach to the problem.

Fractures

Fractures, especially of the femur, ribs, or vertebrae, can be the result of falls or car accidents. Pathologic fractures due to osteoporosis are also common. Other etiologies, such as abuse or metastatic cancer, need to be ruled out. Because of loss of calcium and protein from the bone matrix, the older adult is more vulnerable to fractures. Corticosteroid therapy and chronic diseases are also contributing factors. Signs and symptoms range from severe pain to aching and tenderness upon palpation of the involved body part. You need to investigate any unexplained pain or reports of falls with pain and bruising and refer the person to appropriate health care professionals as indicated.

Health Promotion and Client Education

At the conclusion of the interview and physical assessment, share your findings with the client and answer any questions. Make plans with the client for any follow-up care or referrals to other health care professionals. This is an excellent time for health teaching based on actual problems or risk factors uncovered during the interview and assessment. You also can assess the client's understanding of health-promotion activities and provide teaching based on the client's individual needs. Although a number of risk factors do exist, the variations in older individuals are immense, and it is better to focus on positive health measures to promote well-being than to dwell on the negative aspect of the many risks associated with aging. As you uncover individual problems, develop a teaching plan that focuses on that specific area, taking into consideration the older person's unique situation.

Health promotion includes supporting any physician-prescribed regimen, such as dietary changes to manage hypertension, cardiac disease, and diabetes. Include these in the plan. The following general suggestions promote better health in any older client.

Nutrition

1. Use the new Food Guide Pyramid from the U.S. Department of Agriculture and the U.S. Department of Health and Human Services to plan meals (see Chapter 5).
2. Reduce fat in the diet to 30–35 g per day, and try to get most of fat calories from nonanimal sources. Read labels to get an idea of the fat content of a food item. (See Chapter 5 for a more complete discussion of identifying fat content in food.)
3. Get most of your protein from chicken, fish, legumes, grains, or vegetables. All beans—navy, kidney, black, lima—provide protein and are low in fat and high in fiber.
4. High-fiber foods, which include most vegetables, fruits, whole grains, and legumes, provide satiety and promote good bowel function.
5. Older people often do not tolerate milk well, and milk is not necessary as a nutrient. However, the client must find alternative sources of calcium. Broccoli, cheese, yogurt, and fish with bones (such as sardines) are excellent sources.
6. Reduce salt and sugar intake. Read the labels on prepared and canned foods. Limit salt to 3 g a day, and be aware that it goes by many names, such as sodium chloride, baking soda, baking powder, and others. Some foods, such as celery, are naturally high in salt. Not adding salt during or after cooking reduces sodium intake; a variety of herbs, lemon juice, and chili powder are good salt substitutes. Sugar hides under the names of glucose, sucrose, fructose, maltose, and corn syrup. It is added to many commercially prepared foods as well as cough syrups, cough drops, antacid tablets, and fiber powders.
7. Drink at least four glasses of water a day, spread throughout the day. If you drink caffeinated beverages, drink extra water to replace water lost through the diuretic effects of the caffeine.
8. Local chapters of the American Diabetes Association, American Heart Association, and American Cancer Society provide excellent information on special diets and ways to decrease disease risk. A variety of inexpensive cookbooks and receipes are available.

Exercise

1. Walking is an excellent aerobic exercise that also lifts the spirits. Walking music tapes are available in a variety of paces to accommodate slow, intermediate, and fast walkers.
2. Gentle warm-ups of stretching or walking in place are useful before walking, though starting and finishing with a slower-paced walk has the same effect.
3. Wear warm, layered clothing with a hat and gloves during cold weather and loose-fitting, cool clothing during warmer weather. Walk inside to music or while watching TV if the weather is too cold, stormy, or hot. Mall-walking is an acceptable substitute for outside walking during inclement weather.
4. Proper shoes are very important. They should be lightweight, fit comfortably, and have good arch support and a roomy toe box. Have shoes fitted by a knowl-

edgable person in a store that sells shoes for walkers. Get shoes that can be used for multiple purposes if cost is a concern.

5. Swimming is also an excellent exercise, especially for those older people troubled by arthritis or other joint problems.
6. Many senior centers offer a variety of non-impact or low-impact aerobic exercises for many different levels of ability. This provides socialization as well as professional supervision of exercise.
7. Bicycling is another excellent exercise. It can be done on a stationary bicycle in the home or a recreational center. Three-wheeled bicycles are available. Get a bicycle with a basket and use it to do the daily shopping.
8. Tai chi chuan is a new low-impact exercise that is becoming a favorite with many older people. It is best learned from a master; many recreational and senior centers offer lessons.
9. An exercise partner is very beneficial. Exercise is more fun with a partner and also safer.
10. Learn what the target heart rate should be for your age group. Monitoring for fatigue and inability to talk without breathlessness are good guidelines for determining when the exercise is too strenuous.
11. The time of day is important for exercise. Either early morning or late evening before dark are good times for summer or year-round warm climates. Limit exposure to midday sun and use a sun-screen for any daylight outdoor activities. Figure 21.7 illustrates exercises that can be done at any time.

Hygiene and Skin Care

1. Unless you engage in "dirty" activities or occupations, daily bathing is not necessary for older people. Overly frequent bathing, especially with soap, can result in excessively dry skin and itching. Bathe with moderately warm water no more than every other day. Use soap substitutes or bath gels that contain emolliants. Rinse and dry thoroughly, using lotion afterward as needed.

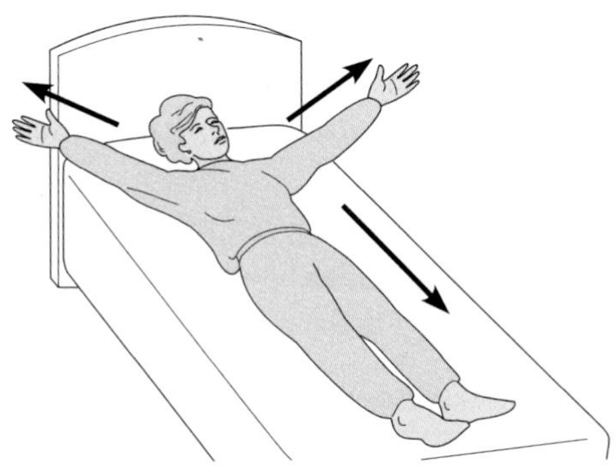

Stretch your arms and legs; breathe deeply.

A

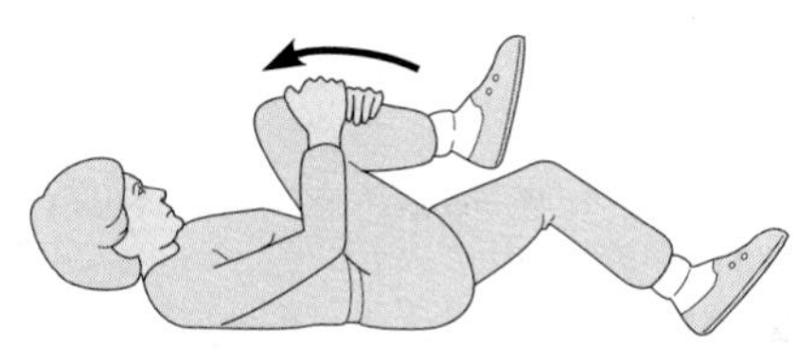

Hold each leg with both hands below the knee and pull toward your chest slowly and gently.

B

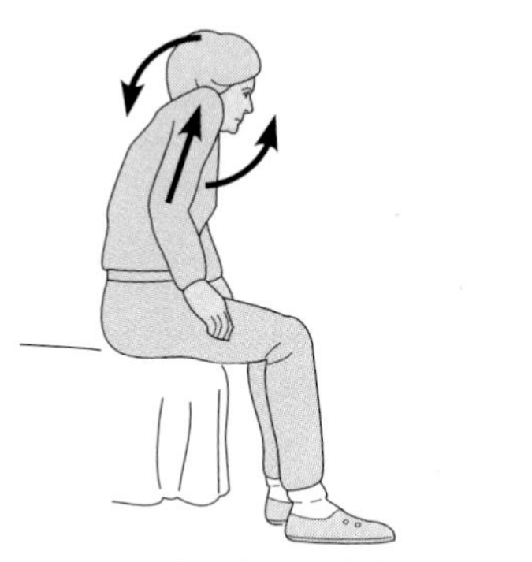

Shrug your shoulders forward, then move them in a circle.

C

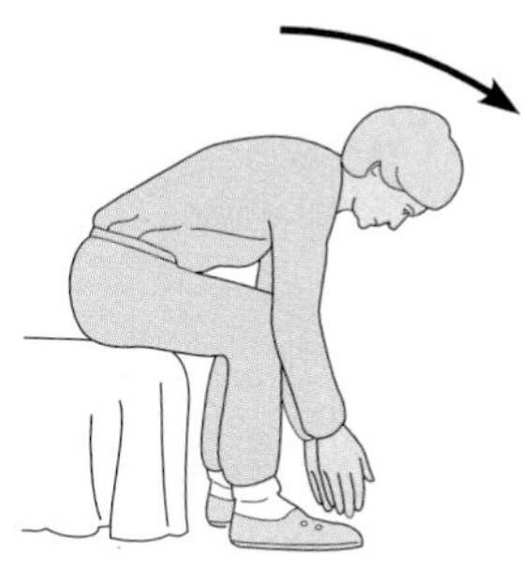

Bend forward and let your arms hang; try touching the floor with your hands.

D

Figure 21.7 Exercises to improve flexibility and muscle tone in the older adult.

Applying baby oil after washing with gentle soap in the shower, then rinsing off throughly is an inexpensive but effective way to prevent dry, itchy skin. Just be sure to rinse all of the oil out of the bottom of the tub or shower to avoid slipping and falling.

2. Inspect skin and feet for any new lesions, accidental injury, or changes in existing skin lesions, such as a change in the color of moles. Use a mirror to check areas you can't see, or ask someone else to check.
3. See the doctor if you notice any suspicious skin changes.
4. No matter the color of your skin, use a sun-screen with a protection factor of at least 12. Reapply frequently when you swim outdoors.

Medications

1. Keep a list of current medications, dosages, and the physician who ordered them. Take the list to any doctor appointments, hospital admissions, or outpatient testing. Review the need for the medications or the need for laboratory testing with the primary physician at least every 6 months or whenever your health status changes.
2. Give a copy of the medication list to a family member or friend—update it as needed.
3. Use a medication box and fill it weekly. This is a good way to separate medications taken at different times of the day and to keep track of medications and check if they were all taken (Figure 21.8).
4. Check the medications for expiration dates with each refill or monthly for those you take infrequently. Return any expired medications to the pharmacy for a new supply.

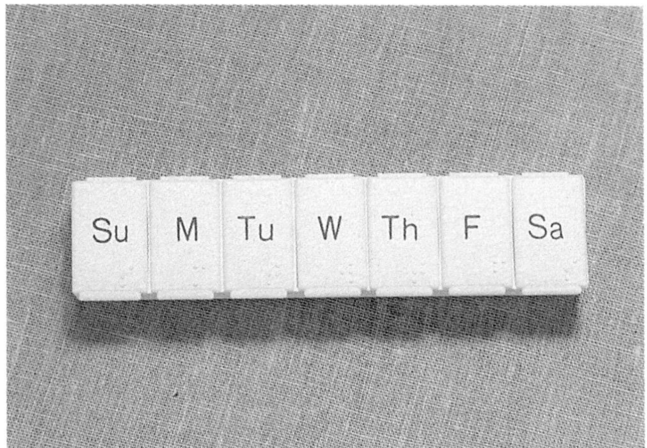

Figure 21.8 A medication box helps clients remember if they have taken all of their medications.

5. Know the adverse reactions and side effects of medications; consult with a nurse or physician if you are concerned.
6. Wear a medic-alert bracelet or medallion for any diseases (diabetes, seizure disorders) or medications (anticoagulants, insulin) that could affect the care to be given during an emergency.

Safety

1. Keep a list of emergency numbers by the phone, or better still, get a memory phone and program important numbers so you can access them by pressing a button.
2. Be sure that smoke alarms are working, and keep a fire extinguisher handy. Have the fire extinguisher recharged yearly. Keep a box of baking soda by the stove for extinguishing grease or other stove fires with a minimum of mess.
3. If you live alone, leave a house key with a trusted relative, friend, or neighbor.
4. Safety-proof the home, as follows:
   - Remove obstacles that you can trip over.
   - Replace throw rugs with wall-to-wall carpeting or tacked-down rugs.
   - Install bars by the toilet and in the shower or tub.
   - Put nonslip decals in the bottom of the tub or shower.
   - Place frequently used objects in the same location.
   - Note furniture, appliances, or walls that can provide support in the event of dizziness or faintness.

Table 21.3 lists extrinsic risk factors contributing to falls.

Working

1. Meaningful work should be as much a part of the daily activities of the older adult as it is for the younger population. Even though you may want or have to retire from a regular job, there is no reason why you cannot continue to contribute to the community or society if physical health permits. There are multiple opportunities for mentoring younger people in similar careers or for providing volunteer service. Many older adults may continue in their chosen careers, opting for a less rigorous or regimented schedule.
2. Arrange work or volunteer schedules so that you can meet the needs of the job without tiring yourself.
3. Do not continue in any job that is excessively stressful or does not provide some measure of satisfaction.

Table 21.3 Extrinsic Risk Factors Contributing to Falls

Category	Discriminator
Clothing	Improper footwear, especially slippers
	Loose, long, or flowing clothing
Furnishings	Inappropriate furniture: too low, soft cusions, with wheels, sharp corners, and susceptible to tipping if grabbed
	Low bed height
	Use of high shelving
	Low-lying objects: footstools, pets, small children
	Trailing electric cords
Structural	Unadapted bathroom: no handrails, elevated toilet seat, safety mats or decals in tub/shower
	Uneven, slippery, waxed, patterned, or glaring floor surfaces; worn carpeting, loose rugs, or throw rugs
	Deteriorated stairs and treads without rails or with insecure handrails; poorly identified and anchored stairway edges
Safety	Clutter and poor storage of items (shoes, clothing)
	Unfamiliar surroundings
	Inadequate lighting, especially of stairs and bathroom
	Worn, broken, or improperly used equipment or adaptive devices

Adapted from: Loftis PA and Glover TL. *Decision Making in Gerontologic Nursing.* (St. Louis, MO: Mosby, 1993).

4. If you need a salary, negotiate one that is commensurate with the value of skills offered and that meets the financial need.

Recreation and Rest

1. Continue with activities that have been enjoyable in the past as long as they are not too tiring or risky.
2. Many older people enjoy travel, especially with groups that provide socialization. Maintaining a relaxed pace is important; do not go on tours that cover five countries in five days.
3. Senior centers can be a good source of ongoing recreational activities, such as card games or arts and crafts. Seek out opportunities for taking community education classes about old or new areas of interest.
4. Consider becoming a college student again or for the first time. Complete that old degree or start a new one. Because interests change with age, take advantage of that momentum. Many community colleges and universities offer reduced fees for the student over 65. You can make new friends and gain new perspectives.
5. Start slowly with any new projects or activities, especially when you move into new environments, and allow additional time for adjustment. Also avoid overdoing.
6. Set aside several hours during the middle of the day for a complete rest, either a nap or just quiet time with feet up.
7. Try to get about 6 to 9 hours of uninterrupted sleep a night. Use rituals that have been successful in the past, and avoid stimulating activities or beverages near bedtime.
8. If you are not sleeping well, try to analyze the reasons why not, such as physical discomfort or worrying.
9. Avoid sleeping medications except in extreme situations, because the rebound effect when you discontinue them creates even more sleeplessness. In addition, sedatives, hypnotics, and alcohol cause a decrease in REM sleep, the stage of deepest relaxation in sleep.
10. A walk or other relaxed exercise, such as tai chi, can promote sleep if done a few hours before bedtime.
11. Try a warm bath 2 to 3 hours before bedtime; a drop in body temperature often induces sleep.
12. If insomnia persists and is affecting the quality of life, ask for a referral to a sleep clinic.

Sexuality

1. There is no reason not to enjoy sexual activity, either alone or with the partner of your choice.

2. Sexual response is slowed with aging, and so partners need to be patient with each other.
3. Some medications, such as antihypertensive drugs, and some diseases, such as diabetes, impair sexual functioning. Consult with the physician regarding a possible change of medication.
4. If overt sexual function is not possible, many older people derive much pleasure from other aspects of sexuality, such as cuddling and touching (Figure 21.9).

Elimination

1. For stress incontinence or dribbling, women benefit from Kegel exercises. If you are incontinent, consult a urologist.
2. If you are taking diuretic medications, try to take them in the morning. If you need to take them two times a

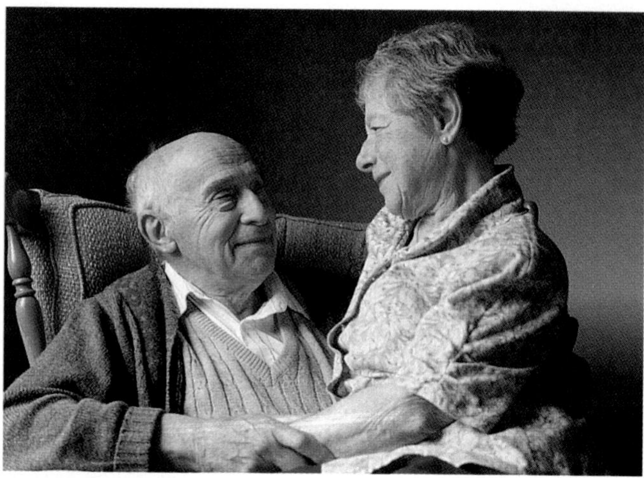

Figure 21.9 Many elderly people find that cuddling and touching help them maintain their sexual intimacy.

Spiritual Perspective Clinical Scale

Directions: A spiritual perspective is that which relates one to a transcendent or nonphysical realm, or to something greater than the self without disregarding the value of the individual. Please answer the following questions by marking an "X" in the space above the group of words that best describes you.

1. In talking with others, how often do you typically mention spirital matters?

______	______	______	______	______	______
Not at all 1	Less than once a year 2	About once a year 3	About once a month 4	About once a week 5	About once a day 6

2. How often do you engage in private prayer?

______	______	______	______	______	______
Not at all 1	Less than once a year 2	About once a year 3	About once a month 4	About once a week 5	About once a day 6

3. To what extent do you agree or disagree that having a spiritual perspective is an important part of your life?

______	______	______	______	______	______
Strongly disagree 1	Disagree 2	Disagree more than agree 3	Agree more than disagree 4	Agree 5	Strongly agree 6

4. To what extent do you agree or disagree that you seek spiritual guidance in making decisions at this time of your life?

______	______	______	______	______	______
Strongly disagree 1	Disagree 2	Disagree more than agree 3	Agree more than disagree 4	Agree 5	Strongly agree 6

day, take the last dose before dinner to decrease the number of times you need to get up during the night.

3. For constipation, increase activity, fiber in the diet, and water intake.
4. Take bulk medications, such as psyllium husks and stool softeners, but avoid cathartics, which cause the bowel to become dependent on that level of stimulus to function.
5. Avoid large-volume water enemas, because they stretch the bowel and can result in permanent dilation, thereby complicating the problem of constipation. If you have persistent constipation, you can use a small-volume "salt" enema, such as a Fleet's phosphosoda enema, but only occasionally.
6. Consult the physician if the constipation is not resolved by the suggested dietary means and activities, especially if nausea, vomiting, or abdominal pain accompanies the constipation.

Spirituality

The accompanying box can be used to assess spiritual needs.

1. People don't need to belong to a specific religious denomination or attend religious services to achieve spiritual fulfillment, but finding a belief system to explain the meaning of life and death can provide support and comfort in times of loss.
2. If you have no particular affiliation, try visiting a number of different services or meetings of religious and secular communities to explore new ideas or find a fit for your own.
3. Reestablish connections with a former belief system.

5. To what extent do you agree or disagree that you feel a sense of connectedness to God or a higher power in your life?

Strongly disagree	Disagree	Disagree more than agree	Agree more than disagree	Agree	Strongly agree
1	2	3	4	5	6

6. To what extent do you agree or disagree that your spiritual perspective helps to answer questions about the meaning of life?

Strongly disagree	Disagree	Disagree more than agree	Agree more than disagree	Agree	Strongly agree
1	2	3	4	5	6

Please feel free to express any views you may have about your spiritual perspective that have not been addressed by these six questions.

___

___

Scoring Instructions

Scores of 4.6 or above indicate a high level of spiritual perspective; scores between 3.0 and 4.5 indicate a middle range; and scores below 3.0 indicate a low level of spiritual perspective. Qualitative data (comments offered by the person) should be used in conjunction with the quantitative results to aid in interpreting the meaning of the score and the implications for intervention.

From Reed PG. Spirituality and mental health of older adults: Extant knowledge for nursing. *Fam Community Health* 1991; 14 (2):14–25.

DIAGNOSTIC REASONING IN ACTION

George Miller is a 76-year-old retired English teacher who lives alone in a one-bedroom apartment in a senior housing complex located in a pleasant urban neighborhood. He socializes with his neighbors and attends many of the functions provided at the senior center. He denies major disabilities, "just slowing down a little," and is seeking a routine checkup at the clinic. During the nursing assessment, his nurse, Sadie Greenwald, discovers no unusual findings except a distended abdomen with palpable firm stool in the area of the sigmoid colon. (Mr. Miller had a normal sigmoidoscopy 2 weeks ago). He also complains of being constipated recently. When Ms Greenwald inquires about his dietary habits, he states, "I'm a meat-and-potatoes man—with normal cholesterol!" He also says he enjoys specialty coffee drinks and never touches water. Since the weather turned cold, he has not been taking his usual 2-mile daily walk. "I hibernate and read in the winter."

Ms Greenwald clusters the information and derives the following nursing diagnoses:

1. *Constipation* related to inadequate dietary fiber, inadequate water intake, and decreased physical activity
2. *High risk for altered health maintenance* related to inappropriate nutritional habits

Ms Greenwald explains to Mr. Miller that his constipation is the result of a natural slowing of the motility of the bowel that occurs with aging but that he can promote normal evacuation of soft stool by changing some of his habits. She discusses the need for fiber in his diet and encourages him to try to include more vegetables, fruits, and whole grains in his daily meals. Also he can add fiber by taking two tablespoons of sugar-free psyllium (such as Metamucil or its generic equivalent) in a full glass of water daily. He can continue to enjoy his coffee drinks, but he would assist his bowel function by drinking a full glass of water each time he has coffee and consuming at least two more glasses spread out during the day. Keeping tap water in the refrigerator often makes it more palatable, but if he really does not like tap water, he can buy several gallons of bottled water to keep on hand. Mineral waters are an acceptable substitute if they do not contain sodium or sugar (fructose, sucrose, or glucose). He could increase his exercise level by walking the halls of the senior complex or going to the nearby mall and walking through it several times, not stopping to shop until he has chalked-up sufficient mileage. He might consider asking one of his neighbors to walk with him to offset boredom.

Regarding his nutritional habits, Ms Greenwald reminds him that even though his cholesterol is normal, his meat-and-potato diet may be depriving him of some vitamins and minerals that he can get only by eating a wide variety of foods, especially fruits and vegetables. She also points out that a high-fat diet, especially one high in animal fat, has been implicated in numerous cancers. He can protect himself by changing the diet.

Ms Greenwald complements Mr. Miller on how he has maintained his health and managed his life. She reinforces his socialization and exercise, and she encourages him to consider volunteering his time helping illiterate adults learn to read at the nearby recreational center. He states that he is interested in the idea and will follow up on it. She makes another appointment with him to review his diet and help him plan new menus based on the Food Guide Pyramid and his individual preferences. She asks him to try making some changes before the next appointment and to bring a diary with him of his daily food and water consumption.

4. Volunteer time to help with community activities, teach, or mentor younger generations.
5. Set up discussion meetings for a peer group striving to understand and expand spiritual meanings of life.

Summary

Aging adults are a diverse group, ranging in age from 65 to over 100, and their physical conditions vary from youthfully healthy to extremely debilitated. Although the physiologic and psychologic changes of aging eventually affect all older adults, it is extremely important to deal with each client, as well as oneself, as an individual with individual needs, preferences, and beliefs. You can use the generalizations about aging as a point of departure when you assess potential problems, but always be on the outlook for the exceptions. The newspapers and magazines are filled with stories of mountain climbers, marathon runners, and sky divers who, well into their seventh and eighth decades, not only take risks but also excel. Maintain a conservative stance in your health-promoting recommendations, but do not discourage those senior citizens who wish to live their final years to the fullest by their own definitions. In her 80s, Hope Cahill wrote a book called *Old Age—A Balance Sheet* (Cahill 1981, p. 59). She sums up the good and not-so-good aspects of old age this way: "It is impossible to put a numerical value on each of the assets and liabilities listed above, but after analyzing them objectively, I think you will agree with me that the assets far outweigh the liabilities. The resultant net worth is a sense of thankfulness, peace of mind, and faith in ultimate good in the mysterious future."

Key Points

- ✓ The aging process affects all body systems in varying degrees over time. Alterations in the DNA that determines consistency in cell reproduction, accumulations of the end products of metabolism, and gradual wearing down of tissues and structures cause a variety of changes in structure and function. However, heredity and lifestyle are also important variables. Effects on immunity make the older adult less resistant to infection, less able to handle stress, and more prone to autoimmune disorders. Changes in cellular reproduction, especially hormones and enzymes, result in changes in skin, sensation, memory, and reflexes as well as cardiac, respiratory, gastrointestinal, and genitourinary functions. With normal aging, mental function, intelligence, creativity, and problem-solving ability actually increase, but unfortunately some elderly fall prey to mentally degenerative diseases such as Alzheimer's or multi-infarct dementia. Additionally, chronic disease from acute episodes occurring earlier in life can mar healthy aging. However, most older persons modify their activities to accommodate physiolgic changes and therefore consider themselves healthy and able within their cohort group.
- ✓ The initial interview includes the regular adult health history and psychosocial profile with specific questions focused on common aging problems, such as mobility, sleep disorders, incontinence, substance abuse, and depression. Questions are also addressed to family members or caretakers to discover problems not noted by the client.
- ✓ The physical assessment includes a careful evaluation of all body systems and a laboratory screening, including a complete blood count, electrolyte studies, and blood chemistry studies. Men should have a yearly PSA, women should have a yearly Pap smear and mammogram, especially if they are on hormone replacement therapy. Both should have a test for occult blood in the stool and a sigmoidoscopy.
- ✓ Nursing diagnoses commonly used for elderly clients include *Body image disturbance, Perceived constipation, Ineffective family coping, Fatigue, Altered home maintenance management, Stress incontinence, Altered nutrition: less than body requirements, Self-care deficit,* and *Impaired social interaction.*
- ✓ The nurse provides information to the aging client about individual diseases, adapted to medical regimen, and health-promoting measures.

Chapter 22

Health Assessment Checklist

Now that you have learned how to perform comprehensive physical assessments of a client's body systems and regions, you may use the following health assessment checklist to guide you through a complete assessment of the adult client. It is not unusual to feel overwhelmed when you perform a complete health assessment for the first time. The successful health assessment requires you to practice effective communication skills; proceed in an organized manner; ensure the comfort, safety, and privacy of your client; draw on a knowledge of anatomy and physiology; perform assessment techniques efficiently and effectively; recognize assessment cues; and interpret and document findings. It's a formidable task, but well worth mastering: A complete health assessment has tremendous health benefits for the client and is the foundation on which you will build the client's plan of care.

Proceeding slowly and methodically helps ensure success. Take time to arrange not only the equipment but also the steps of the exam. This chapter provides one possible exam sequence, which requires a minimum of position changes for the client. But remember that many different sequences are possible. If you forget a step during the exam, you can always insert that assessment at an appropriate time later on. If you forget a step after you have left the examination setting and feel it is important to include it, you may choose to return and perform the assessment. In such a case, you should simply explain to the client that you would like to check one more thing before concluding the exam.

Don't be discouraged if your first exam seems awkward, with many stops and starts. The more assessments you perform, the easier they will become.

The Health History

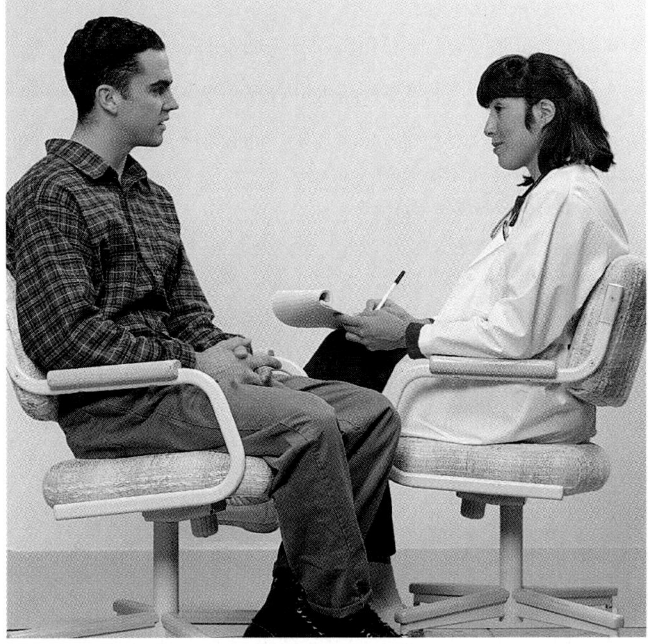

Δ *The client is seated, fully clothed.*

- ❑ Gather the health history by interviewing the client, or review together the health history form that the client filled out.

The General Survey

Appearance and Mental Status

- ❑ Compare the client's stated age with the client's appearance.
- ❑ Observe the client's body build, height, and weight in relation to the client's age, lifestyle, and health.
- ❑ Observe the client's facial expression, posture, and position.
- ❑ Observe the client's overall hygiene and grooming, relating these to the client's activities just before the assessment.
- ❑ Note the client's body odor and breath odor, again relating these to the client's prior activities.
- ❑ Note obvious signs of health or illness (eg, in skin color, breathing, bending over because of abdominal pain, wincing).
- ❑ Assess the client's attitude, attentiveness, affect, and mood, and assess the appropriateness of the client's responses.
- ❑ Listen for the quantity of speech, quality, relevance, and organization.

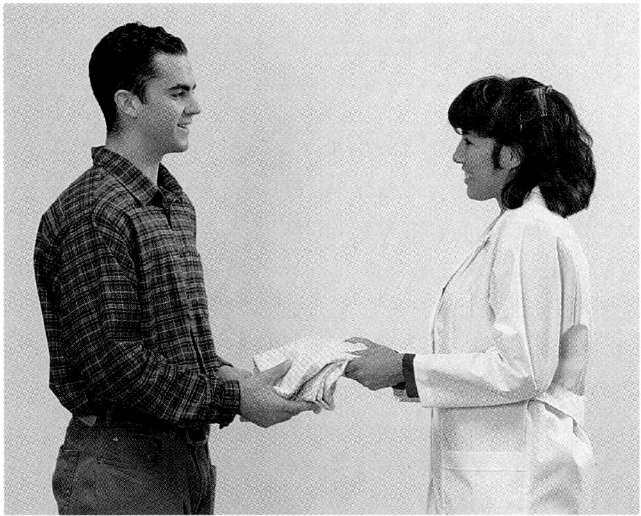

Δ *If the client has not already emptied the bladder, the client should do so now. Provide the client with an examination gown. If appropriate, provide the client with a sterile container and instruct the client in obtaining a clean catch specimen.*

Measurements

- ❑ Measure the client's height.
- ❑ Measure the client's weight.
- ❑ Measure the client's skinfold thickness, if appropriate.

Vital Signs

- ❑ Assess the client's radial pulse.
- ❑ Count the client's respirations.
- ❑ Take the client's temperature.
- ❑ Measure the client's blood pressure.

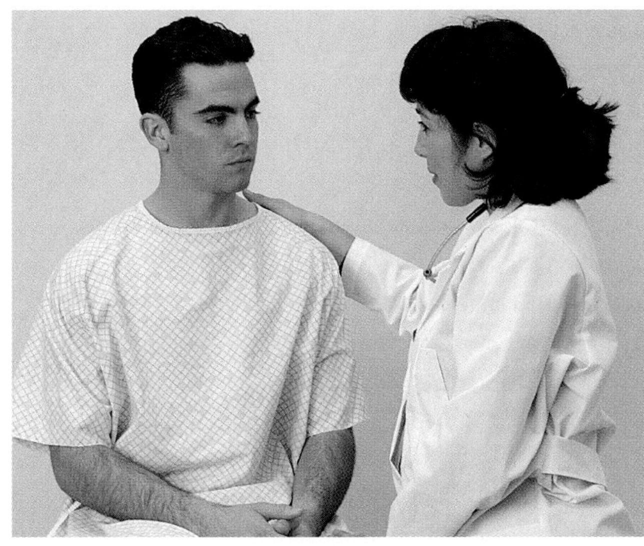

Δ *The client is seated on the examination table, wearing a gown. Stand in front of the client or to the client's side as appropriate.*

The Physical Assessment

Skin, Hair, and Nails

- ❑ Inspect the skin for color and uniformity of color.
- ❑ Observe and palpate skin moisture.
- ❑ Palpate skin temperature.
- ❑ Test for skin turgor.
- ❑ Palpate for edema.
- ❑ Inspect, palpate, measure, and describe skin lesions.
- ❑ Inspect the hair for growth, thickness, texture, moisture, and lesions. Inspect the amount of body hair.
- ❑ Palpate the texture of the hair.
- ❑ Inspect the nail plate for curvature and angle.
- ❑ Inspect and palpate nail texture.
- ❑ Inspect color of nail bed.
- ❑ Inspect tissue surrounding nails.
- ❑ Palpate fingertips to test for capillary refill.

Skull and Face

- ❑ Inspect the skull for size, shape, and symmetry.
- ❑ Inspect the facial features for symmetry.
- ❑ Note facial expressions and the symmetry of facial movements (cranial nerve VII).
- ❑ Palpate the skull for nodules or masses and depressions.
- ❑ Palpate the lymph nodes of the face and head.
- ❑ Palpate the muscles of the face (cranial nerve V).
- ❑ Assess facial response to sensory stimulation (sharp, dull, light touch) (cranial nerve V).

Eyes and Vision

- ❑ Inspect the eyebrows, eyelashes, and eyelids.
- ❑ Inspect the bulbar and palpebral conjunctivae for color, texture, and lesions.
- ❑ Inspect the lacrimal apparatus for edema or redness.
- ❑ Inspect the cornea for clarity and texture.
- ❑ Inspect the anterior chamber for transparency and depth.
- ❑ Inspect the pupils for color, size, shape, and equality.
- ❑ Test the client's vision using the Snellen eye chart (cranial nerve II).
- ❑ Test the visual fields (cranial nerve II).
- ❑ Test extraocular movements (cranial nerves III, IV, VI).
- ❑ Test pupillary reaction to light (cranial nerve III).
- ❑ Test corneal reflex (cranial nerves V and VII).
- ❑ Using an ophthalmoscope, inspect the internal eye structures.
  - ◆ Red light reflex through the pupil
  - ◆ Optic disc and cup for color, size, and shape
  - ◆ Retinal blood vessels for size, color, pattern, and arteriovenous crossings
  - ◆ Retinal background for color and surface characteristics
  - ◆ Macula and fovea centralis for color and surface characteristics

Ears and Hearing

- ❑ Inspect the auricles for color, texture, and symmetry of size, position, and angle.
- ❑ Palpate the auricles for texture, elasticity, and areas of tenderness.
- ❑ Using an otoscope, inspect the external ear canals for cerumen, inflammation, scaling, drainage, foreign bodies, or lesions.
- ❑ Using an otoscope, inspect the internal ear structures.
  - ◆ Tympanic membrane for color and gloss
  - ◆ Appearance of the annulus, pars flaccida, pars tensa, malleus, umbo, and light reflex
- ❑ Test hearing acuity using voice tests and turning fork tests (Weber, Rinne) (cranial nerve VIII).

Nose and Sinuses

- ❑ Test sense of smell (cranial nerve I).
- ❑ Using a speculum, inspect the nasal mucosa for redness, swelling, growths, discharge, and nasal polyps, and the nasal septum for deviation.
- ❑ Palpate the external nose for tenderness.
- ❑ Palpate the maxillary and frontal sinuses for tenderness.
- ❑ Transilluminate the maxillary and frontal sinuses for the presence of air or fluid.

Mouth and Throat

- ❑ Inspect the lips for color, texture, and symmetry.
- ❑ Using a penlight, inspect
  - ◆ The inner and buccal mucosa for color, moisture, texture, and lesions
  - ◆ The teeth for color, presence of fillings, dental caries, partial or complete dentures, and tartar
  - ◆ The gums for bleeding, color, retraction, edema, and lesions
  - ◆ The tongue for color, size, texture, position, mobility, and coating
  - ◆ The hard and soft palates for color, shape, texture, and the presence of bony prominences
  - ◆ The salivary gland openings for swelling and redness
  - ◆ The palatine arches for redness, lesions, and plaques

- The tonsils for color, discharge, and size
- The oropharynx for edema, inflammation, lesions, or exudate

❑ Test the sense of taste (cranial nerve VII).

❑ Wearing gloves, palpate the mucosa, the gums, the tongue, and the floor of the mouth.

❑ Observe the uvula for position and mobility as the client phonates "ah" and test the gag reflex (cranial nerves IX, X).

❑ Observe as the client sticks out the tongue (cranial nerve XII).

Neck

❑ Inspect the neck for symmetry, pulsations, and swellings or masses.

❑ Assess neck movement, range of motion, and strength of muscles against resistance: observe as the client moves the head forward and back and side to side, and shrugs the shoulders (cranial nerve XI).

❑ Palpate the lymph nodes of the neck.

❑ Palpate the carotid pulses one at a time.

❑ Palpate the trachea for position.

❑ Moving behind the client, palpate the thyroid gland for symmetry and masses.

Posterior Chest

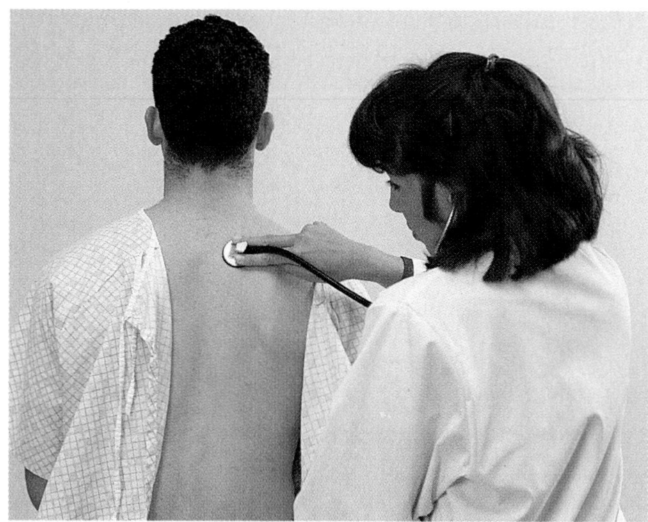

Δ *The client is seated on the examination table with the gown open in the back, exposing the posterior chest. Stand behind the client.*

❑ Inspect the posterior chest for symmetry of shoulders, musculoskeletal development, and thoracic configuration.

❑ Inspect and palpate the scapula and spine.

❑ Palpate and percuss the costovertebral angle, noting any tenderness.

Lungs

❑ Observe the client's respirations for excursion, depth, rhythm, and pattern.

❑ Palpate the client's chest for expansion and tactile fremitus.

❑ Percuss over all lung fields.

❑ Percuss for diaphragmatic excursion.

❑ Auscultate breath sounds, noting adventitious sounds.

Anterior Chest

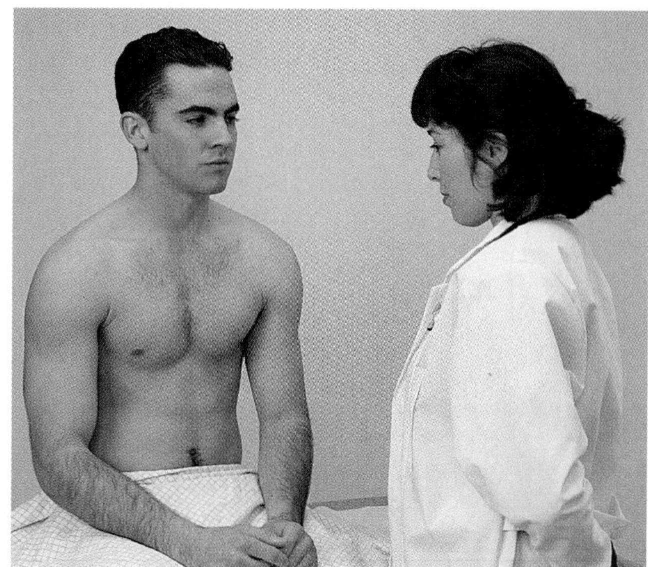

Δ *The client is seated on the examination table. The female's gown is lifted to drape on the shoulders. The male's gown is lowered to the lap. Stand in front of the client.*

❑ Inspect the client's posture.

❑ Inspect the anterior chest for symmetry and musculoskeletal development.

❑ Inspect the supraclavicular and infraclavicular areas.

❑ Palpate the chest for stability, lumps, or tenderness.

Heart

❑ Determine the location of the atria and ventricles of the heart.

❑ Inspect and palpate the aortic, pulmonic, tricuspid, and apical areas for the presence of pulsations or lifts or heaves.

❑ Palpate the chest wall for the presence of abnormal pulsations or lifts or heaves.

- ❑ Use both the diaphragm and the bell of the stethoscope to auscultate for heart sounds at the aortic, pulmonic, tricuspid, and apical areas.
- ❑ Auscultate the aortic, pulmonic, tricuspid, and apical areas for heart sounds.
- ❑ At each area of auscultation, distinguish rate, rhythm, and location of both the S1 and S2 sounds.

Breasts and Axillae

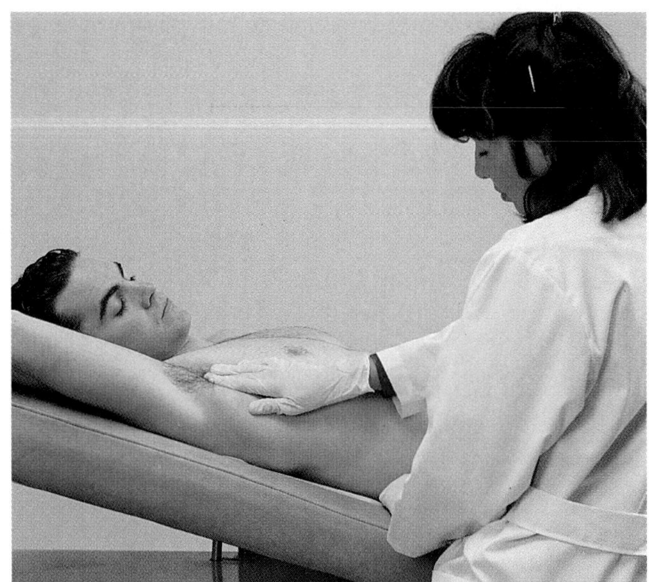

Δ *The client is reclining on the examination table with the head at a 30- to 45-degree angle. The anterior chest is still exposed. A drape is over the client's abdomen. Stand at the client's right.*

- ❑ Inspect the male or female client's breasts for symmetry, mobility, masses, dimpling, and nipple retraction. Ask the female client to lift her arms over her head, press her hands on her hips, and lean forward as you perform the inspection.
- ❑ Palpate the nipples and observe for discharge.
- ❑ Palpate the axillary lymph nodes.
- ❑ Lift each of the female client's arms over her head and palpate each breast, including the tail of Spence and the areola, for masses.
- ❑ Teach the female client breast self-examination.

Neck Vessels

- ❑ Inspect the jugular veins for pulsations and distention.
- ❑ Estimate jugular venous pressure.

Abdomen

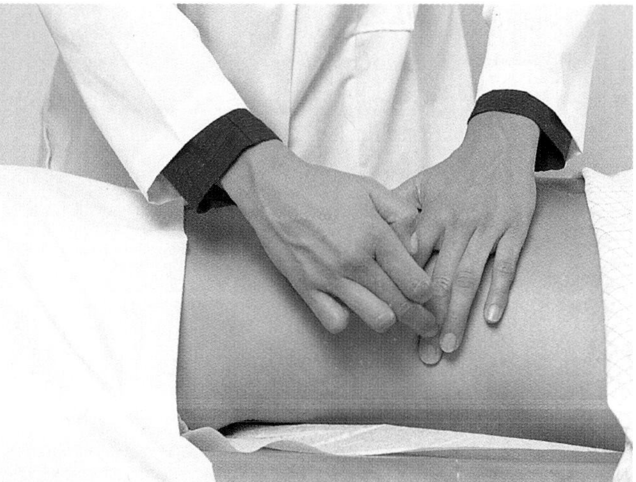

Δ *The client is supine on the examination table, with the abdomen exposed from the nipple line to the pubis and the drape covering the legs. Remain on the client's right.*

- ❑ Inspect the abdomen for skin integrity, contour, and symmetry.
- ❑ Observe any movements associated with respiration, peristalsis, or aortic pulsations.
- ❑ Auscultate the abdomen for bowel sounds, vascular sounds, and any peritoneal friction rubs.
- ❑ Percuss the abdomen for tympany and dullness.
- ❑ Percuss the abdomen to determine liver and spleen size.
- ❑ Percuss the abdomen to detect areas of tenderness over the liver, kidney, and spleen.
- ❑ Percuss the abdomen to define the outline of a distended bladder.
- ❑ Palpate the liver, spleen, and kidneys to determine position and size.
- ❑ Palpate the abdomen to detect tenderness, presence of masses, and distention.

Inguinal Region

- ❑ Palpate for inguinal lymph nodes, pulses, and to detect any hernias.

Lower Extremities

- ❑ Inspect the legs and feet for skin integrity, color, symmetry, and hair distribution.
- ❑ Inspect for muscle mass and musculoskeletal configuration.
- ❑ Palpate for temperature, texture, and edema.

- ❑ Palpate the popliteal, posterior tibial, and dorsalis pedis pulses.
- ❑ Palpate the toes to test for capillary refill.

Musculoskeletal

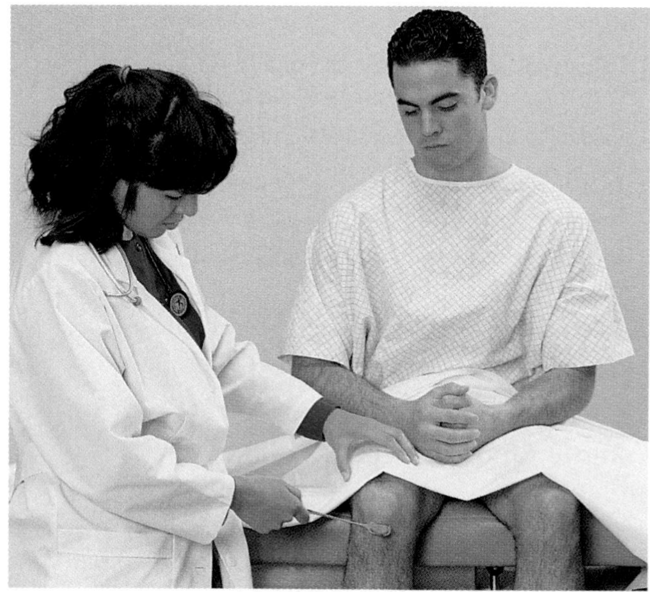

Δ *Assist the client to a sitting position, with the legs dangling off the examination table. Move in front of the client and to the client's right during the following assessments, as appropriate.*

- ❑ Test range of motion and muscle strength in the hips, knees, ankles, and feet.
- ❑ Observe the client's ease of movement, muscle strength, and coordination as the client moves from the supine to the sitting position.
- ❑ Test range of motion and muscle strength in the shoulders, elbows, wrists, and hands.
- ❑ Assist the client to a standing position and observe the client's standing posture.
- ❑ Perform the Romberg test. Stand nearby in case the client begins to fall.
- ❑ Observe the client's natural gait.
- ❑ Observe as the client walks heel-to-toe.
- ❑ Observe as the client stands on the right foot, then the left, with the eyes closed.
- ❑ Ask the client to hold onto the edge of the examination table, then observe as the client performs a right knee bend, then a left knee bend.
- ❑ Standing behind the client, observe the spine as the client touches the toes.
- ❑ Test range of motion of spine.

Neurologic

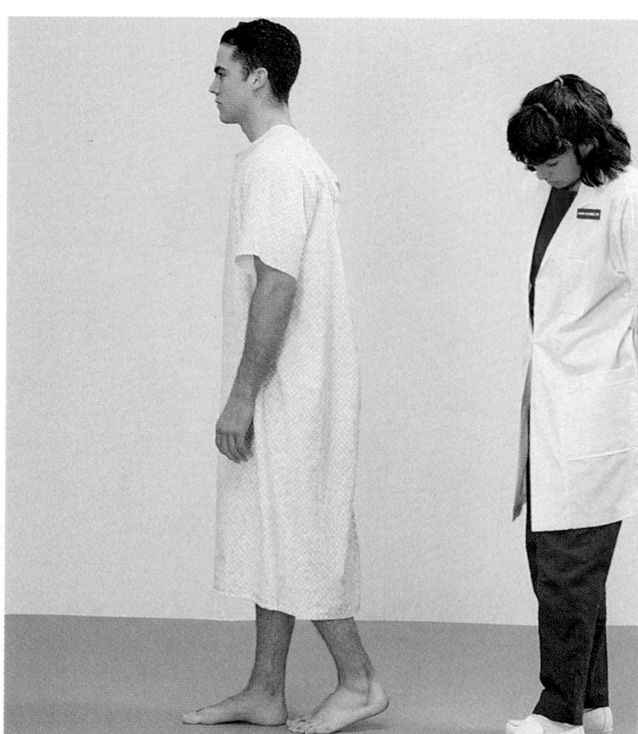

Δ *The client is standing, wearing gown.*

- ❑ Assess the client's sensory function, including
    - ◆ Light touch sensation and tactile location
    - ◆ Pain sensation
    - ◆ Temperature sensation
    - ◆ Vibratory sense
    - ◆ Kinesthetic sensation
    - ◆ Tactile discrimination
- ❑ Assess the client's fine motor function in both the upper and lower extremities.
    - ◆ Client touches nose with alternating index fingers.
    - ◆ Client performs rapid alternating movements.
    - ◆ Client runs heel down opposite shin.
- ❑ Conduct the gross motor and balance tests.
- ❑ Test tendon reflexes bilaterally and compare
    - ◆ Biceps
    - ◆ Triceps
    - ◆ Brachioradialis
    - ◆ Patellar
    - ◆ Achilles
    - ◆ Plantar (Babinski)

Male Genitals and Rectum

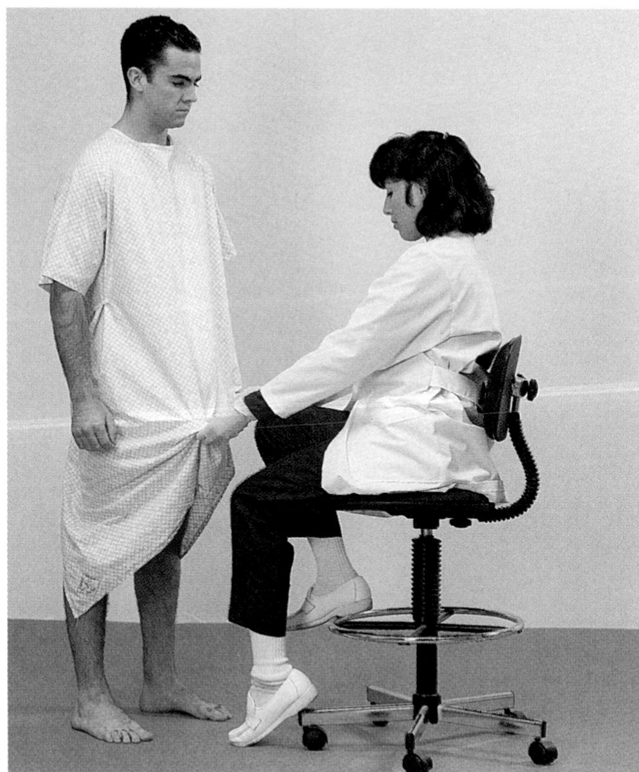

Δ *The male client remains standing. Sit in front of the client and lift the examination gown.*

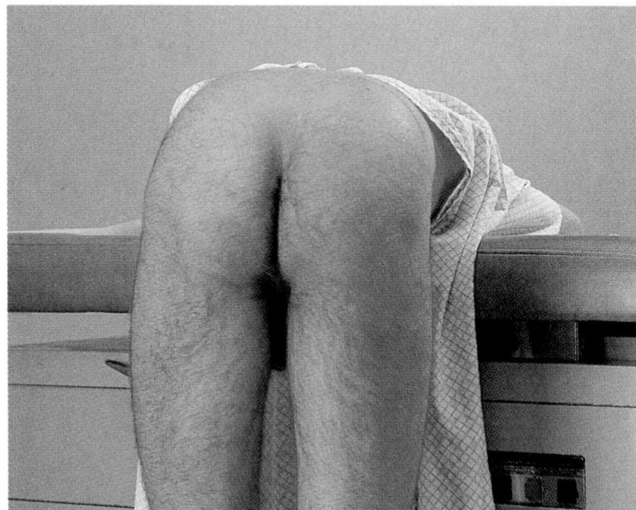

Δ *Assist the male client in leaning over the examination table, with the examination gown draped to expose the sacrococcygeal and perianal regions.*

- ❑ Observe the amount, distribution, and characteristics of pubic hair.
- ❑ Inspect the penile shaft, glans, and urethral meatus for lesions, nodules, swelling, inflammation, and discharge.
- ❑ Observe the color and position of the urethral meatus.
- ❑ Inspect the scrotum for appearance, general size, and symmetry.
- ❑ Palpate the scrotum, testicles, epididymis, and spermatic cord for swelling, irregularities, and tenderness.
- ❑ Palpate to detect any inguinal hernias.
- ❑ Teach testicular self-exam.
- ❑ Inspect the sacrococcygeal and perianal regions.
- ❑ Palpate the rectal walls and prostate gland with the lubricated index finger.
- ❑ Observe any stool on glove and test for occult blood.
- ❑ Wipe the perianal area with tissues.

Female Genitals and Rectum

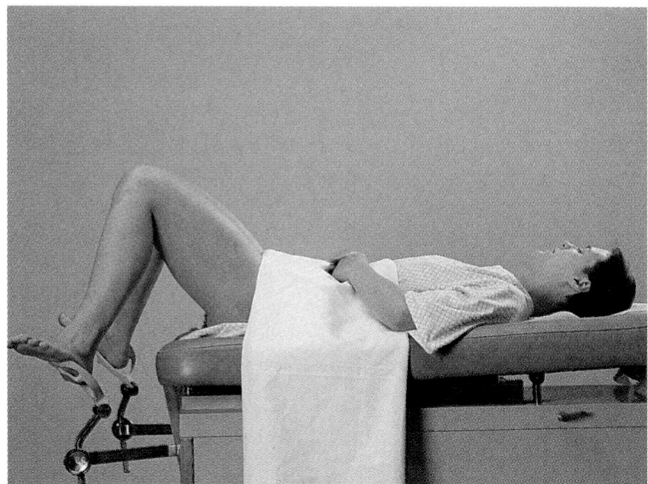

Δ *Assist the female client into the lithotomy position. The client is wearing the examination gown and her lap is draped.*

- ❑ Inspect the amount, distribution, and characteristics of pubic hair.
- ❑ Inspect the pubic skin for parasites, inflammation, swelling, and lesions.
- ❑ Palpate the inguinal lymph nodes for enlargement and tenderness.
- ❑ Inspect the clitoris, urethral orifice, and vaginal orifice for lesions, discharge, and inflammation.
- ❑ Palpate Bartholin's glands.
- ❑ Assess the integrity of the pelvic musculature.

- ❑ Insert a vaginal speculum and examine the internal genitals.
  - ◆ Inspect the cervix for shape of the os, color, size, and position.
  - ◆ Obtain a specimen for a Papanicolaou smear.
  - ◆ Inspect the vaginal walls for color, texture, and secretions.
- ❑ Palpate the rectum and rectovaginal walls.
- ❑ Observe any stool on the glove and test for occult blood.
- ❑ Wipe the perianal area with tissues.

Δ *Assist the client to a sitting position.*

Conclusion

At the conclusion of the health assessment, answer any questions the client might have and provide health teaching as appropriate. Before leaving the room, make sure the client is not experiencing any discomfort from the examination. Record your assessment data as soon as possible, preferably immediately after the exam. See Chapter 1 for information on documenting assessment findings.

Interviewing Strategies for Special Situations

1. Assessing for Domestic Violence 2. Assessing for Substance Abuse 3. Assessing for Child Abuse 4. Assessing for Elder Abuse 5. Interviewing the Homeless Client

Assessing for Domestic Violence

A 1990 study reported that 22%–35% of all injuries treated in emergency rooms are related to on-going domestic abuse (McFarlane et al 1992). Domestic violence annually causes 5400 deaths, 21,000 hospitalizations, and 28,700 emergency room visits, costing $44 million yearly in medical expenses (Colorado Domestic Violence Coalition 1993). Yet only approximately 5% of emergency room injuries are identified as abuse-related in medical records (McLeer and Anwar 1989, Tilden and Shepherd 1987). Currently, many victims of domestic abuse, the majority of whom are women, are overlooked by health care professionals reluctant to bring up such a sensitive topic.

A nurse is often in a position to uncover domestic abuse. By creating a safe environment for women to speak of their situations openly, the nurse provides an opportunity for the woman to seek help. As nurses we may attend to broken bones and bruises, but our treatment must extend beyond the physical. Our role as caregivers may affect whether or not the client feels able to disclose the abuse, and this disclosure affects the success of intervention. There are some important challenges to consider as you prepare yourself to listen.

Understanding the Client Experiencing Abuse

Women who are physically abused are almost always emotionally abused, and the emotional abuse usually appears in the relationship before the physical abuse occurs. Emotional abuse occur in the lives of over 8 to 12 million women (Flitcraft et al 1992). Abused women report they are belittled, interrogated, humiliated in public, yelled at, and made to feel guilty. Many also say their abusive partner tells them that they deserve the abuse. In other cases, the woman may feel shame because she feels she was provocative or verbally abusive during an argument. These feelings of shame and guilt can be very confusing for someone in an abusive relationship. As one woman said, "You know inside that you don't deserve it, but over time it has an effect and you begin to believe you do." When a woman's feelings about her role in the abuse are unresolved, it may be very difficult for her to see a way out of her situation and to marshal the internal resources necessary to make a major life change.

The complex issues that are part of the process of leaving abusive situations are evident in another woman's story. She feared not only for her life but also for the lives of her children, as do many women in abusive relationships. She lived seven miles from a town and did not have a car. Her husband routinely terrorized her, destroying her personal items, and threatened to kill her if she left him. In this kind of frightening situation, the woman may be risking her life when she talks to anyone about the abuse. She also explained that it was difficult for her to seek help because it was humiliating to admit that she was being abused by someone who was supposed to love her. She had "not been brought up to be treated that way" but somehow felt responsible for what was happening. If your intervention is to be useful to a woman such as this one, you must first understand that the reality of being in an abusive relationship is frightening, sometimes paralyzing, and almost always isolating. As a health care provider, you provide women with a window of opportunity to seek help, find support, and gain access to other resources when you assess for abuse.

Examining Your Own Beliefs

Keep in mind that difficult feelings may arise for caregivers connected to abuse in our own lives. Adult caregivers may come to discover and acknowledge the fact that we were abused as children. Others may become aware of abuse that exists within our present relationships. Getting help for these issues is important as you work to facilitate positive change for clients in abusive relationships.

You need to couple this internal reflection with an external evaluation of current societal thoughts and expectations about abusive relationships. Much of the current sociocultural milieu encourages beliefs and practices about abuse that can subtly or overtly support it. Some individuals feel that men wouldn't be abusive if women didn't make them angry, or they may feel obliged to counsel the woman to mollify her partner so that the abuse will stop. When a woman risks sharing this information regarding abuse and her listener responds with subtle accusations or questions that somehow implicate her in the abuse, the woman receives a powerfully negative message. This message perpetuates the abuse instead of offering a potential way out. One woman reported that her employer kept makeup at work for her so that she could cover the marks of the abuse in order to continue her responsible position (Ulrich 1990). This action implies that on some level abuse is acceptable and encourages the woman to endure it and keep silent.

When working with abused clients, understand that you need to find ways to care for yourself, especially when coming face to face with the unpredictability of violence. Caring for yourself includes dealing with emotional stress by taking time for yourself each day, building friendships, and meeting your own needs.

Making a Difference

To determine if abuse exists, you need to ask. There is no way of telling if a woman is abused, so you should ask all women, including women of all ages and cultural groups, heterosexual as well as lesbian women. Screeening for domestic abuse should be a regular part of all health assessments. After you have built trust during an interview, in a sensitive manner, ask her about abusive actions. You can explain that you are inquiring because abuse is common. Specific questions may be more effective than asking, "Have you been abused?" or "Are you battered?" In the beginning, many women may not feel ready to acknowledge the full scope of the problem. The step of labeling oneself as abused or battered usually takes place late in the healing process.

It is better to begin by asking if specific actions have taken place. The following list of questions may elicit some helpful information without forcing the client to identify herself as a battered woman:

- Does the person you love:
  - "Track" all of your time?
  - Constantly accuse you of being unfaithful?.
  - Discourage your relationships with family and friends?
  - Prevent you from working or attending school?
  - Anger easily when drinking or on drugs?
  - Control all of the finances and force you to account for what you spend?
  - Humiliate you in front of others?
  - Destroy personal property or sentimental items?
  - Hit, punch, slap, kick, or bite you or your children?
  - Threaten to hurt you or your children?
  - Have a weapon or threaten to use a weapon against you?
  - Force you to have sex against your will?
- Have you ever had to take out a restaining order?

If a woman says yes to any of these questions, offer reassurance and refer her to resources for domestic abuse in her community. You should ask these questions of pregnant woman as well. A recent study showed that physical abuse during pregnancy occurs twice as often as previous studies had revealed (McFarlane et al 1992).

Be prepared for clients to resent your questions regarding abuse at first. However, women have later said that even though they were angry at the questions, the awareness that they were being abused was a first a first step in the process of ending the abuse. Although the woman may not feel ready to respond in an interview setting, your questions and concern may plant the seed for change.

It is important to provide opportunities for women to discuss abuse, but you should respect the woman's need to work through the problem and make her own decisions. For example, you should help the woman brainstorm about possible solutions to make life improvements, but do not rush in with all the answers. Remember that one of the primary objectives of intervention is to support a woman in her own choices. Only she can decide when it is safe or comfortable for her to leave. You may want to say, "It sounds like that is very difficult for you and your children. What do you think would help you?" The more invested the woman feels in the solution, the more likely she is to carry it out.

Provide privacy. The woman may be too frightened and confused to talk in her husband's or partner's presence. She also may need to prevent her partner from knowing that she has sought help. Assure her of confidentiality, and let her determine how much she feels comfortable revealing.

Build trust. Trust with a client builds over time, but it is possible to establish safety and rapport over a shorter period of time. This begins with your ability to be understanding, respectful, and empathic. Display your confidence in the woman's ability to make changes, and help her identify her strengths. It is important for the client to see that you are both working together for her safety.

Affirm her story. Many women are afraid that no one will believe their story. Sometimes the abusive partner is well known and respected in the community. Perhaps she has not been believed in the past, or perhaps she has never let anyone know what was going on and is afraid that no one will believe her. It is important for you as the listener to consider seriously all that she tells you. Your respect for her will help her to trust you enough to tell her story.

Plan for her safety. Don't be discouraged if the woman plans to return to the relationship. Women describe leaving as a process and may leave many times before they decide to escape the abuse permanently. Leaving any close relationship takes courage. The abused woman needs even greater courage to extract herself from violence.

If the woman chooses to remain in a violent relationship, you should direct your intervention toward planning with her for her own safety and the safety of her children. You can review with her options such as a crisis center, a battered women's shelter, counseling, and victim's rights advocates. Her plan needs to include identifying support that is realistic for her situation and actually accessible to her. Remember that many women stay, in part, because they fear they cannot support themselves and their children financially. Before she can even consider leaving, she will probably need to address these concerns directly and take practical steps to ensure a certain degree of security. She also needs to have keys, clothes, and important documents ready in case she needs to make a quick exit. Concern, appropriate referrals, and documentation can be enough to be effective; there is no rescue.

Women's reports of ending and recovering from abuse point to the importance of a shift in the power balance to a more egalitarian relationship and to personal growth. Nurses who can effectively and systematically assess for abuse may also be fostering the woman's own awareness of her situation. The nurse who can design a care plan tailored to the woman's experience may be fostering the woman's ability to end or leave the abuse. Take some time to familiarize yourself with the resources in your area that provide services to women and children in abusive relationships (crisis hotlines, telephone number for emergency shelters, legal services, district attorney's victim/witness programs and so on).

Remember that you can not single-handedly provide all of the support someone needs to leave an abusive partner. For many women, leaving an abusive relationship is a process, and one that needs to be supported in many different ways. You can play a very important role in this process as a health care provider and a guide to other resources within the community.

Resources

For more information, call National Coalition Against Domestic Violence: 303/839-1852.

If you live in New York State call 1-800-942-6906 (English), 1-800-942-6908 (Spanish).

The videotape "Crime against the Future" is an excellent resource for learning to assess for abuse. It is put out by the March of Dimes Birth Defects Foundation, Materials and Supply Division, 1275 Mamaroneck Ave, White Plains, NY 10605. Other valuable resources include the training video with protocol "Domestic Violence: Recognizing the Epidemic" from The Colorado Domestic Violence Coalition (1-800-368-0406, $75.00) and the training manual "Domestic Violence, A Guide for Health Care Providers," 1993, by the Colorado Domestic Violence Coalition (1-800-368-0406, $40.00).

References

Brendtro M, Bowker LH. 1989. Battered women: How can nurses help? *Issues Mental Health Nurs,* 10:169–180.

Crime against the future (videotape). March of Dimes Birth Defects Foundation, Materials and Supply Division, 1275 Mamaroneck Avenue, White Plains, NY 10605.

Flitcraft AH, Hadley SM, Hendricks-Matthews MK, McLeer SV, Warsaw C. 1992. *Diagnostic and treatment guidelines on domestic violence.* Chicago: American Medical Association.

Goldner V. 1992. Making room for both/and. *Networker* 55–61.

McFarlane J, Parker B, Soeken K, Bullock L. 1992. Assessing for abuse during pregnancy: Frequency and extent of injuries and entry into prenatal care. *JAMA,* 267:3176–3178.

Schlesinger JL, Salamon MJ. 1987–1988. A case of wife abuse in the intermediate care facility. *Clin Gerontol,* 00:163–166.

Trute B, Sarsfield P, Mackenzie DA. 1988. Medical response to wife abuse: A survey of physicians' attitudes and practices. Special Issue: Wife battering: A Canadian perspective. *Can J Community Mental Health* 7(2):61–71.

Ulrich YC. 1990. Battered women who got out. *Wichita Women,* 4(1): 10. The Company of Women, PO Box 742, Nyack, NY 10960.

Domestic violence: A guide for health care providers. (1993). Denver: Colorado Domestic Violence Coalition.

Assessing for Substance Abuse

Substance abuse is an enormous problem in the United States, and its consequences are devastating. According to a new Robert Wood Johnson (1993) report on substance abuse, "there are more deaths, illnesses and disabilities from substance abuse than from any other preventable health condition. Of the two million U.S. deaths each year, more than one in four is attributable to alcohol, illicit drug or tobacco use. Many of these deaths and other losses could be reduced—if not eliminated—by changing people's habits."

Substance abuse negatively affects not only the addict but also everyone in our society directly or indirectly through traffic accidents and deaths, domestic violence, child abuse, increased health care costs, economic cost to employers and families, and the destruction of individual lives. It is estimated that 30% to 50% of all hospital admissions can be attributed to the effects of substance abuse. According to an article in *America,* 57 million people are addicted to nicotine, 18 million are addicted to alcohol, and 10 million are abusing psychotherapeutic drugs. Crack, heroin, and hallucinogens each account for 1 million addicts. Annually, the cost, in health care and loss of productivity, is approximately $600 billion for alcoholism, $60 billion for tobacco-related ailments, and $40 billion for illicit drugs (Lynch and Bolmer 1993).

It is estimated that only 10% of substance abusers are in treatment (Frances and Miller 1991). This alarmingly low percentage indicates a serious gap in identification and referral and in the availability of treatment for people suffering from addictions. Because addictions frequently go unrecognized by health care providers, assessment for substance abuse is an essential component of every thorough nursing health history and interview process. Often, when health care providers identify a pattern of abuse, they minimize or avoid it and focus instead on the illness or injury caused or exacerbated by substance abuse. For example, the provider who treats gastritis with antacids and fails to address the client's drinking habits, or teaches the use of an inhaler to treat asthma without addressing the client's addiction to nicotine or crack cocaine gives the message that, on some level, the addiction is acceptable. In essence, the provider is encouraging the client to keep silent about the substance abuse. Both of these examples illustrate fragmented treatment. Providers need to abandon this "bandaid" approach and adopt instead a more holistic approach to assessment that identifies the problem and allows the client to begin to address the primary issue: addiction.

Definition

Lack of clarity in the definition of substance abuse and addiction can lead to misunderstanding and misdiagnosis. Not all drug and alcohol use is addiction. Although there is no finite point at which the use of drugs or alcohol becomes addiction, you can diagnose addiction when the use of any substance affects a person's physical, psychologic, or spiritual health, compromising employment, relationships, finances, or legal status.

Our society tends to tolerate the use of tobacco, alcohol, diet pills, and prescription drugs to some extent, whereas it typically censors the use of illegal drugs such as heroin, marijuana, and cocaine. You must not jump to the conclusion that any drug use is addicition and therefore a problem for the client. However, if a client indicates use of drugs or alcohol, you should explore further. Addiction to legal drugs is as difficult to treat as addiction to illicit ones. It is very important to remember that both groups of drugs have addictive potential and damaging effects.

Assessment

As a health care professional, you have a responsibility to assess all clients for potential substance abuse. It is not enough to assess only high risk groups or individuals. You cannot recognize addiction or those who may be prone to addiction at first glance; you need to assess carefully. An addict can be old or young, male or female. Addicts come from all socioeconomic, cultural, and racial backgrounds.

When assessing the client for substance abuse, you must first examine your own feelings and preconceptions about addiction. We as nurses may feel underinformed or inadequate to deal with substance abuse and the many difficult issues that surround it, but we must remember that we can solve the secondary medical problems only if we address the primary causes—the addiction and the power it has in the life of the addict. Generally, the addict is extremely sensitive and can readily detect unaccepting attitudes; being nonjudgmental is the first step toward establishing a good rapport. As health care providers, we can best help people when they feel valued or cared for. This attitude ultimately affects the overall care plan in positive ways, because it facilitates more honest and direct communication.

Begin the initial assessment by taking a medication history. Include questions such as these:

- What prescription drugs have you used/are you currently using?
- Do you drink alcohol, smoke cigarettes?
- Have you ever used marijuana, heroin, cocaine, speed, or other drugs?
- Do you use crack cocaine?

Addiction is often referred to as the disease of denial. Denial can distort thinking and is usually one of the primary symptoms of substance abuse. It decreases addicts' awareness of the problems addiction causes in their lives and thus can be a tremendous barrier to identification and treatment of the addiction. With this in mind, remain alert for signs of denial, which frequently manifests itself as minimizing the effects of the addiction, rationalizing, intellectualizing, excusing or avoiding problems that result from drug use, and finally blaming the addiction on external circumstances or other people.

Here are some examples of statements that may indicate denial:

- I can quit anytime.
- I smoke (drink, take drugs) to relax.
- You would drink, too, if you had my problems.
- If only I had a different job (house, boss, wife, partner) I wouldn't drink (smoke, use drugs).
- Once I retire (graduate, get a job), I'll stop.
- I use only once a week; I only had a couple.
- I didn't like that job (girlfriend/boyfriend) anyway.
- I get angry only when I drink (do drugs).

Like anyone trying to hide a problem, substance abusers can become angry or defensive when attention is drawn to their addiction. Defensiveness often masks fear and bolsters the addict's characteristic low self-esteem, helping the addict to avoid disclosure of the problem. Disclosure of an addictive habit is usually very threatening, especially when illegal drugs are involved. The addict undoubtedly fears many things—being turned in to the police; being rejected or abandoned by friends, family, or health care providers; and ultimately being denied health care. You must reassure the client that all information is confidential.

Guilt, remorse, anxiety, despair, depression, isolation, self-pity, and hopelessness are emotions that many substance abusers feel to varying degrees. To temporarily ease the pain of difficult experiences, the addict begins (and continues) to self-medicate with the drug of choice. Once this begins, the cycle of addiction is set in motion: difficult feelings, drugs to ease the pain, more feelings, more drugs. This cycle is often extremely difficult to break, but as a health care provider you must make the addict aware of the many options for treatment.

Defensiveness may serve to keep the nurse from getting too close to the client and the client's addiction. It is important for you to be aware of some of the more typical responses so that you can avoid being intimidated or misled by the client during the interview. Empathic confrontation may help defuse the client's defensiveness. These statements can often divert defensiveness:

- It seems like my questions are making you uncomfortable. Do you want to talk about what's bothering you?
- I sense that you're getting upset. Does it make you uncomfortable to talk about your drinking (smoking, drug use)?

Once you have established any drug use, it is important to ask the following questions:

- What is the name of the drug?
- How long did you/have you been using this drug?
- How often do you use it?
- How much do you use at one time?
- How do you take it (snort, shoot up)?

If the person has taken drugs intravenously, you must also assess for HIV risk.

Like many other assessments, the assessment for substance abuse should include both objective and subjective data obtained from direct questioning and observation of behavior. Pay careful attention to contradictory behavior, because it may give you an opportunity to open up a discussion about substance use/abuse. Often what the client does not say is a clearer indication of what is going on than what the client actually says. For example, someone with two arrests for driving while intoxicated may insist that drinking is not a problem.

The next step of the assessment is to employ a specific substance-abuse screen. A simple and effective tool is the CAGE substance abuse screen. This interview technique is concise and can elicit very useful information on which you can base your overall assessment. The CAGE screening consists of four simple questions that encourage the client to examine general patterns of drug use.

Cut down. Has anyone ever suggested to you that you should, or have you ever tried to, cut down on your drinking (drug use)?

Annoyed. Has anyone ever become angry or annoyed at your behavior when you were drinking (using drugs)?

Guilt. Have you ever felt guilty about something you did when you had been drinking (taking drugs)?

Eye-opener. Have you ever used drugs or alcohol for an eye-opener in the morning?

The client's social history may indicate addiction, such as problems with the law, family, relationships, finances, employment, or an episode of homelessness. The past health history may include many accidents, injuries, falls, fractures, and other illnesses that could be related to substance abuse, such as gastritis, liver disease, pancreatitis, and frequent upper respiratory infections. These problems do not always indicate substance abuse, but you need to remain alert for problems that are commonly seen in cases of substance abuse. Medical diagnoses can often obscure the reality of the client's situation and shift the focus away from the source of the problem (drug use/self-medication) to the secondary problems, namely medical conditions. It is important for health care providers to recognize the necessity of moving beyond this medical model and into a more holistic approach to treatment and nursing care plans.

The final step in assessing for substance abuse is processing what you observe during the actual interview. You must become aware of how to watch for signs without making assumptions. You must learn to trust your own instincts, and note when a client's responses contradict what you observe. You may want to consider the following questions:

- What does the client's body language say to you?
- Is the client oriented and alert?
- Is the client's affect congruent with the substance of the client's words?
- Does the client deny any substance abuse, yet smell of alcohol or cigarette smoke, or appear to be high on drugs?

Once you have made note of these observations, giving feedback to the client indicating what contradictions you observed can often help you break down barriers in communication and move the client out of denial. Try to phrase the feedback in this way:

"What I hear you say is, . . . but this is what I see." For example, "I hear you saying that you don't use drugs, but these marks on your arm look very much like needle tracks."

Intervention

A holistic approach to health care stresses that prevention and wellness are far more suited to identifying and addressing the problems of substance abuse than the medical model, which emphasizes acute and episodic illness. Prevention, identification, and treatment of substance abuse can be addressed at all levels using the nursing model's primary, secondary, and tertiary levels of care.

Primary. Assess for substance abuse as well as provide preventative education about addiction and the impact it has on physical health, relationships, and communities.

Secondary. Identify addiction, work with the client to confront addiction, and plan intervention and treatment. It may take several visits before a client is able to build enough trust to disclose substance abuse and related problems. You must be patient and develop a feel for when confrontation is appropriate and confrontation may drive the client away. Ultimately, the client must make the decision for treatment. Your role must be one of nonjudgmental support. When referring clients to available treatment resources, encourage them to make their own contacts when ready. It is important for the client to take responsibility for treatment as the first step in recovery.

Tertiary. Provide on-going support to the client (and significant others) through recovery and relapse. Relapse is part of recovery. It is vital that you not take responsibility for a client's recovery, but instead listen to the issues the client is facing before, during, and after relapse while providing on-going support throughout treatment. It can be very difficult for clients to continue with counseling and/or other forms of treatment. In these cases, encourage the client to look at what has helped in the past and remind the client of successful periods of sobriety.

Remember that people who are addicted to substances generally do not trust easily. Trust usually evolves over time. As you continue to relate to the client over several visits, you may obtain new information that contradicts earlier information volunteered by the client. It is important to continue to ask questions about substance abuse at each encounter if you suspect the client is using drugs.

The nurse who can assess for addiction, intervene, and serve as a resource for the client to enter into treatment will undoubtedly provide a service, not just to the individual but to a much broader community. Make the effort to learn about treatment options that are available in your community for substance abusers who want to seek help. These resources might include private groups and counseling, detoxification centers, 12-step meetings (Alcoholics Anonymous, Narcotics Anonymous), rehabilitation programs, and halfway houses.

Treatment for substance abuse is difficult and often becomes a lifelong struggle. The addict must first acknowledge and confront the addiction. This confrontation generally comes after a series of negative consequences resulting from the substance abuse (eg, domestic violence, accidents, job loss, health problems). Recovery is typically a cycle of abstention and relapse. Try not to be discouraged by this process and refrain from labeling the client a noncompliant if relapse occurs. Relapse is very common, especially in the early phases of treatment. Recovery is a lifelong process of personal awareness and a constant struggle with the power of addiction.

Summary

- Be in touch with your feelings about substance abuse.
- Become aware of treatment and intervention services available in your area.
- Include substance-abuse assessment in health history interviews for all clients, not just high-risk clients.
- Remember that nicotine, alcohol, and prescription drugs, as well as illegal drugs, are addictive.
- Be alert for subtle signs of addiction and denial.
- Trust your instincts, but don't jump to conclusions.
- Try to understand the circumstances affecting the client.
- Assure the client that the information is confidential.
- Try to determine an overall plan of intervention and treatment.
- Provide the client with appropriate referrals.

References

Ewing JA. 1984. Alcoholism: The CAGE questionnaire. *JAMA* 252 (14):1905–1907.

Frances R, Miller S. 1991. *Clinical textbook of addictive disorders.* New York: Guilford Press.

Lynch G, Bolmer R. 1993. Legalizing drugs is not the solution. *America,* 8:7–9.

Robert Wood Johnson Foundation. 1993. Substance abuse: The nation's number one health problem. Institute for Health Policy, Brandeis University, Waltham, MA.

Assessing for Child Abuse

The subject of child abuse can cause severe anxiety among health care professionals. There is a great need for calm, sequential clinical approach to victims of child abuse. Abuse, whether physical, sexual, or emotional, is considered to impair the child's physical, psychologic, and developmental growth. Nurses play an important, often pivotal, role in the lives of children who are abused and have a responsibility to assess for violence.

According to the National Center on Child Abuse and Neglect (NCCAN), 2.9 million reports of abuse and neglect are made yearly. Last year, 1251 children died of abuse and neglect; this is an average of 3 deaths per day (personal communication, National Child Abuse Hotline, 3/25/1994). The NCCAN further reports that every 13 seconds a child is abused in the United States. This statistic mirrors reports from the Centers for Disease Control that a woman is beaten every 15 seconds in this country. As studies on the prevalence of child abuse unfold, estimates of sexual abuse now range from 27% of girls and 16% of boys (Finkelhor et al 1990), with many cases in middle- and upper-class homes.

Remember, however, that these numbers reflect substantiated cases only; it is believed that these instances represent just the tip of the iceberg, particularly in the area of emotional abuse. Many cases of physical, sexual, and emotional abuse go undetected and unreported. These numbers do not account for underreporting of abuse cases by private practitioners who deal primarily with higher economic groups. This situation creates a "class bias" of child abuse toward lower income groups, which can be played out in detrimental ways, because of stereotyping. Since the passage of the Child Abuse Prevention and Treatment Act of 1974 (PL 93-247), many cases of abuse have been presented in the medical setting. Thus, it becomes the responsibility of nurses to become proficient in detecting and evaluating abuse, planning, and on occasion testifying on behalf of the child victim.

The literature consistently documents that abuse severely affects children irrespective of age, gender, socioeconomic status, or geographic location. Experts in the field of child sexual assault suggest that 1 in 4 girls and 1 in 10 boys will experience some form of unwanted or forced sexual contact before the age of 18 (Finkelhor 1993). The average age for girls to experience abuse is 8 years, whereas boys appear to be more at risk from ages 9 to 13. However, it should be noted that many victims are only 2 and 3 years of age. Retrospective studies have shown that 20% to 30% of females have been sexually victimized in some way before the age of 13 and that abuse by stepfathers is seven times more common than abuse by biologic fathers (Russell 1986).

Only 21% of abusers of females are strangers, and 79% are known, trusted adults and family members; among abusers of males, 40% are strangers (Finkelhor et al 1990). Some clinics devoted to the evaluation of child abuse report even higher percentages of familial perpetrators. Children who are abused by someone external to the family may respond with less emotional trauma than victims of incestuous abuse (Sgori 1982). However, the family's reaction to the discovery, especially if it is disbelief or denial of the assault, can strongly affect how the abuse affects the child at any stage of disclosure. Consequently, health care professionals need to provide services to enhance the physical, psychologic, developmental, and psychosocial well-being of children and their parents. Nurses are in a position to facilitate healthy intervention measures.

In the past, most cases involving children who were sexually abused were inadequately evaluated and managed at every level of care. Those who were responsible for case mangement tended to be overwhelmed by their caseloads and were not aware of the severity of the effects that sexual abuse has upon children. Often they worked for agencies that were reluctant to be responsible for child sexual abuse cases and were unwilling to train their staff properly and to develop and utilize appropriate community resources (Sgori 1982).

Today, extensive research in the field has contributed to educating those who work with victims of sexual abuse, thus enhancing their ability to evaluate, manage, and treat the victims. As the prevalence and incidence of child sexual abuse become known, health care and human service professionals have begun to develop programs that recognize the significant emotional and physical impact of abuse. Helping children and their families to overcome the effects of sexual victimization is not an easy task; however, with proper care and attention, it is possible. Health care providers should familiarize themselves with the issue of child (sexual) abuse through reading literature and becoming familiar with community resources available to children and their families.

The Role of the Nurse

Nurses have begun to educate each other about child abuse through documentation. Because most children who are sexually abused are females and most offenders are male, and because the majority of nurses are women, nurses in general are in a more favorable position than other health care providers for assessing a child who has been sexually abused. A child who has been abused by a male offender is not likely to want to be examined by or trust a male. A male nurse assessing a girl may need to seek help from female colleagues. As they begin to permeate the primary care settings, nurses of both sexes need to become proficient in the assessment, intervention, and prevention of child abuse.

The worst stance adults and health care providers can take with a sexually abused child is to minimize the abuse and its effects or to deny that the abuse is taking place. This reaction may allow the abuse to continue or allow the experience of abuse to take on a new significance. Denial and minimizing may intensify the immediate impact and prolong the long-term effects (Kelley 1990). Therefore, health care professionals who provide services to victims of abuse must be aware of any personal feelings that may affect the victim.

Nurses functioning within a team setting have been trained to assess the child's and family's psychosocial, emotional, spiritual, physiologic, and environmental needs and priorities. A strong working relationship with other members of the health care team enhances the quality of the child's health care. Victims are often experiencing multiple symptoms with a variety of manifestations, such as extreme depression, suicidal feelings, drug abuse, or chronic migraine headaches. This symptom complex implies a need for various services. The many tragedies associated with sexual abuse, eg, runaways, teen pregnancies, STDs, prostitution, exploitation, and eating disorders, highlight the risk factors associated with abuse. Because of the complexity of related issues, a multidisciplinary approach is optimal.

Screening in the Primary Care Setting

PITFALLS is an acronym that helps nurses remember potential obstacles in the assessment of abuse.

P. Personal feelings. Have you yourself experienced abuse? If so, how might your experience affect your ability to work with victims? Who might be able to help you with your own feelings? What are your feelings toward the victim? Are you ready to develop skills in this area that are beneficial to your well-being and the well-being of the client? A self-assessment of your personal feelings may be instrumental in facilitating an effective and therapeutic relationship.

I. Identification. How am I to identify children who have been sexually abused? The most important thing to remember is to be extremely sensitive to the child. Though disclosing the abuse may be a relief to the child on some level, it is almost always a terrifying process. The developmental level of the child dictates the means of identification. With preverbal children, health care professionals need to assess the genital areas for abnormalities. This assessment involves spreading the labia gently apart in girls, as well as conducting a visual examination of the anus of both boys and girls. You can recognize abnormalities only after you become familiar with the norms of young children's genitals. Use your history taking time to build a rapport with the client. The following framework is helpful in eliciting a history of abuse:

Disclaimers:
- I ask all my patients these questions.
- Your safety means a lot to me.

Questions:
- Has anyone been hurting you?
- Do you know your private parts?
- What do you call your private parts?
- Has anyone hurt your private parts?
- Are you afraid of anyone?
- If someone was hurting you, what would you do?
- What do you think about secrets? When is it OK to keep a secret? When is it not OK to keep a secret?
- What do you think is the worst thing that will happen?

Goal: To ascertain what happened, who was involved, when the abuse occurred, and where the assault took place.

Ask open-ended questions:
- Can you tell me what happened?
- What did he/she touch you with?
- What parts of your body did he/she touch?
- What happened after that?

- Who hurt you?
- Where were you when this happened?
- When did this happen? (Before or after your birthday? Was it warm or cold out? Was it around a special holiday, like Christmas, Valentine's Day, Thanksgiving?)

Avoid:

- Questions that will elicit a Yes or No answer.
- Questions framed in the negative; eg, "He didn't force you to touch him, did he?"
- Making promises, eg, "I promise he'll be arrested."
- Asking why, eg, "Why didn't you tell your mother?" Instead, ask, "What are you afraid of?"
- Making suggestions to the child, eg, "Did he force you to touch his penis?"
- Asking "Did he threaten you?" Instead, ask:
  - "What part of his body touched your body?"
  - "Where did that part of his body touch your body?"
  - "How did he scare you?"
  - "What are you afraid of now?"

T. Time. Some clinicians might argue that they "don't have time to be asking these questions." We must find the time. Perhaps it is time to rethink our history-taking questions. Make time in every interview to assess for abuse.

F. Fear. If abuse is reported, how should I respond? What should I say? These are very common questions, and the response of the interviewer is crucial to a successful therapeutic encounter. Abused children often feel intense guilt, shame, fear, betrayal, self-blame, and anger. Given that abuse is often such an intensely emotional issue for children, the following statements may help you provide much needed reassurance and comfort to the child:

- I believe you.
- This was not your fault.
- You did nothing wrong.
- You did nothing to cause this.
- You are so brave for sharing this.
- It is normal to feel afraid when you think about having told the secret.
- I really care about how you feel.

A. Awareness. The need for the awareness of resources is imperative. It is helpful to contact resources prior to beginning screening so that you have a sense of those in the area that provide services to children who have been abused, eg, rap groups for teens, individual therapy for victims, writing or art groups, and legal services. Without support, information, and places at which to seek advice, you cannot do this work.

L. Law. All 50 states have laws related to reporting child abuse. You need to know your state's laws about what findings are considered reportable. Whenever in doubt about reporting, speak with members of your team and consult resources within your organization. The ultimate goal is the child's safety, not necessarily state intervention.

Having representatives and advocates from the legal system as a resource is extremely valuable. Most states have child prosecution units that deal exclusively with abuse and violence. You may be called to testify as an expert witness. In this setting, an expert witness is anyone who possesses a special skill or knowledge beyond that of an ordinary person. Formal titles or qualifications are not a prerequisite for testifying as an expert. Once again, it is important to establish resources to work with you in the event you are called to testify. Testifying on behalf of abused children can be a rewarding experience and offers you the opportunity to be recognized within the legal system as an advocate for children.

L. Lethality. It is crucial to have an understanding of how dangerous a perpetrator is to the victim. You may assess this by asking:

- What are some of the worst things this person has done to you?
- Have you ever needed to go to the hospital?
- What kinds of threats has he/she ever made?
- Does he/she have a gun? Has that or any other weapon/object been used against you?

  When assessing the situation, you need to have a sense of whether the custodial parent will be able to protect the child from the perpetrator. Remember that often the mother is also being abused by the same perpetrator.

S. Safety. Safety must always govern your plan for the child and family. When you are making decisions that have direct bearing on the child, ask yourself:

- Is this a safe plan for the child?
- Is the child in imminent danger?

  Although there are laws for reporting child abuse, it is difficult to fault any nurse whose first consideration is the safety of the child. However, you must report the case after ensuring the child's safety. Whenever in doubt as to a safe plan for the child, consult your resources for support and advice.

  You must always think about your own safety as well. Do not disclose your home address or telephone number. If you suspect danger, never leave work alone. Under no circumstances should you speak with the alleged perpetrator. Always report harassing telephone calls or letters to the police.

Recognizing the PITFALLS is a useful way to begin addressing what must occur to make screening for abuse and violence a standard practice in all settings. Nurses have the capacity and the fundamental skills to incorporate assessment for abuse and violence into their health-taking histories. Living with the secrecy that goes along with abuse, especially when it occurs within the family, is incredibly painful and isolating. Many children have little or no other opportunity to disclose, outside of the health care setting, the abuse they are experiencing. Nurses have the responsibility to provide children with that opportunity.

Nurses can begin to meet the professional and personal challenge by educating themselves. The first step is to institute the measures needed to ensure that abuse evaluations occur routinely. If a child is not being abused, you have a window of opportunity for preventitive education; if a child is being abused, you have the means of initiating interventions on behalf of the child. The numbers of cases reported certainly demand proactive responses from health care providers taking a holistic approach. Nurses play a major role in helping children feel safe and live free of abuse and violence. Helping children and their families overcome the effects of abuse is not an easy task, but it is not impossible.

For futher information, contact:
National Toll-Free Child Abuse Hotline
1-800-4-ACHILD
or
National Child Rights Alliance
(919)479-7130

References

Burgess AW et al. 1985. *Sexual assault of children and adolescents.* Lexington, MA: Lexington Books.

Devlin BK, Reynolds E. 1994. Child abuse: How to recognize it, how to intervene. *Am J Nurs*:26–32.

Elvik S et al. 1986. Child sexual abuse: The role of the NP. *Nurse Pract*:15–22.

Finkelhor D et al. 1990. Sexual abuse in a national survey of adult men and women: Prevalence, characteristics, and risk factors. *Child Abuse Neglect* 14:19.

Finkelhor D. 1993. Epidemiological factors in the clinical identification of child sexual abuse. *Child Abuse Neglect* 17:67–70.

Flynn EM. 1987. Preventing and diagnosing sexual abuse in children. *Nurse Pract* 12(2):47–65.

Kelley SJ. 1986. Learned helplessness in the sexually abused child. *Issues Comprehens Pediatr Nurs* 9:193–207.

Kelley SJ. 1990. Parental stress response to sexual abuse and ritualistic abuse of children in day care centers. *Nurs Res* 39:25–29.

MacFarlane K et al. 1986. *Sexual abuse of young children.* New York: Guilford Press.

Ming JSL. 1990. Responsibilities of primary care providers in child sexual abuse. *Nurse Pract Forum.* 1(2):90–97.

Rhodes AM. 1987. Identifying and reporting child abuse. *Matern Child Nurs* 12(6).

Russell DEH. 1986. *The secret trauma: Incest in the lives of girls and women.* Basic Books.

Ryan MT. 1984. Identifying the sexually abused child. *Pediatr Nurs* 419–421.

Sgori SM. 1982. *Handbook of clinical intervention in child sexual abuse.* Boston: Lexington Books.

Smith D et al. 1988. Pediatric sexual abuse management in a sample of children's hospitals. *Pediatr Emerg Care* 4(3):177–79.

Assessing for Elder Abuse

Elder abuse and mistreatment is a serious problem with potentially fatal outcomes. It is a widespread problem, affecting up to 10% of all elderly people (Bourland 1990). There are no typical victims, although the common descriptors of abused elders are that they are predominantly female, are over 75 years of age, and have major physical or psychologic impairments that affect their activities of daily living.

Elderly people also make up a large percentage of clients whom health care providers perceive as confused, noncompliant and noncooperative. This perception has led to disproportionate use of psychotropic drugs and restraints in the treatment of the elderly population. For this reason, health care providers must challenge themselves to look beyond the surface and to perform a careful assessment of the multiple factors affecting the overall health status of the elderly. Among these factors is, in some cases, elder mistreatment, which cuts across all socioeconomic and ethnic groups. Sadly, the abusers are apt to be family members, although many elders are abused by nonrelated caregivers as well.

It is estimated that by the turn of the century 13.1% of the population will be 65 or older. The fastest growing percentage of that elderly group are the "old/old," or those 85 or older, many of whom are frail and dependent. As the number of elderly people increases, there may be an ever-increasing incidence of elder abuse and mistreatment.

Definitions

Most definitions of elder mistreatment include both abuse and neglect. Neglect is the failure to provide for basic needs. Abuse includes:

- Direct physical contact or actions that cause physical injury
- Financial abuse, which includes threat of misuse or actual misuse of money or property
- Psychologic abuse, which is the infliction of pain through verbal or emotional means.

There are many theories as to why caregivers, or others, abuse elderly individuals, but as of yet none of the theories provides a clear answer to the problem. The following theories are currently proposed:

- Exchange theory. According to the exchange theory, abuse continues when the caregiver derives pleasure, monetary gain, or other rewards from the abusive exchange. If it ceases to benefit the abuser, then the abuse will stop (Pillemer 1986).
- Stressed caregiver theory. This theory is that stress leads to abuse and neglect. The stress can be the result of caring for the elder or can have indirect causes, such as loss of job or marital difficulties. The abuser perceives the elder as a cause of distress (Block and Sinnott 1979).
- Transgenerational violence. In the transgenerational violence theory, violence is seen as a learned behavior that is passed from generation to generation (Straus et al 1980). Thus, an abused child exhibits the same abusive behaviors when placed in the role of the caregiver of the elder parent. There may also be an element of retribution involved.
- Psychopathology of abuser. Some theorists believe that psychiatric illness, substance abuse, and mental retardation may be abuser characteristics that account for an increased rate of abused elders (Lau and Kosberg 1979).
- Impairment (dependency) theory. The debilitated elder is seen as vulnerable to abuse as a result of the increased stress to the caregiver. However, some researchers have found that dependence on the elder for housing, household repairs, finances, and transportation can also lead to abuse (Pillemer 1986, 1990).

Types of Abuse and Neglect

Physical Abuse

Direct physical abuse of elders accounts for many reported cases. Physical abuse is often demonstrated by the presence of unexplained bruises and welts on various body parts. Sometimes the bruises show the outline of the device used, such as rulers or cords. Abuse can also be suspected when there are fractures or bruises in various stages of healing. Sexual abuse of the elderly should be suspected in the presence of genital bruising or venereal disease.

Psychologic Abuse

Psychologic abuse can be seen when elders are demeaned, treated as children, yelled at, or ignored. All forms of psychologic abuse can result in mental health problems for the elder.

Financial abuse

Financial abuse is also common. Caregivers may steal money and resources. The elderly may also be targets of mail fraud or scams. Indicators include evidence of unusual bank account activity, suspicious signatures on checks, unrealistic explanation of financial status, and evidence of theft.

Neglect

Neglect, by others as well as self-neglect, can also occur in the elderly. It can be both intentional or unintentional. Some signs of neglect include poor hygiene, malnutrition, inappropriate dress, and unmet health care needs.

Assessment

History

There are few direct and conclusive observations of abusive behavior, and the elderly themselves rarely, or with great difficulty and hesitancy, report acts of abuse and neglect. The reluctance to discuss mistreatment may be the result of embarrassment, fear, or a concern for privacy. Elders may find it very difficult to tell strangers that a caregiver is neglectful or abusive, especially if the caregiver is a family member. Elders may also fear a loss of autonomy, financial security, or abandonment.

The first and most obvious method of determining abuse is to ask the elder. Because there are different types of abuse, it is important to ask the elder general questions that allude to each type. These can then be followed by more specific questions. Examples of opening questions are

- What would be a typical day for you?
- Have you recently been in any situations that made you uncomfortable?
- Have you been hurt recently?
- Who takes care of your finances?
- Who do you call when you need help?

It is important to speak to the elder person alone as well as in the presence of the caregiver. All too frequently, if the elderly client is cognitively impaired or hesitates to speak out, personnel may rely on the reports given by those who accompany the older person. These same people may be the abusers.

The behavior of the abused person can sometimes be the key to detecting abuse. You should ask yourself the following questions during the interview:

- Does the elderly person appear unduly afraid, withdrawn, or compliant in the presence of the caretaker?
- Does the client appear unwilling to discuss symptoms or injuries, or does the client minimize them?
- Does the client appear depressed or express depression overtly through crying or hand wringing?
- Do the old person's eyes dart continuously, signifying anxiety or fear?
- Does the elder stay as distant from the caregiver as possible?

Other behaviors that may signal abuse are crying and backing off or cringing, as though the elder expects to be struck. Also the elder may huddle when sitting or display other symptoms of nervousness. You must question any display of fear when the older person is in the presence of familiar individuals.

Physical Assessment

A thorough physical assessment is essential for all elderly patients. To assess the older person accurately, you need a thorough knowledge of the normal physiologic and psychosocial changes that occur with aging.

Unfortunately, many of the changes of aging and disease resemble signs of abuse and neglect. Malnutrition or poor nutritional status resulting from neglect, mistreatment, or lack of financial resources can easily be mistaken for lack of appetite due to depression, loneliness, medications, or chronic health problems. Chronic health problems such as joint pain, tenderness, and difficulty in movement can indicate arthritis or an injury sustained during an abusive episode. Cognitive impairment or confusion can easily be attributed to "senility" or old age when in reality it indicates oversedation of the elder. Osteoporosis can result in fractures that are occasionally spontaneous. Although fractures are one of the indicators of abuse in children, more often than not such findings do not suggest abuse in the aged.

The challenge of elder assessment is determining the exact cause of the finding. You must resist the impulse to jump to conclusions. Verification of abuse and neglect is difficult because of physical health problems that confound the assessment, elder refusal to confirm or report abuse, and lack of widespread and systematic screening.

Even when you verify abuse, it can be difficult to find the right solution for the problem. Many health care providers adopt a "paternalistic" attitude, making decisions that they think are in the best interests of the elder but often without consulting the elder. The health provider's choice, however, does not always reflect the elderly person's desires. Even when a situation appears less than optimal to the outsider, the elder may prefer a known situation to an unknown one, and the health care provider has a responsibility to respect those wishes. However, it may still be useful to recommend other resources in the community in case the elderly client decides to try to leave the abusive caregiver.

Intervention

To be effective, professional interventions should include participation by nurses, physicians, social workers, and when applicable, clergy. It is vitally important to engage in multidisciplinary strategizing and problem solving in cases of elder abuse.

Professional intervention strategies should be geared toward individuals and families, including counseling for victims, caregivers, and families. Support groups for victims and for overwhelmed caregivers, and training groups for at-risk groups can all be helpful. Effective nursing intervention requires not only caring for immediate physical injuries but also a thorough knowledge of available resources.

All 50 states now have some form of elder abuse laws, although legislation varies as widely as definitions of abuse, neglect, and exploitation. Some states have legislation that is specific to the elder, while others cover elder abuse under domestic violence legislation or other protective service laws.

In most states professionals are required to report abuse. The verification and follow-up of abuse then become the responsibility of the appropriate state agency. In 71% of the states there are penalties for failing to report abuse. The penalties vary and range from fines to loss of licensure and prison sentences. However, the safety of the elderly person must be the foremost concern.

Use your best judgment to determine what course of action makes the most sense in each specific situation. It may, for instance, be more detrimental to report abuse and risk the abuser finding out, which could lead to more intensified abuse. In these cases, you must find a balance between the client's needs and the requirements of the protective legislation. Consult the other members of your team, along with the elderly person, to find a solution that ensures the client's safety.

References

Block M, Sinnott J, eds. 1979. *The battered elder syndrome: An exploratory study*. College Park, MD: University of Maryland, Center on Aging.

Bourland MD. 1990. Elder abuse: From definition to prevention. *Postgrad Med* 87(2):139–144.

Lau E, Kosberg J. 1979. Abuse of the elderly by informal care providers. *Aging* 228(10):5.

Pillemer KA. 1986. Risk factors in elder abuse: Results from a case-control study. In Pillemer et al, eds. *Elder abuse: Conflict in the family*. Dover: Auburn House.

Pillemer K. 1990. Ten (tentative) truths about elder abuse. *J Health Human Resources Admin* 12:468–481.

Straus MA, Gelles RJ, Steinmetz SK. 1980. *Behind closed doors*. New York: Anchor Books.

Interviewing the Homeless Client

Many health providers have become sensitized to the lack of access to health care for the homeless, most of whom are uninsured. A Columbia University study reveals that over 13.5 million Americans have been on the streets or stayed in homeless shelters at some point in their life ("Safety Network" 1993). Because the homeless population has been increasing and now includes many families and single women with children, health care providers are placing more emphasis on the urgency of their health, social, and financial needs. Initial efforts to address the concerns of the homeless were the result of volunteer programs set up through community centers, churches, and or mobile units. The goal of these programs was to establish alternative systems of care designed to address the specific needs of the homeless. Health care programs for the homeless exist in shelters, mobile vans, and private physicians' offices. In some cities, hospitals are beginning to develop their own health care programs to provide services through the use of emergency rooms and field nurses, while working in coalition with other municipal social service groups.

The health problems of the homeless mirror those of the general society; however, many homeless people neglect health and thus often have multiple, complex, and chronic conditions. Their lack of regular access to health care and inability to follow through with medications and treatments because of lack of money further exacerbate health problems. The rates of both chronic and acute health problems are extremely high among the homeless population. Homeless people suffer from at least one chronic health problem almost twice as often as housed persons (Wright and Weber 1987). As a health care provider, you will find that their problems often include neglected gynecologic conditions, sexually transmitted diseases, lack of prenatal care, skin problems, and stress-related phenomena. There are also growing numbers of people infected with TB and HIV.

Substance abuse is common in homeless populations. Adults in general have increased psychiatric and mental health problems, poor dental hygiene, foot problems due to ill-fitting shoes and excessive walking, skin problems related to exposure to the elements, and trauma due to violence on the streets. Homeless children are frequently malnourished and have a high incidence of upper respiratory infections, delayed immunizations, developmental delays, diarrhea, rashes, and behavioral or school-related problems. As a health care provider, you play a very important role for homeless clients, as one of the few resources available to them for treatment and care and as a guide to other community resources such as soup kitchens, detox centers, clinics, and shelters.

The Setting for Homeless Health Care

It is not unusual for services to be provided in older buildings located in central areas of the city. It is useful to familiarize yourself with facilities and their locations as soon as you can. The host site (which is the homeless shelter) may place more emphasis on feeding and housing the homeless than on health care. Shelters generally don't have the same resources as outpatient clinics or hospitals. In resource-poor facilities, you will have to share resources and space with social workers and other care providers.

As a health care professional, you may be challenged to maintain privacy when interviewing or counseling a client, secure adequate space to provide the care, and follow through with health teaching. In this setting, you will get first-hand experience in negotiating for space to provide client care, respecting another professional's contribution to the client's overall plan of care, and advocating for the client. These circumstances demand collaboration and provide an excellent opportunity for growth. The creativity and flexibility you develop from this experience will be useful to you in many other experiences during your professional career.

Interviewing the Homeless Client

The homeless as a group generally have had negative experiences with health care providers and health care agencies because of stereotypes and the client's inability to pay for services. As a result, they may be reluctant to accept the help. It was once commonly believed that homeless individuals cared little about their health and would not engage in a therapeutic relationship with a health care professional or follow through with a care plan. However, experience with the homeless has proven something quite different. Like all clients, the homeless respond positively to sensitivity and genuine concern, and you can make the health care experience both positive and effective. The first and most important skill is to accept clients as they are by conveying a nonjudgmental attitude.

The homeless population consists of individuals from every walk of life who have certain things in common: lack of money and a regular place to sleep, and few resources to draw upon to change their situation. Homeless people may be of any age. Some have college educations, and others are unable to read or write. Some have no job; others work but are temporarily homeless and unable to sustain themselves without a free meal and a place to sleep. There are as many reasons for homelessness as the individuals you will encounter.

There is a disproportionate number of individuals with psychiatric and emotional problems in the homeless group as well as a significant number of substance abusers, some of whom started using in an attempt to self-medicate. There are also many women with children who generally lack a regular source of health care and therefore have multiple health, financial, and emotional needs.

The timing of the interview may vary, depending on the client. Because of the stresses of living on the street, many clients may find it difficult to stay focused on the interview for an entire 20–60 minutes. Use the time you do have to get the most relevant information; this will take some prioritizing. You need to adjust the interview process to the client's concerns and needs. It is important to accept clients as they present themselves to you. For instance, a young mother may not be able to focus on her family's health needs immediately because of her crisis situation. Her attention span will most probably be short, and the children may be disruptive in the clinic. She may be more concerned with her children's behavior than the fact that their immunizations are incomplete. Take this opportunity to observe the communication and behavior between the mother and her children. Find something positive to say about the children. These individuals are in crisis and need an extra measure of kindness to help them feel secure and to reduce their anxiety.

Remember: Whatever health problems you identify, the homeless person will probably give them a lower priority than housing and financial concerns. Homeless people may arrange their priorities differently than you may expect. Remember that they are evaluating their needs within the context of problems and daily concerns that housed people aren't forced to contend with.

Be Open and Nondirective

When you deal with a population under such stress, a nondirective and open-ended approach yields the best results. You may need to use the interview form as a guide only. Use language that you feel comfortable with, but be sensitive to the client's response. As you would with any client, make sure your homeless clients understand the questions and terminology clearly. If you assume they know what you mean, you may fail to get the information you need to determine a care plan. Additionally, speak to the client softly and in a nonthreatening manner. Smile often and reassure the client with touch when appropriate (eg, a pat on the hand). In this way, you convey that you are sensitive to your client's concerns and you put the client at ease.

Be a Good Listener

When possible, talk to the client a few minutes before proceeding with the interview to establish initial rapport. Ask the person to tell you about the circumstances that led to homelessness. If you ask with concern and empathy, the client will share more information than you originally asked for. Be prepared for powerful stories of what the client has been through. Being a good listener is the important first step to building trust. It is extremely important for the client to participate in mutual goal setting. The client must feel invested in the solution to carry it out.

Tailor the Interview to the Client's Needs

If a mother indicates that she wants the visit to be as brief as possible, respect her wishes, attend to the major concern, and encourage her to return for a complete health assessment. In most cases, the client will respond to the request if possible. If the client is too stressed to answer questions or becomes agitated, consider shortening the interview and focus only on the most pressing concerns.

- What are you most concerned about today?
- How did you come to this shelter/clinic?

- Why are you here?
- What is it that you think you need?
- How long have you had this health concern/problem?
- How will you get your medicine/supplies?
- How will you get back to the shelter/clinic?
- Do you have an appointment for follow-up care? Do you plan to keep it? (Reinforce the importance of follow-up care.)
- How can we contact you after you leave here?
- Where will you sleep tonight? or Where are you going when you leave here?

Reassure the Client

Homeless clients may also appear nervous or distracted and may be unable to remember dates of hospitalization and surgeries or names of medications. Reassure the client that you understand that it is difficult to keep medical records when living arrangements are changed frequently.

Like any disenfranchised group, the homeless can be extremely suspicious of how information obtained during an interview might be used. Clients may be reluctant to give their names or the names of their children, or to share important health history essential to assessment and decision-making. Parents are particularly concerned about being accused of child neglect or abuse and may fear that you will turn them in to child-protection agencies, the shelter administration, or law enforcement officers. Respond by saying that you understand the hesitation, and stress that you are asking questions to help you provide care. Make sure that you tell the client that the information will be used only by health providers at the clinic.

Follow-Up

When providing care to homeless people, follow-up visits and instructions for medications can be difficult to arrange. Though homeless people are often perceived as having enormous amounts of free time, they often must work around the busy schedules of several social services to get their basic needs met. Endless lines and waiting can turn homelessness into a full-time occupation. Because they tend to be very transient, the client may not be available when laboratory results are ready. Try to obtain a phone number or address where she/he can pick up messages. If that is not possible, it is important for you to emphasize that it is necessary for the client to return on a specific date to hear test results. Explain that this information could help prevent additional health problems and minimize the need for future visits. Remember that you may be the only health care provider this person has seen or will see for some time. Homeless clients have many needs. It is often the health care provider's responsibility to serve as an access point into many other services available within the community (welfare agencies, substance abuse clinics/services). As a group, the homeless are in need of comprehensive health and social services, and as a sensitive health care provider, you can be a part of a positive experience for these clients.

Summary

- Be in touch with your own feelings—examine your assumptions
- Determine what social services are available to serve homeless people in your area
- Focus on the client
- Express empathy for the client's problems
- Try to understand circumstances affecting the homeless client
- Be open, warm, friendly, and smile
- Adapt interview to client's needs
- Allow time for mutual goal setting
- Assure that the information is confidential
- Provide client with appropriate referrals
- Try to determine a follow-up plan

For more information, call the National Coalition for Homelessness at (202)775-1322.

References

Safety network: The newsletter of the National Coalition for the Homeless. 1993. Vol. 12, issue 6. Washington, D.C.

Wright JD, Weber E. 1987. *Homelessness and health*. Washington, D.C.: McGraw-Hill.

References

General References

Baird SB, Donehower MG, eds. 1991. *A cancer source book for nurses.* Atlanta: American Cancer Society.

Block G, Nolan JW. 1986. *Health assessment for professional nursing, a developmental approach,* 2nd ed. Norwalk, CT: Appleton-Century-Crofts.

Boyle J, Andrews M. 1989. *Transcultural concepts in Nursing.* Glenview, IL: Boston/Scott/Foresman/Little, Brown.

Carpenito L. 1991. *Nursing diagnosis,* 4th ed. Philadelphia: Lippincott.

Davis-Sharts J. 1989. The elder and critical care. In Bessner BA, Armstrong ML, Rempusheski VF, eds. *Nurs Clin North Am* 224(3): 755–767.

Doenges M, Moorhouse M. 1991. *Nursing diagnosis,* 3rd ed. Philadelphia: FA Davis.

Ignatavicius D, Bayne M. 1991. *Medical-surgical nursing: A nursing process approach.* Philadelphia: Saunders.

Kozier B, Erb G, Blais K, Wilkinson J. 1995. *Fundamentals of nursing,* 5th ed. Redwood City, CA: Addison-Wesley Nursing.

Marieb E. 1992. *Human anatomy and physiology.* Redwood City, CA: Benjamin/Cummings, 1992.

McFarland GK, McFarlane EA. 1989. *Nursing diagnosis and intervention.* St Louis: Mosby.

Phipps WJ et al. 1991. *Medical surgical nursing concepts and clinical practice,* 4th ed. St Louis: Mosby.

Potter PA, Perry AG. 1989. *Fundamentals of nursing: Concepts, process, and practice,* 2nd ed. St. Louis: Mosby.

Tucker SM, Canobbio MM, et al. 1992. *Patient care standards: Nursing process, diagnosis and outcomes,* 5th ed., St. Louis: Mosby.

Swartz MH. 1989. *Textbook of physical diagnosis.* Philadelphia: Saunders.

Chapter 1 Introduction to Health Assessment

Alfaro R. 1990. *Applying nursing diagnosis and nursing process. A step-by-step guide,* 2nd ed. Philadelphia: Lippincott.

American Nurses Association. 1991. *Standards of clinical nursing practice.* Washington, DC: ANA.

American Nurses Association. 1980. *Social policy statement.* Kansas City, MO: ANA.

Barker P. 1987. Assembling the pieces: Assessment is like a jigsaw puzzle. *Nurs Times* 83:67–68.

Black KM. 1967. Assessing patients' needs. In Yura H, Walsh MB, eds. *Evaluating the nursing process: Assessing, planning, implementing.* Catholic University of America Press.

Gebbie K, Lavin MA. 1974. Classification of nursing diagnoses. *Am J Nurs* 74:250–253.

George JB, ed. 1985. *Nursing theories: The base for professional nursing,* 2nd ed. Englewood Cliffs, NJ: Prentice Hall.

Gordon M. 1987. *Nursing diagnosis: Process and application,* 2nd ed. Hightstown, NJ: McGraw-Hill.

Hall LE. 1955. Quality of nursing care. Address given at the Department of Baccalaureate and Higher Degree Programs of the New Jersey League for Nursing, Public Health News, New Jersey State Department of Health, June, 1955.

Henderson V. January/February 1965. The nature of nursing. *Int Nurs Rev* 12:23–30.

Ilyer P, Taptich B, Bernocchi-Losey D. 1986. *Nursing process and nursing diagnosis.* Philadelphia: Saunders.

Knowles L. 1967. *Decision-making in nursing: A necessity for doing:* ANA Clinical Sessions, 1966. Norwalk, CT: Appleton-Century-Crofts.

Kozier B, Erb G, Blais K, Wilkinson J. 1995. *Fundamentals of nursing,* 5th ed. Redwood City, CA: Addison-Wesley Nursing.

Krieger D. 1981. *Foundations for holistic health nursing practices: The renaissance nurse.* Philadelphia: Lippincott.

La Monica EL. 1985. *The humanistic nursing process.* Belmont, CA: Wadsworth.

Lange JT. 1976. Harriet Newton Phillips: The first trained nurse in America. *Image* 8:49–51.

NANDA. 1990. Proceedings of the Ninth National Conference of the North American Nursing Diagnosis Association, March 1990.

Nightingale F. Notes on nursing. 1859. What it is, and what it is not. London: Harrison.

Pletsch PK. 1981. Mary Breckenridge: A pioneer who made her mark. *Am J Nurs* 81:2188-90.

Risner PB. 1986. Analysis and Synthesis. In Grifith JW, Christensen PJ, eds. *Nursing process: Applications of theories, frameworks, and models.* St Louis: Mosby.

Smith MP. 1984. The new frontier, *RNABC* (Registered Nurses Association of British Columbia) *News* 16:5.

Steel JE. 1981. Putting joint practice into practice. *Am J Nurs* 81:964–67.

Weinstein S. 1993. A coordinated approach to home infusion care. *Home Healthcare Nurse* 11(1):15–20.

Western Interstate Commission on Higher Education. 1967. *Defining clinical content.* Graduate Nursing Programs, Medical and Surgical Nursing. Boulder, CO: Western Interstate Commission on Higher Education.

World Health Organization. 1947. Constitution of the World Health Organization. Geneva: WHO.

Chapter 2 The Interview and Health History

Alfaro R. 1990. *Applying nursing diagnosis and nursing process. A step-by-step guide,* 2nd ed. Philadelphia: Lippincott.

Brammer LM. 1988. *The helping relationship: Process and skills,* 4th ed. Englewood Cliffs, NJ: Prentice Hall.

Carkhuff RR, Anthony WA. 1979. *The skill of helping.* Amherst, MA: Human Resource Development Press.

Cormier LS, Cormier WH, Weisser RJ. 1984. *Interviewing and helping skills for health professionals.* Belmont, CA: Wadsworth.

Doenges MA, Moorhouse MF. 1990. *Nursing diagnosis with interventions,* 3rd ed. Philadelphia: Davis.

DeVito JA. 1980. *The interpersonal communication book,* 2nd ed. Scranton, PA: Harper and Row.

Freebairn J, Gwinup K. 1979. *Cultural diversity and nursing practice: Instructor's manual.* Concept Media.

Gordon M. 1990. Toward theory-based diagnostic categories. *Nurs Diagnosis* 1(1):511.

La Monica EL. 1985. *The humanistic nursing process.* Belmont, CA Wadsworth.

Mehrabian, A. 1972. *Nonverbal communication.* Chicago: Aldine-Atherton.

Northouse G, Northouse L. 1992. *Health communication: Strategies for health professionals.* Norwalk, CT: Appleton & Lange.

Orem DE. 1991. *Nursing: Concepts and practice,* 4th ed. St. Louis: Mosby.

Rogers CR. 1951. *Client-centered therapy.* Boston: Houghton Mifflin.

Rogers CR. 1957. The necessary and sufficient conditions of therapeutic personality change. *J Consult Psychol.* Reprinted in *J Consult Clin Psychol,* 1992. 827–32.

Chapter 3
Assessing Growth and Development

Jarvis C. 1992. *Physical examination and health assessment.* Philadelphia: Saunders.

Klaus MH, Kennell JH. 1978. *Maternal-infant bonding.* St. Louis: Mosby.

Kozier B, Erb G, Blais K, Wilkinson J. 1995. *Fundamentals of nursing: Concepts, process and practice,* 5th ed. Redwood City, CA: Addison-Wesley Nursing.

Levine MD, Carey WB, Crocker AC. 1992. *Developmental-behavioral pediatrics,* 2nd ed. Philadelphia: Saunders.

Lowrey GH. 1986. *Growth and development of children,* 8th ed. Chicago: Year Book Medical Publishers.

Phillips Jr JL. 1975. *The origins of intellect: Piaget's theory,* 2nd ed. San Francisco: WH Freeman.

Schuster CS, Ashburn SS. 1980. *The process of human development: A holistic approach.* Boston: Little, Brown.

Chapter 4
Assessing Psychosocial Health

American Psychiatric Association. 1987. *Diagnostic and statistical manual,* 3rd ed, rev. American Psychiatric Association.

Barry PD. 1989. *Psychosocial nursing, assessment, and intervention.* Philadelphia: Lippincott.

Birckhead LM. *Psychiatric/mental health nursing: The therapeutic use of self.* Philadelphia: Lippincott.

Brammer LM. 1988. *The helping relationship: Process and skills,* 4th ed. Englewood Cliffs, NJ: Prentice Hall.

Carkhuff RR, Anthony WA. 1979. *The skill of helping.* Amherst, MA: Human Resource Development Press.

Carson RC, Butcher JN, Coleman JC. 1988. *Abnormal psychology and modern life,* 8th ed. Glenview, IL: Scott Foresman.

Carson VB: *Spiritual dimensions of nursing practice.* Philadelphia: Saunders.

Duska R, Whelan M. 1975. *Moral development: A guide to Piaget and Kohlberg.* Paulist Press.

Erikson EH. *Childhood and society,* 2nd ed. New York: Norton.

Fowler J, Keen S. *Life maps: Conversations in the journey of faith.* Waco, TX: Work Books.

Fox B. 1989. Depressive symptoms and risk of cancer. *JAMA* 262(99):1231.

Freud A. 1966. *The ego and the mechanisms of defense.* New York: International Universities Press.

Goodkin K, Antoni M, Blaney P. 1986. Stress and hopelessness in the promotion of cervical intraepithelial neoplasia to invasive squamous cell carcinoma of the cervix. *J Psychosom Res* 30(1): 67–76.

Haber J, Leach A, et al. 1982. *Comprehensive psychiatric nursing,* 2nd ed. New York: McGraw-Hill.

Hagerty BK. 1984. *Psychiatric mental health assessment.* St. Louis: Mosby.

Harris TA. 1973. *I'm OK—You're OK.* New York: Harper and Row.

Johnson BS. 1990. *Psychiatric-mental health nursing: Adaptation and growth,* 2nd ed. Philadelphia: Lippincott.

Lazarus RS, Folkman S. 1984. *Stress, appraisal, and coping.* New York: Springer.

Lederer J, Marculescu G, Mocnik B, Seaby N. 1993. *Care planning pocket guide,* 5th ed. Redwood City, CA: Addison-Wesley Nursing.

Ornish D et al. July 21, 1990. Can lifestyle changes reverse coronary artery disease? *Lancet* 129–133.

Pelletier K. 1991. A review and analysis of the health and cost effective outcome studies of comprehensive health promotion and disease prevention programs. *Am J Health Promotion* 5(4):311–315.

Pelletier K. 1992. Mind-body health: Research, clinical, and policy applications. *Am J Health Promotion* 6(5):345–358.

Peplau HE. 1952. *Interpersonal relations in nursing.* New York: Putnam's Sons.

Perko JE, Kreigh HZ. 1988. *Psychiatric and mental health nursing,* 3rd ed. Norwalk, CT: Appleton & Lange.

Piaget JP. 1966. *The origin of intelligence in children.* International Universities Press.

Polonsky W, Knapp P, Brown E, Schwartz G. 1985. Psychological factors, immunologic function, and bronchial asthma. *Psychosom Med* 47:114.

Rogers C. 1951. *Client-centered therapy.* Boston: Houghton Mifflin.

Rogers C. 1966. *On becoming a person.* Boston: Houghton Mifflin.

Rogers C. 1975. Empathic: An unappreciated way of being. *Counseling Psychol* 5(2):2.

Smith G, McKenie J, Marmer D, Steele R. 1985. Psychologic modulation of the human immune response to varicella zoster. *Arch Intern Med* 145:2110–2112.

Spiegal D et al. October 14, 1989. Effects of psychosocial treatment on survival of patients with metastatic breast cancer. *Lancet* 888–891.

Stuart GW, Sundeen SJ. 1988. *Pocket nurse guide to psychiatric nursing.* St Louis: Mosby.

Sullivan HS. 1953. *The interpersonal Theory of psychiatry.* New York: Norton.

Sundeen SJ, Stuart GW, et al. 1989. *Nurse-client interaction,* 4th ed. St. Louis: Mosby.

Wilson HS, Kneisl CR. 1988. *Psychiatric nursing,* 3rd ed. Redwood City, CA: Addison-Wesley Nursing.

Chapter 5
Assessing Self-Care and Wellness Activities

Adam K, Oswald I. 1977. Sleep is for tissue restoration. *J R Coll Physicians London* 11:376–88.

Barnett R. 1991. The feds speak out: The USDA recommendations get more specific. *Am Health.*

Canavan T. 1984. The psychobiology of sleep. *Nursing* 84 2:682.

Clenney SL, Johnson SM. 1983. *Back to basics: A handbook of EEG technology.* Anaheim, CA: Beckman Instruments.

Closs S. 1988. Assessment of sleep in hospitalized patients: A review of methods. *J Adv Nurs* 13(4):501–510.

Cohen FL 1988. Narcolepsy: A Review of a common, life-long sleep disorder. *J Adv Nurs* 13(5):546–56.

Emra KL, Herrera CO. 1989. When your patient tells you he can't sleep. *Am J Nurs* 52(9):79–84.

Guilleminault D. 1987. Disorders of arousal in children: Somnambulism and night terrors. In Guilleminault D, ed. *Sleep and its disorders in children.* New York: Raven Press.

Hales D. 1992. *An invitation to health,* 5th ed. Redwood City, CA: Benjamin/Cummings.

Hayter J. 1983. Sleep behaviors of older persons. *Nurs Res* 32(4):242–246.

Hoch C, Reynolds C. 1986. Sleep disturbances and what to do about them. *Geriatr Nurs* 7:25.

Karvey NB, Anderson D. December 1986. Why every patient needs a good night's sleep. *RN* 49:16–19.

Koop TE. 1988. The surgeon general's report on nutrition and health. Bethesda, MD: Department of Health and Human Services.

Kotagal S, Dement WC. 1985. Overview of sleep apnea and its prevalence in the elderly. *Consultant* 25(3):86–105.

Mackenzie E, Shapiro S, Siegal J. 1988, The economic impact of traumatic injuries. *JAMA.*

Marley WP. 1982. *Health and physical fitness.* Philadelphia: Saunders.

Pender NJ. 1987. *Health promotion in nursing practice,* 2nd ed. Norwalk, CT: Appleton & Lange.

Ryan RS, Travis JW. 1981. *Wellness workbook for health professionals.* Berkeley, CA: Ten Speed Press.

Swinford P, Webster J. 1989. *Promoting wellness: A nurse's handbook.* Rockville, MD: Aspen Publishers.

U.S. Centers for Disease Control and Prevention and American College of Sports Medicine. 1993. Summary statement: Workshop on physical activity and health. *Sports Med Bull* 28(4):7.

U.S. Department of Agriculture and U.S. Department of Health and Human Services. 1980. Nutrition and your health: Dietary guidelines for Americans. Home and Garden Bulletin #232. Washington, DC: U.S. Government Printing Office.

Weaver T, Millman R. 1984. *Sleep apnea.* Springhouse, PA: Nursing Books.

Weaver T, Millman R. 1986. Sleep apnea. *Am J Nurs* 86(2):146–150.

Whalley LF, Wong DL. 1989. *Essentials of pediatric nursing,* 3rd ed. St Louis: Mosby.

Chapter 6
Assessing the Family, Culture, and Environment

Bozett FW, Hanson SMH, eds. 1992. *Fatherhood and families in cultural context.* New York: Springer.

Dunn HL. 1959. High level wellness for man and society. *Am Public Health* 49:786–792.

Dunn HL. 1959. What high level wellness means. *Can J Public Health* 50:447.

Friedman MM. 1992. *Family nursing: Theory and practice,* 3rd ed. Norwalk, CT: Appleton & Lange.

McCubbin HI, Thompson AI. 1987 *Family assessment inventories for research and practice,* 2nd ed. Madison: University of Wisconsin.

Muhlenkamp AF, Sayles JA. 1986. Self-esteem, social support, and positive health practices. *Nurs Res* 35:334–338.

Smilkstein G. 1978. The family APGAR: A proposal for a function test and its use by physicians. *J Fam Pract* 6(6):1231–1239.

U.S. Bureau of the Census. 1985. *Statistical abstract of the United States,* 10th ed. Washington, DC: U.S. Government Printing Office.

U.S. Bureau of the Census. 1991. *Census and you* 26(2). Washington, DC: U.S. Government Printing Office.

U.S. Department of Health and Human Services, Public Health Service. 1992. *Healthy people 2000: National health promotion and disease prevention objectives.* Boston: Jones and Bartlett.

Chapter 7
Techniques of Physical Assessment and the General Survey

American Heart Association. 1987. Recommendations for human blood pressure determination by sphygmomanometer. Pub No 701005. American Heart Association.

Chapter 8
Assessing the Integumentary System

Frantz RA, Kinney CK. 1986. Variables associated with skin dryness in the elderly. *Nurs Res* 35:98–100.

Hagermark O. 1985. Pruritis. In Fry L, ed. *Skin problems in the elderly.* Edinburgh: Churchill Livingstone.

Kopf AW. Prevention of malignant melanoma. In *Dermatology clinics,* vol 3(2), pp 351–360. Philadelphia: Saunders.

Roach L. 1977. Dark skins: Recognizing and interpreting color changes. *Crit Care Update* 5–15.

Chapter 9
Assessing the Head and Neck

Blair KA. 1990. Aging: Physiologic aspects and clinical implications. *Nurse Pract* 15(2):14–28.

Boyd-Monk H. 1980. Examining the external eye, part I. *Nursing 80* 10(5):58–63.

Boyd-Monk H. 1980. Examining the external eye, part II. *Nursing 80* 10(6):58–63.

Burrage RL, Dixon L, Sehy A. 1991. Physical assessment: An overview. In Chenitz WC et al, eds. *Clinical gerontolological nursing: A guide to advanced practice.* Philadelphia: Saunders.

Dilorio C, Price ME. 1990 Swallowing: An assessment guide. *Am J Nurs* 90(7):38–46.

Facione N. 1990. Otitis media: An overview of acute and chronic disease. *Nurse Pract* 15(10):11–22.

Gabai IJ, Spierings EL. 1990. Diagnosis and management of cluster headaches. *Nurse Pract* 15(10):32–36.

Overfield T. 1985. *Biological variations in health and illness: Race, age, and sex differences.* Menlo Park, CA: Addison-Wesley Nursing.

Winter J, Brown P, Brown D. 1991. *Adult health nursing: Concepts and skills. Eye and ear health problems.* [Computer disk]. Chapel Hill, NC: Professional Development Software.

Yeomans AC. 1990. Assessment and management of hypothyroidism. *Nurse Pract* 15(11):8–16.

Chapter 10
Assessing the Respiratory System

Anderson L. 1990. ABGs: Six easy steps to interpreting blood gases. *Am J Nurs* 90(8):42–43.

Brenner M. 1990. Pulmonary and acid-base assessment. *Nurs Clin North Am* 25(4):761–770.

Cunha B. 1993. Chronic bronchitis. *Emerg Med* 25(8):111–112.

Della Bella L. 1992. Steroidphobia and the pulmonary patient. *Nursing* 92:26–29.

Doenges M, Moorhouse M, Geissler A. 1992. *Nursing care plans,* 3rd ed. Philadelphia, FA Davis.

Finesilver C. 1992. Respiratory assessment. *RN* 55(2):22–30.

Franklin R. 1992. Smoking. *Nurs Clin North Am* 27(3):631–642.

Gift A. 1993. Dyspnea and fatigue. *Nurs Clin North Am* 28(2):373–384.

Green E. 1992. Solving the puzzle of chest pain. *Am J Nurs* 92(1):32–37.

Jaffe M. 1992. *Medical-surgical nursing care plans,* 2nd ed. Norwalk, CT: Appleton & Lange.

Kersten LD. 1992. *Comprehensive respiratory nursing.* Philadelphia: Saunders.

Kersten LD. 1984. *Respiratory disorders.* Springhouse, PA: Springhouse.

Kersten LD. 1984. *Respiratory emergencies.* Springhouse, PA: Springhouse.

Kuhn JK. 1992. Respiratory assessment of the elderly. *J Gerontol Nurs* 18(5):40–43.

LeBlanc KB. 1990. Assessment of the neonatal respiratory system. *AACN-Clin Issues Crit Care Nurs* 1(2):401–408.

Lederer J, Marculescu G, Mocnik B, Seaby N. 1993. *Care planning pocket guide,* 5th ed. Redwood City, CA: Addison-Wesley Nursing.

Liebler JM. 1991. Respiratory complications in critically ill medical patients with acute upper gastrointestinal bleeding. *Crit Care Med* 19(9):1152–1157.

Marieb E. 1992. *Human anatomy and physiology,* 2nd ed. Redwood City, CA: Benjamin/Cummings.

Mathews P. 1992. Airway monitoring and ventilation: What the future holds. *Nursing 92* 22(2):48–51.

McFarland G, McFarlane E. 1993. *Nursing diagnosis and intervention,* 2nd ed. St Louis: Mosby.

Nelson D. 1992. Interventions related to respiratory care. *Nurs Clin North Am* 27(2):301–324.

Risser NL. 1987. Prevention of lung cancer: Stopping smoking. *Semin Oncol Nurs* 3(3):228–236.

Stephenson J. 1992. Emphysema: Positively breathtaking. *Harvard Health Letter* 18(2):5–7.

Stevens S, Becker K. 1988. How to perform picture perfect respiratory assessment. *Nursing 88,* 18(1):57.

Stockdale-Woolley R. 1993. Overview of lung disease: Screening and preventions. *Nurse Pract Forum* 4(1):11–15.

Stringfield Y. 1993. Back to basics, acidosis, alkalosis, and ABG's. *Am J Nurs* 93(11):43–44.

Weaver T. 1992. Physiological and psychological variables related to functional status in chronic obstructive pulmonary disease. *Nurs Res* 41(5):286–291.

Weilitz P. 1994. Back to basics: Test your knowledge of tracheostomy tubes. *Am J Nurs* 94(2):46–50.

Whitney L. 1992. Chronic bronchitis and emphysema: Airing the differences. *Nursing 92* 22(3):34–42.

Yean E. 1992. How position affects oxygenation: Good lung down? *Am J Nurs* 92(3):27–29.

Chapter 11
Assessing the Cardiovascular System

Auvenshine M, Enriquez M. 1990. *Comprehensive maternity nursing: Perinatal and women's health,* 2nd ed. Boston: Jones & Bartlett.

Bailey C. 1991. *The new fit or fat.* Boston: Houghton Mifflin.

Braunwald E. 1992. The physical examination. In Braunwald E, ed. *Heart disease: A textbook of cardiovascular medicine,* 4th ed. Philadelphia: Saunders.

Bush T. 1991. Women and heart disease. Presented at National conference on Cholesterol and High Blood Pressure Control. April 8–10, Washington, DC.

Cheitlin M, Sokalow M, McIlroy M. 1992. *Clinical cardiology,* 6th ed. Norwalk, CT: Appleton & Lange.

Chiriboga D, Yarzebski J, Goldberg R, Chen Z, Gurwitz J, Gore J, Alpert J, Dalen J. 1993. A community wide perspective of gender differences and temporal trends in the use of diagnostic and revascularization procedure for acute myocardial infarction. *Am J Cardiol* 71:268–273.

Cochrane B. 1992. Acute myocardial infarction in women. *Crit Care Nurs Clin North Am* 4(2):279–289.

Colgan M. 1993. *Optimum sports nutrition: Your competitive edge.* New York: Advanced Research Press.

Connor R. 1983. Coronary artery anatomy: The electrocardiographic and clinical correlations. *Crit Care Nurse* May/June:68–73.

Consumer Reports on Health. 1992. Are doctors neglecting women's hearts? 4(3):17–19.

Dolan J. 1991 *Critical care nursing: Clinical management through the nursing process.* Philadelphia: FA Davis.

Douglas P, Clarkson T, Flowers N, Hajjar K, et al. 1993. Exercise and atherosclerotic heart disease in women. *Med Sci Sports Exercise* 24(6):S266–S276.

Elkayam U, Gleicher N. 1990. Changes in cardiac findings during normal pregnancy. In Elkayam U, Gleicher N, eds. *Diagnosis and management of maternal and fetal disease,* 2nd ed. New York: Alan R. Liss.

Fink B. 1990. Recognition of a congenital anomaly at birth. In Elkayam U, Gleicher N, eds. *Diagnosis and management of maternal and fetal disease,* 2nd ed. New York: Alan R. Liss.

Greenberg M, Mueller H. 1993. Why the excess mortality in women after PTCA? *Circulation* 87(3):1030–1032.

Khanna P, Geller J. 1992. Clinical implications in the elderly. *Top Emerg Med* 14(3):1–9.

Lakatta E. 1990. Normal changes of aging. In Abrams W, Berkow R, eds. *The Merck manual of geriatrics.* Rahway, NJ: Merck & Co.

Levine G, Balady G. 1992. The cardiac examination in athletes: What's normal and what's not. *J Musculoskel Med* 9(11):61–72.

McCance K, Richardson. 1990. Structure and function of the cardiovascular and lymphatic systems. In: McCance K, Huether S, eds. *Pathophysiology: The biologic basis for disease in adults and children.* St Louis: Mosby.

MacPherson K. 1992. Cardiovascular disease in women and noncontraceptive use of hormones: A feminist analysis. *Adv Nurs Sci* 14(4):34–49.

Marieb E. 1992. *Human anatomy and physiology.* 2nd ed. Redwood City, CA: Benjamin/Cummings.

May K, Mahlmeister L. 1990. *Comprehensive maternal nursing: Nursing process and the childbearing family.* 2nd ed. Philadelphia: Lippincott.

Moore K. 1992. *Clinically oriented anatomy.* 3rd ed. Baltimore: Williams & Wilkins.

Olds S, London M, Ladewig P. 1992. Physiologic response of the newborn to birth. In *Maternal-newborn nursing: A family-centered approach.* 4th ed. Redwood City, CA: Addison-Wesley Nursing.

Ornish D. 1990. *Program for reversing heart disease.* New York: Ballantine Books.

Peberdy MA, Ornato JP. 1992. Coronary artery disease in women. *Heart Dis Stroke* 1(5):315–319.

Rengucci L. 1990. Circulation: Implications of abnormalities in structure and pressure. In Mott S, James S, Sperhac A, eds. *Nursing care of children and families.* Redwood City, CA: Addison-Wesley Nursing.

Sims S. 1990. Alterations of cardiovascular function in children. In McCance K, Huether S, eds. *Pathophysiology: The biologic basis for disease in adults and children.* St Louis: Mosby.

Stanley M. 1992. Elderly patients in critical care: An overview. *AACN Clin Issues Crit Care Nurs* 3(1):120–129.

Stanley M. 1991. Physiologic changes of pregnancy. In Harvey C, ed. *Critical care obstetrical nursing.* Rockville, MD: Aspen Publishers.

Wingate S. 1991. Women and coronary heart disease: Implications for the critical care setting. *Focus Crit Care* 18(3):212–220.

Zaret B, Wackers F, Soufer R. 1992. In Braunwald E, ed. *Heart disease: A textbook of cardiovascular medicine,* 4th ed. Philadelphia: Saunders.

Chapter 12
Assessing the Axillae and Breasts

American Cancer Society. A special touch (pamphlet). Atlanta: American Cancer Society.

American Cancer Society. 1992. Cancer facts and figures—1992 (pamphlet). Atlanta: American Cancer Society.

Fink D. 1991 Guidelines for the cancer-related checkup (pamphlet). Atlanta: American Cancer Society.

Gehring P. 1992. Perfecting the art: Vascular assessment. *RN* 55(1):40–47.

Groenwald S, Frogge M, Goodman M, Yarbro C. 1990. *Cancer nursing: Principles and practice.* Boston: Jones and Bartlett.

Hall L. 1992. Breast self-examination: Use of a visual reminder to increase practice. *AAOHN J* 40(4):186–192.

Harrison L. 1989. Life-saving patient education: Breast self-examination. *Matern Child Nurs J* 14:315–316.

Jirovic M, Brink C, Wells T. 1988. Nursing assessments in the inpatient geriatric population. *Nurs Clin North Am* 23(1):219–230.

Kain C, Reilly N, Schultz E. 1990. The older adult: A comparative assessment. *Nurs Clin North Am* 25(4):833–848.

Lederer J, Marculescu G, Mocnik B, Seaby N. 1993. *Care planning pocket guide: A nursing diagnosis approach,* 5th ed. Redwood City, CA: Addison-Wesley Nursing.

Ludwick R. 1988. Breast examination in the older adult. *Cancer Nurs* 11(2):99–102.

Murali M, Crabtree K. 1992. Comparison of two breast self-examination palpation techniques. *Cancer Nurs* 15(4):276–282.

Nielsen B, East D. 1990. Advances in breast cancer: Implications for nursing care. *Nurs Clin North Am* 25(2):365–375.

Olds S, London M, Ladewig P. 1992. *Maternal-Newborn Nursing,* 5th ed. Redwood City, CA: Addison-Wesley Nursing.

Redeker N. 1988. Health beliefs, health locus of control, and the frequency of practice of breast self-examination in women. *J Obstet Gynecol Neonatal Nurs* 17(1):45–51.

Rudolph A, McDermott J. 1987. The breast physical examination: Its value in early cancer detection. *Cancer Nurs* 10(2):100–106.

Chapter 13
Assessing the Abdomen

Barthel J. 1990. Gastritis and peptic ulcer disease. *Consultant* 30(8):61–62.

Beachley M. 1993. Abdominal trauma: Putting the pieces together. *Am J Nurs* 93(1):26–34.

Bender JS. 1989. Approach to the acute abdomen. *Med Clin North Am* 73(6):1413–22.

Berk J. 1985. *Gastroenterology,* 4th ed. Philadelphia: Saunders.

Bryant G. 1992. When the bowel is blocked. *RN* 55(1):58–67.

Burkhart C. 1992. Guidelines for rapid assessment of abdominal pain indicative of acute surgical abdomen. *Nurse Pract* 17(6):39.

Cole-Arvin C. 1994. Identifying and managing dysphagia. *Nursing 94* 24(1):48–49.

Cooke DM. 1991. Inflammatory bowel disease: Primary health care management of ulcerative colitis and Crohn's disease. *Nurse Pract* 16(8):27.

Feliciano D. 1991. Diagnostic modalities in abdominal trauma. *Surg Clin North Am* 71:241–256.

Finelli L. 1991. Evaluation of the child with acute abdominal pain. *J Pediatr Health Care* 5(5):251–256.

Gilbert G. 1991. Peptic ulcer disease: How to treat it now. *Postgrad Med* 89(4):91–93.

Greenberg L. 1994. Emergency: Fast action for splenic rupture. *Am J Nurs* 94(2):51.

Haicken BN. 1991. Laser laparoscopic cholecystectomy in the ambulatory setting. *J Post Anesthesia Nurs* 6(1)33–39.

Holmgren C. 1992. Abdominal assessment. *RN* 55(3):28–34.

Lail LM. 1990. Risks of endoscopic retrograde cholangiopancreatography and therapeutic applications. *Gastroenterol Nurs* 12(4):239–245.

Lawrence DM. 1993. Gastrointestinal trauma. *Crit Care Nurs Clin North Am* 5(1):127–140.

McConnell E. 1994. Loosening the grip of intestinal obstructions. *Nursing 94* 24(3):34–41.

McKinney S. 1992. The nurse who listened. *Nursing 92* 22(5):71.

Miller D. 1986. Cancer prevention: Steps you can take. In Holleb AI, ed. *The American Cancer Society cancer book.* Garden City, NY: Doubleday.

Murrey RB, Zentner JP. 1989. *Nursing assessment and health promotion strategies through the life span,* 4th ed. Norwalk, CT: Appleton & Lange.

Perucca R. 1992. Understanding Crohn's disease. *J Intravenous Nurs* 15(3):164–169.

Roberts M. 1992. Assessing and treating volvulus. *Nursing 92* 22(2):56–57.

Weber J. 1988. *Nurse's handbook of health assessment.* Philadelphia: Lippincott.

White JH. 1991. Feminism, eating and mental health. *Adv Nurs Sci* 13(3):68–80.

Young R. 1993. Helicobacterpylori: A cause of chronic abdominal pain in children. *Gastroenterol Nurs* 15(6):247–251.

Chapter 14
Assessing the Urinary System

Baird SB, Donehower MG, eds. 1991. *A cancer source book for nurses.* Atlanta: American Cancer Society.

Dodds P, Hans AL. 1990. Distended urinary bladder drainage practices among hospital nurses. *Appl Nurs Res* 3(2):68–69.

Frank A, Murray SM. 1988. A no-guess guide for urinary color assessment. *RN* 51(6) 46.

Ignatavicius D, Bayne M. 1991. *Medical-surgical nursing: A nursing process approach.* Philadelphia: Saunders.

Jirovec MM, Brink CA, Wells TJ. 1988. Nursing assessments in the inpatient geriatric population. *Nurs Clin North Am* 23(1):219–230.

Kain CD, Rielly N, Shultz ED. 1990. The older adult: A comparative assessment. *Nurs Clin North Am* 25(4):833–48.

Lockhart-Pretti PA. 1990. Urinary incontinence. *J Enterostomy Ther* 17(3):112–119.
McDowell BJ, Burgio KL, Candib D. 1989. Assessment of urinary incontinence in the elderly, part1. *J Am Acad Nurse Pract* 1(1):24–29.
Mott S, James S, Sperhac A. 1990. *Nursing care of children and families,* 2nd ed. Redwood City, CA: Addsion-Wesley Nursing.
Murrey R, Zentner. 1993. *Nursing assessment and health promotion: Strategies through the life span.* Norwalk, CT: Appleton & Lange.
Ruff CC, Reaves EL. 1989. Diagnosing urinary incontinence in adults. *Nurs Pract* 14(6):8.
Stark JF. 1988. A quick guide to urinary tract assessment. *Nursing* 18(7):56–58.
Walsh P, Retik A, Stamey T, Vaughn E, eds. 1992. *Campbell's urology,* 6th ed. Philadelphia: Saunders.
Wells T. 1990. Conquering incontinence. *Geriatr Nurs* 11(3):133–35.
Wilson J, Braunwald E, Isselbacher K, Petersdorf R, Martin J, Fauci A, Root R, eds. 1991. *Harrison's principles of internal medicine,* 12th ed. New York: McGraw-Hill.
Wyman JF. 1988. Nursing assessment of the incontinent geriatric outpatient population. *Nurs Clin North Am* 23(1):169–187.

Chapter 15
Assessing the Reproductive System

American Cancer Society. 1992. Cancer facts and figures—1992. Atlanta: American Cancer Society.
Butler R, Lewis M. 1990. Sexuality. In Abrams W, Berkow R, eds. *The Merck manual of geriatrics.* Rahway, NJ: Merck & Co.
Custodio D, Henschen R. 1991. Sexually transmitted diseases. *Top Emerg Med* 13(1):66–74.
Felten B. 1990. The lingering tragedy of DES. *RN* 36–41.
Fontanarosa P, Hellman M. 1991. Pediatric genitourinary emergencies. *Top Emerg Med* 13(1)84–92.
Harward M. 1991. Evaluation of sexual dysfunction in women. *Hosp Pract*:53–54, 56–57.
Hembree D. 1986. High-tech hazards. *Ms.* March 14, 1986.
Lederer J, Marculescu G, Mocnik B, Seaby N. 1993. *Care planning pocket guide: A nursing diagnosis approach.* Redwood City, CA: Addison-Wesley Nursing.
Marieb E. 1995. *Human anatomy and physiology,* 3rd ed. Redwood City, CA: Benjamin/Cummings.
Mason D. 1989. Erectile dysfunctions: Assessment and care. *Nurse Pract*:23.
McCann M. 1989. Sexual healing after heart attack. *Am J Nurs* 89(9):1132–40.
McGuire E, Delancey J, Elkins T. 1990. Female genitourinary disorders. In Abrams W, Berkow R, eds. *The Merck manual of geriatrics.* Rahway, NJ: Merck & Co.
Morrison-Beedy D, Robbins L. Sexual assessment and the aging female. *Nurse Pract* 14(12):35.
Nettina S, Kauffman F. 1990. Diagnosis and management of sexually transmitted genital lesions. *Nurse Pract* 15(1):20–39.
Olds S, London M, Ladewig P. 1992. Physiologic response of the newborn to birth. In *Maternal-newborn nursing: A family-centered approach,* 4th ed. Redwood City, CA: Addison-Wesley Nursing.
Ott M, Jackson P. 1989. Precocious puberty: Identifying early sexual development. *Nurse Pract* 14(11):21.
Wasson J, Bruskewitz. 1990. Disorders of the lower genitourinary tract: Bladder, prostate, and testicles. In Abrams W, Berkow R, eds. *The Merck manual of geriatrics.* Rahway, NJ: Merck & Co.

Chapter 16
Assessing the Peripheral Vascular System

Baker JD. 1991. Assessment of peripheral arterial occlusive disease. *Crit Care Nurs Clin North Am* 3:493–98.
Bilodeau ML, Capasso VC. 1990. Peripheral arterial thrombolytic therapy. *Crit Care Nurs Clin North Am*:673–80.
Blank CA, Irwin SH. 1990. Peripheral vascular disorders: Assessment and intervention. *Nurs Clin North Am* 25:777–94.
Dean E. 1988. Arterial assessment of the hand. *Br J Occup Ther* 51:163–67.
Draszkiewicz C. 1992. Comprehensive care of the diabetic foot. *Orthoped Nurs* 11(2):79–82.
Gehring PE. 1992. Vasclar assessment. *RN* 55:40–48.
Haas LB. 1993. Chronic complications of diabetes mellitus. *Nurs Clin North Am* 28:71–78.
Harvard Medical School Health Letter. 1987. Alcohol and blood pressure. 12(12):1–2.
Harvard Medical School Health Letter. 1988. High blood pressure: A new look. 14(2):1–4.
Harvard Medical School Health Letter. 1989. High blood pressure: Newer treatments. 14(3):1–4.
Herman JA. 1986. Nursing assessment and nursing diagnosis in patients with peripheral vascular disease. *Nurs Clin North Am* 21:219–31.
Johns Hopkins Medical Letter. 1993a. The best treatment for varicose veins. 5:6–7.
Johns Hopkins Medical Letter. 1993b. Pay attention to "mild" hypertension. 5(6):1–2.
Lederer JR, Marculescu GL, Mocnik B, Seaby N. 1993. *Care planning pocket guide.* Redwood City, CA: Addison-Wesley Nursing.
Merry JA. 1988. Take your assessment all the way down to the toes. *RN* 51:60–63.
Miller RA, Evans WE. 1988. Nurse and patient: Allies preventing amputation. *RN* 51:38–42.
Norris MKG, Persky JM. 1992. Popliteal artery entrapment syndrome: Implications for nursing care. *Heart Lung: J Crit Care* 21(3):250–54.
U.S. Department of Health and Human Services. 1990. *Healthy People.* Washington, DC: U.S. Government Printing Office.
Zorb SL. 1991. *Cardiovascular diagnostic testing: A nursing guide.* Rockville, MD: Aspen Publishers.

Chapter 17
Assessing the Musculoskeletal System

American Academy of Orthopaedic Surgeons. 1965. *Joint motion: Method of measuring and recording.* Chicago: The Academy.
Ebersole P, Hess P. 1994. *Toward healthy aging: Human needs and nursing response,* 4th ed. St Louis: Mosby.
Epstein O, Perkin GD, de Bono DP, Cookson J. 1992. *Clinical examination.* London: Gower Medical Publications.
Gibbs J, Hughes S, Dunlop D, Edelman P, Singer R, Chang R. 1993. Joint impairment and ambulation in the elderly. *J Am Geriatr Soc* 41:1212–1218.
Hogstel MO. 1994. *Nursing care of the older adult,* 3rd ed. Albany, NY: Delmar.
Jones-Walton P. 1990. Orthopaedic nursing: Assessment. *Adv Clin Care* 5(3):22.
Lederer JR, Marculescu GL, Mocnik B, Seaby N. 1993. *Care planning pocket guide: A nursing diagnosis approach,* 5th ed. Redwood City, CA: Addison-Wesley Nursing.
Maas M, Buckwalter KC, Hardy M. *Nursing diagnosis and interventions for the elderly.* Redwood City, CA: Addison-Wesley Nursing.

Milde FK. 1988. Impaired physical mobility. *J Gerontol Nurs* 14(3):20–24.

Nevitt MC, Cummings SR, the Study of Osteoporotic Fractures Research Group. 1993. Type of fall and risk of hip and wrist fractures: The study of osteoporotic fractures. *J Am Geriatr Soc* 41:1226–1234.

Olson E, Johnson B, Thompson L. 1990. The hazards of immobility. *Am J Nurs* 90(3):43–44, 46–48.

Swartz MH. 1994. *Textbook of physical diagnosis: History and examination,* 2nd ed. Philadelphia: Saunders.

Chapter 18
Assessing the Neurologic System

Ackerman L. 1992. Intervention related to neurologic care. *Nurs Clin North Am* 27(2):325–346.

Bagley S. 1991. The effects of visual cues on the gait of independently mobile Parkinson's disease patients. *Physiotherapy* 77(6):415–420.

Barker E. 1992. Neurological assessment. *RN* 55(4):28–35.

Bonema JD. 1992. Syncope in elderly patients: Why their risk is higher. *Postgrad Med* 9(1):129–132, 135–136.

Bryant G. 1992. When your patient needs back surgery. *RN* 55(7):46–52.

Chitty K. 1991. The primary prevention role of the nurse in eating disorders. *Nurs Clin North Am* 26(3):789–800.

De Young S. 1983. *The neurological patient: A nursing perspective.* Englewood Cliffs, NJ: Prentice Hall.

Dilorio C. 1993. Learning needs of persons with epilepsy: A comparison of perceptions of persons with epilepsy, nurses and physicians. *J Neurosci Nurs* 25(1):22–29.

Doenges M, Moorhouse M, Geissler A. 1992. *Nursing care plans,* 3rd ed. Philadelphia: FA Davis.

Everson LJ. 1993. Improving care for the patient with epilepsy. *J Nurs Care Quality* 7(3):46–50.

Gaffney S. 1990. Seizure disorder and pregnancy. *NAACOG's Clin Issues Perinat Women's Health Nurs* 1(2):146–153.

Grainger R. 1991. Dealing with feelings: Managing stress. *Am J Nurs* 91(9):15–16.

Guyton A. 1993. *The textbook of medical physiology.* Philadelphia: Saunders.

Herr K. 1992. Interventions related to pain. *Nurs Clin North Am* 27(2):347–370.

Jaffe M. 1992. *Medical-surgical nursing care plans.* 2nd ed. Norwalk, CT: Appleton & Lange.

Kozier B, Erb G, Blais K, Wilkinson J. 1995. *Fundamentals of nursing, concepts, process, and practice,* 5th ed. Redwood City, CA: Addison-Wesley Nursing.

Lederer J, Marculescu G, Mocnik B, Seaby N. 1993. *Care planning pocket guide,* 5th ed. Redwood City, CA: Addison-Wesley Nursing.

Lilley C. 1993. A 43 year old man with syncopal episode and bradycardia 2 weeks after a motor vehicle crash: Splenic rupture. *J Emerg Nurs* 19(2)83–85.

Mariciello MA. 1993. Magnetic resonance imaging related to neurologic outcome in cervical spinal cord injury. *Arch Phys Med Rehabil* 74(9):940–946.

Marieb E. 1995. *Human anatomy and physiology,* 3rd ed. Redwood City, CA: Benjamin/Cummings.

Marr J. 1991. The experience of living with Parkinson's disease. *J Neurosci Nurs* 23(5):325–329.

Mayo N. 1991. Observer variation in assessing neurophysical signs among patients with head injuries. *Am J Phys Med Rehabil* 70(3):118–123.

Neatherlin J. 1990. Neurologic assessment: You can make a difference in cost. *J Neurosci Nurs* 22(5):317–318.

Paulson G. 1993. Management of the patient with newly-diagnosed Parkinson's disease. *Geriatrics* 48(2):30–34, 39–40.

Sander E. 1992. Olfaction:The neglected sense. *J Neurosci Nurs* 24(5):273–280.

Stewart-Amidei C. 1991. Assessing the comatose patient in the intensive care unit. *AACN: Clin Issues Crit Care Nurs* 2(4):613–622.

St. George C. 1993. Spasticity: Mechanisms and nursing care. *Nurs Clin North Am* 28(4):819–828.

Stolley J. 1993. Managing the care of patients with irreversible dementia during hospitalization for comorbidities. *Nurs Clin North Am* 28(4):767–782.

Sullivan J. 1990. Neurologic assessment. *Nurs Clin North Am* 25(4):795–809.

Chapter 19
Assessing Infants, Children, and Adolescents

Barnes L. 1991. *Manual of pediatric physical diagnosis,* 6th ed. St Louis: Mosby.

Bates B. 1991. *A guide to physical examination and history taking,* 5th ed. Philadelphia: Lippincott.

Boynton RW, Dunn ES, Stephens GR. 1994. *Manual of ambulatory pediatrics,* 3rd ed. Glenview, IL: Scott Foresman.

Carpenito LJ. 1989. *Nursing diagnosis: Application to clinical practice,* 3rd ed. Philadelphia: Lippincott.

Carpenito LJ. 1991. *Handbook of nursing diagnosis,* 4th ed. Philadelphia: Lippincott.

Engle J. 1989. *Pocket guide to pediatric assessment.* St Louis: Mosby.

Green M, Haggarty RJ. 1990. *Ambulatory pediatrics,* 4th ed. Philadelphia: Saunders.

Malasanos L, et al. 1990. *Health assessment,* 4th ed. St Louis: Mosby.

Park M. 1991. *The pediatric cardiology handbook.* St Louis: Mosby.

Sperhac AM. 1990 Physical assessment. In Mott S, James S, and Sperhac AM, eds. *Nursing care of children and families.* Redwood City, CA: Addison-Wesley Nursing.

Swartz MH. 1994. Textbook of physical diagnosis: *History and examination,* 2nd ed. Philadelphia: Saunders.

Chapter 20
Assessing the Childbearing Client

Alexander JM, Grant AM, Campbell MJ. 1992. Randomized controlled trial of breast shells and Hoffman's exercises for inverted and non-protractile nipples. *Breastfeeding Rev* 2(6):272–275.

Billett J. 1992. A closer look at pregnancy sickness. *Prof Care Mother Child* 2(10):310–311.

Brouillard-Pierce C. 1993. Indication for induction of labor. *Matern Child Nurs J* 18:14–12.

Bryant CA, Coreil J, D'Angelo SL. 1992. A strategy for promoting breastfeeding among economically disadvantaged women and adolescents. *NAACOGS Clin Issues Perinat Women's Health Nurs* 3(4):723–730.

Caffeine use and pregnancy outcomes. 1993. *Nurses Drug Alert* 17(3):24.

Ceyhan B, Celikel T, Ceyhan N. 1993. Adult respiratory distress syndrome during pregnancy: A case report. *Respir Care* 38(9):993–996.

Cohen MP. 1992. Pregnancy in women with diabetes. *J Women's Health.* Spring:81–87.

Cunningham FG, Lindheimer MD. 1992. Hypertension in pregnancy. *N Eng J Med* 326:927–932.

Delorio C. Patterns of nausea during first trimester of pregnancy. *Clin Nurs Rev* 1(2):127–143.

Freda MC, Mikhail M, Mazloom E. 1993. Fetal movement counting: Which method? *Matern Child Nurs J* 18(6):314–321.

Fuschino W. 1992. Physiologic changes of pregnancy: Impact on critical care. *Crit Care Nurs Clin North Am* 4(4):691–701.

Giotta MP. 1993. Nutrition during pregnancy: Reducing obstetric risk. *J Perinat Neonat Nurs* 6(4):1–12.

Gottesman MM. 1992. Maternal adaptation during pregnancy among adult early, middle, and late childbearers: Similarities and differences. *Matern Child Nurs* 20(1):93–110.

Jimenez, SLM. 1992. Pregant and uncomfortable? *Am Baby* 54(10):38.

Kemp WH, Halmaker DD. 1993. Health practices and anxiety in low-income, high and low-risk pregnant women. *J Obstet Gynecol Neonat Nurs* 22(34):266–272.

Lee KA Rittenhouse CA. 1992. Sleep disturbances, vitality, and fatigue among a select group of employed childbearing women. *Birth* 19(1):208–213.

Lilford RJ, Kelly M, Baines A. 1992. Effects of using protocols on medical care: Randomised trial of three methods of taking an antenatal history. *Br Med J* 1184.

Mashburn J, Graves BW, Gillmor-Kahn M. 1992. Hematocrit values during pregnancy in a nurse-midwifery caselo *J Nurs Midwife* 37(6):404–410.

Mawn B. Standards of care for high-risk prenatal clients: Community nurse case management approach. *Public Health Nurs* 10(2):78–88.

Nandi C, Nelson MR. 1992. Maternal pregravid weight, age, and smoking status as risk factors for low birth weight births. *Public Health Rep* 107(6):658–662.

Omar MA, Schiffman RF. 1993. Prenatal vitamins: A right of passage. *Matern Child Nurs J* (6):322–324.

Palmore S, Millar K. 1990. An interview for pregnant teens: Identifying special needs in school setting. *School Nurse* 6(4):18–21.

Queenan JT. 1991. Prenatal care incentives: When all else fails. *Women's Health Issues* 1(3):127–128.

Sibai BM. 1992. Hypertension in pregnancy. *Obstet Gynecol Clin North Am* 19(4):615–632.

Warrick L, Christianson JB, Walriff J. 1993. Educational outcomes in teenage pregnancy and parenting program: Results from a demonstration. *Family Planning Perspect* 25(4):148–152.

Zeanah M, Schlosser SP. 1993. Adherence to ACOG guidelines on pregnancy outcomes. *J Obstet Gynecol Neonat Nurs* 22(4):329–335.

Chapter 21
Assessing the Older Adult

Bernbaumer DM. 1993. Abdominal emergencies in later life. *Emerg Med* 25(5):74.

Breitung JC. 1987. *Caring for older adults: Basic nursing skills and concepts.* Philadelphia: Saunders.

Burggraf V, Donlon B. Assessing the elderly: System by system. *Am J Nurs* 85(9):973–84.

Cahill HL. 1981. *Old age—a balance sheet.* San Carlos, CA: Wide World Publishing/Tetra House.

Cowgill DC. 1986. *Aging around the world.* Belmont, CA: Wadsworth.

Deakins DA. 1994. Teaching elderly patients about diabetes. *Am J Nurs* 94(4):38–42.

Doenges ME, Moorhouse MF. 1993. *Nurse's pocket guide: Nursing diagnoses with interventions,* 4th ed. Philadelphia: FA Davis.

Eliopoulos C. 1990. *Health assessment of the older adult,* 2nd ed. Redwood City, CA: Addison-Wesley Nursing.

Eliopoulos C. 1993. *Gerontological nursing,* 3rd ed. Philadelphia: Lippincott.

Fraser D. 1993. Patient assessment: Infection in the elderly. *J Gerontol Nurs* 19(7):5–11.

Giordano M. 1992. Clinical assessment of the geriatric patient. *AARC Times* 16(12):42–45.

Guralkik JM, Simonsick EM, Ferrucci L, Glynn RJ, Berkman LF, Blazer DG, Scherr PA, Wallace RB. 1994. A short physical performance battery assessing lower extremity function: Association with self-reported disability and prediction of mortality and nursing home admission. *J Gerontol Med Sci* 49(2):85–94.

Hays AM, Borger F. 1985. Assessing the elderly: A test in time. *Am J Nurs* 85(10):1107–11.

Heckheimer EF. 1989. *Health promotion of the elderly in the community.* Philadelphia: Saunders.

Henderson ML. 1985. Assessing the elderly: Altered presentation. *Am J Nurs* 85(10):1104–1106.

Janz M. 1990. Clues to elder abuse. *Geriatr Nurse* 11(5):220–22.

Kimmel DC. 1980. *Adulthood and aging,* 2nd ed. New York: Wiley.

Levinson DJ. 1978. *The seasons of a man's life.* New York: Ballantine Books.

Loftis PA, Glover TL. 1993. *Decision making in gerontologic nursing.* St Louis: Mosby.

Lusis SA. 1993. Nursing assessment of mental status in the elderly. *Geriatr Nurse* 14(15):255–59.

Matteson MA, McConnell ES. 1988. *Gerontological nursing: Concepts and practice.* Philadelphia: Saunders.

Mehta SM. 1993. The road back to independence: Applying Orem's self-care framework. *Geriatr Nurse* 14(4):182–85.

Mellillo KD. 1994. Interpretation of abnormal laboratory values in older adults, part I. *J Gerontol Nurs* 19(1):39–45.

Mellillo KD. 1994. Interpretation of abnormal laboratory values in older adults, part II. *J Gerontol Nurs* 19(2):35–40.

O'Rourke CM, Britten F, Gatschet CA, Krien TL. 1993. Effectiveness of a hearing screening protocol for the elderly. *Geriatr Nurse* 14(2).

Osato EE, Stone JT, Phillips SL, Winne D. 1993. Clinical manifestations: Failure to thrive in the elderly. *J Gerontol Nurs* 19(8):28–34.

Parzick JA, Triebsch HC, eds. 1988. Home health care rehabilitation. *J Home Health Care Pract* 1(1).

Parzick JA, Triebsch HC, eds. 1989. Care of the geriatric patient in the home setting. *J Home Health Care Pract* 2(1).

Schuster CS, Ashburn SS. 1986. *The process of human development: A holistic life-span approach,* 2nd ed. Boston: Little, Brown.

White MW, Karem S, Cowell B. 1994. Skin tears in frail elders: A practical approach to prevention. *Geriatr Nurse* 15(2):95–99.

Woodlei MA. 1993. Assessing urge incontinence in elderly women. *Geriatr Nurse* 14(1).

Art and Photography Credits

Art Credits

Unit and chapter opening illustrations: Kristin N. Mount.

Chapter 1: 1.2: Betty Gee. 1.3: Romaine LoPrete. 1.4: Nea Hanscomb.

Chapter 2: 2.1, 3, 5: Romaine LoPrete.

Chapter 5: 5.1: Kristin N. Mount. 5.2: Robert Voigts.

Chapter 6: 6.1: GTS Graphics. 6.3, 4: Betty Gee.

Chapter 7: 7.7b, 15, 16, 17: Romaine LoPrete. Table 7.2: Precision Graphics.

Chapter 8: 8.1, 17, 18, 19, 20: Kristin N. Mount. 8.2: Biomed Arts Associates/Wendy Hiller Gee. 8.4: Barbara Cousins. 8.13: Romaine LoPrete. Table 8.3, Table 8.4: Kristin N. Mount.

Chapter 9: 9.1, 48, 49, 50: Kristin N. Mount. 9.2: Biomed Arts Associates. 9.3, 7, 12: Biomed Arts Associates/Wendy Hiller Gee. 9.5, 13, 15: Barbara Cousins. 9.6, 14, 22, 29, 31, 42: Romaine LoPrete. 9.8, 10, 11: Todd A. Buck. 9.40b, 41b: Precision Graphics. Table 9.5: Kristin N. Mount.

Chapter 10: 10.1, 2: Kristin N. Mount. 10.3, 5: Barbara Cousins. Table 10.2, Table 10.6: Kristin N. Mount. 10.4: Romaine LoPrete.

Chapter 11: 11.1, 10, 11, 12, 25: Kristin N. Mount. 11.2, 3: Biomed Arts Associates/Wendy Hiller Gee. 11.4, 5, 7: Todd A. Buck. 11.6: Barbara Cousins. 11.8, 9, 17: Romaine LoPrete. 11.23, 24: Courtesy of Johanna K. Stiesmeyer. Table 11.13: Romaine LoPrete.

Chapter 12: 12.1, 15: Kristin N. Mount. 12.3: Biomed Arts Associates/Wendy Hiller Gee. 12.4, 5, 18, 19, 20: Romaine LoPrete. 12.21: Precision Graphics.

Chapter 13: 13.1, 13, 20, 21, 28: Kristin N. Mount. 13.2: Todd A. Buck. 13.3: Biomed Arts Associates/Wendy Hiller Gee. 13.6, 15, 27: Romaine LoPrete. Table 13.1: Kristin N. Mount.

Chapter 14: 14.1: Kristin N. Mount. 14.2, 3: Biomed Arts Associates/Wendy Hiller Gee.

Chapter 15: 15.1, 20, 21, 22, 23, 28, 29, 33, 34, 35, 38, 39, 40: Kristin N. Mount. 15.2, 5: Barbara Cousins. 15.3, 4, 6: Biomed Arts Associates/Wendy Hiller Gee. 15.9, 12: Romaine LoPrete. Table 15.1, Table 15.2, Table 15.6: Romaine LoPrete. Table 15.5: Kristin N. Mount.

Chapter 16: 16.1: Kristin N. Mount. 16.2, 3, 4, 5, 6: Biomed Arts Associates/Wendy Hiller Gee. Table 16.2: Romaine LoPrete.

Chapter 17: 17.1 Kristin N. Mount. 17.2, 7, 10, 13, 14: Biomed Arts Associates/Wendy Hiller Gee. 17.3, 5, 8, 9, 11, 12: Barbara Cousins. 17.4, 6: Todd A. Buck. Table 17.1, Type of Joint: Kristin N. Mount. Type of Movement: Precision Graphics.

Chapter 18: 18.1, 5, 6: Kristin N. Mount. 18.2: Biomed Arts Associates/Wendy Hiller Gee. 18.3, 4, 7, 14, 36: Romaine LoPrete.

Chapter 19: 19.1, 4, 16, 17: Kristin N. Mount. 19.2, 3, 14: Romaine LoPrete.

Chapter 20: 20.1, 2, 5, 7, 8, 10, 11, 12, 13, 14, 15, 16, 17: Kristin N. Mount. Table 20.1: Kristin N. Mount.

Chapter 21: 21.2: Kristin N. Mount. 21.7: Romaine LoPrete.

Photography Credits

Chapter 1: 1.1: © FPG International.

Chapter 2: 2.2: © Medical Images Inc. 2.4: Alain McLaughlin.

Chapter 3: 3.1, 2, 4: Kim Raftery. 3.3: Peter Fox. 3.5: Elena Dorfman. 3.6: © Tom Wilson/FPG International. 3.7: Tony Freeman/PhotoEdit. 3.8: Alain McLaughlin.

Chapter 4: 4.1, 2: Alain Mclaughlin. 4.3: Elena Dorfman.

Chapter 5: 5.3: © Westlight. 5.4: Elena Dorfman.

Chapter 6: 6.2a: Alain McLaughlin. 6.2b: Robert Brenner/PhotoEdit. 6.2c, 2d: Elena Dorfman.

Chapter 7: 7.1, 2, 3, 4, 5b, 12, 13, 18, 20: Richard Tauber. 7.6, 14, 19: Elena Dorfman. 7.9, 10, 11: Alain McLaughlin. Table 7.1: Elena Dorfman.

Chapter 8: 8.3, 21, 29: SPL/Photo Researchers. 8.5, 9, 10, 14: Richard Tauber. 8.6, 23: Copyright © 1994, Carroll H. Weiss. All rights reserved. 8.7: Custom Medical Stock Photography. 8.8: Biophoto Associates/Photo Researchers. 8.11, 12, 16: Alain McLaughlin. 8.15: Elena Dorfman. 8.22, 24: NMSB/Custom Medical Stock Photography. 8.25: Scheichkorn/Custom Medical Stock Photography. 8.26: Zuber/Custom Medical Stock Photography. 8.27: Levy/Phototake. 8.28: Leonard Lessin/Peter Arnold. Table 8.2: page 144, top to bottom: SPL/Photo Researchers. NMSB/Custom Medical Stock Photography. Biophoto Associates. S. Lissau/Medichrome. page 145, top to bottom: Mike English, MD/Medical Images, Inc. Copyright © 1994, Carroll H. Weiss. All rights reserved. De Grazia/Custom Medical Stock Photography. SPL/Custom Medical Stock Photography. Table 8.6: page 153, top to bottom: Biophoto Associates/Photo Researchers. NMSB/Custom Medical Stock Photography. NMSB/Custom Medical Stock Photography. NMSB/Custom Medical Stock Photography. page 154, top to bottom: NMSB/Custom Medical Stock Photography. Harry J. Prezekop Jr./Medichrome. NMSB/Custom Medical Stock Photography. Biophoto Associates/Photo Researchers. page 155, top to bottom: Rotker/Phototake. Custom Medical Stock Photography. American Academy of Dermatology. American Academy of Dermatology. page 156, top to bottom: Custom Medical Stock Photography. Zeva Delbaum/Peter Arnold. Copyright © 1994, Carroll H. Weiss. All rights reserved. Leonard Morse/Medical Images, Inc.

Chapter 9: 9.17, 18, 19, 20, 21, 23, 24, 25, 26, 27, 28, 32, 33, 34, 36, 37, 38, 39, 40a, 41a, 43, 44, 45, 46: Richard Tauber. 9.35: Dr. Richard Buckingham. Table 9.2: page 210, top to bottom, left column: University of Illinois/Custom Medical Stock Photography. NIH/Phototake. top to bottom, right column: Biophoto Associates/Photo Researchers. Erika Stone/Photo Researchers. University of Washington, Seattle. page 211, top to bottom, left column:

Copyright © 1994, Carroll H. Weiss. All rights reserved. University of Illinois/Custom Medical Stock Photography. right column: NMSB/Custom Medical Stock Photography. Table 9.3: page 212, top to bottom: NMSB/Custom Medical Stock Photography. Custom Medical Stock Photography. Buddy Crofton/Medical Images, Inc. page 213, top to bottom: SPL/Photo Researchers. SPL/Photo Researchers. Copyright © 1994, Carroll H. Weiss. All rights reserved. SPL Photo Researchers. page 214, top to bottom: Leonard Lessin/Peter Arnold. Copyright © 1994, Carroll H. Weiss, All rights reserved. Table 9.4: page 215, top to bottom: SIU/Peter Arnold. SPL/Custom Medical Stock Photography. Janet Hayes/Medical Images, Inc. Custom Medical Stock Photography. page 216, top to bottom: SPL/Photo Researchers. Courtesy of Brenda Spriggs, MD FACP. Xomed.Treace/Goode T.Tube. Table 9.5: Biophoto Associates/Photo Researchers. Table 9.6: page 218, top to bottom: Custom Medical Stock Photography. Copyright © 1994, Carroll H. Weiss. All rights reserved. SPL/Photo Researchers. page 219, top to bottom: © Michael English, MD/Medical Images, Inc. Copyright © 1994, Carroll H. Weiss. All rights reserved. Custom Medical Stock Photography.

Chapter 10: 10.13, 14, 17a, 19: Richard Tauber.

Chapter 11: 11.13, 15, 19, 20, 21: Richard Tauber. 11.14: Dr. Michael Hawke. 11.16: American Academy of Dermatology.

Chapter 12: 12.7, 10, 11, 12, 13, 16, 17: Richard Tauber. 12.8: CNRI/Phototake. 12.9: Copyright © 1994, Carroll H. Weiss. All rights reserved.

Chapter 13: 13.7, 8, 12, 14, 16, 17, 18, 19, 22: Richard Tauber. 13.23: Myrleen F. Cate/PhotoEdit. 13.24: Craig Lorenz/Photo Researchers. 13.25: © William Thompson/Picture Cube. 13.26: SPL/Photo Researchers.

Chapter 14: 14.8, 11, 12: Richard Tauber.

Chapter 15: 15.7, 8, 10, 11, 13, 14, 15, 16, 17, 18, 19, 24, 25, 27, 30, 31, 36, 37: Richard Tauber. 15.26: Michael English, MD/Custom Medical Stock Photography. 15.32: SIU/Custom Medical Stock Photography. Table 15.4: page 450, top to bottom: Courtesy of National A/V Center. Fred J. Fleury, MD. Biophoto Associates/Photo Researchers. Courtesy of the National A/V Center. page 451, top to bottom: Courtesy of the National A/V Center. Biophoto Associates/Photo Research. NMSB/Custom Medical Stock Photography. Table 15.5: page 452, top to bottom: Rotker/Phototake. Biophoto Associates/Photo Researchers. page 453, top to bottom: Copyright © 1994, Carroll H. Weiss. All rights reserved. Courtesy of Dr. Anderson/Cancer Center.

Chapter 16: 16.7, 8, 9, 10, 11, 12, 13a, 14, 15, 16, 17, 18, 19, 20, 21: Richard Tauber. Table 16.3: page 483, top to bottom: Dr. P. Marazzi/Science Photo Library. Copyright © 1993, Carroll H. Weiss. All rights reserved. Alex Bartel/Science Photo Library. Copyright © 1992, Science Photo Library.

Chapter 17: 17.15, 22, 23, 26, 28, 34, 37, 38, 41: Richard Tauber. 17.45, 46, 49: Elena Dorfman. 17.47: Judy Braginsky. 17.48: Walter Hodges/West Light. Table 17.3: page 535, top to bottom: Custom Medical Stock Photography. Biophoto Associates/Photo Researchers. Duncan/Medical Images, Inc. page 536, top to bottom: NMSB/Custom Medical Stock Photography. Copyright © 1994, Carroll H. Weiss. All rights reserved. Biophoto Associates/Photo Researchers. page 537, top to bottom: Custom Medical Stock Photography. Sunset/Peter Arnold. NMSB/Custom Medical Stock Photography.

Chapter 18: 18.8, 9, 11, 12, 13, 15, 16, 17, 18, 19, 20, 21, 22, 23, 24, 25, 27, 28, 29, 30, 31, 32, 34: Richard Tauber.

Chapter 19: 19.6, 9, 10, 11, 12, 13, 15: Richard Tauber.

Chapter 20: 20.3, 4, 6, 9, 18, 19: Elena Dorfman.

Chapter 21: 21.1a: Biophoto Associates/Photo Researchers. 21.1b: Amethyst/Custom Medical Stock Photography. 21.1c, 1d: SPL/Photo Researchers. 21.1e: Levy/Phototake. 21.1f: Copyright © 1994, Carroll H. Weiss. All rights reserved. 21.3, 4, 5, 6, 9: Richard Tauber. 21.8: Elena Dorfman

Chapter 22: 22.1, 2, 3, 4, 5, 6, 7, 8, 9, 10, 11, 12, 13: Richard Tauber.

Composite Photography and Art Credits

Chapter 7: 7.5a, 7.7a, 7.8, Table 7.1: Elena Dorfman/Nea Hanscomb.

Chapter 9: 9.4, 9, 16, 47: Richard Tauber/Nea Hanscomb. 9.30: Don Wong/Photo Researchers/Nea Hanscomb.

Chapter 10: 10.4, 10.6: Richard Tauber/Biomed Arts Associates/Wendy Hiller Gee. 10.7, 8, 9, 10, 11, 12, 15, 16, 17b, 18, 20, 21, 22: Richard Tauber/Nea Hanscomb.

Chapter 11: 11.18, 22: Richard Tauber/Nea Hanscomb.

Chapter 12: 12.2: Richard Tauber/Biomed Arts Associates/Wendy Hiller Gee. 12.6: Richard Tauber/Kristin N. Mount. 12.14: Richard Tauber/Nea Hanscomb.

Chapter 13: 13.4, 5, 9, 10, 11: Richard Tauber/Nea Hanscomb.

Chapter14: 14.4, 5: Richard Tauber/Biomed Arts Associates/ Wendy Hiller Gee. 14.6, 7, 9, 10: Richard Tauber/Nea Hanscomb.

Chapter 16: 16.13b: Richard Tauber/Nea Hanscomb.

Chapter 17: 17.16, 17, 18, 19, 20, 21, 24, 25, 27, 29, 30, 31, 32, 33, 35, 36, 39, 40, 42, 43, 44: Richard Tauber/Nea Hanscomb.

Chapter 18: 18.10, 26, 33, 35: Richard Tauber/Nea Hanscomb.

Index

NOTE: Page numbers followed by *f* refer to illustrations appearing separate from accompanying text; page numbers followed by *t* refer to tables.

(continued)

(continued)

(continued)

(continued)

(continued)

(continued)

(continued)

(continued)

(continued)